The Psychosocial Aspects
of Pediatrics

O let me e'er behold in the afflicted
and the suffering only the human being.

(Moses Maimonedes,
Prayer for Physicians)

Some patients, though conscious that their condition is perilous,
recover their health simply through their contentment
with the goodness of the physician.

(Hippocrates, Precepts)

Medicine is a science of uncertainty
and an art of probability.

(Sir William Osler)

The Psychosocial Aspects of Pediatrics

Dane G. Prugh, M.D.

Professor of Psychiatry and Pediatrics
University of Colorado School of Medicine
Denver, Colorado

Lea & Febiger   *1983*   *Philadelphia*

Lea & Febiger
600 Washington Square
Philadelphia, Pa. 19106

Library of Congress Cataloging in Publication Data

Prugh, Dane G.
  The psychosocial aspects of pediatrics.

  Bibliography: p.
  Includes index.
  1. Pediatrics—Psychological aspects. 2. Sick
children—Psychology. 3. Children—Diseases—Social
aspects. I. Title. [DNLM: 1. Child development
disorders. 2. Mental disorders—In adolescence.
3. Mental disorders—In infancy and childhood.
4. Child psychology. 5. Pediatrics. WS 350 P971]
RJ47.5.P75 1983   618.92′0001′9   81-8289
ISBN 0-8121-0614-8   AACR2

PRINTED IN THE UNITED STATES OF AMERICA

Print Number   2   1

This book is dedicated to my father, Wallace E. Prugh, M.D., a practicing physician for more than forty years. His wise and dedicated example and his unrelenting concern for the welfare of his patients first gave me an understanding of the challenges and satisfactions of the art of medicine.

Foreword

This is a remarkable book both in scope and depth as well as in timeliness. It fills an important niche in the rich history of modern pediatrics. This requires some explanation.

Modern pediatrics has always been concerned with the study and care of the child in health and in disease. During the early decades of this century, there existed a fitting preoccupation with life-threatening, acute diseases that resulted in so much morbidity and mortality. The rapidity with which so many of these diseases have been controlled is one of the spectacular stories of modern medicine. The world-wide eradication of smallpox and the virtual elimination of measles, rubella, diphtheria, tetanus, pertussis, and poliomyelitis from the United States, along with the nutritional deficiency syndromes that consumed the pediatrician's time and energy in training and practice, are examples of this transformation. Striking reductions in the infant mortality rate and in the incidence of the diarrheal disorders were concomitant developments.

It is logical, therefore, for the historical concerns with the psychosocial aspects of the child's development and aberrations in this process to assume greater prominence now for pediatric health care workers. It is fortunate that this coincides with a rapid expansion of our knowledge of the psychosocial aspects of child development. The behavioral sciences have undergone unprecedented growth in recent decades; thus, the fields of child psychiatry, psychology, sociology, cultural anthropology, social work, special education, and other related fields have contributed increasingly to our understanding of child and family development. New journals have appeared and new training programs developed. Efforts to improve the lot of families rearing children has been evident through new child care programs such as Head Start, Day Care, Early Periodic Screening, Diagnosis and Treatment, and others of the past two decades. These are efforts to respond to the changes in the sociology of the family as well as to meet, in a more sensitive way, the special needs of children and parents.

Pediatric training programs in psychosocial pediatrics have emerged in order to more adequately prepare tomorrow's practitioners. Other child health professionals have followed suit. The recent Report of the Task Force on Pediatric Education defined such training as an important need in pediatrics.

These trends bespeak the importance of this volume. The task for child health workers has been to integrate the knowledge of the physical, psychologic, social educational, and cultural aspects of the life of the family in order to meet the needs of the child more fully and effectively. This integrative task is not readily accomplished; hitherto, we have not had adequate teaching aids to help us achieve our goals.

We are fortunate that a person who has lived through these transitions has undertaken the task of integrating for the clinician our knowledge in child development. Dr. Prugh brings to this task a rich background, which is reflected throughout the text, in pediatrics and in child psychiatry. The bibliographies for the various chapters also reflect a respect for the rich history of the field, which helps the reader understand the roots of our knowledge while at the same time presenting recent advances.

The text has remarkable balance, being rich in theory without in any way lacking in practical applications for the clinician. It is encyclopedic without losing the forest for the trees. The focus is always on what is useful in the clinical setting. This is particularly evident in the case presentations that are scattered throughout the chapters to add to the lucidity of the text.

Most importantly, this volume sets a conceptual tone for all of medicine that is much needed. It is an integrative view of biologic and psychosocial development important not only for child health professionals, but for all health professionals as well. Dr. Prugh, along with Dr. George Engel and others, has been one of the architects of a biopsychosocial approach to medicine, which is the conceptual basis for the future of medicine and pediatrics. We are much in his debt for having accomplished this monumental task of bringing to us an integrated, comprehensive view of the child and family on such an optimistic note. This is a source book that should not be permitted to become outdated.

Julius B. Richmond, M.D.
Professor of Health Policy
Harvard University
Cambridge, Massachusetts

Preface

As a child psychiatrist and psychoanalyst with training and experience in pediatrics, I have long felt the need for a comprehensive textbook that would relate modern concepts of dynamic psychology to the understanding, prevention, and treatment of illness in children. This volume is a step in that direction. It is a step taken in all humility, as I know that capable people have made somewhat similar offerings in the past. This book has been designed to provide broad insights into the psychosocial aspects of pediatrics; practical suggestions are included as to how these insights can be applied to the management of children and adolescents who have predominantly physical disorders with psychosocial components or who show milder forms of developmental or psychologic disorders. It is therefore addressed primarily to the student of medicine, the pediatrician, the internist, the family physician, the nurse, the child health associate, and other health professionals who work with such patients and their families. (Where the word "pediatrician" is used, it is often, though not always, interchangeable with "the physician" and sometimes with "the child health associate.") I hope the book will also be of value to child psychiatrists and other mental health professionals who work in pediatric settings or who may be called upon for consultation or collaboration by pediatricians or other health professionals, as is often the case today.

In selecting the topics discussed in each chapter, I have limited myself to illnesses and disorders commonly encountered in pediatric practice, and I have restricted myself to discussing the basic principles of diagnosis and treatment, with suggestions as to the management of the psychosocial aspects of the problems that may be encountered. A number of case examples and summaries of interviews are included to clarify points of technique or management, and numerous references and an extensive bibliography are provided for those who wish to investigate certain subjects in greater detail.

Obviously, in preparing this manuscript, I have drawn upon the wisdom of many other professionals who, like myself, have experienced the joy of cooperating with parents in helping their children to grow and develop to maturity. I am particularly indebted to my former teachers, whose inspiration and example have influenced my professional development. These include Dr. Bronson Crothers (now deceased), former professor of neurology at Harvard Medical School and chief of the Neurology Division of the Children's Hospital in Boston; Dr. John Romano, distinguished professor of psychiatry and former chairman of the Department of Psychiatry at the University of Rochester School of Medicine; Dr. George L. Engel, professor emeritus of Psychiatry and Medicine and former head of the Medical Liaison Division of the University of Rochester; Dr. Reginald Lourie, former director of the Department of Psychiatry at the Children's Hospital National Medical Center in Washington, D.C.; Dr. Charles A. Janeway (recently deceased), formerly Emeritus Thomas Morgan Rotch Professor of Pediatrics at Harvard Medical School and chairman of the Department of Medicine at the Children's Hospital in Boston; Dr. Grete Bibring, who was, at the time of her recent death, emeritus professor of psychiatry at Harvard Medical School and who had been head of the Department of Psychiatry at Beth Israel Hospital in Boston, and Dr. Milton J. E. Senn, Emeritus Sterling Professor of Pediatrics and Psychiatry at Yale University School of Medicine. I am particularly grateful to Dr. Senn, since it was he, as a pediatrician with training in child psychiatry, who helped me plan my training and gave generously of his vast knowledge as my mentor.

I am also grateful for the assistance of my colleagues in Denver, Dr. Kent Jordan (now in California), Dr. Anthony Kisley, and Dr. Lloyd Eckhardt, and others elsewhere who have collaborated with me in the writing of other publications that have been drawn upon in this book, and to Drs. Barkley Clark, Alan Levine, William Loomis, and Douglas Robbins, and to Mrs. Erlyne Cooper, for permission to publish, in several chapters, summaries of cases they evaluated or treated. I am grateful to Dr. Jay Tarnow, assistant professor of psychiatry and pediatrics in the Department of Psychiatry at Baylor University School

of Medicine, who kindly reviewed the discussion of diabetes in Chapter 2, and to Dr. John Sadler, former director of the Children's Behavioral Sciences Division at the National Jewish Hospital in Denver, who was kind enough to review the discussion of asthma in Chapter 21. Dr. Charles Spezzano, assistant clinical professor of psychiatry (psychology) at the University of Colorado School of Medicine, offered valuable suggestions after reading the section on behavior therapy.

Additionally, I wish to acknowledge the invaluable contributions of Mrs. Corinne Copeland, Mrs. Tilli Urban, and Mrs. Rita Taylor, my secretaries during the years this book was in preparation, who gave unstintingly of their time and energy, typing and retyping the manuscript through its many revisions and offering helpful suggestions as to its format. The use of masculine pronouns throughout the text was prompted by a desire for conciseness on my part and not by a disregard of the substantial contribution of women in pediatrics, child psychiatry, and other fields.

I am boundlessly grateful to my wife, Anne Davison Prugh, whose faith in my work and compassionate support have bolstered me in many trying hours; I also appreciate the tolerance of my children, Joan and Wallace, with my preoccupation during the preparation of this book.

Denver, Colorado   Dane G. Prugh

Contents

I
Background Concepts

Art is long, life short,
judgment difficult,
occasion transient.
(Goethe)

1
Modern Trends in Pediatrics

*The practice of medicine affords scope
for the exercise of the best faculties
of the mind and heart.*
(Osler)

Over the past 30 years, pediatrics has changed greatly. Chemotherapy and antibiotics have brought many infectious diseases under control although some bacterial infections still resist treatment. The work of obstetricians and pediatricians has lowered infant mortality and morbidity. The refinement of prophylactic measures has virtually eliminated smallpox, diphtheria, pertussis, poliomyelitis and tetanus in urban areas. However, immunity acquired to those diseases is limited, and the antibodies provided by immunization must be stimulated throughout one's life. Preventive medicine has eradicated many communicable diseases. It has become possible to detect and prevent deleterious effects of inborn errors of metabolism.

Despite new knowledge, however, many problems have not been solved, especially problems related to viral diseases, mental retardation, neoplastic disease, congenital anomalies, collagen diseases, and other chronic disorders. When one problem is solved, another may appear, such as the handicaps of some surviving premature infants, sensitivity to antibiotics and other drugs, adverse reactions to smallpox vaccination, and the increased susceptibility to infection caused by steroids.

Of even greater concern is the fact that new knowledge cannot immediately help millions of children (e.g., those suffering from kwashiorkor, a distressing phenomenon in many underdeveloped parts of the world).

Many people do not benefit from preventive or therapeutic treatment because they do not know how to obtain treatment, because they cannot reach a medical facility, or because they mistrust or dislike impersonal, crowded public medical facilities. About 25% of the children in the United States (and a larger percentage of black children in the South) have until recently received little or no health care, and so the infant mortality in the United States is higher than in a number of other countries.

3

Tuberculosis is still a widespread problem, even in urban areas, despite new methods of detection and early treatment. If the advances of medical science are to benefit children and adolescents fully, the distribution of health care must be wider and public education about health must be more effective. Public education must be directed particularly toward people who live in ghettos, because the rate of infant morbidity and mortality among them is significantly higher than among the general population.

The problems of the children and adolescents who are seen by pediatricians have been categorized (most of the children are from middle-class families). Many pediatricians estimate that they see 95% of their patients on an ambulatory basis. They see most of their patients in the office; they see perhaps 2% to 3% at home and no more than 3% to 4% in the hospital. About 40% to 45% of the pediatrician's patients have physical illnesses. About 30% of the physical illnesses are infections of the throat and the respiratory tract. Other illnesses (e.g., contagious diseases, allergies, and skin diseases) make up the other 70%. Only about 5% (at the most) of the physical illnesses are serious. At least 20% to 25% of the pediatrician's patients have emotional or behavioral problems and learning difficulties, without any related physical illnesses. Well infants and children, mostly newborns and very young children, make up about 35% (or even 50%) of some pediatricians' practices. Many of the patients who have physical illnesses, particularly those who have chronic illnesses or handicaps, have psychologic problems as well. Also, the health supervision of well children has psychosocial implications. So the estimate of the number of problems that involve significant psychosocial factors increases to 60% or 70% or even more—a figure comparable to similar estimates made by physicians who treat adults.

For various reasons, the patients now seen in teaching hospitals by medical students and residents have many more difficult diagnostic and therapeutic problems than did patients seen in the past. One estimate shows that 50% of the children and adolescents on a pediatric ward are there for diagnostic study of inborn errors of metabolism or for evaluation or reevaluation of other chronic illnesses or handicaps rather than for treatment of acute illness. A large percentage of patients who have chronic illnesses may be seriously ill. The illnesses of many of them have psychologic components, and the illnesses of all of them have psychosocial effects on their families.

At least 75% of pediatric residents go into private practice. Unfortunately, most of the residents leave the hospital expecting to encounter rare and exotic syndromes quite often in their practices. They have relatively little interest in children's health and development and in the psychosocial issues pertinent to children's health. Since residents are not well trained in the continuing care of ambulatory patients (only one recent textbook concerning ambulatory pediatrics exists), many young pediatricians have, as several recent publications attest, experienced surprise and disillusionment when they began to practice. They often wish that they had had more training in the treatment of emotional and developmental problems, parent counseling, and work with adolescents and their families and that they had greater knowledge of resources in their communities which could help them treat such problems—as well as more experience in treating allergic, dermatologic, and orthopedic problems.

Other studies show that parents emerge from their pediatricians' offices with many unanswered questions about their children's behavior and development. They have not asked questions because they are unwilling to take the time needed to talk to the pediatrician or because they feel that the pediatrician may not be interested. In one study, physicians were shown to record complaints about bodily dysfunctions more often than they recorded complaints about behavior. A recent survey made in California showed that 28% of a large group of parents were "seriously concerned" about their children's behavior even though the behavior problems were often not objectively serious ones. (A survey made recently by the Joint Commission on Mental Health of Children shows that at least 8% to 12% of the children in the United States have problems that require mental health services; therefore, some of the parent's concerns are probably valid.) The public has expressed dissatisfaction with methods of hospital care and other aspects of medical treatment. People apparently want a comprehensive approach to medical treatment, an approach that includes, in addition to the technical advances made in medical science, a lasting personal relationship between the patient and the physician. Such relationships spring up only rarely because of the current approach to medical treatment. Technologic advances are not enough, and inpatient pediatric practice is no longer the "real" pediatrics. The effects of the current approach to medical treatment are apparent in the emergency rooms of public hospitals; the poor and minority groups use public hospitals as their main medical resource, but public hospitals are set up to give care only in a crisis, not to maintain patients' health continuously.

The pediatrician must develop a balanced, comprehensive approach to treatment, an approach that includes the evaluation of the psychologic as well as the physical factors in both acute and chronic illnesses, and he must promote the psychologic as well as the physical health of the child and his family. A "new" idea of the role of the pediatrician that is now presented in some training programs can help pediatricians to find challenge and satisfaction in their practices.*

*The recent Report of the Task Force on Pediatric Education, under the leadership of C. Henry Kempe, has called for more teaching in the biosocial aspects of pediatrics, among other recommendations.

The functions of the pediatrician, as adapted from Romano's concepts of the functions of the general (or family) practitioner, are:

1. Diagnostic. The pediatrician identifies illness patterns, considers the relative importance of the physical and the psychologic factors in illnesses, and makes initial decisions about the appropriate type of care.
2. Preventive. The pediatrician employs all the available methods of science to prevent physical or psychologic illness and to promote actively the child's physical and psychologic growth and development.
3. Therapeutic. The pediatrician provides intensive treatment for the acutely ill child and continuous care and rehabilitation for the chronically ill child. The pediatrician considers the child's psychologic and social needs and the feelings and reactions of his parents.
4. Integrative. The pediatrician correlates and coordinates the care given the child by other professionals, such as specialists, health associates, hospital workers, and the personnel of community agencies.
5. Investigative. The pediatrician pursues clinical and epidemiologic studies, formally or informally, on his own or in collaboration with others. He also studies the effect of illness on each child and his family.
6. Educational. The pediatrician gives parents and older children information about a child's illness and corrects any misconceptions they have about the illness. He shares his knowledge of the nature and course of the particular illness and its impact on family life with students and residents as a part-time teacher in hospitals or clinics, and serves as an educational source for the community at large, including organizations and legislative bodies.

Much has been made recently of the "new pediatrics," which provides for a comprehensive approach to pediatric care. The new pediatrics is not new, but its value has been recognized only recently in many academic centers. The core of pediatric practice (like that of general medicine) has always been the relationship between the pediatrician and the child he treats, together with the child's parents. It is within the framework of this relationship, with its human, humanistic, and humanitarian qualities, that any therapeutic, preventive, or rehabilitative measures must be taken if they are to succeed. The new pediatrics is so called because it uses new knowledge of children's behavior and personality development and of the psychosocial factors that affect behavior and development. New techniques of treatment accompany the new knowledge. Now pediatrics can be considered "unscientific" if it fails to consider the effect of the emotions on the body's functioning.

With training and experience, the pediatrician can refine and develop his intuitive perceptions of the emotional forces within a family and their effect on a child's illness. He can make his perceptions more accurate by studying human coping or adaptive behavior and the psychosocial aspects of children's development. He can learn to employ his intuitive emotional responses to the behavior of sick or troubled children (and to their parents) to achieve a constructive and controlled empathy with the children's feelings. The pediatrician's empathy enables children and parents to reveal their feelings to him and to themselves; such revelation helps them cope with their problems. The pediatrician can learn to offer supportive psychologic help to children and families who are undergoing acute emotional crises. The pediatrician's help may prevent psychosocial decompensation or disorder in the family's members.

Recognizing the signs and symptoms of depression (as they appear differently in children of different ages), perceiving the intensification of a child's asthma during his parents' marital crisis, and recognizing the need for satisfying educational and social experience of a child who has chronic rheumatoid arthritis all require that the pediatrician understand specific phenomena and techniques. Such measures as the referral of a severely disturbed child for psychiatric treatment or the use of psychiatric or psychologic consultations require from the pediatrician both diagnostic skill and a recognition of his own limitations. In order to make referrals and arrange for consultations, the pediatrician must understand

thoroughly the functions of various facilities in the community and be able to collaborate with many specialized professionals.

Whether the pediatrician should become a consultant able to deal with the physical, behavioral, and developmental problems of children (as in Britain and some other countries) or should remain a "general practitioner of medicine in childhood" remains to be determined in the United States. In either case, the pediatrician must learn about the development of and adaptation by the child who lives in a multiple-person field. The pediatrician should learn about the family and about the psychology, sociology, and epidemiology of illnesses of all kinds; he should be able to use effectively his relationship with the child and the child's parents. He must also increase his capacity for critical observation in order to collect the verbal and behavioral data which he requires, in addition to laboratory tests, to reach his diagnoses and to take the appropriate therapeutic or preventive measures.

The psychosocial or behavioral aspects of pediatrics are now vitally important because child psychiatrists and other mental health professionals cannot possibly treat all the psychosocial disorders of children and adolescents. The pediatrician need not—indeed, should not—become a child psychiatrist. His practice should center on his specialized knowledge of the physical aspects of the illnesses and of the growth and development of the child. Nevertheless, he must broaden his skills and understanding in order to practice "comprehensive pediatrics" effectively and satisfyingly.

Since about 60% of the children seen by physicians in the United States are treated by primary care practitioners, such as internists, general practitioners, or family physicians, rather than by pediatricians, knowledge of comprehensive pediatrics must be available to the undergraduate student of medicine so that he can treat children in his future practice, whether or not he specializes in pediatrics.

The remainder of the book discusses the various topics that are related to the achievement of the above-mentioned goals for pediatricians. The book presents a conceptual framework and goes on to discuss the essential features of diagnosis, treatment, and prevention in a psychosocial approach to pediatrics. It relates the psychosocial aspects of illness to the physical aspects. The book discusses the principles underlying successful psychiatric referral and collaboration with child psychiatrists, psychologists, social workers, educators, courts, and other community workers and agencies. It also discusses direct work with adolescents, habilitative and rehabilitative techniques used to help the mentally retarded and other handicapped children, the pediatrician's role in dealing with juvenile delinquency and his role as a consultant to camps, schools, and community agencies, and other recent developments in pediatric practice.

No written work, however, can do justice to the complexities of the psychosocial aspects of pediatrics. Supervised experience during undergraduate medical education and in pediatric residency, involvement in postgraduate courses offered by the Academy of Pediatrics or other groups (such as the Academy of Family Practice) and by university centers, and day-to-day collaboration with psychiatrists and other mental health professionals are necessary for the pediatrician to assimilate the knowledge available and to apply it confidently and satisfyingly for the benefit of his patients. The book supports the idea that the physician can assimilate and use well all the knowledge available to him.

Suggested References

Blum, R.H.: *The Management of the Doctor-Patient Relationship.* New York, McGraw-Hill, 1961.

Brees, B.B., Disney, F.A., and Talpey, W.: The nature of a small pediatric group practice. Pediatrics, *32*:246, 1966.

Commentary. The clinician's art: Some questions for our time. Pediatrics, *43*:157, 1969.

Deisher, R.W., et al.: Changing trends in pediatric practice. Pediatrics, *25*:711, 1960.

Friedman, S.B.: The challenge in behavioral pediatrics. J. Pediatr., *77*:172, 1970.

Green, M.: Integration of ambulatory services in a children's hospital. Am. J. Dis. Child., *10*:178, 1965.

Green, M., and Haggerty, R.J., Eds.: *Ambulatory Pediatrics.* Philadelphia, Saunders, 1967.

Hessel, S.J., and Haggerty, R.J.: General pediatrics: A study of the practice in the mid-1960's. J. Pediatr., *73*:271, 1968.

Korsch, B.M.: Pediatric out-patient departments. Pediatrics, *23*:162, 1959.

Lengthening Shadows. A Report of the Council on Pediatric Practice of the Academy of Pediatrics on the Delivery of Health Care to Children. Evanston, Ill., American Academy of Pediatrics, 1970.

Menkes, J.H.: A new role for the school physician. Pediatrics, *49*:803, 1972.

Peabody, F.W.: The care of the patient. JAMA, *88*:67, 1927.

Pediatric Residency Training. Proceedings of an Institute Sponsored by the American Board of Pediatrics at Atlanta, Georgia, on September 17–19, 1965. Pediatrics, *38*:Suppl., 1966.

Pediatrics in general practice (editorial). Pediatrics, *23*:369, 1959.

Plunkett, D.C.: Military pediatric out-patient care: Report of experiences in a large army hospital. Milit. Med., *131*:711, 1966.

Rogers, K.D.: A teaching program in community pediatrics. Pediatrics, *25*:336, 1960.

Romano, J.: Basic orientation and education of the medical study. JAMA, *143*:409, 1950.

Rose, J.A.: The dimensions of comprehensive pediatrics. Pediatrics, *26*:729, 1960.

Shatkin, E.P.: Comprehensive care. Pediatrics, *47*:141, 1971.

Silver, G.A.: *Family Medical Care.* Cambridge, Harvard University Press, 1963.

Solnit, A.J.: A need for pediatric guidance. Pediatrics, *47*:325, 1971.

Somers, A.R.: The missing ingredient. Med. Opin. Rev., *5*:27, 1969.

Starfield, B., and Borko, S.: Physicians' recognition of complaints made by parents about their children's health. Pediatrics, *43*:168, 1969.

Starfield, B., and Sharp, E.: Ambulatory pediatrics: The role of the nurse. Med. Care, *6*:507, 1968.

Thorpe, H.S.: Behavioral pediatrics in private practice. J. Pediatr., *78*:181, 1971.

2
Current Concepts of Health and Disease*

*For this is the great error of our day. . .
that physicians separate the soul
from the body.
(Plato)*

The development of medical science can be studied through an examination of the various explanations of the causes of disease offered since medical science began. The causes of disease have been explained by the magical and supernatural beliefs of witch doctors, by the naturalistic observations of the ancient philosopher-physicians, by Western methods of scientific inquiry, and finally by the concept of the bacterial causation of disease.

No disease has a single cause. The host's immunity and the virulence of the invading organism both affect an infectious disease. The study of ecology shows that man's relationship to his environment affects diseases. The study of psychology

shows that emotional conflict can precipitate or perpetuate disease. Ideas about the causes of diseases have been influenced by new ideas in other scientific fields. Most scientists no longer believe that any phenomenon has a single cause. Instead they believe that the interaction of several factors usually explains phenomena more satisfactorily. Multiple causality is now an established concept in medicine.

The term disease (dis-ease) means an impairment of health. Until recently, health has frequently been defined as the absence of disease. In the fields of pediatrics, child psychiatry, psychology, and child development, it is now believed that a child's health has positive features which must be understood in order to maintain health. Advances made in immunology provide a good example of that belief. Current psychosomatic concepts provide another example that is discussed more fully later in the book.

---

*Some of the material in this and the following two chapters is adapted from D.G. Prugh: Towards an understanding of psychosomatic concepts in relation to illness in childhood. In: *Modern Perspectives in Child Development*. (A.J.Solnit and S.A. Provence, Eds.). New York, International Universities Press, 1963.

Health and Disease: A Unitary Concept

The modern unitary theory of health and disease comes from the work of Bernard,[2] Cannon,[3] and Freud,[12] and has been most explicitly stated by Romano[21] and Engel.[10] The unitary theory considers health and disease as "phases of life" which depend on the balance maintained by the organism, through the use of genetically and experientially determined devices, in satisfying his needs and in mastering stresses that come from within or without. Health is the phase of successful adaptation (and, in children, of growth and maturation) in which the child is able, within the limits of his development, to master his environment and in which he is reasonably free from pain, disability, or limitations in his social capacity. Disease is the phase in which the organism fails to adapt or is unable to maintain an adaptive equilibrium or "dynamic steady state." In disease, failures or disturbances occur in the growth, development, functioning, or adjustment of the organism as a whole or of any of its systems.

Levels of Organization

In recent years, Engel,[11] Grinker,[15] Mirsky,[18] and others have developed a conceptual approach to the human organism that recognizes 3 basic levels of organization: physiologic, psychologic, and social or interpersonal. The interrelationships of the 3 levels of organization involve multiple feedback operations at "nodal" points of interaction. The feedback operations are carried out through the neuroendocrine system and its relationships with the brain and the mental apparatus as well as the various organ systems. Biologic systems that are so organized are "open," as opposed to the "closed" systems of the physical universe. Alterations in an organism's function that occur at any level of its or-

ganization cause reverberations throughout the related systems. Alterations and reverberations occur constantly; the reverberations maintain an adaptive equilibrium. The contemporary systems theory, first articulated by Von Bertalanffy,[26] describes the subsystems within the 3 levels, beginning with cells and tissues at the physiologic level and ending with transactional or mutually reciprocal social interactions within the family, peer group, and community (and beyond).

The Concept of Stress

As Engel[11] has pointed out, stress for the human organism may be caused by any influence, internal or external, that interferes with the satisfaction of the person's basic needs or disturbs the adaptive equilibrium. Stresses may frustrate the person's basic drives or needs (from the intake of oxygen to sexual activity), damage organs or parts of his body, or limit the capacities of the systems that are involved in growth, development, or adaptation. Physiologic or psychologic changes in the internal dynamics of the human organism (e.g., the changes that occur during puberty) may operate individually, conjointly, sequentially, or summatively within the external environment as stresses. To an extent, stress is relative rather than absolute. A person's past experience, his physical, psychologic, and social nature, interacting with his genetic endowment, his developmental capacities, the reactions of his family to him, and the noxious influence of the stimulus affecting him all help to determine what stresses exist that may strain his adaptive capacity.

Physical stresses include noxious physical or chemical agents; substances or forces formed or developed within the body, such as excess insulin or increased intracranial pressure, a lack of oxygen, water or vitamins, and insufficiency states, such as hormone deficiencies. Invading microorganisms and parasites have various effects, depending on the virulence of the organism and the host's resistance; the latter is influenced by the host's past immunologic experience, among other variables. Damage to molecules, cells, tissues, or organs may arouse physiologic defenses or compensatory mechanisms in order to maintain or reestablish homeostasis. The effect of physical stresses on the biochemical or physiologic systems, as well as the action of defenses or compensatory mechanisms, may affect a person's psychosocial functioning.

Psychologic stresses in the older child or adult affect the central regulating system (the brain and the mental apparatus, discussed later in the chapter). Psychologic stresses arise from thoughts or feelings that are unacceptable to or produce conflict within a person and are closely linked with social stresses. *Social* stresses arise from the loss (or a threat of the loss) of important persons or relationships, the presence of real or fantasied danger, or the frustration of a drive or need. Psychologic or social stresses must be registered by the perceptual systems and receive conscious or unconscious central symbolic representation in the mental apparatus. Whether the representation (and the mental associations, memory traces, or emotions connected with it) becomes a stress depends on the person's past experience, personality development, and current situation, including such factors as the emotional support given him by other persons and the condition of his central nervous system.

When psychologic or social stimuli become stressful, the central symbolic representations of them produce signal-anxiety in the ego. Signal-anxiety arouses psychologic defense mechanisms, such as projection and denial, in order to maintain the adaptive equilibrium. Signal-anxiety may produce other unpleasant and often conflicting emotions, such as fear and guilt. It may also arouse behavioral and social coping devices, such as withdrawal or ag-

gressive attack in order to alter the source of the stressful stimulus or to resolve in another way the conflicting emotions. Murphy[19] and Cobb,[6] among others, have made a distinction between adaptation (internal change to improve a person's fit with his environment) and coping (change or manipulation of a person's environment).

Physical stimuli may affect the mental apparatus directly by altering brain tissue or indirectly by changing its perceptual threshold. Physical stimuli include external damaging forces, such as trauma or infection, or changes within the organism, such as hormonal excesses or deficiencies. Disturbances in the mental representation of a person's body image may be caused by gross damage to his brain or to his organs or body parts. It is unlikely, however, that central symbolic representation occurs with changes that take place first on the cellular level in the internal organs that maintain physiologic homeostasis. Physical stimuli may produce, intensify, or compound psychologically or socially stressful stimuli and so arouse physiologic or psychologic defenses or social coping behavior in any combination. Psychologic or social stimuli may change the functioning of physiologic systems and so affect growth, development, or adaptation.

Variations in the adaptive capacity of the human organism, caused by genetic, constitutional, developmental, or experiential factors affect the organism's vulnerability to potentially stressful stimuli. Other biologic factors, such as gender, racial background, and periodic rhythms that involve circadian systems or biologic clocks, may also affect vulnerability (although their action is poorly understood). The season and the climate may also affect vulnerability. Depending on the person's adaptive capacity at the time that he receives stressful stimuli and on the nature, duration, and intensity of the stimuli, the stimuli may have a variety of effects, as Engel[11] lists: (1) a new and successful adaptive equilibrium may be established with the help of physiologic, psychologic, or social defense mechanisms, (2) the organism's functioning (or growth and development) may be partially restricted; the importance of the physiologic or of psychologic components varies, (3) temporary marked decompensation may occur; it may be physiologic, psychologic , or both, (4) a complete breakdown in adaptation may occur, leading ultimately to death from physical damage or depletion or from psychologic malfunctioning (as in self-starvation or suicide).

Disease Pictures

Restriction of the functioning (or of the growth and development) of, decompensation by, or adaptive breakdown of the organism are states of disease. Many of the signs and symptoms, such as fever or regressive behavior, may result from attempts made by the organism to adapt, to compensate, to make restitution, or to satisfy basic physiologic, psychologic, or social needs, rather than from the action of the stressful stimuli. Under severe stress, the organism may go through phases of response that resemble impact, recoil, and restitution. Each phase includes particular physiologic, psychologic, or behavioral and social defenses or adaptive devices (see Chap. 24).

If a stressful stimulus is primarily physical, the changes that it causes in physiologic systems may have a transactional influence on the psychologic and social levels of a human being's organization. Reverberating responses often occur at the physiologic level in systems other than the one originally affected by the stimulus. When the stimulus is primarily psychologic or interpersonal (and such stimuli are usually accompanied by conflicting emotions), the signal-anxiety or other emotions aroused by the stimulus may cause physiologic changes (called concomitants of emotions) in many organ systems. Such changes are ordinarily reversible although they may last

as long as the emotional conflict lasts. Such physiologic changes may, however, further strain an already damaged organ, such as the heart—as Chambers and Reiser[4] have indicated—or may precipitate, accelerate, or enhance preexisting or latent pathologic processes at a biochemical level or at an organ system level, with the appearance of so-called psychophysiologic disorders, such as peptic ulcer, asthma, or diabetes (see Chap. 21). Psychophysiologic disorders may affect the mental apparatus either directly, as in diabetic coma, or indirectly, by arousing psychologic or social adaptive devices. Failure of an adaptive device may cause the sick person to use his psychologic defenses inappropriately and so cause further decompensation, as does the child who denies he is ill with diabetes and overeats heavily, for example, or the child who refuses to take the medication that he needs for his asthma.

If an emotional conflict remains unresolved and unpleasant emotions persist, the psychologic defenses or social coping mechanisms used by a human being may develop to unhealthy and maladaptive extremes (discussed in detail in later chapters). In people who are predisposed by past experience and by constitution, the extreme development of defenses and coping mechanisms may lead to psychoneurotic disorders or personality disorders, or psychotic disorders (which represent severe decompensation or adaptive breakdown). In infants and young children, such crystalized psychologic states are rare; they usually exhibit symptomatic behavioral or psychologic reactions (reactive disorders). Maladaptive behavior that is used to deal with stressful stimuli may cause physiologic reverberations, such as a nutritional deficiency caused by the refusal of food by a chronically depressed child or the exposure to physical injury by a child who is struggling to deny intense fears.

The symptoms experienced by the patient and even the signs noted by the physician may not have an obvious relationship to the stressful stimuli first experienced and to the level of organization that was originally affected. Indeed, the symptoms reported by the patient (or, in the case of a younger child, by his parents) may vary widely even when caused by similar original stresses at the same level of organization. Characteristic patterns of response, traditionally called syndromes, commonly occur. Nevertheless, each person responds differently to potential stresses, and the physician should keep that in mind.

Developmental Factors

In a child, the dynamic steady state that reflects his adaptive equilibrium is only relatively stable, existing at hypothetical points on a continuum of time during his growth and maturation. During a child's development, certain "sensitive" phases (rather than "critical" phases, as Wolff[29] has put it) in the child's biologic progress appear to make him more vulnerable to potentially stressful stimuli. Intrauterine infections that occur during the early months of embryonic development, for example, produce congenital anomalies more often than those that occur later. Gastrointestinal disturbances that can cause severe dehydration occur most often in early infancy. In the second half of the first year of its life, an infant can easily be damaged by a significant and prolonged lack of adequate mothering; the infant experiences serious depression, a failure to thrive, intellectual and physical retardation, or marked personality distortions. Recent studies of animals and humans suggest that particular patterns of behavior in infants and young children must be aroused by certain social stimuli that occur in a certain configuration during certain phases of development. If a child does not receive these stimuli from an appropriate care-taking figure, those patterns may be seriously blunted, and the child may suffer irreversible defects in his intellectual development or in some other aspect of his development. In infancy and early childhood the central nervous system has a greater tendency to respond with seizures to a variety of stimuli. Allergic responses change in nature and severity during different stages of a child's development. Psychologic development during the late preschool phase that deals with the issues of social integration and sexual differentiation is another "sensitive" phase. Adolescence, during which the child should develop a satisfying self-concept and become fully independent, is another.

Special features of a child's physical development also influence his immune responses and susceptibility to illness. For example, the frequent occurrence of otitis media in infants appears to be related to the shape, position, and size of the eustachian tubes. The gradual increase and later decline in the total mass of lymphoid tissue during childhood is partly responsible for the more frequent occurrence of tonsillitis and adenoiditis in childhood. Infectious disease tends to produce more generalized, severe, and widespread reactions in infants, whereas it tends to produce more localized and mild responses in older children and adults. Tuberculosis affects the meninges more readily in infancy than in later childhood (and quiescent pulmonary lesions are often reactivated during puberty); school-age children have rheumatic fever and other collagen diseases more often than do infants. The infant responds to disturbing psychologic and interpersonal stimuli with relatively global and undifferentiated patterns of disturbed behavior, while the preschool-age child has more restricted, differentiated, and frequently shifting responses. Crystalized syndromes resembling adult neuroses or personality disorders rarely appear before the school-age period, at a time when most of a child's personality structure has been laid down and he has acquired certain defensive and adaptive capacities.

Vulnerabilities and Strengths

In certain early stages of development, the human organism tolerates certain stresses more readily than in the later stages. The capacity of the fetus to withstand hypoxia during delivery and immediately after birth is a case in point. The effects of contagious diseases are milder in young children than in adults. The impetus toward growth and maturation that is characteristic of the human organism provides children with remarkable resiliency and powers of recuperation and compensation, even when they have very serious illnesses.

Differences in a child's reactions to noxious stimuli during different stages of his development have many causes. The causes include changes in his anatomic structure and metabolic activity, the maturation of his organ systems, tissue tropism, and changes in his immunologic responses to neuroendocrine integration, the patterning of his neural organization, the level of development of his mental apparatus, and his available social capacities. Other causes are his genetic potentialities, constitution, gender, and previous exposure to stimuli.

Constitutional Factors

The contemporary concept of constitution is a dynamic one. A person's constitution is the sum total of his structural and functional qualities or potentialities as they interact with his physical environment and the different levels and kinds of his experience, beginning with his intrauterine environment. A person's hereditary endowment is modified by his environment and experience throughout his development; these 3 factors influence his physique, his intellectual capacity, his autonomic functioning, his patterns of immunologic response, certain qualities of his temperament and his adaptive capacity. One's constitution is a "process"—as Witmer[28] says—not a "given." A person's inborn characteristics may produce some developmental deviation which may be en-

hanced or mitigated by experience. The effect on behavior of variations in persons' levels of hormones is not fully understood.

The Mental Apparatus

The central regulating system (the brain and the mental apparatus) has integrating relationships with the autonomic and endocrine systems—and through them with the organ systems—and with the striated musculature and somatosensory apparatus. The mental apparatus, an operational construct conceived by Freud, is a concept of the "mind," as linked with but transcending the neurophysiologic functioning of the brain. Although both cognitive, or thinking, processes and the neurophysiology of the cerebral cortex (which is connected to the subcortical structures that integrate thoughts and feelings) are better understood now than in Freud's time, the problem of the difference between the brain and the mind still exists. The flashbacks experienced by patients given electric stimulation in the temporal lobe by Penfield[20] and others justify the conclusion that the nerve cells and the junctions that preserve a memory can respond to excitation for most of a person's lifetime. Cognitive-ideational factors affect the brain's functioning, as evoked electroencephalographic responses show. However, despite recent studies of the role of ribonucleic acid in learning, it is still not understood how learning and retention take place at the cellular or molecular level, nor is there more than a vague cybernetic concept of the mechanisms of association and retrieval.

The mental apparatus is a combination of three psychic structures or systems. The first system, the id, is the instinctual part of the mind (one's basic drives). It operates on the unconscious level. Unconscious thinking influenced by instinctual drives is primitive and prelogical. Magical, omnipotent, and wishful thinking, like that of the very young child, is characteristic.

The ego, the executive or adaptive "organ" of the mind that is responsible for consciousness and for the discrimination and integration of stimuli, is the most important psychic system in the mental apparatus. The ego "tests reality" by distinguishing between external perceptions, experiences, and thoughts and inner fantasies. Other functions of the ego are memory, abstract and rational thought, decision making, learning, speech and other means of symbolic communication, self-awareness, the control of instinctual drives, the use of skills and creative capacities, the regulation of tension, the use of psychologic defense mechanisms and social coping devices, and the synthesis of all the functions previously mentioned to produce a smoothly operating adaptive equilibrium. The ego seems to rely on stimuli from the external world for its orientation in time and for the support of rational thought and reality testing, as the extensive literature on sensory deprivation indicates.

The third system, the superego, is a special aspect of the ego that is concerned with control and censorship. It develops from the internalization of parental and societal standards and prohibits and limits the instinctual drives. It is also concerned with the development of abstract ideals and models. The conscience is the conscious part of the superego.

The id, ego, and superego are functional or structural systems within the mental apparatus. Part of all 3 systems is a "topologic" or topographic set of constructs that refer to the dimensions or degrees of a person's conscious awareness of his mental activity. Conscious activity is characterized by perceptions, thoughts, memories, feelings, or sensations of which a person is fully aware. Other perceptions, thoughts, and so on are preconscious; they are available to conscious recall only under certain circumstances. Still others are unconscious; they have been fully excluded from awareness and are not subject to conscious recall.

Much of the activity of the ego is conscious, but a certain part is preconscious or unconscious. The ego's functions in dealing with the signal-anxiety aroused by intense or conflicting emotions have been discussed earlier, and its use of defense mechanisms and coping devices has been mentioned. Psychologic defense mechanisms work unconsciously and automatically. They relate to the function of repression, a central defense on which other defenses depend. Repression automatically blocks or removes from awareness the unpleasant or conflicting thoughts and feelings. (In suppression, blocking and removal are accomplished through conscious effort.) Unpleasant reality is frequently denied in children. The defense of projecting one's unacceptable feelings of blame onto others is often used and is often associated with the displacement of such feelings onto other situations. A person often rationalizes in favor of his own views.

Obviously, the psychic structures or systems in the mental apparatus, because they are operational constructs, cannot be assigned to any particular region of the central nervous system. It appears, however, that many of the executive, or governing, functions of the ego are carried out (or at least integrated) by the cerebral cortex and particularly by the frontal or associational areas of the cortex, drawing on other parts of the nervous system, on the sense organs, and on the musculoskeletal system. Most of the instinctual drives, together with their mental derivatives, the impulses and the ideational and emotional components of the impulses, can appear in people who lack functioning or effective cerebral cortical processes. The control and utilization of the drives and impulses in adaptation seem to be impaired in those people, however; the impairment is obvious in some people who have serious brain damage.

The subcortical areas of the brain can be conceptualized, in an oversimplified way, as the parts of the organism from which the instinctual drives (the id) receive their impetus and energy. The newborn's brain is principally equipped with the subcortical parts before the cortical inhibition of primitive reflexes and the cortical control and regulation of other subcortical functions develop. Brain damage in infancy may interfere with the development of cerebral cortical controls, while such damage in later life may remove those controls, both neurologically and psychologically.

In this view, the functions of the ego can be correlated with those of the cerebral cortex, the functions of the superego with those of the brain's frontal areas, and the id, the source of the instinctual drives, with subcortical areas. One can speak metaphorically of the "anatomy of the personality" if one recalls that the terms used to describe the personality cannot yet be closely linked with anatomic localities. Other terms can be and have been used to discuss the various aspects of personality functioning. Nevertheless, the conceptualizations of the id, the ego, and the superego can be helpful in the understanding of personality development and adaptation.

Instincts

The term instinct usually refers to the potential patterns of unlearned behavior which predominate in the lower animals (although recent studies indicate that much behavior in many species is actually produced by much social learning). At birth, the human infant is also equipped with potential patterns of unlearned behavior which may require certain social configurations to evoke them. The use of the term instinct to describe such behavior, as well as other aspects of human functioning, has caused much confusion and controversy among different schools of psychologic and psychoanalytic thought. Several ideas about instinct have some validity. Perhaps the broadest definition of instinct is that of Engel, who defines "an instinct as an internal force which acts as an impetus to

some action involving the external world." Engel's definition transcends the definition of an instinct as a bit of unlearned behavior, such as the nest building pattern of a bird. In unlearned behavior, a number of reflex patterns, the simplest responses to stimuli, may be involved; they often operate in clusters.

Instincts range from simple needs, such as the need to find water in order to satisfy thirst, to the complicated core of the sexual needs of adults. The energy of instinctual forces (or drives) comes from within the organism; it has a predominantly physiologic source. Ethologists have used the term "environmentally stable behavior" to describe drives. The expression of drives in human beings, however, in contrast to that in most of the lower animals, can be delayed or diverted by the action of the central nervous system and the mental apparatus in the service of rational behavior and adaptation. Much learned behavior may "long-circuit" an immediately perceived drive.

The expression of a newborn's drives centers on the satisfaction of his hunger and other basic physical needs. The infant does not consciously perceive such needs; its mother must perceive and satisfy them. The drives of the older child and the adult are more numerous and complex. Much controversy exists as to how many drives human beings have. Lists of human drives have ranged in number from 2 to a great many, depending on how much one defines particular drives. When Freud reduced the number of human drives to 2, the sexual and the aggressive, he attached to each drive a cluster of related drives, such as the drives that are related to reproduction of the species, which he attached to the sexual drive, and the drives that are related to self-preservation and mastery of the environment and often include competition, which he attached to the aggressive drive. Sexual and aggressive drives, as Freud saw them, have the highest emotional charge of any in civilized society. Freud considered all other drives as derivatives of the sexual and aggressive drives; the aggressive drive subserves physiologic needs. Other investigators have seen the drive toward mastery of the environment or toward competence as separate from the competitive parts of the aggressive drive, while still others, such as Dollard and his colleagues,[8] have seen aggression as the result of the frustration of other drives, such as the drives for dependency and love. Freud's view of the sexual drive has often been misinterpreted because many commentators have read only his earlier writings, in which he decried the repressive and destructive attitudes of his day toward sexuality. They may not be aware of his later writings about the mental apparatus and its necessary control and channelling of the sexual impulses, nor that he gave equal weight to the sexual and the aggressive drives. Freud's idea of the innate and ubiquitous character of (destructive) aggression was probably influenced by the thinking of his times, particularly by Darwinian concepts of the "struggle for existence" (which he used only metaphorically), but which Spencer applied, somewhat inappropriately, to human society. Eisenberg[9] has pointed out that human nature is not a "biological invariant." He cites the examples of the Eskimos who abhor war and of the Pueblo Indians who repress aggression.

The Tasaday, a recently discovered tribe that has an isolated existence like that of Stone Age peoples and lives in caves in the forests of the Philippines, may show man as he was before the population increased and competition for food began (at least as he was in a setting where there were no large predatory animals). The Tasaday have no words for anger, hostility, weapon, or war. Spencerian concepts of or recent theories about man's innate territoriality, propounded by Lorenz[17] and others, seem to be inaccurate; even gorillas and other higher primates are not territorial in the wild, as Schaller[24] and others have shown. If man shows concern for the "social qualities of intelligence," as Eisenberg indicates, he can free himself from fixed ideas about human nature and draw on his cultural virtuosity to make society's aspirations and behavior more peaceful.

The basic human drives as I see them are listed in the following paragraphs, albeit with much overlapping:

1. A cluster of physiologic drives that includes the needs for oxygen, food, water, and heat; the satisfaction of those drives is necessary for basic survival, whatever the circumstances and regardless of the intensity of other drives, although other drives may influence the level of the expression or the quality of the satisfaction of those physiologic needs.

2. The drive toward social interaction that is manifested initially in the first few months of a person's life in the mother-infant relationship and includes the social smile, attachment behavior, love and dependence, and, later, cooperative play and needs for social companionship.

3. The drive toward mastery of the environment that is manifested initially by activity, curiosity, the need to explore, learning, and constructive aggression and that is transformed later into learning, competence, competition, and self-preservation. The marked frustration of the drive toward mastery (or of other drives) can lead to destructive aggression.

4. The sexual drive that is manifested initially in the bodily pleasures of the infant and the young child and gradually evolves toward its goal of sexual union and reproduction of the species.

If the approach just described is followed, a distinction must be made among drives, impulses, needs, emotions, and motivations. Drives, the internal forces that impel certain actions and have physiologic sources, cannot be thought of as receiving representation in the mental apparatus. Impulses, the mental derivatives of drives, can be thought of as the forces in the mental apparatus pushing toward expression and conscious awareness through momentary upsurges in the urgency of the drives. The impulses may or may not receive conscious representation; they ordinarily operate at the unconscious level but evoke an accompanying emotion or feeling-state, which is then associated with a certain ideational or fantasy-thought content (such as the wish to imitate a friend for whom one feels affection). If the emotion evoked by an impulse conflicts with another emotion and especially if the impulse is an unacceptable one, the evoked emotion and/ or thought or fantasy may cause signal-anxiety in the ego and may be repressed or suppressed.

There are many human emotional needs that are related to different drives and impulses. The emotional needs include needs for love, security, acceptance, dependency, intimacy, admiration, self-esteem, self-realization, and success experience. Awareness of the emotional needs is ordinarily experienced at the conscious level; positive emotions (such as pleasure and satisfaction) may be aroused when emotional needs are satisfied. Tension builds up when emotional needs are not satisfied, and tension is relieved when they are satisfied. The infant and the young child require immediate satisfaction of their immediate and basic emotional needs (the *pleasure principle*). Older children and adults can postpone satisfactions in favor of more distant and enduring rewards (the *reality principle*). Such rewards include the satisfaction of others' needs. The drives, the impulses, and the emotions and needs that accompany them can be transformed into more complex motivations and value systems that have conscious as well as unconscious elaborations.

Emotions

Emotions (or feelings)* may be aroused by impulses or by needs. Emotions usually are felt by a person in a particular social or interpersonal context. They may be pleasant or unpleasant and be intensified when

*I prefer the terms *emotions* and *feelings* to the colder term *affect*.

drives are frustrated or two needs conflict. If unpleasant emotions are sufficiently intense, they may become stressful stimuli that affect the person's psychologic or social levels of organization and are registered, perceived, and given central psychic representation in the mental apparatus.

Cobb[5] and others have pointed out that an emotion characteristically has 3 components:

1. The subjective mental content, that is, the ideational thoughts or fantasies associated with the emotion. The thoughts or fantasies may be consciously registered or may remain unconscious.

2. The physiologic component or concomitant, which involves changes in the nerves, viscera, glands, and muscles. The changes can be conditioned to occur in situations that arouse the subjective component.

3. The behavioral expression, which may involve various adaptive actions, such as communicating the emotion to other persons verbally or nonverbally.

Behavioral expressions of emotions may be facilitated, altered, or inhibited by the mental apparatus. For example, appropriate control of the emotions that are aroused by sexual and aggressive drives is demanded of every person in society. The degree of control and the form of the behavioral expression of emotions vary from culture to culture; for example, the mourning rituals, such as the wake, which promote the release and working through of feelings about the dead person differ in different cultures. A person's behavior or communication of his emotions may provoke responses from other people which act as feedback and so modify the person's emotional experience, physiologic state, or behavioral expression.

Emotions seem to range along a continuum, from the more pleasant and positive emotions of love, joy, tenderness, contentment, optimism, trust, confidence, curiosity, and sexual satisfaction to the more unpleasant and negative emotions of anxiety, anger, fear, sadness, despair, helplessness, depression, and hopelessness. Darwin[7] was among the first to point out the adaptive character of emotions in animals and man. As Cannon[3] suggested, certain emotions, such as anger or fear, probably had greater significance in primitive societies, in which the associated physiologic preparation for "fight or flight" was essential to survival. In more advanced societies, such responses are less necessary for adaptation. (No attempt is made here to discuss the classifications of the subjective components of emotions that writers such as Cobb and Engel have offered, nor to associate individual emotions with particular drives or needs in other than the general way suggested in the preceding discussion.)

As has been mentioned, when the mental apparatus deals with the emotions aroused by drives and impulses, the subjective or ideational parts of the emotions may be repressed. The physiologic concomitant of the emotion lasts as long as the emotion remains intense, however, and behavioral expression of the emotion may occur that is dissociated, as is the physiologic concomitant, from the emotion itself. Conflicting emotions occur frequently, as when a child feels anger toward a parent whom he loves. Indeed, there is some ambivalence, or mingled quality in the emotions that are involved in every human relationship. In a mentally healthy person, conflicts of emotions are usually resolved fairly easily by psychologic means, such as the automatic exclusion from awareness of the negative feelings or the conscious working through of the conflicting emotions to a point of resolution, or by behavioral coping devices, such as withdrawal from the situation that is producing the conflict. The resolution of conflicting emotions ends the physiologic concomitant or the behavioral expression. When a person's unconscious emotional conflicts are not resolved and the conflicting emotions become psychologically stressful stimuli,

they may affect the person's dynamic steady state. Obviously, some successful resolution of the partially conflicting clusters of emotions that are aroused by the sexual and aggressive drives is necessary, as in the aggressive competition with others of the same sex that is usually carried on by the adolescent or young adult in order to win the affections of someone of the opposite sex.

Anxiety is a vague apprehension, uneasiness, or tension, without specific conscious content, which may signal the mental apparatus that the dynamic steady state of the ego is about to be disrupted. Anxiety may appear acutely during sudden, intense emotional conflicts, or it may exist chronically in people who have unresolved and unconscious conflicts and a fear of the unknown that includes a fear of some challenge to which they might not be equal. In contrast to anxiety, fear usually occurs when some actual external danger arises; young children may fear the strange or the unknown. Older children who constantly guard against any threat from the world, which they do not trust because of their experience, often have chronic fear. The actual, threatened, or symbolic loss of a loved or needed person, most often a parental or supportive figure, often causes depression. Engel has suggested that anxiety may have a biologic anlage in the reaction of a living cell with irritability to any stimulus, and that depression may derive from the tendency of primitive organisms to conserve energy when undergoing continuing stimulation by slowing down the rate of their responses to the stimuli.

The Social Field of Illness

The social or interpersonal level of a person's functioning is elaborated here in regard to the psychosocial field of forces within which a child may fall ill. Adults as well as children exist in a network of interpersonal relationships; changes in the network can cause changes in a person's adaptive equilibrium at his psychologic or his physiologic level of organization. Children are more dependent on the close caretaking figures in their environment, however, and are more vulnerable to many socially stressful stimuli than are adults.

At birth, the infant is equipped with reflex mechanisms that operate primarily at the subcortical level. The infant does not show conscious psychologic and social levels of organization. It appears that for the first several months of his life, the infant's physiologic level is most important; his mother is the external representative of his psychologic level. Social interaction between the mother and infant consists largely of contacts concerning the infant's physiologic needs, which he communicates to his mother by crying or restlessness. Recent research suggests that during the neonatal period certain physiologic systems of the infant show sensitive responses to feeding and other contacts with his mother, particularly in his autonomic functioning and motor behavior.

As true social transactions between the parent and the infant become possible, beginning in the infant's second or third month with his first social response, the smile, the infant's rapidly developing capacities soon (at least by the second half of his first year) bring him to the point at which he may perceive and respond sensitively to social stimuli.

Parent-Child Relationships

The interpersonal contacts of the infant and young child include the initial two-person relationships: mother-child, father-child, sibling-child, and the like. The importance of those relationships, particularly of the mother-child relationship, for the psychologic aspects of the development and adaptation of the young child has been recognized for many years. Recent studies show that actual, threatened, or symbolic disruptions of the early mother-

child relationship, as well as other vicissitudes in parent-child interaction, act as predisposing, contributing, precipitating, and perpetuating factors in many childhood diseases. The diseases range from psychologic disorders (such as depression, "environmental" retardation in psychomotor development, psychoneuroses, psychoses, and antisocial personality disorders) to diseases in which psychologic and physiologic disturbances coexist (such as hospitalism, peptic ulcer, marasmus, or failure to thrive, ulcerative colitis, and asthma). Our knowledge of the precise character and degree of the influence of a disturbance in the parent-child relationship on a child's disease is limited. The deleterious effects of such gross disturbances as marked overprotection, overpunitiveness, and overpermissiveness or, more rarely, open rejection or neglect that occasionally leads to willful injury or inadequate nutrition are well documented. Evidence is accumulating to support the view that markedly unhealthy parental attitudes (that are often unconscious) are more crippling to a child's personality development and his health than is any single child-rearing technique.

Although the concept of a parent's or parents' "doing" or "failing to do" something for a child has been a popular one, the current view is that of an interreacting, mutually reciprocal or transactional relationship between parents and child.[1] That concept holds that the developmental characteristics of a child at particular points, beginning with his first feeding response after his birth, act as feedback and so may affect his parents. The nature of the relationship between parents and child is influenced at least partly by the child's contributions to it. Thus the personality structures of each parent, the natures of their previous experiences, their attitudes toward child rearing and toward the particular child, the events that occur during the pregnancy and neonatal period, their ability to work together harmoniously in rearing the child, and their capacities to perceive the child's needs as a developing person, interact with the child's physical and behavioral characteristics, his unfolding genetic and constitutional potentialities, and with fortuitous events, such as illness, to determine the quality of the parent-child relationship and its effect on the child's adaptive capacity and, consequently, on his health.

Even though the tone of the parent-child relationship may be set by its early transactions, those transactions may help to form but not completely fix the child's personality and ultimate psychologic health and maturity. Later events may offset initial difficulties. Indeed, as Erickson has pointed out, subsequent psychosocial interactions may compensate considerably for earlier deficiencies or distortions. In spite of initial problems, parents may develop in their capacities as parents or in their abilities to deal with a particular child.

Family Influences

The relationship between a child and his parents exists within the nuclear family. The nuclear family exists in all societies (there are differences in its organization and function in different societies). The transactional balance between parent and child must be enlarged to include other members of the family. Family members carry on their transactions with one another as individuals, pairs, or other subgroups; the family as a unit or a group of persons also carries on transactions. The tone of the relationship between the parents has an important effect on their handling of one child, for example; the physical or behavioral characteristics of another child may evoke "preferential" responses in one or both parents. The degree of a family's intactness and cohesiveness, its patterns of communication, role operations, and leadership, its values, and the nature and extent of its integration into the community, together with the operations of the subgroups that exist among its members, affect the maintenance of a "family adaptive equilibrium" or a balance of interpersonal forces in the family.

Disruptions in the family adaptive equilibrium may affect parent-child relationships and, indirectly, the adaptive capacity of a particular child by acting as a stressful stimulus at the social level of organization. If a parent withdraws support as a result of physical illness or depression, the withdrawal can be a stressful stimulus that affects a child who is in a vulnerable phase of his development and produces reverberations at either the psychologic or the physiologic level or at both. The child's altered behavior (altered in response to the stressful stimulus) may act as feedback and affect unfavorably one or both parents or other family members. The illness and hospitalization of a child, followed by regressive behavior, may alter the parents' patterns of handling the child because the parents feel anxiety, guilt, or other emotions. Overprotectiveness or overpermissiveness toward the child by one or both parents may cause jealousy or regressive behavior, in a sibling with a predisposition toward psychologic or physical illness patterns, producing adaptive breakdown and disease in the sibling.

Crises such as a child's illness may, in a healthy family, temporarily alter the family's patterns of communication, interpersonal transactions, and role operations. But the flexibility and cohesiveness of the family is not destroyed, and a new and different family adaptive equilibrium is soon established. The new equilibrium may be either temporary or permanent; it may produce some emotional growth in family members and often does produce a higher, more adaptive level of "family development." In the family which fails to achieve a new equilibrium, a crisis may cause decompensation and disorganization or various types of "schism and skew" in role operations or subgroups. The sick child may be made a scapegoat for a family's tensions, or if he is temporarily sick, he may unconsciously be kept in the role of a chronic invalid, permitting a tenuous and unhealthy equilibrium to be maintained in the family at the cost of the psychologic health of the child. The breakdown or disintegration of a family may be caused by several factors, including death or marital incompatibility. The breakdown of a family often has a strong effect on the personality development or health of young children.

Family members who have serious psychologic illnesses may influence adversely the family's patterns of response and may serve as "carriers" of disturbed behavior over several generations if their illness influences the family's children. In certain deeply pathologic and precariously poised family equilibria, unhealthy relationships of an intensely complementary nature may occur between parent and child or may involve other two-person units, triangular relationships, or even the whole family. The adjustment of the persons involved is so deeply dependent, in an interlocking fashion, upon that of the specific partner or partners that the death, illness, or even improvement during psychologic treatment of one of the partners may disrupt the adjustment of the other or others. Decompensation that is manifested by illness at a physiologic level, marked depression, or even psychosis may occur in the people concerned. Such families are rare; they are seen often enough, however, to contraindicate active psychotherapeutic treatment at times or at least to contraindicate the treatment of one member without the careful simultaneous treatment of the others.

Sociocultural Factors

In addition to immediate reverberations within the social field of the family, other phenomena involving social interaction within the community, state, and national society must be considered in considering a person's response to stressful stimuli at the social level of organization.

That social contacts outside the home can influence the form of a person's psychologic illness has long been known. Historical accounts indicate that epidemics of "dancing frenzy" or other group behavior have occurred periodically in particular subcultural groups. In modern times, small epidemics of hysterical conversion symptoms have been observed on pediatric wards; in the epidemics, the "contagion" has been touched off by such events as the death of one patient, for example. Until recently, epidemics of hysterical weakness or paralysis in adolescent girls were common during the poliomyelitis season. A variety of symptoms including asthma, increased difficulty in breathing, and respiratory infections, have been noted in a group of patients in a respiratory poliomyelitis center immediately after the discharge of a beloved and supportive patient. Recent studies of normal people suggest that such psychophysiologic responses as skin potentials and levels of free fatty acids may be affected by social variables, such as sociometric relations in small groups and increased pressure to conform.

Patterns of child rearing are strongly influenced by parents' socioeconomic backgrounds, although it is difficult to attach value judgments to the differences, except under extreme circumstances. Attitudes toward feeding and discipline may differ among families that have different ethnic or national origins. Feeding problems occur more frequently and juvenile delinquency and alcoholism less frequently in particular subcultural groups; the groups' attitudes and family structure apparently cause the differences in incidence.

Recent observations imply that socioeconomic factors may affect the incidence of various illnesses. How they affect the incidence of illnesses is not clear. Higher incidences of mental illnesses and certain types of psychosomatic illnesses have been reported in groups that are lower on the socioeconomic scale in North American society, particularly in members of those groups who live in central urban areas.[16] Some evidence suggests that population shifts or migrations from rural into urban areas may be associated, at least temporarily, with an increased incidence of disorders in function of certain organ systems, particularly in the cardiorespiratory system, and, in certain countries, with changes in the types of mental illness found in the population. The incidence of illnesses such as hypertension and diabetes, which differ among different ethnic groups (perhaps partly as the result of inbreeding) may be altered or more often may increase when people are first exposed to the stresses—physical, psychologic, and social—that affect them in urban areas. Such stresses include changes in dietary patterns and encounters with social discrimination, for example. In different countries, the incidence of some psychologic disorders has increased in semirural communities that are disintegrating. Some investigators think that members of North American families that are moving from the lower to the middle class are more susceptible to psychologic illnesses. Gadjusek[13] identifies sociocultural factors as some of the causes of kuru in isolated populations in New Guinea.

The incidence of rheumatic fever in the North American population is higher in groups that are lower on the socioeconomic scale. Perhaps the higher incidence is caused by frequent exposure and even lowered resistance to streptococcal infections as a result of poorer nutrition and living conditions. Differing attitudes toward prenatal care as the result of limited education may be responsible in part for the fact that complications of pregnancy and premature deliveries occur more frequently in women from underprivileged socioeconomic backgrounds. Differences in suicide rates have been found in groups that differ in age, sex, and nationality, and in different seasons. Differences in attitudes toward pain

and in localization of pain have been found in different socioeconomic and ethnic groups. Studies of adults have shown that a relatively small number of people in a city accounted for many of the illnesses that are reported; psychologic and interpersonal factors affect many of those illnesses. The children of a core of multiproblem families often contribute heavily to the figures on the incidence and prevalence of children's disorders, especially delinquency. Since the turn of the century in Western society, for reasons which are obscure but which may be related to changes in child-rearing practices, family structure, and social patterns, the incidence of certain diseases has changed. The incidence of hysterical disorders seems to have decreased, for example, while disturbances in gastrointestinal function seem to have increased.

The interplay between human biology and the socially relevant components of the ecosystem is just beginning to be understood. Recent studies[14] have been made of the effect of noise, both predictable and unpredictable, on human behavior, physiology, and task performance. Other studies are going on that deal with the effects of contacts with strangers and of crowding; the latter has been shown to have disastrous effects on certain animals beyond a certain point. Habitat may have effects on biology and behavior which range from the ecologic relationships among hosts, parasites, and their environment to the effects of crowding, noise, social stress, and ways of living on the adaptation of groups and individuals to their surroundings.

The causes of the relationships that seem to exist among many of the variables mentioned remains to be clarified. Artifacts may have been introduced by different methods of study by different investigators. In different studies, there are differences in the populations that are available in clinical facilities, in samples, and in other factors. Whatever the contributions of sociocultural factors to the causes of illness, however, they definitely affect attitudes toward sick people,[25] physicians and other helping persons, and community agencies. Research suggests that families from different sociocultural backgrounds react differently to illness in their children. Healthy patterns of reaction predominate, but unhealthy patterns exist that range from overprotection of a sick child to isolation and even ostracism of the child from the family. Differences appear to exist also in the reactions of families to the need for medical treatment and, in particular, for hospitalization. Families from rural parts of southern Europe, for example, may resist the admission of a child to the hospital because they regard the hospital as a death house, to be used only for the terminally ill. Chicano and Indian families in the American Southwest distrust hospitals staffed by white people and may prefer to ask the help of their own practitioners of folk medicine.[23]

Attitudes toward the sick person may vary from society to society. In Western society, the role of patient is more comfortably assigned to a person who is physically ill than to one who is mentally ill. Stereotypes of social classes that are held by physicians may unconsciously affect the nature of the treatment that the physicians offer, particularly to the mentally ill.

The Family As the Unit of Study

Consideration of the social level of organization must include consideration of the forces that affect a person as a result of his membership in his family, in his social class and ethnic group, and in his local community, region, and national society. The pediatrician must accept the family, rather than the child alone, as the unit for study, treatment, and prevention of disease. The genetic and constitutional potentialities of family members, the developmental level of each, the history of the family and its members in relation to its state of development, the parenting capac-

ities of the adults, the nature of the family's physical environment, the current patterns of interaction within the family, and the family's sociocultural setting, are pertinent to the occurrence and nature of any illness in one or more family members. When a child becomes acutely or chronically ill, his illness both affects and is affected by his family's interpersonal equilibrium in the family's community, society, and culture.

Bibliography

1. Benedek, T.: The psychosomatic implications of the primary unit: Mother-child. Am. J. Orthopsychiatry, 19:642, 1949.
2. Bernard, C.: *An Introduction to the Study of Experimental Medicine.* New York, Macmillan, 1927.
3. Cannon, W.B.: *The Wisdom of the Body.* New York, Norton, 1932.
4. Chambers, W.N., and Reiser, M.F.: Emotional stress in the precipitation of congestive heart failure. Psychosom. Med., 15:38, 1953.
5. Cobb, S.: *Emotions and Clinical Medicine: With an Introduction on Semantics and Definitions.* New York, Norton, 1950.
6. Cobb, S.: Social support as a moderator of life stress. Psychosom. Med., 38:300, 1976.
7. Darwin, C.: *Expression of Emotion in Man and Animals.* New York, Philosophical Library, 1955.
8. Dollard, J., et al.: *Frustration and Aggression.* London, Kegan Paul, 1944.
9. Eisenberg, L.: Can human emotions be changed? Bull. Atomic Scientists, 22:27, 1966.
10. Engel, G.L.: Homeostasis, Behavioral Adjustment, and the Concept of Health and Disease. In: *Mid-Century Psychiatry: An Overview* (R.R. Grinker, Ed.). Springfield, Ill., Thomas, 1953.
11. Engel, G.L.: A unified concept of health and disease. Perspect. Biol. Med. 3:459, 1960.
12. Freud, S.: *An Outline of Psychoanalysis.* New York, Norton, 1949.
13. Gadjusek, D.C., et al.: Isolated and migratory population groups: Health problems and epidemiologic studies. Am. J. Trop. Med. Hyg., 19:127, 1970.
14. Glass, D.C., and Singer, J.F.: *Urban Stress: Experiments on Noise and Social Stressors.* New York, Academic Press, 1972.
15. Grinker, R.R., Ed.: *Toward a Unitary Theory of Human Behavior.* New York, Basic Books, 1959.
16. Hollingshead, A.B., and Redlich, F.C.: *Social Class and Mental Illness.* New York, Wiley, 1958.
17. Lorenz, K.: *On Aggression.* New York, Harcourt, Brace & World, 1963.
18. Mirsky, I.A.: The psychosomatic approach to the etiology of clinical disorders. Psychosom. Med., 19:424, 1957.
19. Murphy, L.: Coping styles. In: *The Widening World of Childhood.* New York, Basic Books, 1962.

20. Penfield, W., and Roberts, L.: *Speech and Brain Mechanisms*. Princeton, N.J., Princeton University Press, 1959.
21. Romano, J.: Basic orientation and education of the medical student. JAMA, *143*:409, 1950.
22. Rome, H.P.: Emotional problems leading to cardiovascular accidents. Psychiatr. Ann., *5*:259, 1975.
23. Saunders, L.: *Cultural Difference and Medical Care*. New York, Russell Sage Foundation, 1954.
24. Schaller, G.B.: *The Year of the Gorilla*. Chicago, University of Chicago Press, 1964.
25. Twaddle, A.C.: The concepts of the sick role and illness behavior. In: *Psychosocial Aspects of Physical Illness* (Z.J. Lipowski, Ed.). Basel, S. Karger, 1972.
26. Von Bertalanffy, L.: The theory of open systems in physics and biology. Science, *111*:23, 1950.
27. Wilson, E.O.: *Sociobiology: The New Synthesis*. Cambridge, Harvard University Press (Bellknap), 1973.
28. Witmer, H.L., and Kotinsky, R., Eds.: *Personality in the Making*. New York, Harper, 1952.
29. Wolff, P.H., and Feinbloom, R.: Critical periods in cognitive development in the first two years. Pediatrics, *44*:999, 1969.

General References

Benjamin, J.D.: The innate and the experiential in child development. In: *Childhood Psychopathology*. (S.I. Harrison, and J.F. McDermitt, Eds.). New York, International Universities Press, 1972.

Bliss, E.L., Ed.: *Roots of Behavior: Genetic, Instinct, and Socialization in Animal Behavior*. New York, Harper, 1962.

Engel, G.L.: *Psychological Development in Health and Disease*. Philadelphia, Saunders, 1962.

Engel, G.L.: The need for a new medical model: A challenge for biomedicine. Science, *196*:129, 1977.

Erickson, E.: *Childhood and Society*. New York, Norton, 1950.

Fried, M., and Lindemann, E.: Sociocultural factors in mental health and illness. Am J. Orthopsychiatry, *31*:87, 1961.

Halliday, J.L.: *Psychosocial Medicine: A Study of the Sick Society*. New York, Norton, 1948.

Harrison, S.I., et al.: Social class and mental illness in children: Choice of treatment. Arch. Gen. Psychiatry, *13*:411, 1965.

Hinkle, L.E., and Wolff, H.G.: Ecological investigations of the relationship between illness, life experience, and the social environment. Ann. Intern. Med., *49*:1373, 1958.

Opler, M.K., Ed.: *Culture and Mental Health*. New York, Macmillan, 1959.

Parsons, T.C.: *The Social System*. Glencoe, Ill., Free Press, 1951.

Prugh, D.: Towards an understanding of psychosomatic concepts in relation to illness in childhood. In: *Modern Perspectives in Child Development*. (A.J. Solnit and S.A. Provence, Eds.) New York, International Universities Press, 1963.

Rennie, T.A.C., and Srole, L.: Social class preference and distribution of psychosomatic conditions in an urban population. Psychosom. Med., *18*:449, 1956.

Scott, J.P.: *Animal Behavior*. New York, Doubleday Doran, 1963.

Seguin, C.A.: Migration and psychosomatic disadaptation. Psychosom. Med., *18*:404, 1956.

Sheldon, W.H., Stevens, S.S., and Tucker, W.B.: *The Varieties of Human Physique: An Introduction to Constitutional Psychology*. New York, Harper, 1940.

Spiegel, J.P.: Mental health and the family. N. Engl. J. Med., *251*:843, 1954.

Syme, S.L., and Berkman, L.F.: Social class, susceptibility, and sickness. Am. J. Epidemiol., *104*:1, 1976.

Thomas, A., and Chess, S.: *Temperament and Development*. New York, Brunner/Mazel, 1977.

Wittkower, E.D., and Fried, J.: Some problems of transcultural psychiatry. Int. J. Soc. Psychiatry, *3*:245, 1958.

3
Toward a New Physiology

*These changes—the more rapid pulse,
the deeper breathing, the increase
in the sugar from the blood, the secretion
from the adrenal gland. . . seemed unrelated.
Then, one wakeful evening. . . the idea
flashed through my mind that they could
be. . . conceived as bodily preparations for
supreme effort as in flight or in fighting.*
(Walter B. Cannon)

The physiologic concomitants of emotions have recently been carefully studied. Most reports about the physiologic concomitants use facts obtained in laboratory situations in which psychologic stresses have been induced. The stresses are usually conscious and are induced in normal subjects, usually adults. The negative emotions have been studied most carefully; outstanding exceptions are Stevenson's[78] and Levi's[44] studies of pleasurable experience and Cobb's[18] summary of his impressions of the physiologic concomitants of heterosexual attraction or love. Wolf[90] and Wolff,[93] and many others, have made many similar studies that Applezweig[5] has summarized and that have added much to our understanding of the physiologic concomitants.

A brief list of some of the physiologic concomitants of emotions follows; they are listed in relation to the organ systems.

1. *Cardiovascular:* variations in the heart rate and rhythm (including the appearance of extrasystoles) and in its stroke volume, in cardiac output, arterial blood pressure, peripheral resistance, and arteriovenous oxygen difference, in electrocardiographic patterns; in tolerance for exercise; in capillary activity; and in coronary blood flow.

2. *Respiratory:* variations in the respiratory rate, rhythm, and amplitude, in tidal volume, CO_2 tension, and oxygen exchange, in bronchiolar action; the activity of the diaphragm and the accessory muscles of respiration, and in the secretory responses, which are associated with changes in the vascularity of the mucous membranes of the nose and other parts of the respiratory tree.

3. *Gastrointestinal:* changes in the motor, vascular, and secretory activity of the esophagus,

the stomach (including the cardiac and pyloric sphincters), and the large intestine; changes in the amounts of hydrochloric acid, pepsin and lysozyme that are produced, changes in the functioning of the external anal sphincter, variations in the pH, viscosity, and total amount of secretion of the salivary glands, changes in the bacterial flora of the oropharynx, and changes in the absorption of iron.

4. *Genitourinary:* changes in vesical functioning and external sphincter control, changes in the renal blood flow and filtration rate, in urine flow and in the amount of uropepsin excreted, changes in the muscular activity of the uterus and in menstrual functioning, and changes in penile tumescence.

5. *Hemic and lymphatic:* variations in the blood levels of leukocytes, lymphocytes, and circulating eosinophils, changes in the values for relative blood volume and viscosity, clotting time, hematocrit, and sedimentation rate, and changes in pH values and oxygen saturation.

6. *Musculoskeletal:* variations in the muscles' electrical potentials, and changes in the coordinating activity of muscle groups.

7. *Skin:* changes in the skin's temperature, psychogalvanic skin responses, thermal sweat production, the secretion of sebum and fatty acids, cutaneous vascular responses and patterns of wheal formation and exudation, and changes in the skin's vulnerability to inflammatory reactions.

8. *Endocrine:* variations in the amount of the steroids secreted by the adrenal cortex (including plasma hydrocortisone, plasma cortisol, urinary hydroxycorticosteroids, and 17-ketosteroids), variations in the amounts of male and female hormones secreted by the gonads (such as testosterone and estrone), changes in the thyroid's activity that cause changes in plasma-bound iodine and thyroxin; variations in secretion of insulin, changes in the level of aldosterone, and changes in the levels of growth hormone and prolactin.

9. *Central nervous system:* changes in the electroencephalographic measurements of cortical activity, nerve reaction time, sedation threshold, pain perception and response, activity level, the response to various drugs and anesthetic agents; variations in perceptual accuracy and in cognitive functions, such as memory and reasoning.

In addition to those specific responses of the organ systems, broader metabolic changes occur. Some of the broader changes are related to changes in hormonal balance, including variations in the amounts of water, electrolytes, catecholamines, ketone bodies, creatinine, hippuric acid, uric acid, and coproporphyrins found in the blood and urine, changes in basal metabolism and body temperature, variations in the blood glucose levels, and changes in the values of plasma lipids, such as free fatty acids and cholesterol.

Little is known about any immediate changes that occur in enzymatic activity in the biochemical or other processes of metabolism that occur at the tissue, cellular, or molecular levels, although some studies of animals were done by Henry and his colleagues[37] concerning the effect of stress on the enzymes that are involved in the biosynthesis and metabolism of the catecholamines. Chapman and his colleagues[15] have described the changes in tissue vulnerability that hypnosis produces, but it is not understood how those changes occur. The roles of cyclic adenosine monophosphate (AMP) and of prostaglandins in the regulation of hormones at the cellular and tissue levels are being studied.

The levels of gastric pepsin and lysozyme vary in relation to the emotions. The variations seem to be caused by changes in the secretory activity of the exocrine cells, which secrete those enzymes and exist in the mucosal wall of some parts of the gastrointestinal tract. Psychologic stresses probably cause such variations at the cellular level. Some recent clinical studies indicate that people who are depressed or who have conflicting emotions have poor wound healing and delayed convalescence. Full documentation must await the development of new and more refined methods of psychophysiologic investigation.*

---

*Most of the specific references that concern the studies mentioned so far in Chapter 3 are included in the review article by D.G. Prugh: Towards an understanding of psychosomatic concepts in relation to illness in childhood. In: *Modern Perspectives in Child Development* (A.J. Solnit and S.A. Provence, Eds.). New York, International Universities Press, 1963. Some are also included in some of the review works cited in Chapters 2 and 4. Several references concerning more recent studies of particular physiologic functions are included in the bibliography for Chapter 3.

Sleep physiology and sensory deprivation have been investigated by Usdin,[84] Luby and his colleagues,[47] Laties,[43] Zuckerman,[94] and Solomon.[76] Developmental changes in sleep patterns begin in early infancy; arousal systems may differ in men and women. Dreaming or rapid eye movement (REM) sleep is associated with psychophysiologic activity in many organ systems. In persons who have peptic ulcers, most nighttime acid secretion comes during REM periods. Sleep deprivation can cause irritability, paranoid thinking, visual hallucinations, and episodic rages. Man may also need his dreams. Man needs external stimuli; the results of sensory deprivation experiments are similar to those of sleep deprivation—temporary psychotic disorientations. Patients who are in respirators, are blindfolded, or are in certain types of intensive care units may react badly to their treatment if they do not receive compensatory sensory stimulation. Transcendental meditation has been shown to produce a physiologic state of restful alertness that differs from sleep, waking, dreaming, or hypnosis; and meditators have been found to be more stable on several autonomic indices, such as the galvanic skin response (GSR), than nonmeditators.[62]

Some of the studies from which the material just described is drawn are preliminary; they use very small numbers of subjects. Usually, in such correlative studies, scientists can study only one or two physiologic responses to stressful psychologic stimuli at a time. The complex and constantly varying interrelationships among the various organ systems and metabolic processes can often only be inferred, although Mason[53] and others are investigating interrelationships among hormonal processes. It now seems clear that many endocrine systems participate in psychoendocrine responses (a subject that is discussed more fully in Chapter 4). Polygraphic techniques that can record changes in many physiologic parameters have recently been developed, but analysis of the large amounts of complex data they provide is difficult and at times misleading. It is difficult to define a stressful stimulus. In some instances, as Reiser and others[67] have noted, the stressful stimuli may result from the laboratory situation and not from the experimental psychologic stimulus; in other instances, the stimulus or the situation may be a significant stress for some people and not for others. It is now difficult to determine the exact degree and nature of psychophysiologic events, even though the studies that have been done prove that they occur. Exceptions include such studies as the study of Benedek and Rubenstein,[7] who predicted estrogen and progesterone levels in women by using psychoanalytic data, and the study of Dongier and his colleagues[20] who predicted the rate of thyroid secretion in people who had anxiety neuroses (see Chap. 4) using the rate of decay of radioactive iodine, on the basis of a cluster of personality traits.

Certain physiologic phenomena, such as the hormonal changes that occur during the menstrual cycle (that Benedek and Rubenstein and others have studied)[7] affect psychologic functioning. (Recent studies suggest that women's expectations and social learning affect the emotional and cognitive effects of the hormonal changes.) Because mental activity depends on the biochemical milieu of the central nervous system, changes in certain physiologic values, such as the levels of thyroid hormone, calcium, and magnesium, can produce definite changes in mentation, as in hypothyroidism and hyperparathyroidism. Correcting the changes in values reverses many of the changes in mentation. The effects of stressful stimuli that are predominantly physical must also be considered. Pain from a traumatized part of the body or malaise caused by a viral infection may cause physiologic changes which may be intensified or changed by the physiologic concomitants of the emotions that are aroused by the experience of becoming ill. As Mason[60] has indicated, many of the physiologic changes mentioned may be caused by intense muscular effort during exercise that is performed in response to a crisis and might be mingled with the changes caused by the emotional response to the crisis.

The Question of Specificity

The question of the specificity of the physiologic concomitants of particular emotions is still open. The results of some studies of the concomitants of particular emotions conflict with the results of others. Such conflicts may be caused partly by difficulties in categorizing the particular emotions being studied. The emotions studied in artificial laboratory situations are usually conscious; the experiments seem to evoke emotions separately (to evoke "pure" emotions). But most real situations evoke mixed, often conflicting emotions; a person often feels emotions like grief and anger at the same time. Unconscious emotions often conflict with conscious ones. Margolin's[51] studies suggest that unconscious emotions may strongly affect physiologic function. Data from animal studies, which are valuable because they stimulate studies of human beings, cannot help answer the question of specificity.

It has long been known that blushing accompanies shame or embarrassment and that nausea accompanies disgust. Some investigators still hold that specific physiologic changes are caused in particular organs or organ systems by particular emotions. The data collected so far indicate that no specific physiologic change accompanies each emotion. Exceptions like the blushing and nausea that accompany shame and disgust exist; however, general patterns of responses seem to exist.

The first general pattern of response is the "emergency reaction" to real or imagined danger, which includes the physiologic preparations for "fight or flight" that are associated with anxiety, fear, or rage

(as described originally by Cannon[14]). Increased mental alertness, increased muscular activity and physiologic changes (e.g., increased cardiac rate and output, increased blood pressure, the redistribution of the blood flow to essential areas, an increased number of leukocytes, the mobilization of glucose, and an increase in the respiratory rate and amplitude) characterize the emergency reaction. Some of the physiologic changes are caused by epinephrine, which is secreted by the adrenal medulla; others are caused by the activity of the sympathetic nervous system.

Recent research has indicated that in animals, stimulation of the anterior part of the hypothalamus, which is interconnected with the reticular formation of the brain stem, produces the emergency reaction (or "defense alarm reaction" as Folkow and Rubenstein[27] have termed it). The emergency reaction has also been produced by Brod and his colleagues[12] in an experiment performed with human subjects under stress (the subjects were doing mental arithmetic while listening to a metronome). Sympathetic arousal increased the subjects' arterial pressure, cardiac output, and heart rates. The increased cardiac output was handled by increased blood flow in the skeletal muscles, which was shown by diminished resistance to blood flow through the muscles of the forearm in the face of reduced renal blood flow. Recent studies of animals by Bliss and Zwanziger[9] have shown that the amount of epinephrine in the brain decreases significantly during emotional stress although other amines in the brain remain constant.

Cannon described a reparative pattern that follows the mobilization of energy that prepares for muscular exertion. Selye's[75] studies have indicated that more long-range metabolic preparations for the repair of tissue injury that include the action of corticosteroids begin during the emergency phase of what he termed the general adaptation syndrome. In his studies of rhesus monkeys, Mason[59] extended Selye's reparative pattern. Mason has postulated an integrated, biphasic, reciprocally innervated catabolic-anabolic sequence that occurs in response to psychologic disturbances. The first phase of the sequence includes the secretion of hormones that have a catabolic effect (such as cortisol, thyroid hormone, and the growth hormones) and epinephrine and norepinephrine. During the catabolic phase, the secretion of anabolic hormones (e.g., insulin, estrogen, and androgen) is suppressed. In the anabolic phase that follows the cessation of stress, the production of the anabolic hormones resumes, and the levels of some of them become higher than the basal levels, while the catabolic hormones return to the basal levels. The catabolic-anabolic sequence is modifiable at times, and, although some studies of humans support the idea of the sequence, its existence has not been fully confirmed. Nevertheless, it provides a frame of reference that is useful in describing the organization and "overall balance" of psychoendocrine responses to stress.[54]

Much information about biologic or circadian rhythms has been accumulated recently. Both the relationships of a person's rhythmic processes to his responses to drugs and the relationships between deranged rhythms and disease have been studied. Curtis[19] has shown that 6 of the variables that affect Mason's catabolic-anabolic sequence have large diurnal variations. The variables include urinary corticosteroids, epinephrine, norepinephrine, aldosterone, urinary volume, and plasma growth hormone. Curtis believes that the amount of androgen that is secreted probably varies diurnally and that the amounts of estrogen, insulin, and thyroid hormone that are secreted may also vary diurnally. He points out that the organization of the daily neuroendocrine cycle differs significantly from Mason's psychoendocrine sequence.

Curtis believes that changes in the normal phases of the endocrine rhythms that are caused by an unusual living schedule or by an impairment of a person's capacity for synchronization could affect the person's overall hormonal balance as much as or more than does his psychoendocrine response. He points out that more nervous activity is needed to synchronize a person's internal rhythms with his environmental cycles, and that the person's capacity for synchronization depends on the structural and functional integrity of his brain. In addition to the possible effect of diurnal activity on hormonal balance, several studies (e.g., Stroebel's[79]) suggest that emotional stress can significantly disrupt the organizational patterns of the circadian rhythms.

The second general pattern of response has been described by Engel and Reichsman[24] and has been recently termed by Engel[23] the "conservation-withdrawal" pattern. Although there are few specific physiologic data, emotional states that include feelings of helplessness and hopelessness and that arise in situations that involve the loss of a significant figure or from an inability to deal with real or imagined threats of loss are apparently accompanied by a general slowing of physiologic activity. The slowing includes a reduction of motor activity and of the secretory activity of the gastrointestinal tract, and an increase in sleep. The slowing is related to the clinical phenomena of slowed motor responsiveness, poor appetite, constipation, and other physiologic signs of prolonged grief or depression. Recent studies by Engel,[22] by Sachar,[70] and by others indicate that psychoendocrine responses in clinical depression and experimentally induced sadness include changes in the levels of growth hormone, corticosteroids, and catecholamines. Sachar[71] predicted that in a group of depressed patients undergoing psychotherapy, a person's corticosteroid secretion would be highest when he suffered an actual or a symbolic loss. A person's constitutional tendencies may determine whether he exhibits the withdrawal-conservation pattern or the emergency reaction.

No full physiology of the emotions as yet exists. The study of physiologic responses to social interaction includes Richmond's and Lipton's[69] study of the newborn and the study of the mother-infant interaction by Kulka and her colleagues.[41] Malmo[50] and others have reported that the muscle tension, skin temperature, and electrocardiographic tracings of patient and therapist vary during interviews, showing an "interpersonal physiology." Shottstaedt[74] has reported changes in heart rate and in the patterns of renal excretion of water and electrolytes during vicissitudes in the doctor-patient relationship. Wolf[89] and others have reported variations in the responses of patients to drugs in similar situations. Nonverbal and verbal communication appear to occur in interpersonal emotional exchanges and to affect their physiologic concomitants. Thaler-Singer[81] has suggested that the degree and nature of "engagement-involvement" (transactional involvement with other people) may be the relevant variable for correlation with physiologic phenomena, rather than the verbal content of interviews. She and Mason predicted the levels of plasma 17-hydroxycorticosteroids (OHCS) that would be found in preoperative patients from the estimated levels of the patients' "distress-involvement."

The physician must consider his patients' emotional states when he assesses mild deviations in physiologic values, such as their blood pressure, heart rates, or levels of plasma-bound iodine; thus he can avoid the iatrogenic effects of overcautious handling. Success or failure in producing the effects expected from drugs in a child may be related to changes in the child's threshold of response that are caused by his emotions. The child's emotions are affected by the reactions of his parents (as well as his own reactions) to events surrounding his illness, and by the degree of his parents' confidence in his pediatrician.

The Mechanisms of Psychophysiologic Interrelationships

The exact nature of the psychophysiologic mechanisms has not been discussed; those mechanisms are not fully understood. Recent studies, however, have provided an understanding of most of the mechanisms; the studies' results have been well summarized by Cobb,[18] Cleghorn,[17] Engel,[23] Prugh,[66] Mason,[54] and Weiner.[85]

The physiologic effects of psychologic or social stresses resulting from interpersonal or intrapsychic events that have emotional or symbolic significance are mediated by the neural interconnections of the cerebral cortex, which receives stimuli from the external world that the thalamus passed on to it, and the hypothalamus, in which lie controls for the autonomic and endocrine systems. There is such a close relationship between functions of the cerebral cortex and the hypothalamus that some scientists term them the *neuroendocrine system*. The studies of MacLean[48] and Papez[63] have indicated that the limbic (paleo) cortex, or "visceral brain," has a close relationship with the temporal cortex and so plays an important role in integrating and regulating external and internal perceptions, in determining whether nervous impulses are inhibited or are transmitted to the hypothalamus, and in the experiencing of emotions. The studies of Magoun[49] and others have indicated that the ascending reticular activating system acts as an alerting center and has many rich interconnections with the cerebral cortex, so that it affects the motor and autonomic responses that are involved in states of consciousness or arousal. Reciprocal influences appear to operate by proprioceptive input on reticular, thalamic, and hypothalamic activity. Henry and his colleagues[36] believe that the instinctual drives, or environmentally stable behavior, have their roots in the limbic system and the brain stem, where they are experienced as emotions. Henry also believes that (at least in animals) such responses are inhibited or facilitated by the neocortex because of the learning experiences that are part of social maturation.

Following Cannon's[14] pioneering studies, the activities and interrelationships of the autonomic nervous system have been widely studied. The direct effects of the hypothalamus on the activity of the sympathetic and parasympathetic parts of the autonomic nervous system have been well summarized by Gellhorn;[32] his summary included a description of their neuro-humoral action on the cardiovascular system and respiratory mechanisms, on the gastrointestinal system and other viscera, and on certain aspects of the metabolism of carbohydrates. Although the sympathetic and parasympathetic parts still seem to act reciprocally on the viscera, it is now known that their effects overlap. Their action now seems much more complex, as recent reviews by Mason,[55] Weiner,[86] and Hofer[38] indicate.

The posterior hypothalamic-sympathetic-adrenal medullary neural linkage causes the secretion of both epinephrine and norepinephrine. Earlier studies by Funkenstein[31] and others suggested that anger directed "inward," in a situation in which a person held his emotions in check and did not respond actively to outer danger (with a so-called anxious reaction) was associated with a predominant secretion of epinephrine. Anger directed "outward" (in a so-called aggressive reaction) was associated with a predominant secretion of norepinephrine. More recent studies do not fully support that suggestion. Frankenhauser and her colleagues[28] have shown that certain pleasant states, such as sexual arousal, are associated with higher levels of catecholamines, as are unpleasant states and states of understimulation as well as overstimulation. Subjects whose excretion rates of both hormones are high perform better than subjects whose rates are low in certain tests of cognitive functioning during psychologic stress.

The actions of acetylcholine and norepinephrine in autonomic neurotransmission have been more fully studied recently. The role of the autonomic afferent fibers in the regulation of visceral and hormonal interrelationships and of the autonomic visceral reflexes is beginning to be understood. In addition, many physiologic stimuli apparently can affect autonomic afferent activity; the resulting feedback affects the central regulatory processes of the higher nervous system.

Simple concepts of sympathetic or parasympathetic overactivity are no longer tenable. The conditioning of autonomic responses and the effects of transcendental meditation and biofeedback, indicate that the autonomic nervous system can learn and that its "involuntary" mechanisms can be voluntarily controlled to some extent. Finally, the effects of the hypothalamus on temperature regulation, appetite control, fat metabolism, the extrapyramidal system, and the reactivity of the somatic musculature under voluntary control have been described, although some of its effects are incompletely understood.

The posterior pituitary is influenced by the hypothalamus through neural interconnections, thus affecting the secretion of vasopressin and antidiuretic hormone, affecting water balance and renal mechanisms, and of oxytocin (thus affecting parturition). An increase in the amount of epinephrine that is secreted appears to inhibit the action of vasopressin. The influence of the hypothalamus on the anterior pituitary seems to be a neurohumoral one, through the hypothalamo-hypophyseal portal capillary system. By means of such interrelationships, psychologic stimuli from the cerebral cortex can affect the secretion of adrenocorticotropic hormone (ACTH), brought about by corticotropin-releasing hormone (CRH) that affects the adrenal cortex. Thus CRH affects the secretion of cortisol and other adrenal cortical steroids;

it may affect the cerebral cortex and behavior. The action of the other tropic hormones that affect the gonads (FSH and LH) and the thyroid (TSH) can be affected by "minihormones," such as the thyroid-releasing hormone (TRH), which is elaborated in the anterior pituitary and by other releasing factors, such as FSHRF and LHRF. Regulating action is apparently furnished by neural and humoral feedback mechanisms. Psychologic stimuli can affect both the secretion of the growth hormone, which is one of the nontropic hormones of the anterior pituitary, and probably the secretion of prolactin. Greene's[33] studies indicate that the secretion of the growth hormone can be activated independently by the pituitary-adrenocortical axis; Greene's[33] studies support the studies of others that indicate that the secretion of the growth hormone is caused by a separate releasing factor (GHRF) and that the secretion of prolactin is caused by an inhibiting factor (PIF).

Figure 3–1 shows the location of the diencephalic "alarm center" in the hypothalamus. The reticular formation (dotted area) sends stimuli to the cortex (solid lines). Specific afferents to the cortex from the brain stem and spinal cord (represented by the heavy shaded line with offshoots) strongly influence the reticular formation. The cortex itself has both activating and deactivating effects (broken lines) on the alarm center. Interconnections among the hypothalamus, the pituitary, and the reticular activating system are shown by short, solid, two-directional lines. Relationships with the endocrine, autonomic, and somatosensory systems (the 3 "effector" systems of the brain) are not represented.

Although psychoendocrine responses in the pituitary-adrenal cortical system seem to be sensitive indicators of emotional arousal from baseline states, they do not seem to differentiate qualitatively among different emotional states (as Mason has indicated). The adrenal responses of human subjects to stressful stimuli have proved in recent studies to be less consistent and less intense than the adrenal responses of animals. The difference in re-

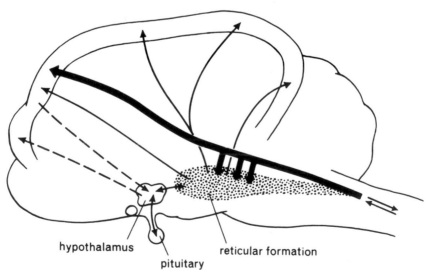

hypothalamus

pituitary

reticular formation

Fig. 3–1. Schematic representation of the interrelationships within the mammalian brain (Adapted from Henry, J.P., Ely, D.L., and Stephens, P.M.: Mental factors and cardiovascular disease: Psychosocial factors facilitating and inhibiting the neuroendocrine alarm response upon the course of cardiovascular disease. Psychiatr. Ann., 2:25, 1972.) (This adaptation in turn is modified from that of Charvat, Dell, and Folkow.[16])

sponses seems to stem from man's highly developed system of psychologic coping devices, which include defense mechanisms. Thus the higher centers apparently can inhibit as well as initiate psychoendocrine responses, and human beings can defend themselves from the emotional effects of stressful stimuli with less intense adrenocortical responses. Differences in different people's responses are significant, however, and shifts in one person's ability to cope are associated with changes in his patterns of adrenocortical response.

Starting from the observation that in a group of parents of leukemic children, a few parents who had low 17-OHCS secretion had effectively denied their children's illnesses, Wolff, Friedman, Mason and their colleagues[91,92] and Hofer[39] predicted the degree of adrenocortical response in that group of parents by assessing the effectiveness of their coping mechanisms. Other studies support that idea. A release of the growth hormone that is caused by stress usually occurs in fewer people than do adrenal secretory responses. The studies of Greene and his colleagues[33] suggest that the degree of a person's self-involvement may be related to his growth hormone response; the study of Brown and Heninger[13] partly corroborates that suggestion. They found that the degree of a person's field independence is also related to his growth hormone response. The effect of interpersonal stimuli on physiologic responses has been mentioned earlier, in relation to the work of Thaler-Singer,[81] Malmo,[50] and others. Finally, from animal studies, Mason[59] suggests that adrenal cortical responses are affected by a person's past life and environmental experience and by his own perception of the current stressful events that affect him (in addition to the nature of the stressful events and to constitutional factors, such as the person's body size and weight). Similar factors may affect the autonomic responses, as Weiner[86] points out, as may genetic predisposition and early conditioning.

Although the major ideas about the action of the psychoendocrine system have been developed mostly from studies of the pituitary-adrenal cortical[55] and sympathetic-adrenal medullary systems,[57] Mason[58,59] believes that only through further study of the pituitary-thyroid,[56] pituitary-gonadal, and other neuroendocrine systems[58]—and of the overall balance[54] of their responses—can psychoendocrinology be fully understood.

The drawing in Figure 3–2 shows in greater detail the points of anatomic contact between the nervous and endocrine systems. It is clear why Henry and his colleagues assume that the emergency, or defense alarm, reaction (described by Cannon and elaborated by Folkow) forms the neurogenic part and that the Selyean general adaptation syndrome (as elaborated by Mason) forms the endocrine part of the neuroendocrine alarm response to psychosocial stimuli. Knowledge of these interrelated systems and of their patterns of response, which are affected by such factors as diurnal rhythms and individual differences, helps greatly in understanding the central mechanisms that integrate the in-

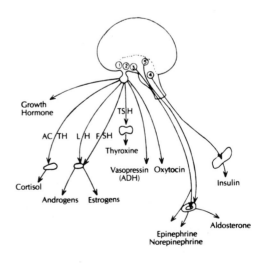

Fig. 3–2. Points of anatomic contact between the nervous system and the endocrine system. (From J.W. Mason: The scope of psychoendocrine research. Psychosom. Med., *30*:565, 1968.)

ternal environment and maintain the homeostatic equilibrium of the organism.

Developmental Considerations

The studies cited so far have been made mostly with adult subjects. Their validity for infants and young children has not been determined. Newborn infants are equipped with potential patterns of neural organization and regulation that have been studied in adults. For the first several months of a child's life, however, the physiologic parts of his emotional responses and of his reactions to stressful stimuli seem not to be smoothly integrated, particularly in regard to his autonomic functioning. Migeon[61] has shown that the enzyme systems of the newborn that are involved in the catabolism of cortisol seem to be less active than are those of adults, although plasma cortisol levels do vary with behavioral state (Anders,[4] Tennes,[80] Ader,[1] and Franks[29]). Other studies indicate that newborns have higher thyroxin uptake and thyroid-stimulating hormone (TSH) values than do adults (Marks[52]). The newborns' metabolism of catecholamines seems to have special characteristics, as do their hormonal and metabolic responses to the external temperature (Fisher and colleagues[26]). Newborns have limited capacities to metabolize certain drugs (Brazelton[10]). Such findings, however limited, suggest that neuroendocrine patterns of response to stressful stimuli may be different at birth than during later stages of development.

Lipton, Steinschneider, and Richmond[46] have summarized well what is known of the neurophysiology of the newborn, including autonomic activity, motor activity, and sensory response patterns. Their studies, which deal principally with changes in the heart rate that occur as responses to airstream, stroking, and thermal stimulation, indicate that a normal distribution curve can be found for a single physiologic

parameter that reflects autonomic activity among a group of healthy infants, with the use of regression coefficients and with due consideration for the "law of initial values" or baseline state. In such studies, differences among infants within the first few days of their lives in regard to a particular physiologic parameter can be identified, an observation confirmed by Bridger and Reiser.[11] Differences in the heart rates of newborns of different races have been found; black newborns have significantly higher rates (though not higher blood pressure) than do white newborns (Schachter[73]).

The studies of Grossman and Greenberg[34] have indicated that newborns may vary in their responsiveness within partitions of the autonomic nervous systems, without necessary correlations even among valid indices of individual parameters of functioning. Grossman and Greenberg have suggested that each newborn may have at least one "vulnerable" component of the autonomic nervous system. The responses of this vulnerable part to environmental stimuli, which begin with his contacts with his mother, may be more labile and thus participate more intensively in his later emotional responses. Changes in a child's autonomic response patterns occur during his development. The stability of his responses increases after the first 2 to 3 months of his life. The studies of Harper and his colleagues[35] have suggested that there are several phases in the ontogenetic sequence of cardiac rate and variability during infancy and that the nature of cardiac regulation during infancy may be a function of a state maturation. Harper believes that a child's autonomic balance shifts during his development, and thus makes him more vulnerable to stressful stimuli during certain phases of his development (although no data as yet support this belief).

Fries[30] has studied levels of activity in infants and children. She has found individual differences in infants' responsiveness to a standard stimulus that evokes the startle response: those differences correspond with others in their levels of activity. Wolf[88] has observed the apparent effects of endogenous neural stimuli on newborns' patterns of activity; Brazelton[10] has observed the patterns of reaction of normal newborns. Bergman and Escalona[8] have observed differences in the sensitivity of very young infants to external stimuli. Their studies have suggested that an individually characteristic "stimulus barrier" or threshold of response exists. Differences in infants' patterns of sleep and sucking and in their sensory patterns have been observed by Bergman and Escalona,[8] Parmalee,[64] and Pratt.[65] Apparent differences in infants' drive endowments have been observed by Alpert and her colleagues;[3] differences in biochemical patterns have been observed by Williams,[87] and differences in infants' patterns of stable reactions in regard to their mood responses, biologic rhythms, and other temperamental reaction patterns have been observed by Thomas and Chess.[82]

The emotional responses of the infant in the first several months of his life are less well studied; they seem to be relatively undifferentiated. The responses range from apparently pleasurable to unpleasurable states; many autonomically innervated organ systems participate in a more or less global type of physiologic concomitance. As the infant develops psychologic and interpersonal levels of organization, beginning with his first social response at 2 to 3 months of age, more fully differentiated patterns of emotional response that are associated with voluntary behavior become available to him. Some significant integration in REM sleep and other dimensions occur at the latest by 3 or 4 months, according to Emde and his colleagues,[21] Parmalee and his colleagues,[64] and Sostek and his colleagues.[77] By the beginning of the second year, the infant shows joy, anxiety, contentment, anger, fear, sadness, and depression. Data are not available, but many investigators believe that the phys-

iologic concomitants of emotions become more limited and involve fewer organ systems. The studies of Engel, Reichsman and Segal[25] showed changes in hydrochloric acid secretion in an infant in the second year of her life in association with the emotions aroused during her interpersonal contacts. The infant's level of gastric hydrochloric acid rose during states of positive relatedness and of anger; they fell during depression-withdrawal phenomena. Animal studies done by Reite and his colleagues[68] seem to confirm some of the observations cited above.

Tjossem and his colleagues[83] have systematically demonstrated temperature changes in the skin of young children in relation to the anxiety generated by separation from their mothers. Hospitalization has been reported to raise the blood pressure of preschool-age children. Lacey and his colleagues[42] have described, in older children and adults, overall patterns of autonomic responsiveness ("autonomic response specificity") that vary from person to person. Genetic factors may affect those patterns, as Jost and Sontag have suggested.[40] Cortisol levels in infancy and later childhood have been studied in relation to behavior by Tennes and her colleagues[80] and by Franks,[29] but there are few studies of corticosteroid, catecholamine, and other psychoendocrine responses,[45] at other levels of development. It is not known whether children's early experiences can cause the individual differences that exist in their later patterns of psychoendocrine response (although Mason,[59] from certain data on animals and human beings, feels that the question should be studied). Sander[72] is studying the effect of caretaking experience in the neonatal period on autonomic patterns, biologic rhythms, and the like. Although differential responses are clear, the question of long-term effects remains unanswered.

The few data available seem to indicate that progression from less organized to more organized modes of psychophysiologic response occurs during children's development. Individual differences in autonomic and other parameters of response apparently exist in newborns and older children. The idea that the molecules of epinephrine, cortisol, and perhaps other neurohumoral substances are small enough to cross the placental barrier suggests that the mother's neuroendocrine system may affect the fetus. The methods of study are promising but primitive and the results obtained so far are meager (Ader[1]). Although exciting vistas lie ahead, much work remains to be done before a full understanding of developmental psychophysiology is possible.

Bibliography

1. Ader, R.: Early experiences accelerate maturation of the 24-hour adrenocortical rhythm. Science, *163*:1125, 1969.
2. Ader, R., and Deitchman, R.: Effects of prenatal maternal handling in the maturation of rhythmic processes. J. Comp. Physiol. Psychol., *71*:492, 1970.
3. Alpert, A., Neubauer, P.B., and Weil, A.P.: Unusual variations in drive endowment. Psychoanal. Study Child, *11*:125, 1956.
4. Anders, T.F., et al.: Behavioral state and plasma cortisol levels response in the human newborn. Pediatrics, *46*:532, 1970.
5. Appelzweig, M.H.: *Psychological Stress and Related Concepts: A Bibliography.* New London, Conn., Connecticut College Press, 1957.
6. Benedek, T.: *Psychosexual Functions in Women.* New York, Ronald Press, 1952.
7. Benedek, T., and Rubenstein, B.B.: Correlations between ovarian activity and psychodynamic processes. Psychosom. Med., *1*:245, 461, 1939.
8. Bergman, P., and Escalona, S.: Unusual sensitivities in very young children. Psychoanal. Study Child, *3/4*:333, 1949.
9. Bliss, E.L., and Zwanziger, J.: Brain amines and emotional stress. J. Psychiatry Res., *4*:189, 1966.
10. Brazelton, T.B.: Psychophysiologic reactions in the neonate. I. The value of observation of the neonate. J. Pediatr., *58*:508, 1961.
11. Bridger, W.H., and Reiser, M.F.: Psychophysiologic studies of the neonate. An approach toward the methodological and theoretical problems involved. Psychosom. Med., *21*:265, 1959.
12. Brod, J., et al.: Circulatory changes underlying blood pressure elevation during acute emotional stress (mental arithmetic) in normotensive and hypertensive subjects. Clin. Sci., *18*:269, 1959.
13. Brown, W.A., and Heninger, G.: Stress-induced growth hormone release: psychologic and physiologic correlates. Psychosom. Med., *38*:145, 1976.
14. Cannon, W.B.: *Wisdom of the Body.* New York, Norton, 1963.
15. Chapman, L.F., Goodell, H., and Wolff, H.G.: Changes in tissue vulnerability induced during hypnotic suggestion. J. Psychosom. Res., *4*:99, 1959.
16. Charvat, J., Dell, P., and Folkow, B.: Mental factors and cardiovascular disease. Cardiologia (Basel), *44*:124, 1964.
17. Cleghorn, R.A.: The interplay between endocrine and psychological dysfunction. In: *Recent Development in Psychosomatic Medicine.* (E.D. Wittkower and R.A. Cleghorn, Eds.). Philadelphia, Lippincott, 1957.
18. Cobb, S.: *Emotions and Clinical Medicine: With an Introduction on Semantics and Definitions.* New York, Norton, 1950.
19. Curtis, G.C.: Psychosomatics and chronobiology: Possible implications of neuroendocrine rhythms. Psychosom. Med., *34*:235, 1972.
20. Dongier, M., et al.: Psychophysiological studies in thyroid function. Psychosom. Med., *27*:497, 1965.
21. Emde, R.N., Gaensbauer, T.J., and Harmon, R.J.: *Emotional Expression in Infancy.* New York, International Universities Press, 1976.
22. Engel, G.L.: General concepts of adrenocortical function in relation to response to stress. Psychosom. Med., *15*:565, 1953.
23. Engel, G.L.: Anxiety and depression–withdrawal: The primary affects of unpleasure. Int. J. Psychoanal., *43*:89, 1962.
24. Engel, G.L., and Reichsman, F.: Spontaneous and experimentally induced depressions in an infant with gastric fistula. J. Am. Psychoanal. Assoc., *4*:428, 1956.
25. Engel, G.L., Reichsman, F., and Segal, H.L.: A study of an infant with a gastric fistula. I. Behavior and rate of total hydrochloric acid secretion. Psychosom. Med., *18*:374, 1956.
26. Fisher, D.A., Oddie, T.H., and Makoski, B.S.: The influence of environmental temperature on thyroid, adrenal, and water metabolism in the newborn human infant. Pediatrics, *37*:583, 1966.
27. Folkow, B., and Rubenstein, E.H.: Cardiovascular effects of acute and chronic stimulations of the hypothalamic defense area in the rat. Acta Physiol. Scand., *28*:28, 1966.
28. Frankenhauser, M., et al.: Catecholamine excretion as related to cognitive and emotional reaction patterns. Psychosom. Med., *30*:109, 1967.
29. Franks, R.C.: Diurnal variation of plasma 17-hydroxycorticosteroids in children. J. Clin. Endocrinol. Metab., *27*:75, 1967.
30. Fries, M.E., and Woolf, P.J.: Some hypotheses on the role of the congenital activity type in personality development. Psychoanal. Study Child, *8*:48, 1953.
31. Funkenstein, D.H.: Norepinephrine-like and epinephrine-like substances in relation to human behavior. J. Nerv. Ment. Dis., *124*:58, 1956.
32. Gellhorn, E.: *Principles of Autonomic-Somatic In-*

tegrations. Minneapolis, University of Minnesota Press, 1967.

33. Greene, W.A., et al.: Psychologic correlates of growth hormone and adrenal secretory responses of patients undergoing cardiac catheterization. Psychosom. Med., *32*:599, 1970.

34. Grossman, H.J., and Greenberg, N.H.: Psychosomatic differentiation in infancy. I. Autonomic activity in the newborn. Psychosom. Med., *19*:293, 1957.

35. Harper, R.M., et al.: Polygraphic studies of normal infants during the first six months of life. I. Heart rate and variability as a function of state. Pediatr. Res., *10*:945, 1976.

36. Henry, J.P., Ely, D.L., and Stephens, P.M.: Mental factors and cardiovascular disease: Psychosocial factors facilitating and inhibiting the neuroendocrine alarm response upon the course of cardiovascular disease. Psychiatr. Ann., *2*:25, 1972.

37. Henry, J.P., et al.: Effect of psychosocial stimulation on the enzymes involved in the biosynthesis and metabolism of noradrenaline and adrenaline. Psychosom. Med., *33*:227, 1971.

38. Hofer, M.A.: The principles of autonomic function in the life of man and animals. In: *American Handbook of Psychiatry*, 2nd Ed., Vol. 4. (S. Arieti, Ed.). New York, Basic Books, 1975.

39. Hofer, M.A., et al.: A psychoendocrine study of bereavement. I. 17-hydroxycortico-steroid excretion rates of parents following death of their children from leukemia. Psychosom. Med., *34*:481, 1972.

40. Jost, H., and Sontag, L.W.: The genetic factor in autonomic nervous system function. Psychosom. Med., *6*:308, 1944.

41. Kulka, A.M., Walter, R.D., and Fry, C.P.: Mother-infant interaction as measured by simultaneous recording of physiologic processes. J. Am. Acad. Child Psychiatry, *5*:496, 1966.

42. Lacey, J.I., Bateman, D.E., and Van Lehn, R.: Autonomic response specificity. An experimental study. Psychosom. Med., *15*:8, 1953.

43. Laties, V.G.: Modification of affect, social behavior and performance by sleep deprivation. J. Psychiatr. Res., *1*:12, 1961.

44. Levi, L.: The urinary output of adrenaline and noradrenaline during pleasant and unpleasant emotional states. Psychosom. Med., *27*:80, 1965.

45. Levine, S.: The pituitary-adrenal system and the developing brain. In: *Progress in Brain Research*, Vol. 32. (D. DeWied and J. Weijnen, Eds.). New York, Elsevier, 1970.

46. Lipton, E.L., Steinschneider, A., and Richmond, J.B.: The autonomic nervous system in early life. N. Engl. J. Med., *273*:147; 201, 1965.

47. Luby, E.D., et al.: Sleep deprivation: Effects on behavior, thinking, motor performance, and biological energy transfer systems. Psychosom. Med., *22*:182, 1960.

48. MacLean, P.D.: Contrasting function of limbic and neocortical systems of the brain and their relevance to psychological aspects of medicine. Am. J. Med., *25*:611, 1958.

49. Magoun, H.W.: *The Waking Brain.* Springfield, Ill., Thomas, 1958.

50. Malmo, R.B., Boag, T.J., and Smith, A.A.: Physiological study of personal interaction. Psychosom. Med., *19*:105, 1957.

51. Margolin, S.G.: The behavior of the stomach during psychoanalysis. Psychoanal. Q., *20*:349, 1951.

52. Marks, J., Wolfson, J., and Klein, R.: Neonatal thyroid functions: Erythrocyte T3 uptake in early infancy. J. Pediatr., *58*:32, 1961.

53. Mason, J.W.: Organization of psychoendocrine mechanisms. Psychosom. Med., *30*:565, 1968.

54. Mason, J.W.: "Over-all" hormonal balance as a key to endocrine organization. Psychosom. Med., *30*:791, 1968.

55. Mason, J.W.: A review of psychoendocrine research on the pituitary-adrenal-cortical system. Psychosom. Med., *30*:516, 1968.

56. Mason, J.W.: A review of psychoendocrine research on the pituitary-thyroid system. Psychosom. Med., *30*:666, 1968.

57. Mason, J.W.: A review of psychoendocrine research on the sympathetic-adrenal medullary system. Psychosom. Med., *30*:631, 1968.

58. Mason, J.W.: The scope of psychoendocrine research. Psychosom. Med., *30*:565, 1968.

59. Mason, J.W.: Clinical psychophysiology: Psychoendocrine mechanisms. In: *American Handbook of Psychiatry*, 2nd Ed., Vol. 4. (S. Arieti, Ed.). New York, Basic Books, 1975.

60. Mason, J.W., et al.: Plasma cortisol and norepinephrine responses in anticipation of muscular exercise. Psychosom. Med., *35*:406, 1973.

61. Migeon, C.J.: Cortisol production and metabolism in the neonate. J. Pediatr., *55*:280, 1959.

62. Orme-Johnson, D.W.: Autonomic stability and transcendental meditation. Psychosom. Med., *35*:341, 1973.

63. Papez, J.W.: A proposed mechanism of emotion. Arch. Neurol. Psychiatry, *38*:725, 1937.

64. Parmalee, A., Wenner, W., and Schulz, H.: Infant sleep patterns from birth to 16 weeks of age. J. Pediatr., *65*:576, 1964.

65. Pratt, K.C.: The neonate. In: *Manual of Child Psychology*, 2nd Ed. (L. Carmichael, Ed.). New York, Wiley, 1954.

66. Prugh, D.G.: Towards an understanding of psychosomatic concepts in relation to illness in childhood. In: *Modern Perspectives in Child Development*. (A.J. Solnit, and S.A. Provence, Eds.). New York, International Universities Press, 1963.

67. Reiser, M.F., Reeves, R.B., and Armington, J.: Effect of variations in laboratory procedure and experimenter upon the ballistocardiogram, blood pressure, and heart rate in healthy young men. Psychosom. Med., *17*:185, 1955.

68. Reite, M.L., et al.: Depression in infant monkeys: Physiological correlates. Psychosom. Med., *36*:363, 1974.

69. Richmond, J.B., and Lipton, E.L.: Some aspects of the neurophysiology of the newborn and their implications for child development. In: *Dynamic Psychopathology of Childhood*. (L. Jessner and E.

Pavenstedt, Eds.). New York, Grune & Stratton, 1959.

70. Sachar, E.J., Finklestein, J., and Hellman, L.: Growth hormone responses in depressive illness. Arch. Gen. Psychiatr., 25:263, 1971.

71. Sachar, E.J., et al.: Corticosteroid responses to the psychotherapy of reactive depressions. II. Further clinical and physiological implications. Psychosom. Med., 30:23, 1968.

72. Sander, L.V., et al.: Continuous 24-hour interactional monitoring in infants reared in two caretaking environments. Psychosom. Med., 34:270, 1972.

73. Schachter, J., et al.: Heart rate and blood pressure in black newborns and in white newborns. Pediatrics, 58:283, 1976.

74. Schottstaedt, W.W.: *Psychophysiological Approach in Medical Practice*. Chicago, Yearbook, 1960.

75. Selye, H.: The general adaptation syndrome and the diseases of adaptation. Am. J. Med., 10:549, 1951.

76. Solomon, P., et al.: Sensory deprivation: A Review. Am. J. Psychiatry, 114:357, 1957.

77. Sostek, A.M., Anders, T.F., and Sostek, A.J.: Diurnal rhythms in 2- and 8-week-old infants: Sleep-waking state organization as a function of age and stress. Psychosom. Med., 38:250,1976.

78. Stevenson, I.: Physical symptoms during pleasurable emotional states. Psychosom. Med., 12:98, 1950.

79. Stroebel, C.F.: The importance of biological clocks in mental health. In: *Behavioral Sciences and Mental Health* (E.A. Robinson and C.V. Coelho, Eds.). U.S. Public Health Service Publication No. 2064. Washington, Government Printing Office, 1971.

80. Tennes, K., Downey, K., and Vernadakis, A.: Urinary cortisol excretion rates and anxiety in normal 1-year-old infants. Psychosom. Med., 39:178, 1977.

81. Thaler-Singer, M.T.: Engagement-involvement: A central phenomenon in psychophysiological research. Psychosom. Med., 36:1, 1974.

82. Thomas, A., and Chess, S.: *Temperament and Development*. New York, Brunner/Mazel, 1977.

83. Tjossem, T.D., et al.: Psychophysiological studies of 2- to 4-year-old children. Psychosom. Med., 17:476, 1955.

84. Usdin, G.: *Sleep Research and Clinical Practice*. New York, Brunner/Mazel, 1973.

85. Weiner, H.: Some recent neurophysiological contributions to the problem of brain and behavior. Psychosom. Med., 31:457, 1969.

86. Weiner, H.: Autonomic Psychophysiology: Peripheral autonomic mechanisms and their central control. In: *American Handbook of Psychiatry*, 2nd Ed., Vol. 4. (S. Arieti, Ed.). New York, Basic Books, 1975.

87. Williams, R.V.: *Biochemical Individuality*. New York, Wiley, 1956.

88. Wolf, P.H.: The causes, controls, and organization of behavior in the neonate. Psychol. Issues, 5:1, 1966.

89. Wolf, S.G.: Effects of suggestion and conditioning on the action of chemical agents in human subjects: The pharmacology of placebos. J. Clin. Invest., 29:100, 1950.

90. Wolf, S.G.: Report of the committee on psychosomatic relationships in gastroenterology. Gastroenterology, 18:55, 1951.

91. Wolff, C.T., et al.: Relationship between psychological defenses and mean urinary 17-hydroxycorticosteroid excretion rates. I. A predictive study of parents of fatally ill children. Psychosom. Med., 26:576, 1964.

92. Wolff, C.T., Hofer, M.A., and Mason, J.W.: Relationship between psychological defenses and mean urinary 17-hydroxycorticosteroid excretion rates. II. Methodological and theoretical considerations. Psychosom. Med., 26:592, 1964.

93. Wolff, H.G.: *Stress and Disease*. Springfield, Ill., Thomas, 1953.

94. Zucherman, M., Levine, S., and Biase, D.V.: Stress response in total and partial perceptual isolation. Psychosom. Med., 26:250, 1964.

General References

Axelrod, J.: The pineal gland. Endeavor, 29:144, 1970.

Bardwick, J.M.: *Psychology of Women: A Study of Bio-Cultural Conflicts*. New York, Harper & Row, 1971.

Benjamin, J.D.: *The Innate and the Experiential in Development*. In: *Lectures in Experimental Psychiatry*. (H.W. Brown, Ed.). Pittsburgh, University of Pittsburgh Press, 1961.

Brown, G.M., and Reichlin, S.: Psychologic and neural regulation of growth hormone secretion. Psychosom. Med., 34:45, 1972.

Bunney, W.E.,Jr., et al.: A psychoendocrine study of severe psychotic depressive crises. Am. J. Psychiatr., 122:72, 1965.

Cathro, D.M.: The adrenal cortex and medulla. In: *Paediatric Endocrinology*. (D. Hubble, Ed.). Philadelphia, Davis, 1969.

Coelho, G.V., et al.: *Coping and Adaptation: A Behavioral Sciences Bibliography*. U.S. Public Health Service Publication No. 2087, Washington, Government Printing Office, 1970.

DiMascio, A., Boyd, R.W., and Greenblatt, M.: Physiological correlates of tension and antagonism during psychotherapy: A study of interpersonal physiology. Psychosom. Med., 19:99, 1957.

Dreyfuss, E., and Czaczkes, J.W.: Blood cholesterol and uric acid of healthy medical students under the stress of an examination. Arch. Int. Med., 103:708, 1959.

Dudley, D.L., et al.: *The Psychophysiology of Respiration in Health and Disease*. New York, Appleton-Century-Crofts, 1969.

Duffy, E.: The psychological significance of the concept of arousal or activation. Psychol. Rev., 64:265, 1957.

Elmadjian, F.J., Hope, F.M., and Lamson, E.T.: Excretion of epinephrine and norepinephrine in various emotional states. J. Clin. Endocrinol., 6:117, 1965.

Engle, G.L.: Selection of clinical material in psychosomatic medicine: The need for a new physiology. Psychosom. Med., *16*:368, 1954.

Engle, G.L.: Is grief a disease? Psychosom. Med., 23:18, 1961.

Folkow, B., and Rubenstein, E.H.: Cardiovascular effects of acute and chronic stimulations of the hypothalamic defense area. Acta Physiol. Scand., *28*:14, 1953.

Frank, G., et al.: Circadian periodicity, adrenal corticosteroids, and the EEG of normal man. J. Psychiatr. Res., 4:73, 1966.

Funkenstein, D.H., King, S.H., and Drolette, M.E.: *Mastery of Stress*. Cambridge, Harvard University Press, 1957.

Gatewood, J.W., Organ, C.H., and Mead, B.T.: Mental changes associated with hyperparathyroidism. Am. J. Psychiatry, *,132*:129, 1975.

Gershon, E.S., et al.(Eds.): *The Impact of Biology on Modern Psychiatry*. New York, Plenum, 1977.

Hamburg, D.A.: Plasma and urinary corticosteroid levels in naturally occurring psychologic stresses. Proc. Acad. Res. Nerv. Ment. Dis., *25*:426, 1962.

Hamburg, D., et al.: *Endocrinology and Human Behavior*. New York, Oxford University Press, 1968.

Heim, E., Blaser, A., and Waidelich, E.: Dyspnea: Psychophysiologic relationships. Psychosom. Med., 34:405, 1972.

Levi, L. Ed.: *Emotions—Their Parameters and Measurement*. New York, Raven Press, 1975.

Mason, J.W., et al.: Corticosteroid responses to hospital admission. Arch. Gen. Psychiatry, 16:461, 1967.

Meites, J., Nicoll, C.S., and Talwalker, P.K.: The central nervous system and the secretion and release of prolactin. In: *Advances in Neuroendocrinology*. (A.V. Malbandor, Ed.). Urbana, Ill., University of Illinois Press, 1963.

Mirsky, I.A., Kaplan, S., and Broh-Kahn, R.: Pepsinogen excretion (uropepsin) as an index of various life situations on gastric secretion. Res. Publ. Assoc. Res. Nerv. Ment. Dis., *29*:625, 1949.

Notterman, J.M.: Experimental anxiety and a conditioned heart rate response in human beings. Trans. N.Y. Acad. Sci., 16:24–33, 1953.

Orme-Johnson, D.W.: Autonomic stability and transcendental meditation. Psychosom. Med., *35*:341, 1973.

Poe, R.O., Rose, R.M., and Mason, J.W.: Multiple determinants of 17-hydroxycorticosteroid excretion in recruits during basic training. Psychosom. Med., *32*:369, 1970.

Pribram, K.H.: Emotion: Steps toward a neuropsychological theory. In: *Neurophysiology and Emotion*. (D.C. Glass, Ed.). New York, Rockefeller University Press, 1967.

Reichlin, S.: Neuroendocrinology. N. Engl. J. Med., *269*:1182, 1963.

Reimann, H.A.: Periodic disease. Medicine, *30*:219, 195.

Reiser, M.F., Ed.: Organic disorders and psychosomatic medicine. In: *American Handbook of Psychiatry*. Vol. 4. (S. Arieti, Ed.). New York, Basic Books, 1975.

Richmond, J.B., and Lipton, E.L.: Some aspects of the neurophysiology of the newborn and their implications for child development. In: *Dynamic Psychopathology of Childhood*. (L. Jessner and E. Pavenstedt, Eds.). New York, Grune & Stratton, 1959.

Richter, C.P., and Rice, K.K.: Experimental production in rats of abnormal cycles in behavior and metabolism. J. Nerv. Ment. Dis., *124*:393, 1956.

Rose, R.M.: Androgen responses to stress. I. Psychoendocrine relationships and assessment of androgen activity. Psychosom. Med., *31*:405, 1969.

Rose, R.M., et al.: Androgen responses to stress. II. Excretion of testosterone, epitestosterone, androsterone, and etiocholanolone during basic combat training and under threat of attack. Psychosom. Med., *31*:418, 1969.

Rubin, R., et al.: Luteinizing hormone, follicle stimulating hormone, and growth hormone secretion in normal adult men during sleep and dreaming. Psychosom. Med., *35*:309, 1973.

Sachar, E.J.: Psychological factors relating to activation and inhibition of the adrenocortical stress response in man. A review. In: *Progress in Brain Research, Vol. 32*. (D. DeWied and J. Weijnen, Eds.). New York, Elsevier, 1970.

Sachar, E.J.: Some current issues in psychosomatic research. Psychiatr. Ann., *2*:22, 1972.

Sachar, E.J., et al.: Corticosteroid excretion in normal young adults living under "basal" conditions. Psychosom. Med., *27*:435, 1965.

Spiegel, J.P., and Machotka, P.: Messages of the body. New York, Free Press, 1974.

Steinschneider, A., and Lipton, E.L.: Individual differences in autonomic responsivity: Problems of measurement. Psychosom. Med., *27*:446, 1965.

Stone, W.N., et al.: Stimulus, affect, and plasma free fatty acid. Psychosom. Med., *31*:331, 1969.

Verney, E.B.: The antidiuretic hormone and the factors which determine its release. Proc. R. Soc. Med., *135*:25, 1947.

Wallace, R.K., and Benson, H.: The physiology of meditation. Sci. Am., *226*:84, 1972.

Weiner, H.: Some recent neurophysiological contributions to the problem of brain and behavior. Psychosom. Med., *31*:457, 1969.

Wolff, C.T., et al.: Relationship between psychological defenses and mean urinary 17-hydroxycorticosteroid excretion rates. I. A predictive study of parents of fatally ill children. II. Methodological and theoretical considerations. Psychosom. Med., *26*:576, 1964.

Wolff, H.G.: *Stress and Disease*. Springfield, Ill., Thomas, 1953.

Wolff, H.G.: Man's nervous system and disease. Arch. Neurol., 5:235, 1961.

Wolff, H.G., Wolf, S.G., Hare, C.C., Eds.: *Life Stress and Bodily Disease*. Baltimore, Williams & Wilkins, 1950.

Zimmerman, E., Smyrl, R., and Critchlow, V.: Suppression of pituitary-adrenal response to stress with physiological plasma levels of corticosterone in the female rat. Neuroendocrinology, *10*:246, 1972.

4

Psychosomatic Concepts: Clinical and Therapeutic Considerations

The term psychosomatic-somatopsychic continuum is often used in discussing disorders of bodily function that occur in children and adults. Despite the limitations of the term, the ideas that underlie the term should be discussed because they relate to clinical syndromes. In this chapter, disorders in which disturbances in bodily function are important, and that are either caused by predominantly psychologic or interpersonal stresses or have accompanying psychologic reactions will be discussed. The foregoing qualifications of the multiple causes of disorders apply in the discussion of disorders, despite the arbitrary separation of categories. (The word predominantly should be understood whenever psychologic or physical disorders are mentioned.) The following list of categories is arbitrary; many categories overlap. (The list is not a classification of the psychopathologic disorders of children; such a classification will be offered later.)

1. Psychologic reactions that lead to self-inflicted injuries or disorders.
2. Psychologic reactions that are accompanied by changes in bodily function.
3. Psychophysiologic (vegetative) disorders.
4. Mixed conversion and psychophysiologic disorders.
5. Psychologic reactions to physical disorders.

The physiologic concomitants of emotions will hereafter be mentioned only as they occur during anxiety states or as they pertain to the precipitation, intensification, or perpetuation of other disease pictures. Physiologic concomitants occur in healthy as well as psychologically or physiologically ill children. They are usually reversible and usually cause no structural or permanent changes in the organ systems or metabolic processes.

Psychologic reactions are sometimes accompanied by a preoccupation with bodily functions but not by a disturbance in bodily function. Such reactions occur in severely disturbed children who are usually of school age or older and who have obsessive fears of a physical dysfunction or abnormality, the compulsive need to touch parts of their bodies to reassure themselves of their intactness, hypochrondriacal reactions, or somatic delusions. Such preoccupation may occur briefly in a less disturbed child, who fears that he has abnormal genitals or an abnormal stomach, or in an adolescent, who is troubled when he notices an extrasystole or borborygmi, during a temporary threat to his adaptive equilibrium.

Psychologic Reactions That Lead to Self-Inflicted Injuries

Self-inflicted bodily injury or mutilation occurs rarely during childhood but occurs during adolescence during psychoses, deep personality disorders, or acute and sweeping psychologic decompensations. In less severe form, self-inflicted injuries may occur in preschool-age children who bite their own hands or arms, often because of conflicts about the handling of their aggressive impulses toward their parents. Children who have severe psychoneuroses or depression may pick open wounds, usually because they have unconscious needs for self-punishment or an unhealthy enjoyment of pain, and thus interfere with the healing process and prevent their return to competitive or other conflict-producing situations. (These clinical pictures will be discussed more fully later, as will other types of self-injury, such as suicidal attempts and accident proneness.)

Psychologic Reactions That Are Accompanied by Changes in Bodily Functions

Manifest Anxiety

Children who show manifest anxiety, whether because of normal developmental fears that occur while they are of preschool age or because of more severe chronic psychoneurotic and phobic disorders that occur while they are of school age and during adolescence, have physiologic concomitants of their emotions that are related to the fight-or-flight biologic pattern. Startle reactions, increases in blood pressure and heart rate, marked sinus arrhythmias, a slight increase in the sedimentation rate, changes in the respiratory rate and a tendency to hyperventilate, slight-to-moderate increases in body temperature, increased perspiration with cold, moist palms, and nightmares or other sleep disturbances often occur. Those symptoms sometimes cause manifest anxiety to be confused with essential hypertension, rheumatic fever, or thyrotoxicosis. The symptoms are usually reversible when the child is relaxed.

Depression

Depression in children and adolescents may be different from that in adults. (It is discussed later in more detail.) Disturbances of eating or sleeping, hyperactivity, or other phenomena may mask depression in children. When children have marked grief reactions or overt and prolonged depression, the symptoms of depression may resemble the slowing of physiologic responses that is characteristic of the withdrawal-conservation pattern. Apathy, anorexia, slowed motor activity, constipation and other symptoms may occur and may complicate mild physical disorders that are associated with emotionally significant events within the family.

Conversion Disorders

Changes in function, usually changes that cause diminution or loss or that occur in parts of the body that are innervated by the voluntary parts of the central nervous system, mostly affect the striated muscles and somatosensory apparatus. Disturbances in motor function, changes in sensory perception, disturbances in mental

function and consciousness, and disturbances of specific organ systems often occur in children and adolescents (and sometimes in children of preschool age).
Disturbances of the organ systems may include: (1) disorders of the upper end of the
gastrointestinal tract (including the throat
and mouth), such as vomiting, trismus,
globus hystericus, dysphonia, disorders of
the appetite (anorexia, hyperphagia, and
bulimia), and abdominal distention, (2)
disorders of the lower end of the gastrointestinal tract, such as encopresis and certain types of constipation, (3) disorders of
the voluntary components of respiration,
as in hyperventilation, certain types of
dyspnea, breath holding, respiratory tics,
certain types of coughing and hiccoughs,
yawning, and sighing respirations, and (4)
disorders of the genitourinary tract, such
as certain types of urinary retention or sudden incontinence, and certain types of enuresis, dysuria, and urinary frequency.
(Genital dysfunctions, such as impotence,
frigidity, and dyspareunia, may occur in
older adolescents.)

Most of the disorders of the voluntarily
innervated parts of the organ systems overlap the involuntarily innervated parts. (The
involuntarily innervated parts will be discussed later with certain severe and generalized types of weakness, paralysis, or
other symptoms of marked psychologic invalidism. The distinction between conversion disorders and psychophysiologic (or
vegetative) disorders, which is a conceptual and clinical distinction that has been
emphasized by Alexander[4] and others and
that has been recognized in the past in the
AMA nomenclature[6] will be emphasized.)

Conversion disorders usually do not follow patterns of anatomic distribution or
motor or sensory innervation. Rather, they
are related to the central symbolic representation of a particular bodily function,
such as walking, hitting, speaking, or
seeing, or to the individual's (often erro-
neous) subjective idea of the boundaries of
a part of his body. The exact neurophys-

iologic mechanisms that cause conversion
disorders are not yet known. Probably a
functional change in the activity of the cerebral cortex occurs in response to psychologic or interpersonal stimuli during a repressed and unresolved conflict, as a result
of which the muscular components or sensory organs act "as if" their function were
suspended or blocked. Local structural
changes in the parts of the body that are
affected cannot be demonstrated; nonspecific electroencephalographic changes that
disappear when the symptom disappears
have been described. Distortions in the
perception of pain, touch, and other sensations may occur in reverse, as if such
stimuli were perceived centrally without
the existence of specific sources in the sites
involved. Secondary changes in structures
may occur, such as the development of
contractures as the result of continued conversion paralysis or changes in the metabolism and excretion of calcium as the result
of a bedridden existence.

Freud[41] has clarified the psychodynamic
meaning of the classic hysteric conversion
symptom. A person's conversion symptom, such as paralysis of an arm or blindness, appears to have an unconscious symbolic meaning for him. The meaning may
be, for example, punishment for a wish to
hit a loved person or an unwillingness to
see disturbing sexual acts. The emotional
conflict between the wish to hit and the
fear of punishment or loss of love (or between the wish to see and the fear of seeing)
is automatically repressed by the mental
apparatus. The symptom resolves the conflict temporarily albeit unhealthily. The intrapsychic conflict is unconsciously "converted" to a somatic dysfunction or a
disturbance in innervation, and the anxiety
aroused by the conflict is apparently
"bound" with the symptom. The person
has no conscious insight into the origin and
the meaning of his symptom, and he experiences little or no anxiety subjectively—
leading to *la belle indifference* (that has been

described in nineteenth-century French literature on hysteria).

Conversion symptoms may often be removed (or sometimes be produced) by suggestion, hypnosis, or narcohypnosis. Unless the underlying conflict can be resolved, however, the symptom may return or be replaced by another symbolically equivalent one.* A person can maintain an unhealthy adaptive equilibrium for a long time and so avoid an unbearable amount of tension or anxiety that might cause decompensation and an adaptive breakdown.

The specific unconscious determinants of a child's conversion symptom seem to come from the child's previous experience and his current situation. As Engel[34] has emphasized, the determinants may originate in: (1) a translation into body language of an unacceptable wish and the defense against it (unconsciously, "I wish to see; I should not see; therefore, I cannot see"), (2) the revival of a memory trace of a previous physical experience, usually involving painful sensation, that often comes from a mild physical illness or a sexually exciting contact, (3) identification with an important figure, most often a parent, who has suffered from a particular symptom now experienced by the child in the distorted fashion in which children perceive such symptoms and their bodies, and (4) punishment for an unacceptable wish or impulse directed against a loved person, usually a parent, in which the child suffers "magically" what he wished on the other.

Different combinations of specific unconscious determinants may occur; other factors may also affect the genesis of a conversion symptom. Unconscious conflicts that all children have seem to be intensified in children who have conversion symptoms by disturbing events that occur in their families and their social lives outside their families. Precipitating events, such as a loss, the distortion of an important relationship, another emotionally traumatic experience, or a change in his family's adaptive equilibrium apparently operate to bring about an adaptive need in a child for a conversion symptom. Traumatic situations within the child's family or social life often continue and so make his symptom necessary on a continuing basis. The child's unconscious "secondary gain" from his symptoms is unhealthy but vital.

It is not known why one child has a conversion symptom and another has an anxiety reaction, depression, or a phobia or acts out his hostile or rebellious impulses directly against his parents or society. Many different factors probably work together to determine each child's reaction to a traumatic event. For example, the constitutionally determined capacity of a child's mental apparatus for greater repression of unacceptable feelings and impulses might predispose the child to conversion symptoms. No systematic research on predisposing factors has as yet been made although Witkin[122] and others have related field independence or dependence and other innate qualities of the mind to the patterns of emotional expression of people and their families (and to other factors).

I believe that true conversion symptoms do not usually occur in children under 7 or 8 years old. Conversion symptoms can occur in younger children; disorders in bodily functions that have psychologic causes often occur in preschool-age children. Conversion symptoms and earlier disorders seem to differ in important ways, perhaps because the child's mental apparatus, including his capacity for active repression that seems necessary for the development of the conversion symptom to occur, is not sufficiently developed until the early school-age period.

Clinical studies show that conversion disorders usually occur in older children and adolescents who have established hysteric personality disorders, are overdramatic and suggestible, and have conflicts over sexual adjustment and a propensity

---

*Major conversion disorders seem to occur less often now, and conversion symptoms that have been removed seem to be replaced less often.

for expressing conflict in bodily disturbances. (The children are usually female.) But conversion symptoms can occur in children whose personalities vary widely; the children may have neuroses, personality disorders, or psychoses, and be males.

As Brazelton[14] has pointed out, the pediatrician sees many mild-to-moderate transient conversion symptoms in children of school age, in prepubescence, or early adolescence. Such symptoms often occur during convalescence from a physical disorder. Such a disorder may, for example, temporarily block a child's need to achieve scholastically, athletically, or socially, or it may cause a conflict between a child's regressive wish to be cared for and the pressure to return to the competition of his peer group. The symptoms of the physical disorder often become unconsciously incorporated into the conversion symptoms, as when a "memory" of pain, vomiting, headaches, weakness, a tendency to fatigue, or mild catatonia continues after the disorder has ended. Many such conversion symptoms end in a few days or weeks, either spontaneously (as when a child works out his lesser conflicts) or therapeutically (with the help of the child's parents and physician). A healthy child's developmental capacities and impetus toward maturation may give him great flexibility of adaptive responses, even to great interpersonal stresses.

Other Reactions

Infants and preschool-age children respond to psychologic or interpersonal stresses with various disturbances in their bodily functions. Their responses fluctuate and lack the structural quality of true neuroses or personality disorders presumably because the adaptive capacities of their mental apparatus (including the fully developed functions of the ego, such as repression, and the intrapsychic functions of the superego) do not seem to crystalize until the end of the preschool period. Such

disturbances of bodily functions are usually caused by stimuli from a child's environment, including external and largely conscious conflicts between his wishes or feelings and those of his parents. Unlike those of older children, such disturbances are rarely caused by internal or intrapsychic, unconscious conflicts between the child's wishes or feelings and his conscience. The disturbances (called symptomatic reactions or reactive disorders) of younger children often disappear when the external conflicts with their parents are resolved. In older children, internalized conflicts may continue in a self-perpetuating or repetitive way, even when their interpersonal situations have changed.

Such disturbances in bodily function in young children rarely occur alone. They are usually accompanied by other reactive responses in the child's behavior. Such disturbances are listed and described briefly (the list follows the list of symptoms drawn up by the Group for the Advancement of Psychiatry)[52]:

1. Disturbances of bodily functions, including disturbances in eating (e.g., the refusal of food, rumination, pica, vomiting, and failure to thrive), sleeping, bowel and bladder control, speech, patterns of motor activity, rhythmic patterns (e.g., rocking, head rolling, and head banging), habit patterns (such as thumb sucking, nose picking, and masturbation), and sensory disturbances.
2. Disturbances of the cognitive functions, including learning failures, distortions of perception, and disorders in thinking.
3. Disturbances in social behavior, such as overaggressiveness, negativistic or oppositional behavior, disturbed sexual behavior, isolated or withdrawn behavior, and overly dependent or overly independent behavior.
4. Disturbances in emotional behavior, such as chronic anxiety, marked fears, states of acute panic, depression, and feelings of inadequacy.
5. Disturbances in integrative behavior, such as repeated tantrums, impulsive behavior, or disorganized behavior.

Other disturbances include compulsive, ritualized, or overperfectionistic behavior, and transient hypochondriacal behavior. All of those disturbances may occur in older children; they may be caused by new stresses or they may continue from earlier stages of development. Disturbances in bodily function will be focused on briefly, although such disturbances often overlap reactive disorders in the other areas mentioned.

Such disturbances in young children may resemble conversion symptoms, but they have important differences. Because the capacities of young children's mental apparatus are less fully developed, young children's symptoms are not so strongly symbolic as are conversion symptoms. Many of their symptoms are regressive. They are usually temporary abandonments of more fully developed functions (as when an 18-month-old infant stops speaking and walking after a physical disorder) or returns to earlier, familiar modes of satisfaction (as when a 3-year-old begins to suck his thumb again when a sibling is born). Other disturbances are the physiologic concomitants of anxiety. The greatest anxiety of a child under 4 years old is that of separation from his mother. Prolonged or frightening separation causes anxiety and often regression, which usually includes several of the aforementioned disturbances of bodily functions.

A child's developmental capacities may also affect his responses to stresses. True separation anxiety does not occur in infants less than 6 or 7 months old because they cannot distinguish between themselves and the outside world. An infant of that age responds to inappropriate stimulation from his mother with disturbances in eating and sleeping and gastrointestinal disorders. (Those responses are in keeping with the very young infant's tendency to respond in a relatively undifferentiated and global fashion.) Tension or neglect on the part of his mother may cause an older child to ruminate; his capacity (acquired at about 3 months) for voluntary hand-to-mouth activity and movements of his tongue, pharynx, and abdominal muscles make rumination possible. By the second half of his first year, the infant's capacity to relate to his mother and to perceive himself as separate from her has developed, and so sudden or prolonged separations may cause depression. Other disturbances in eating, sleeping, gastrointestinal function, growth patterns, and other bodily functions that are caused by separation continue at times until the infant fails to thrive.

Disturbances may arise from a persistence of developmental patterns beyond their usual point of disappearance. Head rolling and rocking usually occur by the end of the first year and stop before the third year, as does the intense motor activity which begins in the second year. Because of unhealthy parent-child relationships or disruptions in the family's equilibrium, any of those patterns may persist beyond the preschool period. A delay in the appearance of maturational patterns may be caused by similar circumstances and may include lags in psychomotor development, memory, reasoning, and other learning capacities. Uneven or fragmented development may occur; it includes variations in a child's inherent capacities that interact with inconsistent treatment by his parents that includes overstimulation toward development in some areas and understimulation or blockage in others. It is not known whether precocity of a child's psychologic development may be stimulated constructively by his parents or anyone else. A child who is precocious in his physical growth, sexual maturation, or intellectual development certainly has important adaptive challenges (as do his parents).

Symptomatic reactions may have secondary physiologic reverberations; for example, a child may fail to grow or may develop nutritional anemia because he refuses food while experiencing negativism or depression. Pica seen in emotionally deprived infants and young children may cause lead intoxication or (when it occurs with thumb sucking) such conditions as the formation of a hairball (trichobezoar). A physical illness may precipitate or intensify symptomatic reactions, as when a young child who has a chronic infection becomes irritable and hyperactive. A symptomatic reaction that is caused by interpersonal stresses may disappear when the stresses stop or when the child (with the help of his parents) becomes able to adapt without his symptomatic reaction.

Psychophysiologic (Vegetative) Disorders

Psychophysiologic disorders, so called because psychologic and interpersonal factors are prominently involved, usually occur in involuntarily innervated visceral organs or organ systems that are supplied by the autonomic nervous system, particularly by the parasympathetic branch. In psychophysiologic disorders, the symptoms of the disturbance of bodily function have no symbolic significance because they operate at a vegetative level (as originally pointed out by Alexander[4]) and thus presumably do not receive central symbolic representation. Structural changes often occur during psychophysiologic disorders. Such changes are sometimes reversible, but such a disorder may result in chronic and irreparable damage to the organ or organ system that is affected. Physiologic reverberations often occur in other systems; and the organism's homeostasis may be seriously upset.

The term psychophysiologic autonomic and visceral disorder, until recently employed in the official AMA nomenclature,[6] has limitations. The term can imply that psychologic factors, through the action of the physiologic concomitants of the emotions, are the major causes of psychophysiologic disorders. The term was used that way by some early proponents of the psychosomatic view who assumed that changes in bodily function, if they continued for a long time during unresolved emotional conflicts, could cause structural changes. More recent information has indicated that predisposing physiologic factors must exist in order for a psychophysiologic disorder to appear and that the physiologic concomitants of emotions act only to precipitate, intensify, or perpetuate the disorder. Some investigators, such as Engel,[34] call those disorders somato-psychic-psychosomatic disorders, emphasizing the importance of physiologic predisposition. The term psychophysiologic (or vegetative) disorder will be used here, to refer to disorders that involve both psychologic and physiologic factors. Each factor has its own reverberations at other levels of organization.

Many disorders have recently been said to be strongly affected by psychologic and interpersonal factors. No list of those disorders can be complete or up-to-date. The following list categorizes those disorders according to the organ system that they affect, even though such a categorizing does not describe the complex interrelationships and the overlapping of the bodily processes involved. (For more specific discussions of each disorder, see Chapter 21 and the original references.)

1. *Cardiovascular*. In adults, essential hypertension, eclampsia, vasodepressor and related syncopal reactions (as distinct from hysterical fainting or conversion syncope), various peripheral vascular disorders (from central angiospastic retinopathy to Raynaud's disease), angina pectoris and coronary thrombosis. In adults and children, migraine and paroxysmal tachycardia.

2. *Respiratory*. In adults and children, bronchial asthma, allergic rhinitis, and certain types of chronic sinusitis. In children, breath-holding spells.

3. *Gastrointestinal*. In adults and children, peptic ulcer, certain types of gastritis, cardiospasm, pylorospasm, ulcerative colitis, mucous or spastic colitis (the "irritable bowel syndrome"), certain types of constipation, regional enteritis, certain types of dental malocclusion, bruxism, and periodontal disease, anorexia nervosa, obesity, and pernicious vomiting of pregnancy. In children, megacolon (nonaganglionic type), certain types of polydipsia, idiopathic celiac disease, certain cases of failure to thrive and

persistent colic, and certain disorders in salivation.

4. *Genitourinary.* In adults and adolescents, disturbances in menstruation, including dysmenorrhea, dysfunctional uterine bleeding, and premenstrual tension. In adults, certain types of sterility, certain types of urethral and vaginal discharges, habitual abortion, certain types of polyuria, and vesical paralysis.

5. *Hemic and lymphatic.* Most of the vegetative disorders studied thus far are reversible and have been listed earlier under the physiologic concomitants of emotions.

6. *Musculoskeletal.* In adults and children, rheumatoid arthritis, certain types of low back pain, and "tension" headache.

7. *Skin.* In adults, seborrheic dermatitis, neurodermatitis, psoriasis, certain types of pruritus, and certain types of alopecia and rosacea. In adults and children, certain atopic reactions, such as eczema, urticaria, and angioneurotic edema, verruca vulgaris, herpes simplex, and acne.

8. *Endocrine.* In adults and children, thyrotoxicosis, diabetes, hyperinsulinism, and pseudocyesis. In children, certain types of growth disturbances.

9. *Central nervous system.* In adults and children, idiopathic epilepsy (including petit mal, grand mal, psychomotor, and other equivalents), narcolepsy, sleep disturbances, dizziness and vertigo, asthenic reactions, motion sickness, and recurrent fever. In children, hyperactivity.

10. *Organs of special sense.* In adults, glaucoma, asthenopia, phlectenular keratitis, Meniere's syndrome, and certain types of tinnitus and hyperacusis.

The list is not exhaustive. It cites only representative studies and mostly the more recent ones in the English literature. Compilations of original papers edited by Wolff,[128] Alexander,[4] Wittkower and Cleghorn,[124] Deutsch,[27] and Jores and Freyberger[64] (the latter covering recent European studies), and monographs by Grinker,[50] Schottstaedt,[107] and others should be consulted for more detailed surveys of each area covered in the list. Most of the papers and monographs concern studies of adults. Reviews of psychophysiologic disorders in children are more rare, although publications by Sperling,[113] Finch,[39] Sontag,[111] Gerard,[45] Carpentieri and Jensen,[21] Wolff and Bayer,[127] Garner

and Wenar,[44] Mohr,[87] Bruch,[16] and more recently Prugh[94] and Lipton and his colleagues[72] concern those disorders.*

Psychologic Observations

Over the past 40 years, investigators have used many different concepts in order to understand and explain the psychologic aspects of the disorders just listed. Early investigators, particularly psychoanalysts, thought that the physiologic disturbances were conversion reactions or "organ neuroses" involving the visceral organs and that a kind of unconscious "organ language" was substituted for feelings that could not be expressed verbally or behaviorally. Although the verbal associations of some people who had those disorders supported that view, studies have not demonstrated any symbolic meanings of the physiologic disturbances at the organ level. Exacerbations of symptoms, however, as in ulcerative colitis, can be associated with symbolic fantasies that come from unconscious, unresolved conflicts.

Personality Patterns

Later studies by Dunbar[31] and others have suggested that specific personality patterns that were produced by common developmental experiences were associated with specific disorders, as when someone who has the driving executive type of personality develops a peptic ulcer. Certain personality patterns are present with some consistency in people who have certain disorders; people who are passive-dependent and somewhat compulsive often have ulcerative colitis. Such patterns are not present in all people who have cer-

*Most of the specific references concerning each area are included in the review article by D.G. Prugh: Towards an understanding of psychosomatic concepts in relation to illness in childhood. In: *Modern Perspectives in Child Development* (A.J. Solnit, and S.A. Provence, Eds.). New York, International Universities Press, 1963. Other references dealing with more recent approaches to treatment are included in Chapter 21.

tain disorders, however, and the personality disorders reported by many investigators are not type specific, because they also occur in people who have other psychophysiologic disorders, in disturbed people who do not have physiologic disturbances, and sometimes in people who have chronic physiologic disorders. Sometimes one person has as many as 3 or 4 psychophysiologic disorders;[15,94] the disorders often develop one after another, but sometimes they develop simultaneously.

Young children may develop some of those disorders before their personalities crystalize into a specific personality structure; crystalization usually does not occur until at least the early school-age period. Finally, since the studies mentioned are retrospective, it is hard to distinguish between the influence of personality patterns on disorders and the effect of a chronic disorder on someone's personality.

Conflicts

Later work by Alexander[4] introduced the idea that specific, mostly unconscious conflicts that occurred in people who had been predisposed to conflict by dissatisfying early experiences (and whose predisposition was physiologic) helped to precipitate some disorders. A conflict about a wish to receive dependent gratifications that developed around feeding in infancy was thought to be specific for peptic ulcer, for example. The secretory activity of the stomach (as if the stomach prepared for the original feeding) that occurred later during frustration and heightened conflict was thought to provide "vegetative" discharge of tension. A conflict about a wish to hold back or to extrude the stool that developed during toilet training was said to involve "vectors" that characterize people who later have constipation or diarrhea. The vectors were said to be associated with the personality traits of stinginess or generosity, respectively (as earlier psychoanalysts suggested).

Although this view may have some validity,[5] more recent studies that tested it have not confirmed it.[78] People who have the appropriate disorders often have such conflicts, but such conflicts are also present in many people who do not have those disorders. The simultaneous occurrence of multiple disorders in one person and the effects on the personality of a chronic disorder are not accounted for by Alexander's concepts. Although confirmation of his views seems to me to be unlikely, they have stimulated other ideas.

Parent-Child Relationships and Early Experience

Those who study children have described conflicts in the relationship between the mother and her infant who later develops a psychophysiologic disorder. For example, Gerard[45] believed that asthma occurs in children who have demanding and controlling mothers who make their children overly dependent; the symptoms of asthma appear when the child's dependence is threatened. Other investigators believe that children who have asthma and eczema have been rejected by their mothers. The mother's reaction to a particular symptom (e.g., vomiting or diarrhea) has been thought to be relatively specific, and the symptom is enhanced by the child's unconscious symbolic response. A number of investigators believed that early and coercive toilet training was the most important cause of bowel disorders. Sperling[112] has suggested that the mothers of children who have psychophysiologic disorders handled their infants overanxiously and developed a symbiotic relationship with their infants because of their own needs to deal in this way with serious emotional or mental disturbances of their own. Parents have been described who have unconscious needs to keep their children ill so that they may care for the children and thus deny unconscious hostile or destructive feelings that they have for the children. Families that have dominating mothers and passive, retiring fathers also have been said to produce children who have such psychophysiologic disorders as asthma, peptic ulcer, and ulcerative colitis.

Studies of parent-child and family relationships are very complicated; very few have been made using instruments of measurement that permit comparisons or contrasts that are at all quantitative to be made. It is very hard to separate, in a retrospective study, the parents' original attitudes and child-rearing techniques from those produced by their child's disorder. Garner and Wenar,[44] for example, found some significant differences in the reactions and attitudes of the mothers of children who have ulcerative colitis and other disorders when they systematically compared them with those of the mothers of physically ill and healthy children (who were studied in control groups). Those reactions and attitudes are not, however, specific for the families of children who have psychophysiologic disorders. The parents of children who have ulcerative colitis and those of children who have peptic ulcers have been observed to show relatively similar personality patterns. Fitzelle,[40] in a controlled study, did not find significant differences in the mothers' attitudes when he compared groups of children who had asthma and children who had chronic physical disorders. Neuhaus[89] had a similar difficulty in a similar study. My investigations indicate that the parents' attitudes and handling of their child may change somewhat from the beginning of the child's disorder to its later chronic stages.

The studies published support the idea of pathology in parent-child relationships, early child-rearing practices, the nature of the family's equilibrium, and other important early experiences of children who have certain psychophysiologic disorders. However, the early experiences of many children who have psychoneurotic reactions but not vegetative disorders may show

considerable similarity. When the research instruments that are now being developed for measuring family interactions and parent-child relationships have been refined, more type-specific features may possibly be found.

Specificity

With few exceptions, the studies mentioned are retrospective. Most are studies of small groups of patients and do not attempt to compare those groups with other groups of ill or healthy people. Admittedly, it is very hard to make anterospective and controlled studies. Nevertheless, in my opinion, hypotheses implicating specific pathogenic emotions, personality profiles, conflicts, early experiences, parental attitudes, child-rearing techniques, or family patterns as the exclusive causes of specific psychophysiologic disorders have not been even partially confirmed.

Although some competent investigators, such as Graham,[46] still believe that specific emotions or attitudes are characteristically associated with specific disorders, Kubie,[69] Grinker,[51] Mirsky,[84] Engel,[33] Prugh,[94] and others have seriously questioned the validity of the idea of specificity in its strict form. The critical reviews of Mendelson,[80] Wittkower,[123] and Brown[15] support that questioning. The ubiquity of the observations cited, however, indicated that all the variables mentioned can be significantly involved in predisposing, contributory, and perpetuating fashion. Thus, as Engel[34] has emphasized, the variables may be "necessary but not sufficient" conditions for the development of a psychophysiologic disorder.

Theories About Physiologic Mechanisms

Many theories or physiologic models have been put forth to explain the nature and degree of the structural changes that occur in colitis, peptic ulcer, rheumatoid arthritis, and other disorders, as these may be affected by psychologic and interpersonal stimuli. Most of the earlier theories that postulated hereditary influences, constitutional types, or the operation of a *locus minoris resistentiae* as the main causes of disorders have been abandoned as too general and insufficient by themselves. Although some investigators still adhere to the early psychoanalytic view that the visceral organs may express conflicting emotions symbolically, as in conversion reactions, most now believe that physiologic disorders cannot be explained in psychologic terms and that the two levels of organization, although they are interconnected through the mental apparatus and neuroendocrine pathways, have different laws of operation.

Weiss and English[120] and others have developed a model from Cannon's[18] theory of emergency responses and the fight-or-flight pattern. In their model, the physiologic concomitants of emotions, if they continue for a long time during an unresolved conflict, can cause structural end-organ changes and characteristic disorders as the result of the continuing activation of the sympathetic or parasympathetic components of the autonomic nervous system. Other investigators have used Pavlov's[90] idea of conditioned reflexes to explain local structural changes. More recently, Selye[109] has developed a model of the general adaptation syndrome and the "diseases of adaptation." He has produced (in animals) disorders that resemble colitis, arthritis, nephritis, and other disorders by injecting ACTH or cortisone.

Although each of the 3 models that deal with responses at the autonomic or hormonal level has stimulated other good ideas, the available evidence does not fully support any one model. Cannon's emergency responses (or the defense alarm response) by themselves explain little more than the anxiety reaction and such reversible end-organ disturbances as diarrhea. Many changes in the end-organs that are innervated mostly by the parasympathetic component of the autonomic nervous system can be produced in animals by stressful experiences or by the injection or local application of parasympatheticomimetic substances. Such experiments do not, however, reproduce the structural changes that occur in many vegetative disorders in humans.

Pavlov's conditioned responses do not explain local structural changes. Recent studies have indicated, however, that many physiologic phenomena (including some that occur in humans as well as in animals), such as the galvanic skin response (GSR), vasomotor responses, systolic blood pressure, diuresis and inhibition of urine flow, electroencephalographic (EEG) patterns, bronchiolar constriction, gastrointestinal contractions, and the gastrocolic and defecation reflexes, may be conditioned to various types of stimuli in a type of "instrumental learning" by the autonomic nervous system. The biofeedback techniques used by Miller[83] and others[8] have shown that humans can be taught to control their EEG patterns, heart rates, amounts of muscle tension, and blood pressure levels. Stoyva[116] has summarized the recent therapeutic applications of these observations.

Selye's[109] theory of the diseases of adaptation has not been confirmed. The studies on which it was based were all studies of animals, and the local and systemic changes produced in those studies are not the same as those produced by chronic disorders in humans. Furthermore, some confusion arose from this view between stress as a response of the body and the existence of stressful stimuli. (However, the significance of Selye's general adaptation syndrome, as extended by Mason,[76] has been referred to in the previous chapter as part of the neuroendocrine alarm response.) Thus mechanisms related to each of the 3 models have validity and are involved in various ways in responses to stressful stimuli. None taken alone, however, seems to adequately explain the disorders.

Several other theories should be cited.

Deutsch[26] suggested that a physical disorder that occurs in a particular organ (e.g., the lung) at the time of an important emotional conflict during the early development of the personality might somehow sensitize that organ to later dysfunction, (e.g., asthma) when the conflict reappears. Michaels,[82] Szasz,[118] Margolin,[74] and others have believed that a type of physiologic regression or "regressive innervation" that coincides with psychologic regression may occur during a conflict. The regression continues until the level of physiologic functioning of the newborn is reached. They see in the symptoms of the disorder the emergence of undifferentiated, fluctuating, primitive responses that are appropriate to a newborn's physiologic state but that cause pathologic organ functioning in a child or an adult.

Other psychoanalysts have believed that fixations of conflicts at early points in psychosexual development, engendered by traumatic experiences, may provide focal points to which the individual may regress physiologically in response to later stresses and may inappropriately affect organs whose functioning was important at the time of the original fixation. Hendrick[58] has suggested that "physiologic infantilism" may continue in people who later develop psychophysiologic disorders. Garner and Wenar[44] feel that a disruption in the patterns of physiologic integration that is caused by a disturbed mother-infant relationship may be partly responsible for the vulnerability to such disorders.

Margolin[74] and others believe that people who develop ulcerative colitis or certain other vegetative disorders are severely disturbed and regress psychologically during stress to infantile levels that are close to psychosis. That view is close to that of Sperling,[112] who has suggested that vegetative disorders, because they seem to have their roots in very early physical and psychologic development, may adaptively ward off psychosis. Other observers believe that psychosis alternates with such disorders as asthma, peptic ulcer, and colitis in one person; that idea suggests that there are substitutive or interchangeable adaptive operations between the psychologic and physiologic levels of organization. Kepecs and his colleagues[66] have suggested that in skin disorders, changes in the fluid compartments of the body that occur during exudation or transudation may be correlated with psychologic changes. Engel[32] has found that headaches sometimes occur when the gastrointestinal symptoms of ulcerative colitis begin to subside during treatment. He thinks that such headaches may be conversion mechanisms that occur when the person begins to deal with his conflicts at a higher adaptive level, in contrast to the more primitive conflicts originally mobilized in response to the interpersonal stresses which helped precipitate his disorder.

Some of the theories just discussed have not yet been confirmed. Many people have psychologic and behavioral regressions, and the regressions may be affected by the effects of the pathophysiologic states themselves on people's bodies, as well as by the precipitating psychologic and interpersonal stresses. But there is no substantial evidence that physiologic regression does occur in such disorders. Even if physiologic regression did occur, it would not explain the abnormal tissue responses that occur in peptic ulcer, ulcerative colitis, or rheumatoid arthritis (for example) because there is no physiologic paradigm for those responses in the healthy human infant, even in the newborn (as Grossman and Greenberg[53] have indicated). The fixation of psychologic conflicts at early levels of psychosexual development undoubtedly has an important effect on the person's later personality patterns. A disorder in an organ that occurs during its early development might well sensitize the organ to produce an abnormal type of tissue response. Repeated environmental stimulation, such as from the many suppositories or enemas administered during toilet training by the bowel-conscious parents of children who later have bowel disorders, might predispose the end-organ that was stimulated to have conditioned reflex responses during the reactivation of the conflicting emotions that the child experienced at this early level. Such experiences affect but do not by themselves explain a pathophysiologic disorder, including chronic structural changes. People who do not develop vegetative disorders also have such experiences.

Although many patients with ulcerative colitis, peptic ulcer, or other disorders show serious psychopathology, even of psychotic proportions, others have milder personality disorders. Most of the patients studied have been seen after they were referred for hospital study, which skews the group of people studied so that it includes more seriously ill people. Practicing physicians may see many people outside the hospital who have milder pathophysiologic disturbances and respond more readily to supportive therapy than do the people usually studied. Alternation of psychosis with psychophysiologic disorders does occur. Statistical studies by Ross[101] and others, however, do not confirm that such alternation occurs often nor that psychotic people always have fewer psychophysiologic disorders than the general population. No precise correlation between the severity of the psychologic disturbance and the pathophysiologic disturbance has been confirmed although several studies suggest that such a correlation sometimes exists.

Family Interaction

Ruesch[102] has done studies of verbal and nonverbal communication that have led him to believe that a breakdown in verbal communication between 2 people (or in a family) may result in physical symptoms that take the place of verbal communication. Berblinger and Greenhill[10] have reported such phenomena in the family relationships of people who have ulcerative colitis, similar to those seen at times within the family relationships of asthmatic children. Some differences in verbal communications between children who have conversion disorders and children who have psychophysiologic disorders have been described. Nonverbal communication through physical patterns occurs often in conversion disorders, as Engel[34] and others have emphasized. Such communication is also part of some of the psychologic and behavioral manifestations of psychosis. Conceptualizations of this nature, although they help at the psychologic and interpersonal levels, are difficult to substantiate at the physiologic level.

Although symbolic nonverbal communication in bodily terms between the ill person and members of his family may not occur in psychophysiologic disorders, some evidence has been offered by Lindemann[71] and Grinker[50] that changes in the family's adaptive equilibrium can help to precipitate ulcerative colitis. The work of Prugh and Tagiuri[96] supports the idea that, in people who have damaged respiratory systems, bronchial asthma may be precipitated by similar changes in interpersonal forces that involve other patients and staff members in a hospital ward. Such evidence does not necessarily support the theory of nonverbal communication at the somatic level; it also does not define the nature of the pathophysiologic process.

Wolff[126] has elaborated his earlier idea of protective patterns of physiologic responses to stressful stimuli. He cites patterns of riddance of noxious agents by vomiting, defecation, secretion of mucus in the respiratory tree, and other mechanisms. Wolff believes that hyperemia, hypersecretion, and hypermotility occur in all vegetative disorders. He believes that such methods of riddance have become associated with particular attitudes and feelings and may be characteristic of each person (possibly because of constitutional or genetic factors). Wolff's ideas deal with physiologic phenomena in appropriate terms.

The generality of his ideas, however, makes them open to some question, and they do not explain chronic and abnormal tissue responses.

A Comprehensive View of Psychophysiologic Disorders

In the summary of psychologic observations and theories about the causes of pathophysiologic processes, the concepts of biologic predisposition (by constitutional or genetic factors), the effects of early experiences, and psychologic and social precipitating factors often recur; many investigators have different ideas about the relative importance of each idea. Today most investigators agree that multiple etiologic factors of somatic, psychologic, and social nature are involved in psychophysiologic disorders (and all disorders, as the unitary theory postulates). Engel,[33] Mirsky,[85] and Grinker[51] (in his field theory) have recently discussed that idea with cogency and originality. Mirsky has developed a comprehensive theory that has led to hypotheses that can be tested. Engel[37] and Prugh[95] have recently called for a new bio-psycho-social model to replace the current biomedical model.

Mirsky's[85] studies of patients who have peptic ulcers showed that most have high levels of blood pepsinogen, principally caused by increased gastric secretory activity. His studies also showed that the general population has a normative distribution of blood pepsinogen levels that begins in early infancy. Mirsky also observed (as Alexander[4] did earlier) that people who have peptic ulcers usually have strong wishes to please and to be taken care of by others, even though those wishes may be unconscious and unacceptable to them. Drawing on these physiologic and psychologic data, Weiner, Thaler, and Reiser, working with Mirsky,[119] predicted that in a large group of men in Army basic training, peptic ulcers would develop in those who showed high serum pepsinogen levels (hypersecretors) and, in this potentially stressful situation, high levels of conflict over dependent wishes. (The conflicts were studied in psychologic tests that Thaler administered.) The study's results seemed to confirm their prediction. Later studies by Mirsky[86] showed that children who later develop peptic ulcer are gastric hypersecretors from infancy. Ader's[1] studies of animals lend support to Mirsky's general thesis.

Mirsky's[84] conceptual model includes the postulate that all physiologic values follow a normal distribution curve from birth or very early infancy. Mirsky hypothesizes that newborns who have high blood pepsinogen levels and thus high gastric secretory activity may have greater needs to be fed (representing the biologic substrate of strong oral needs) than do newborns who have moderate or low gastric activity. Newborns who have high gastric secretory activity may demand feeding more often and strongly than others; their demands may affect their mothers differently. Some mothers may respond comfortably to such demands and may be gratified by such a need for their ministrations. Others may be frustrated by their infants' constant demands. A cycle of transactional responses between mother and infant may be set; the pattern may be positive or negative. Depending on the relationship between the child's parents and his family's situation at the time of his birth, and on later events, the child may have a conflict over the satisfaction of his dependent, receptive needs during his development. Although anterospective studies of those ideas have not been done systematically, Mirsky's ideas have clarified the interaction of innate biologic characteristics and the early experiences of the child who later develops a peptic ulcer; his ideas have implications for the study of other psychophysiologic disorders.

The work of Mirsky and his colleagues has left some things about peptic ulcer and its causes unexplained. Not everyone who develops a peptic ulcer has a high blood pepsinogen level; there may be different subforms of peptic ulcer. Not everyone who has either a high blood pepsinogen level or increased levels of conflict over dependent wishes necessarily develops a peptic ulcer. The sex difference in the incidence of gastric ulcer as opposed to that of duodenal ulcer has not been explored, although that difference may be a biologic difference in the responses of men and women.* Finally, as Mirsky realized, his studies have not fully explained the pathophysiologic processes by which people develop chronically ulcerative lesions. In addition to the hypersecretion of acid and pepsin, other factors that may contribute to the development of a peptic ulcer include mechanical trauma to the gastric mucosa (caused by diet or smoking) and the petechial hemorrhages and minute ulcerations that were found by Wolf and Wolff[125] to occur during gastric hyperemia, hypersecretion, and hypermotility, in response to strong emotions.

In spite of the limitations mentioned, Mirsky's work has confirmed that predisposing biologic and psychologic factors act predictably and with some specificity if both types of factors are present to produce a peptic ulcer during significantly stressful events. It has also stimulated other anterospective studies of disorders for which biologic "tags" can be obtained. Such studies include, for example, studies of people who, as Dongier and Wittkower[29] have shown, have a high uptake of radioactive iodine but do not yet have any of the signs of thyrotoxicosis. Mirsky[84] has suggested that people who have low blood pepsinogen levels and who might later develop pernicious anemia, people who do not have clinical diabetes but have diabetic glucose-

tolerance curves after a standard dose of corticosteroids, and women who develop diabetes some years after giving birth to infants who weigh over 10 pounds should be studied. Some of Mirsky's evidence suggests that people who do not yet have those disorders have psychologic characteristics that are relatively similar to those of patients who have developed those disorders.

In addition to the physiologic predispositions that are related to the distribution curve of physiologic values (which may include levels of activity and other values not yet studied), other predisposing factors have been found. The biologic characteristics of people who develop bronchial asthma offer one example; another is the lowered convulsive threshold that is characteristic in epileptic patients. Inborn errors of metabolism, many of which are hereditary, have been studied recently. Probably many disorders have such biologic predispositions, and the people who have the metabolic defect but do not develop the disorder may not have had sufficiently stressful experiences.[93] Diabetes represents such a defect, with strong hereditary influences; it may be provoked by metabolic changes that occur in response to stressful stimuli. A presumed enzymatic defect in the handling of the gliadin fraction of wheat glutens seems to combine with psychologic factors and interpersonal stresses to precipitate and perpetuate idiopathic celiac disease in children (Prugh[92,93]). Although the mechanisms of obesity are poorly understood, recent studies of animals have suggested that obesity is often predicated upon a derangement in the dynamics of fat metabolism together with the psychologic and interpersonal factors identified by Bruch[17] in overeating and underactivity. Finally, it is possible that disorders such as ulcerative colitis, rheumatoid arthritis and others that may be precipitated by psychologic and interpersonal stresses may have as a predisposition enzymatic abnormalities that can lead to auto-

---

*Such differences in the incidence of psychophysiologic disorders in men and women need to be studied again. Recent studies have suggested that the incidence of peptic ulcer, hypertension, and myocardial infarction, which has always been higher in men, has begun to rise in women, possibly because more women now work outside the home.

immunization and resulting abnormal tissue responses.

Some of the types of predisposing or contributing factors mentioned earlier are the innate patterns of autonomic response, the operation of conditioned reflexes, and other factors that may affect the immediate functioning of the end-organs as well as more long-range neuroendocrine changes. Contributing factors, such as concurrent bacterial infection and mechanical trauma, may exist in addition to any of the predisposing or precipitating factors.

Many factors, such as secondary infection or lowered resistance to infection, may help to perpetuate a lesion that already exists. An increase in the secretion of hormonal substances that is caused by psychologic factors in biologically predisposed people may, as in thyrotoxicosis or hyperinsulinism, affect behavior and so further disrupt the dynamic steady state and increase susceptibility to physical, psychologic or social stresses. The general debilitation caused by other psychologic disorders may also help the disorder continue. Finally, the features of the ulcer may be in part determined by the patterns of responses to noxious stimuli of the end-organs that are affected, as when a discrete ulcer characteristically occurs in the stomach and duodenum and small, scattered ulcers occur in the large bowel. Disorders such as ulcerative colitis seem to have generalized features that affect many organ systems, suggesting that a vascular or immunologic defect may be the basic somatic one.

Mirsky[86] has described his model of the factors that cause a psychophysiologic disorder as follows: (1) predisposing biologic factors, (2) developmental psychologic (or psychosocial) factors, and (3) current precipitating stress.

Some people may be biologically predisposed to more than one psychophysiologic disorder. Also, recent studies by Schmale[104] and others have indicated that conflicts over dependent needs may act, both as developmental psychosocial factors and, by intensifying the response to an actual or symbolic loss of an important relationship (or sometimes the "anniversary"[59] of such a loss), as current precipitating factors in a number of psychophysiologic disorders.

Prugh's studies of children who have ulcerative colitis, mucous colitis (recurrent diarrhea, or the "irritable bowel syndrome"), and idiopathic celiac disease support the fact that actual or symbolic losses occur in a large percentage of the onsets and exacerbations of those disorders.[94] Other studies of similar factors that occur in the lives of people who have diabetes, thyrotoxicosis, asthma, and obesity also support that idea. The intense frustrations of needs or actual or fantasied danger may also act as stresses at the social level of organization.* Many people who have those disorders have the feelings of being let down, angry, helpless, deserted, or alone. The prevalence of such feelings may comment on our urbanized society, in which it is hard to satisfy our dependent needs, particularly because of our historic and economic ethos of independence.

Developmental Factors. Most psychophysiologic disorders in children resemble in general those in adults. Peptic ulcer and ulcerative colitis have occurred (rarely) in infants and have even occurred at birth or in the neonatal period. The occurrence of such disorders at birth suggests that they are responses to physical stressful stimuli that provoke neuroendocrine mechanisms and seems to support the idea of a char-

---

*More anterospective, controlled, and experimental studies are needed because of the problems of retrospective studies. A recent review of the conditions that are present at the onset of psychosomatic symptoms that Luborsky and his colleagues[73] made contrasts the relatively few "immediate-context" (direct observation) with the "broad-context" (largely retrospective) studies and finds that the same types of psychologic antecedents have been reported by both types of studies and that both occur about the same number of times, with one exception. Frustration was more often reported in the immediate-context studies and separation more often in the broad-context studies.

acteristic end-organ reaction to nonspecific stimuli.

Developmental factors may influence the responses of organs. Infantile colic, in which tension in the family and allergies and other factors appear to be involved, ordinarily disappears by the infant's third or fourth month. The disappearance suggests that the infant takes an integrative step in autonomic functioning at that time and develops a more effective monitoring shield or barrier against stimuli. Failure to thrive (often associated with depression) usually occurs in early infancy, when responses to stress are usually global. Bronchial asthma, without an accompanying infection, rarely occurs until after the second half of the infant's first year; it usually appears after eczema disappears in allergic infants. It is not known whether such a change in responses results from a developmental difference in the capacity for sensitization of the two organ systems (the lungs and the skin) or may also be related to the effect on the respiratory system of the appearance of anxiety over separation from the mother (which usually begins toward the end of the first year). Usually chronic psychophysiologic diarrhea and idiopathic celiac disease also begin toward the end of the infant's first year.

Most severe psychophysiologic disorders seem to occur less often in young children than in adults. Most of them seem to first appear when children are in the middle school-age period. If that is true, it may result from changing patterns of tissue response, perhaps associated with developmental changes in the mental apparatus that include an increase in the repression of emotions and in the internalization of conflict. (Other ideas discussed in Chapter 3, in the section on the developmental aspects of the physiology of emotions, may be relevant to those issues.)

Disturbances in growth patterns (that are not completely understood but seem to involve neuroendocrine responses and insufficient nutrition based on food refusal)

are specific to childhood. Innate or developmental biologic characteristics may affect a child's behavior and the emotional feedback of the parent-child relationship. The possibility also exists that the biochemical systems of the infant or the young child may be affected by his early experiences through neuroendocrine mechanisms and the effect that they may have on the production of catecholamines or growth hormone, for example, in a way that may later render him more vulnerable psychophysiologically. The monitoring of infant caretaking during the first months of life that was done by Sander and his colleagues[103] supports that idea. Mason[76] and Prugh[94] share the belief that a longer-term vulnerability may result under certain circumstances. Finally, certain psychophysiologic disorders, such as diabetes, may become more severe during adolescence, possibly because of the emotional (as well as the metabolic) changes that occur then.

Mixed Conversion and Psychophysiologic Disorders

Although conversion disorders and psychophysiologic or vegetative disorders are usually distinct, symptoms of both types of disorders may occur in the same person, sometimes simultaneously. For example, a child who has asthma may develop a coughing tic; a child who has idiopathic epilepsy may also have episodes of fainting of a conversion nature. The physical sensations that the child experiences during the active phase of his vegetative disorder may determine his conversion disorder.

The symbolic and nonsymbolic mechanisms in the organ systems that are innervated by both the voluntary and involuntary parts of the central nervous system overlap. Kubie[68] has classified the types of bodily functions that are disturbed in psychologic conflicts.

The Organs That Help a Person Relate to His External Environment

The exteroceptive sense organs, the striated muscles (which have proprioceptive controls), and the organs of speech facilitate external relationships. They give a person orientation in space, the ability to communicate with others, the reception and organization of sensory impressions from the outside world, and the conscious orientative faculties. They all have central representations in the mental apparatus, have a place in conscious thought, and are innervated mostly by the voluntary somatomuscular and somatosensory apparatus. (The involuntary nervous system has a secondary synergic or supportive role.) Such organs are the objects of complex ideational processes; the organs themselves can represent those processes symbolically. During times of conflict, the symbolic significance of those organs can lead to conversion disorders in predisposed people.

The Organs of Internal Economy

The organs of internal economy are inside the body and are innervated by the autonomic or involuntary nervous system. Thus they have very limited central representation. Their place in conscious thought is often based on misconceptions, such as the misconception of young children who think that the stomach and the uterus are directly connected and that a "seed" may be swallowed and grow into a baby. Disorders of those organs that are caused by psychologic conflicts are usually vegetative.

The Organs of Instinctual Function

The organs of instinctual function have direct apertural connections to the outside world. They include the organs for the intake and output of food and air and the output of excrement, the swallowing mechanism, the organs of appetite, and the genital organs. Those organs act reflexly in early infancy. Later, the voluntary nervous system initiates their functioning. At some point in their functioning, the autonomic nervous system takes over the more automatic secondary steps. Their combined voluntary and involuntary innervation permits disturbances in their functioning to be both symbolic and vegetative.

Involvement of The Body Image

These include sweeping distortions in the body image, as in chronic invalidism with widespread conversion paralyses and states of extreme weakness or marked fatigability. Many people who have disturbances in their body images pass through phases that represent the involvement of each of their other organ groups. Conscious central representation is present; the somatosensory and the higher conceptual and symbolic systems are most important.

Kubie[69] has suggested that the relationship between the temporal cortex and the visceral brain is responsible for the integration of the symbolic process because it provides a mechanism for integrating the past and the present and the external and the internal environments of the central nervous system (which are subserved by the phylogenetically and ontogenetically "new" and "old" parts of the brain, respectively). In this way, all the data that link the organism to the world of experience, both external and internal, may be coordinated. Kubie believes that "the translation into somatic disturbance of those tensions which are generated on the level of psychological experience" is mediated through these mechanisms.

Kubie's ideas are supported by the work of MacLean and Penfield, cited in Chapter 3, and by the work of Meissner.[79] (Meissner recently reviewed the functions of the hippocampolimbic system in learning.) Kubie's formulation clarifies the balance of the symbolic (or voluntary) parts and the vegetative (or involuntary) parts of the disorders of particular organs or combinations of organs.

The disturbances in bodily function that occur during psychologic conflicts and affect both the organs that help a person relate to his external environment and the systems that maintain the body image are usually symbolic and seem to be characterized by conversion disorders. Rheumatoid arthritis may be an exception because its initial causes are partly symbolic, such as the inhibition of an angry wish to hit someone else. Involuntarily innervated structures may participate in the response, together with bacterial infection or sensitization phenomena. Disturbances of the organs of internal economy are usually nonsymbolic vegetative or psychophysiologic disorders. Disturbances in the function of the organs of instinctual function are puzzling.

The functions of the organs of instinctual function (which are not necessarily the same as the organ systems) include swallowing (deglutition), respiration, urination and defecation, and the functions of the external genitalia. (Probably the functions of the skin should also be included.) Disorders of each of these organ functions are briefly discussed. Some of the disturbances that are mentioned have already been listed as either conversion or vegetative disorders, but that listing did not establish a fixed or arbitrary categorization.

Swallowing

Conversion disorders in swallowing, such as globus hystericus, seem to affect those parts of the swallowing mechanism that are part of the somatomuscular system: the tongue, the myohyloid muscle, and the associated muscles. Other conversion disorders in swallowing, such as vomiting and cardiospasm, may affect the esophagus. The esophagus contains in its upper two-thirds some striated muscles, but its lower one-third contains only smooth muscle. Symbolic conversion dis-

orders may affect the upper two-thirds of the esophagus; involuntary components may be caused by a lack of coordination of the automatic movements of the lower one-third of the esophagus and the cardiac sphincter.

Psychologic stimuli may produce vomiting by a true conversion mechanism, by the hypersensitivity of the gag reflex to excitement, or possibly by a conditioned reflex of the involuntary parts of the swallowing mechanism. Infection or disease in another organ may initially stimulate cyclic vomiting; later conversion mechanisms, together with enhanced dependence on parents and other secondary gains, perpetuate the vomiting pattern. Cyclic vomiting sometimes results in serious dehydration and alkalosis. Rumination that occurs in emotionally deprived infants as a substitute for basic satisfactions may be caused initially by a voluntary hand-to-mouth movement that leads to regurgitation. Rumination can later involve both voluntary and involuntary components, the latter perhaps rendered more feasible by the physiologic chalasia of young infants. In disorders of appetite, a person may eat for symbolic reasons rather than because he is hungry. If he eats for symbolic reasons and has physiologic predisposing factors, he may develop obesity. In anorexia nervosa, the initial suppression of appetite may be a voluntary symbolic act. Later, neuroendocrine changes have psychophysiologic effects in addition to the physiologic effects of starvation.

Respiration

Voluntary control of respiratory movements comes from the action of the accessory muscles, including the abdominal muscles; all those muscles are striated. Changes in the rate and amplitude of respiration may occur as physiologic concomitants of emotions. Changes in respiration may acquire symbolic significance and become conversion disorders; hyperventilation is such a disorder. (Hyperventilation has associated metabolic changes that lead to tetany.) Respiratory coughing, snorting, or barking tics, which often are initially reflexive responses to respiratory infection, may acquire unconscious symbolic meanings. A cough may become an attempt to cough up or breathe out some fantasied harmful substance. Breath-holding spells, common during the second year of life, appear to involve an initial voluntary component related to intense crying over frustration. An involuntary component then takes over and leads to cyanosis, syncope, or even convulsions. Convulsions probably occur more often in infants who have lowered convulsive thresholds.

In bronchial asthma, the basic response is at the level of the terminal bronchioles, predicated upon an allergic diathesis. Psychologic stimuli may intensify the response through cortical-hypothalamic-parasympathetic interconnections, through the triggering of a conditioned reflex, or through conversion disturbances in the accessory muscles, as when a child suppresses his crying over a feared separation from his mother.

Urination

Reflexive voiding in the infant gradually gives way to voluntary control of urination. Voluntary control requires contracting the external sphincter muscle in the male and the perineal muscles in the female and inhibiting the action of the detrusor muscle of the bladder. Enuresis (nocturnal or diurnal) is a failure to maintain such voluntary muscular tone; that tone usually can be maintained even during sleep by conditioned reflexes. A failure in the function of a child's external sphincter mechanisms, based on feelings of rebellion toward his parents or deeper conflicts about his sexual development that are initially conscious and later repressed may thus be symbolically involved. Nocturnal enuresis often occurs during dreams about conflicts. Enuresis often (though not always) occurs in children who underwent coercive bladder training. Enuresis may indicate a developmental lag in a child's capacity for voluntary control, or, more rarely, other physiologic factors. Enuresis may occur in children who have widely differing personalities and family patterns; it may be an encapsulated symptom in a child who has only a slight personality disturbance, or it may be one of many symptoms in a child who has a serious personality disorder or psychosis. It may occur as a failure to develop control or as a symptom of regression.

A negativistic preschool-age child may consciously disregard the pressure of his distended bladder during the daytime. Recurrent anxiety may have involuntary physiologic concomitants, such as urinary frequency or urgency or the inhibition of urination. Conditioned reflexes may play a role in situations involving specific fears.

Defecation

Infants defecate automatically although they can acquire conditioned reflexes to the use of suppositories in their first few weeks of life. Voluntary control of defecation can be achieved before the end of the first year. It requires voluntarily maintaining the tone of the external anal sphincter, assisted by the levator ani muscles, so that the sphincter can resist the defecation reflex that ordinarily operates as the pressure of a fecal mass within the rectum grows.

The preschool-age child who consciously resists training may extrude or withhold his stool. He often associates feelings of rebellion with pleasurable stimulation of his anorectal mucous membrane. In some cases, unconscious conflicts of this nature that persist or recur in the older child may lead to soiling that seems to be caused by conversion mechanisms of the external muscles. Encopresis, like enuresis, may be a developmental failure to achieve control or a symptom of regression provoked by stressful stimuli, as when it occurs in a school-age child who is separated from his hospitalized mother. Coercive bowel training may be a predisposition acquired through experience. A developmental lag in a child's capacity for voluntary control, conditioning of the defecation reflex to certain emotions, local disease during the training period, or overfrequent stimulation of the anorectal region with suppositories or enemas may also be involved. Temporary loss of bowel control, such as that caused by infectious diarrhea, may cause anxiety and guilt in the young child and may be a precipitating factor in persistent soiling. Encopresis, even more than enuresis, may cause resentment or guilt in a child's parents and lead to a struggle for control with the child which may spread from bowel control into other areas of behavior.

If the child, during the training period or later, suppresses his defecation reflex, his bowel may bcome temporarily unresponsive. Some children may continue such suppression in response to coercive toilet training, the pain of an anal fissure, the fear of explosive release that they associate with hostile fantasies, or the need to obtain unhealthy substitute satisfactions from the pleasurable sensation of stopping the extrusion of the stool after it begins. Such voluntary withholding, together with the necessary involuntary readjustments in the peristaltic action and the action of the internal anal sphincter (possibly including conditioning of the intestinal contractions), may cause chronic constipation, even though the associated feelings are no longer conscious. In some children who have such predisposing experiences, the sigmoid may become distended and alterations in its propulsive action (such as those seen in the nonaganglionic type of megacolon) may occur.

Diarrhea that occurs during psychologic conflict ordinarily involves physiologic concomitants of anxiety, with perhaps a hyperactive gastrocolic reflex, or increased motility resulting possibly from the overwhelming of sympathetic by parasympathetic discharges in the emergency response. Situations that provoke symbolic fantasies and the feelings associated with them may, however, evoke conditioned responses that trigger the defecation reflex and other involuntary mechanisms, as in some cases of ulcerative colitis.

The External Genitalia

The functions of the external genitalia are rarely disturbed in childhood. In adolescent and adult males, priapism and impotence are mostly conversion disorders that are caused by sexual conflicts. Priapism and impotence involve disturbances in the action of the bulbocavernosus muscle and associated alterations in the functions of the involuntarily innervated urethra, seminal vesicles, and venous supply. Frigidity in females who have sexual conflicts may be caused by spasms of the striated perineal muscles, although involuntary mechanisms may also be involved.

Skin

The skin is innervated by the sympathetic nervous system, except for the sebaceous glands (which seem to have no autonomic innervation). Thus the vascular, sweating, and pilomotor functions of the skin appear to have no central representation although the responses of the skin to heat, cold, pain, and touch do have central representation. In the usual sense, only the disturbances that occur in sensory perception in response to psychologic or social stimuli would be regarded as conversion disorders. Eczema, urticaria, and so-called neurodermatitis, for example, are considered vegetative disorders; eczema and urticaria have the predisposing physiologic factors of allergies. In addition to its functions of protection, sensation, and excretion, however, the skin is also an organ of sexual attraction and emotional expression. Its external appearance is part of the body image. Some studies support the idea that some changes in the skin have functions of discharge that symbolically express psychologic conflicts and thus represent intermediate phenomena between vegetative disorders and conversion disorders. The production of skin lesions through hypnosis, and Seitz's[108] substitution by hypnosis of skin disorders for symbolically equivalent nondermatologic psychologic syndromes support that idea. Clinical studies of chronic skin disorders that have psychologic components have indicated that people who have such disorders also have symbolic conflicts over unconscious exhibitionistic and self-punishing needs. Some of the self-punishing needs are satisfied by painful scratching. The effectiveness of hypnosis, and of other methods involving suggestion, in treating verruca vulgaris, a lesion known to involve a filtrable virus, is also pertinent but not yet understood.

Conversion disorders and psychophysiologic disorders overlap and may be mixed with other types of psychologic reactions. Most of the more severe and chronic psychophysiologic disorders seem to occur, among older children and adults, in people who have chronic obsessive-compulsive, passive-dependent, or other types of personality disorders. But it is my observation that vegetative disorders may be seen in children who have milder psychologic problems (perhaps because those children have a greater somatic predisposition) or, more rarely, in children who have near-psychoses.

Psychologic Reactions to Predominantly Physical Disorders

In recent years, an abundance of observations have been made about psychologic reactions to predominantly physical disorders. Physical disorders that affect mainly the central nervous system and those that affect mainly the rest of the body are dis-

cussed separately, although that distinction is artificial. (A fuller discussion of each category is given in later chapters.)

Reactions to Physical Disorders That Affect Mainly the Central Nervous System

Such disorders have been called acute and chronic brain syndromes. (Many such disorders affect other organ systems.) Disorders such as poliomyelitis, which affects mainly the motor neurons of the spinal cord, and mumps, which causes prominent pathology in the salivary glands, usually also cause meningoencephalitis that is sometimes severe. The disturbances in behavior that are caused by brain syndromes, such as hypothalamic lesions, may be very similar to those caused by psychologic conflicts. Disturbances in behavior are often caused by both brain syndromes and psychologic conflicts.

Acute Brain Syndromes. Little is known about the reactions of children to acute insults to the central nervous system, except to head injuries. Romano and Engel[100] pointed out that in adults delirium is characteristic of the acute brain syndrome. Delirium is a disturbance in awareness that is caused by disordered cerebral metabolism, brought about by noxious stimuli of infectious, traumatic, or other nature. Delirium often occurs in children in response to head injury, meningitis, encephalitis, or high fever and as a result of cerebral metabolic changes caused by pneumonia, heart disease, and other illnesses outside the central nervous system. Delirium shows certain features that are affected by the child's state of development, personality, and past experience. In younger children, delirium may be masked by marked withdrawal, anxiety, or aggression. Delirious reactions to drugs occur particularly in children because children's responses to drugs vary in relation to their developmental level.

Children often respond with great resiliency to insults to the central nervous system. But disturbances in perceptual or visuomotor functioning that are caused by such insults may persist even without obvious delirium or gross neurologic lesions. Crothers and Meyer[25] have described difficulties in perceiving and arranging patterns or forms that showed up on the Bender-Gestalt test or similar tests. Those difficulties lasted as long as several months after meningitis or encephalitis without apparent neurologic sequelae. Such disturbances may occur after pneumonia and other febrile diseases that do not directly affect the central nervous system. Resulting lags in the achievement of such perceptual-motor tasks, together with regression, may lead to learning difficulties in the early school-age child if these are not recognized and dealt with in planning for the child's return to full academic performance.

Chronic Brain Syndromes. Insults to the central nervous system that cause structural changes may occur during intrauterine existence as the result of viral infection, toxoplasmosis, erythroblastosis, eclampsia, or placenta previa. They may occur during birth, as the result of hemorrhage or anoxia, or after birth, as the result of infections, or traumatic, neoplastic, heredodegenerative, vascular, metabolic, or other noxious influences. Sometimes gross neurologic lesions occur, as in the cerebral palsies. In other cases, only EEG abnormalities, perceptual-motor defects, and certain behavioral changes can be found; if that is the case, diagnosis is difficult. Mental retardation may accompany such defects. Most children who have more mild and diffuse damage to the cerebral cortex are not mentally retarded, although their learning capacity is often limited.

Brain syndromes, conversion disorders, and other patterns that include chronic personality disorders are often mixed in older children. Children who have uncontrolled idiopathic epilepsy may develop brain damage as a result of status epilepticus, and later conversion mechanisms may complicate the epilepsy. Sydenham's chorea may begin during psychosocial stress. Children with this disorder may show conversion mechanisms of dystonic or other type, superimposed upon the choreiform movements and at time perpetuating the disability.

Damage to the brain that occurs at different levels of development may have different effects; the effects of brain damage are not always predictable. The newborn's brain can withstand considerable hypoxia during and immediately after birth. It can also compensate, with its undamaged parts, for diffuse damage caused by petechial hemorrhages or hypoxia even though no brain tissue is regenerated. The clinical signs of brain damage may improve during maturation, as Graham[47] and Keith[65] have shown. Children have compensated remarkably for extensive lacerations of the cerebral cortex, congenital porencephalic cysts, and congenital absence of the corpus callosum, for example. Some few of those children have shown very little cerebral dysfunction on psychologic tests later in development. The prognosis of children who have arrested hydrocephalus (whether or not the hydrocephalus is related to meningomyelocele) is much better now than it was formerly believed to be. Older children compensate less well although better than do adults. But some functions that have not yet developed may be affected more seriously in infants than in older children who sustain brain damage, as Graham has indicated. Functions that have developed recently may be in a critical or vulnerable state, in contrast to more solidly established ones, as Hebb[56] and Birch[11] have suggested. Longitudinal and controlled studies now going on may answer such questions.

Reactions to Physical Disorders Outside Affect the Central Nervous System

Any illness or injury may have a decompensating effect on a child's dynamic steady state or on his family's equilibrium.

Reactions to Acute Illness or Injury. An illness or injury often causes manifestations of regression. The misinterpretation of an illness or accident as a punishment, the fear of bodily mutilation during medical or surgical procedures, and other "magical" ideas about pain or illness are characteristic of children of preschool age or early school age. The parents often assign blame for their child's illness; they feel guilt (or self-blame) or blame teachers, physicians, or a hostile world for the illness. Manifestations of regression by a young child, such as a return to bed wetting or soiling, may cause guilt or anxiety on the part of the child and anger or guilt on the part of the parents. In older children and adolescents, pain that has a physical cause may be intensified or perpetuated by conversion mechanisms by which the child unconsciously atones for his feelings of guilt. The greater care that an ill child needs may be a burden on his parents, with resentment underlying willingness. There may be rivalry or other reverberations on the part of the ill child's siblings. Such influences may slow a child's convalescence.

Since many children are hospitalized during treatment of a serious illness, it is often hard to separate the effects of the illness from the effects of hospitalization on the child and his family. In addition to separation anxiety, regression, depression, and other situational responses (that have been described by a number of investigators[94]), Robertson and Bowlby[99] have described phases of the response to illness of the older infant and young child. The phases of response are (1) protest, (2) despair, and (3) detachment and other coping mechanisms that the child uses to deal with separation from his mother.

Reactions to Chronic Illness or Handicap. Children's reactions to chronic illness or handicaps have their origins in the outcome of the generic type of human responses to catastrophic illnesses or injuries. Those generic responses include the adaptive mechanisms that people use dur-ing the phases of impact, recoil, and restitution. Richmond[98] has described somewhat parallel phases in the responses of parents to a child's illness during which the parents learn to accept their child's physical state and the uncertainty of his return to health. The lack of anticipation of or preparation for such devastating experience makes the immediate effect of a child's illness on the child and his parents overwhelmingly strong. In order to treat a catastrophic illness or injury, a physician must know about the phases of response and know how to adapt treatment and rehabilitation to them. He must also be aware of the personalities and needs of the child and the child's family as residual defects or handicaps appear.

Although chronic disorders do affect personality development and social adjustment, many children (and adults) who have chronic illnesses or congenital or acquired handicaps cope with their disabilities and adapt very well to their limitations. The timing of a handicap's appearance is important, as with a sensory handicap (e.g., blindness or deafness) that is congenital rather than acquired. But handicaps that appear at the same time, relatively, have different effects on different children and parents. Most children who have chronic disorders find it difficult to establish or maintain a body image. The child's parents have much influence on the development of his conscious and unconscious awareness of his body and its characteristics. Children who have chronic disorders often have disturbed body images, but children who have no physical disfigurement also may have disturbed body images.

Specific personality disorders are not associated with chronic brain syndromes or with chronic bodily illnesses or handicaps. The development of the child's personality is affected by the severity of his defect, the level of development at which it occurred, the child's previous adaptive capacity, the nature of the parent-child relationship, the psychologic meaning of the illness to the child and his parents, the family's equilibrium, and other factors, such as the quality and nature of medical treatment and educational planning. The capacity of the child's family to accept and nurture him in ways appropriate to his capacities probably affects the development of his personality most.

Psychosocial factors may precipitate disorders that include infectious, toxic, or traumatic noxious stimuli. Pediatricians are now concerned about accidents and poisoning in childhood, such as the lead intoxication sometimes caused by pica, because they are aware that the child's developmental state, degree of activity, and biologic capacities, the type of supervision or discipline offered by his parents, his family's equilibrium, and his internal psychologic conflicts all affect the child who often has accidents or shows self-injuring behavior.

Host Resistance to Disease

Many predominantly physical disorders occur at the same time as important psychologic or social stressful stimuli; other psychologic reactions are caused by the experience of being ill. Such disorders range from infectious hepatitis and the common cold,[94] in people who are undergoing acute emotional conflict, to streptococcal infections, in families that are experiencing stressful events.[81] The psychophysiologic and immmunologic mechanisms triggered by such stimuli that lower immunity or host resistance are not understood. Studies of animals by Jensen and Rasmussen[63] and by Friedman, Ader, and Glasgow[42] support the idea that such stimuli can lower immunity in humans (although they do not confirm it). Ader and Cohen[2] have shown that immunosuppression can be behaviorally conditioned. Friedman and his colleagues have studied the relative suscep-

tibility to encephalomyocarditis virus of mice that lived alone and mice that lived in groups. The mice that lived alone had a mortality rate that was nearly twice that of the mice that lived in groups. In another study, they put adult mice in environments that produced different degrees of stress. Neither stress nor the inoculation of Coxsackie B2 virus alone made the mice ill. But the combination of stress and Coxsackie B2 virus resulted in a significant loss of weight. They have considered that study as a model for what Engel[34] has called the "multifactorial approach to etiology." They have suggested that the changed susceptibility to the virus involves the central nervous system-pituitary-adrenocortical axis; they have cited the fact that cortisone lowers the normal resistance of adult mice to various strains of Coxsackie virus but have admitted that they do not understand the exact nature of the physiologic process that causes the change in susceptibility. Whybrow,[121] Kiely,[67] Amkrant,[7] and others have made similar studies of animals and humans. Mason[75] has offered the working hypothesis (based on some supporting evidence but as yet unconfirmed) that stress-related, multiple changes in "overall hormonal balance," operating on both a short- and a long-term basis, may change host resistance to infectious disorders. That hypothesis recalls Engel's[33] designation of disease as a disorder in the integration of the "dynamic state."

Friedman and his colleagues observe that people are exposed to a great number of microorganisms every day and that many of those microorganisms can cause disease. They commented that it is thus surprising that illness occurs as an exception rather than as a rule. Other studies of humans that should be made about the defense mechanisms that resist infectious disorders include studies of the functional barrier of the skin and other membranes, the vascular and cellular reactions that occur during local inflammation, specific immune mechanisms, and nonspecific responses, such as interferon production. Friedman and his colleagues believe that psychosocial factors do affect host resistance in humans. They quote Dubos,[30] who has pointed out that "each host-parasite relationship is an expression of the genetic make-up of both components of the system, and is affected by temperature, humidity, diet, external stimuli—induced by each and every factor of the total environment." Figure 4–1 represents schematically the interaction of such factors.

Psychosocial factors have been observed clinically to contribute to and sometimes precipitate some chronic disorders, although physical predisposing or perpetuating factors may predominate. Such observations have been reported in relation to disseminated lupus erythematosus (McClary and Meyer[77]), infectious disorders such as tuberculosis (Holmes and colleagues[60]) and brucellosis (Harris[55]), degenerative disorders such as multiple sclerosis (Philippopolous and colleagues[91]), and

Parkinsonism (Booth[13]) and others, including pernicious anemia (Lewin[70]), herpes simplex (Blank and Brody[12]), and fungus infections (Harris[54]).

Other studies have shown that life crises often precede disorders. Studies in Great Britain and the United States indicate that the death of a loved one, particularly a spouse, is followed within a year by a high incidence of disorders and even death among the survivors; widowers are most vulnerable.[22] Wyler, Masada, and Holmes[61,129] have found some correlation between the intensity of the crisis (as ranked by them) and the duration and intensity of the following disorder.

Engel and his colleagues have studied the concept of separation-depression, arising as a result of the actual or symbolic loss of an important relationship and sometimes causing feelings of helplessness and hopelessness or even a complex of "giving up–given up."[35] They believe that a person who acquires that complex may become

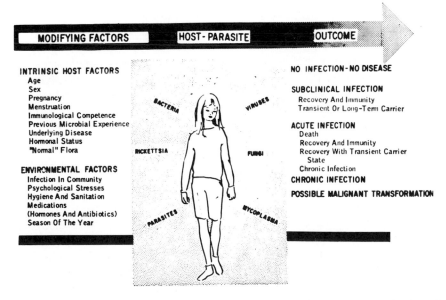

Fig. 4–1. The intrinsic host and environmental factors that may interact to influence the host's response to potentially pathogenic microorganisms, and the possible outcomes of the relations between the host and a parasite. (From S.B. Friedman and L.A. Glasgow: Psychological factors and resistance to infectious diseases. Pediatr. Clin. North Am., *13*:315, 1966.)

mentally or physically ill; the physical illness is the result of a physiologic process that involves immunologic and neuroendocrine systems. Or the person may become socially deviant. Improvement in a person's life situation may help rid him of that complex, but some people who have particular biological predispositions may develop irreversible or even fatal disorders. "Anniversaries"[59] of losses may cause disorders to worsen or recur.

Engel developed the concept of separation-depression as a result of his studies of ulcerative colitis and his studies (with Reichsman and others) of an infant who had a gastric fistula.[97a] Following Engel's approach, Greene[48] has reported that leukemia and lymphoma in adults and children may begin during depression over the actual or symbolic loss of an important supportive figure. The time of onset of leukemia in adults is often difficult to determine, although leukemia's course was formerly very rapid in young children. I have known 3 preschool-age children who developed leukemia and died within several months after the death of a parent. Schmale and Iker,[105,106] using a blind approach, predicted in a high percentage of cases the development of cancer in women who had cervical cytology suspicious for cancer on the basis of the presence or absence in the women whom they interviewed of criteria defined as a high hopelessness potential and/or recently experienced feelings of hopelessness. Ader and Friedman[3] showed that rats that were shocked or handled during the first week of life died more quickly from transplanted carcinosarcoma tumors than did the members of a control group. But several other studies have shown contradictory results, and much clarifying work needs to be done.[117]

Schmale[104] and others have observed the relation of separation-depression to the onset of disorders in a large percentage of patients in a general hospital population. Mutter and Schleifer[88] have found that children who were hospitalized for various physical illnesses came from more disorganized families that had more recent losses or other disruptive changes than did a comparison group of healthy children. Using a "life event score," Coddington and his colleagues[24] found that recent major "life changes" had been experienced by twice as many children who had physical illnesses as would have been expected in a control group of healthy children. Holmes and Rahe,[62] using a more or less calibrated social readjustment scale, have shown in adults that major life changes can predict health changes. Other studies have shown that psychologically vulnerable people are more likely than nonvulnerable people to seek care for physical symptoms and that premorbid indicators of unresolved life stress can accurately predict who will seek care for disorders.[20,28,97,114] As Cobb[23] has emphasized, the availability and effectiveness of social support systems may help determine a person's response to life stresses.

In such studies of humans, it is hard to set up controls in a clinical setting; most of those studies have comparison groups rather than control groups.* Still, such studies support the separation–depression, helplessness–hopelessness, giving up–given up complex, its adverse effect on mental, physical, and social functioning, and its precipitation of some predominantly physical disorders. That conceptual approach is compatible with Mirsky's model of psychophysiologic disorders, as has been implied earlier, although the predisposing biologic factors in separation–depression are more difficult to ascertain and study. It is also possible that some of the patients studied by Engel and his colleagues, most of whom are adults, have had some developmental psychosocial experiences that made them more vulnerable to separation–depression and to

---

*"Life event" and similar scales are difficult to weight, in order to deal with different intensities of stress for different persons.

tendencies to give up when they feel help-less. Rahe concedes that a person's earlier experiences and methods of coping may affect his susceptibility to life changes. Some studies of children have been made about vulnerability to stressful psychoso-cial stresses, whether or not such stresses precipitate physical disorders.

Death Related to Psychosocial Stress

People who are fatally ill may not die as the result of their disorders themselves. Some people who feel hopeless about a ma-lignancy die before their disorder has be-come physically fatal. Engel,[36] Greene,[49] and others have discussed deaths that oc-cur during a "lethal life situation," char-acterized by intense emotion, a fear of los-ing control over what happens, and a feeling of hopelessness about being able to change the situation. Cannon[19] gave cred-ibility to the concept of "voodoo death" that exists in some primitive societies; lethal catatonia ("exhaustion death") has been described in excited patients. Richter[98a] ob-served death in wild rats who found them-selves in a hopeless situation. Beecher[9] has presented evidence that fear itself can cause death.

The physiologic mechanisms by which emotional states, especially states of hope-lessness or intense fear, can cause death are not understood. Some investigators, like Cannon, have thought that sympa-thetic overactivity causes death. Others, like Richter, have believed that parasympa-thetic or vagal overactivity caused death. Richter's later observations and some more recent studies of monkeys have suggested that overactivity of both systems may cause death. The initial increase in heart rate is a sympathetic response; the following bra-dycardia that leads to death is a vagal dis-charge.

Experienced surgeons (e.g., Halstead) have refused to operate on a person who is convinced that he will die or who is se-riously depressed (see Chapter 27). It also seems likely, as Solnit and Green[110] have suggested, that the fear resulting from an authoritative, trusted person's prediction that death will soon come can worsen the course of a fatal illness.

The Relative Importance of Factors That Affect Disorders

The multiple factors that cause the break-down of adaptation or failure in develop-ment and the appearance of disorders include genetic, constitutional, develop-mental, environmental, and experiential factors that bring significantly stressful stimuli to act initially on 1 of a person's 3 basic levels of organization. The traditional arbitrary classification of disorders as either predominantly physical or predominantly psychologic comes from an awareness of the initial effect of stressful stimuli on the organism. Such a classification implies an emphasis on the level of organization that is most seriously (though not always ini-tially) involved in the restriction of function or development, decompensation, adap-tive breakdown, or attempts to maintain or regain equilibrium.

From the approach described, there is no room for artificial dichotomies of wholly somatic or completely psychologic disease, no true characterization of illness as either organic or functional, no valid diagnosis of a psychologic disorder by ruling out so-matic influences. As Engel[34] has said, "There can be no linear concept of etiology, but rather the pathogenesis of disease in-volves a series of negative and positive feedbacks with multiple, simultaneous, and segmented changes potentially affecting any system of the body." A valid diagnosis must consider all the predisposing, con-tributing, precipitating, and perpetuating factors, whether physical, psychologic, or social, that operate in each disorder. The weighting of such positive evidence and the interrelationships of those factors will lead to a plan of treatment that balances the physical, psychologic, and social or environmental methods of therapy or treatment.

In that same conceptual framework, there can be no room for a medical specialty or scientific discipline called psychosomatic medicine. All disease may be said to be psychosomatic, if the mind and the body are considered as integrated forces, in line with the unitary theory of health and illness just described. The psychosomatic approach is a conceptual one; it considers the balance of the physiologic, psychologic, and social factors that affect the onset and perpetuation of disorders.

The term psychosomatic disorder has often been used to designate those disorders in which the predisposing, precipitating, and perpetuating factors are psychologic and social. The term somatopsychic disorder has often been used to designate disorders that are caused mainly by pathophysiologic factors and have psychologic contributing or perpetuating factors or cause secondary psychologic and social reactions. Such terms, however useful operationally, have the obvious limitation of implying the selective involvement of psychologic or somatic factors in certain syndromes only. Both factors are involved in varying degrees in every disease. Psychosomatic concepts thus fit comfortably into the purview of comprehensive pediatrics.

A positive and dynamic approach is as essential to the assessment of health as to the evaluation of disease. As every pediatrician knows, the traditional ruling out of disease does not constitute a valid health examination. The pediatrician must also appraise the child's current level of development in physiologic, psychologic, and social dimensions as well as the social characteristics, equilibrium, and expectations in the child's family. The support of healthy developmental patterns in all areas and the prevention of adaptive breakdown or dis-

ease, whether predominantly physical or predominantly psychologic, must be based on such understanding and knowledge.

Bibliography

1. Ader, R., Beels, C.C., and Tatum, R.: Blood pepsinogen and gastric erosions in the rat. Psychosom. Med., 22:1, 1960.
2. Ader, R., and Cohen, N.: Behaviorally conditioned immunosuppression. Psychosom. Med., 37:333, 1975.
3. Ader, R., and Friedman, S.B.: Differential early experiences and susceptibility to transplant tumor in the rat. J. Comp. Physiol. Psychol., 59:361, 1965.
4. Alexander, F.: Psychosomatic Medicine. New York, Norton, 1950.
5. Alexander, F., French, T.M., and Pollock, G.H., Eds.: Psychosomatic Specificity. Chicago, University of Chicago Press, 1968, Vol. I.
6. American Psychiatric Association: Diagnostic and Statistical Manual of Mental Disorders. 2nd Ed. Washington, D.C., 1968.
7. Amkrant, H., and Solomon, G.F.: From the symbolic stimulus to the pathophysiologic response: Immune mechanisms. Int. J. Psychiatry Med., 5:541, 1974.
8. Barber, T.X., et al., Eds.: Biofeedback and Self-Control. Vols. I. and II. New York, Aldine-Atherton, 1970 and 1971.
9. Beecher, H.K.: Non-specific forces surrounding disease and the treatment of disease. JAMA, 179:437, 1962.
10. Berblinger, K.W., and Greenhill, M.H.: Levels of communication in ulcerative colitis: A case study. Psychosom. Med., 16:156, 1954.
11. Birch, H.G.: Brain Damage in Children: The Biological and Social Aspects. Baltimore, Williams & Wilkins, 1964.
12. Blank, H., and Brody, M.W.: Recurrent herpes simplex: A psychiatric and laboratory study. Psychosom. Med., 12:254, 1940.
13. Booth, G.: Psychodynamics in parkinsonism. Psychosom. Med., 10:1, 1948.
14. Brazelton, T.B.: The pediatrician and hysteria in childhood. Nerv. Child., 10:306, 1943.
15. Brown, F.A.: A clinical psychologists perspective on research in psychosomatic medicine. Psychosom. Med., 21:174, 20:174, 1958.
16. Bruch, H.: Psychosomatic approach to childhood disorders. In: Modern Trends in Child Psychiatry. (D.C.N. Lewis and B.L. Pacella, Eds.) New York, International Universities Press, 1945.
17. Bruch, H.: Eating Disorders. New York, Basic Books, 1973.
18. Cannon, W.B.: The Wisdom of the Body. New York, Norton, 1932.
19. Cannon, W.B.: "Voodoo" death. Amer. Anthropol., 44:169, 1942.
20. Canter, A., Imboden, J.B., and Cluff, L.E.: The frequency of physical illness as a function of prior

psychological vulnerability and contemporary stress. Psychosom. Med., *28*:344, 1966.

21. Carpentieri, J., and Jensen, R.A.: Psychosomatic medicine and pediatrics. Quart. J. Child Behavior, *1*:72, 1949.

22. Clayton, P.J.: The clinical morbidity of the first year of bereavement: A review. Compr. Psychiatr., *14*:151, 1973.

23. Cobb, S.: Social support as a moderator of life stress. Psychosom. Med., *38*:300, 1976.

24. Coddington, R.D.: The significance of life events as etiological factors in the diseases of children: II. A study of a normal population. J. Psychosom. Res., *16*:205, 1972.

25. Crothers, B., and Meyer, E.: The psychologic and psychiatric implications of poliomyelitis. J. Pediatr., *28*:324, 1946.

26. Deutsch, F.: The choice of organ in organ neurosis. Int. J. Psychoanal., *20*:252, 1939.

27. Deutsch, F., Ed.: *The Psychosomatic Concept in Psychoanalysis.* New York, International Universities Press, 1953.

28. Dohrenwend, B.S., and Dohrenwend, B.P., Eds.: *Stressful Life Events: Their Nature and Effects.* New York, Wiley-Interscience, 1974.

29. Dongier, M., et al.: Psychophysiologic studies in thyroid function. Psychosom. Med., *18*:310, 1956.

30. Dubos, R.: *Man, Medicine, and Environment.* New York, American Library, 1968.

31. Dunbar, H.F.: *Emotions and Bodily Changes.* New York, Columbia University Press, 1946.

32. Engel, G.L.: Studies of ulcerative colitis: IV. The significance of headaches. Psychosom. Med., *18*:334, 1956.

33. Engel, G.L.: A unified concept of health and disease. Persp. in Biol. & Med., *3*:459, 1960.

34. Engel, G.L.: *Psychological Development in Health and Disease.* Philadelphia, Saunders, 1962.

35. Engel, G.L.: A life setting conducive to illness: The giving-up–given-up complex. Ann. Intern. Med., *69*:293, 1968.

36. Engel, G.L.: Sudden and rapid death during psychological stress: Folklore or folk wisdom. Ann. Intern. Med., *74*:771, 1971.

37. Engel, G.L.: The need for a new medical model: A challenge for biomedicine. Science, *196*:129, 1977.

38. Engel, G.L., Reichsman, F., and Segal, H.L.: A study of an infant with a gastric fistula. I. Behavior and rate of total hydrochloric acid secretion. Psychosom. Med., *18*:374, 1956.

39. Finch, S.M.: Psychosomatic problems in children. Nerv. Child., *9*:261, 1952.

40. Fitzelle, G.T.: Personality factors and certain attitudes toward child-bearing among parents of asthmatic children. Psychosom. Med., *21*:208, 1959.

41. Freud, S.: *An Outline of Psychoanalysis.* New York, Norton, 1940.

42. Friedman, S.B., Ader, R., and Glasgow, L.A.: Effects of psychological stress in adult mice inoculated with coxsackie B viruses. Psychosom. Med., *27*:361, 1965.

43. Friedman, S.B., and Glasgow, L.A.: Psychological factors and resistance to infectious disease. Pediatr. Clin. North Am., *13*:315, 1966.

44. Garner, A.M., and Wenar, C.: *The Mother-Child Interaction in Psychosomatic Disorders.* Urbana, Ill., University of Illinois Press, 1959.

45. Gerard, M.W.: Genesis of psychosomatic symptoms in infancy. The influence of infantile traumata upon symptom choice. In: *Psychosomatic Concept in Psychoanalysis.* (F. Deutsch, Ed.) New York, International Universities Press, 1953.

46. Graham, D.T., et al.: Specific attitudes in initial interviews with patients having different "psychosomatic" diseases. Psychosom. Med., *24*:257, 1962.

47. Graham, F.K., et al.: *Development Three Years After Perinatal Anoxia and Other Potentially Damaging Newborn Experiences.* Psychological Monograph No. 76. Washington, American Psychological Association, 1962.

48. Greene, W.A.: The psychosocial setting of the development of leukemia and lymphoma. Ann. N.Y. Acad. Sci., *125*:794, 1966.

49. Greene, W.A., Goldstein, S., and Moss, A.J.: Psychosocial aspects of sudden death. Ann. Intern. Med., *129*:725, 1972.

50. Grinker, R.R.: *Psychosomatic Research.* New York, Norton, 1953.

51. Grinker, R.R., Ed.: *Toward a Unitary Theory of Human Behavior.* New York, Basic Books, 1959.

52. Group for the Advancement of Psychiatry. *Psychopathological Disorders in Childhood: Theoretical Considerations and a Proposed Classification.* Vol. 6, Report No. 62, New York, 1966.

53. Grossman, H.J., and Greenberg, N.H.: Psychosomatic differentiation in infancy. I. Autonomic activity in the newborn. Psychosom. Med., *19*:293, 1957.

54. Harris, H.J.: Fungus infection of feet. A case report illustrating a psychosomatic problem. Psychosom. Med., *6*:336, 1944.

55. Harris, H.J.: *Brucellosis: Clinical and Subclinical.* New York, Hoeber, Hoeber, 1950.

56. Hebb, D.O.: *The Organization of Behavior.* London, Chapman & Hall, 1949.

57. Heisel, J., et al.: The significance of life events as contributing factors in the diseases of children. III. A study of pediatric patients. J. Pediatr., *83*:119, 1973.

58. Hendrick, I.: *Facts and Theories of Psychoanalysis.* New York, Knopf, 1947.

59. Hilgard, J.R., and Newman, M.F.: Anniversaries in mental illness. Psychiatry, *22*:113, 1959.

60. Holmes, T.H., et al.: Psychosocial and psychophysiologic studies of tuberculosis. Psychosom. Med., *19*:134, 1957.

61. Holmes, T.H., and Masuda, M.: Life change and illness susceptibility. In: *Stressful Life Events.* (B.S. Dohrenwend and B.P. Dohrenwend, Eds.). New York, Wiley, 1974.

62. Holmes, T.H., and Rahe, R.H.: The social readjustment rating scale. J. Psychosom Res., *11*:213, 1967.

63. Jensen, M.N., and Rasmussen, A.F.: Stress and susceptibility to viral infections. J. Immunol., *90*:21, 1963.

64. Jores, A., and Freyburger, H., Eds.: *Advances in Psychosomatic Medicine: Symposium of the Fourth European Conference on Psychosomatic Research.* New York, R. Brunner, 1961.
65. Keith, H.M., and Gage, R.D.: Neurological lesions in relation to asphyxia of the newborn and factors of pregnancy. Long-term follow-up. Pediatrics, 26:616, 1960.
66. Kepecs, J.G., Robin, M., and Brunner, M.: Relationship between certain emotional states and exudation into the skin. Psychosom. Med., 13:10, 1951.
67. Kiely, W.F.: From the symbolic stimulus to the pathophysiological response: Neurophysiological mechanisms. Int. J. Psychiatry Med., 5:517, 1974.
68. Kubie, L.S.: The central representation of the symbolic process in relation to psychosomatic disorders. In: *Recent Developments in Psychosomatic Medicine* (E.D. Wittkower and R.A. Cleghorn, Eds.) Philadelphia, Lippincott, 1957.
69. Kubie, L.S.: The problem of specificity in the psychosomatic process. In: *Recent Developments in Psychosomatic Medicine* (E.D. Wittkower and R.A. Cleghorn, Eds.). Philadelphia, Lippincott, 1957.
70. Lewin, K.K.: Role of depression in the production of illness in pernicious anemia. Psychosom. Med., 21:23, 1959.
71. Lindemann, E.: Modifications in the course of ulcerative colitis in relationship to changes in life situations and reaction patterns. In: *Life Stress and Bodily Disease* (H.G. Wolff, S.G. Wolf, and C.C. Hare, Eds.). Baltimore, Williams & Wilkins, 1950.
72. Lipton, E.L., Steinschneider, A., and Richmond, J.C.: Psychophysiological disorders in children. In: *Review of Child Development Research*, Vol 2. (M.L. Hoffman and L.W. Hoffman, Eds.). New York, Russell Sage Foundation, 1966.
73. Luborsky, L., Docherty, J.B., and Penick, S.: Onset conditions for psychosomatic symptoms: A comparative review of immediate observation with retrospective research. Psychosom. Med., 35:187, 1973.
74. Margolin, S.G.: Psychotherapeutic principles in psychosomatic practice. In: *Recent Developments in Psychosomatic Medicine.* (E.D. Wittkower and R.A. Cleghorn, Eds.). Philadelphia, Lippincott, 1957.
75. Mason, J.W.: "Over-all" hormonal balance as a key to endocrine organization. Psychosom. Med., 10:791, 1968.
76. Mason, J.W.: Clinical psychophysiology: Psychoendocrine mechanisms. In: *American Handbook of Psychiatry*, 2nd Ed., Vol. 4 (S. Arieti, Ed.). New York, Basic Books, 1975.
77. McClary, A.R., Meyer, E., and Weitzman, E.L.: Observations on the role of the mechanism of depression in some patients with disseminated lupus erythematosus. Psychosom. Med., 17:311, 1955.
78. Mednick, S.A., Garner, A.M., and Stone, H.K.: A test of some behavioral hypotheses drawn from Alexander's specificity theory. Am. J. Orthopsychiatry, 29:592, 1958.
79. Meissner, W.W.: Hippocampal functions and learning. J. Psychiatr. Res., 4:235, 1956.
80. Mendelson, M., Hirsch, S., and Webber, C.S.: A critical examination of some recent theoretical models in psychosomatic medicine. Psychosom. Med., 18:363, 1956.
81. Meyer, R.J., and Haggerty, R.J.: Streptococcal infections in families. Pediatrics, 29:539, 1962.
82. Michaels, J.J.: A psychiatric adventure in comparative pathophysiology of the infant and the adult. J. Nerv. Ment. Dis., 100:49, 1944.
83. Miller, N.E.: Learning of visceral and glandular responses. Science, 163:434, 1969.
84. Mirsky, I.A.: The psychosomatic approach to the etiology of clinical disorders. Psychosom. Med., 19:424, 1957.
85. Mirsky, I.A.: Physiologic, psychologic and social determinants in the etiology of duodenal ulcer. Am. J. Dig. Dis., 3:285, 1958.
86. Mirsky, I.A.: Physiologic, psychologic, and social determinants of psychosomatic disorders. Dis. Nerv. Syst., 21:50, 1960.
87. Mohr, G.J., Garner, A., and Eddy, E.J.: A program for the study of children with psychosomatic disorders. In: *Emotional Problems of Childhood.* (G. Caplan, Ed.). New York, Basic Books, 1955.
88. Mutter, A.Z., and Schleifer, M.J.: The role of psychological and social factors in the onset of somatic illnesses in children. Psychosom. Med., 28:333, 1966.
89. Neuhaus, E.C.: A personality study of asthmatic and cardiac children. Psychosom. Med., 20:181, 1958.
90. Pavlov, I.P.: *Lectures on Conditioned Reflexes.* (W.H. Gantt, trans.). New York, International Publications Service, 1928.
91. Philippopolous, S.G., Wittkower, E.D., and Cousineau, A.: The etiological significance of emotional factors in onset and exacerbations of multiple sclerosis: A preliminary report. Psychosom. Med., 20:458, 1958.
92. Prugh, D.G.: Role of emotional factors in idiopathic celiac disease. Psychosom. Med., 13:220, 1951.
93. Prugh, D.G.: Psychophysiologic aspects of inborn errors of metabolism. In: *The Psychological Basis of Medical Practice.* (H. Lief, N. Lief, and V. Lief, Eds.). New York, Hoeber, 1963.
94. Prugh, D.G.: Towards an understanding of psychosomatic concepts in relation to illness in childhood. In: *Modern Perspectives in Child Development.* (A.J. Solnit and S.A. Provence, Eds.). New York, International Universities Press, 1963.
95. Prugh, D.G.: Psychosocial disorders in childhood and adolescence: Theoretical considerations and an attempt at classification. In: *The Mental Health of Children: Services, Research, and Manpower.* (Reports of Task Forces IV and V and the Report of the Committee on Clinical Issues by the Joint Commission on Mental Health of Children.) New York, Harper & Row, 1973.
96. Prugh, D.G., and Tagiuri, C.K.: Emotional as-

pects of the respiratory care of patients with poliomyelitis. Psychosom. Med., 16:104, 1954.

97. Rahe, R.H., and Holmes, T.H.: *Life Crisis and Disease Onset. II. A Prospective Study of Life Crises and Health Changes.* Seattle, University of Washington School of Medicine, 1966.

97a. Reichsman, F., and Segal, H.L.: A study of an infant with a gastric fistula. I. Behavior and rate of total hydrochloric acid secretion. Psychosom. Med., 18:374, 1956.

98. Richmond, J.B.: The pediatric patient in illness. In: *The Psychology of Medical Practice.* (M.H. Hollender, Ed.) Philadelphia, Saunders, 1958.

98a. Richter, C.P.: On the phenomenon of sudden death in animals and man. Psychosom. Med., 19:191, 1957.

99. Robertson, J.: *Young Children in Hospitals.* New York, Basic Books, 1958.

100. Romano, J., and Engel, G.L.: Physiologic and Psychologic Considerations of Delirium. Med. Clin. North Am., 28:629, 1944.

101. Ross, W.D.: Psychosomatic disorders and psychoses. In: *Recent Developments in Psychosomatic Medicine.* (E.D. Wittkower and R.A. Cleghorn, Eds.). Philadelphia, Lippincott, 1957.

102. Ruesch, J.: Infantile personality: The core problem of psychosomatic medicine. Psychosom. Med., 10:134, 1948.

103. Sander, L.W., et al.: Continuous 24-hour interactional monitoring in infants reared in two caretaking environments. Psychosom. Med., 34:270, 1972.

104. Schmale, A.H., Jr.: Relationship of separation and depression to disease. I. A report on a hospitalized medical population. Psychosom. Med., 20:124, 1958.

105. Schmale, A.H., and Iker, H.: The psychological setting of uterine cervical cancer. Ann. N.Y. Acad. Sci., 125:807, 1966.

106. Schmale, A.H., and Iker, H.P.: Hopelessness as a predictor of cervical carcinoma. Soc. Sci. Med., 5:95, 1971.

107. Schottstaedt, W.W.: *Psychophysiologic Approach in Medical Practice.* Chicago, Yearbook, 1960.

108. Seitz, P.F.D.: Symbolism and organ choice in conversion reactions: An experimental approach. Psychosom. Med., 13:254, 1951.

109. Selye, H.: The general adaptation syndrome and the diseases of adaptation. J. Clin. Endrocrinol., 6:117, 1946.

110. Solnit, A.J., and Green, M.: Psychologic considerations in the management of death in pediatric hospital services. I. The doctor and the child's family. Pediatrics, 24:106, 1959.

111. Sontag, L.W.: Psychosomatic aspects of childhood. In: *Contributions Toward Medical Psychology.* (A. Weider, Ed.). New York, Ronald Press, 1953.

112. Sperling, M.: The role of the mother in psychosomatic disorders in children. Psychosom. Med., 11:377, 1949.

113. Sperling, M.: Psychosomatic medicine and pediatrics. In: *Recent Developments in Psychosomatic Medicine.* (E.D. Wittkower and R.A. Cleghorn, Eds.). Philadelphia, Lippincott, 1957.

114. Spilken, A.Z., and Jacobs, M.A.: Prediction of illness behavior from measures of life crisis, manifest distress, and maladaptive coping. Psychosom. Med., 33:251, 1971.

115. Staub, E.M., et al.: A study of emotional reactions of children's families to illness and hospitalization. Am. J. Orthopsychiatry, 23:78, 1953.

116. Diamond, S., et al.: Biofeedback: Therapy with electronic teaching aids. Pat. Care, 9:164, 1975.

117. Surawicz, F.G., et al.: Cancer, emotions and mental illness: The present state of understanding. Am. J. Psychiatry, 133:1306, 1976.

118. Szasz, T.S.: Oral mechanisms in constipation and diarrhea. Int. J. Psychoanal., 32:196, 1951.

119. Weiner, H., et al.: Etiology of duodenal ulcer. I. Relation of specific psychological characteristics to rate of gastric secretion (serum pepsinogen). Psychosom. Med., 19:1, 1957.

120. Weiss, E., and English, O.S.: *Psychosomatic Medicine. The Clinical Application of Psychopathology to General Medical Problems.* Philadelphia, Saunders, 1943.

121. Whybrow, P.C., and Silberfarb, P.M.: Neuroendocrine mediating mechanisms from the symbolic stimulus to the physiological response. Int. J. Psychiatr. Med., 5:531, 1974.

122. Witkin, H.A.: Psychological differentiation and forms of pathology. J. Abnormal Psychol., 5:317, 1965.

123. Wittkower, E.D.: Twenty years of North American psychosomatic medicine. Psychosom. Med., 22:308, 1960.

124. Wittkower, E.D., and Cleghorn, R.A.: *Recent Developments in Psychosomatic Medicine.* Philadelphia, Lippincott, 1957.

125. Wolf, S.G., and Wolff, H.G.: *Human Gastric Function: An Experimental Study of Man and His Stomach.* New York, Oxford University Press, 1947.

126. Wolff, H.G.: *Stress and Disease.* Springfield, Ill., Thomas, 1953.

127. Wolff, H.G., and Bayer, L.M.: Psychosomatic disorders of childhood and adolescence. Amer. J. Orthopsychiatry, 22:510, 1952.

128. Wolff, H.G., and Hare, C.C., Eds.: *Life Stress and Bodily Disease.* Baltimore, Williams & Wilkins, 1950.

129. Wyler, A.R., Masada, M., and Holmes, T.H.: Magnitude of life events and seriousness of illness. Psychosom. Med., 33:115, 1971.

General References

Cannon, W.B.: *Wisdom of the Body.* New York, Norton, 1963.

Cassel, J.: The contribution of the social environment to host resistance. Am. J. Epidemiol.,104:107, 1976.

Ciba Foundation Symposium No. 8 (New Series): *Physiology, Emotion, and Psychosomatic Illness.* Amsterdam, Elsevier, 1972.

Darwin, C.: *Expression of the Emotions in Man and Animals.* New York, D. Appleton, 1872.

Deutsch, F., Ed.: *The Psychosomatic Concept in Psychoanalysis.* New York, International Universities Press, 1953.

Engel, G.L.: *Psychological Development in Health and Disease.* Philadelphia, Saunders, 1962.

Engel, G.L.: The psychosomatic approach to individual susceptibility to disease. Gastroenterology, *67*:1085, 1974.

Engel, G., and Schmale, A.: Psychoanalytic theory of somatic disorder. J. Psychoanal. Assoc., *15*:344, 1967.

Freud, S.: *An Outline of Psychoanalysis.* New York, Norton, 1940.

Hill, O.W.: *Modern Trends in Psychosomatic Medicine,* Vols. 1, 2. New York, Appleton-Century, 1970.

Lief, H.J., Lief, V.F., and Lief, N.R., Eds.: *Psychological Basis of Medical Practice.* New York, Harper & Row, 1963.

Lipowski, Z.J.: Psychosomatic medicine in the seventies: An overview. Am. J. Psychiatry, *134*:233, 1977.

Lipowski, Z.J., Lipsitt, D.R., and Whybrow, P.C., Eds.: *Psychosomatic Medicine: Current Trends and Clinical Applications.* New York, Oxford University Press, 1977.

Prugh, D.G.: Psychological and psychophysiological aspects of oral activities in children. Pediatr. Clin. North Am., *3*:1049, 1956.

Reiser, M.F., Ed.: Organic Disorders and Psychosomatic Medicine. *American Handbook of Psychiatry.*

2nd Ed., Vol. 4. (S. Arieti, Ed.). New York, Basic Books, 1975.

Richter, C.P.: *Biological Clocks in Medicine and Psychiatry.* Springfield, Ill., Thomas, 1965.

Schmale, A.H.: Giving up as a final common pathway to changes in health. In: *Psychosocial Aspects of Physical Illness.* (Z.J. Lipowski, Ed.). Basel, S. Karger, 1972.

Solomon, G.F.: Emotions, stress, the central nervous system, and immunity. Ann. N.Y. Acad. Sci., *164*:335, 1969.

Stein, M., Schiavi, R.C., and Camerino, M.: Influence of brain and behavior on the immune system. Science, *191*:435, 1976.

Thomas, C.B., and Greenstreet, R.L.: Psychobiological characteristics in youth as predictors of five disease states: Suicide, mental illness, hypertension, coronary heart disease, and tumor. Johns Hopkins Med. J., *132*:16, 1973.

Wallace, R.K.: Physiologic effects of transcendental meditation. Science, *167*:1751, 1970.

Wittkower, E.D., and Lipowski, Z.: Recent developments in psychosomatic medicine. Psychosom. Med., *28*:722, 1966.

Wittkower, E.D.: Historical perspective of contemporary psychosomatic medicine. Int. J. Psychiatry Med., *5*:309, 1974.

Wittkower, E.D.,and Cleghorn, R.A.: *Recent Developments in Psychosomatic Medicine.* Philadelphia, Lippincott, 1957.

Wolff, H.G., Wolf, S.G., and Hare, C.C., Eds.: *Life Stress and Bodily Disease.* Baltimore, Williams & Wilkins, 1950.

5
The Development of
the Child's Personality

He who watches a thing grow has
the best view of it.
(Heraclitus)

Freud's discovery of the importance of the
experiences of early infancy for the subsequent
development of the personality has profoundly
influenced our conception of human nature, and
has had lasting effects on ethics.
(W. Russell,
Lord Brain)

Of all aspects of human biology, development may be the most remarkable and the least understood. Although development is part of the human condition, its source, the "built-in life plan," is not understood despite recent advances in genetics. But pediatrics, child psychiatry and psychology, and child development have recently gained much knowledge about the development of the child. The development of the child is affected by interpersonal and cultural forces. The idea of the 3 levels of organization of the human being—the physiologic, psychologic, and social levels—is useful in discussing the development of the child's personality.

Personality

The terms psychologic development, emotional development, and personality development are used loosely in the literature that deals with studies of personality.

73

The idea of personality refers to all the patterned aspects of a person's functional behavior—his intellectual capacities, physical characteristics, social behavior, motivations, and potentialities, mental and emotional experiences, and his awareness of himself as an individual who has a past, a present, and a future. Allport[4] describes personality as "the dynamic organization within the individual of those psychophysical systems that determine his characteristic behavior and thought." There are 4 important aspects of personality development: the intellectual, the emotional, the physical, and the social. The psychologic aspect of personality development includes both the intellectual and emotional aspects, leaving 3 basic dimensions of development—the physical, the psychologic, and the social—which correspond with the 3 levels of organization.

The terms character and temperament are sometimes used interchangeably with the term personality. The terms character, character traits, character structure, and character development have been used in psychoanalytic and other terminologies. Those terms correspond with the terms personality, personality traits, personality structure, and personality development. Popular ideas about character are often affected by moral standards and value judgments, such as the judgments implied in the phrases good character and bad character. For this reason, I prefer to use the term personality to refer to the unique patterns that characterize each person. (A person's ideals and values are also important parts of his personality, as is the social appropriateness and acceptability of his behavior.)

The term temperament refers to certain aspects of a person's constitution, from which his personality develops (using the more modern and dynamic idea of the constitution that was referred to in Chapter 2). Allport and others believe that a person's level of activity, his susceptibility to sensory and emotional stimulation, his strength and speed of response, his prevailing mood, his rhythms of biologic functioning, and other characteristics make up his temperament. A person's temperament may be affected by his experience. Chess, Thomas, and Birch[18] have recently identified and measured some characteristics or "reaction patterns" in infants that usually last throughout the preschool period. Reaction patterns are different from simple conditioned reflexes, habits (or "integrated systems of conditioned reflexes"), and other characteristics of the integrated personality.

The terms growth, development, and maturation have all been applied to the psychologic and social aspects as well as to the physical aspects of development. Although a child can be said to grow in his capacity to adapt to and control the world about him and in his understanding of himself and others, the term growth is used here only in its physical sense to mean the increase in size of the human organism as a whole or any of its parts or tissues. Growth includes permanent changes in tissues and it occurs during the child's maturing. The term maturation refers to the physical and psychologic progress that occurs according to the sequence of specific steps toward maturity. The sequence follows a timetable that is assumed to arise from largely biologic or inborn sources.

The term development refers to the increasing differentiation, complexity, and ultimate integration of structure, function, and behavior. Development includes the interaction of maturational patterns and experience or learning. The maturational timetable may be changed by physical, psychologic, or social stimuli. Within the general pattern of development of humans, each person has his own pattern. Differences in development can be healthy. Some precocious or retarded development is pathologic because it is inappropriate for the stage of development at which it occurs or is out of phase with other aspects of development. The idea of developmental deviations that are outside the range of normal individual variations can be applied to psychologic and social as well as to physical development.

The Basic Principles of Personality Development

Some characteristics of personality development occur often enough to be considered principles. Although there are some parallels between the principles of physical development and the principles of psychologic and social development, the laws operating for phenomena belonging to these differing dimensions are very different, and the parallels between them are not exact.

Continuity and consistency are the most important principles of personality development, as Ausubel[9] has pointed out. Each stage of development is affected by the preceding stages while preparation for future stages is going on. The personality's patterns of response become more organized and consistent. The patterns of response are individual despite the tendency of clusters of the same personality traits to emerge in particular groups of people during later childhood and adulthood. Personality development usually follows a certain sequence; the rate of personality development is fairly consistent, but it may vary considerably in different people and in different stages in the same person. The stages of development, which sometimes overlap, are separated by transitional periods. A transitional period is a developmental crisis that must be resolved so that the child can go on to the next stage.[23]*

Although progress toward the crystalization of an inner psychic structure is usually gradual, development during childhood is ordinarily uneven. Spurts, plateaus, and lags often occur; they usually affect only part of the personality at any time. Noxious stimuli may cause tempo-

*The concept of "sensitive" phases in development has been discussed in Chapter 2.

rary behavioral regression to more familiar levels of adaptation, or they may cause arrest or fixation in different aspects of psychologic or social development. Either hereditary or environmental factors can cause a developmental lag, a serious retardation, or a blunting of or distortion in one or another aspect of personality development.

The dimensions of personality development are interrelated. Parallel progress may occur, but the development of different aspects of the personality may occur at very different rates and still be healthy. Lags or distortions in 1 aspect of development, as in the development of the emotional part of the psychologic aspect, may affect another part within the same dimension and so cause a lag in intellectual growth. Erikson[25] and others have suggested that each child has a basic ground plan of personality development. Within this overall framework (which has maturational underpinnings), each part or function has its own special time of ascendency. Each stage is based on preceding stages and is a response to a particular configuration of environmental stimuli. The personality progresses from global, undifferentiated, diffuse, and uncoordinated responses in early infancy toward the differentiation of the functions of its different aspects. Finally, the differentiated functions of the personality are integrated by the constant interplay between the organism and its environment. Integration results in a functioning personality that is more than the sum of its parts—the "epigenetic model."[24]

Although anxiety and conflict may harm a child's development, mild anxiety and conflict may spur the development of new and more mature coping mechanisms, thus promoting adaptation, individuation, mastery, and creativity. The balance of internal and external influences that occurs in the interaction between the "innate and the experiential" creates a balance between the progressive and regressive forces of development.[29] These forces may be affected positively or negatively by anxiety and conflict, depending on the intensity of the anxiety and conflict, the child's developmental capacities, the responses of people who are important to the child, and other factors.

Maturity and the Healthy Personality

Since development involves maturation, the concept of maturity as the goal of development should be defined. Physical maturity is easy to define, even though the time at which it is attained may vary considerably within the healthy range.[77] Psychologic or emotional maturity remains more difficult to define. Personality development continues, or should continue, throughout a person's life. A person's psychologic and social characteristics need not cease to develop when he becomes physically mature. Those characteristics need not deteriorate seriously with advancing age.

Psychosocial maturity represents the point at which fundamental developmental tasks are completed, the personality's structure is fully consolidated, and the person can function independently and effectively. The characteristics of the psychologically mature or healthy person differ in different cultures and times. For example, among the Indians in northwestern North America, young men who had visions during tribal initiation ceremonies were considered mature and healthy. But in most urban parts of the world, having visions is considered pathologic. And although adaptation, the capacity to maintain a dynamic steady state or a balance of one's personality while coping with potentially stressful external and internal stimuli, and adjustment, the comfortable fit of the person into a particular set of social circumstances, are characteristics of a healthy personality, they are not always the same as psychologic or social maturity.

Jahoda,[41] Allport,[4] Erikson,[25] Riesman,[65] and others have defined a person who has a healthy personality as one who: (1) actively, flexibly, and rationally copes with and masters his environment most of the time, (2) has unity and integrity of personality, (3) correctly perceives the world and himself, including the needs of others as well as his own feelings and needs, (4) has capacities for friendship, more intimate love, work, and play, (5) has mental well-being, emotional security, a zest for life, the capacity to accept himself, and senses of perspective, detachment, and humor, (6) has values or goals that permit him to organize, unify, and improve his life and work, while accepting the values of others.

A person who has a healthy personality can maintain a balance at all 3 levels of organization and can adjust to most situations; he tolerates some tensions and sometimes postpones immediate gratifications for long-term ones. A truly mature person, however, has values[5] or goals that may make him sacrifice his own interests for the welfare of others. Thus a mature person may at times forsake adjustment and conformity in order to contribute to or change his world creatively. As Erikson[24] and others[4,20] have said, a mature person's personality continues to develop throughout his life. His insight, judgment, social awareness, and perception of the needs of others increase; his spiritual development continues. He becomes more able to change himself constructively.

The Origins of Behavior: Heredity and Environment

Besides the phylogenetic characteristics of humans, the human infant has inherited potentialities that are determined by his parents and their ancestors. Anthropologic research has found that all inherited potentialities (except those related to physical appearance) among members of different racial groups are equivalent.[8] It is not known whether each infant is born with the potentiality for the development of a particular type of personality.

Before modern methods of scientific investigation were used, most investigators (with some notable exceptions) believed that heredity caused both deviant and healthy personality development. But psychologic and psychoanalytic studies of child development made in the last 50 years emphasized the influence of environment on personality development. Watson and other behaviorists in the 1930s believed that environment and education could produce any characteristics in a child's personality. Scientific methods and industrialization have changed man's environment. Such changes support the idea that heredity has little influence on personality development.

Although the nature-versus-nurture controversy has diminished, some investigators who deal with dynamic psychology disregard (or treat lightly) the influence of heredity on children's behavior. Those investigators consider each newborn a *tabula rasa*. They have established goals for the rearing and treatment of children that are sometimes unrealistic and have developed narrow theories about disturbances in behavior. Other investigators believe that heredity alone (or almost entirely alone) influences development. Both of these extreme ideas about development must be regarded as invalid. Today, development is explained by the reciprocal interaction or transaction between heredity and environment. Both are thought to affect personality development. The following discussion considers the relative influences of heredity and environment.

Genetic Influences

Although Mendelian laws apply to human genetics, knowledge of human genetics is limited because of the complexity of human endowment and experience. The genes inherited by man determine his phy-logenetic patterns of development and his individual characteristics, such as sex, size, build, other physical features, racial characteristics, and to some extent the rate of physical development. There are approximately 100 abnormal conditions that seem to be influenced by heredity; they include hemophilia and sickle-cell anemia as well as inborn metabolic defects, such as phenylketonuria and galactosemia. But even in the inheritance of basically physical traits, the original model of single major genes that always control the development of specific characteristics has proved to be oversimplified.

It is now known that the effects of many single genes are modified by those other genes; it is thought that constellations of polygenes exist. Although genes are usually not modified by the environment (except by unusual influences, such as direct radiation), the environment may affect the expression of genes. The clinical expression of hereditarily determined defects in metabolism, for example, is caused by a complex interaction of genetic, metabolic, and environmental influences; the interaction includes diet, endocrine function, diseases, and psychologic stresses. Some hereditarily determined defects are present at birth. Others do not appear until later in life; they are brought out by contact with particular foods or by stressful circumstances. Some defects may appear under most environmental circumstances, while others appear only under particular environmental influences. It is probable, though not yet proven, that psychologic stresses may, because they change physiologic patterns of response, cause metabolic compounds to be produced in excess of the available supply of enzymes, leading to the appearance of a particular enzymatic defect in heterozygous people who have partial defects. Finally, the chronic disability caused by some defects may have psychologic or interpersonal effects on the disabled person and his family; the effects include personality distortion, heightened invalidism, or even intensification of metabolic derangements.

Modern genetics supports the idea that the influence of genes on ontogenetic development always reflects the influence of the intracellular, the gestational, and the external environments. A person's phenotype is always the result of the interaction between his genotype and his environment. Genetic influences must be couched in terms of potentialities. Birch[14] believes that all phenotypic expression is caused by the continual biochemical and physiologic interaction of the gene complex cytoplasm, the internal milieu, and the external environment. Dubos[21] has said, "Life experiences determine the extent to which the genetic endowment is converted into the functional attributes that make a person what he is and behave as he does." The ideas of Birch and Dubos and the polygenetic determination of most hereditary defects render certain eugenic concepts, whether negative (e.g., legalized sterilization) or positive (e.g., selective mating) naive and unscientific.

The Effects of Genes on Personality Characteristics

Studies of identical twins indicate that physical characteristics, except for weight and muscular development, are less affected by environment and experience than are intellectual performance and other personality characteristics. Little is known of genetic influences on the psychologic and social aspects of personality development and functioning. There are, of course, uniquely human predispositions toward specific kinds of developmental patterns and psychologic and social functioning. Heredity strongly affects basic intellectual capacity. But the achievement of intellectual potentialities may vary widely in relation to environmental stimulation, the opportunity to learn, parental motivation, and other kinds of experience, including

chronic physical disorders. Heredity seems to strongly affect talents in music and art, but learning and motivation seem also to strongly affect those talents.

The recent "authoritarian backlash" (led by Jensen and Shockley, among others) has revived the nature-versus-nurture controversy by attributing persistent differences in intelligence (as measured by scores on intelligence tests) to differences in genetic endowment and racial or ethnic background. The eminent behavioral scientist Herbert Birch said (in a symposium held at Columbia University) that such views show both limited knowledge of heredity and unsound judgment.[13] Birch believes that differences in learning achievements, whether measured by intelligence tests or by achievement in school, are caused by differences in the adjustment of the learner, the task, and the instrumental mode to each other.[14] Mercer recently applied statistically 7 sociocultural factors to differentiate among the test scores of groups of blacks, Mexican-Americans, and whites.[56,57] Her methods accounted for sociocultural differences; she found no significant residual difference in the groups' scores. Mercer believes that Jensen used fallacious logic when he used information derived from studies of white people to judge the cause of the lower test scores made by blacks. Behavioral geneticists (e.g., Vandenberg[79]), anthropologists (e.g., Ashley-Montagu[8]), child psychiatrists (e.g., Eisenberg[22]), and others (e.g., Golden and Bridger[32]) agree.

The incidence of schizophrenia and, to a lesser degree, of manic-depressive psychosis in adults has been shown in studies of twins to be influenced by genetic potentialities. The data from different studies conflict, however, and diagnostic and methodologic problems make it hard to draw final conclusions about inherited mental disorders. Kallmann's[45] figures for the risk of a child born of 2 schizophrenic parents to be schizophrenic were 68% but a more recent review by Rosenthal[68] of studies by Kahn, Schulz, and Elsasser has lowered the figure to about 35%. Kall-mann's figures for the concordance of schizophrenia in monozygotic twins have also been lowered markedly by a recent study by Kringlen[47] of an unselected sample drawn from all the twins in Norway. In the Norwegian study, the figures for concordance in monozygotic twins were about 35%; they were 10% for dizygotic twins. However, a recent study by Allen, Hoffer, and Pollin[3] lowers the age-corrected figures for concordance in monozygotic twins in the United States to 15.5% and for dizygotic twins to 4.4%.

A study of children of schizophrenic parents who were adopted before the end of their first year was made by Rosenthal, Kety, and Wender[69] in Denmark. Comparing those children with a group of adopted children of normal parents, they concluded that the risk of schizophrenic-type illness is 3 times as great for the children of schizophrenic parents as for the children of normal parents. Anthony[6] says that the possibility is about 18%. Stabenau and Pollin[76] studied 15 pairs of monozygotic twins who were discordant; they concluded that the twin who later became schizophrenic had had greater difficulty in breathing and other difficulties at birth, including susceptibility to infection.

Most investigators now agree that heredity is much less important as a cause of schizophrenia than it was formerly believed to be. Several investigators agree that it is not schizophrenia that is inherited, but that the genes involved may cause a vulnerability to schizophrenia. Experience, such as the coddling of the weaker twins by their parents, was important as a cause of schizophrenia in the study of Stabenau and Pollin. The threshold of psychologic distress that must be exceeded in order for schizophrenia to appear may never be exceeded in many people who are predisposed to schizophrenia.

Psychoses that appear during early childhood, especially in infancy and the early preschool period, show little hered-itary influence.[46] But there is some biologic predisposition that interacts with experience to cause such psychoses. Mental retardation may be caused by heredity or by physical factors, such as chromosomal aberrations, or by inborn metabolic defects, as in phenylketonuria. Experience, especially a lack of appropriate social and intellectual stimulation, however, may be more important than genetic endowment in many cases of retardation in which there is no specific metabolic defect. Such experience may also strongly affect the degree of retardation of people who have such defects by causing them to perform below the limits of their already limited intellectual potentialities. For example, some heredodegenerative diseases of the central nervous system, including Huntington's chorea, familial amaurotic idiocy, and Heller's disease, result in serious behavioral and intellectual deficits by causing gross brain lesions. Even in these diseases, the reaction of the child and his family to his disorder may affect the course of the disease and the degree of disability that it causes in its early stages.[55]

Many ideas about genetic influences on personality development and functioning are theoretic and speculative. The results of studies of animals, although they stimulate human research, cannot be used directly to draw conclusions about humans. Jung[44] first suggested that there may be an inherited predisposition to a particular personality pattern (e.g., introversion or extroversion). Recent studies of twins seem to support such ideas but do not establish them as facts. In, for example, Sheldon's[71] studies, particular somatotypes have been said to be associated with particular personality patterns. Methodologic problems and the problem of interpreting psychologic data make it hard to prove that association. I think the association is partially valid, but there are many exceptions to its rules. A person's somatotype may be affected by experiential factors, such as diet, exercise, and the stage of his life. A child's physical build and its "emotional signifi-cance" may cause reactions in his parents; the reactions may affect the development of the child's personality. (Abnormal sex chromosomes may possibly affect person-ality development, a topic that will be dis-cussed later.)

Specific personality traits, as some have suggested, might be affected by heredity, as in the case of the intellectually preco-cious child who has a strong need to or-ganize his environment and behaves com-pulsively. No data support such ideas, though. In the areas of intellectual devel-opment, even studies of identical twins may have limited value.[3] The personality development of each twin[16,81] is affected by the fact that he is a twin and is treated by his parents as a twin. Each twin faces con-siderable challenges in developing his in-dividual self-concept. Thus identity in the behavior even of proven monozygotic twins does not absolutely prove a genetic influence on behavior. (Of course, no two people are ever identical, since the intra-uterine experiences of monozygotic twins may differ slightly and since parents never handle twins in absolutely identical fash-ion.)

Although lower species of mammals can be selectively bred to produce particular characteristics (e.g., tameness and aggres-siveness), the likelihood that selective breeding affects human behavior is slight. Studies of testosterone levels in relation to behavior in males are as yet inconclusive. Studies by Jost and Sontag,[43] however, support the idea that newborns have in-dividual differences in their autonomic pat-terns of response; identical twins have sig-nificantly greater concordance in those patterns. That conclusion suggests that a genetic factor affects the autonomic ner-vous system functioning. Genetic factors may contribute to patterns of bodily dys-function that are associated with emotional responses to stress during later stages of development. A genetic predisposition might also affect the ease or nature of con-ditioning responses in early infancy and temperamental qualities, such as emo-tional reactivity and rhythm.

Current knowledge, although limited, indicates that there are strong genetic in-fluences on particular physical character-istics. Those influences affect a person's personality development mostly by their importance to his family and society, and so to the person himself, as they affect his self-concept. Intellectual capacity and the potentialities for some talents are partially affected by heredity, although motivation to develop and opportunity for developing these potentialities are very important. Ge-netic factors also affect some tempera-mental qualities (although less clearly). The evidence indicates that genetic factors as well as environment (beginning at concep-tion) affect one's temperament.[18] Some dis-eases are strongly affected by genetic fac-tors. But environment and experience also affect (in various and complex ways) those diseases. (It is useful to underline the state-ment made earlier regarding supposedly "simple" inheritance: The phenotype is al-ways the result of complex interactions be-tween the genotype and the environment.)

The Origins of Experience: The Intrauterine Environment

Because the intrauterine environment is relatively stable, a person's genetic poten-tialities can strongly affect his development before his birth. (The Chinese used to date one's age from the time of one's concep-tion; they recognized that experience be-gins in the womb.) The early development of the fetus follows phylogenetic patterns. Neural maturation follows the cephalocau-dal principle that was recognized long ago. As Coghill[19] observed, the fetus first en-gages in diffuse mass activity. Next the part response patterns of the fetus are indivi-dualized. Finally those patterns are inte-grated into a coordinated total response system. Ontogenetic development is usually affected only by extreme changes in the intrauterine environment that occur when particular organ systems of the fetus are in a vulnerable stage of development. Usually the fetus draws on his mother's nutritional stores to meet his parasitic needs.

There is a wide range of important changes that may occur in the intrauterine environment. The changes include uterine abnormalities that interfere with the implantation of the ovum or cause the premature separation of the placenta, serious omissions in the mother's nutrition, the effects of drugs such as thalidomide, the results of diseases of the mother, such as infection, eclampsia, and rubella, the appearance of Rh sensitization or other antigenic effects, and exposure to x rays. Many of these changes have gross effects, such as death in utero, stillbirth, severe anemia, or a congenital malformation or other abnormality of the fetus. Malnourished mothers may produce children of small stature whose ability to learn is impaired. The age of the mother and the number of her previous pregnancies may also (presumably because of some changes in her metabolism) decrease the chances that the newborn will live or increase the incidence of congenital abnormalities. Studies of animals have suggested that certain substances, such as aflatoxin, can cause chromosomal abnormalities. Some changes in the intrauterine environment may be caused by chance events, such as exposure to x rays or a severe famine. Other such changes may be caused by changes in the psychologic state of the mother, such as in a dietary deficiency that is caused by depression, by the intensification of hypertension, or by vomiting caused by emotional stress. Social or cultural influences, such as religious fasts or special patterns of eating food or using drugs, may cause other changes.

A gross physical abnormality or deformity in the fetus may affect the later development of his personality and his adaptive capacity. It may handicap the child, intellectually or in his motor capacities, or give him an abnormal appearance, or change his parents' reactions to him.

Subtler changes in the uterine environment may occur. A startle-like response, associated with an acceleration in the heart rate, has been produced in fetuses by loud noises or external vibrations, which can condition the fetal heart rate.[73] Other auditory, tactile, or proprioceptive stimuli may be transmitted to the fetus through spontaneous, irregular, rhythmic activity by the uterine musculature; it has been shown that such activity occurs. The movements of the mother's diaphragm or her own heart beat, transmitted from the aorta, may also rhythmically stimulate the fetus, as Greene[35] has indicated. Imprinting of the mother's heart beat might occur during pregnancy and may cause positive responses by the infant after his birth to certain kinds of rhythmic stimulation. Mann[54] and others have shown that emotional conflicts strongly affect (by causing unusual contractions of the uterus) the occurrence of early miscarriages, habitual abortion, and certain cases of premature labor.

The passage of neurohumoral or hormonal substances across the placental barrier has recently been studied. Epinephrine and norepinephrine, when injected into the circulation of pregnant women, have different effects on the heart rate of the fetus. Other studies by Sontag[73] suggest that fetal activity increases in proportion to the level of maternal anxiety. Studies of animals indicate that cortisol (and possibly other substances) can cross the placental barrier. Such results suggest that extreme psychologic conflict or fatigue in the mother may expose the fetus to the neurohumoral and endocrine products that are called out by its mother's neuroendocrine response to social or psychologic stressful stimuli. Such exposure may lower the infant's threshold of response to some stimuli after its birth. The newborn may have, for example, greater irritability of response and a higher level of activity. Ader's[1] studies of animals indicate that handling the mother while she is pregnant can affect the emotional responses of her offspring.

Few such possibilities have been proved for humans. Clinically, it seems that infants who are more active in utero remain more actively physically and possibly autonomically for some months after their birth. Mothers who are more anxious often report greater activity of their unborn infants after the fifth month of gestation. Newborns who show more motor activity often show more gastrointestinal activity and less storage of fat in their first few months of life. They resemble the thin hypertonic infants who have more attacks of "paroxysmal fussing" (so-called colic). All these are only clinical impressions; there have been few systematic studies in that difficult and elusive but very important area of research.

Despite the lack of concrete evidence, the impressions, partial data, and inferences about the intrauterine environment definitely suggest that many stimuli (both normal and pathologic in degree and nature) can affect the fetus through metabolic, sensory, or other pathways. The intrauterine experience of the fetus also includes some proprioceptive stimuli that come from within the fetus itself in relation to its movements, whether its movements are spontaneous or induced by stimulation. The constitutional characteristics with which the newborn enters the world have already been affected by much contact with the intrauterine environment, as well as by its original genetic endowment. Whether prenatal experience can, as some have suggested,[34] cause a predisposition to anxiety or tension in early infancy or in later stages has not been proved, although it is likely.

The Birth Experience

Birth ends the physiologic aspect of the parasitic existence of the fetus. But, in a psychologic sense, the parasitic relationship of the infant to his mother continues. The infant is helpless at birth, equipped with only a few reflex patterns, such as the crying response, rooting, sucking, and grasping reflexes, startle responses and vestigial righting reflexes. The birth experience can influence the infant's capacity to use these rudimentary reflexes and his primitive sensory capacities.

Birth traumata, such as cerebral hemorrhage or laceration, the results of anoxia caused by respiratory difficulties, or the effects of obstetrical anesthetics or analgesics on the infant's immediate functioning and adaptive capacities have been well summarized by others and are considered later in relation to their influence on the parents' feelings about their child and the child's personality development.

Damage to newborns, caused by late complications of pregnancy or abnormalities in the birth process, can cause a "continuum of reproductive casualty." The continuum ranges from stillbirth and prematurity through mental retardation to brain damage. Such damage is more common in the infants of women who belong to lower socioeconomic groups and who receive little prenatal care. It is hard for the child and his family to adapt to such major defects. Some disturbed children have a history of difficult or prolonged delivery. Many later problems in adaptation and disturbances in behavior should not be attributed without adequate evidence to "difficult delivery" that caused "minimal brain damage."

Much has been written, particularly by Rank,[63] about the possibility of psychologic trauma caused by the birth. No evidence now indicates that birth—the sudden transition from a relatively stable life in the uterus to a world full of new stimuli—causes lasting psychologic imprints. The fact that the newborn's behavior is mostly at a subcortical level suggests that any such subjective response is unlikely. As Greene[35] has suggested, it is possible that the intrauterine environment may not be quiet or inactive, considering the different stimuli just described that may affect the fetus. But as Greenacre[34] and others have pointed out, the length or the degree of difficulty of the birth process might sensitize the infant's cardiorespiratory apparatus to later stimuli, including psychologic stimuli. Such sensitization may affect his later symptoms. However, there is now no evidence of such sensitization. As Freud[28] said, birth and the infant's first cry may be a physiologic prototype of his later attacks of anxiety; they may set the pattern of the infant's response to anxiety without having a perceptible effect on him.

Recent studies show that marked hyperventilation by an anxious woman who is undergoing a cesarean section apparently can cause severe acidosis and delay the onset of spontaneous respiration in the newborn. Emotional disturbance in the mother can also make her labor more difficult and prolonged and so increase the chance of complications.[61]

No matter what other effects delivery has on the normal newborn, the use of even moderate amounts of medication has been shown to affect the newborn's responsiveness to early feedings and to delay his early weight gain. Those effects have no important influence on the newborn's survival or later functioning. But they may have an important effect on the newborn's mother if she needs evidence that she can satisfy her infant's hunger in order to increase her confidence in her capacity to be a mother.

Personality Development

The stages of development that lead to maturity are designated as (1) infancy, from birth to 2 years of age, (2) the preschool-age period, or early childhood, from 2 through 5 years of age. (The preschool-age period is divided into the early and late preschool-age stages.), (3) the school-age period, or later childhood, from 6 years of age until the onset of puberty (at approximately 11–13 years of age in girls and 13–15 years of age in boys). (The school-age period includes the pre-pubertal stage.), and (4) adolescence, from the onset of puberty until the completion of biologic maturity. (Adolescence is divided into early, middle, and late stages.)

The division of development into the 4 stages, which are defined mostly according to the pediatric nomenclature, is arbitrary. The stages do not correspond exactly with the psychosexual and psychosocial stages of development, particularly in relation to the achievement of psychosocial maturity, but also in relation to the overlapping of infancy and the preschool-age period. But now professionals in many fields understand the division and can discuss development in terms of it. Although the division is based on physical development, its 4 stages also correspond sufficiently with psychologic and social development.

Theories about Development

The discussion of personality development includes ideas drawn from many schools of thought. These areas include dynamic psychology (which has drawn on psychoanalytic theory), learning theory, neurophysiology, child development, social science, and ethology. An eclectic approach that treats the ideas of all these areas equally without supporting one idea in particular would, in my opinion, be tedious and of little value. In addition, some conceptual framework is necessary, in the absence of final facts, in order to approach the immediate problems of treatment and the establishment of hypotheses in order to test the ideas. Textbooks by Mussen, Conger, and Kagan,[61] Lindzey,[51] Brenner,[15] Carmichael,[17] and others thoroughly discuss the theories of personality development and cite the original sources of the theories.

As Lindemann[50] has pointed out, there are now at least 3 theories that can offer explanatory principles for human behavior and personality development. They are (1) the reflex theory, which considers behavior as a series or a set of clusters of conditioned responses, (2) the field theory, which considers behavior as motion in a field of force, and (3) the dynamic theory, which assumes that humans have inner drives or needs and that they may have emotional conflicts over the handling of these in interpersonal situations. The 3 theories overlap; among these theories, each alone is incomplete. All 3 may help to explain behavior. (There are of course other theories, such as Luria's;[53] most of them are variations on the 3 most important theories.)

Pavlov first put forth the *reflex*, or conditioning, theory. It explains some psychophysiologic phenomena, both normal and pathologic (as mentioned in Chapter 2). It explains some avoidance phenomena, as in the case of a child who has had a frightening experience with a dog and avoids situations in which he might see a dog. Miller and Dollard[59] later added the ideas of social learning and motivation. Skinner[72] has shown the power of reward and reinforcement given for certain kinds of behavior or learning, which can lead to an "operant conditioning" effect. Modern learning theory, behavior therapy, and biofeedback derive from this theoretical base.

The orientation to a single or a specific situation (that includes some motivation as Miller[58] indicated) does not explain more complex motivating needs and driving forces that produce behavior that is broadly goal directed. The *field theory*, first put forth by Lewin,[48] considers a person as a reflection of the social forces around him that motivate his social movement within his "life space" and that may act as barriers of varying difficulty to his goal-directed behavior. Differences between the child's reactions to punishments and rewards may be explained by the field theory, which largely emphasizes conscious wishes and decisions. Modern sociologic theory draws on the field theory; it emphasizes each person's social, occupational, heterosexual, and other role operations, as society defines his roles for him, but with frequent conflict among roles.

The *dynamic theory* is derived largely from psychoanalytic thought with various modification. It explains the effects of unconscious forces and internal conflicts on a person's behavior, as well as the effects of conscious conflicts with external forces, such as social forces. The dynamic theory's explanations must be supplemented by contributions from the reflex and field theories, however, as well as by other theories. There is no theory that completely explains behavior and development. The reflex theory is most closely related to the physiologic level of organization, the dynamic theory to the psychologic level, and the field theory to the social level. The dynamic theory can most easily integrate the other 2 theories. The unitary theory of health and disease draws on the dynamic theory although it also includes elements of the reflex, field, and other theories.

In relation to the personality development of the child, a dynamic theory of behavior must consider the interaction between innate and experiential factors during the child's development, as his growing mental apparatus integrates the forces of his external environment with his intrapsychic perceptions and adaptive operations. Thus what defensive, adaptive and coping[60] mechanisms that the child uses depends on his inherent characteristics and the capacities that he has at his level of development. Support of or interference with such mechanisms occurs as a result of the child's interaction with his parents or other members of his social milieu. Thus the balance between internal and external forces is always very important and should be considered in diagnosis and treatment planning for a child and his family.

Erikson's organizing framework[24] for considering personality development is probably the most useful and balanced one.

(Erikson is a child psychoanalyst. He has experience in education and anthropology. He originally prepared his framework for the 1950 White House Conference on Childhood and Youth. Witmer and Kotinsky[83] elaborated his framework in important ways.) His framework is based on psychoanalytic theory, but it considers the contributions of other fields, such as anthropology and the other social sciences, including history. It tries to integrate the psychologic and social aspects of personality development, but it is broad enough to integrate physical development also. Erikson considers personality development "from the point of view of the conflicts, inner and outer, which the healthy personality weathers, emerging and re-emerging with an increased sense of inner unity, with an increase in good judgment, and an increase in the capacity to do well, according to the standards of those who are significant to him." (The idea of "doing well" is relative, of course.) The child learns that the impressions of and expectations about his behavior and personality of important people in his life change as the stages of his development change. Such impressions and expectations may differ in different societies. That idea agrees with the idea set forth earlier in this chapter about maturity and the healthy personality.

Erikson draws on Freud's ideas. Freud first described the adaptive functioning of the mental apparatus, including the ego and the super-ego, or conscience. Freud introduced the idea of emotional conflict, conscious and unconscious levels of thought and feeling, repression, the response of other psychologic defense mechanisms to signal anxiety, and the importance of "object" (human and inanimate, as opposed to "subject") relations, with their vicissitudes. Those ideas are very important in modern dynamic psychology. Freud also developed the idea of different and progressive stages of psychosexual development. He pointed out that psychosexual development begins in infancy and early childhood and culminates at the end of adolescence and the attainment of biologic and psychologic maturity, which includes readiness to have true heterosexual relationships and to reproduce. Freud emphasized the importance of personality development in early childhood. That emphasis brought scrutiny to bear upon the nature and efficacy of the child-rearing methods used by a child's parents or other caretaking figures in these early phases, in relation to the strong emotional experiences for the child that can be associated with them.

Psychoanalytic theory was developed by Freud out of his clinical experience and has been amplified and modified by later investigators. The most significant recent trend in psychoanalytic theory has been influenced by the ideas of Anna Freud,[29] Hartmann,[37] Spitz,[74] Rapaport,[64] Erikson,[25] Murphy,[60] and others. That trend emphasizes "ego psychology," or the study of the more conscious adaptive and coping functions of the personality in its interactions with external forces, without ignoring internal unconscious forces. The trend has brought psychoanalytic theory into closer harmony with some of the earlier work of Jung[44] and Adler[2] and with the ideas of Sullivan,[78] Horney,[39] Fromm,[31] Lewin,[48] and others, who have all been more concerned with the study of interpersonal relations, from different points of view, than with intrapsychic phenomena. Thus in dynamic ego psychology, the balanced consideration of the effects of internal and external forces on human behavior is finally being achieved.

In attempting to implement such a conceptual balance, Erikson adds to personality development what he calls a "psychosocial" aspect. He includes the stages of psychosexual development, with their intrapsychic reverberations, but adds to each of them the need for the child to complete particular psychosocial "tasks" in development, in his relationships with his parents, the rest of his family, and his society. Erikson describes the psychosocial conflicts that occur during each stage of development. He believes that the child, with the help of his parents and of other people who appear later within his expanding "social radius," must resolve the conflicts that occur at each stage, and in so doing undergo a "developmental crisis" and go to the next stage. He believes that the child works on the developmental task of his current stage while he also works to prepare for the next task and works to complete any tasks not completed during his previous stage.

In 2 other ways, Erikson's theory of personality development is very unusual. Because Erikson believes that the child can work on several tasks at the same time and that each child is born with a "ground-plan" of personality development, he concludes that during development, psychosocial tasks not completed during earlier stages may be completed during later stages. Erikson's optimistic theory recognizes (as Freud did) the formative influences of the child's early relationships and experiences on his personality development, but he believes that those influences do not always determine his personality development. Because of his experience in longitudinal research, Erikson has developed "the greatest respect for the resiliency and resourcefulness of individual children who. . . (have) learned to compensate for grievous early misfortunes of a kind which in our clinical histories would suffice to explain malfunctioning rather convincingly." I share Erikson's view, and I think that the later completion of psychosocial tasks that were not completed during earlier stages depends on the child's inherent capacities and maturational forces, his later experiences, and how his parents and his family as a whole develop.

Erikson is the only major personality theorist who has developed a scheme of personality development that continues

beyond the end of adolescence and supposed maturity. Others, such as Allport,[4] have recognized that psychologic maturity comes later in life, but Erikson was the first to formulate specific stages of the personality development of adults. His scheme supports the idea of the need for a "fit" between continued completion by a child's parents of later psychosocial tasks and the child's developing psychosocial needs. If the needs of both are not satisfied, a developmental "push" or "drag" or other conflicting pressures upon the child may result, deriving from the parents' unresolved needs. Their needs are related to their own early experiences. Erikson's belief that personality development continues throughout life agrees with Bibring's[12] belief that pregnancy and motherhood comprise a "maturational" or developmental task and with the belief of Benedek[10] that parenthood is a "developmental phase."

Erikson's theory accommodates many learning and behavior theories, including operant conditioning, the ideas of Piaget and others about intellectual development, theories about small groups and families (see Chap. 6), sociologic theories, such as the field theory and the role theory, social anthropologic theory, general systems theory, communication theory, the theory of psychosexual development, drive theory, ego psychology, and more recent psychoanalytic theories. The greater vulnerability of the child during a developmental crisis—"openness" to leaps forward or to damage to his ego—agrees with the "critical" periods of ethologic theory that Wolff[84] recently modified to "sensitive" periods for humans. Erikson's theory also accommodates the interaction between genetic endowment and the environment (or between the innate and the experiential, as Benjamin has put it[11]).

A Schematic Representation of Personality Development

Table 5–1 is based on Erikson's stages of development. It provides orientation for the following discussion. The psychosocial "crises" that it refers to are needs to complete psychosocial tasks, such as that of establishing a "sense of trust" and mastering a conflicting "sense of mistrust" that must be completed by the infant at about 1 year of age, for example. The psychosocial "modalities" are the orientations or approaches to life that are characteristic of each stage. Each modality depends on all the previous ones and affects future modalities. The approaches to life that are characteristic of a person's parents, of his family, and of his society largely determine which of the modalities the person uses when he becomes an adult and how that modality is expressed. The "modes" of the first 3 psychosexual stages (modified from Freud's ideas) are the specific attitudes of the child toward his physical functions as they give him pleasure when he interacts with the members of his family who care for him. Modes are "bodily process" thinking and are characteristic of the young child. The central "value orientations" of each stage are Erikson's ideas of the values (or "virtues," when they are applied to a person's social functioning) that a person can achieve at each stage at his development. Each value becomes more consolidated during each stage; finally all the values are integrated into a system or set of values. Each person has his own system of values, but his system is related to the values of his society.

In order to discuss personality development in terms of the 3 major levels of organization that correspond to the three major aspects of development (the physical, the psychologic, and the social), the table includes other aspects of development.

The stages of intellectual adaptation or development, as described by Piaget,[26,62] are shown in relation to the psychosocial and psychosexual stages of development. Correlations with important stages of physical development and growth, maturation of the central nervous system, and EEG de-

velopment are shown. Those correlations are particularly important in studying the psychomotor development of the infant and young child; psychomotor development strongly affects the intellectual, emotional, and social aspects of development. The table includes developmental "landmarks," important developmental "lines" (as suggested by Anna Freud[30]), and the developmental problems that are associated with each stage. (Although the visual correlations of the table may be helpful, the more basic correlations must be established in the mind of the clinician.)

This book does not fully discuss the behavioral patterns, adaptive mechanisms, psychosocial interactions, sensitive phases, and everyday developmental problems of the infant, child, and adolescent. Thus it cannot discuss the approach to health supervision that is used to deal with common developmental problems. The management of some special problems that occur in the family and during development is discussed in Chapter 28, while other problems are discussed in the chapters on clinical disorders. A fuller treatment of such health supervision can be found in the works of Arnold,[7] Green and Haggerty,[33] Harper,[36] Illingworth,[40] Jensen,[42] Lewis,[49] Lourie and Werkman,[52] Richmond,[66,67] Senn and Solnit,[70] Spock,[75] Stuart and Prugh,[77] Wessel,[80] Wishik,[82] and Work and Call.[85]

Bibliography

1. Ader, R., and Deitchman, R.: Effects of prenatal maternal handling in the maturation of rhythmic processes. J. Comp. Physiol. Psychol., 71:492, 1970.
2. Adler, A.: *The Neurotic Constitution: Outlines of a Comparative Individualistic Psychology and Psychotherapy.* New York, Dodd Mead, 1926.
3. Allen, M.G., Pollin, W., and Hoffer, A.: Parental, birth, and infancy factors in infant twin development. Am. J. Psychiatry, 127:1597, 1971.
4. Allport, G.W.: *Pattern and Growth in Personality.* New York, Holt, Rinehart, and Winston, 1961.
5. Allport, G.W., Vernon, P.E., and Lindzey, G.: *Study of Values.* Boston, Houghton-Mifflin, 1952.
6. Anthony, E.J.: Developmental antecedents of schizophrenia. In: *Transmission of Schizophrenia.* (S.

Katz and D. Rosenthal, Eds.). London, Pergamon Press, 1968.

7. Arnold, L.E.: *Helping Parents Help Their Children*. New York, Brunner/Mazel, 1978.

8. Ashley-Montagu, M.F.: *Man's Most Dangerous Myth: The Fallacy of Race*. New York, Columbia University Press, 1945.

9. Ausubel, D.P.: *Theory and Problems of Child Development*. New York, Grune & Stratton, 1958.

10. Benedek, T.: Parenthood as a developmental phase. J. Am. Psychoanal. Assoc., 7:389, 1959.

11. Benjamin, J.C.: The innate and the experiential in development. In: *Lectures on Experimental Psychiatry* (H. Brosin, Ed.). Pittsburgh, University of Pittsburgh Press, 1961.

12. Bibring, G.L., et al.: Pregnancy as crisis and maturational process: Theoretical considerations. Psychoanal. Study Child, 16:9, 1961.

13. Birch, H.G.: Personal communication.

14. Birch, H.G.: Boldness and judgment in behavior genetics. In: *Science and the Concept of Race*. New York, Columbia University Press, 1968.

15. Brenner, C.: *An Elementary Textbook of Psychoanalysis*. New York, International Universities Press, 1955.

16. Burlingham, D.: *Twins*. New York, International Universities Press, 1952.

17. Carmichael, L.: *Manual of Child Psychology*. New York, Wiley, 1946.

18. Chess, S., Thomas, A., and Birch, H.: Characteristics of the individual child's behavioral responses to the environment. Am. J. Orthopsychiatry, 29:791, 1959.

19. Coghill, G.E.: The early development of behavior in amblystoma and in man. Arch. Neurol. Psychiatry, 21:989, 1929.

20. Datan, N., and Ginsberg, L.H.: *Life-Span Developmental Psychology: Normative Life Crises*. New York, Academic Press, 1975.

21. Dubos, R.: *Man Adapting*. New Haven, Conn., Yale University Press, 1965.

22. Eisenberg, L.: Social class and individual development. In: *Crosscurrents in Psychiatry and Psychoanalysis*. (R.W. Gibson, Ed.). Philadelphia, Lippincott, 1967.

23. Erikson, E.H.: Growth and crises in the healthy personality. In: *Identity and the Life Cycle*. New York, International Universities Press, 1959.

24. Erikson, E.H.: *Identity and the Life Cycle. Selected Papers*. New York, International Universities Press, 1959.

25. Erikson, E.H.: *Childhood and Society*, Rev. Ed. New York, Norton, 1963.

26. Flavell, J.H.: *The Developmental Psychology of Jean Piaget*. The University Series in Psychology. Princeton, N.J., Van Nostrand, 1963.

27. Freud, S.: *New Introductory Lectures in Psychoanalysis*. New York, Norton, 1933.

28. Freud, S.: An outline of psychoanalysis. Int. J. Psychoanal., 21:27, 1940.

29. Freud, A.: *The Ego and the Mechanisms of Defense*. New York, International Universities Press, 1955.

30. Freud, A.: The concept of developmental lines. Psychoanal. Study Child, 17:245, 1962.

31. Fromm, E.: *Escape from Freedom*. New York, Rinehart, 1941.

32. Golden, M., and Bridger, W.: A refutation of Jensen's position on intelligence, race, social class and heredity. Ment. Hygiene, 53:648, 1969.

33. Green, M., and Haggerty, R.J.: *Ambulatory Pediatrics*. Philadelphia, Saunders, 1968.

34. Greenacre, P.: The predisposition to anxiety. Psychoanal. Q., 10:66, 1941.

35. Greene, W.A.: Process in psychosomatic disorders. Psychosom. Med., 28:150, 1956.

36. Harper, P.: *Preventive Pediatrics (Child Health and Development)*. New York, Appleton-Century-Crofts, 1962.

37. Hartmann, H.: *Ego Psychology and the Problem of Adaptation*. New York, International Universities Press, 1958.

38. Hoffer, A., and Pollin, W.: Schizophrenia in the NAS-NRC Panel of 15,909 Veteran Twin Pairs. Arch. Gen. Psychiatry, 17:723, 1967.

39. Horney, K.: *The Neurotic Personality of Our Time*. New York, Norton, 1939.

40. Illingworth, R.H.: *The Development of the Infant and Young Child, Normal and Abnormal*, 3rd Ed. Edinburgh, Livingstone, 1966.

41. Jahoda, M.: *Current Concepts of Positive Mental Health*. New York, Basic Books, 1958.

42. Jensen, G.D.: *The Well Child's Problems: Management in the First Six Years*. Chicago, Yearbook Medical Publishers, 1962.

43. Jost, H., and Sontag, L.W.: The genetic factor in autonomic nervous system function. Psychosom. Med., 6:308, 1944.

44. Jung, C.G.: *Psychological Types*. Princeton, N.J., Princeton University Press, 1971.

45. Kallmann, F.: *Heredity in Health and Mental Disorder*. New York, Norton, 1953.

46. Kanner, L.: Early infantile autism. J. Pediatr., 25:211, 1944.

47. Kringlen, E.: *Heredity and Environment in the Functional Psychoses*. London, Heinemann, 1968.

48. Lewin, K.: *Field Theory in Social Science*. New York, Harper, 1951.

49. Lewis, M.: *Clinical Aspects of Child Development*. Philadelphia, Lea & Febiger, 1971.

50. Lindemann, E.: The ingredients of personality. In: *The Healthy Child: His Physical, Psychological and Social Development*. H. Stuart and D.G. Prugh, Eds. Cambridge, Harvard University Press, 1960.

51. Lindzey, G., Ed.: *Handbook of Social Psychology*. Cambridge, Mass., Addison-Wesley, 1952.

52. Lourie, R.S., and Werkman, S.L.: Normal psychological development and psychiatric problems. In: *The Biological Basis of Pediatric Practice*. (R. Cooke, Ed.). New York, McGraw Hill, 1968.

53. Luria, A.R.: *The Role of Speech in the Regulation of Normal and Abnormal Behavior*. New York, Pergamon Press, 1961.

54. Mann, E.C.: The role of emotional determinants in habitual abortion. Surg. Clin. North Am., 37:447, 1957.

55. Mattsson, A.: Long-term physical illness in childhood. A challenge to psychosocial adaptation. Pediatrics, 50:801, 1972.

56. Mercer, J.R.: *Labelling the Mentally Retarded: Clin-*

ical and Social System Perspective on Mental Retardation. Berkeley, University of California Press, 1973.

57. Mercer, J.R.: A policy statement on assessment procedures and the rights of children. Harvard Educ. Rev., 44:125, 1974.

58. Miller, N.E.: Experiments on motivation. Studies combining psychological, physiological, and pharmacological techniques. Science, 126:1271, 1957.

59. Miller, N.E., and Dollard, J.: Social Learning and Imitation. New Haven, Conn., Yale University Press, 1941.

60. Murphy, L.B.: The Widening World of Childhood: Paths Toward Mastery. New York, Basic Books, 1962.

61. Mussen, P.H., Conger, J.J., and Kagan, J.: Child Development and Personality, 2nd Ed. New York, Harper & Row, 1963.

62. Piaget, J.: The Origins of Intelligence in Children. New York, Norton, 1963.

63. Rank, O.: The Trauma of Birth. London, Kegan, Trench, & Truber, 1929.

64. Rapaport, D.: A historical survey of psychoanalytic ego psychology. In: Identity and the Life Cycle. Selected Papers (E.H. Erikson, Ed.). New York, International Universities Press, 1959.

65. Riesman, D.: The Lonely Crowd. New Haven, Conn., Yale University Press, 1950.

66. Richmond, J.B.: The pediatric patient in illness. In: The Psychology of Medical Practice (M.H. Hollender, Ed.). Philadelphia, Saunders, 1958.

67. Richmond, J.B.: The role of the pediatrician in early mother-child relationships. Clin. Proc. Children's Hosp., 15:101, 1959.

68. Rosenthal, D.: The offspring of schizophrenic couples. J. Psychiatr. Res., 4:169, 1966.

69. Rosenthal, D., et al.: Schizophrenics' offspring reared in adoptive homes. In: The Transmission of Schizophrenia (D. Rosenthal and S. Kety, Eds.). London, Pergamon Press, 1968.

70. Senn, M.J.E., and Solnit, A.J.: Problems in Child Behavior and Development. Philadelphia, Lea & Febiger, 1968.

71. Sheldon, W.H., Stevens, S.S., and Tucker, W.B.: The Varieties of Human Physique: An Introduction to Constitutional Psychology. New York, Harper, 1940.

72. Skinner, B.B.: A new method for the experimental analysis of the behavior of psychotic patients. J. Nerv. Ment. Dis., 120:403, 1954.

73. Sontag, L.W.: Differences in modifiability of fetal behavior and physiology. Pyschosom. Med., 6:151, 1944.

74. Spitz, R.A.: A Genetic Field Theory of Ego Formation: Its Implications for Pathology. New York, International Universities Press, 1959.

75. Spock, B.: Avoiding behavioral problems. J. Pediatr., 27:363, 1945.

76. Stabenau, J.R., and Pollin, W.: Early characteristics of monozygotic twins discordant for schizophrenia. Arch. Gen. Psychiatry, 17:723, 1967.

77. Stuart, H., and Prugh, D.G., Eds.: The Healthy Child: His Physical, Psychological, and Social Development. Cambridge, Mass., Harvard University Press, 1960.

78. Sullivan, H.S.: Psychiatry: Introduction to the study of interpersonal relations. Psychiatry, 1:121, 1938.

79. Vandenberg, S.: Personal communication.

80. Wessel, M.A.: Value of prenatal pediatric visit. Pediatrics, 32:926, 1963.

81. Winestine, M.E.: Twinship and psychological differentiation. J. Am. Acad. Child Psychiatry, 8:436, 1969.

82. Wishik, S.M.: Parents' group discussions in a child health conference. Am. J. Public Health, 43:888, 1953.

83. Witmer, H.L., and Kotinsky, R., Eds.: Personality in the Making: The Fact-Finding Report of the Mid-Century Conference on Children and Youth. New York, Harper & Row, 1952.

84. Wolff, P.H., and Feinbloom, R.I.: Critical periods and cognitive development in the first 2 years. Pediatrics, 44:999, 1969.

85. Work, H.H., and Call, J.D.: A Guide to Preventive Psychiatry: The Art of Parenthood. New York, McGraw-Hill (Blakiston), 1965.

General References

Allee, W.C.: The Social Life of Animals. New York, Norton, 1938.

Allport, G.W.: The open system in personality theory. J. Abnorm. Soc. Psychiatry, 61:301, 1960.

Anderson, S., and Messick, S.: Social competency in young children. Dev. Psychol., 10:282, 1974.

Anthony, E.J.: The significance of Jean Piaget for child psychiatry. Br. J. Med. Psychol., 29:20, 1956.

Aries, P.: Centuries of Childhood. New York, Knopf, 1962.

Bandura, A., and Walters, R.H.: Social Learning and Personality Development. New York, Holt, Rinehart, & Winston, 1963.

Benjamin, J.: Further comments on some developmental aspects of anxiety. In: Counterpoint: Libidinal Object and Subject (H.R. Gaskill, Ed.). New York, International Universities Press, 1963.

Benjamin, J.D.: The innate and the experiential in child development. In: Childhood Psychopathology (S.I. Harrison and J.F. McDermott, Eds.). New York, International Universities Press, 1972.

Bertelanffy, L.V.: General systems theory and psychiatry. In: American Handbook of Psychiatry, Vol. 3. (S. Arieti, Ed.). New York, Basic Books, 1966.

Blos, P.: Prolonged adolescence: The formulation of a syndrome and its therapeutic implications. Am. J. Orthopsychiatry, 24:733, 1954.

Blos, P.: On Adolescence: A Psychoanalytic Interpretation. New York, Free Press, 1961.

Bornstein, B.: On latency. Psychoanal. Study Child, 6:279, 1951.

Bowlby, J.: Symposium on the contribution of current theories to an understanding of child development. I. An ethologic approach to research in child development. Br. J. Med. Psychol., 30:230, 1957.

Brackbill, Y., Ed.: Behavior in Infancy and Early Childhood: A Book of Readings. New York, Free Press, 1967.

Brazelton, T.B.: *Infants and Mothers: Differences in Development*. New York, Dell, 1969.

Brazelton, T.B.: *Toddlers and Parents*. New York, Dell, 1974.

Bremer, R.H., Ed.: *Child and Youth in America*. Cambridge, Mass., Harvard University Press, 1970.

Brim, O.J.,Jr.: *Education for Child Rearing*. New York, Russell Sage Foundation, 1959.

Bronfenbrenner, U.: *Two Worlds of Childhood; U.S. and U.S.S.R.* New York, Russell Sage Foundation, 1970.

Caldwell, B.M., and Ricciuti, H.N.: *Review of Child Development Research*, Vol. 3. Chicago, University of Chicago Press, 1974.

Campbell, J.D.: Peer relations in childhood. In: *Review of Child Development Research*, Vol. 1. (M.L. Hoffman and L.W. Hoffman, Eds.). New York, Russell Sage Foundation, 1964.

Caplan, G., Ed.: *Prevention of Mental Disorders in Children*. New York, Basic Books, 1961.

Caplan, G., and Grunnebaum, H.: Perspectives on primary prevention: A review. Arch. Gen. Psychiatry, 17:331, 1967.

Chess, S., and Thomas, A.: *Temperament and Development*. New York, Brunner/Mazel, 1977.

Cooper, M.M.: Evaluation of the Mothers' Advisory Service. Monogr. Soc. Res. Child Dev., No. 12, 1947.

Eisenberg, L.: The relationship between psychiatry and pediatrics: A disputatious view. Pediatrics, 39:645, 1967.

Erikson, E.H.: *Identity: Youth and Crisis*. New York, Norton, 1968.

Fairbairn, W.R.D.: *An Object-Relations Theory of Personality*. New York, Basic Books, 1954.

Fraiberg, S.: *The Magic Years*. New Year, Scribner's, 1959.

Freedman, D.G.: Behavioral differences between Chinese-American and European-American newborns. Nature, ,224:1127, 1969.

Freud, A.: *The Ego and the Mechanisms of Defense* (1939). New York, International Universities Press, 1946.

Freud, A.: *Normality and Pathology in Childhood: Assessments of Development*. New York, International Universities Press, 1965.

Goulet, L.R., and Battes, P.B.: *Life-Span Developmental Psychology: Theory and Research*. New York, Academic Press,1970.

Harms, E.: The development of religious experience in children. Am. J. Sociol., 50:112, 122, 1944.

Hilgard, E.R.: *Theories of Learning*, 2nd Ed. New York, Appleton-Century-Crofts, 1959.

Hinde, R.A.: *Animal Behavior: A Synthesis of Ethology and Comparative Psychology*. New York, McGraw-Hill, 1968.

Hoffman, L.W., and Hoffman, M.L.: *Review of Child Development Research*. New York, Russell Sage Foundation, 1966.

Ivan, F., and Hoffman, L.N.: *The Employed Mother in America*. Chicago, Rand McNally, 1963.

Jacobsen, E.: Development of the wish for a child in boys. Psychoanal. Study Child, 5:139, 1950.

Jersild, A.: *Child Psychology*. New York, Prentice-Hall, 1950.

Josselyn, I.: *Psychosocial Development of Children*. New York, Family Service Association of America, 1948.

Josselyn, I.: Psychological effect of the menarche. In: *Psychosomatic Obstetrics, Gynecology and Endocrinology*. (W.S. Kroger, Ed.). Springfield, Ill., Thomas, 1963.

Kagan, J.: The child's perception of the parent. J. Abn. Social Psychol., 53:257, 1956.

Mahler, M.S.: *On Human Symbiosis and the Vicissitudes of Individuation*. New York, International Universities Press, 1968.

Mahler, M.S., Pine, F., and Bergman, A.: *The Psychological Birth of the Human Infant: Symbiosis and Individuation*. New York, Basic Books, 1957.

Maier, H.W.: *Three Theories of Child Development: The Contributions of Erik H. Erikson, Jean Piaget, and Robert*R. Sears and Their Applications*. New York, Harper and Row, 1965.

McGraw, M.B.: *The Neuromuscular Maturation of the Human Infant*. New York, Hafner, 1966.

McLearn, G.: Genetics and behavior development. In: *Review of Child Development Research*, Vol. 1. (M.L. Hoffman and L.W. Hoffman, Eds.). New York, Russell Sage Foundation, 1964.

Mead, M.: The implication of culture change for personality development. Am. J. Orthopsychiatry, 17:663, 1947.

Mead, M.: Technological change and child development. Understanding the Child, 21:109, 1952.

Mead, M., and Wolfenstein, M., Eds.: *Childhood in Contemporary Culture*. Chicago, University of Chicago Press, 1955.

Moustakas, C., Ed.: *The Child's Discovery of Himself*. New York, Ballantine Books, 1972.

Murphy, L.B.: Preventive implications of development in the preschool years. In: *Prevention of Mental Disorders in Children* (G. Caplan, Ed.). New York, Basic Books, 1961.

Neubauer, P.: The one-parent child and his oedipal development. Psychoanal. Study Child, 7:95, 1952.

Opler, M.K., Ed.: *Culture and Mental Health*. New York, Macmillan, 1959.

Parsons, T.: Social structure and the development of personality: Freud's contribution to the integration of psychology and sociology. Psychiatry, 21:321, 1958.

Prugh, D.G.: Psychophysiological aspects of prepuberty. J. Am. Psychoanal. Assoc., 12:600, 1964.

Richmond, J.: Health supervision of infants and children. J. Pediatr., 40:634, 1952.

Rosenthal, D.: *Genetics of Psychopathology*. New York, McGraw-Hill, 1971.

Sarnoff, C.: *Latency*. New York, Aronson, 1976.

Senn, M.J.E., and Hartford, C.: *The Firstborn*. Cambridge, Mass., Harvard University Press, 1966.

Spock, B.: *The Middle-Aged Child*. Penn. Med. J., 50:1045, 1947.

Tennes, K., and Lampl, E.E.: Stranger and separation anxiety in infancy. J. Nerv. Ment. Dis., 139:247, 1964.

Wallder, R.: The psychoanalytic theory of play. Psychoanal. Quart., 2:208, 1933.

Washburn, A.H.: The child as a person developing.

I. A philosophy and program research. Am. J. Dis. Child., 9:46, 1957.

Washburn, A.H.: The child as a person developing. II. More questions raised than answered. Am. J. Dis. Child., 9:54, 1957.

Werner, H.: *Comparative Psychology of Mental Development*, Rev. Ed. New York, International Universities Press, 1957.

White, R.W.: Ego and reality in psychoanalytic theory. Psychol. Issues, 3:1, 1963.

Winnicott, D.W.: Transitional objects and transitional phenomena. In: *Collected Papers.* New York, Basic Books, 1958.

Wolff, P.H.: Psychoanalytic research and infantile sexuality. Int. J. Psychiatry, 41:64, 1967.

Wolff, P.H.: Review of psychoanalytic theory in the light of current research in child development. J. Am. Psychoanal. Assoc., 19:565, 1971.

6
The Child in the Family

The Joys of parents are secret, and
so are their griefs and fears.
(Francis Bacon)

The childhood shows the man
as morning shows the day.
(John Milton)

Although lower species show family behavior, human children spend a much longer time as members of a family. The human child's longer dependence on the adults in his family gives him affection and nurturing and lets him develop to the point of independent functioning and acquire skills and knowledge. It also lets him develop his concept of himself as an individual and as a member of a family in a particular society that has its own characteristic mores and cultural patterns.

Anthropology has found the nuclear family unit in all societies, at all levels of the societies' development, although the family unit's structure and shape vary considerably. The patriarchal and matriarchal units are the two types of family units that exist in primitive societies. Both types have specific patterns of functioning; the patterns include ways of handling the inheritance of property and patterns of kinship that extend beyond a family's household to its clan or tribe. Their forms of marriage include monogamy, polygamy, and polyandry. In nomadic and some agrarian societies, the patriarchal and matriarchal units prevail; the patriarchal unit is more common. In modern urban society, the patriarchal and matriarchal units still exist. Urbanization and industrialization have increased the mobility of families' members; the extended system of kinship has broken down in the middle class (although not in certain ethnic groups), and the large households that contain several generations of a family have largely broken up. (But such households can still be found in rural areas.)

The family probably originated in the relationship between the mother and her child. That relationship is a primary social bond. The intimate and affectionate attachment of a husband and his wife should transcend their sexual desire or their urge to reproduce. That desire and that urge cannot be the only foundation of the complex behavior and functioning of the family. As Kluckhohn and Spiegel[70] have pointed out, the family can be viewed as a group of individuals, each of whom has certain patterned but also unique characteristics, needs, goals, and roles, such as those of parent, child, worker, and housewife, that they assume inside and outside of their families. The family members form a social unit or a group of individuals that has particular patterns of functioning as a group and as several subgroups. The family is also an economic unit, originally one that produced. Also, it transmits its culture's values. These values begin in the family itself, the community, the region, the nation's society, and the sociocultural environment, which all affect the methods of child rearing and education that the parents use. Finally, the family is a unit in a particular time and place; those units range from the nomadic family of a primitive time to the urban family of today. The family has its own continuity that comes from the influence of successive generations on each other—the "history of the family."

Today more and more families (who live in larger and larger cities) have patterns of living, systems of values, and economic goals that are very different from past ones and from those of the contemporary rural family. With the growth of industrialization and the number of job opportunities, the family has more geographic mobility. In democratic societies, the family has more social mobility; families tend to move from lower-class to middle-class values and behavior. As a result of both kinds of mobility, 1 out of 5 families in U.S. cities moves every year; that is, each family moves once every 5 years on the average. So, the continuity of a middle-class family's generations tends to be broken up. There are now smaller family units that consist largely of 2 generations, parents and children, or one-generation units that consist of older people or of a young married couple.

The change in the family's structure and location has caused other changes in patterns of authority and of the transmission of property, and in other aspects of the family's functioning. Fewer "institutional" families, in which someone has firm authority, exist. Now, in many families, husbands and wives share authority and companionship. Many marriages are not patriarchal. During periods of rapid social change, particularly in cities, social patterns are disorganized and reorganized; families temporarily lose stability. Also, methods of child-rearing have changed;[105,113] there is still some difference among the methods of child-rearing of some socioeconomic groups.[56,67]

Other important social changes, including the increases in the political and economic freedom of women, affect the changes in the family's structure and functioning. With the trend toward earlier marriage has come a growing divorce rate. More than 1 out of 3 marriages in the United States ends in divorce; most of the couples who divorce are very young and do not have children. One out of 6 children in the United States lives in a single-parent family; most single-parent families are headed by women and are white. Yet a slightly greater proportion of the adult population is married today than was at the turn of the century, despite changes in the form of the family and in the nature of the relationships between parents and their children.[83] So no grounds for fear of the decline of the family as an institution in U.S. society exist, apparently, despite problems seen in the family, as Clausen[32] and Kluckhohn[69] have pointed out. Until recently, studies of the family have concentrated on the mother. But recent studies have concentrated on the father also.[18,72]

The Relationship Between Parents and Their Children; Methods of Child Rearing; and the Parents' Capacities

A discussion of the relationships between parents and their children, methods of child rearing, and the parents' capacities must examine several ideas. The concept of transactional responses or feedback between the parent and the child, as developed by Benedek[16] and elaborated on by Brazelton[23] (among others), was discussed in Chapter 2. Also, methods used by the parents may be appropriate to the child's needs at one stage of his development and inappropriate at another stage. So the idea of the parents' development, described by Benedek[17] and elaborated on by Friedman[47] and others, is very important. Different parents have different "sensitive" stages. The continuation of personality development during an adult's life, as described by Erikson,[40] is also very important. It leads to the idea that the parents' completion of their later psychosocial tasks must synchronize with their child's developing psychosocial needs. Finally, different parents respond differently to different children during different stages of their development. The parent (as well as the child) has needs.

Interpersonal Dimensions

The family can be looked at from the point of view of the types of relationships among its members.

1. The nature of the marital relationship (whether it is healthy, balanced, and mutual, or unhealthy, immature and unbalanced).
2. The nature of the relationships between the parents and the child and the degree of the parents' development.
3. The nature of other relationships within the family (with siblings and grandparents, for example).
4. The nature of the family as a unit or a small group of people and of its development.

Social and Cultural Dimensions

The family can also be looked at from the point of view of its functioning as a unit in society.

1. The composition of the family (that is, the people who are involved in the family's behavior).
2. The origin and growth of the family (the family unit's original form and the changes of that form).
3. The methods of child-rearing of the parents and of the other parenting figures in the family.
4. The family's living situation (the physical characteristics of its home and the home's immediate surroundings).
5. The socioeconomic background, status, and values of the family.
6. The ethnic and/or religious background of the family.

Children characteristically need from their parents solicitous care, protection, unconditional love, guidance, and discipline. Besides children's needs for security, acceptance, intimacy, sharing, dependence, individuation, self-realization, and satisfaction in a social group, some studies show that children need to know what they are allowed to do, what is expected of them, and what limits are to be set on their actions. Permissiveness can be carried too far; liberty should not become license. Children not only need but want to be controlled reasonably and kindly, although they often need to test the limits of that control during early childhood and especially during adolescence. Finally, the capacity of the parents to "let go" of their children and to let the older child and the adolescent grow away from them and become mature and independent requires understanding and restraint from the parents. Those qualities are very important—and often difficult to achieve. The majority of parents, however, try very hard to meet their children's needs and to rear and guide them lovingly.

Since the studies of Levy,[74] Newell,[90] and others, most investigators who study the mental health of children believe that certain *extreme* methods of child-rearing have a pathologic effect on the child, as Anthony[6] has pointed out. Those methods include extreme overdomination, marked overprotection, complete permissiveness, total rejection, physical abuse of the child, and marked emotional neglect of the child. (Some of those methods are discussed in more detail in later chapters.) Even if the behavior of 1 parent becomes pathologic, the child may be able, through his relationship with his other parent or with one of his grandparents or with another person who is close to his family, to gratify his basic needs and to have normal personality development, depending on such factors as his temperament and the balance of his family's operations, for example.

Discontinuity, insufficiency, or distortion in the relationship between the parent and the child should be avoided.[4,92] It is hard to predict the psychopathologic effects of those qualities in the relationship, as the few longitudinal studies that have been made indicate.[41,62,82] It is easier to understand why some children decompensate than to understand why others do not under comparable circumstances.

Many parents can adjust their treatment of their children's needs at different stages of the children's development and their treatment of different children who have different characteristics as the family grows. The idea of "family development," first set forth by Lindemann[79] and divided into developmental stages by Solomon,[102] is in harmony with this approach and with the concept of "family crisis." Table 6–1 integrates the child's development, the parents' development, and the family's development. The table is based on the ideas of Erikson (discussed in Chapter 4) and, with slight changes, on the ideas of Fried-

man and Solomon, mentioned earlier in the chapter.*

The term parental skills implies that such skills can be acquired or learned and so can be taught. Some of the skills of a parent can be learned, such as setting limits for and praising children. But some of a parent's attributes, such as showing empathy or accepting a child as a separate and independent person, may be hard to learn and teach intellectually. Some parents may find it hard to learn some child-rearing techniques, such as using a positive approach to discipline, because they have problems with their jobs or their marriages or because they were deprived of something early in life.

Most studies have indicated that parents' attitudes toward and expectations for their children may affect the children's personality development more than the particular methods of child-rearing that they use. As Caldwell[28] and Richmond[95] have indicated, the parents' attitudes may even determine what methods of child-rearing they use, and the parents' attitudes and methods of child-rearing together may affect their children's personality development more than either does separately. Thus the term parental skills would seem to embrace parental attitudes, behavior, and child-rearing practices, which are all interrelated. The broader term parental capacities seems more appropriate than the term parental skills, implying also the important potential for change during parent and family development.

The parents' attitudes and behavior can be described in relation to several dimensions of the relationship between the parents and the child. Table 6–2 outlines the

---

*The tables and much of the other material in Chapter 6 come from a paper I gave at a workshop on the assessment of parental skills. The workshop was part of a conference that dealt with the relation of mental health care to the care given by a primary care physician. The American Medical Association and the National Institute of Mental Health sponsored the meeting. It was held in Chicago, Illinois, in November, 1976.

Table 6-1. *Child Development, Parent Development, and Family Development*

Child's Developmental Stages	Individual Developmental Tasks (Erikson)	Parent Development (Friedman)	Family Development (Solomon)
			The marriage
Infant	Trust vs. mistrust	Learning the cues	The birth of the first child and of the rest of the children—solidification of the marriage and establishment of the parents' roles
Toddler	Autonomy vs. shame and doubt	Learning to accept the child's growth and development	
Preschool age	Initiative vs. guilt	Learning to separate	The separate growth of the family members' personalities—continual changes in their roles and the growing independence of each one
School age	Industry vs. inferiority	Learning to accept temporary rejection and to "let go" of the child without deserting him	
Adolescence	Identity vs. diffusion of identity	Learning to build a new life	The departure of the children—reworking of the parents' roles because their children are now adults
Young adulthood	Intimacy vs. isolation	Helping the child without holding on to him or ignoring him	
Middle adulthood	Generativity vs. stagnation		
Late adulthood	Integrity vs. despair and disgust	Grandparenthood—loving their grandchildren without interfering with their children's roles as parents	The integration of loss—the acceptance of the social, economic and physiologic changes that old age brings

Adapted from: The physician and the mental health of the child. 1. Assessing development and treating disorders within a family context. (H.J. Grossman, et al., Eds.) Chicago: American Medical Association, 1979.

Table 6–2. *Dimensions of Parent-Child Relationships*

	The Child's Position on Scale	
The Parents' Attitude or Behavior	*Upper Extreme*	*Lower Extreme*
The parents' acceptance of the child	Accepted	Rejected
Whether the parents value the child for himself or in terms of their own needs	Intrinsically valued	Extrinsically valued
How important the child is to the parents	Overvalued	Undervalued
How the parents express affection (are they loving, warm and nurturing, or detached or hostile?)	Positive	Negative
The parents' communication with the child (is it verbal, or appropriate to the child's level, or is it nonverbal or conflicting?)	Appropriate	Inappropriate
The parents' protectiveness (do they show care and solicitude, or neglect?)	Overprotected	Neglected (underprotected)
The parents' indulgence or frustration of the child's needs	Overindulged	Overfrustrated (underindulged)
The parents' appreciation or recognition of the child's competence	Overappreciated	Underappreciated (depreciated)
The parents' dominance (their self-assertiveness in control, or deference to the child's will)	Overdominated	Underdominated
The parents' control of the child (how restrictive or permissive they are)	Overrestricted	Underrestricted (overly permitted)
The parents' criticism of the child (whether it is overt or implied)	Overcriticized	Undercriticized
The parents' aspiration for the child	Overmotivated	Undermotivated

Adapted from D.P. Ausubel: *Theory and Problems of Child Development.* New York, Grune & Stratton, 1958.

dimensions of parent-child relationships, adapted from Ausubel,[9] with some modifications. Many of the dimensions in the table overlap one another. Different dimensions could be added to the table or substituted for the dimensions already in the table; such dimensions are the degrees of relatedness, stimulation, nurturance, the satisfaction of needs, consistency, approval, and punishment. Those belong to several dimensions. Some studies of how some aspects of the parents' behavior relate to each other use factor analysis to analyze the correlations. Schaefer and Bell[98] translated one such model of the parents' behavior into a research scale. The scale is called the Parent Attitude Research Instrument (PARI). That scale includes all the parents' attitudes in 2 dimensions: (1) love versus rejection and (2) autonomy versus control. The 2 dimensions form a diagram (the circumplex model, shown in Fig. 6–1) in order to plot the relationship between the parent and the child. An equation is used to transfer the results of a questionnaire onto the model. The relationship of these factors is still hypothetical and should be tested further.

More recently, Becker[13] has used studies that use factor analysis to expand such a model into 3 dimensions. He has changed the dimension love-versus-rejection to warmth-versus-hostility, and has subdivided the dimension control-versus-autonomy into restrictiveness-versus-permissiveness and anxious-involvement versus calm-detachment.

On the basis of his model, Becker has suggested a typology of parents' attitudes and behavior that are within the normal range. The typology includes the democratic parent, who is warm, permissive, calm, and detached and who gives the child autonomy; the organized-effective parent, who is warm, restrictive, and somewhat detached; the indulgent parent, who is loving, permissive, and very involved emotionally with the child; and the protective

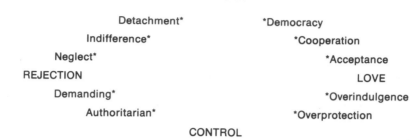

Fig. 6–1.   The circumplex model. (From Schaefer, E.S.: A circumplex model for maternal behavior. J. Abnorm. Soc. Psychol., *59*:226, 1959.)

parent, who is warm, restrictive, and emotionally involved with the child. Other types of parents, such as the autocratic parent who is cold, restrictive, and detached, the authoritarian parent, the perfectionistic parent, and the accepting or the rejecting parent have been suggested in studies that use other methods. Different typologies could be constructed using various different dimensions of parents' attitudes and behavior.

Sears and his colleagues,[100] Baldwin,[11] and Radke[93] made other studies of the effects on a child of the behavior of both his parents in the home. Those studies showed democratic, indulgent, and intellectual types of parents. Since those studies used different kinds of approaches to methodologies and different populations, it is hard to compare them to each other. In one of Baldwin's studies, the children of parents who were warm and democratic and who gave their children autonomy were considered more outgoing in both friendly and hostile ways, more active in their participation in activities at school, and generally assertive, successful, and popular. The children of indulgent parents tended to be inactive, unaggressive, and socially unsuccessful; other studies have shown that some of those children are more demanding and controlling. Radke described the children of autocratic parents as more

unpopular, quarrelsome, daring, and uninhibited than the children of democratic parents. Sears found that cold, punitive parents produced high aggressiveness in their children.

Such studies have some methodologic limitations. The long-term effects of parents' attitudes toward their children's behavior are not clear. All such typologies applied to the healthy range of parent-child relationships have significant limitations. Individual parents often do not fit one or any of the types. However, as Conger[34] has pointed out in his studies of adolescents, some generalizations do apply in North America. With respect to a child's adjustment to and competence in his or her male or female role and in dealing with his or her environment while living away from home, the most effective parents are democratic ones. They encourage discussion of issues related to the family, but although they are warm, they are not too permissive. Such parents encourage the growth of a child's independence without relinquishing all control of the child. They are authoritative but not authoritarian. They discuss values with the child and do not use their control of him for its own sake. Children best accept authority that is based on a rational concern for their welfare, and they often reject authority that is based on control. "Love-oriented" approaches (in which a parent shows love with limits) seem more likely than "power-oriented" approaches to produce children who can cope with life easily and effectively and have developed their own values.

Of course parents with attitudes other than those have reared children successfully, and children differ in their responses to authority in part because they have different temperaments. Also, the relationship between the parents and the child changes at different stages of the child's development. The above picture is also based largely on studies of white middle-class families. In other cultures, the parents' attitudes are different but equally effective[112] in producing mature adults. The physician should try to assess the attitudes and behavior of the parents he deals with in terms of the different dimensions and should recognize that no parents are always consistent.

The Family As a Unit

There is now no generally accepted model of the family's structure, functioning, and adaptive equilibrium. But there are some criteria for the optimal functioning of the family that can be generally formulated, as Josselyn[61] indicated. The family maintains an interpersonal adaptive equilibrium; crises in the family may weaken or strengthen its equilibrium. Also, the family develops as a unit. While the family maintains its equilibrium and develops, its members function as individuals, in dyads (e.g., the marital relationship), triads, or other subgroups, and in relation to the transactions of the family as a unit.

Criteria for Evaluating the Family's Functioning

Each family is unique; it has its own history, and it is made up of interacting personalities. Each personality is also unique.

As Clausen[32] points out, cohesiveness is desirable for any family. Mutual respect may make a family more cohesive than mutual dependency. Directness and openness in communication is also desirable. It may be more important, however, that a family's members show each other affection and understand each other than that they discuss their feelings in depth, because cultural norms can affect what people feel comfortable discussing. Some roles must be complementary and must not conflict (e.g., the parents' roles as husband and wife and as parents) and authority and leadership must be balanced. Finally, a family's members should have consonant goals and values in order for the family to function best.

Since the family must exist economically, its members must be able to perform tasks. Therefore, the family must be part of the external community. The family's values and goals must harmonize with those of its neighborhood, community, and culture (at least enough to let its members survive). The family is also an agent of socialization. Although different families give their children different role models and precepts, and those models and precepts differ in different strata of society, perhaps, as Clausen[32] has indicated, the best test of a family's socialization is its children's capacity to function effectively in society.

Following the thought of Clausen,[32] Spiegel and Kluckhohn,[70] Bell and Vogel,[15] and Ackerman[1] and drawing on 2 recent studies of healthy families by Lewis and his colleagues[75] and Senn and Hartford,[101] there are at least 9 dimensions of the family's functioning that can be classified as effective or ineffective. (The classification includes other qualifications.)

The dimensions are:

1. *The performance of tasks* (e.g., how efficiently, smoothly, and effectively the family's members care for the home, rear the children, handle money, and perform at home and in school).

2. *The complementary quality of roles* (e.g., the

comfort of the family members in their roles as worker and supporter of the family outside the home or as husband, wife, father, mother, son, daughter, or sibling, and the balance of the several roles of one person with the several roles of others).

3. *Patterns of leadership* (e.g., the availability of decision-making processes as to which parent assumes authority under what circumstances, the clarity of the difference in leadership and authority between the parents and the children, and the balance of the use of power and authority for the needs of each person and the needs of the whole family).

4. *Patterns of communication* (e.g., how clear and open the channels of communication are, the balance between verbal and nonverbal communications, and the appropriateness of the linguistic symbols that the family's members use for shared thinking).

5. *Patterns of expressing and handling affection and other emotions* (e.g., how mutual the affection among the family's members is and how well each member of the family perceives the mutual quality of the affection, and how comfortable and effective the family's members are in expressing and dealing with negative feelings, such as anger and jealousy, and with sexual feelings).

6. *Patterns of the fulfillment of needs* (e.g., how clearly the family's members perceive each other's needs and their comfort and balance in patterns of satisfying needs, control, and limit-setting in relation to needs for dependency, self-esteem, independence, sharing, competitive striving, sexuality, privacy, and identity between parents and toward children, and in the capacity to balance the satisfaction of one person's needs with those of others).

7. *Systems of values* (e.g., how clear, consistent, and consonant the family members' shared values and goals are, and the balance between the family's values and those of each of its members).

8. *Integration and solidarity* (e.g., how cohesive the family unit is, the balance of its capacity to work together as a group, and its recognition of each member's contributions, and the flexibility of the family's responses to crises).

9. *Relationship to the external community* (e.g., to what extent the family as a group is integrated into its neighborhood, community, nation, and society, the capacity of its members to function effectively in their roles in the community without losing their identity as members of the family, and the ability of its members to share values with people who are outside the family without giving up their own values.

Other dimensions of the family structure, functioning, and adaptation could be added. The dimensions listed overlap each other. They could be applied equally well to the marital relationship and the parent-child relationship since they apply to any "primary group" (face-to-face) social unit. Such a typology of the dimensions can encompass the intrapsychic conflicts of each member of the family and the conflicts between members, but, as a cross-sectional picture, it does not focus on the development of the child, his parents, or his family. Anthony[8] has recently discussed the need for a developmental-transactional model of the family's functioning.

Classification of the Family's Functioning

Many classifications of the family's functioning and dysfunction have been made during the past 20 years. As Fisher[44] has pointed out, some of these classifications are based on the family's *style of adaptation*. They include families that unconsciously try to solve their conflicts internally by failing to communicate,[15] making one child a scapegoat,[110] developing a "symbiosis" between a parent and a child,[38] oversexualizing relationships,[1] giving a child verbal and nonverbal messages that conflict (as in a double-bind[12]), a child's acting out a parent's unconscious conflicts,[94] or developing patterns of "localized neurotic interaction"[43,92] between a parent and a child, in which the child is driven unconsciously to repeat a parent's earlier problem. Other families in this category have externally "power-aligned," delinquent, or paranoid life-styles.[1]

Other classifications are based on the family's *developmental stage*. Solomon's[102] is one of the most clinically helpful. It relates types of family pathology to the family's inability to complete (negotiate) particular tasks in its development. Role reversal, failure to individuate, and intense rivalry are examples of family pathology. Still other classifications are based on the initial problem of one of the family's members or the *diagnosis of the referred patient*. They assume that some types of family or marital pathology, such as the transmission of irrationality,[78] "pseudo-mutuality" in relationships,[115] or the development of patterns of "schism and skew"[77] in marital relationships, are associated with the decompensation of one of its members. That decompensation sometimes represents the symptom of the family's dysfunction.

The broadest approach to family classification was one of the earliest, typified by Ackerman's.[1-3] Ackerman's classification is based on themes or *dimensions in family dysfunction*. His classification includes some of the dimensions discussed earlier, particularly the dimension of the family's integration into its community. The extremes of that dimension are isolation or a nomadic life involvement in external activities. Others, such as Voiland and Buell, have concentrated on the degree of cohesiveness[111] or chaos[27] in the family's reactions to emotional conflicts or of external stress. The classifications overlap; none is generally accepted or used in the fields of mental health, sociology, or related fields.

Tseng, Arensdorf, and McDermott[109] have offered the most interesting and helpful recent approach to classification of family dysfunction. That classification combines elements of 3 of the basic criteria of approaches mentioned earlier: (1) style of adaptation, (2) stage of family development, and (3) the dimensions of its functioning. It follows (though it does not quite fulfill) the model that Anthony called for. That classification is based on a developmental history of the family that traces the occurrences of psychopathology in parents and children, a current "mental status" of the family based on a clinical evaluation of it that uses group task-oriented situations, and a brief diagnostic separation of the child from the family group (Fig. 6–2).

Using that model, Tseng and his colleagues have identified 6 categories of family pathology. They have made operational definitions of and suggested methods of treatment for each type. They point out that their "focus-oriented" diagnostic scheme does not replace individual diagnosis, but supplements the diagnosis by clarifying the deficiencies of the families' interactions. It can also facilitate appropriate therapeutic interventions along a continuum of pathology, ranging from that of the family's members to those of the family as a unit.

Figure 6–3 summarizes schematically Tseng's 6 types of family pathology. Tseng and his colleagues point out that they have not listed all the types of family pathology. They also point out that probably no case fits exactly any of the described 6 categories and that one family may have problems that are classified under different types of pathology.

In the "child-reactive" family, the child's problems may be developmental, psychoneurotic, psychotic, or physical; the family's interactions center on them. The interactions of the "parent-reactive" family is dominated by the problems of one parent. Usually the parent has a severely psychoneurotic personality or a psychosis, even though the family's interactions may result in identifying a child as the patient. In the "marital-reactive" family, both parents may function normally as individuals, although the child's problems result from his being caught in the chronic marital conflict. In the "unresolved triangular" family, one of several children is unconsciously involved in the unresolved conflicts of both parents. A chronic dysfunction may become a family crisis when the child reaches a level of development that is particularly relevant to one or both the parents' conflicts. The interactions of the "special-theme" family are dominated by family myths, secrets, "family romances," or sometimes cultural beliefs. The parents usually develop the theme, and a child is unconsciously selected by the family's

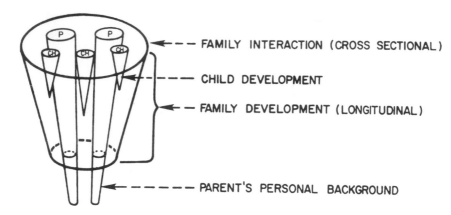

Fig. 6–2. Dimensions of family development, individual development of family members, and family interaction at a particular time. (From W.-S. Tseng, et al.: Family diagnosis and classification. J. Am. Acad. Child Psychiatry, *14*:15, 1975.)

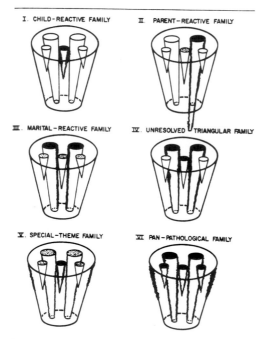

Fig. 6–3. Classification of disorders in family functioning in relation to disturbances in development in individuals and nature of psychopathologic interactions. (From W.-S. Tseng, et al.: Family diagnosis and classification. J. Am. Acad. Child Psychiatry, *14*:15, 1975.)

members to carry the theme in the family. The theme may last for generations.

The "panpathologic" family is the only type that Tseng and his colleagues have divided into subtypes (although they admit that the others may also have sub-

types). In the panpathologic family, role functions, patterns of communication, performance of tasks, integration into the community, and other dimensions of the family's functioning are pathologic, poorly defined, or inadequate for coping. The subtypes are (1) the inadequate family; all its members have dysfunctions, (2) the unintegrated family; it has role problems, conflicting functioning in several dimensions, a lack of cohesiveness, or chaotic dysfunction, and (3) the pathologically integrated family; some of its interactions are integrated, but it has pathologically interlocking or complementary relationships.

The classification offered by Tseng and his colleagues accommodates most of the types of family dysfunction mentioned earlier. It permits the use of different ideas about the dynamics of the behavior of individuals or small groups and of the idea that many factors work together to cause children's disorders. It can also relate easily to family crises because in a crisis, family members may react temporarily in ways that are reminiscent of all the categories, from the patterns of children's accidents that occur in relation to the family's moves,[85] the increased susceptibility to streptococcal infections of the children of families that are under external stress,[86] and the temporary disruptions of the family's interpersonal equilibrium (that may produce greater strength when the crisis has been overcome).[78] Tseng's classification can help resolve the problem relating to the indications for individual and/or family therapy. Only the last 2 types of pathology, the special-theme and panpathologic, need total and intensive family therapy, according to Tseng and his colleagues, although individual, residential, or other types of treatment may be required.[49] In the other types (e.g., the child-reactive, parent-reactive, and unresolved triangular types), therapy is given to the people who are most centrally involved (although they are not always the ones who were initially identified as patients) and although other people who take part in the family's interactions may need help. Parent therapy may be called for, especially in the child-reactive and triangular families. Sometimes therapy for the whole family may help, as may residential treatment for children who have been severely affected, especially children in marital-reactive families. The different methods of treatment of pathology in children, therapy for parents, pediatric counseling in milder cases, how to refer patients and their families, and some methods of preventing problems are discussed later.

Clinically Assessing Parents' Capacities

Many investigators have developed methods of assessing or measuring parents' capacities. The Parent Attitude Research Instrument (PARI) of Schaefer and Bell[98] and some of the other studies mentioned earlier contain typologies of parents' attitudes and behavior. Some investigators have developed methods of analyzing the interactions of parents and children. Some of the methods are designed to be used during infancy[5,24,25,33,97] and some when the children are older.[7,26,50,84,88,108] Most of the methods are designed to study healthy interactions, but some are designed to study pathologic interactions.[14,57,74,91]

Other interpersonal interactions within the family have been studied. Levy[73] first studied sibling rivalry systematically. Sibling rivalry can cause serious problems, but it may not be pathologic as often as it has been believed.[106] A child's ordinal position in his family can cause problems, but reviews by Anthony,[6] Ausubel,[9] and Clausen[32] indicate that although an only child often has problems, these problems are not inevitable. More systematic studies of the effects of ordinal position should be made.

The serious and chronic physical illness of a parent[19,54] has been shown to occur in association with a high incidence of delinquent, neurotic, and other disturbances in children, although a parent's illness alone does not cause a child's disturbance. Dalton[36] has shown that children have more behavioral difficulties, accidents, and hospitalizations during their mother's menstrual periods while she is young.

Many studies[35,37,96,104,114] have indicated that disturbed families often produce disturbed children, especially families that have depressed mothers,[42] marital conflicts,[81] and reciprocal or complementary neurotic patterns.[87] But some children seem to be constitutionally less vulnerable to problems caused by their family's problems.[32] Other factors may mitigate the effects of the family's problems on its children. In most cases, it is hard to define and establish the correlation between the nature of the family's pathology and that of the child,[2] even though neurotic interactions and other forms of pathology may continue over several generations of a family in a pseudo-hereditary way.[39,45]

The separation of a child in early childhood from his parents and inadequate substitute parenting (that often occurs in institutions) has been known to be a serious problem, even leading to death (see Chapter 27), since Chapin's study (made in 1909[30]) that Bakwin,[10] Spitz,[103] and Bowlby[21] followed in the 1930s and 1940s. But often such cases of separation are affected by many factors, including the nature of the child's relationship with his mother before the separation, the nature as well as the length of the separation, the type of substitute parenting, the events that occurred after the separation, and the characteristics of the child's constitution or temperament, as Clarke and Clarke,[31] Yarrow,[116] and others have pointed out. In his later studies,[22] Bowlby has reconsidered some of his earlier generalizations. Prugh and Harlow[92] have pointed out that "masked deprivation" can occur without any separation even in intact families.

Deprivation is now being carefully studied. Both maternal deprivation and paternal deprivation[18] have been too easily equated with separation. Separation under unhealthy circumstances certainly does not benefit a child, though the outcome for the child may vary considerably. Young children may even need practice in being separated from their parents under healthy circumstances, as can be arranged by working parents (see Chapter 28).

Many of the studies of separation have used different methodologies and different populations. Even the definitions of healthy behavior in children and of maturity, the goal of personality development, still pose problems. Other factors, such as the child's temperament, affect his development and behavior, as Thomas and Chess[107] have pointed out.

All of the approaches just described have important implications for the clinician, although some still need to be validated. None of those methodologies is as yet suitable for practical clinical use.

How to Make a Clinical Assessment

The clinician, during his contacts with parents and children, should use check points to make observations that he can use to make qualitative or semi-quantitative assessments of the parents' capacities and the stage of the parents' and the family's development. Some of the implications of studies just mentioned and to be mentioned may be used in practice. (Ethnic and sociocultural differences must be considered in the assessment.)

Ways to assess the parents' capacities at different stages in their development, rather than ways to intervene, are discussed here. Observations made at the check points that follow help to assess the parents' strengths, as well as their problems and limitations. Supporting the parents' strengths is just as important as intervening clinically by treating their pathology.

Assessment During Pregnancy and at Delivery

The ideas of Bibring and her colleagues,[20] who consider pregnancy and motherhood a maturational task, are very helpful. Much of the pregnant woman's behavior and apparent symptoms can be considered healthy rather than pathologic. The father must go through certain steps in maturation as the husband of his pregnant wife and as a father-to-be, as Jessner[60] and others[52,53,59] have indicated. Benedek's[16] and Caplan's[29] ideas that the mother becomes attached to her unborn child (as a person-to-be) during her pregnancy and around the time of quickening, and that there is a "maternal time lag" after the child's birth are also very helpful. Klaus and his colleagues[68] have studied events that occur in the hospital which may interfere with the healthy development of the parents' attachment to their child after it is born.

Clinical methods are being developed for assessing the parents' capacities and so determining the probability that the parents' relationship with their infant will be troubled. A recent study[48] suggests that women who lost a parent (through separation, divorce, or death) before they reached the age of 11 have more complaints during pregnancy and more feeding and sleeping problems with their infants in the first year of life than do women who did not lose a parent. The following is a list, adapted from Klaus and Kennell[67] and others, of circumstances that often (though not always) produce "high-risk" relationships between the parents and their infant. In such relationships there are problems in the parents' attachment to the infant (as well as other problems). The relationship between the parents and their infant will probably be troubled if:

1. The mother is teen-aged, particularly if she is primiparous and less than 17 years old.
2. The mother is unwed, whether or not she plans to keep the child.
3. The child is premature and particularly if there are complications during the delivery.
4. The infant has any congenital abnormalities.
5. The infant has any illness or defect and needs continued hospitalization that causes an extended separation of it from its mother.
6. The parents have had problems with previous pregnancies, particularly the loss of an infant, an abortion (whether therapeutic or illegal), habitual abortions, fertility problems, or miscarriages, or the parents have waited a long time for a child and feel that they will have no other chance to have a child.
7. The parents have experienced serious problems during the pregnancy. The problems can be medical (such as toxemia, diabetes, or Rh incompatibility) or psychosocial (such as a death in the family, a marital separation, or a disturbing move).
8. The parents have had serious marital problems before the pregnancy, such as a dispute about the infant's paternity or desertion by the father.
9. The mother lives in a ghetto or barrio, particularly if she received limited prenatal care, is very poor, and is sensitive to racial or economic discrimination.
10. Either of the parents (but particularly the mother) lost a parent in early childhood.

Kempe and his colleagues[64] and others[58] are developing questionnaires and methods of observation that may help to evaluate the parents' attachment to their child and to predict battering or child abuse. Kennell and Klaus[67] have developed a

broad clinical approach to studying the parents' attachment. Prugh has developed a set of 5 questions that elicit some information about the progress of the parents' attachment in an interview that lasts about 20 minutes and is held during pregnancy or shortly after the child's birth. Harmon and his colleagues[55] have shown that the 5 questions are reliable, but their validity has not yet been established. The likelihood that a high-risk relationship between the parents and their infant will develop can be estimated. (Prugh's questionnaire appears in the appendix.) Fletcher[46] is developing a similar questionnaire, and Goldson[51] is working on an assessment of the family.

Assessment During Early Infancy

Many investigators, including Spitz, Kempe, Call, and others, have experimented with the use of movies, videotapes, and other methods in studying the relationships of mothers and their infants while the mothers are feeding their infants. Electromyographic measures of the mother's muscle tension during the feeding and other measures of the infant's autonomic responses have been made.[71] The measures suggest that there is an "interpersonal physiology" between the mother and the infant. Such studies can show the strengths and problems of the relationship between the mother and the infant. Studies such as Sander's[97] infant caretaker studies, mentioned earlier, may suggest methods of intervention. But interest in and support of the mother (and the father) may help the mother to be happy and relaxed while she feeds and cares for her infant as much as or more than specific counselling techniques.

Two studies help assess the parents' capacities to deal with premature infants or infants who have other problems and who must stay in the hospital's nursery for some time. One of the studies, made by Kaplan and Mason,[63] follows Caplan's view of prematurity as a family crisis. The study predicted problems in the relationship between parents and their infant if the mother's visits to the infant were not regular or became fewer during the last 2 weeks of the infant's hospital stay. Klaus and Kennell[66] believe that fewer than 3 visits in 2 weeks to the infant or fewer than 5 telephone calls and visits in 2 weeks indicates the likelihood of a "mothering" disorder. Intervention made by visiting the mother at home during the first week after she leaves the hospital, in the study of Kaplan and Mason, resulted in fewer problems in the relationship between the mother and the infant during the first year of life.

Finally, home visits help to assess parents' capacities to perceive their infant's needs. Kempe, Prugh, and others believe that a home visit should always be made by a health care professional within the first week after the mother and infant leave the hospital (as is done by health visitors in the health care systems of some countries). That week causes new parents much anxiety. The mother's office visit 1 month after the child's birth is routine; but it gives no observations about feeding and other kinds of care given the infant as well as the support that the father gives the mother and the way that the husband and wife are assimilating their roles as parents. Permission and encouragement to call the physician at any time, as a sort of "telephone lifeline," between visits, can be revealing by the number and nature of the calls. Brazelton and Prugh believe that encouraging the parents to call can give them greater confidence and independence.

Assessment During Early Childhood

During early childhood, the physician often has several opportunities to assess the parents' capacities. If a secretary or a nurse, for example, observes the parents and their child while they are in the physician's waiting room, that observation can give the physician important information about the parents' capacity for empathy and their ability to support their child's autonomy while setting limits for him or to accept beginning separation-individuation. Observing the interaction between the parents and their child in a nursery school or day care center and during home visits can give the physician more information about the parents' capacities.

Home visits by the physician, the health associate, or the public health nurse made during a child's acute minor illnesses can show the parents' capacities to tolerate regression and greater dependence on the part of the young child. Such observations of the parents' capacities can be made during a family crisis such as the serious illness and hospitalization of a child. The physician can learn about the parents' capacities for performing tasks, the complementary quality of their roles, and their patterns of decision-making, leadership, communication, need-fulfillment, and expressing their emotions within the family.

Assessment During Later Childhood and Adolescence

During later childhood and adolescence, the most important capacities of the parents are those to support the child's continuing separation-individuation involved in going off to regular school, to give the child increasing responsibility,[99] and to permit the child's independence and attachment to his teachers and his peer group to grow. Next, the parents' capacity to tolerate their child's search for identity and greater independence in his adolescence while they give him guidance and set limits for him becomes important. (In later adolescence, the child can participate with his parents in arriving at such limits.) Finally, the child leaves home when he needs to establish a new life. Then his parents must take on new roles.

The physician can add to the observations that he makes in his office and his home visits by consulting the school teacher

Table 6-3. *Check-Points for Clinical Assessment of Parental Capacities*

Points in Child Development	Parental Capacities to Be Assessed	Where Assessment Possible
Pregnancy and delivery	The beginning of the mother's attachment to the child; both parents' readiness for parenthood	Contact with the parents before the delivery, an interview with the mother (and the father and other important members of the family) in the hospital's obstetric unit
Early infancy	The capacities to learn cues, to perceive the child's needs, and to develop an attachment to the child	Observation of the mother's feeding of the infant in the hospital or at home, and of the mother's (and father's) patterns of visiting if the infant stays in the hospital
Late infancy and the level of the toddler	The capacities to accept the child's growth and development, to empathize, and to perceive the child as a separate person; the development of the capacities to support the child's independence and the beginning of his individuation, and to set limits for him	Observation of the parents and the child in the physician's waiting room, during home visits, and in a day care center
The preschool-age level	The capacities to accept separation, to support the child's continuing individuation and his attraction to the parent of the opposite sex, and to tolerate the child's dependence and regression; the development of roles and capacities in the family, including the capacity to mourn losses	Observation of the parents and the child in the physician's waiting room, the nursery school, or the day care center, during home visits made during minor illnesses, and during the hospitalization of the child for a serious illness
The school-age level	The capacities to accept the child's growing independence, his need to engage in activities with the parent of the same sex and his interest in his teachers and his peer group, to give the child increasing responsibility and to perceive and support actively the child's need for mastery and a sense of competence	Observation of the parents and the child in the physician's waiting room, during office visits, home visits and hospitalization, and communication with teachers and school health personnel
Adolescence	The capacities to support the child's search for identity and greater independence, to offer the child guidance and set limits for him (and to let the adolescent help to set those limits), to develop further roles and capacities in the family, to let the child leave the family, and to begin to build a new life and new roles for themselves	Observation of the parents and the child during office visits, home visits and hospitalization, and communication with teachers, school health personnel, and other important people in the child's life (e.g., a clergyman)

Adapted from: The physician and the mental health of the child. 1. Assessing development and treating disorders within a family context. (H.J. Grossman, et al., Eds.) Chicago, American Medical Association, 1979.

during telephone conversations and school conferences. The newly developed roles of the school nurse and the school physician may bridge the gap betwen the physician and the teacher. The representatives of community agencies can also help the physician to assess the parents' capacities.

The positive capacity to mourn losses, whether the losses are real or symbolic, always shows that the parents and the family have strength (as pointed out by Lewis and his colleagues[75]). Knowing how the family has handled losses caused by death or separation can be very helpful. For example, Natterson and Knudson[89] have suggested that mourning over a child who has been diagnosed as having a fatal illness usually takes about 4 months. However, their studies were made in a supportive hospital setting. Others have found that the time of mourning over a death in the family varies considerably, but often lasts for 6 to 12 months. Mourning often occurs later, on the anniversary of the loss, and is usually shorter then. It can be helpful to know how the parents have reacted to any catastrophic illness, accident, or other experience and how they cope with problems. A family's system of values, its degree of integration and cohesiveness, its relationship to the external community, and its patterns of communicating and expressing emotions are very important.

It is not yet clear whether such clinical information can be collected systematically. If a list of the variables to be considered in assessing the parents' capacities could be assembled, together with a way of rating the resultant categories in a semiquantitative fashion, such an approach would at least make assessment of the parents' capacities more organized, if not more accurate. Several investigators are studying how to assess a family's strengths and problems in order to study children who have chronic illnesses. Prugh has offered a rough categorization of the family's operations that is based on levels of function and dysfunction.[92a] There is much work to

be done in learning how to assess the parents' capacities. Many studies of assessing the parents' capacities are now being made in the United States and other countries.

Bibliography

1. Ackerman, N.: *The Psychodynamics of Family Life.* New York, Basic Books, 1958.
2. Ackerman, N.W., and Behrens, M.L.: Child and family psychopathy: Problems of correlation. In: *Psychopathology of Childhood* (P.H. Hoch and J. Zubin, Eds.). New York, Grune & Stratton, 1955.
3. Ackerman, M., and Behrens, M.: A study of family diagnosis. Am. J. Orthopsychiatry, 26:66, 1956.
4. Ainsworth, M.D.: The effects of maternal deprivation: A review of findings and controversy in the context of research strategy. In: *Deprivation of Maternal Care: A Reassessment of Its Effects.* New York, Schocken Books, 1966.
5. Ainsworth, M., and Bell, S.: The development of infant-mother attachment. In: *Review of Child Development Research*, Vol. 3. (B.M. Caldwell and H.N. Ricciuti, Eds.). Chicago, University of Chicago Press, 1974.
6. Anthony, E.J.: Behavior disorders of childhood. In: *Carmichael's Manual of Child Psychology*, 3rd Ed. Vol. 2. (P. Mussen, Ed.). New York, Wiley, 1970.
7. Anthony, E.J.: A working model for family studies. In: *The Child in His Family: The Impact of Disease and Death* (E.J. Anthony and C. Koupernik, Eds.). New York, Wiley, 1973.
8. Anthony, E.J., and Bene, E.: A technique for the objective assessment of the child's family relationships. J. Ment. Sci., ,103:541, 1957.
9. Ausubel, D.P.: *Theory and Problems of Child Development.* New York, Grune & Stratton, 1957.
10. Bakwin, H.: Emotional deprivation in infants. J. Pediatr., 35:512, 1949.
11. Baldwin, A.L., Kelhorn, J., and Breese, F.H.: The appraisal of parent behavior. Psychol. Monogr., 63:4, 1949.
12. Bateson, G., et al.: A note on the double bind—1962. Fam. Process, 2:154, 1963.
13. Becker, W.C.: Consequences of different kinds of discipline. In: *Review of Child Development Research*, Vol. 1. (M.L. Hoffman and L.W. Hoffman, Eds.). New York, Russell Sage Foundation, 1964.
14. Behrens, M., and Sherman, A.: Observations of family interaction in the home. Am. J. Orthopsychiatry, 29:2, 1959.
15. Bell, N.W., and Vogel, R., Eds.: *A Modern Introduction to the Family.* Glencoe, Ill., Free Press, 1960.
16. Benedek, T.: Adaptation to reality in early infancy. Psychoanal. Q., 7:200, 1938.
17. Benedek, T.: Parenthood as a developmental phase. J. Am. Psychoanal. Assoc., 7:389, 1959.

18. Benedek, T.: Fatherhood and providing. In: *Parenthood: Its Psychology and Psychopathology* (E.J. Anthony and T. Benedek, Eds.). Boston, Little, Brown, 1970.

19. Bennett, I.: *Delinquent and Neurotic Children*. London, Tavistock, 1960.

20. Bibring, G.: A study of the psychological processes in pregnancy and of the earliest mother-child relationships. Psychoanal. Study Child, 16:9, 1961.

21. Bowlby, J.: *Maternal Care and Mental Health*. (WHO Report.) New York, Schocken Books, 1966.

22. Bowlby, J., et al.: The effects of mother-child separation: A follow-up study. Br. J. Med. Psychol., 29:211, 1956.

23. Brazelton, T.B., Koslowski, B., and Main, M.: The origins of reciprocity: The early mother-infant interaction. In: *The Origins of Behavior: The Effect of the Infant on its Caregiver*. (M. Lewis and L.A. Rosenblum, Eds.). New York, Wiley, 1974.

24. Brody, S.: *Patterns of Mothering*. New York, International Universities Press, 1956.

25. Broussard, E.R.: Neonatal prediction and outcome at 10/11 years. Child Psychiatry Hum. Dev., 7:85, 1976.

26. Brown, G.W., and Rutter, M.: Measurement of family activities and relationships—A methodological study. Hum. Relat., 19:241, 1966.

27. Buell, B., et al.: *Classification of Disorganized Families for Use in Family Oriented Diagnosis and Treatment*. New York, Community Research Association, 1953.

28. Caldwell, B.M.: The effects of infant care. In: *Review of Child Development Research*, Vol. 1. (M.L. Hoffman and L.W. Hoffman, Eds.). New York, Russell Sage Foundation, 1964.

29. Caplan, G.: Emotional implications of pregnancy and influences on family relationships. In: *The Healthy Child. His Physical, Psychological, and Social Development* (H.C. Stuart and D.G. Prugh, Eds.). Cambridge, Mass., Harvard University Press, 1960.

30. Chapin, H.P.: A plan for dealing with atrophic infants and children. Arch. Pediatr., 25:491, 1908.

31. Clarke, A.D.B., and Clarke, A.M.: Some recent advances in the study of early deprivation. J. Child Psychol. Psychiatry, 1:26, 1960.

32. Clausen, J.A.: Family structure, socialization, and personality. In: *Review of Child Development Research*, Vol. 2. (M.L. Hoffman and L.W. Hoffman, Eds.). New York, Russell Sage Foundation, 1966.

33. Coleman, R.W., Kris, E., and Provence, S.: The study of variations of early parental attitudes. Psychoanal. Study Child, 8:20, 1954.

34. Conger, J.J.: *Adolescence and Youth: Psychological Development in a Changing World*, 2nd Ed. New York, Harper & Row, 1977.

35. Craig, W.: The child in the maladjusted household. Practitioner, 177:21, 1956.

36. Dalton, K.: The influences of the mother's health on her child. Proc. R. Soc. Med., 59:1014, 1966.

37. Downes, J., and Simon, K.: Psychoneurotic patients and their families. Psychosom. Med., 15:463, 1953.

38. Dunbar, F.: Symbiosis of parent and child. Am. J. Orthopsychiatry, 22:809, 1952.

39. Ehrenwald, J.: Neurotic interaction and patterns of pseudo-heredity in the family. Am. J. Psychiatry, 115:134, 1958.

40. Erikson, E.H.: *Identity and the Life Cycle*. New York, International Universities Press, 1959.

41. Escalona, S., and Heide, G.: *Prediction and Outcome*. New York, Basic Books, 1959.

42. Fabian, A.A., and Donohue, J.F.: Maternal depression: A challenging child guidance problem. Am. J. Orthopsychiatry, 26:400, 1956.

43. Finzer, W.F., and Kisley, A.: Localized neurotic interaction. J. Am. Acad. Child Psychiatr., 3:265, 1964.

44. Fisher, L.: On the classification of families: A progress report. Arch. Gen. Psychiatry, 34:424, 1977.

45. Fisher, S., and Mendell, D.: A multi-generation approach to the treatment of psychopathology. J. Nerv. Ment. Dis., 126:523, 1958.

46. Fletcher, K.: Assessment and Prediction of Parenting: A Research Need. (Paper presented at the Second National Conference on Peri-Natal Social Work on March 15, 1978, in Denver, Colorado.)

47. Friedman, D.B.: Parent development. California Med., 86:25, 1957.

48. Fromm, E.: Mothers who were deprived in childhood. Br. Med. J., 1:113, 1971.

49. Geismar, L.: Three levels of treatment for multiproblem families. Soc. Casework, 42:124, 1961.

50. Glidewell, J.C.: *Parental Attitudes and Child Behavior*. Springfield, Ill., Thomas, 1961.

51. Goldson, E.: Personal communication.

52. Green, M.: Paternal deprivation—A disturbance in fathering. Pediatrics, 30:91, 1962.

53. Gurwitt, A.R.: Aspects of prospective fatherhood: A case report. Psychoanal. Study Child, 31:237, 1976.

54. Hare, E.H., and Shaw, G.K.: A study in family health: A comparison of the health of fathers, mothers, and children. Br. J. Psychiatry, 111:467, 1965.

55. Harmon, R.H.: Personal communication.

56. Havighurst, R.J.: Child development in relation to community social structure. Child Dev., 17:85, 1946.

57. Hollander, L., and Karp, E.: Youth psychopathology and family process research. Am. J. Psychiatry, 130:814, 1973.

58. Hunter, R.S., et al.: Antecedents of child abuse and neglect in premature infants: A prospective study in a newborn intensive care unit. Pediatrics, 61:629, 1978.

59. Jarvis, W.: Some effects of pregnancy and childbirth in men. J. Am. Psychoanal. Assoc., 10:689, 1962.

60. Jessner, L., Weigert, E., and Foy, J.L.: The development of parental attitudes during pregnancy. In: *Parenthood, Its Psychology and Psychopathology* (E.J. Anthony, and T. Benedek, Eds.). Boston, Little, Brown, 1970.

61. Josselyn, I.M.: The family as a psychological unit. Soc. Casework, *34*:336, 1953.
62. Kagan, J., and Moss, H.A.: *Birth to Maturity: A Study in Psychological Development*. New York, Wiley, 1962.
63. Kaplan, D., and Mason, E.: Maternal reactions to premature birth viewed as an acute emotional disorder. Am. J. Orthopsychiatry, *30*:539, 1960.
64. Kempe, C.H.: Personal communication.
65. Klatskin, E.H.: Shifts in child care practices in three social classes under an infant care program of flexible methodology. Am. J. Orthopsychiatry, *22*:52, 1952.
66. Klaus, M.H., and Kennell, J.H.: Mothers separated from their infants. Pediatr. Clin. North Am., *17*:1015, 1970.
67. Klaus, M.H., and Kennell, J.H.: *Maternal-Infant Bonding*. St. Louis, Mosby, 1976.
68. Klaus, M., et al.: Maternal attachment: Importance of the first post-partum days. N. Engl. J. Med., *286*:460, 1972.
69. Kluckhohn, F.R.: Variations in the basic values of family systems. Soc. Casework, *39*:63, 1958.
70. Kluckhohn, F., and Spiegel, J.P., Eds.: *Integration and Conflict in Family Behavior*. Group for the Advancement of Psychiatry, Report No. 27, August, 1954.
71. Kulka, A.M., Walter, R.M., and Fry, C.P.: Mother-infant interaction as measured by simultaneous recording of physical processes. J. Am. Acad. Child Psychiatry, *5*:496, 1966.
72. Lamb, M.E., Ed.: *The Role of the Father in Child Development*. New York, Wiley, 1976.
73. Levy, D.M.: *Studies in Sibling Rivalry*. The American Orthopsychiatric Association, 1937.
74. Levy, D.: *Maternal Overprotection*. New York, Columbia University Press, 1943.
75. Lewis, J.M., et al.: *No Single Thread: Psychological Health in Family Systems*. New York, Brunner/Mazel, 1976.
76. Liebenberg, B.: Expectant fathers. Am. J. Orthopsychiatry, *37*:358, 1967.
77. Lidz, T., et al.: The interfamilial environment of schizophrenic patients. II. Marital schism and marital skew. Am. J. Psychiatry, *114*:241, 1957.
78. Lidz, T., et al.: Intrafamilial environment of the schizophrenic patient. VI. The transmission of irrationality. Arch. Neurol. Psychiatry, *79*:305, 1958.
79. Lindemann, E.: Symptomatology and management of acute grief. Am. J. Psychiatry, *101*:141, 1944.
80. Mason, E.A.: A method of predicting crisis outcome for mothers of premature babies. Public Health Rep., *78*:1031, 1963.
81. Mahler, M.S., and Rabinovitch, R.: The effect of marital conflict on child development. In: *Neurotic Interaction in Marriage* (V.W. Eisenstein, Ed.). New York, Basic Books, 1956.
82. McFarlane, J.W., Allen, L., and Honzick, M.P.: *A Developmental Study of Normal Children Between Twenty-One Months and Fourteen Years*. Berkeley, Calif., University of California Press, 1954.
83. Mead, M.: Changing patterns of parent-child relationships in an urban culture. Int. J. Psychoanal., *38*:369, 1957.
84. Merril, B.: A measurement of mother-child interactions. J. Abnormal Soc. Psychol., *41*:37, 1946.
85. Meyer, R.J., Roclofs, H.A., Bluestone, J., and Redmond, S.: Accidental injury to the preschool child. J. Pediatr., *63*:95, 1963.
86. Meyer, R.J., and Haggerty, R.J.: Streptococcal infections in families: Factors altering individual susceptibility. Pediatrics, *29*:539, 1962.
87. Mittelman, B.: Analysis of reciprocal neurotic patterns in family relationships. In: *Neurotic Interaction in Marriage* (V.M. Eisenstein, Ed.). New York, Basic Books, 1956.
88. Moustakas, C.E., Segal, I.E., and Shalock, H.D.: An objective method for the measurement and analysis of child-adult interaction. Child Dev., *27*:109, 1956.
89. Natterson, J.M., and Knudson, A.G.: Observations concerning fear of death in fatally ill children and their mothers. Psychosom. Med., *22*:456, 1960.
90. Newell, H.W.: A further study of maternal rejection. Am. J. Orthopsychiatry, *6*:576, 1936.
91. Pavenstedt, E.: A study of immature mothers and their children. In: *Prevention of Mental Disorders in Children* (G. Caplan, Ed.). New York, Basic Books, 1961.
92. Prugh, D.G., and Harlow, R.G.: "Masked deprivation" in infants and young children. In: *Deprivation of Maternal Care: A Reassessment of its Effects*. New York, Schocken Books, 1966.
92a. Prugh, D.G.: Psychosocial disorders in childhood and adolescence: Theoretical considerations and an attempt at classification. In: The mental health of children: Services, research, and manpower. (Reports of the Task Forces IV and V and the Report of the Committee on Clinical Issues by the Joint Commission on the Mental Health of Children.) New York, Harper & Row, 1973.
93. Radke, M.: Relation of parental authority to children's behavior and attitudes. (Monograph No. 62.) Minneapolis, University of Minnesota Press, 1946.
94. Rexford, E., and Van Amerongen, S.: The influence of unsolved maternal conflicts upon impulsive acting out in young children. Am. J. Orthopsychiatry, *27*:75, 1957.
95. Richmond, J.B., and Caldwell, B.M.: Child-rearing practices and their consequences. In: *Modern Perspectives in Child Development*. (A.J. Solnit and S. Provence, Eds.). New York, International Universities Press, 1963.
96. Rutter, M.: *Children of Sick Parents*. London, Oxford University Press, 1966.
97. Sander, L.W.: Adaptive relationships in early mother-child interaction. J. Am. Acad. Child Psychiatry, *3*:231, 1964.
98. Schaefer, E.S., and Bell, R.Q.: Development of a parental attitude research instrument. Child Dev., *29*:339, 1958.
99. Schmidt, B.D., Jordan, K., and Hamburg, F.L.: The role of the pediatrician in helping children

develop a sense of responsibility. Clin. Pediatr., 11:509, 1972.

100. Sears, R.R., Maccoby, E.E., and Levin, H.: *Patterns of Child Rearing.* New York, Harper and Row, 1957.

101. Senn, M.J.E., and Hartford, C.: The Firstborn: Experiences of Eight American Families. Cambridge, Harvard University Press, 1968.

102. Solomon, M.A.: A developmental conceptual premise for family therapy. Family Process, 12:179, 1973.

103. Spitz, R.A.: Hospitalism. Psychoanal. Study Child, 1:53, 1945.

104. Stachowiak, J.G.: Psychological disturbances in children as related to disturbances in family interaction. J. Marr. Fam., 30:123, 1968.

105. Stendler, C.B.: Sixty years of child training practices. J. Pediatr., 36:122, 1950.

106. Sutton-Smith, B., and Rosenberg, B.: *The Sibling.* New York, Holt, Rinehart, & Winston, 1970.

107. Thomas, A., and Chess, S.: *Temperament and Development.* New York, Brunner/Mazel, 1977.

108. Thompson, R.J., and Finscheid, T.R.: Adult-child interaction analysis: methodology and case interaction. Child Psychiatry Hum. Dev., 7:31, 1976.

109. Tseng, W.-S., et al.: Family diagnosis and classification. J. Am. Acad. Child Psychiatry, 14:15, 1975.

110. Vogel, E.F., and Bell, N.W.: The emotionally disturbed child as the family scapegoat. In: *A Modern Introduction to the Family.* (N.W. Bell, and E.F. Vogel, Eds.). New York, Free Press, 1960.

111. Voiland, A.L., et al.: *Family Casework Diagnosis.* New York, Columbia University Press, 1962.

112. Whiting, J.W.M.: *Child Training and Personality: A Cross-Cultural Study.* New Haven, Conn., Yale University Press, 1953.

113. Wolfenstein, M.: Trends in infant care. Am. J. Orthopsychiatry, 23:120, 1953.

114. Wolff, S., and Acton, W.P.: Characteristics of parents of disturbed children. Br. J. Psychiatry, 114:593, 1968.

115. Wynne, L.C., et al.: Pseudo-mutuality in the family relations of schizophrenics. Psychiatry, ,21:205, 1958.

116. Yarrow, L.J.: Separation from parents during early childhood. In: *Review of Child Development Research,* Vol. 1. (M.L. Hoffman and L.W. Hoffman, Eds.). New York, Russell Sage Foundation, 1964.

General References

Ackerman, N.W., and Sobel, R.: Family diagnosis: An approach to the pre-school child. Am. J. Orthopsychiatry, 20:244, 1956.

Anthony, E.J., and Benedek, T., Eds.: *Parenthood: Its Psychology and Psychopathology.* Boston, Little, Brown, 1970.

Anthony, E.J., and Koupernik, C., Eds.: *The Child in His Family.* New York, Wiley, 1970.

Anthony, E.J., and Koupernik, C., Eds.: *The Child in His Family: Children at Psychiatric Risk.* New York, Wiley, 1974.

Aries, P.: *Centuries of Childhood.* New York, Knopf, 1962.

Atkin, E., and Rubin, E.: *Part-time Father.* New York, Vanguard Press, 1976.

Behrens, M.: The home visit as an aid in family diagnosis and therapy. Soc. Casework, 37:1, 1956.

Benedek, T.: Parenthood during the life cycle. In: *Parenthood: Its Psychology and Psychopathology* (E.J. Anthony and T. Benedek, Eds.). Boston, Little, Brown, 1970.

Benedek, T.: The psychology of pregnancy. In: *Parenthood: Its Psychology and Psychopathology* (E.J. Anthony and T. Benedek, Eds.). Boston, Little, Brown, 1970.

Benedict, R.: *Patterns of Culture.* Boston, Houghton Mifflin, 1945.

Block, J.: Personality characteristics associated with father's attitudes toward child-rearing. Child Dev., 26:41, 1955.

Bossard, J.S., and Boll, E.S.: *The Sociology of Child Development.* New York, Harper & Row, 1966.

Brim, O.G.,Jr.: *Education for Child Rearing.* New York, Russell Sage Foundation, 1959.

Byhan, W.C., and Katzell, M.F.: Women in the Work Force: Confrontation with Change. New York, Division of Personal Psychology of the New York State Psychological Association, 1971.

Caplan, G.: Emotional implications of pregnancy and influences on family relationships. In: *The Healthy Child: His Physical, Psychological, and Social Development* (H.C. Stuart and D.G. Prugh, Eds.). Cambridge, Mass., Harvard University Press, 1960.

Coppolillo, H.P.: The questioning and doubting parent. J. Pediatr., 67:371, 1965.

Eisenstein, V.W.: *Neurotic Interaction in Marriage.* New York, Basic Books, 1956.

Elder, R.A.: Traditional and developmental conceptions of fatherhood. Marriage and Family Living, 11:98, 1949.

English, O.S., and Foster, C.J.: *A Guide to Successful Fatherhood.* Chicago, Science Research Associates, 1954.

Fisher, S., and Mendell, D.: Approach to neurotic behavior in terms of a three-generation model. J. Nerv. Ment. Dis., 123:171, 1956.

Fisher, S., and Mendell, D.: The communication of neurotic patterns over two and three generations. Psychiatry, 19:41, 1956.

Galdston, I., Ed.: *The Family in Contemporary Society.* New York, New York Academy of Medicine, 1960.

Gardner, L.P.: A survey of the attitudes and activities of fathers. J. Genet. Psychol., 63:15, 1943.

Glidewell, J.: *Parental Attitudes and Child Behavior.* Springfield, Ill., Thomas, 1961.

Gordon, T.: *P.E.T.—Parent Effectiveness Training. The Tested New Way to Raise Responsible Children.* New York, Peter Wyden, 1970.

Green, M., and Beall, P.: Paternal deprivation—A disturbance in fathering. Pediatrics, 30:91, 1962.

Grunebaum, H., and Christ, J., Eds.: *Contemporary*

Marriage: Structure, Dynamics, and Therapy. Boston, Little, Brown, 1976.

Haley, J., and Glick,I.: *Psychiatry and the Family. An Annotated Bibliography Published 1960–64.* Palo Alto, Calif., Family Process Publications, 1966.

Hetherington, E.M., and Barclay, M.: Family interaction and psychopathology in children. In: *Psychopathological Disorders in Children* (H.C. Quay and J.S. Werry, Eds.). New York, Wiley, 1972.

Jacobsen, E., and Bychowski, G.: Interaction between psychotic partners. In: *Neurotic Interaction in Marriage* (V.W. Eisenstein, Ed.). New York, Basic Books, 1956.

Josselyn, I.M.: Cultural forces, motherliness, and fatherliness. Am. J. Orthopsychiatry, 26:264, 1956.

Josselyn,I.: Psychology of fatherliness. Smith Coll. Stud. Soc. Work, 26:1, 1956.

Kantor, M.B., Ed.: *Mobility and Mental Health.* Springfield, Ill., Thomas, 1965.

Kleinman, A.K.: Clinical relevance of anthropological and cross-cultural research. Am. J. Psychiatry, 135:427, 1978.

Kohlberg, L.: Development of moral character and moral ideology. In: *Review of Child Development Research* (M.L. Hoffman and L.W. Hoffman, Eds.). New York, Russell Sage Foundation,1964.

LaBarre, M., Ussery, L., and Jessner, L.: Significance of the grandparents in the psychopathology of children. Am. J. Orthopsychiatry, 30:175, 1960.

Lasko, J.K.: Parent behavior toward first and second children. Genet. Psychol. Monogr., 40:97, 1954.

Leighton, A.: Psychiatric disorder and social environment: An outline for a frame of reference. Psychiatry, 18:367, 1955.

Levy, D.M.: Psychosomatic studies of some aspects of maternal behavior. Psychosom. Med.,4:223, 1942.

Levy, D.M.: *The Demonstration Clinic.* Springfield, Ill., Thomas, 1959.

Liebman, S., Ed.: *Emotional Forces in the Family.* Philadelphia, Lippincott, 1959.

Lynn, D.B.: *The Father—His Role in Child Development.* Berkeley, Calif., Brooks/Cole, 1974.

Mittelman, B.: Complementary neurotic reactions in intimate relationships. Psychoanal. Q., 13:479, 1944.

Mussen, P., and Distler, L.: Masculinity, identification and father-son relationships. J. Abnorm. Soc. Psychol., 59:350, 1959.

Neubauer, P., Ed.: *Institute on Child Development in Kibbutzim, Oranim, Israel, 1963. Children in Collectives.* Springfield, Ill., Thomas, 1965.

Parad, H.J., and Caplan, G.: A framework for studying families in crisis. Soc. Work, 5:5, 1960.

Parsons, T.C.: *The Social System.* Glencoe, Ill., Free Press, 1951.

Parsons, T.: Social structure and the development of personality. In: *Studying Personality Cross Culturally.* (B. Kaplan, Ed.). Evanston, Ill., Row, Peterson, 1961.

Parsons, T., and Bales, R.F.: *Family, Socialization, and Interaction Process.* Glencoe, Ill., Free Press, 1955.

Parsons, T., and Fox, R.C.: Illness, therapy, and the modern urban American family. In: *A Modern Introduction to the Family* (N.W. Bell and E.F. Vogel, Eds.). Glencoe, Ill., Free Press, 1960.

Plotsky, H., and Shereshefsky, P.M.: An isolation pattern in fathers of emotionally disturbed children. Am. J. Orthopsychiatry, 30:780, 1960.

Psychiatric Disorder and the Urban Environment. (Report of the Cornell Social Sciences Seminar.) New York, Behavioral Publications, 1971.

Reiss, F.E.: The extended kinship system: Correlates of and attitudes on frequency of interaction. Marr. Fam. Liv., 24, 1962.

Rosenthal, M.J., et al.: Father-child relationships and children's problems. Arch. Gen. Psychiatry, 7:360, 1962.

Ross, J.M.: The development of paternal identity: A critical review of the literature on nurturance and generativity in boys and men. J. Am. Psychoanal. Assoc., 23:783, 1975.

Ryder, R.G.: A Topography of Early Marriage. Fam. Proc., 9:385, 1970.

Sabbath, J.C.: Infantilization of a pre-school child. In: *Emotional Problems of Early Childhood* (G. Caplan, Ed.). New York, Basic Books, 1955.

Sloman, S.S.: Emotional problems in "planned for" children. Am. J. Orthopsychiatry, 18:523, 1948.

Spencer, S.W., and McLarnan, G.: Fostering spiritual values in family life. Soc. Casework, 44:575, 1963.

Spiegel, J.P.: The resolution of role conflict within the family. Psychiatry, 20:1, 1957.

Spiro, M.E.: *Children of the Kibbutz: A Study in Child Training and Personality.* New York, Schocken Books, 1961.

Switzer, R.E., et al.: The effect of family moves on children. Ment. Hyg., 45:528, 1961.

Towne, R.D., and Afterman, J.: Psychosis in males related to parenthood. Bull. Menninger Clin., 19:19, 1955.

Von Mering, O.O.: Forms of fathering in relation to mother-child pairs. In: *The Significance of the Father.* New York, Family Service Association of America, 1959.

Waldrop, M.F., and Bell, R.Q.: Effects of family size and density on newborn characteristics. Am. J. Orthopsychiatry, 36:544, 1966.

Winch, R.F.: Complementary needs in mate selection. Am. Sociol. Rev., 20:1, 1955.

Yarrow, L.J., and Goodwin, M.S.: Some conceptual issues in the study of mother-infant interaction. Am. J.Orthopsychiatry, 35:3, 1965.

II
General Clinical Considerations

If he (the physician) enlarges his study to cover life as affected by disease and masters the psychology of the individual sick in body, he will widen his usefulness.
(Sir John Parkinson)

7

General Principles of
Clinical Examination

*In the last analysis, we see only what we are
ready to see, what we have been taught to see.
We eliminate and ignore anything that is not a
part of our prejudices.*
(Jean Martin Charcot)

The pediatrician can and must develop a comprehensive method of evaluating the psychosocial as well as the physical aspects of diseases. Physicians who have been trained in hospitals often rely too much on laboratory data when they evaluate sick children. If they do so, they may not use clinical impressions and information about behavior that they can obtain by carefully observing the children and the interactions between parents and their children.

For example, flaring of the nostrils, shallow breathing and grunting during expiration, listlessness, suprasternal and substernal retractions, and visible disturbances of the peripheral circulation may indicate an impending cardiorespiratory collapse in an infant who has serious tracheobronchitis when the disease is in an early stage but is rapidly advancing. The physician may find such signs by inspecting the infant be-

fore physical, roentgenographic and laboratory data tell him how serious the disease is. Failure to recognize the early signs of serious disease often lets diseases progress when they might have been stopped. Similarly, if a physician relies on the absence of abnormal physical and roentgenographic data in the case of a 3-year-old child who has a history of persistent, nonproductive cough, he may order a strenuous and expensive course of laboratory study of the child, or he may make an unhelpful diagnosis of "no disease." If the physician had more carefully observed the interaction between the mother and the child and investigated the family's history, he might have learned that the cough began during a slight cold that the child caught when another child was born in his family and occurred later only when the mother picked up the younger child. Such information can reveal the psychophysiologic component of such a symptom and may help the physician treat the symptom more rationally.

Since the parents cannot assess accurately the physician's technical competence, the physician's manner most affects the parents' confidence in him. The parents may have confidence in the physician whether or not he gives the child medication or any other treatment. Some parents unconsciously attribute almost magical powers to the physician; other parents have an unhealthy dependence on the physician and cannot take simple and obvious steps without consulting him. Negative attitudes of parents toward physicians include fear of criticism, distrust or suspicion, fear of domination, and resentment. A few parents who have such attitudes may be unable to use the physician's services effectively. Most parents, however, can establish an effective relationship with the physicians who are caring for their children.

The attitudes of the child toward his physician are affected by his parents' attitudes toward and his own experiences with the physician. Most emotionally healthy children can overcome their anxieties about seeing the physician and learn to trust him. A child who is acutely ill, however, may regress emotionally and behave like a much younger child, even when he is with a physician whom he knows. Fears of pain, of the unknown, of going to the hospital, and of being separated from his parents are important to an acutely ill child.

The wise and experienced physician learns to see the behavior of the parents and their child as information about their personalities and their interactions; such information is a part of his clinical findings and may be important to him when he decides how to treat the child. The physician develops capacities for sympathy and understanding and also empathy—the ability to put himself in the places of the parents and their child and to see things from their points of view. The physician who has

those capacities is less likely to interpret a depressed parent's apathy as unconcern about his child's condition or to label parents as uncooperative, unreliable, or rejecting on the basis of his first impressions of them.

The physician's manner is most valuable in establishing a good relationship with the parents and obtaining accurate information about the family's history. He communicates nonverbally his interest and confidence in the parent through his facial expression, tone of voice, and posture. The physician must seem unhurried, accepting, respectful, and noncritical, even if time is limited. And privacy is essential when the physician talks with the parents. The physician should be as prompt as possible; a system of individual appointments can work in a clinic, and is most important. The physician should learn the parents' names and should not call a woman "mother" to save himself the trouble of learning her name. If he often encounters parents whom he considers "troublesome" and with whom he cannot get along, he should examine his own attitudes and behavior toward the parents or consult a psychiatrist. Occasionally he may have to suggest to certain parents that they might feel more comfortable with or be better served by another physician.

Parents' demands for quick advice and easy solutions usually show their own anxieties. They soon lose confidence in physicians who quickly draw conclusions from insufficient information. Parents do not lose respect for physicians who say that they do not yet know what is wrong or what to do, and that their child's conditions needs further investigation and thought. The physician should not give advice too quickly or make premature promises that treatment will succeed because he can promote overdependence or disappointment by doing so.

The physician usually sees infants and children of preschool age with their mother. The physician may give the child a toy that is appropriate for a child of his age from a supply of toys that he should keep in his office, or he may give him another object as a toy (e.g., a throat stick). Giving the child a toy shows the parents the physician's interest in their child and helps to make the physician's first contact with the child a positive one. If the parents are worried about the child's behavior or talk too freely about the child's personality, the physician may want the nurse or the secretary to interest the child in play in the waiting room while the physician talks with the parents.

The physician can learn a good deal in a few moments of casual observation of the young child's play while he talks with the parents. The physician can learn about the child's level of development from the degree of the complexity and organization of his play and the length of his span of concentration, for example. The child's attitude toward the physician often reflects his parents' anxiety. He may show that such attitudes in his drawings, his play with toys, and his demeanor, including his emotional and behavioral responses.

In the cases of older children and young adolescents, it is best to see the parents and the child together during the first interview since an anxious or suspicious child may fear that the parent is giving the physician secret information about him. If the physician must see the parents alone so that they can freely discuss emotional problems, he may see them alone after the first interview. Occasionally, if the parents want to discuss a very disturbing aspect of their child's behavior, the first interview may take place without the child's knowledge. During that interview, the parents and the physician can decide whether or not the physician should see the child alone. Older adolescents may be seen alone during the first interview. Preferably, the physician should see both parents together (with or without the child). By doing so, he may obtain valuable impressions about their relationship, their attitudes as parents, and their attitudes toward their child and his disease or problems in adjustment.

Observing the Child and the Parent

Physicians frequently overlook information that is available from careful observation of the child and the interactions between parents and their children. From the moment that the parents and their child enter his office, the physician can obtain clinical impressions, as can an alert nurse, secretary, or health associate, about how the parents relate to their child and how the child relates to his parents, the interaction between the parents, and the child's patterns of play and reactions to strangers. Some parents cannot let the child play independently in the waiting room or answer a question by himself; they show that they have a need to dominate the child or the situation. Other parents constantly correct the child or require that he stay perfectly still; they show that they have unrealistically high standards of behavior and conformity. A mother and her child may huddle together; that shows that one (or both) of them finds it hard to be separated from the other. Inactivity, hyperactivity, disturbances in gait, and some other physical characteristics can be assessed more easily and accurately while the physician casually observes the child's play than during a formal examination.

If the physician interviews the child's parents together, they may reveal to him their disagreements about methods of child-rearing. Their posture or gestures may reveal anger toward each other. A 2-year-old child usually stays nearer to his mother than to his father in a strange situation, but he may cling to his father if his mother is angry or overly critical of him. A few parents may pay little attention to their children; for example, the physician may see a mother who does not stand close enough to her infant to keep him from falling off the examining table. Disturbed parents who have unconscious needs to deny the extent or the seriousness of the child's disease may belittle the child or urge him to act as if he were well.

The physician should record such observations and consider them with his later observations. The physician can make many such observations if he visits the home and has continuous contact with the parents and their child. The physician can assess the parents' standards of care and the family's patterns of living and functioning more easily during home visits than in the office.* A nursery school teacher, recreational therapist, or trained volunteer, who gives children the chance to play individually and in small groups in a clinic waiting room can also make such observations.

Interviews with the Parents

At first it is important for the physician to let the parents talk freely about what concerns them most. Usually, the physician can begin by asking what seems to be the matter. The physician should not ask leading questions or prematurely probe into sensitive subjects. Even if the physician's time is limited and the parents' first comments seem confused, too detailed, or irrelevant to the child's obvious condition, the physician should let the parents talk freely and reveal private things at their own pace (at least for a little while). Letting the parents talk freely strengthens their impression that the physician values their observations. Also, the act of talking helps them to discharge their initial tensions and thus to overcome their anxiety or fear about the physician's findings or opinion. Giving the parents a few extra minutes to talk dur-

*Although physicians now are often unable to make home visits, certain situations may call for them. Social workers and public health nurses have often made home visits, and nurse practitioners and child health associates are beginning to make home visits.

ing the first interview saves time later. The physician can learn a good deal in 20 to 30 minutes, and he can make another appointment for a longer interview with the parents if he thinks that is necessary. If the physician seems unhurried, he may learn sooner that the stated reason for the parents' visit or their stated complaint may not be the source of their concern. For example, the mother of a mildly obese 9-year-old boy who consults a physician about his weight may admit with some embarrassment during a relaxed interview that her real concern is that his genitals seem too small.

As the interview proceeds, the physician may ask questions about important details or about subjects that the parents have not discussed. Rather than asking rapid-fire questions or asking questions from a checklist that elicit only a "yes" or "no" and do not encourage the parents to elaborate on their answers, the physician can ask general or open-ended questions such as, "Can you tell me a little more about his difficulty in breathing?" or "How about his toilet training?" and ask the parents to elaborate if that is necessary. The physician may sometimes repeat an emotionally powerful word or phrase, using his inflection to encourage the parent to elaborate. Such an approach lets the parents tell the physician many important facts that they might otherwise forget to mention or omit as unimportant. In the health examination, the parents may tell the physician pertinent facts or ask him important questions about feeding, weaning, toilet training, discipline, and accident prevention, for example. Some parents may become oversensitive or suspicious if the physician focuses too closely on their own behavior or background (at least if he does so in the first interview, before he has developed a trusting and secure relationship with the parents). What the parents do not say may also be important. The observant physician often asks himself what the parents may feel toward him and what they may expect of him. They may decide whether he is interested in their child according to how sympathetic, tolerant, and respectful his attitude is.

Some parts of their history may affect the parents emotionally. It may be painful and difficult for them to talk about those parts. The history of familial illnesses and emotional disturbances usually has a great deal of emotional effect on the parents. For example, the parents of children who have seizures sometimes cannot reveal during the first interview that one (or more) of their close relatives has epilepsy because they fear that they have been guilty of transmitting the disease. Parents also recognize that their feelings about the child may play a part in disturbances in his behavior. So when the physician tries to find out whether the parents have any psychologic problems or when he asks questions about their behavior, he must be very tactful. The anxious parent may misinterpret his questions as a critical attack. Questions such as, "Did you want this child?" "Do you spend time with your children?" "Was she jealous of the new baby?" and "Is your marriage happy?" if asked during the first interview, usually elicit conventional and socially acceptable replies or provoke defensive indignation.

Such information is important, but the physician must obtain it at first by inference or by asking questions that are more indirect and less judgmental, such as "Were you able to plan the pregnancy for this child?" "What is it like to be the parent of a 4 year old?" "How much time do you get to spend with the children?" "How did she seem to take the new baby's arrival?" and "How do you work out differences between you?" Before asking emotionally charged questions that may imply value judgments, such as questions about the child's sexual activity, the physician can make the parents more comfortable about answering by saying that all children show some sexual curiosity and usually ask questions about sex (e.g., about the differences

between boys and girls). Later, when the physician has established a good relationship with the parents, he can obtain more detailed and accurate information about such matters. The physician should not forget to ask about positive, pleasant aspects of the family's functioning, such as how they have fun together, thus emphasizing its strengths as well as its problems. He should ask what things about the child please the parents and what they praise in him, as well as what displeases them.[12]

The parents may sometimes not answer a question, especially if it is an emotionally charged one. If they do not answer, the physician should wait for a moment or two, or repeat an emotionally charged word and then wait. Such an approach may give the physician much important verbal or behavioral information; if the physician changes the subject or reassures the parents too quickly, he may not acquire that information. Nonverbal behavior, such as blushing, crying, nailbiting, or signs of neuromuscular tension, may show the physician what subjects he should investigate. The physician must learn to wait silently even if the parents seem to be about to cry. The physician can, with practice, curb his social impulse to stop the parents from expressing strong emotion (by crying, for example). It may help the parents to release emotion in a sympathetic atmosphere and may strengthen their relationship with the physician. The physician may tell them that he understands, offer them some tissues, and not try immediately to assuage their emotions.

When the physician ends the first interview, he should return to the problem that the parents identified as their major concern; that problem is not always the same as their stated complaint. Returning to the parents' major concern lets the physician ask questions that have arisen from the information that he obtained during the interview. If the physician ends the interview in that way, he shows the parents that he fully understands their concern and will try to deal with it constructively.

Interviews with the Child

The physician often cannot obtain factual information by talking with a pre-school-age child or with a child who is acutely ill. But he probably can obtain valuable information by talking with older children. An older child can tell the physician how he sees his disease, any physical limitation caused by his disease, or his health in general. Occasionally only the child can give the physician any pertinent information; for example, the child can tell the physician what toxic substance he ingested or can describe the quality and the location of his pain or discomfort. While the physician interviews the parents, he can also ask the child questions and so make him feel that he takes part in solving the problem.

When the physician interviews older children and adolescents, he can conduct the first interview in different ways under different circumstances. If the parents call the physician about what they think is an emotional problem, it may be best for him to see them together first without the child so that they can talk more freely. On the other hand, if the physician learns that there is a bitter struggle between an adolescent and his parents, it may be best for him to see the adolescent first in order to assure the adolescent that he has a chance to tell his story. (But the adolescent should know that when the physician tries to help, he cannot take sides.) If the child is anxious or suspicious, the physician should see the parents and the child together first. He can see the parents and the child separately later. When the physician has made his evaluation, it may be best for him to see the parents and the child together.

During the evaluation, the physician should see the child alone, if he can separate the child from the parent. The physician can see the child alone in an office more easily than in his examining room because the child will be less anxious. The physician should have told the parents before the interview to tell the child why he is going to see the physician. If it is in relation to an apparent emotional problem, they can tell the child that the physician is interested in problems which may make children worried or unhappy, because of some problem of which the child is aware, such as losing his temper, particular fears, or difficulty in getting along with other children at school. This can help to prevent overanxious or confused parents from deceiving or threatening the child, which will only cause mistrust. The mother of an older preschool-age child who is anxious about separation can bring him into the physician's office. Often she can leave a few minutes later, unless she has trouble separating from the child.

Whether or not the parents have been able to tell the child the truth about why they are bringing him to the physician, the physician should ask the child why he thinks he has come to see the physician. If the child says that he does not know why, which often happens, the physician can ask him whether he is aware that he has any problems or worries. If the child says that he is not aware that he has any problems, the physician should tell the child briefly and sympathetically, so that the child does not have to confirm or deny his problem, that he knows that the child has a problem (e.g., that he wets his bed or he loses his temper); he can add that he and the child can work together to solve the problem, but that he understands that the child may have trouble talking about his problem during the first interview. If the child has an emotional problem, the physician may tell him (if he is an older child or adolescent) that his problem does not mean that he is "crazy."

The physician may obtain a larger amount of more accurate information from an older child after he has established a good relationship with the child. A school-age child or an adolescent may be inhibited and withdrawn during the first interview because he is anxious, even if he does not have a serious emotional problem or limited intelligence. A wise physician does not judge too quickly a child's capacity to adjust or his intelligence.

A physician who is relaxed and friendly and who keeps his conversation at the child's level (without talking down to the child) can quickly win the child's cooperation and confidence. The physician may show the child toys on a table and suggest that they can talk while he plays. When the child is absorbed in playing, he may talk spontaneously, or the physician may start a conversation by commenting on his play.

By observing the child's play, the physician can learn a great deal about his emotional conflicts or anxieties. For example, a 4-year-old boy who makes a smaller boy doll beat up a larger boy doll shows his feelings toward his 6-year-old brother. The physician should not interpret the child's feelings immediately because that may make the child anxious. The physician may bring up the subject of the child's feelings about his brother later. He may recall the boy's play incident and suggest that the boy feels like the smaller boy doll. The physician should gently and firmly limit aggressive or destructive play. He may let the child do or say things things he would not do or say at home, but he should not be completely permissive.

With the child who talks freely, the physician should gain impressions of the meaning to the child of his symptoms or disability, if there is a physical component. The physician should ask the child how his problem affects his experiences at school, his status in his peer group, and his status in his home, for example. The physician can first ask general questions, such as "How do you like school?" "How about your family?" and "Do you play with any kids who live near you?" He can ask more specific questions later. The physician may have to obtain such information from frightened or withdrawn children by asking them what they want to do or be when they grow up. If a school-age child cannot name anything that he wants to do when he grows up, the physician can usually infer that the child has fears or feelings of hopelessness about growing up. The physician may learn about the family's functioning from the child's feelings about getting married and having children. The physician can ask the child what 3 things he most wishes for. The child's wishes may tell the physician something about him; for example, a seriously depressed child may not be able to wish for anything. A dream that the child has had recently may show his fears or aggression. If the child cannot recall a dream, the physician may ask him what he would like to dream about or if he had a bad dream what it might be about. The child's first memory (whether it is happy or sad) and his favorite (or least favorite) animal, book, or television show can tell the physician something about him. A child who has conflicts about growing up may say that he is younger than he really is. If a child who is physically ill does not say, when he is asked what he wishes for, that he wants to get well, he usually has a conflict about returning to school or another fear, often an unconscious one.

The physician can ask a sick child what he would do if he were well or a child who cannot talk easily about himself what a hypothetical child would wish for or do in a particular situation. Most school-age children cannot talk easily at first about subjects that provoke anxiety (e.g., their feelings of hostility toward their parents or their sexual activity). The physician should not bring up such subjects during the first interview. If he does, the child may become more inhibited or deny any such feelings, for example. The physician who takes his time in learning about a child can usually (if the child has reached the late preschool-age stage) help the child to understand his symptoms or his behavior as a problem that can be helped.

Interviewing the Adolescent

The physician should use a different approach when he interviews late preadolescent and adolescent children.* They usually understand why they are seeing the physician. If their parents adequately prepare them to see the physician, they may openly ask him for help with their problems. If the parents have treated the visit to the physician as a punishment or if the referral has come from school or judicial authority, the physician should first ask the adolescent to explain the situation from his point of view. If the physician seems authoritarian and gives lectures and unsolicited advice, he will have trouble establishing a good relationship. He should put a frightened adolescent at ease. Hostile or defensive adolescents usually have reasons for being hostile or defensive; a physician who can see how they feel and accept their attitudes without criticizing them can usually learn what those reasons are. If the physician's attitude is open and neutral and if he shows an interest and a desire to help, but does not side either with him or his parents, he can usually convince even the most suspicious adolescent that he is sincere.

Physicians sometimes use current slang in order to show young people that he understands them. But the physician who uses slang often sounds like he is "talking down" to a young person. Adolescents know that adults are different from them and have more experience than they do, and so can help them. Adolescents usually prefer to be treated with respect, as young adults. They may not want to use slang when they talk to the physician. The phy-

sician's attitude toward, interest in, and acceptance of him are most important to the adolescent.

The physician uses different techniques when he interviews adolescents and children. For example, most adolescents do not respond seriously when the physician asks them to make 3 wishes. Most adolescents do not want to draw during the first interview; they may be ashamed of their ability to draw or they may feel that the physician is testing them. They talk easily about their interests, hobbies, social activities, friends, and sometimes about their experiences at school. (The physician can ask them what things they like most or least about school and how they feel about their teachers and fellow students.) Adolescents can usually tell the physician their important dreams; if not, he can ask them what they would like or would not like to dream about. The physician can learn about them by asking them what they would do if they had a million dollars or whom they would choose to be with them if they were marooned on a desert island. They can usually tell the physician about their early memories. An adolescent may bring up his sexual concerns early in the interview. If he does not, the physician should not bring up the subject of sex or masturbation during the first interview although the physician should ask him about friends of the opposite sex.* An adolescent is usually concerned about his future; he often talks about what he would like to be or what he may be able to do.

The physician can learn about an adolescent's attitudes toward his family by asking him whether he wants to marry, how many children he wants to have, and what sex he wants his children to be. The adolescent who says that he will never get married because marriage is "only fight-

---

*Some pediatricians have entrances and examining rooms for adolescents that are separate from the ones for children, like the separate adolescent clinics that exist in some teaching programs in hospitals.

*The adolescent's sexual concerns may appear in relation to a physical examination; the physician should tactfully ask older adolescents about their sexual activity in order to decide whether or not to make certain examinations, such as a pelvic examination.

ing" and that he does not want to have children because children "only bring trouble" clearly describes his family's life, as does the adolescent girl who says she wants to have only male children because "boys get everything they want." The physician can often learn about the adolescent by asking him how he sees himself and what kind of a person he thinks he is, what things he can and cannot do, and what things about himself he would change. The adolescent who says, "I can't do anything right," or says, "I haven't got any good points" shows not only how he sees himself but also how his parents see him. Adolescents often have concerns about lags in growth, menstruation, and the onset of puberty.

The physician may have to wait a few minutes for an inhibited or generally quiet adolescent to answer a question. An adolescent may misinterpret a long silence as disinterest or hostility on the physician's part, however; the physician should not wait too long to ask another question. If an adolescent continues to be silent, the physician should not push him to talk. The physician should tell the adolescent that he understands that the adolescent may find it hard to talk at that point but may want to talk later. The physician can show an overtly hostile or angry adolescent that he understands the adolescent's feelings by making a direct statement, such as, "I think that you're angry today." He may put a suspicious adolescent at ease by saying, "It seems to be hard for you to trust adults."

Adolescents often worry about the intensity of their fantasies and feelings. If an adolescent has an emotional problem, the physician should reassure him that he is not "crazy" and that there is nothing wrong with the way his mind works.

The physician should help the adolescent state his problem in simple terms when the interview ends. For example, the physician may say, "Your feelings about yourself seem to be mixed up," or, "You and your parents seem to have trouble understanding each other." The physician should

tell the adolescent that he can help the adolescent deal with his problem, or he should say "We'll talk more about things next time."

The physician should tell an adolescent what he will tell the adolescent's parents. The physician can use the statement of the adolescent's problem that he and the adolescent made at the end of the first interview as a summary of what he will tell the adolescent's parents. For example, he may say, "I'm going to tell your parents that I think you've got a lot going for you, but that you seem to be mixed up about yourself and that I think that you need some help to sort things out." Or he may say, "I'm going to tell your parents that it seems hard for you and them to understand each other and talk things over but that I think that problem can be solved." Some adolescents may want to be present at talks with their parents.

Case Example. A 7½-year-old boy was referred to a pediatric clinic by his school because the school's staff thought that he might be hyperactive. The boy had been restless, had trouble concentrating in class, and showed outbursts of aggressive behavior toward other children. Tests made at the school showed that he was of above average intelligence. The boy's problems had appeared when he began second grade (he had had no problems when he was in the first grade). He had developed normally; he had no physical abnormalities. His family's history showed that his mother had rheumatic heart disease. She had had a recurrence of congestive heart failure (and she was recovering from it) late in the summer after the boy had finished first grade. The boy's father was often away on business.

When the physician interviewed the boy alone, he sat quite still and did not want to play. He said little about school; his 3 wishes all concerned his mother's getting well. He would not talk about the future but said, "How can they let a mother be sick? It makes me angry." When the physician repeated the word angry, the boy burst into tears, and said "something terrible might happen to my mother any minute if something isn't done."

Case Example. A 15-year-old girl was brought to the pediatrician because her room was always messy. When her mother asked her (and often threatened and shouted at her) to clean her room, she made her room even messier. The girl's mother said that she feared that the girl would turn out to be an irresponsible adult, "like my younger sister." The father took the girl's side; he said that the mother was "picking on my daughter." The parents said that they had occasionally quarreled about the problem, but neither thought the quarrels were serious. When the physician saw the girl alone, she said that she had come "because my mother thinks my room's a mess." When the physician asked her how she felt about the problem, she first said "It's my room; it's the only place where I can do what I want." When he asked her what she wanted to be or do, her answer was vague. When he asked her whether she wanted to marry, she began to cry and said, "It isn't safe." When he asked her why marriage was unsafe, she told him about the divorce of a couple who were friends of her parents, and said, "I'm no good; I make my parents quarrel, and they might get divorced too."

Confidentiality

Although the physician should give the parents an evaluation of their child and the child's problems, he must keep the details of the child's revelations about himself confidential in order to encourage trust and openness on the child's part. But he may have to tell the parents certain things because they are responsible for the child's welfare. The physician may have trouble deciding what he must tell the parents during his diagnostic study of the child, and even more trouble during his treatment of the child. If a child tells the physician that he has stolen something or that he is doing something that is illegal or that may put him in serious physical danger, the physician must tell the parents what the child has told him. The physician should usually tell a child (or an adolescent) during or at the end of the interview, "I'll have to tell your parents what I think the problem is, and how it can be helped, but the kinds of things we talk about will be just between us." In that way the physician can assure the child that he will keep what the child

says confidential and still be able to communicate with the parents. Adolescents usually find it easier to trust a physician who does not take notes during the interview. Also, taking notes often interferes with listening actively and responding quickly.

If the child tells the physician something that his parents must know, the physician should encourage him to tell them himself; he should promise to help them understand and work things out the best way possible. If the child cannot tell his parents, the physician must tell the child that he must, because they must know in order to help. He can offer to help the child tell them by conducting an interview with the child and the parents. Or if the child cannot face this, the physician can tell the child exactly what he will tell the parents. When the child tells the physician something he has done, he usually is asking the physician for help. He would feel guilty and not trust the physician if the physician did not respond to what the child told him. Although laws recently passed giving minors the right to be treated for such problems as drug abuse and to have abortions[1] can affect the physician's decision about what he must tell the parents, he usually can and should help the parents understand and help plan treatment.

Evaluation of Mental Status

A formal examination of the type used to evaluate the mental status of adults (which includes questions regarding orientation, information about awareness, serial subtractions, proverbs, and tongue-twisters) is hard for children and sometimes demeaning for adolescents. (It also has some cultural bias toward the knowledge of middle-class white people.) The physician can evaluate mental functioning with reasonable accuracy by using the observations that he makes during his interview with the child, his observation of the child's play, the child's answers to questions about his school, his siblings, where he lives, his future, and his dreams and daydreams, and the child's ability to write his name and draw a picture, and the results of brief tests, such as those for right-left orientation and finger agnosia. The physician can evaluate the child's mental status more easily when he has begun to establish a relationship with the child.

When the physician evaluates the child's mental status, in the informal way suggested, he should consider the following areas of the child's functioning. (The physician should of course consider the child's level of development.)

1. *Appearance and behavior:* his composure in manner and organization in dress, any fear, anxiety, apprehensiveness, restlessness, hyperactivity, hypoactivity, or psychomotor retardation that he shows, any tics that he has, or any grimaces or bizarre movements of his head, hands, or body.

2. *Orientation:* his orientation in time, space, and person, the clearness of his sensorium, and any confusion or disorientation that he shows.

3. *Memory:* the intactness of both his recent and remote memory, any gaps or blocks in his memory, and any amnesia.

4. *Thought content and thought process:* how understandable, relevant, and logical his thoughts are, his capacity for forming concepts, how concrete his thought is, his capacity for abstract thought, his capacity to distinguish fantasy from reality, how appropriate his reasoning and judgment are, his capacity for symbolic play, any obsessive, ruminative, or bizarre thoughts that he has, any loosening of associations and loss of logical sequence that he shows, and any illusions, hallucinations, or delusions.

5. *Speech:* how intelligible and articulate it is, its volume and rhythm, the child's capacity for communicating his thoughts and feelings, how well he understands syntax, any pressure, rambling, or distorted sounds, and any neologisms or bizarre expressions that he uses.

6. *Emotionality:* his capacity for relating to people, how warm he is, how appropriate his emotions are to the content of his thoughts and his speech, any feelings of unreality or marked depersonalization that he has, his capacity for controlling his feelings and impulses, degree of frustration tolerance and any depression, over-

elation, rage, quick changes of mood, or inhibition that he shows.

7. *Perceptual-motor capacities:* his span of attention, his capacity for perceiving objects correctly, his capacity for understanding and reproducing symbols in drawing or writing, his motor skills, and his patterns of coordination.

When he considers the information that he has obtained about the different areas of the child's functioning, the physician should be aware that all children are more restless and circumstantial in their thinking than are adults. Young children often become momentarily confused in their thought and speech, particularly when they are anxious because they are in an unfamiliar setting. Signs of perceptual-motor difficulty are not necessarily diagnostic of brain damage. The physician should also consider that most adolescents have quickly changing moods, occasional feelings of depersonalization, and confusion or blocks in thinking when they feel strong emotions (those signs are more serious when they occur in adults). (Specific diagnostic considerations related to various syndromes, which may draw upon data from the mental status examination, are discussed elsewhere.)*

Considering the Child's Cultural Background

When the physician makes his diagnostic study of the child and particularly when he evaluates the child's mental status, his own cultural background can influence and even distort his perceptions of the child and the child's family if they belong to an ethnic or a socioeconomic group that is different from his.[11] For example, some Hispanic, American Indian, and some black and white people who live in rural areas in the South may have hallucinatory experiences during religious rites.[8] Some peoples' beliefs may seem to middle-class white people to be delusions, such as the

---

*A special set of tests that can be used if delirium is suspected is discussed in Chapter 22.

tradition of folk medicine and the voodoo and "evil eye" convictions regarding illness.[20]

Deep mistrust or suspicion of the members of the majority by members of a minority may seem to members of the majority to be signs of paranoia. Members of minorities who do not know the language of the majority well may wrongly be diagnosed as being mentally retarded, a label that disappears promptly if an interpreter is employed.[18] If a member of a minority remains silent during an interview with a member of the majority because he does not trust the interviewer, or if he has a limited education or a different cultural idiom, he also may be diagnosed as being mentally retarded, as may people who live in rural areas (as Loof[16] has shown). Familiarity with other cultures, along with caution and humility, are vital to the clinician involved in diagnostic study. Until these are acquired, he may have to rely on other persons more knowledgeable about patients' cultural backgrounds. Programs of affirmative action and protection of patients' rights are contributing importantly to the solution of this very real problem.

Evaluating the Child's Development: Methods of Screening

The physician can form some picture of the child's general level of intelligence during the interview.* But evaluating intelligence is a very complex process and should be done only by a clinical psychologist who has been trained to work with children. The pediatrician must evaluate the child's level of development; now one of his health associates can also make such an evaluation. In the past few years, developmental

---

*In a study by Korsch and Cobb,[13] pediatricians' evaluations of the levels of functioning of infants and preschool-age children were mostly accurate, but they often overestimated the capacities of retarded children, and underestimated those of children who had chronic diseases.

screening tests have been designed that can be given by pediatricians, nurses, child health associates, nurse practitioners, nursery school teachers, and paraprofessionals. The Denver Developmental Screening Test (DDST) is based on the Provence modification of the Gesell Developmental Schedules and has been standardized for middle-class and working-class children by Frankenburgh and Dodds.[5] It can be given in the context of continued health supervision; it takes only a short time, and it evaluates the child's language skills, his fine motor–adaptive skills, gross motor skills and the personal-social aspects of his development during the preschool-age period. The DDST helps to assess the tempo and evenness of the child's development; it shows any lags, prolonged plateaus or regressions, and wide discrepancies between attainments in different dimensions.

The DDST and several other developmental screening tests have recently been used to screen large groups of children (e.g., in the Head Start program). Title XIX, the early periodic screening program of diagnosis and treatment, has required developmental screening as part of the health screening of children who are recipients of welfare (although many of the problems or handicaps identified have not received treatment). As Thorpe[22] has pointed out, the DDST and other developmental screening tests (including her own test, the Thorpe Developmental Inventory [TDI]), all have limitations. The tests' norms are based on relatively small groups of children who often do not represent the children who are screened later. Longitudinal studies of children who have different socioeconomic, ethnic, and educational backgrounds must be used to design such tests before the tests can be considered to have predictive potential. When people who have been adequately trained give the tests, however, they can be considered as narrative-descriptive instruments, without a numerical score, for use in planning health management and education for preschool children. (The TDI is the only test that has a recording form in Spanish and norms for the children of migrant farm workers.)

The physician who sees a child when he cannot immediately use a developmental screening test can make a quick, rough evaluation of the child's level of development by asking him to copy simple figures (like those that are included in the DDST, the TDI, and other tests) and using the following rules when he makes his evaluation. (He should always make a more complete evaluation at a later point.)

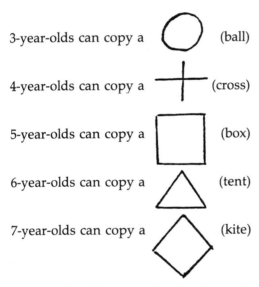

3-year-olds can copy a   (ball)

4-year-olds can copy a   (cross)

5-year-olds can copy a   (box)

6-year-olds can copy a   (tent)

7-year-olds can copy a   (kite)

Some pediatricians use the Goodenough Draw-A-Person Test[6]; it is easy to give and to score. It can be given to children who are between 3 and 11 years old. The child is asked to draw a person. If he draws a circle, he is scored at 3 years. One year is added to his score for each additional 4 details that he adds to the circle. (There are 51 possible details.)

The tests of a child's level of development do not measure his intelligence or provide evidence for diagnoses of mental retardation, brain damage, or any other clinical disorder. If a test shows any deviation in one of the aspects of development that it studies, a clinical psychologist who

has been trained to work with children should make a complete study of the level of development of the child who was tested. (The book discusses the tests that clinical psychologists use to make such a study later.)

Willoughby and Haggerty[24] and others[14] have designed methods of screening for developmental and psychosocial problems in children. They give parents questionnaires about their children's behavior. Metz and his colleagues[17] have reported that a psychosocial phase has been added to a pediatric multiphasic examination in a prepaid medical program that is operated by the Kaiser Permanente Foundation. The methods of screening included questionnaires about the child's behavior and stress in the family and shorter versions of standard psychologic tests that are given to children. Trained aides gave the questionnaires and tests; the child's pediatrician received the test results after the questionnaires and tests had been processed by a computer. The examination showed that about 7% of about 1000 children who were screened were at high risk for problems. Boys, black children, and the children from families of lower educational backgrounds had more problems than the average child. (However, the validity of the examination has not yet been confirmed.) In another study by Tasen and his colleagues,[21] 70% of the parents who were given a behavioral questionnaire by allied health personnel said their children had had developmental or behavioral problems or problems in school. But in routine histories that were taken before, only 6% of the parents said that they had had such problems.

Although such methods of screening can help a physician study a child, Metz and his colleagues have pointed out that different pediatricians in the program used such reports differently and that the impersonal nature of the results given by the computer, based on routine examinations, gave those results less influence on the pediatrician's studies of children than the information that they obtained by examining the children themselves. As Korsch and her colleagues[4] have pointed out, a person more often follows advice that he has received directly from someone to whom he has explained his problem. If the physician obtains psychosocial information directly from the child and his parents, he can learn what problem the child has without using special methods of screening. The physician's relationship with the child and the child's parents helps them to accept his evaluation of the child and the child's problems.

Chapter 5 discussed the criteria for the successful development of a sense of trust, autonomy, initiative, industry, and identity at the different levels, and it included a table that listed the physical, psychologic, and social aspects of development. (The reader is referred also to the texts on development and behavior referred to in Chapter 5.) The following is a list of signs of incipient psychosocial deviance—danger signals observable in the office setting. (The list has been adapted from Provence[19] and from Jordan.[9])

0–1 years	1. Failure to smile at the parent.
	2. Failure to make anticipatory gestures before being picked up.
	3. Failure to distinguish between adults who are familiar to him.
	4. Absence of stranger anxiety or of separation anxiety.
	5. Absence of normal negativism.
	6. Inability to accept familiar parent substitutes.
1–3 years	7. Failure to ask adults for appropriate help.
	8. Failure to play appropriately.
	9. Failure in modulation and control of his activity.
	10. Absence of normal fears and phobias.
	11. Inability to separate from his parents or to function

4–6 years	independently when he goes to school.
	12. Inability to move independently around his neighborhood.
	13. Failure to develop a sense of what is right and what is wrong.
	14. Inability to find pleasure in mastering skills.
6–12 years	15. Isolation from his peer group in his neighborhood or at school.
	16. Failure to make friends of his own age.
	17. Sudden drop in grades.
	18. Failure to develop sex-typed behavior.
12–18 years	19. Failure to show some struggle for his identity and independence.

None of these danger signals is diagnostic in itself, but each represents a failure to show crucial signs of positive personality development. Each calls for prompt investigation into family and environmental circumstances. Other "high risk" indicators are discussed in Chapter 28.

Evaluation of Reading Ability

Most tests of a child's ability to read, such as the Gray Oral Reading Paragraphs and the Gates Primary Reading Tests, are complex and long. The physician can study first-, second-, and third-grade readers and have 1 of each in his office. Kanner and Eisenberg[10] have suggested the following short reading tests; the tests give a quick and rough evaluation of the child's ability to read.

First grade:	40 seconds; 4 errors A little boy had a cat; she ran away; she said, "I want some milk."
Second grade:	25 seconds; 2 errors A man took me to see his large barn. There was a horse in the yard; its tail was black.

Third grade: 30 seconds; 2 errors
One of our favorite birds is
the robin. He is a very useful
bird. He eats many insects and
worms. The robin is less afraid
of people than most birds.

A short sample of the child's writing may
show how well the child can perceive, interpret, and reproduce written symbols.
Children may reverse letters, (e.g., a child
may write "was" for "saw") or write "d"
instead of "b". If a child has trouble reading or writing (and such a child often has
trouble in arithmetic also[3]), the physician
should talk with the child's teacher, who
may know about his problem. The physician can evaluate the child further or visit
the child's school (with the parents' permission and the child's knowledge) to talk
with the principal, the child's teacher, and
other people at the school.[3]

Assessment of possible visual, hearing,
and speech defects may help the physician
understand what causes the child's problems although most defects in vision contribute to rather than cause such problems.
The diagnosis and management of problems in these areas are discussed in Chapter 28.

History Taking

The leads that the physician obtains
when he takes the history during the first
interview will determine in large part the
points of emphasis in the physical examination and the selection of laboratory tests.
Thus there is no substitute for a well taken
history. Of equal importance is the opportunity to begin the establishment of a positive relationship with parents and child.
The quality of his relationship with them
affects both the accuracy of the information
that he obtains and their response to his
treatment of the child or to anticipatory
guidance. The first interview helps to establish the psychotherapeutic aspect of the
physician's role. During later interviews,

the physician expands and corrects his first
impression of the parents and the child. Of
course, different physicians use the principles of interviewing[12] in different ways.
The physician should develop a technique
of interviewing that puts him at ease rather
than try to copy someone else's technique
too closely. Regardless of his technique, he
must always respect the parents' dignity.

The appendix includes an outline of the
information that the physician should obtain for the history. The outline has been
modified from the traditional one; it should
only guide the physician. Such outlines are
necessary, but they often lead the medical
student to use a checklist of questions when
he takes a history. Using a checklist may
keep the parents from commenting spontaneously and in more detail. Even questionnaires that the parents fill out before
they visit the physician may keep the parents from commenting spontaneously on
their child's behavior and can give the physician wrong impressions because the parents feel and act defensively. Questionnaires cannot substitute for a sensitive and
thorough history.

The tendency to record the family or social history as "noncontributory" is a pernicious one, arising in part from the checklist practice. The circumstances of the family's life, their position as members of a
particular minority group, the father's
chronic depression caused by an unsatisfying job, and the part-time work of a
mother that begins at the child's bedtime,
for example, may affect the child's health
status as much as do factors related to a
physical disease. The physician should
learn whether there is or has been a disease
in the family that may be relevant to the
child's disease. The experienced physician
will avoid, however, the monotonous listing of all possible illnesses. Such a listing
often confuses the parents and may make
them feel resentful or guilty. The physician
should ask instead about the symptoms
that accompanied the illness of a member
of the family or preceded his death.

When the physician asks for details about the child's birth, growth and development, and past diseases, and about the parents' child-rearing, he should remember that most parents have trouble remembering such details accurately. The parents may remember more details later or find them in other sources of information, such as baby books; details that the physician learns later may expand or correct what the parents first remember. If the parents first have blocks in their memories of feeding or toilet training the child, for example, they may have had some trouble or conflict then; what they remember later may show what the trouble was. The physician should not rely too much on such data secured during the first interview. Several studies have shown that information about a child's early development, even information that was obtained from the parents of preschool-age children, is not very accurate. That information includes information about psychomotor milestones in the child's development[23] and particularly about the child's behavior.[2]

The physician cannot (and does not have to) obtain the information that the outline contains during his first interview with the parents. When he records the family's history, he should list all the pertinent negative items to show that he has considered all of the factors that may affect the child's problem.

The history that an experienced physician takes may resemble an expanded summary more than it resembles the outline, but the person in training needs to use some such outline. By using the general approach indicated, the physician can obtain psychologic and social information about the family while he explores the history of physical factors. If the physician finds that a problem proves more complex than it seemed before he talked to the parents, he can make a second, longer appointment to see them, perhaps on a half-day set aside for such purposes. But even during a short interview the physician can

learn something about the problem, and about how the child functions at home, at school, and in his peer group.

If the child is acutely ill, the physician should take only a short history that is relevant to the child's illness before he does a physical examination of the child. He can complete the history after he finishes the examination.

The Physical Examination of the Child

The Approach to the Child

While he takes the history the physician forms impressions about the child's general physical and emotional state, the nature of his disease, and the interaction between him and his parents. He can invite the child to actively participate in the examination; however, the child may show resigned submission, passive resistance, or, more rarely, active resistance or violent battle. The rapport that the physician has already established with the child and his parents may determine the diagnostic success of the examination. The physician cannot hear subtle changes in the child's heart or lung sounds, for example, when the child is crying or squirming; nor can he assess the child's ocular fundi or deep tendon reflexes accurately. Sometimes the physician must examine acutely ill children while they are crying or resisting him. Only experience, skill, and good judgment can help the physician at such times. If the child is seriously ill, the physician can do the physical examination while he takes the latter portion of the history in order to save time and so lessen the suspense of the anxious child and the parents.

The child should usually be undressed by his mother or by a nurse before the physician examines him. The physician should remember that preschool-age children who refuse to remove certain items of clothing may be anxious about being so completely exposed rather than sexually modest. The physician should respect their anxiety; it usually does not last. Older children may keep their underpants on and remove them for a short time when they feel more at ease so that the physician can examine their genitals.

No matter how the child acts, the physician should always be relaxed and unhurried. If the physician spends a few minutes talking with the child about a toy he has or about his birthday, for example, and uses the child's first name or nickname several times, the child may cooperate much more during the examination. But the physician must not spend too much time talking with the child; to postpone the examination too long makes both the child and his parents tense. The physician should explain each step of the examination, such as when he examines the child's throat or darkens the room before he examines the child's eyes. He should use terms that the child can understand. Although the physician must be able to relate to the child, he should not descend to the child's level; he should behave like a sympathetic adult. He must tell the child truthfully (and make sure that the child understands what he says), when something that he must do during the examination will cause the child discomfort. Not to do so makes the child trust or cooperate with the physician less. Asking the child about his concepts about parts of his body and how they work may show the physician any misconceptions and anxieties that the child has that he can correct or remove while he makes the physical examination.[15]

The physician may let the young child examine instruments such as his stethoscope before he uses them. A child may enjoy pretending to use the instrument on himself or a doll, a method that may help overcome apprehension about the examination. (Many pediatricians let toddlers blow out the light of the otoscope, for example.)

The physician should handle infants and children differently at different levels of their development.

Infants. The physician usually has little trouble examining the very young infant if the mother is relaxed and trusts the physician. The physician may give the infant a pacifier to lessen his crying or restlessness. If it is time to feed the infant, the physician can complete much of the examination while the mother holds and feeds the infant; the physician can see how she feeds the infant and the mother can ask him questions or express any fears that she has about the infant's physical condition or development.

Infants who are in the second half of their first year usually show some fear of the physician because they have stranger or separation anxiety, even if he has examined them regularly. The physician may give the mother some object (a throat stick, for example) that she can give the infant to play with while he sits in her lap and she talks with the physician. During their talk, the infant can study the physician. If he is crawling or toddling, the infant may move toward the physician while the physician is taking the history and make friendly overtures to him; letting the child make such overtures rather than the physician better establishes rapport between them.

The infant often resists examination when he lies on his back or on the examining table; it may be easier to examine him while he sits on his mother's lap. She can hold his head against her shoulder while the physician examines his ears and throat. An older infant may fear a female nurse less than he fears a male physician at first. If the infant shows anxiety or even terror at first, that is usually not a sign of failure by the physician.

During the period of normal negativism that occurs during the late part of the second year and the early part of the third year, representing a healthy movement of the child toward autonomy and self-assertion, the physician should not ask the child to do anything (e.g., to open his mouth) during the examination because the child may refuse. The physician must be very patient with the child. A stubbornly negativistic child, diverted to some other activity, may later become able to cooperate. If the physician uses force to make the child do something, the child loses trust in him.

Preschool-Age and School-Age Children. The physician can usually examine a preschool-age child on a table. Most preschool-age children are anxious when they have to lie down to be examined because they feel exposed or helpless. They feel less anxious when they are sitting up.

When he examines a school-age child (or an older preschool-age child), the physician can learn a great deal during the physical examination about the child's feelings about himself and his development—his feelings about himself or herself as a developing boy or girl, his feelings about his body and its adequacy, and his fears or misconceptions about parts of his body and how they work.[15] If the child feels comfortable with the physician, he may bring up his fears or concerns about his body. If he does not, the physician can ask him such questions as where he thinks his stomach is and where swallowed food goes.* The parents may also bring up fears or concerns during an unhurried examination.

Adolescents. Preadolescents and adolescents often show modesty when the physician examines them. The physician should respect their modesty and their concerns about their minor blemishes and other aspects of their bodies while their bodies are changing. Adolescent boys may fear that a lag in growth may affect their masculinity or fear that they have some physical abnormality. Adolescent girls may be concerned particularly about the onset of their menses and the development of their secondary sex characteristics. The physician should always examine adoles-

*More specific discussion of children's concepts and misconceptions about their bodies, particularly their internal organs, is offered in Chapter 25.

cent girls with a woman present (a nurse or another assistant); the girls should always be draped.

Approach to the Parent

Some physicians prefer to examine a child without his mother if she is anxious because the child often submits more passively in her absence. This approach carries with it not only the pain of separation for the young child but also the implication of punishment by the physician. The child's mother may feel guilty or resentful, concerned that the physician thinks that she is not a good mother. The physician should almost always let the mother of an infant or a young child stay with him.

If the mother is apprehensive and wants to leave during the examination the physician should usually let her leave, but it is better that she leave before rather than during the examination. If the mother leaves, the physician should tell the child where she is going and when she will return.

Methods of Examining Children

When the physician examines a child, he should make sure that the instruments that he applies to the child's skin are warm. He may (especially if he is examining a young or an anxious child) rinse his hands in warm water before he begins the examination because if he touches the child with cold hands, the child may show more fear or resistance.

The usual order of procedures in the examination of adults is not appropriate for children. When he examines young children, the physician should begin by examining a peripheral part of the child's body, examining more sensitive parts, such as the head, later so that he does not frighten the child or cause the child to resist. The order of procedures that the physician follows may vary according to the age of the infant or the young child and according to the circumstances of the examination. The physician may begin to examine an older infant by testing his deep tendon reflexes. Some physicians may find it more effective to use the stethoscope playfully on the child's legs, then on his abdomen, and finally on his chest. The physician may begin to examine a pre-school-age child by listening to his chest. An occcasional child may become anxious when the physician waits too long to examine his throat, an examination that the child anticipates, and dislikes. When the physician must restrain the child, he should tell the child why he is doing it and then examine the child as quickly as is commensurate with gentleness and thoroughness.

The pulse and respiratory rates and the blood pressure levels of infants and young children vary; fear can increase them. Only persistent deviations can be relied upon. The temperature of children, particularly young children, can be increased by fear or activity. Active exercise can increase a child's rectal temperatures by as much as 1 degree Fahrenheit (although it usually does not increase his oral temperature). Ingesting hot or cold substances may change a child's oral temperature. A child's rectal temperature is usually 1 degree higher than his oral temperature. Rectal temperatures are ordinarily employed in infants and small children. Older infants and pre-school children may resist this approach, although not yet able to retain the thermometer safely by mouth. (An occasional pneumoperitoneum can be produced by rectal thermometers in the newborn, as Greenbaum and his associates have observed.[7]) In such a situation, an axillary temperature, about a degree lower than an oral reading, will suffice for the moment.

Examining the heart and lungs of infants and young children is hard because the walls of their chests are thin and so their breathing sounds loud. The physician often hears what sounds like bronchial breathing over the right upper lobe of the chest of a healthy child. The physician must learn to listen quickly and accurately while the child is not crying or making any other vocal noise. Many young children cannot easily follow the physician's directions during tests for tactile fremitus or vocal resonance. So the physician must listen to the child's spoken words, play a "blowing" game with him or even listen to him crying.

When the physician examines a child's abdomen, he must spend considerable time in putting the child at ease so that the child relaxes his abdominal muscles. The physician can divert and help him relax by talking with him. If the child is old enough to cooperate when the physician asks him to take a deep breath, the physician can gently increase the pressure of his hand during each deep breath without making the child tense his muscles.

Rectal examinations often may disturb children who have passed early infancy. The physician does not always have to include a rectal examination in his routine examination of the child. Instead he can inspect a child's rectum and genitals routinely and make a rectal examination only if there is a particular reason to do so. The physician should make rectal examinations gently and explain them to the child; the same is true of vaginal examinations of pre-adolescent or early adolescent girls, since they may have extreme fear and misconceptions about a vaginal examination. If a girl has a history of a daily vaginal discharge or regular sexual activity, the physician should give her a pelvic examination. He should fully explain the examination to the girl and give her a chance to ask questions about it. A female nurse should drape her before the examination begins. The physician should make a vaginal examination slowly and gently, explain each step in the examination as he performs it, and warn the girl when she may feel any discomfort.

After the physician has examined the child he should give the child time to ask questions about the examination (for example, about the procedures or the instruments that the physician used). The physician should always end the examination by giving the child a friendly and personal farewell—that is more important than giving him a gift, such as a balloon or a piece of candy.

Laboratory Diagnostic Studies of the Child

When the physician considers making laboratory studies of the child other than routine blood studies, a urinalysis, and a tuberculin test, he should choose the studies very carefully according to their relevance to the child's problem. Many physicians think that a child who is seriously ill should be disturbed as little as possible by venipuncture or by other tests that require vigorously moving the child or making him anxious. Of course, the physician should make whatever tests are necessary to diagnose the child's disease and determine the course of the treatment. Nevertheless, a battery of tests can have detrimental effects upon a child who has cardiac failure, by causing fatigue and anxiety that tax his cardiorespiratory system. Possible secondary effects of tests, such as the subdural effusion that the pneumoencephalogram can cause, should also be considered. Physicians usually make femoral or other types of puncture rather than physically and psychologically traumatic jugular punctures when they take blood from infants. Microlab procedures that require less blood are physically and psychologically less traumatic. The physician must explain carefully the need for laboratory studies to anxious parents.

Multiphasic screening that uses automated laboratory procedures has some advantages. It may detect an unsuspected disease, and it may cost less (and require less blood and pain) than a number of sequential tests. However, multiple test results must be interpreted, and automated procedures (like others) are not free from error. (Chapter 3 discussed the effect of anxiety on certain laboratory results.) If a single test has an abnormal result, the physician should repeat the test before he makes other tests or plans treatment for the child. Even a persistent slightly abnormal finding calls for clinical judgment in order to avoid treating the test results instead of the illness. Finally, if the physician relies too much on laboratory tests, his diagnostic acumen can atrophy as well as his ability to make clinical judgments that are based on his observations.

Preparing the Child for Painful Tests

When painful procedures are involved, such as throat cultures, venipunctures, blood cell counts, and intradermal tests, the child should be told briefly what will happen, in terms he can understand. He can be told that a finger prick or venipuncture is necessary in order to choose the right medicine to help stop his throat hurting. He should be told truthfully that it will hurt "a little." The child should be given enough time to ask questions, but too long a period of anxious questioning may make the child too anxious. The physician should also explain the test to the parents, even if the test is brief and simple. If the child must be restrained, the physician should tell the child that someone will hold his arm (or another part of his body) in order to help him hold still so that the test will hurt less. Many parents cannot hold their children during painful tests during which they may see blood; and a nurse may hold the child, but the parents should stay in the room if they can.

After the procedure, many younger children (and even children of school age) cry briefly. (A clever laboratory technician may tell a young child to cry as loudly as he can and finish the test while the child is expanding his lungs.) The child should not be made to feel that he should not cry or that it is "bad" to do so. If a child's parents try to stop him from crying (and many do because they fear criticism by the physician), it is wise to indicate that it is difficult for the child not to cry. The physician can also tell the child that he knows that the child may be angry at him momentarily, thus helping the child to avoid complete suppression of negative feelings.

Portions of this chapter have been adapted from Prugh, D.G., and Kisley, A.J., Psychosocial aspects of pediatric and psychiatric disorders, in *Current Pediatric Diagnosis and Treatment*, 6th Edition, C. Henry Kempe, H.K. Silver, and D. O'Brien, Eds., Los Altos, CA, Lange Medical Publications, 1980. In addition, some elements of this chapter have been adapted from Prugh, D.G., Clinical appraisal of infants and children, in *Textbook of Pediatrics*, 9th Edition, W.E. Nelson, V.C. Vaughan, and R.J. McKay, Eds., Philadelphia, Saunders, 1969.

Bibliography

1. American Academy of Pediatrics: The implications of minor's consent legislation for adolescent health care: A commentary. Pediatrics, 54:481, 1974.
2. Chess, S., Thomas, A., and Birch, H.G.: Distortions in developmental reporting made by parents of behaviorally disturbed children. J. Am. Acad. Child Psychiatry, 5:226, 1966.
3. Eisenberg, L.: Office evaluation of specific reading disability in children. Pediatrics, 23:997, 1959.
4. Francis, V., Korsch, B., and Morris, M.: Gaps in doctor-patient communication: patients' response to medical advice. N. Engl. J. Med., 280:535, 1969.
5. Frankenburgh, W.K., and Dodds, J.B.: The Denver Developmental Screening Test. J. Pediatr., 71:181, 1967.
6. Goodenough, F.L.: *Measurement of Intelligence by Drawings*. Chicago, World Book, 1926.
7. Greenbaum, E.J., et al.: Rectal thermometer-induced pneumoperitoneum in the newborn: Report of two cases. Pediatrics, 44:539, 1969.
8. Henry, J.: Environment and symptom formation. Am. J. Orthopsychiatry, 17:628, 1947.
9. Jordan, K.: Signs of deviant development. Unpublished material.
10. Kanner, L., and Eisenberg, L.: Childhood problems in relation to the family. Pediatrics, 20:155, 1957.
11. Katz, M.M., Cole, J.D., and Lowery, H.A.: Studies of the diagnostic process: The influence of symptom perception, past experience, and ethnic background on diagnostic decisions. Am. J. Psychiatry, 125:937, 1966.
12. Korsch, B.M.: Practical techniques of observing, interviewing, and advising parents in pediatric practice as demonstrated in an attitude study project. Pediatrics, 18:467, 1956.
13. Korsch, B.M., Cobb, K., and Ashe, B.: Pediatricians' appraisals of patients' intelligence. Pediatrics, 27:990, 1961.
14. Krajecek, M.J., and Tearney, A.I.: *Detection of Developmental Problems in Children: A Reference Guide for Community Nurses and Other Health Care Professionals*. New York, University Park Press, 1976.
15. Levy, D.: A method of integrating physical and psychiatric examination, with special studies of body interest, overprotection, response to growth and sex differences. Am. J. Psychiatry, 9:121, 1929.
16. Loof, D.H.: *Appalachia's Children*. Lexington, Ky., University Press of Kentucky, 1971.
17. Metz, J.R., et al.: A pediatric screening examination of psychosocial problems. Pediatrics, 58:595, 1976.
18. Oakland, T.: *Psychological and Educational Assessment of Minority Children*. New York, Brunner/Mazel, 1977.
19. Provence, S.: Danger signals in development. Unpublished material.
20. Saunders, L.: *Cultural Difference and Medical Care*. New York, Russell Sage Foundation, 1954.
21. Tasen, W.M., Dasteel, J.C., and Goldenberg, E.B.: Psychiatric screening in a pediatric program utilizing allied health personnel. Am. J. Orthopsychiatry, 44:568, 1974.
22. Thorpe, H.S., and Werner, E.E.: Developmental screening of preschool children: A critical review of inventories used in health and educational programs. Pediatrics, 53:362, 1974.
23. Wenar, C.: The reliability of developmental histories: Summary and evaluation of findings. Psychosom. Med., 25:505, 1963.
24. Willoughby, J.A., and Haggerty, R.J.: A simple behavior questionnaire for preschool children. Pediatrics, 34:798, 1964.

General References

Anthony, E.J.: Communicating therapeutically with the child. J. Am. Acad. Child Psychiatry, 3:106, 1964.

Anthony, E.J.: The talking doctor has begun to shoot. Proc. Inst. Med. Chicago, 25:274, 1965.

Balint, M.: *The Doctor, His Patient, and the Illness*, 2nd Ed. London, Pitman, 1964.

Brody, S.: Signs of disturbance in the first year of life. Am. J. Orthopsychiatry, 28:362, 1958.

Brown, S.L.: Clinical impressions of the impact of family group interviewing on child and adolescent psychiatric practice. J. Am. Acad. Child Psychiatry, 3:688, 1964.

Chamberlain, R.W.: Social data in evaluation of the pediatric patient: Deficits in out-patient records. J. Pediatr., 78:111, 1971.

Chance, E., and Arnold, J.: The effect of professional training, experience, and preference for a theoretical system upon clinical case description. Hum. Relat., 17:195, 1965.

Davidson, P., et al.: Diagnostic services for maladjusted rural children. J. Psychol., 69:237, 1968.

Diesing, L.: Observations on interactions between

mothers and their children in the waiting room of an outpatient child psychiatric clinic. J. Am. Acad. Child Psychiatry, 6:226, 1967.

Frankenburg, W.K., and Camp, B.W., Eds.: *Pediatric Screening Tests*. Springfield, Ill., Thomas, 1975.

Freud, A.: Assessment of childhood disturbances. Psychoanal. Study Child, 17:149, 1962.

Freud, A.: *Normality and Pathology: Assessment of Development*. New York, International Universities Press, 1965.

Freud, A.: *Normality and Pathology in Childhood*. New York, International Universities Press, 1965.

Gesell, A., and Amatruda, C.S.: *The Evaluation and Management of Normal and Abnormal Neuropsychologic Development in Infancy and Early Childhood* (H. Knobloch, and B. Pasamanick, Eds.). New York, Harper & Row, 1974.

Goodman, J.D., and Sours, J.A.: *The Child Mental Status Examination*. New York, Basic Books, 1967.

Green, M.: The clinician's art: Some questions for our time. Pediatrics, 43:157, 1969.

Group for the Advancement of Psychiatry: *The Diagnostic Process in Child Psychiatry*. Report No. 38. New York, Group for the Advancement of Psychiatry, 1957.

Hersh, S., and Rojcewicz, S., Eds.: Health Care Screening and Developmental Assessment. National Institute of Mental Health. Washington, U.S. Government Printing Office, 1974.

Holden, R., et al.: Relations between pediatric, psychologic, and neurological exams during the first year of life. Child. Dev., 33:719, 1962.

Hollingshead, A.B., and Redlich, F.C.: *Social Class and Mental Illness: A Community Study*. New York, Wiley, 1958.

Jason, H., Kagan, N., and Werner, A.: New approaches to teaching basic interview skills to medical students. Am. J. Psychoanal., 127:1404, 1971.

Knobloch, H., Pasamanick, B., and Sherard, E.S.: A developmental screening inventory for infants. Pediatrics (Suppl.), 38:1095, 1966.

Korsch, B.: Pediatrician-patient relations. In: *Ambulatory Pediatrics* (M. Green and R.J. Haggerty, Eds.). Philadelphia, Saunders, 1968.

Layman, E.M., and Lourie, R.S.: Waiting room observation as a technique for analysis of communication behavior in children and their parents. In: *Psychopathology of Communication* (E. Hock & Zubin, Eds.). New York, Grune & Stratton, 1958.

Levy, D.M.: *The Demonstration Clinic*. Springfield, Ill., Thomas, 1967.

Luborsky, L.: Clinicians judgments of mental health. Arch. Gen. Psychiatry, 7:407, 1962.

Morgan, W.L., and Engel, G.L.: *The Clinical Approach to the Patient*. Philadelphia, Saunders, 1969.

Oakland, E.: *Assessing Minority Group Children*. New York, Behavioral Publications, 1974.

Richmond, J.B., and Green, M.: *Pediatric Diagnosis*, 2nd Ed. Philadelphia, Saunders, 1962.

Richmond, J.B., and Green, M.: The pediatric history. In: *Pediatric Diagnosis*, 2nd Ed. Philadelphia, Saunders, 1962.

Van Amerongen, S.T.: Initial psychiatric family studies. Am. J. Orthopsychiatry, 24:73, 1954.

8
Special Methods of Evaluation

*To know what kind of a person has a disease is
as essential as to know what kind of disease
a person has.*
(Francis Scott Smyth)

Chapter 7 discussed the principles of history-taking and interviewing parents, children, and adolescents, and the evaluation of a child's mental status and developmental capacities, including his ability to read. It also discussed the psychologic aspects of the approach to physical examinations and laboratory procedures. The emphasis was upon the achievement of a balanced appraisal concurrently of both the physical and the psychosocial aspects of the child's problems. But sometimes the child's initial history, interviews with him and his parents, and a physical examination of him show the physician that the child has complex psychosocial problems and that the physician needs much more time than is usual to evaluate the child's problem.

If the physician thinks that he needs more time than usual to evaluate the child's problems, he should make another appointment to interview the parents and the child more extensively and for a longer

time. Some physicians keep open a half day each week or take time in the evening to talk to children and parents who have complex or obscure problems. When the physician holds more extensive interviews, he can use the same principles that he uses when he makes routine interviews. When the physician studies a family closely, he often obtains information during play interviews and from children's drawings. Though discussed separately, these two techniques are often employed concurrently (during routine interviews, the physician may of course use such techniques in abbreviated form).

The Play Interview

The physician can carry out a play interview with a child who can verbalize his thoughts and feelings and can separate from his parents. Many 3-year-olds can do so, although some may need their mothers to be present during at least part of the interview. (A child who is 3 years old or younger and shows no stranger or separation anxiety when his mother leaves him alone with the physician often is evincing a failure to differentiate between his mother and a stranger or between himself and his mother, with a lack of attachment, which may occur for various reasons.) Sometimes the parents cannot easily leave their child. The physician can observe the play of children who are less than 3 years old readily while he takes the family's history. For example, if a 2-year-old is very aggressive or inhibited when he plays, the physician should consider the child's behavior when he evaluates the child's problems. The physician can carry on play interviews even with older children who do not talk for differing reasons.

If the physician offers an adolescent a game when the interview begins, the adolescent may take this as an insult if he wants the physician to talk with him as though he were an adult, or the offer may make the adolescent feel as though he has no control during the interview. (Even taking off his coat may make an adolescent feel vulnerable.) Later in the interview, a game may help draw out a silent adolescent, and some adolescents may want to draw.

The physician should keep special equipment in his office for play interviews. (He does not need a great deal of equipment.) He should have a small chair and a low table that preschool-age children can use to color on, for example. A school-age child can use an adult-sized chair, but an adult-sized desk (such as the physician's desk) may be too high for him. A fold-out table with a Formica surface can easily be installed, at an appropriate height, and folded away when it is not being used. The physician should keep play materials for children of different ages in a closed cupboard.

Preschool-age girls may play with white (or black) baby dolls that they can feed and change. Preschool girls and boys may play with a family of plastic dolls that has enough members to represent the members of the child's family. (The physician may keep doll furniture or a doll house, but children can imagine those accessories.) They may also play with a set of animals and color with crayons and paper. Older preschool boys may like to shoot a dart-gun. The physician should keep a target and set limits to make sure that the children shoot or throw only at the target. (Children may feel anxious and guilty if they can throw wildly and hit a person.) A toy gun that does not shoot can be used in fantasy; a withdrawn child may communicate with the physician if they play with 2 toy telephones. The physician and the child can play together with a small rubber ball. Children may also play with sets of blocks or of toy cars and trucks.

School-age girls will often use the same dolls and the doll family; early school-age boys may show open or covert interest in the doll family and may play with them if encouraged gently. School-age boys like dart-guns; rubber throwing darts may be of equal value. Simple short games, like checkers, interest both sexes. A spinning-type of game gives the physician information about the child's fine motor movements. Children may also play with puppets, particularly animal puppets, and both sexes can be encouraged to draw or use crayons.

Adolescents may play games like checkers or occasionally darts, may draw with pencils and paper, or, sometimes may play with equipment that the physician keeps for younger children. Some adolescents like to play chess, but chess requires much concentration and time and makes it hard to talk. Gardner[10] has developed a "mutual storytelling technique" that uses a tape recorder and which may help some older children and early adolescents to begin to talk comfortably.

Thus the total equipment necessary for the play interview does not exceed 2 baby dolls, a family of dolls, toy animals, crayons, pencils, paper, a toy gun or rubber darts, a car, a truck, puppets, blocks, 2 telephones, a ball, and 2 or 3 games, plus appropriate chairs and play surfaces. The physician can use the ball as part of the equipment that he uses when he gives the Denver Developmental Screening Test. He can keep the equipment in a cupboard. It is hard for preschool-age children to choose a toy if the physician shows them all the toys. He should set out a few simple toys when they begin to play and bring out other toys later, 1 toy at a time.

In general, as Finzer[9] has pointed out, the physician should carry out a play interview with a child under circumstances that let the child express himself freely, comfortably, and safely and let him communicate in every way that he can while he plays (for example, through verbal, behavioral, interactional, or fantasy play). Werkman[23] has identified 3 phases of the play interview. During the first phase, the physician observes how easily the child separates from his parents and begins to play. In the first phase, the child plays freely and expresses his fantasies and conflicts. During the second phase, the physician asks the child questions to draw out more information about his fantasies. The physician then asks the child direct questions about his problems and daily life, his dreams, what 3 things he most wishes for and other questions like those discussed in Chapter 6. During the third phase the physician observes the child's attitude toward leaving and returning to his parents; he also talks to the child about future plans. Throughout the interview the physician should observe the child's attitudes toward separating from and returning to his parents, how he relates to the physician (for example, how much he trusts or mistrusts the physician) and how much anxiety he shows, including physiologic signs of anxiety, such as changes in skin color and in activity or the appearance of tics), how well the child concentrates and controls his impulses, how much the child tests the limits that adults set for him, to what level of development his behavior is appropriate, the quality of his thinking, and his awareness of himself as a person, (as well as what he says, his fantasy play, and his behavior).

In the diagnostic phase, the physician is wise not to probe the child's feelings toward his parents or other highly charged topics. The physician must limit the child's aggressive play. A very anxious child may become wild or disorganized in his play; the physician may have to gently and firmly stop the play. He may suggest a quieter activity for the child or talk with the child.

The physician in general should accept the feelings that a child shows in his fantasy play as fantasy. The child usually displaces his feelings, giving them to objects or situations in his play. He identifies with symbolic figures. Those are the child's way of dealing with his feelings "at arm's length." Occasionally, the physician may suggest that the child feels angry, like an alligator puppet that bites, or afraid, like a doll that runs away. He may ask about situations that the child creates in a family of dolls, saying, "What's going to happen next?" or, "How do the kids feel when the mother and father fight?" When the physician plays checkers with an adolescent, he may make comments, such as, "It's certainly important for you to win" or, "You could have taken me there; you say you don't play well, but I think you're kind of hard on yourself."

This approach is based on the establishment of a relationship with the child, exploration and clarification of problems or conflicts, and occasionally gentle confrontation, without significant interpretation of connections between events in the family or elsewhere and the child's feelings. (The appropriate use of such principles in a supportive psychotherapetic approach is discussed in Chapter 12). Occasionally the child or adolescent himself will make such insightful connections. It may help the child to express his feelings through his play to a sympathetic adult who does not belong to his family (such as the physician), even if he and the adult do not discuss exactly what his play means.

Case Example. A 4½-year-old-boy who had a history of unruly and aggressive behavior visited a pediatrician for the first time. His family history showed that his behavior began when his 2-year-old sister was born, about whom it was said only that she had been born a month prematurely. When the pediatrician saw him during a play interview, the boy set up a doll play situation in which the mother and father dolls were playing with a baby in the living room. The boy doll was off by himself—"in his room." When asked how the boy doll felt, the child said he was "sad and mad." Upon inquiry as to why the doll felt that way, the boy answered, "Because nobody pays any attention to him." When the pediatrician asked the parents more about the boy's sister, the mother told him that the sister had had frequent respiratory infections since she was born. The mother had not told the pediatrician about the infections because she feared that she had not taken good care of the boy's sister.

Case Example. An 8-year-old boy who was an only child had had frequent nightmares and enuresis since he was 5 years old. Nothing in the family's history seemed unusual. During a play interview, the boy built a fort out of blocks. He put a cow and a calf in the fort. He made a male horse try to knock down the fort's walls. When the pediatrician asked the boy what might happen, the boy said the horse wanted to "beat up" the cow and the calf. When the pediatrician asked the parents more about their relationship, a serious marital problem was revealed. The father committed no violent acts, but the mother feared his temper and spent most of her time with the boy, which made the father angry.

Using the Child's Drawings

When the physician uses a child's drawings as a diagnostic instrument, he should not make conclusions about a drawing because the drawing resembles one that the physician has seen in a book about the drawings of children and adolescents. Each drawing has its own symbolic meaning; and drawings that are similar may have entirely different meanings if they are made by different children. The physician can easily make a mistake when he looks for symbolic meaning in a drawing; he must know the child's association to the drawing or the story that the child tells about it in order to understand its symbolic meaning. As Bender[3] has emphasized, a diagnosis cannot be made on the basis of drawings alone. The Goodenough Draw-a-Person Test,[11] or the House-Tree-Person Test[4] can give valuable information about the child's development and emotional maturity. Machover developed the idea that a child's drawing of a human figure can be a projection of his own body image—a picture of himself. Koppits used an interpersonal theoretical approach when he studied children's drawings. More recently, Di Leo,[7] Kellog,[13] and others have drawn diagnostic conclusions from children's drawings, as have Schildkraut and his colleagues[19] from adolescents' drawings. Burns and Kaufman[5,6] have developed the Kinetic-Family-Drawing Test. That test can show the child's conscious and unconscious feelings about the interactions that take place in his family. The physician can learn how to give these tests; but they are complex and take much time to interpret. They are generally best left to the well trained child psychologist to administer.

The physician can get very good results by first asking the child to draw whatever he wants to draw. He may need to encourage the child by telling him that his drawing does not have to be perfect. Most children and early adolescents want to draw although negativistic, overly anxious, or overly inhibited ones may not want to do so. The physician should not push them to draw. He should give overeager or compulsive children enough time to finish their drawings. If a child cannot choose something to draw, the physician can suggest something to him. If children have such reactions when the physician asks them to draw, they give him diagnostic clues regarding the anxiety, passivity, inhibition, or perfectionism that they show.

Children draw all kinds of things. Many boys may draw cars, tanks, or rockets, but a child who draws rockets, for example, over and over in great detail clearly does not want to express feelings about other people. Well-adjusted children of both sexes usually include people in their drawings. A late school-age or an early adolescent child often draws a young person of his or her own sex. Children may draw animals. Young preschool-age children may scribble but they can copy simple figures.

The style of a child's drawing may show his personality traits. Compulsive emphasis on detail is easy to recognize. Inhibited children often draw small, constricted pictures; children who have trouble controlling their impulses often draw disorganized, sprawling pictures. Some children show creativity and artistic talent.

When the child has drawn something, usually something that the physician can recognize, the physician should not comment on the drawing's content or ask leading questions about it at first. He can avoid making qualitative judgments about the drawing while he explores the child's associations if he says, "That's an interesting picture; tell me about it." If the child cannot easily talk about his drawing, the physician can ask him about or comment on a specific object or person in the drawing; for example, the physician can say that the picture seems happy (or sad), can ask who lives in a house that the child has drawn, or can ask why there are no people in the drawing and ask where they might be. If the physician draws the child out, the child's fantasies may be added to the drawings' immediate associations.

If a child cannot choose something to draw (or if he has already chosen and drawn something), the physician can ask him to draw any person that he chooses. A school-age child usually draws a person of his or her own sex and age. The phy-sician can say, "Tell me about that boy (or girl)." If the child cannot answer easily, the physician can say, "Let's pretend we know about that boy. How old is he?" He can then ask such questions as, "Where does he live?" "Does he go to school?" "What about his family?" and "What does he want to be when he grows up?" Asking a child to draw a person of the opposite sex next may help the physician learn more about the child.

The physician can then ask the child to draw a picture of his family "doing things." Some children refuse to draw such a picture; if the child refuses, the physician can ask him to draw a more impersonal picture—of a "house, a tree, and a person." (Often the child draws more than 1 person.) The physician can ask the child for associations by saying, for example, "Tell me about that" or, "What does that make you think of?"; or he can ask the child to make up a story about the drawing to learn more about what fantasies the child expresses in the drawing.

By studying and talking with the child about his drawing, the physician can learn about not only about the child's developmental level* and the content and style of his drawings but also the symbols, themes, and action dynamics of them. By projecting and displacing his fantasy and feelings onto his drawings, the child can deal with emotionally charged subjects from a distance. Ordinarily, the physician should not try to tell the child what thoughts or feelings his drawings show or make immediate interpretations of his behavior based on his drawings. But sometimes the physician can do that superficially and cautiously by saying, for example, "Maybe that's the way you feel sometimes."

If a child draws what he calls a "war" and shows violent fighting and people being killed, what he sees on television may have influenced the drawing, but he is not

---

*Very primitive or very advanced drawings may suggest but are not tests of a child's level of intelligence.

following the usual tendency of children to fulfill their wishes by showing a happy or ideal situation. The physician probably can infer that members of the child's family often have fights or that the child is trying to control anger or hostility. If the child later draws a small, weak boy and huge, angry parents who have big teeth, those drawings strengthen the physician's inferences. If an 8-year-old boy draws a girl, he usually shows that he feels uncertain about being a boy or becoming a man. If a 9-year-old girl draws a picture of a 2-year-old baby girl, she usually shows that she has a conflict about her level of development; she may want to be a baby like her sister or fear to be her own age because her parents protect her too much. A child who draws an animal may show a monster that reflects his fears, a small, helpless creature that represents himself, or a kind animal who loves him.

The child who draws a dark picture that has clouds or rain usually expresses sadness or depression, especially if he remarks about the drawing that the people in it have all "left home." The child who draws a family that is divided into 2 groups that are fighting each other often tells something about his family's functioning, as does the child who draws a father or a mother who is isolated from the rest of the family or draws each of the family's members separately. The child who says that a person of his or her own sex lives alone usually expresses loneliness or anger, as does the adolescent who draws a very small, thin, or fat and sad person with whom he identifies. If an adolescent's drawing of himself is smaller or uglier, for example, than his drawing of a parent or another person of his (or her) own sex, he may be revealing that he feels inferior to others.

Confusion about reality or intense fears of loss of control of aggressive impulses may also be communicated through hazy or partial figures or pictures of explosions. If older school-age children draw people who are missing hands or feet, they may

show their own fears of being mutilated or feelings of being incomplete. Children who are about to have operations or who have chronic illnesses or handicaps often show in their drawings that they have misconceptions about their body image, particularly about where their organs are, and fears that their genitals or other very sensitive parts of their bodies may be harmed or that they may die.

When children draw freely, their drawings may show that they have perceptual-motor problems more clearly than do the drawings that they make when they are copying drawings, or making a stylized drawing; they often have better control when they make those kinds of drawings. Children who have mild delirium that is caused by a metabolic disorder may show subclinical or intermittent confusion in thinking in drawings and their associations to them. Distortions of reality or body image may emerge, or the child may try to control his confusion by making small, constricted drawings.

Winnicott has developed a way of encouraging a child to draw freely; he calls it the Squiggle Game.[24] He begins the game by closing his eyes and drawing a "squiggle," a line that usually has 2 or more curves; then asks the child to finish the drawing by turning the squiggle into something. When the child has finished the drawing, he asks the child questions about or comments on what the child has drawn. Winnicott keeps the child drawing by adding to the squiggles or making new squiggles. Winnicott at first talks mostly about the drawing, but then gradually brings up what the child has shown in his drawing about himself and his feelings. Winnicott (who was a pediatrician and a child psychoanalyst and who had an intuitive gift for dealing with children) could bring up what the child has shown in his drawings without upsetting him and could help inhibited children tell him about very private things. If a less experienced and less well trained person plays the Squiggle Game with a child, he should talk only about the child's drawings (at least while he is making a diagnostic study of the child).

Case Example. A 9-year-old boy visited a pediatrician because he had chronic aches and pains and what he called "trouble breathing." His mother had been seriously ill with pneumonia when the boy was 18 months old. After she recovered, she was constantly worried about the boy's health, fearing that she had neglected him while she was ill. She constantly asked him how he felt, and she kept him home from school if he mentioned even the slightest discomfort, getting his homework and tutoring him. Other physicians had suggested that the boy had viremia, but his problems had never been definitively diagnosed. The father had at first criticized the mother for being overprotective of the boy, but then he became caught up in her anxiety. The boy had no physical abnormalities, but he was anxious, inhibited, and afraid to leave his parents. At first he spoke only in a whisper. He could not talk freely, and he could not tell the pediatrician any of his wishes or dreams. When the pediatrician asked him to draw, he drew two pictures.
The boy's first drawing:

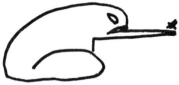

When the pediatrician asked him about that drawing he said that it was a frog that had a fly on its tongue.
The boy's second drawing:

The boy said that the second drawing was of a "happy baby—about 3 years old." When the pediatrician asked him about the baby's feet, he said that the baby was "hobbled, like a horse." When the pediatrician pointed out that the baby had no fingers, the boy drew only 4 fingers on

each hand, implying that the baby's hands were defective.*

Case Example. A 14-year-old girl visited a pediatrician because during the past 2 years she had withdrawn from her peers and her academic performance had declined sharply. The family's history showed that her problems began when her father died although at that time she had mourned only briefly. Physical examination was within normal limits. The girl had trouble talking to the pediatrician. She agreed to draw, and she drew a picture of a girl who had a sad face and who was "hugging herself."

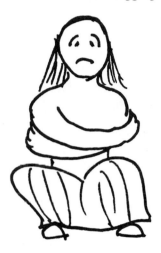

When the pediatrician asked her about the girl in the picture, she said that the girl was "sad because she didn't show her father that she loved him before he died. Her mother cries to herself all the time."

The Psychologic Appraisal

Psychologic tests can be of great diagnostic assistance when administered by a clinical psychologist who has been trained to work with children and adolescents. Like laboratory tests, however, psychologic tests alone cannot be used to make a diagnosis; thorough study and the exercise of wise clinical judgment are necessary, as such

---

*The family seemed to be a family with hypochondriacal concerns like the families described in Chapter 10. Dr. Alan Levine, who was then a Fellow in Child Psychiatry, studied the family. He recommended that the pediatrician follow a certain course of treatment. The treatment had good results after several months.

clinical child psychologists as Engel,[8] Ross,[17] and others[1] have emphasized. Also, a single test may not be accurate if the child is tired, anxious, or ill, for example, when he takes the test. Only a well-trained psychologist can evaluate tests that show the personality dynamics of adolescence; it is easy to misinterpret those tests and conclude from them that an adolescent is more disturbed than he really is.

The uses of tests vary widely. For example, some clinics use tests routinely; others use them only for special reasons. The results of testing are more helpful if the physician asks the psychologist who gave the test specific questions. A physician should not use a test only to confirm something that he already knows from interviewing the child. He should also consider whether testing can help him counsel the parents or plan therapy. Occasionally the need arises to reevaluate the functioning of the child's personality during the child's therapy; retesting may show changes in that functioning.

The physician who wants a child tested should structure the child's problem for the psychologist who tests the child, as Harlow and Salzman[12] have pointed out. Asking for a "personality workup" (a complete battery of tests) is too broad a request to permit focused study by the psychologist. On the other hand, if a physician asks the psychologist to give the child just an I.Q. test, he may be limiting the psychologist's study of the child's personality too much. If the physician tells the psychologist something about the child's problem (whether he tells the psychologist by telephone or letter, or when he sees the psychologist), the psychologist can choose tests that show more about the problem. The physician should decide in advance whether he wants the psychologist to discuss the test's results with the child's parents. In complicated cases, this may be best, but often parents who have a good relationship with the physician can accept his recommendations more comfortably.

A psychologist may test a child several times before he can assess the child's intelligence accurately. Such children may be borderline retarded children, may be from disadvantaged backgrounds, may have suffered emotional deprivation, or show great losses (or gains) in intellectual functioning. (Such losses or gains usually accompany changes in a child's motivation or in the functioning of his personality.) The psychologist may not be able to test children who have psychotic disorders before they are treated. A test given to a child who is in the hospital may give the physician a general idea of his intelligence; it should never be used by itself to plan a child's educational program. The child should be tested again after he leaves the hospital in case he scored lower than his potential because of physical discomfort or emotional regression.

Intelligence Testing

Psychologists have given developmental tests to infants and very young children for some time. Those most often used are the scales of Cattell and Bayley and the Provence modification of the Gesell. Although they are not predictive with certainty of later intellectual development,[2,16,21] these examinations can show the child's current level of development. They are useful in the study of children who may have brain damage, mental retardation, or syndromes of social and emotional deprivation. (The DDST, the TDI, and other screening tests draw on some of the items in the scales just discussed and can show the physician lags or other problems in the child's development. But they do not test children's intelligence.)

To children who have passed infancy, psychologists most often give the Stanford-Binet test and the Wechsler Intelligence Scale for Children (WISC). The Stanford-Binet test yields a range of intellectual functioning by age levels (basal and ceiling). A variety of functions, including memory, reasoning, social comprehension, spatial relations, verbal facility, and numerical concepts, are tested in each range. The tasks are primarily verbal in content; however, nonverbal scales have been developed. The WISC is used more often than any other test; it gives a child's Verbal I.Q., his performance I.Q., and his Full Scale I.Q. The Full Scale I.Q. is weighted and not simply averaged. The results of intelligence tests overlap, but the Stanford-Binet test is more useful for assessing the intelligence of late preschool-age and early school-age children, and the WISC for assessing that of late school-age children and adolescents. The Leiter International Performance Scale, the Raven Progressive Matrices, and other tests have been designed for nonverbal children. Special tests have also been designed for blind or deaf children (although these have some limitations and should be interpreted cautiously). While he tests a child, the psychologist can assess the child's actual and potential levels of intellectual functioning and can make many valuable clinical observations, as Waite[22] has pointed out, including the effects of drugs on the child's performance.[18] Intelligence tests have some cultural bias; care should be taken in their interpretation in order not to underestimate the intelligence of children who belong to differing ethnic groups or children who live in isolated rural areas.

Group I.Q. tests have been used widely in the United States, particularly by schools. The value of a group I.Q. test is limited by its nature; being in a group of children affects each child's performance. But group I.Q. tests can be used to screen children. Children who show problems in the results of a group I.Q. test should be evaluated individually by a child psychologist before conclusions are drawn. Recently, some schools have used group or individual tests that were given by teachers too freely and have based important decisions on the results.

Projective Tests

Projective tests help show a child's personality patterns and psychodynamics. Sometimes only a projective test can find a mild disorder in thinking. The Rorschach Inkblot Test is the most popular and begins to be appropriate for children at about 8 years of age. Studies have shown that on this test, the child shows many of the same personality traits that he shows when he confronts special situations in his life. The Rorschach test helps the psychologist find out how strong (or impaired) the child's ego is. It can show how well the child tolerates tensions and perceives reality, and can evaluate the nature of his psychologic defenses. Other projective tests, such as the Thematic Apperception Test (TAT) and the Children's Apperception Test (CAT) let the children tell stories about sets of pictures. The children's stories often show that they feel depression or anger or emotional conflicts.

Other Tests

The Bender Visual-Motor Gestalt Test can show that a child has perceptual-motor problems and that he may have brain damage. Brain damage may make the child see and copy a geometric design in a distorted way. The psychologist who gives the Bender test must have a keen awareness of developmental factors; a child who makes a "pathologic" drawing may have a lag in the development of his perceptual-motor abilities, may be emotionally immature, or may be anxious. Tests, such as the Frostig test are also useful, but their results should also be interpreted carefully.

Preparing the Child to Take a Test

It is very hard to give a psychologic test to a child who does not cooperate. A child who has been referred to the psychologist to be tested has little choice about coming. If no one has prepared him to take the test, he may show resentment or fear. The child and his parents often need much help to face a psychologic test and its results with a favorable attitude.

When the physician prepares the child, he uses terms that are appropriate to the child's age and previous experience. He should tell the child that this will help the physician understand the child's problems. The physician should not use the words "test" and "examination" when he talks with a school-age child so that the test has no negative or anxiety-arousing associations for the child. He can tell a child who is less than 7 or 8 years old that he will be "doing puzzles" and "playing games[11]." He should tell older children more about the experience; he can describe it as "doing things with your hands" or "looking at pictures and making up stories," for example. The physician can tell an older child that the psychologist will want to know what the child knows, but he should tell the child that this evaluation cannot be passed or failed like a test in school. He should tell adolescents that personality tests cannot read their minds.

When the physician discusses the results of psychologic testing that a child took with the child's parents, he should not use technical terms. He should tell them the range of the child's I.Q. rather than the child's specific score. The parents should not be shown the report because it may confuse or upset them. They may want a copy; if they insist on having a copy, the psychologist or the physician can give them a brief summary of it. The child should be permitted to ask the physician questions about the test; children usually complain about parts of the test that they thought hard to do or inkblots that confused them. If possible, the physician should assure the child (and particularly the adolescent) that the test showed that his mind is working as it should or that he is not "crazy," but that the test helped him understand the child's (or the adolescent's) problems.

The Judicious Use of Electroencephalopathy

The electroencephalogram (EEG) records the brain's electrical activity. Its elec-

trical activity represents the potentials of the neurons in the cerebral cortex. (The EEG records only the sum of the inhibitory and the excitatory potentials of large groups of neurons.) In order to record those potentials, the EEG machine must greatly amplify them. When he interprets a tracing, the electroencephalographer evaluates all the tracings on each page as 1 picture rather than evaluating each wave by itself. So the interpretation of EEGs is in large part subjective although scientists are developing computers that can analyze frequencies. But even a computer's evaluation depends on what samples of EEGs it is given.

To analyze the EEG, electroencephalographers and computers must consider 3 things: (1) the frequency, form, and amplitude of individual waves, (2) the locations of waves (e.g., in regard to differences between cerebral hemispheres), and (3) cerebral electrical activity will be altered with changes in the conscious state of the patient in response to stimuli, and will vary from childhood to adult life.

Epileptiform activity does not by itself make a diagnosis of epilepsy or any other disorder. Virtually no disease except for classic petit mal causes a characteristic EEG pattern. The cerebral electrical activity can only change in a few ways in response to any injury. The nature of the injury (i.e., whether it is anatomic or pathophysiologic) ordinarily has little effect on the response of the brain's electrical activity. After the child has been injured, the EEG shows that the brain's activity slows. Usually, the activity is slowest when the lesion is most severe. Focal spike activity may mean that an old lesion has become epileptogenic. Focal slow activity usually means that the child has a lesion, but the lesion is not always in the place where the EEG finds the most abnormal activity. A lesion that is in 1 of the cerebral hemispheres will often be associated with slow activity predominantly in the occipital lobes of children. However, children may show shifting foci of activity without underlying pathology.

Certain techniques are available to the electroencephalographer to help bring out abnormalities not previously evident in the resting record. Hyperventilation, photic stimulation, sleep induced by sedation, and Metrazol activation have all been used to provoke underlying abnormalities.

Because the EEG can only record the brain's activity in a relatively crude way, it cannot measure the psychologic phenomena that represent the highest integrative function of the central nervous system (although several studies have shown that anxiety can affect the EEG's pattern). Some investigators have thought that people whose EEGs have particular patterns have particular personality types; this area remains to be evaluated. The normal patterns of a child's EEG can be recorded most accurately when the child's cortex is least activated (as when the child rests comfortably and closes his eyes and his mind is unstimulated). If high cerebral function is activated, it disrupts the EEG's pattern. Particular abnormalities in the EEG do not correlate with particular emotional disorders. Although many studies have indicated that a larger percentage of patients who have emotional and behavioral disorders also have abnormal patterns in their EEGs, investigators have found recently that children who are developing normally have a surprisingly high percentage of so-called abnormal patterns in their EEGs. The psychopathologic disorders of children cause no consistent abnormalities in the patterns of the children's EEGs.

Although rather discrete descriptions of abnormal waves have appeared in the literature, such as the 14-per-second and 6-per-second positive spikes in the EEGs of patients who have behavioral disorders, headaches, and abdominal pain, there is now much controversy about whether such disorders had anything to do with those patterns, which have also been found in the EEGs of normal children and adolescents.[20] The longitudinal studies of normal children carried out by Metcalf and Jordan[15] indicate that many children who have no

symptoms may have these and other apparently abnormal patterns in their EEGs while they are growing, especially between the ages of 5 and 10.* So these so-called abnormal patterns may really be transient and may occur during "sensitive" periods of the development of the integrative functions of the central nervous system (see fold-out table in Chapter 5).

The EEG is usually not a definitive test. The physician should assess it only when he also assesses all the other information that he has about a child so that he can diagnose and treat the child's problems.[14] Table 5–1 (see Chapter 5) gives a child's EEG findings as he develops normally from his birth to the end of his adolescence.

It is important to prepare the child for EEG testing. The machine and its wires may make the late preschool-age child afraid of electricity and the early school-age child afraid of being electrocuted. The physician may need to tell an older child that the machine cannot read his mind.

Some elements of this chapter have been adapted from Prugh, D.G., Clinical appraisal of infants and children, in *Textbook of Pediatrics*, 9th Edition, W.E. Nelson, V.C. Vaughan, and R.J. McKay, Eds., Philadelphia, Saunders, 1969.

Bibliography

1. Anastasi, A.: Psychological testing of children. In: *Comprehensive Textbook of Psychiatry* (A.M. Freedman and H.I. Kaplan, Eds.). Baltimore, Williams & Wilkins, 1967.
2. Bayley, N.: Values and limitations of infant testing. Children, 5:129, 1958.
3. Bender, L.: *Child Psychiatric Techniques*. Springfield, Ill., Thomas, 1952.
4. Buck, J.N.: *House-Tree-Person Technique: Manual*, Rev. Ed. Los Angeles, Western Psychological Services, 1966.
5. Burns, R., and Kaufman, S.: *Action, Styles, and Symbols in Kinetic Family Drawings (K-F-D): An Interpretative Manual*. New York, Brunner/Mazel, 1972.
6. Burns, R.C., and Kaufman, S.H.: *Kinetic Family Drawings (K-F-D): Understanding Children Through Kinetic Drawings*. New York, Brunner/Mazel, 1970.
7. DiLeo, J.H.: *Children's Drawings as Diagnostic Aids*. New York, Brunner/Mazel, 1970.
8. Engel, M.: Some parameters of the psychological

*Approximately 70% showed 14 and 6 positive spikes; more than 50% exhibited "epileptiform" sleep patterns, including spike-slow wave paroxysms, with nearly half of these showing similar findings in the awake or drowsy state.

evaluation of children. Arch. Gen. Psychiatry, 2:593, 1960.

9. Finzer, W.F.: Unpublished material.

10. Gardner, R.A.: *Therapeutic Communication with Children: The Mutual Storytelling Technique.* New York, Science House, 1971.

11. Goodenough, F.L.: *Measurement of Intelligence by Drawings.* Chicago, World Book, 1926.

12. Harlow, R.G., and Salzman, L.F.: Toward the effective use of the psychological consultation. Am. J.Psychiatry, *115*:228, 1958.

13. Kellog, R.: *Analyzing Children's Art.* Palo Alto, Calif., Mayfield, 1970.

14. Lewis, D.V., and Freeman, J.M.: The electroencephalogram in pediatric practice: Its use and abuse. Pediatrics, *60*:324, 1977.

15. Metcalf, D.R., and Jordan, K.: EEG ontogenesis in normal children. In: *Drugs, Development, and Cerebral Function* (W.L. Smith, Ed.). Springfield, Ill., Thomas, 1971.

16. Oppenheimer, S., and Kessler, J.: Mental testing of children under three years. Pediatrics, *31*:865, 1963.

17. Ross, A.P.: *The Practice of Clinical Child Psychology.* New York, Grune & Stratton, 1959.

18. Santostefano, S.: Psychologic testing in evaluating and understanding organic brain damage and the effects of drugs in children. J. Pediatr., *62*:766, 1963.

19. Schildkraut, M., Shenker, J.R., and Sonnenblick: *Human Figure Drawings in Adolescence.* New York, Brunner/Mazel, 1971.

20. Small, J.G., and Small, J.F.: Fourteen and six per second positive spikes. Arch. Gen. Psychiatry, *11*:645, 1964.

21. Stott, L.H., and Ball, R.S.: Infant and preschool mental tests: Review and evaluation. Monogr. Soc. Res. Child Dev., *101*:30, 1965.

22. Waite, R.R.: The intelligence test as a psychodiagnostic instrument. J. Projective Techniques, *25*:90, 1961.

23. Werkman, S.: The psychiatric diagnostic interview with children. Am. J. Orthopsychiatry, *35*:764, 1965.

24. Winnicott, D.W.: The squiggle technique. In: *Therapeutic Consultations in Child Psychiatry.* New York, Basic Books, 1971.

General References

American Academy of Pediatrics: *A Guide to School Health Professionals.* Chicago, American Academy of Pediatrics, 1977.

Beiser, H.R.: Psychiatric diagnostic interviews with children. J. Am. Acad. Child Psychiatry, *1*:656, 1962.

Bird, B.: *Talking with Patients.* Philadelphia, Lippincott, 1955.

Conn, J.H.: The Play-interview: A method of studying children's attitudes. Am. J. Dis. Child., *58*:1199, 1939.

Simmons, J.E.: *Psychiatric Examination of Children.* Philadelphia, Lea & Febiger, 1969.

Lippman, H.S.: The thorny youngster. Minn. Med., *41*:813, 1958.

9
Diagnostic Formulation and Treatment Planning

> *"Diagnosis" is the physician's total conception of
> the relationships between the patient as a
> person, the disease as a part of the patient,
> and the patient as a part of the world in which
> he lives.*
> *(Thomas Addis)*

The diagnosis and treatment of a child's problem are usually considered as separate processes. But they often overlap; during emergency situations, a physician may have to treat a child before he has time to get all the information he needs to make a diagnosis. When the physician evaluates a child's psychosocial problem or the psychologic factors that affect a child's physical illness, as Finzer[1] has pointed out, the search for the nature of the problem and its treatment may proceed concomitantly. Thus improvement may occur during the process of diagnosis and evaluation. For example, the parents may learn during the course of evaluation that their quarreling upsets the child. Thus they may be able to modify their interaction so that their quarrels become less intense, and the child's problem may improve simultaneously. But

the physician must be careful to finish his evaluation even when he thinks that he knows what the child's problem is. For example, if a child has a learning disorder and lapses in attention, the physician should not try to treat the learning disorder before considering whether the child has petit mal seizures.

When he evaluates a child who has a psychosocial problem, the physician must make certain inferences based on the verbal and behavioral communications from the parents and the child that he observes while he is making his diagnostic study. The physician may ask the parents and the child questions about what he has observed. As he the physician learns more about the family, however he must be willing to change some of his inferences. When parents ask a physician to help their child they may really want help for themselves (although they cannot recognize or admit that they do). The physician may realize that the parents may want help, but he usually should focus his initial study on the child. Even if he suspects (or thinks he learns) that the family has problems that are more important than the child's problem, it is hard for him to shift the focus onto those problems in the early diagnostic phase. He should also realize that the child's problems are often related to pathologic interactions between the child and one or both of his parents (whether those interactions are taking place now or took place in the past).

When a child's parents consult the physician because they believe that their child has a problem, the physician is faced with a central diagnostic question. On the one hand, he must try to find out whether the child has internal conflicts that are self-perpetuating and relatively independent of the child's current interactions with his parents (although they may derive from pathological interactions that took place in the past). If the child has such repressed unconscious conflicts that affect his thoughts or behavior, he may have a psychoneurotic disorder. (Psychoneurotic disorders are discussed more fully in Chapter 18.)

The physician on the other hand must try at the same time to ascertain whether the parents' current handling of the child (related perhaps to disagreement about how to discipline the child) is causing the child to have a more superficial reactive disorder. If the child does have a reactive disorder, the diagnosis, prognosis, and plan for treatment that the physician makes are very different from those that he makes if the child has a psychoneurotic disorder. If the physician arrives at this inference later in the diagnostic process, he must, as Finzer suggests, interact with the data as they become available to him. He can test his inferences by mentally feeding them back into his interviews with the parents and

their child in the form of questions or by using other techniques of interviewing.) If the parents give the physician feedback that confirms his inferences, the therapeutic potential of evaluation may be enhanced and the degree of modifiability can at least partially be evaluated.

The chapter has so far implied the following things that the physician should consider during the diagnostic and evaluative process: the child's behavior and related problems, the nature of the parent-child interaction, and the nature of the interactions between the parents—all of these in terms of current and past problems and strengths. The next thing that he should consider, the family's interactions, may be harder to understand. The family's interactions include the interactions of the child and his parents with his siblings and other members of his family. The physician may find certain "core" conflicts in the family. For example, a family may prohibit its members from expressing even mild aggression. A child of that family who accepts and follows the family's mode of behavior may (as Finzer suggests) be inhibited when he competes at school (even when he competes in learning) and may be the target of other children's aggression. But another child of that family (perhaps because of historical, developmental, or constitutional factors) may not follow the family's mode of behavior. If he does not, the other members of his family may unconsciously channel their aggression toward each other and toward the world through him. Because he expresses their aggression for them, they can follow their mode of behavior strictly and still keep a family interpersonal balance. Other sources of symptoms may arise from "contagion" from other family members, as Finzer puts it, through identification or other mechanisms (see Chapter 6).[2]

When he evaluates what is clearly a disorder of the child's physical functioning, the physician should consider the child's history (that includes information about the child's health, development, social functioning and functioning at school), the family's history (that includes information about the family's development and functioning, and about important events in the lives of its members), the results of the physical and neurologic examinations of the child, his observations of the child's behavior and the child's interactions with the parents, and interviews that he had with the child.

Again, the physician must consider all the possible causes of the child's problem before arriving at a diagnosis and plan of treatment. For example, if the physician first sees the child when the child has an initial attack of bronchitis, he plans treatment on the basis of his inference that the bronchitis was a nonrecurring acute infectious disorder. But if the child's bronchitis recurs several times or continues, the physician must look for factors that *predispose* the child to bronchitis, factors that *contribute* to the bronchitis, and factors that *precipitate* and *perpetuate* the attacks of bronchitis. For example, the physician may learn that the child has a predisposing allergic diathesis of familial nature. The child may have chronically diseased adenoids or may be chronically undernourished because he had a feeding problem since early infancy; these factors contribute to his bronchitis. Precipitating factors may derive from incidental infections of the upper respiratory tract or from episodes of exposure to cold (that occurred when the child went outside without enough clothing on), as the result of rebellion against parental overconcern. The child may have chronic sinusitis that perpetuates his bronchitis. In arriving at the conclusion that the clinical picture represents the so-called bronchosinusitis syndrome, the physician has considered the psychologic and interpersonal factors (the child's undernourishment and defiance of his parents) that affect the child's physical illness.

In such a comprehensive evaluation, the physician studies the relation of the phys-ical factors to the psychosocial factors. If the child's symptoms always recur when important events occur in his life, the physician may be able to find important clues to psychophysiologic influences, involving multiple etiologic forces, in many illnesses such as ulcerative colitis, asthma, peptic ulcer, and hyperthyroidism. If he considers both the physiologic and the psychologic factors that affect a child's disorder, the physician can see how much each type of factor affects the disorder and thus avoid overemphasizing one factor.[10] Instead of "either-or-," the question is often "how much of which." If the physician finds nothing physically wrong with a child who has abdominal pain and mild problems at school and with his family, he should not rely on the "ruling out" of physical sources and immediately conclude that the problems cause the abdominal pain. He must find positive psychologic data that explain why the child has abdominal pain. (For example, if the child fears going to school, the pain begins before the child leaves his house to go to school. Usually the child is overdependent and the parents are overprotective, and a precipitating event often occurred just before his pain first began.) If the physician cannot find such positive data, he must make sure he has not overlooked something that is physically wrong with the child. This question is discussed more fully in relation to conversion disorders in Chapter 18.

Prognosis

This is discussed in later chapters in relation to the diagnosis and treatment of specific psychopathologic disorders. If a problem is caused by a specific stress or precipitated by a specific event (or events), the prognosis usually appears to be good in children and adolescents. A child's problems may be caused by both the stress (or event) and the child's efforts to deal with it. Such a child's conflicts are usually external and easy to see. The conflicts occur between the child and his parents, his peers, or his teachers or other adults, as do the conflicts of children who have re-active disorders. Most children who have such conflicts are of preschool-age and early school age (although some of them are in later childhood or adolescence). Help for the parents in dealing with the child's needs, with support for the child as needed, generally is sufficient to deal with these. The physician can handle many of these problems successfully by himself (although he sometimes must consult a child psychiatrist). By the time the child has reached middle or late school age, he may have repressed and internalized his conflicts. It is harder for the physician to see and treat such conflicts. Even if the child's parents begin to treat him differently, his conflicts may continue (as they do in children who have psychoneurotic disorders). The physician may be of help in milder problems, but many children who have repressed and internalized conflicts need intensive and long-term mental health care. Children whose behavioral patterns (e.g., overdependence, rebellious behavior, or acting out) have become fixed by later childhood and seem to be "calcified" personality traits generally need such care, as in chronic personality disorders. Adolescents may have emotional fixations that occurred at an early level of development or may show sweeping regression to such a level. It is hard for the physician to treat such problems, though they will respond to psychiatric treatment. The nature of the disorder often affects the prognosis (a psychosis that has bizarre symptoms or a severe case of anorexia are examples of such disorders). When a child's disorder involves a strong symbiotic relationship or another kind of unhealthily close relationship with one of his parents, or if his disorder is part of a pervasive disorder in his family's functioning, the prognosis (even for successful psychiatric treatment) is more guarded.

Other factors that affect the overall prog-nosis are the severity and duration of the disorder, the degree of multiplicity and pervasiveness of symptoms, and the degree of psychosocial dysfunction or "crippling" (which may not correspond exactly with the diagnosis). Two longitudinal studies[5,7] support the idea that the child who has many problems at 1 level of his development is likely to have many problems at later levels. If the child's disorder is mild or moderate, did not appear too long ago, and involves chiefly only one symptom, and the child can function at school and when he plays, the prognosis for a fairly prompt response to immediate intervention is generally good. The child's capacity to relate to other people (e.g., his parents, peers, and the physician) may be the best single criterion for a potentially positive response to therapeutic measures.

Diagnosing and Planning the Treatment of Children's Disorders

When the physician has enough information, he can make an initial diagnosis of a disorder in psychosocial functioning or of the effects of psychosocial factors on a disorder that is mostly physical. Making a tentative diagnosis of the types of disorders that later chapters discuss can be more helpful clinically than the use of vague categories such as "emotional problem," "learning disorder," "family problems," or "functional overlay."

As Jordan and Schmitt[4] (a child psychiatrist and a pediatrician, respectively) have suggested, the physician can diagnose children's disorders specifically as healthy situational or developmental crises, developmental deviations, reactive disorders, psychoneurotic disorders, personality disorders, or other disorders (see Chapters 15 through 23). He can specify the psychosocial factors that affect a physical disorder according to the type of psychosocial disorder or mechanisms involved (conversion, reactive, or psychophysiologic, for example). He can also specify the way in which these mechanisms or other factors predispose the child to, precipitate, contribute to, or perpetuate the child's physical disorder. He can specify whether a learning problem involves a developmental deviation, a reactive disorder, anxiety or inhibition arising from a psychoneurotic or personality disorder, or brain damage or mental retardation, alone or admixed. Family problems are harder to specify. They can be indicated as domination by the parents, overpunitiveness on the part of the father, the parents' preoccupation with their marital problems, their use of the child as a scapegoat for those problems, and lack of cohesiveness in the family, drawing on some of the principles discussed in Chapter 6. The physician hopefully can indicate how the family's problems are related to the child's emotional problem or psychosocial disorder.

The foregoing discussion suggests that a diagnostic formulation drawing upon clinical, developmental, familial, and other factors, can be more helpful than a simple diagnosis.* In making the diagnostic formulation, the physician can get some of the information about the child from the child's history, his clinical examination of the child, and the observations about the child that other professionals, such as the nurse or the teacher, make. The physician can get special information from a child psychiatrist consultant, a speech or hearing therapist, a child clinical psychologist who tests the child, or a social worker who interviews the child's parents.

The following outline suggests an approach to a diagnostic formulation.† It includes different categories of information that the physician should consider. Of course not all the categories pertain to the study of every child; the physician may not be able to get all of the information in all the categories. The outline also helps the physician arrive at a plan for treatment or referral. The types of children's disorders that are best referred are discussed in Chapter 11.

I. Personality characteristics of the child and his parents
  A. Functioning of the child's personality
    1. Clinical picture.
       His symptoms and behavior; his interaction with his parents; his ability to relate to the physician; his mental status (including his emotionality, his speech, his perceptual-motor ability, and his appearance, orientation, memory, thought content and thought processes).
    2. Evaluation of his intellectual ability and functioning (based on clinical information about him, the results of psychological tests and screening tests that he takes, and his work at school).
    3. Basic personality picture (e.g., whether he is overly dependent, rebellious, or overly inhibited), if not included in clinical diagnosis.
    4. His main conflicts and whether they are predominantly external or internal.
    5. How his ego functions.
       a. His capacity for social relations and functioning (e.g., with his parents, his peers, and his teachers).
       b. His self-concept, body image, self-esteem, and sense of his own identity.
       c. The functioning of his conscience or superego and his

---

*As the discussion implies, I see little indication for "computer diagnosis." Computers have been used to diagnose physical disorders. Some investigators are trying to use computers to diagnose psychosocial disorders. Computers can only describe categories of disorders; they cannot describe individual children.

†The outline is adapted from an outline that was included in a report of the Committee on Child Psychiatry of the Group for Advancement of Psychiatry[3] on the classification of children's disorders. (Chapter 14 discusses the classification more fully.)

ability to feel such emotions as shame and guilt.

d. His cognitive capacities (e.g., his abilities to pay attention and to concentrate, his sense of time, his self-awareness, and his abilities to fantasize, to form concepts, and to understand abstractions.

e. His psychologic defenses (e.g., denial and projection; See fold-out table on development in Chapter 5).

f. His current developmental level (his psychosocial and psychosexual levels, and any fixations, regressions, or developmental deviations).

g. His overall adaptive capacity, including his coping skills, his ability to master situations, his strengths and his weaknesses, how he handles competition, degree of frustration tolerance, his ability to sublimate, his social competence, and the balance of the progressive and the regressive forces that affect his personality.

h. How effective or impaired his psychosocial functioning is (including his abilities to develop, play, learn and socialize, for example): whether it is optimal, functioning but vulnerable (high risk), incipient dysfunction (mild), moderate dysfunction, severe dysfunction.*

6. Assessment regarding physical health and energy level and relationship to psychopathologic picture (if not included in clinical diagnosis).

*In a tentative classification of the levels of psychosocial functioning that Prugh has written for the Joint Commission on Mental Health of Children, he defines the 5 levels that are listed here.[8]

B. Parents' personalities
Their ability to relate to the physician, each parent's ability to function socially and at work, their emotional maturity, and what the physician can learn about their intellectual abilities and other characteristics of their personalities during his interviews with them. The physician should get information about their lives (e.g., about their lives with their own families, their educational opportunities, and their experience with illness and death, and how adequately they mourn).

II. The interpersonal situation
A. Marital relationship
Capacity of parents for mutual acceptance and positive evaluation of each other, how effectively they communicate, how easily they express affection and their other emotions, whether they share each other's interests and meet each other's needs, how effectively they cooperate in raising the child, how they divide their work, how much their roles complement each other, and whether they have a mature relationship, an immature one, an unbalanced one (in which one depends too much on or dominates the other) or one that is interlocking (in which both depend too much on each other).

B. Parent-child relationships
1. Each one's parenting capacity, including ability to gain the child's trust, support his independence, reinforce his initiative, encourage his work, and let his identity develop. Each one's ability to change his or her role as a parent when the child's development reaches a new stage and to cooperate with and support the other.

2. Their attitudes toward the child, including each one's ability to respect the child as an individual and to accept, nurture, protect, control, and appreciate him. Either may give the child too much protection, control, freedom, punishment, abuse him, fail to appreciate him or reject him. How the child's interacts with each parent (i.e., whether the child complies with the parent in a healthy way, depends too much on the parent, acts withdrawn or rebellious when he is with the parent, or manipulates the parent, for example). The child's influence on each parent.
3. The relationship between each parent and the child. For example, the relationship beween 1 parent and the child may be healthy, discontinuous, insufficient or distorted in relatedness, unbalanced (e.g., either the parent or the child may dominate the relationship), sexualized, undifferentiated (for example, it may be symbiotic, parasitic, or a *folie à deux*), conflicting (e.g., it may be ambivalent or may involve localized neurotic interaction), or interlocking (e.g., it may be symbiotic, mutually antagonistic, or hostile-dependent).
C. The other relationships between the family members
1. The relationships between the child and each of his siblings. They may accept or rival each other. One may dominate or depend on the other. The relationship may be parasitic, interlocking, or based on the sharing of their parents.
2. The relationships between the child and each of his grandpar-

ents. For example, the degree to which the grandparent accepts, nurtures, protects, or controls the child. How effectively the grandparents cooperate with the parents.
D. The family's functioning
1. How cohesive or integrated the family unit is (i.e., whether it is balanced, cohesive, too closely knit, disorganized, or broken, for example).
2. Subgroups in the family. Healthy alignments. Triangular subgroups (in a triangular subgroup, the mother and child may ally against the father (or vice versa); there may be a double bind, between parents and child, or the child may be a scapegoat for the parents or other family members.
3. The family's equilibrium-disequilibrium balance. Its patterns of leadership and dominance, the complementary quality of the roles of its members, or the "fit" between family members. The family's ability to handle crises and regain its interpersonal equilibrium or to establish a new and better equilibrium.
4. Its members' patterns of communication and expressing their emotions. For example, those patterns may be open, comfortable, mutual, inhibited, blocked, distorted, or displaced.
5. How effectively the family has integrated itself into the community. For example, the family's integration may be balanced, or some of its members may be overcommitted, or it may be isolated or nomadic.
6. Other characteristics of the family (e.g., its values and beliefs)
7. The family's ability to develop.

Its ability to handle the developmental tasks of adding children, supporting their children's development as individuals within the family and letting the children become independent and leave the family.

E. The family's sociocultural setting
1. Its home and neighborhood.
2. Its socioeconomic status.
3. Its ethnic background.
4. Its religious affiliation(s).
5. Its members' occupation(s).
6. Its members' education(s).

III. Clinical diagnosis(es)

IV. Summary of developmental-etiological considerations

A. Precipitating factors
An event (or events) that impinge stressfully upon the child's adaptation, psychosocial functioning, or ability to develop; the child's conscious and unconscious perceptions and misperceptions, or sudden changes in the child's relationship with either of his parents or in his parents' relationship, for example.

B. Predisposing factors
The relationship between each parent and the child, family patterns, the child's personality, his hereditary endowment, his biologic constitution, his adaptive capacity, previous events in his life, fixations, and any chronic illness that he has, for example.

C. Contributory factors
Any intercurrent or related physiologic disorder that the child has, any limitations in his mental endowment, and illness or depression in another member of his family, for example.

D. Perpetuating factors
The child's unconscious secondary gain, 1 parent's use of the child as a vicarious object, and an unhealthy or partial solution of conflicts by the symptoms of the child or parents, for example.

V. Prognostic statement
Based on the nature, severity, and duration of the problem, as well as the information that the physician has about the child and his family, and what the physician learns about them while he is making his diagnostic study (e.g., the ability of the child and his parents to relate to the physician or other professional staff, their psychologic awareness, the motivation to change of important members of the family unit, how well the family functions, and the parents' previous efforts to get help for the child).

VI. Management and treatment plan
The physician can state his recommendations for therapy (e.g., counseling, supportive work, psychotherapy, crisis intervention counseling with drug therapy) and the realistic goals of the therapy. Or he can refer the child and the family for intensive psychotherapy to a community mental health facility or to a psychiatric inpatient facility or placement service. He may recommend pediatric hospitalization with further psychiatric consultation, or remedial education or speech therapy for the child. He may recommend other environmental steps such as activity groups or homemaker services. He should consider any cautions or contraindications to any particular treatment.

An example of such a diagnostic formulation and treatment plan follows, drawing also upon the outline for history and physical examination in the Appendix. For purposes of clarity, it is recorded in more detail than a busy physician's time might allow.

Informants. The child's parents. They give a coherent history but seem anxious (particularly the mother).

Presenting problem. Inability of child to attend school, of 4 months' duration.

Present illness or disorder. The patient is a 7-year-old white boy. He has been unable to attend school most of the time since school began 4 months ago because of marked nausea and abdominal discomfort and occasional vomiting early in the morning. He had symptoms that were similar (but milder) when he started the first grade last year, but they lasted for only a few weeks. His family moved last summer; he feels that he has no friends in his new neighborhood. He does not like his teacher, who is much stricter than his first-grade teacher. His parents have tried encouragement, punishment, and other methods to get him off to school, with no results. At first his parents feared that he was physically ill; but another physician examined him and found no abnormalities. An hour or 2 after school starts, he feels better until the next morning. His parents are desperate, worried, half-angry; they fear criticism for having failed. The child's teacher and his principal have been patient and have sent his homework to his home; he has done his homework adequately. Recently, they have begun to put more pressure on his parents to make him go to school.

In the *developmental survey*, his birth and neonatal history reveal no abnormalities, and his developmental milestones were within normal limits. His patterns of growth have been adequate; he has had no apparent problems in feeding, sleeping or toilet training, and no unusual habits. In regard to sexual development, the parents say that he has asked no questions about babies or sexual differences, and has not masturbated. His parents have used occasional deprivation and sent him to his room as methods of discipline. They say that he has been very obedient during the last few years. His school adjustment, when he has been at school, has been adequate; his teachers say that he is very quiet but performs well academically. He showed much anxiety when he had to separate from

his mother around nursery school at 3 years, and his mother had to stay with him for several weeks. He showed anxiety again when he began to go to kindergarten. In his social development, he is described as shy and sensitive; he has 1 or 2 friends in his neighborhood. He showed anxiety when his parents have left him with sitters. (They have done so infrequently.)

The child's *medical survey* reveals no serious illnesses. He has had only a few respiratory infections, with no injuries and no operations. Systems review showed nothing abnormal except for his gastrointestinal symptoms.

Physical examination was within normal limits. An upper G.I. series was also normal. Routine laboratory studies revealed no abnormalities. No other special tests seemed indicated.

The *family survey* indicates no pertinent familial illnesses. Maternal and paternal grandparents are in good health. Mother is the oldest child in her family, with one female sibling, well, age 28, unmarried. She was close to her mother and afraid of her father's temper, but recalls generally happy childhood. Father has no siblings, feels his mother was rather controlling; his father drank heavily and was rather distant. Parents are both of middle European descent; both were born in this country. Both parents finished high school. They had some delay in conceiving the patient and have not been able to conceive another child. They have not had fertility studies done and recently have talked of adopting a child.

Clinical Evaluation of Child and Parents. The boy seemed anxious during the examination, and he clung to his mother. He had trouble separating from his mother for an individual interview. During the interview, he spoke very quietly; he spoke only when he was answering questions, and on the first contact he refused to play with anything. He indicated that he felt lonely because he had no friends, and that it upset him when his teacher "yelled at the kids." During the second interview, he talked more freely and said that he feared going to school, but did not know why. Later he indicated that he worried that he would fall behind in school. He played briefly with a car and a truck, but did not show any interest in darts or toy soldiers. He refused to draw a picture, saying that he could not draw well. The first of his 3 wishes was to "be good"; his second and third wishes were for toys. At first he could not think of what he would like to do when he grew up; later he said that he might like to be a policeman. He was not sure whether he wanted to marry or have children. His mental status seemed within normal limits and his developmental level seemed to be age-appropriate, except for his social and emotional immaturity. He did not seem to have a reading problem or any other learning problem.

The boy's clinical picture seems to be that of a school phobia. His gastrointestinal symptoms seem to be psychophysiologic, of the type often associated with school phobias. He seems to be of above average intelligence from his vocabulary, his ease in reading, and his teacher's reports about his work. He seems to be overdependent and anxious; he particularly shows a conflict about separation from his mother. He projects his problem onto his teacher; his parents mildly support this. His cognitive capacities seem to be intact, but he shows no confidence that he can function on his own. He seems to be isolated from his peer group, although he relates well to his parents and warmed up somewhat with me during the second interview. He seems emotionally immature; his behavior and play are more like the behavior and play of a 4-year-old or a 5-year-old. His parents said that he "acts like a baby" when he stays home from school. Aside from his anxieties about separation from his mother, he seems to have been able to cope with his peers in his neighborhood and at school until second grade, although new experi-

ences have always made him a little anxious. Although his adaptive capacity seems somewhat limited now, he has some social skills and can perform well in a structured learning situation. But now his psychosocial functioning is impaired; he is unable to go to school or to socialize with his peers. His mother, age 34, seems to be intelligent and in good health; she does not work outside the home. She seems rather overprotective of the boy but is also rather controlling with him, insisting that he sit quietly and straightening his shirt several times. His father, age 35, is more retiring than his mother and says little, although he is concerned that the boy will "lose out" in school. He works as a mail carrier and is in good health. They have no other children, and there are no other family members in the home. They related well and want help very much. The parents seem to have a warm relationship, and they seem satisfied with their roles as husband and wife and as parents. The family's members seem to have trouble expressing even appropriate anger in the home, but aside from the mother's overprotective and overcontrolling tendencies and the father's passivity, the family seems to be cohesive and well integrated into the community. They own a house in a quiet, residential neighborhood; the boy has his own bedroom.

Clinical Diagnosis. Developmental crisis, acute, moderately severe, manifested by school phobia in a somewhat dependent anxious boy with a rather overprotective mother and a passive father.

Summary. The boy's school phobic picture seems to have been precipitated by a family move to a new neighborhood, with a change of schools, a stricter teacher, and the loss of former friends. The boy seems to be in a developmental crisis over separation and individuation, which was intensified by regression and enhanced separation anxiety in the face of the move. His mother's overprotective tendencies, combined with his father's passivity in the home, seem to have encouraged some overdependence on the boy's part in the past; these seem to be predisposing factors to the present crisis, with further intensification of the boy's anxiety and the mother's overprotective behavior resulting from his response to the move. Moving increased both the boy's anxiety and his mother's overprotectiveness. The fact that he is an only child may represent a contributory factor. The unconscious secondary gain from the boy's remaining home seems to be a perpetuating factor, but he seems to feel some guilt as his parents' frustration increases.

Prognosis. The boy's school phobia is of recent onset and, although rather severe, is clearly related to the family move in the context of a developmental crisis. The parens seem to want help very much, and the prognosis should be good.

Treatment plan. Reassurance regarding absence of physical problems, discussion of problem with parents and child, counseling and crisis intervention of supportive nature, contact school and arrange for parents to take child to school firmly. When crisis resolved, further counseling to encourage boy's independence.*

---

*The summary is not difficult to harmonize with the currently popular problem-oriented records.[6,9] A problem-oriented record, however helpful, represents a tool, not a philosophy.

Bibliography

1. Finzer, W.F.: Unpublished material.
2. Finzer, W.F.: Symptom contagion in children's emotional disorders. Clin. Pediatr., 4:18, 1965.
3. Group for the Advancement of Psychiatry, Committee on Child Psychiatry: Psychopathological Disorders of Childhood: Theoretical Considerations and a Proposed Classification. Report No. 62. New York, Group for Advancement of Psychiatry, 1966.
4. Jordan, K., and Schmitt, B.: Unpublished material.
5. Kagan, J., and Moss, H.A.: *Birth to Maturity: A Study in Psychological Development.* New York, Wiley and Sons, 1962.
6. Margolis, C.Z., Sheehan, T.J., and Stickley, W.T.: A graded problem oriented record to evaluate clinical performance. Pediatrics, 51:980, 1973.
7. McFarland, J.W., Allen, L., and Honzick, M.P.: *A Developmental Study of Normal Children Between 21 Months to 14 Years.* Berkeley, University of California Press, 1954.
8. Prugh, D.G.: Psychosocial Disorders in Childhood and Adolescence: Theoretical Considerations and an Attempt at Classification. In: *The Mental Health of Children: Services, Research, and Manpower.* (Reports of Task Forces IV and V and the Report of the Committee on Clinical Issues by the Joint Commission on Mental Health of Children.) New York, Harper & Row, 1973.
9. Weed, L.L.: Medical records that guide and teach. N. Engl. J. Med., 278:593; 652, 1968.
10. Weissberg, M.P., and Friedrich, E.V.: Sydenham's chorea: Case report of a diagnostic dilemma. Am. J. Psychiatry, 135:607, 1978.

General References

Group for the Advancement of Psychiatry, *Committee on Child Psychiatry: From Diagnosis to Treatment: An Approach to Treatment Planning for the Emotionally Disturbed Child.* Report No. 87. New York, 1973.

10

Implementing the Results of the Clinical Evaluation

*[Technological success in medicine]. . . has
tended to blind us to those human and spiritual
values which determine the quality of
relationships between people—doctor and
patient, parent and child.*
(Charles A. Janeway)

Discussing the Diagnosis and the Treatment Plan

Once the physician has completed a balanced appraisal of the child and his family, he must communicate his plan of therapy to them effectively. He should talk with both parents together if possible. He should be confident, at times authoritative, in presenting his formulation and recommendations, but humility, patience, and understanding are the most appropriate and helpful attitudes. In discussing the child's condition, the physician should remember that the parents may have come to the interview with great apprehension. He should present his diagnosis and recommendations in simple, nonmedical terms, omitting unnecessary details. He should repeat his suggestions for therapy, and he

should put in writing detailed or complicated instructions for care. Many parents are so anxious during the final interpretive interview that they may indicate that they understand when in fact they are too confused to retain details or to grasp the implications of what they have been told. Giving the parents a chance to talk freely about their reactions may reveal that they have misconceptions. The physician must deal with those misconceptions patiently if the therapeutic or preventive measures he suggests are to succeed.

Before the end of the interview, the physician should ask the parents whether they have any questions, even if they have already asked some. Their response may reveal that because of their confusion and anxiety they have understood little of what they have been told. This is particularly true if the child has been diagnosed as having a serious illness or the diagnosis comes at a time when the parents are already under stress. (An example is a congenital disorder in a newborn, whose parents are adjusting to the birth of the child and are unprepared to assimilate the meaning of a defect.) In such a situation, the parents usually feel shocked or stunned when they are first told of the diagnosis. After the shock they may feel anger and try to handle the problem by denial or disbelief ("I can't believe this has happened"). Later they may have feelings of self-blame and guilt, along with a need to mourn the loss of their child and his future—the "loss of the child that was to be." (The phases of responses to serious stresses, as well as special techniques the physician may use to deal with them, are discussed more fully in Chapter 24.)

Even in less overwhelming situations, the parents' questions may reveal that they have feelings of guilt ("Was there anything that we could have done to prevent it?") which the physician can deal with effectively at such an early stage. Even if the parents do not ask questions that indicate they feel guilty, it is wise to mention, if at all possible, that the child's problem could not have been prevented or that it is not anyone's fault. The parents' guilt feelings usually surface again later as they begin to understand the ramifications of the child's problems. But once the way has been laid open for questions, those feelings are easier to deal with.

Studies by Korsch,[15] Kennell,[13] Pratt and his colleagues,[20] and others have documented gaps in communication and discrepancies between the physician's expectations and the parents' understanding of the problem, resulting from brief discussions of diagnoses without opportunity for questioning. As Ordonez-Plaja and his colleagues[19] have shown, this is particularly the case if the socioeconomic, educational, or ethnic background of the parents differs from that of the physician. Even

the diagnosis and disposition can be influenced by such factors.[9] In a study of the discussion of the diagnosis of a child's congenital heart problem between pediatric residents and the child's parents, Finklestein and Walker[25] have shown that parents had a fuller understanding of the diagnosis and its treatment if the interview lasted 15 minutes or longer and the parents were asked whether they had questions, than following shorter (or longer) interviews in which the parents were not asked whether they had questions. Even if it takes more time, good communication can prevent many problems and may save time in the long run.

In a recent systematic study in a pediatric cardiology clinic by Schulman and his colleagues,[23] different intervention strategies were used to help parents cope with the implications of a diagnosis of congenital heart disease in their child. Using a team approach, involving a psychiatric social worker, strategies for intervention that involved (1) clarification of medical information, (2) a discussion of psychologic issues (including recognition of the parents' feelings), and (3) a combination of both approaches, were found to be significantly more effective than no intervention in helping the parents understand the diagnosis and related medical information. Parents in the 2 groups in which psychologic issues were discussed asked significantly more questions about diagnosis and prognosis than did parents in the other 2 groups. That finding supports the idea that parents who actively seek information can cope better with stressful situations. A less formal approach, utilizing the part-time consultative services of a child psychiatrist or another type of mental health professional has also proved to be valuable in other specialized types of pediatric clinics and to pediatricians in group practice.

The Approach to Emotional Problems

In discussing a child's emotional problem with his parents, the physician must not imply that the parents have caused the problem. Sometimes the parents are aware at the first interview that their child's problem is emotional and that their handling of the child is involved—or they may come to those conclusions during the study. However, if the parents had thought the child's problem was physical, the physician can begin by saying he is happy to assure them that no serious physical abnormalities have been found. He can then add that the symptoms could be caused by emotional tension and ask the parents whether they have noticed evidence of any such tension. This approach keeps the focus on the child as the parents try to recall any evidence or are able to ask what they have "done wrong" or can do to help the child. Whether or not the parents ask, the physician should indicate that such problems are nobody's fault, and he should mention some of the child's strengths. When the parents respond with their observations, he can bolster these with his own, regarding the child's difficulty in dealing with fears or lack of confidence. He can suggest that there are ways of helping them help their child overcome his difficulties. He can also tell them that after they "think out loud" with him for a time they themselves may see things they can do to help their child. If the parents ask what they have done wrong, the physician should avoid a judgmental answer. He might say to them that no one thing causes such a problem, perhaps adding that after a time, they may see certain things in their handling of the child which they might, in hindsight, want to change about their ways of handling the child.

After some initial defensiveness, most parents will respond positively to such an approach, and the physician can then help them develop further insight into their child's problem. In the presence of the child's parents or alone with the child, the physician should explain the problem and the plan for treatment briefly to the child.

He should take care to use language that the child can understand.

If the parents have considered their child's disorder as an exclusively physical one for some time, they may not find it easy to "shift gears" to a view of the disorder as psychosocial in nature. This is especially the case if physicians the parents previously consulted ascribed the child's symptoms to a disease of obscure physical origin or if the disorder does have a physical component as well as the heretofore unrecognized emotional component. But in any event, parents may encounter guilt feelings about their involvement if they permit themselves to recognize the emotional problem or component, and some may feel more comfortable in clinging to the physical origin of the disorder.

In many cases, using a model to explain how emotional factors can produce physical symptoms and helping the parents deal with their guilt feelings will suffice. The model can be a very simple one; for example, the "butterflies in the stomach" most people have experienced before taking an examination or giving a speech or a description of how one's stomach or the bowels can "tie up in knots" in tense situations and cause discomfort, nausea, or diarrhea. The physician can tell the parents that everyone has his own way of experiencing tension in bodily terms when under pressure—through headaches, fatigue, bowel symptoms, or other manifestations. If the child's history permits, the physician may allow the parents, if they need it, the fact that the symptom may have begun with a virus infection or some other mild physical disorder and was "aggravated" by emotional tension. Although such explanations may deal a little loosely with the physiologic truth, they are essentially honest, and many parents can understand them without difficulty.

Problems in Compliance with Medical Recommendations

Recently, attention has focused on problems patients and parents of patients may have in following the physician's recommendations. Difficulties regarding medication[2] or other types of therapeutic regimens recommended[7] (including self-medication and dropping out of treatment[1,4]) may arise due to gaps in communication, emotional blocks, a language barrier, or an excess of information. Problems may also occur because the physician and parents hold different theories of illness as in the view of illness as "God's will" held by some religious groups or the magical belief system of some ethnic groups.[3,22] In such cases, it would be wise for the physician to work closely with the family's clergyman, or with a representative of folk medicine, such as the curandero or curandera,[21] whom some Chicano families may consult, or the medicine man for some Native Americans.[11] A chaplain on the hospital's staff may be helpful if the family has no contact with a clergyman in the area. (Several medical centers in the Southwest have brought representatives of folk medicine into their clinics.)

Recent studies have indicated that people who are socially isolated or do not have available social support systems in the family or neighborhood often have trouble complying with therapeutic regimens or may tend to drop out of treatment.[4] Both Korsch[14] and Haggerty[10] have suggested that in pediatric practice such problems may occur in the context of a relationship with the physician that is perceived as noncommunicative or nonsupportive. This seems to support the idea that an empathic attitude on the part of the physician may be the key to improving patient and parent compliance. Warmth, understanding, patience, and concern seem to be the characteristic attitudes of the physicians who are most successful in helping patients and their parents understand the illness and follow medical recommendations. Compliance seems to be better also if the physician discusses his recommendation with both parents. It is the physician's responsibility to secure the compliance of the patient and his parents.

Management of Hypochondriacal Concerns of Parents

A few parents of children who have emotional problems may find it difficult, even impossible, to accept the idea that their child's illness has an emotional origin. Such parents often "telegraph" the views they need to hold in comments they make during the discussion of their child's history ("It couldn't be anything emotional, Doctor" or "One doctor said it was all in her head but we left him.") These parents often have made records of their child's temperature and his bodily functions, which sometimes indicate that they have displaced their own hypochondriacal concerns onto their child. Such parents only become angry and argumentative if the physician tries to convince them that their fears about the child's physical health are groundless. If the physician feels compelled to tell the parents the whole truth, he had better advise them to consult another physician. But if he can settle for partial truths and can exercise great patience, he can help some of these parents and their children significantly.

Such parents experience anguish over their child. The parents themselves are often seriously disturbed, and they may have a deep unconscious need to perceive their child as being physically ill and even to suffer themselves in the process. An example is the mother who "devotes her life" to her child in a sacrificial way perhaps to avoid thinking of a marital problem or to give meaning to her life. The parents may be giving the child the physical care and nurturing which they did not receive as children, or 1 parent, usually the mother, may unconsciously regard the child as an extension of herself and her own physical problems. The child of such parents is usually overcontrolled and seriously overdependent, and he is at least on the way to adopting his parents' hypochondriacal concerns. Often he has missed much school, and may be becoming an emotional invalid. But if he is still in the early school-age period, he may not yet be seriously disturbed.

The only way that the physician can help the parents loosen their control of the child is to settle for partial truth. He should do a thorough physical examination of the child and have the appropriate laboratory studies made (he may have to resist the parents' pressure to do unnecessary tests or to redo some tests). Then he should select 1 physical symptom from the array presented by the parents—preferably a vague symptom (e.g., "a weak stomach," "run-down physically," or a "low-grade anemia"). The physician should concede that the problem requires treatment although fortunately it is not deeply serious, and he should indicate that he is aware that the parents must have been very worried. He might add that the child's condition and the medical treatment he may have undergone must have made the child tense and worried about himself and that such emotional tension can aggravate the child's basic disorder, making the symptom worse. The parents will often cautiously accept such a formulation (which is usually more than just partially true) and the recommended treatment program, particularly if the program is explained in considerable detail, preferably in writing. The formulation and plan should always be discussed with both parents together, and they should be seen together in each subsequent interview, if possible, both before and after the child is seen.

The physician should tell the parents that the treatment program will be a long and arduous one for both the child and his parents. The physician should not promise a cure or quick results, as this may upset an already unhealthy family equilibrium, which may be unconsciously based on the need for the child to be sick. Parents in such families will usually resist promises of quick results. If a rapid change should occur, the family's equilibrium may be so threatened that the parents feel impelled

to seek another physician. The physician should rather hold out only the possibility of "getting this problem under control," with the likelihood of very slow, gradual improvement, at the very least to the point where the child can learn to live with his symptoms. Appointments should be made once a week at first, so that the physician and the parents can "work closely together" in carrying out the treatment program.

Among other things, the program should involve some planned but mild restriction of activity at first. If the child has missed much school or has had a "homebound teacher," as is often the case, a new arrangement should be worked out with the school for the child to attend school for part of the day, so that he can get "sufficient rest." But the physician should stress that it is important that the child go to school each day, in order to gradually "build up his strength." Other "building-up" measures should include some sort of innocuous "tonic" to be given regularly at an exact time in order to meet the parents' often intense need to give their child meticulous care.

(Physicians today are taught that tonics have no place in most treatment regimens. But they have an important psychologic meaning to hypochondriacal parents, who need to do something active to help the child, a need that, because of their unconscious conflicts, goes far beyond the placebo effect. Some physicians can use a placebo effectively. I feel diffident about using them to treat hypochondriacal families.)

Small doses of vitamins (if the parents are not giving the child high doses already), diluted doses of elixir of ferrous gluconate if the red blood cell count is low normal, or some other mild agent that has a definite pharmacodynamic effect on the symptoms chosen, will at least not harm the child. And it might help him physically, and it will certainly help him and his parents psychologically. The use of such a medication makes it possible for the physician to answer the parents' questions honestly if they ask its nature and expected effect (they frequently do) and avoids the catastrophic loss of trust that can occur if the parents somehow find out that a placebo has been prescribed.

The management approach just described has several advantages. It allows for the parents' limitations but takes advantage of their strengths. Also, it introduces to them an acceptable concept of emotional tension in their child that can be slowly elaborated in future sessions. It meets the parents' need for action on behalf of their child but permits the emphasis to be gradually shifted from worry about the child himself to concern about the details of his management program, which can be discussed fully on each visit. It gets the child back in school and to healthier and more independent activities, thus removing him from the constant attention of his parents for some time each day. It permits the physician and the parents to cooperate in a limited sense, and the physician can more sympathetically accept the parents' concerns about details of treatment.

As the program continues, the child's time in school can be gradually increased as his "building-up" continues. Although the focus of concern should remain on the child's symptom for some time, the physician's sympathetic acknowledgment of the parents' worries may lead one or both of the parents to reveal their concerns about their own health. The physician may find that over a number of months the child gradually begins to feel "a little better." The parents may begin to permit the child more independence, gradually speaking less of his physical symptom and more of their own symptoms. They may become more aware of the child's emotional difficulties, and, if the difficulties persist, they may be able after a year or more to accept the fact that the child should be treated at a child mental health facility to help relieve his tension. Some parents over a long period of time may even be able to see their own need for help. They may gradually permit the focus of treatment to shift to their own personal problems and eventually accept consultation or referral for appropriate therapy.

The physician who undertakes such an approach with a hypochondriacal family must be patient as well as flexible, and he must be prepared to follow up such a family closely for several years if necessary, accepting the possibility of failure along the way. Not all such families will even accept this type of approach at the outset, but even those who discontinue treatment may return later, after having thought it over or having tried other approaches. If accepted, this approach will be successful in a number of cases of the type described.* In addition, various modifications of the approach can be applied to the management of families of children who have chronic illnesses or handicaps, in which strong emotional components are present, who see the child as much sicker than he is but cannot accept the idea of psychiatric consultation or treatment for him. This approach is somewhat similar to the way general practitioners and at least some psychiatrists (e.g., Lyons[16]) manage patients who have chronic hypochondriacal concerns. The physician probably sees enough such cases to make it worth his while to try such an approach, preferably after discussing the family's situation informally with a child psychiatrist who is familiar with the approach and accepts it.

Collaborating with Mental Health Professionals

Whether in private practice or in working with children and their families in a hospital setting, the pediatrician should know how to collaborate with child psychiatrists or other mental health profes-

*One such family is described in Chapter 8.

sionals in ways that use their specialized knowledge effectively. Although there are similarities in the procedure for working with a consultant in any field, the complexity and sensitivity of mental health problems necessitates some special consideration. The ethical considerations involved in the use of consultants have been well summarized in *Standards of Child Health Care*,[24] published by the American Academy of Pediatrics.

The Use of Mental Health Consultation

The physician should, as a basic principle, complete a comprehensive diagnostic evaluation before referring a patient to a mental health professional for consultation. The physician should take psychologic as well as physical considerations into account in his initial evaluation. He may find that, contrary to his early impression about an apparently psychologic problem, he is still able to offer sufficient help if the problem is a relatively mild one or is not a long-standing one. The physician who has a good deal of information can make a more appropriate referral and that information may be extremely valuable to the consultant or specialist.

The physician should not make a referral to rule out a psychologic problem nor simply because he has not found a physical problem and cannot explain the child's presenting symptoms. If the physician finds it hard to elicit positive psychologic information, he may wish to seek the help of a child psychiatrist or other mental health professional as a consultant in evaluating the child. But he should have some hunches about the child's problem, based on the information he has collected.[18] Otherwise, the consultant may find no evidence of a psychologic problem and may suggest further physical studies. The consequences may be loss of valuable time for the patient who has an underlying but obscure medical problem and embarrassment for the physician if he diagnosed a psychologic problem without having positive supporting information. In some cases, the physician may have omitted some pertinent physical studies because of his too-hasty conviction that the child's problem was not organic or because he wanted to pass the problem on to someone else. Even if the physician has obtained a psychiatric consultation, he may have to work with the child and his family himself, either on an interim basis while awaiting an opening for psychiatric treatment or if there is no appropriate psychiatric treatment facility in his community. Thus his own diagnostic impressions and the quality of his relationship to the child and his family are of vital importance, whether or not he chooses to make a referral.

Studies have shown that the recommendations of a psychiatric consultant are more likely to be carried out if both parents and the child are involved, if the child is brought to the consultant or clinic, if the child is less than 9 years old, and (most important) if the parents' view of the problem tends to agree in some measure with the psychiatrist's.[6] These considerations, particularly the last one, underscore the importance of a careful preparation for the referral by a physician who knows the family and has gained their confidence during his studies of their child.[8]

If the pediatrician is not certain what step to take in a particular situation, he may talk to a child psychiatric consultant informally even before discussing the possibility of referral with the child and his parents. During this preliminary consultation, the pediatrician can give his findings on the immediate problem and his observations on the child's developmental status and adaptive capacity, the child's relationship with his parents, the family's equilibrium, and other characteristics. He may then ask the consultant whether he thinks that a formal consultation with the child and his parents would be helpful or whether he thinks that referral to another source, such as a family agency which deals with marital problems, might be appropriate. The consultant may be able to offer suggestions about another kind of referral or to suggest other techniques of examining the child (e.g., collecting certain kinds of information or having the child evaluated by a clinical psychologist) before deciding whether he should see the child. In some such "curbstone" consultations, the consultant may be able to make suggestions about treatment approaches without seeing the child and family.

If the physician and the consultant both agree that a formal consultation would be helpful, the physician should discuss the decision with the parents and the child in language that is appropriate to the parents' level of education and the child's level of development. The physician should reassure the parents that the child has no serious physical illness, and they can be told that he has the impression that emotional tension or an emotional problem is involved in the child's difficulties. The physician can then say that he would like to have the opinion of a child psychiatrist to help him evaluate the child's problem fully and decide on the best treatment for it. He can give the parents the names of several consultants or he can recommend one he knows particularly well. If the parents prefer to consult someone else, he can discuss that possibility if he knows the specialist they mention. If the parents insist on their choice, he should usually go along with it.

Responsibilities of the Consultant

Through the efforts of Senn, Spock, Richmond, and others, child psychiatrists are becoming increasingly aware that they must learn more about the challenges and difficulties facing the pediatrician if they are to offer consultative help that has practical value. Experience has shown that mental health specialists, are of little help if they simply take over the child's treatment without knowing or considering the pediatrician's role.[18]

Even when intensive psychiatric treatment is the approach of choice for a child, his family continues to consult the pediatrician for the medical care of the child's siblings, as well as the child's intercurrent medical problems. Thus the pediatrician and the mental health specialists must communicate and coordinate their efforts. The referring pediatrician may for good reasons not want the mental health specialist to take over the care of the child, particularly if the child has a mild problem. He may prefer to use the diagnostic knowledge the specialist offers as the fulcrum of his own approach to treatment. The recommendations of the consultant (e.g., for intensive psychotherapy) may not be practical if the family lives in an area where the treatment he recommends is not available, and the pediatrician must still continue to help them in some way.

With these considerations in mind, the consultant must first try to obtain from the referring pediatrician a clear idea of what the pediatrician expects from the consultation. A diagnostic evaluation only, with a referral of the family back to the pediatrician, and a report of the evaluation, can be reasonably requested. A plan for diagnostic services and provision of whatever treatment is deemed necessary (to be given by the consultant or by someone to whom he has referred the family) can also easily be arranged, without concerns over "stealing" patients, if the consultant asks the pediatrician at the outset what he wishes to be done about the treatment he recommends. Often the pediatrician wishes the arrangements for treatment to be made by the consultant, but may understandably resent it if such arrangements are made without his knowledge and consent. The same principles apply to referrals to mental health clinics or other facilities. The pediatrician can be invited to attend a brief intake or coordinating conference, scheduled flexibly, at which plans and roles could be clarified.

As implied, the pediatrician may sometimes want only a confirmation of his own diagnostic impressions before he begins the treatment approach he has chosen. He has that right. But sometimes he may want to transfer a difficult family to someone else's care; or, without realizing it, he may be asking for help in dealing with his own feelings or attitude toward provocative or hostile parents. It is the consultant's responsibility to help the pediatrician express his wishes as explicitly as possible and to offer him help as it becomes apparent where he needs it.[1,12] If the pediatrician indicates that he is seeking a treatment procedure that will suddenly transform the child or his parents, the consultant should be sympathetic but straightforward in pointing out that such an approach would be unrealistic. He should have sufficient knowledge of pediatric practice to understand that the pediatrician feels impelled to do something to help, even if help principally involves protracted listening to desperate and confused parents. The consultant can help him to learn to do this by affording him the opportunity for periodic brief discussions.[5]

In achieving the various goals of consultation, which may include help in the management of child and family in a hospital setting as well as on an outpatient basis, the psychiatric consultant must be mindful of the need to communicate clearly with the pediatrician (and the nurses and other staff members if the patient is hospitalized). In doing so, he may be torn by his responsibility to maintain the confidentiality of the information the child or his family reveals to him and which they divulge because of their intimate professional relationship with him and because he is skilled in helping people unburden themselves.

Some child psychiatrists regard the information they are given in an interview as too personal to be revealed in any form to anyone, including the pediatrician. It is true that some of this material could, if revealed to anyone outside the psychiatric consultative or treatment situation, be misunderstood or misused, even by well-meaning professional persons and thus lead to anguish for the family.[17] But the consultant can discuss some of the child's problem areas with the referring physician if the consultant is given some assurance that the material will be handled discreetly with the child or his parents. The fact that a few pediatricians have misguidedly read or quoted to the parents part or all of reports from a consultant or clinic, or even reports of psychologic tests, has increased the reluctance of some child psychiatrists to send detailed reports to the referring physician. But most pediatricians realize that giving the parents the details of a highly technical report can only confuse parents or, sometimes, make them feel guilty or resentful.

It is the responsibility of the consultant or the clinic to provide the referring pediatrician with a concise, comprehensive and prompt report written in nonpsychiatric terminology. The report should contain a brief diagnostic formulation, together with any pertinent results of tests done, a concise statement about any dynamic trends (those that shed light on the consultant's diagnosis and recommendations), some statement of prognosis, and concrete recommendations about the best therapeutic approach. The report should not recapitulate the patient's history, but it should include any new and significant historical data that may have emerged during the consultative study. Confidential material of a disturbing nature that parents or the consultant consider irrelevant to the child's overall picture may be omitted from the report or presented in the form of a reference to certain broad problem areas for the enlightenment of the pediatrician.

Ideally, before the written report—and within a day or so after the consultation is completed— the consultant should discuss his findings and recommendations with the pediatrician by phone, thus giving the pediatrician the chance to ask any questions he has. If the question has not been settled before, the consultant should ask the pediatrician whether he wishes to discuss the contents of the report with the parents himself or would prefer the consultant to do so in an interpretive interview. In a clinic setting, the pediatrician can be invited to a brief conference, scheduled flexibly, to discuss findings and future plans. Unfortunately some consultants and some clinics fail to provide prompt, helpful reports to pediatricians. No matter how busy the consultant (or the clinic staff) is, a written report should go to the pediatrician within a week—sooner if the problem is urgent.

The report should be brief and to the point, as in the following example.

Dear Dr. _____:

Your patient, Johnny H., and his parents have been seen by our clinic staff in consultation [or for diagnostic study] as you requested. Our impression is that Johnny's rebellious and defiant behavior at home and at school represents a reactive disorder of moderate degree. We could see no evidence of the psychotic trends about which the parents were concerned, and the prognosis seems to be relatively good.

The disorder basically seems to represent Johnny's need to express his conscious resentment over his parents' demands and aspirations, which exceed his or any other child's capacities, and his unconscious need to invite punishment because of guilt over his angry feelings. The parents seem to expect Johnny to live up to the idealized image of his older brother, who died several years ago. In addition, Johnny's behavior has become a battleground on which his parents seem to be struggling over marital difficulties, which they had previously felt they could not discuss.

Although Johnny is of above-average intelligence and has many strengths, particularly in athletic and social areas, his reactions to the family's developmental block has reached crisis proportions. We feel that the parents and Johnny both wish for help, and that focal interview therapy, including family interviews, over a period of several months could help all of them to see and accept each other more clearly and comfortably. We would be able to provide such therapy within the next few weeks.

We have not discussed our findings with the family, as we understand that you wish to discuss this report with them. They are looking forward to talking with you as soon as possible. If, after your discussion with them, the family wishes to undertake therapy here, please ask them to call Ms. _____ to arrange for an appointment.

Thank you for referring this family to us. If you have any questions, please do not hesitate to get in touch with us.

If, as sometimes happens, a family comes to a psychiatric consultant or mental health facility for help with a child's problem without the knowledge of their family physician, certain ethical considerations apply. Before an interview is set up, the family should be asked to discuss the matter with their physician and to obtain a report from him. Once the family physician is aware of the problem, which the parents have been ashamed to discuss with him, he may be happy to have consultative help. Or he may wish to take other steps first or recommend a psychiatric professional he is accustomed to call on for consultation. The parents may indicate that they have already tried to communicate their concern to their physician but that he has not seemed responsive or has assured them that the problem is minor or that the child will grow out of it. Nevertheless, they should be encouraged to again contact their physician for a frank discussion of their feelings, including their wish for mental health consultation. If they still demur, the consultant can offer to call the physician and apprise the physician of the situation and perhaps invite him to a conference. If this offer is rejected, the family should be told that it would be very difficult to offer them help without their physician's support and that it is not ethical to do so without his knowledge. Most families will agree to contact their family physician, and most physicians will support or agree to a consultation. A few physicians will oppose a request for consultation, and a few families will thereupon change their physicians—which is their right. Tactful handling and open communication will resolve most problems of this type and will result in positive collaboration among the family, their physician, and the psychiatric personnel.

Responsibilities of the Pediatrician

Besides providing adequate and helpful referral information after a comprehensive workup, the pediatrician has the responsibility to use the consultative appraisal as constructively as possible. As indicated earlier, he should not read or quote the report directly to the parents. Rather, the pediatrician should give the parents a brief oral outline in nontechnical language. Recent legislation has given parents a legal right to see reports or records concerning their children. Parents who have confidence in their pediatrician and the consultant, do not ordinarily ask to see the report, but sometimes they ask the consultant or the pediatrician for a written report, which can be very brief and couched in sensitive and tactful terms.

Sufficient time, usually at least 30 minutes, should be set aside for the interview during which the consultant's report is discussed with the parents, in order to permit them to ask questions freely. If the parents ask questions which are not answered in the verbal or written reports, the pediatrician should discuss these questions further with the consultant. Scheduling another, briefer interview with the parents within a few days gives them time to assimilate the consultant's findings and recommendations as well as another opportunity to use their relationship with the pediatrician as they work through their often conflicting feelings.

In implementing the results of the consultation, the confidence of the pediatrician in his consultant and of the parents in their pediatrician is of paramount impor-

tance. The pediatrician cannot implement a recommendation if he is uncertain about its validity. Parents cannot cooperate effectively with recommendations for psychotherapy unless their confidence in the pediatrician is bolstered by his confidence in the consultant. The approach, "I'm not sure whether there's anything in it, but you might give it a try" is virtually certain to produce a treatment failure, for obvious reasons. If the pediatrician is not convinced of the value of a consultation, he should probably not suggest one. If he decides to do so, even if he is not convinced of its value—or if the parents, school, court, or community agency insists on such a step— he can at least say, "I don't know very much about such an approach myself, but I think it's best to follow the recommendation." That attitude frees the parents to follow through with the consultation and/or treatment, while the pediatrician awaits results with an open mind.

Indications for Referral to a Mental Health Professional or Facility

The kinds of psychosocial disorders in children and adolescents a pediatrician can be expected to treat with success can be summarized as follows:

1. Developmental problems (e.g., in feeding, sleeping).
2. Developmental and situational crises.
3. Developmental deviations of mild degree.
4. Disorders in which:
    a. Conflicts are largely external (e.g., between child and parent or between siblings).
    b. A precipitating factor is evident.
    c. A disorder of mild degree is present.
    d. The onset is fairly recent (i.e., is of brief duration).
    e. The clinical picture involves only one or a small cluster of symptoms.

f. The disturbance in behavior is localized (i.e., is confined to the family and home or occurs only in the
classroom). (This group includes
mainly reactive disorders of mild
degree, and a few incipient and
mild psychoneurotic disorders in
which the conflicts are not yet fully
internalized.)

5. Disorders in which both physical and
psychologic components are present
   a. Reactions to physical illness—
   mainly milder reactive disorders,
   situational crises, and mild personality disorders.
   b. Psychophysiologic disorders of
   mild degree.

The types of disorders best suited for referral include:*

1. Disorders of marked severity, particularly psychotic disorders involving
bizarre behavior, moderate-to-severe
personality disorders, and marked reactive disorders with sweeping
regression.
2. Disorders of long duration (1 year to
several years), particularly if the
symptoms have proved intractable.
3. Disorders in which conflicts are fully
internalized, particularly moderate-to-
severe psychoneurotic disorders and
some personality disorders involving
"calcified" personality traits.
4. Disorders in which no precipitating
factors are evident—particularly
moderate-to-marked personality disorders with evidence of fixation at
early levels of development.
5. Disorders in which the clinical picture
involves multiple symptoms or large
clusters of symptoms, particularly
marked reactive disorders and near-
psychotic disorders.
6. Disorders in which marked social im-

pairment is evident (e.g., a crippling
psychoneurotic disorder, a disorder
that brings a child in intense conflict
with society or the law, and a disorder
involving psychotic or markedly regressive behavior).
7. Disorders in which the child shows
marked inner suffering, a condition
often overlooked by parents, teachers, and physicians. Also in this category is the well-behaved but quite
inhibited child who is not achieving
in the classroom.
8. Disorders involving a marked discrepancy between the child's age and
his behavior (e.g., the persistence of
particular habits such as head rolling
or head banging far beyond the developmental stage in which they are
usually given up).
9. Disorders in which the child has a
markedly unsatisfactory or deleterious home environment (e.g., a severely handicapping or dangerous
home environment, seriously disturbed parents, markedly impaired
parent-child relationships, serious
marital conflicts or impending divorce, and pervasive disorders in
family functioning).

The Referral Process

Once the pediatrician has decided that
referral is necessary, his preparation of the
child and parents can pave the way to a
successful outcome.[18] Parents are often unduly apprehensive of the unknown and
may be afraid of the words "psychiatry" or
"mental illness," which still carry a stigma.
They may also fear that they will be lec-
tured or possibly condemned because they
have failed as parents.

There are several steps involved in the
referral process. The physician must first
explain to the parents why their child needs
help. He can do that by describing the emotional difficulties he has observed, and how

---

*The need for some referrals, particularly of adoles-
cents, is immediately obvious as in the case of major
suicidal attempts, serious drug abuse, or markedly
violent behaviour.

those difficulties differentiate their child from other children his age. To forestall the parents' feelings of guilt, the pediatrician must give the information tactfully and empathetically, showing genuine concern for the child's discomfort and describing his symptoms as indications of "lack of confidence," or of "being mixed up about himself," or of worries "buried in the back of his head, which he can't get at." An emphasis on the child's inner feelings also helps to convince the parents the physician is not rejecting the child by referring him.

The referring physician should then give the parents a realistic idea of what psychiatric therapy can accomplish. He should indicate to the parents that help is both needed and available, but he should not make extravagant promises or make specific predictions. The main object is to instill in the parents an empathy with the disturbed child, not merely to get them to the clinic. Once the physician is convinced that the parents understand the situation, he should suggest that they talk it over, and let him know what their decision is. If they decide to take the step, he should suggest that they themselves make the appointment with the consultant. Taking this initiative can solidify the parents' motivation to seek help.

In discussing the possibility of a referral, the terms child psychiatrist, child psychiatry clinic, child psychologist, child therapist, and mental health center should be used (as appropriate), not such euphemisms as neuropsychiatrist, a doctor who has an interest in emotional problems, or a counseling center (unless that is the name of the facility). The honest use of terminology not only avoids resentment on the part of the parents when they discover the truth (as they inevitably will), but it also helps them accept emotional and mental illness as another form of disability which can be treated. A few parents may not be able to accept a referral to a psychiatrist because of the possible stigma or because they are unable to admit the existence of an emotional problem, which they fear is their fault alone. But most parents who have confidence in their pediatrician can accept such a referral. Conversely, if the physician is reluctant to suggest the referral because he is skeptical about its value or a result of his own difficulty in admitting the need for help, his negative attitude may deter the parents and make it more difficult for them to seek appropriate treatment for their child.

If parents object to referral, the physician should inquire why they feel as they do. If he questions them in a sympathetic, nonjudgmental way, he may learn that they have had a relative with a mental illness and are afraid that referral means that their child has a similar problem. Once revealed, this fear is usually fairly easy to deal with. The physician can point out that children are different, and that many different factors play a role in the development of problems. He should assure the parents that the information they or the child give will be kept confidential. The pediatrician may add that the mental health professional will help them to understand their child's problem more fully so that they can help him work it out more effectively. With this approach, many parents can accept referral comfortably once they have had time to think it over and discuss it.

But if the parents are still reluctant about the referral, the pediatrician can suggest that they consult with a child psychiatrist to see whether he agrees that a referral is indicated. Often such a consultation will help the parents accept the recommendation for referral.[1] If parents refuse such a consultation, the pediatrician can indicate that he still recommends the referral, but that he is willing to try to help work out the problem first but may have to reopen the question of referral at a later date.

If the problem appears to be of major psychologic proportions, such as a serious suicide attempt, significantly antisocial behavior, or flagrant psychosis, and the parents refuse to permit necessary professional help, the pediatrician must decide where he must draw the line out of concern for the patient and for his own integrity. If he feels that the line has been breached, he can observe, without criticism, that since the parents seem to have some difficulty in accepting his advice, perhaps they would feel happier if they had the opinion of another pediatrician, and he can give the names of several pediatricians. It is impossible for the pediatrician not to feel some anger in such a situation. But he must control his feelings. Often a nonjudgmental, nondefensive attitude permits the parents to sense the physician's sincere concern for their child, and they may accept his recommendation. Even if the parents choose to seek another opinion, they may come back to the original physician with greater confidence. He should therefore not close the door to their return.

Referral for Marital Problems

Marital problems are ordinarily too complicated and difficult for a pediatrician to handle without special training. He can identify such problems, however, and he can also help parents to recognize them and accept referral for help. The existence of marital problems often surfaces during a discussion of the parents' child-rearing methods, particularly the handling of discipline. The pediatrician can point out that the parents seem to disagree on some issues, and he can ask whether they also have disagreements in other areas. Occasionally one parent will reveal that a marital problem exists. The physician should not take one parent's disclosure at face value, however; he should try to see both parents together or at least try to arrange to see the other separately. Once a frank discussion has brought a marital problem out into the open, the physician can suggest a mental health consultation or referral to a marital counseling agency, a family agency, or a mental health professional who offers marriage counseling. Experience has shown that this type of therapy often proceeds best if the same therapist sees both partners, individually or together, although treatment by separate therapists is sometimes necessary. Occasionally 1 parent may feel that he or she needs help for a personal problem and will ask for referral to a therapist who treats adults.

In discussing marital problems with the parents together, a good argument between the parents, with the physician as the referee, sometimes clears the air. More often, the physician must take a more active role, stepping in firmly to prevent the parents' expression of explosive feelings and then confronting the parents with their need for consultation and help. Needless to say, the physician should do this in a kindly and nonjudgmental way and without taking sides.

Telling the Child about the Referral

The physician should be open and honest with the child who is to be referred. He should tell the child where he is going and why. Despite the fact that the child's symptom may have been discussed openly (sometimes critically) at home, the child should know as clearly as possible what his basic problem is, and that other children also have problems like his. This approach can be reassuring to the child rather than threatening. The explanation should take into consideration his age and his level of understanding. If the physician sets an honest pattern of communication at the outset, the child will be better able to respond to therapy.

Ongoing Collaboration During Psychotherapy

After the parents have decided to consult the mental health professional they may have conflicts in themselves or confusion about changes in their child's behavior that may lead them to return to the pediatrician for advice. During the course of therapy, they may be confused or disturbed about shifts in the child's behavior and question the advisability of continuing treatment. The pediatrician must be in a position to deal with such problems as they arise. After the initial communication of his impressions, the mental health professional should communicate with the referring physician (by phone, letter, or brief personal contacts) at least every several months during the course of treatment to keep him aware of the major trends and developments. If this is done, the referring physician will be equipped in advance to help the parents understand the need for patience and trust if they come to see him during what appears to be a plateau in therapy, a temporary behavioral regression, or a misunderstanding with the therapist. In his dealings with the parents, the pediatrician should be sympathetic with their concerns, indicating that ups and downs occur in the often difficult process of psychotherapy, and suggesting that they discuss their concerns with the therapist, which they may have previously feared to do. This approach will usually encourage the parents to continue treatment.

If, for any reason, he himself is also confused, the physician should clarify the situations through a call or in a conference with the therapist or clinical staff. It is well known that parents, particularly conflicted or disturbed parents, may frequently unconsciously distort what is discussed with them in a psychotherapeutic setting. (Of course, the child may do so also.) While empathizing with the parents' concern, it is probably wiser for the pediatrician to take nothing for granted, much less act solely on his intuition or on impulse.

Under no circumstances should the pediatrician suggest that treatment be discontinued for a while to test the child's improvement or to "let the air clear." He can, however, discuss the parents' concerns with the therapist; he may well learn that they or the child are just beginning to face certain troubling or conflicting feelings or thoughts of which they had been previously unaware. They may thus be seeking a way to avoid their feelings and the pain of working them out by discontinuing treatment with the blessing of the pediatrician, just when they are on the verge of constructive steps. Equipped with this knowledge, the pediatrician can compassionately help most such families continue treatment. In a word, a sympathetic and gentle push back into the arena of emotional conflict from a trusted and supportive family physician can often result in rich and even rapid rewards for the family. Permission or encouragement to end the treatment prematurely can cost the family much in terms of wasted effort and money. From a psychologic point of view, an abrupt termination of therapy may result in serious repercussions for the child and/or his parents. The original symptom if quickly removed, may at times be replaced by another, even more painful or incapacitating symptom, if the underlying conflicts have not been worked out. A more common effect of terminating treatment before the family's emotional conflicts have been worked out is at least a period of heightened conflict, accompanied at times by added resentment on the part of the child at having been abruptly removed from a satisfying relationship and source of help.

From the foregoing, it is obvious that collaboration between the referring physician and the psychotherapist may be crucial to the success of treatment, especially if there is a physical component in the child's symptoms, and both medical and psychologic treatment are necessary. Collaboration is needed even if the child's disorder is predominantly psychologic since the pediatrician will continue to supervise his physical health and may be called on to treat an illness or accident, or arrange for an operation which will affect the psychotherapy program.

Unfortunately, it sometimes happens that the psychotherapist first learns that the child is to undergo elective surgery (e.g., a tonsillectomy) right before the operation (perhaps from the child himself). Or a child psychiatry clinic sometimes makes recommendations to the child's family about putting the child in a foster home without having contacted the referring physician. In either instance, the chance to plan the step jointly, to prepare the child and his parents for the step, to work through any conflicts about the step, and to take the step at the best time has been lost.

The time spent on communication is well spent. Good communication usually results in good collaboration and coordination. Although mental health professionals operate largely by appointment and although privacy is one of their therapeutic tools, they should arrange to set aside time for brief communications with the referring physician, either by telephone or in short conferences at a mutually convenient time. Pediatricians are very busy, but they should make it a practice to contact the psychiatric clinic regarding a medication for a child undergoing therapy or if an operation is indicated, and to respond to invitations to meet for brief conferences. In almost all cases, collaboration is not a luxury; it is the fulcrum of successful treatment for the child and his family.

Bibliography

1. Adams, P.: Techniques for pediatric consultation. In *Handbook of Psychiatric Consultation.* Edited by J.J. Schwab. New York, Appleton-Century Crofts, 1968.
2. Arnhold, R.G., et al.: Patients and prescriptions: Comprehension and compliance with medical instructions in a suburban pediatric practice. Clin. Pediatr., 9:648, 1970.
3. Baca, J.E.: Some health beliefs of the Spanish-speaking. Am. J. Nurs., 69:2172, 1969.
4. Baekeland, F., and Lundwell, L.: Dropping out of treatment: A critical review. Psychol. Bull., 82:738, 1975.
5. Caplan, G.: Types of mental health consultation. Am. J. Orthopsychiatry, 33:470, 1963.
6. Davidson, P.O., and Shrag, A.R.: Factors affecting the outcome of child psychiatric consultations. Am. J. Orthopsychiatry, 39:774, 1969.
7. Francis, V., Korsch, B., and Morris, M.: Gaps in doctor-patient communication: Patient's response to medical advice. N. Engl. J. Med., 280:535, 1969.
8. Gath, D.: Child guidance and the general practitioner: A study of factors influencing referrals made by general practitioners to a child psychiatric department. J. Child Psychol. Psychiatry, 9:213, 1968.
9. Gross, H., and Herbert, M.: The effect of race and sex on variations of diagnosis and disposition in a psychiatric emergency room. J. Nerv. Ment. Dis., 148:638, 1969.
10. Haggerty, R.J., and Roghmann, K.J.: Non-compliance and self-medication—two neglected aspects of pediatric pharmacology. Pediatr. Clin. North Am., 19:101, 1972.
11. Jilek, W.G.: Indian healing power: Indigenous therapeutic practices in the Pacific Northwest. Psychiatr. Ann., 4:13, 1974.
12. Kaufman, I.: The role of the psychiatric consultant. Am. J. Orthopsychiatry, 26:223, 1956.
13. Kennell, J.H., et al.: What parents of rheumatic fever patients don't understand about the disease and its prophylactic management. Pediatrics, 43:190, 1969.
14. Korsch, B.: Pediatrician-patient relations. In *Ambulatory Pediatrics* (M. Green and R.J. Haggerty, Eds.). Philadelphia, Saunders, 1968.
15. Korsch, B., Gozzi, E., and Francis, V.: Gaps in doctor-patient communication: I. Doctor-patient interaction and patient satisfaction. Pediatrics, 42:855, 1968.
16. Lyons, J.: The treatment of hypochondriacal patients. Unpublished material.
17. Malmquist, C.: Problems of confidentiality in child psychiatry. Am. J. Orthopsychiatry, 35:787, 1965.
18. Moskowitz, J.: The pediatrician calls for psychiatric referral. Clin. Pediatr., 7:733, 1968.
19. Ordonez-Plaja, A., Cohen, L.M., and Samora, J.: Communication between physicians and patients in outpatient clinics: Social and cultural factors. Milbank Mem. Fund Q., 56:191, 1968.
20. Pratt, L., Seligman, A., and Reader, G.: Physician's views on the level of medical information among patients. Am. J. Public Health, 47:1277, 1957.
21. Ruiz, P.: Folk healers as associate therapists. Curr. Psychiatr. Ther., 16:269, 1976.
22. Saunders, L.: *Cultural Differences and Medical Care: The Spanish-Speaking People of the Southwest.* New York, Russell Sage Foundation, 1954.
23. Kupst, M.J., Blatterbauer, S., Westman, J., Schulman, J.L., and Paul, M.H.: Helping parents cope with the diagnosis of congenital heart defect: an experimental study. Pediatrics, 59:266, 1977.
24. Standards of Health Care, 3rd Ed. (Committee on Standards of Child Health Care.) Evanston, Ill., American Academy of Pediatrics, 1975.

25. Walker, C., and Finklestein, M.: Study of committee re: Diagnosis of congenital heart disease. Unpublished material.

General References

Action against Mental Disability: The Report of the President's Task Force on the Mentally Handicapped. Washington, U.S. Government Printing Office.

Balint, M.: *The Doctor, His Patient, and the Illness,* 2nd Ed. London, Pitman, 1964.

Beller, E.K.: *Clinical Process: A New Approach to the Organization and Assessment of Clinical Data.* New York, Free Press, 1961.

Bender, L.: *Child Psychiatric Techniques.* Springfield, Ill., Thomas, 1952.

Bernard, V.W.: Interracial Practice in the Midst of Change. Am. J. Psychiatry, *128*:978, 1972.

Caplan, G., Ed.: *Prevention of Mental Disorders in Children.* New York, Basic Books, 1961.

Children and Clinics: A Survey of the American Association of Psychiatric Clinics for Children. (Mimeograph) New York, American Association of Psychiatric Clinics for Children, 1968.

Clarke, C.: The family as an integral part of management: The physician's role in guidance. Tex. Med., *65*:60, 1969.

Conrad, F.A., et al.: Need for collaboration of pediatrician and orthodontist. Pediatrics, *29*:349, 1962.

Eisenberg, L., and Gruenberg, E.: The current status of secondary prevention in child psychiatry. Am. J. Orthopsychiatry, *31*:355, 1961.

Finzer, W.F.: Symptom contagion in children's emotional disorders. Clin. Pediatr., *4*:18, 1965.

Finzer, W.F., and Waite, R.R.: The relationship between accumulated knowledge and therapeutic techniques. J. Am. Acad. Child. Psychiatry, *3*:709, 1964.

French, A.: *Disturbed Children and Their Families: Innovation in Evaluation and Treatment.* New York, Human Sciences Press, 1977.

Freud, S.: *New Introductory Lectures on Psychoanalysis.* London, Hogarth Press, 1933.

Group for the Advancement of Psychiatry, Committee on Child Psychiatry: *From Diagnosis to Treatment: An Approach to Treatment Planning for the Emotionally Disturbed Child.* GAP Report No. 87. New York, 1973.

Harms, E.: *Handbook of Child Guidance.* New York, Child Care Publishing Company, 1947.

Hobbs, N.: Helping disturbed children: Psychological and ecological strategies. Am. Psychol., *21*:1105, 1966.

How They Were Reached: A study of 310 children and their families known to referral units. In: *Family-Centered Project of St. Paul* (C.J. Birt, Ed.). Soc. Work 1: 1956, p. 89.

Korner, A.F., and Opsvig, P.: Developmental considerations in diagnosis and treatment. J. Child Psychiatry, *5*:594, 1966.

Kupft, M.J., et al.: Helping parents cope with the diagnosis of congenital heart defect. An experimental study. Pediatrics, *59*:266, 1977.

Lippman, H.: *The Treatment of the Child in Emotional Conflict.* New York, McGraw-Hill, 1956.

McDermott, J.F.,Jr., and Harrison, S.J.: *Psychiatric Treatment of the Child.* New York, Jason Aronson, 1977.

McTaggart, A.N.: The psychiatric care of children in a teaching hospital. Can. Psychiatr. Assoc. J., October, 1965.

Menninger Clinic, Children's Division: *Disturbed Children.* San Francisco, Jossey-Bass, 1969.

Peabody, F.W.: The care of the patient. JAMA, *88*:877, 1927.

Penningroth, P.W.: A Study of Programs for Emotionally Disturbed Children in Selected European Countries. Washington, U.S. Department of Health, Education, and Welfare, 1963.

Pollak, O.: *Social Science and Psychotherapy for Children.* New York, Russell Sage Foundation, 1952.

Prugh, D.G., and Eckhardt, L.O.: Mentally Handicapped Children. (Mimeograph.) Working Paper for White House Conference on Handicapped Children. Washington, D.C., National Institute of Health, 1975.

Redl, F.: *When We Deal with Children: Selected Writings.* New York, Free Press, 1966.

Sabshin, M., Diesenhaus, H., and Wilkerson, R.: Dimensions of institutional racism in psychiatry. Am. J. Psychiatry, *127*:787, 1970.

Shapiro, E.T., and Pinker, R.H.: Shared ethnic scotomata. Am. J. Psychiatr., *130*:1338, 1973.

Trieschman, A.E., Whittaker, J.K., and Brendtro, L.K.: *The Other 23 Hours.* Chicago, Aldine, 1969.

Winnicott, D.W.: *Therapeutic Consultations in Child Psychiatry.* New York, Basic Books, 1971.

11

Types of Treatment for Emotional and Mental Disorders

One of the essential qualities of the clinician is humanity, for the secret of the care of the patient is in caring for the patient.
(Francis W. Peabody)

Formal Psychotherapeutic Approaches

Child psychotherapy is generally considered to have begun in 1905 with Sigmund Freud's famous case report on little Hans, a 5-year-old child. Hans' father, a physician, acting under Freud's direction was the psychotherapist. The major impetus for the subsequent development of therapeutic interventions with children was provided by the pioneering work of Anna Freud and Melanie Klein. Klein's[128] theoretical assumptions formed the basis of a therapeutic technique that substituted the child's free play for the adult's free associations. Anna Freud[77] developed her approach emphasizing the child's inevitable dependence on and interaction with his parents. In the 1920s and 1930s, the development of child guidance clinics under the auspices of the National Committee for Mental Hygiene and the Commonwealth Fund widened the scope of psychotherapy available for children and adolescents in the United States.

Today there are many different approaches to psychotherapy. However, Frank, Strupp, and others,[76,224] including the writer, agree that the success of all approaches seems to depend on the therapeutic relationship (the "therapeutic alliance"). In other words, the patient accepts some dependence for help because he trusts the therapist and develops a confiding, emotionally charged relationship with the therapist, who has an accepting and respectful attitude toward the patient. Thus psychotherapy is a process by which a socially sanctioned healer seeks to help persons with psychologic distress, who have certain expectations of his help—hopes that are supported by the privacy of the relationship and the nature of the setting in which it develops.

177

The therapist must have formed some conceptual scheme that to him explains the cause of the patient's problems and is acceptable to the patient. The therapist must also be skilled in a procedure that requires the active participation of both the patient and the therapist. Such an approach enables the patient to discover new information about himself and his behavior that helps him to handle his feelings more effectively and, ultimately, to change his behavior in a more self-fulfilling and socially adaptive direction.

Karasu,[124] in attempting to classify the various approaches to psychotherapy, found that 1 of 3 themes has usually predominated in their development: (1) a *dynamic theme,* evolving from Freudian psychoanalysis, (2) a *behavioral theme,* originating in the "classical" conditioning of Pavlov and later influenced by the "operant" conditioning of Skinner and by numerous reality, rational, and problem-solving approaches, or (3) an *experiential theme,* primarily based on European existentialist thinking but also influenced by Eastern mysticism (the search for one's spiritual center), focusing on a basic concern for issues involving man's being or becoming.

Therapies based on the *experiential theme* view the patient as a person striving to find meaning and fulfillment in life and seek to help him in the process of growth and self-affirmation. The emphasis is on immediate experience in order to enhance strengths and to reduce the blocking of potential arising from an estrangement from self and alienation from society. The need for a direct experiencing, and at times abreaction, of strong emotions is often stressed. I believe that most experiential approaches are not suited for children but that some may have application for older adolescents.

Dynamic Therapy

Therapies based on the dynamic theme emphasize the resolution of inner emo-

tional conflicts or crises arising as a result of vulnerability to stress which is often in large part related to early experience. They include a number of more or less analytically oriented technical approaches which vary in their emphasis on dealing with the relationship between inner psychic experience and interpersonal interaction. Some approaches to dynamic therapy involve a supportive or nondirective posture and others one which is exploratory and ventilative.

Dynamic psychotherapy can also be described in terms of its depth, duration, and intensity; but since each of these factors is present to some degree in every psychotherapeutic relationship involving children, perhaps a better way to define methods of therapy in terms of their relative importance to the approach would be to identify the position of each factor on a continuum ranging from the supportive end, where little uncovering or interpretation of deeper conflicts occurs, to the intensive insight-promoting end, where conflict-resolving, uncovering, and interpretative activity predominate.

Dynamic therapy may be offered to individuals, families or groups of individuals.

Individual Psychotherapy

Although Levitt[143,144] and others have questioned the effectiveness of child psychotherapy, early studies of treatment results in child guidance clinics by Witmer[238] and a later review of studies involving some elements of control by Heinecke and Goldman[107] have supported the conclusion that the large majority of children can be helped by various psychotherapeutic approaches. More recent studies by Heinecke[106] of long-term psychoanalytically oriented treatment with neurotic children, a controlled study by Eisenberg and his colleagues[63] of the effectiveness of short-term supportive psychotherapy, and critical reviews by Anthony[16] and Kellner[127] of these and other available studies support the following conclusion. As Anthony puts it, in spite of methodological problems in sampling and the use of diverse assessments, the various individual dynamic psychotherapies are effective with disturbed children, and different techniques may lead to changes of differing kinds. Nevertheless, much more research along the lines suggested by Heinecke and Goldman[107] and Rosenfeld and his colleagues[201] remains to be done.

The problem of obtaining data from controlled studies is a serious one, as Strupp[225] and Frank[75] have pointed out, and systematic comparative studies of the various approaches to therapy are badly needed. Luborsky and his colleagues[152] have carried out the most extensive of several recent comparative evaluations of the (sometimes inadequately controlled) studies of the effects of dynamic therapy with some of the other approaches mentioned (also often poorly controlled). The results of the evaluation indicated that the type of approach had little effect on the degree of improvement in adults; the majority of patients receiving each type of therapy have benefited. But the investigators noted that qualitative differences in response were especially difficult to evaluate, that the studies reviewed involved largely short-term treatment approaches (2 to 12 months in length), and that the treatment goals often differed. At present, the dynamic therapist seems justified in believing that his approach will be effective for the majority of patients he treats, but little additional wisdom is as yet available.

A study conducted by the Kaiser Permanente Foundation[56a] showed that members of its prepaid program (adults and some older adolescents) who received psychotherapy for emotional disturbances exhibited a significant decline in utilization of clinic or hospital services, in comparison with an emotionally disturbed group who for various reasons did not receive psycho-therapy. The decline in the use of medical facilities continued for at least 5 years. Replications of this study are now underway in the United States and in Germany.[58a]

Psychotherapy for children may be *psychoanalytically oriented*, aimed at self-understanding that will enable the child to develop his full potential. Such a goal implies liberating for more constructive use the psychic energy that the child uses to defend himself against his inner conflicts. The child is generally unaware of such conflicts and of the psychologic defenses he uses to avoid recognizing them. When he becomes aware of them and when he gains insight into their origin (particularly his conflicts with his parents and siblings), the child can be more readily helped to resolve his symptoms and the unhealthy behavior arising from his conflicts. Helping the parents understand their child's problems and to change their interactions with the child is an integral part of such psychotherapy. Of course, the approach to therapy must be adapted to each patient's level of development.

Play therapy is based on the fact that younger children have difficulty in expressing their feelings and ideas in words but are able to communicate in the symbolic language of play. Thus in play therapy children can recreate past situations involving anxiety or conflict, play out their current feelings, and develop an understanding and mastery of their problems. There are 2 major types of play therapy: the psychoanalytically oriented type, reviewed by Buxbaum,[41] and the nondirective or client-centered type used by Axline.[18] (Both types of approaches and their adaptation to pediatric practice are discussed in Chapter 12.)

Psychoanalytically oriented individual psychotherapy is to be distinguished from child psychoanalysis, although it is not always easy to differentiate intensive psychotherapy (which involves interviews more than once a week) and child analysis (which involves 3 to 4 or more interviews a week).[29,56] Child analysis generally takes longer (often covering 2 or more years), and has as its goal a more deep-seated and far-reaching reorganization of the child's personality.[132,241] It is therefore exceedingly expensive in terms of time and money. Nevertheless, it may be the approach of choice for certain children who have severe obsessive or phobic psychoneurotic disorders or deep-seated personality disorders. Heinecke's studies[106] have shown child analysis to be more effective than psychoanalytically oriented psychotherapy in treating children who have marked neurotic learning disorders. If psychoanalysis is used with adolescents, special adaptations may be needed.[64] Child analysis is beginning to be offered in university clinics that have training centers,[196] but if it is to reach many of the children who could benefit from it, it must be made more widely available at low cost. Therapeutic work with parents is also necessary with this approach.

A growing awareness of the needs of millions of children and families has resulted in the development of briefer methods of psychotherapy, in order to provide more immediate help with the limited mental health facilities available. In the 1930s Rogers, influenced by Rank, was developing brief "client-centered" therapy, while Allen,[9] who also was influenced by Rank, was using brief psychotherapy with children and parents at the Philadelphia Child Guidance Clinic. Senn, a student of Allen, was teaching the principles of such therapies in the 1940s to fellows in "pediatric psychiatry," and Axline, influenced by Rogers and Rank, was using brief nondirective or client-centered therapy in her practice. Bruch[39] described the use of brief psychotherapy by a psychiatrist in a pediatric clinic in 1949, and, in the 1950s, Alpern,[11] (also a student of Allen) advocated its use in a child guidance clinic. At about the same time, Waldfogel and his colleagues[232] described a type of brief intervention with children who had school phobia. With the emergence of the community mental health movement in the 1960s, brief psychotherapy for adults became widely accepted, but it was not until late in the decade that the successful use of brief psychotherapy with children was reported with any frequency. Its efficacy during therapy and follow-up as compared to long-term psychotherapy was not documented systematically until the controlled study by Eisenberg and his colleagues[63] in 1965, the results of which were confirmed more recently by Rosenthal and Levine[202] and in a large-scale study by Leventhal and Weinberger.[141] In 1966, Egan and Robinson[65] applied the principles of brief psychotherapy in dealing with home situations. Visits to the child's home can be valuable diagnostically and therapeutically, as Freeman[80] has emphasized. They often involve drawing on the resources of the community; for example, to provide foster grandparents to work with emotionally disturbed children.

The use of brief psychotherapy calls for a balance between courage and caution on the part of the therapist. The therapist must be flexible in shifting to a longer-term approach if the need becomes evident, and he must provide follow-up to evaluate the effectiveness of the therapy and to determine whether the child needs further help. (Several of the studies previously cited indicated that from 30% to more than 50% of the children who had undergone brief therapy required referral for longer-term treatment.) Finzer and Kirkpatrick[71] developed an approach to brief therapy that proved successful in the management of selected patients (e.g., a reasonably healthy child who showed what seemed to be a developmental or situational crisis or an acute reactive disorder, a family in apparent crisis, and a child with chronic personality disorder who had suddenly decompensated). The therapy Finzer and Kirkpatrick used was family oriented and restricted to 5 to 7 interviews, and the goal was limited to restoring the patient's and his family's equilibrium to their previous states.* Time-limited approaches (1 to 8 interviews) have also been reported by Shulman,[213] Proskauer,[188] and others.[101]

In the foregoing discussion, reference has been made to children in developmental or situational crises, to family crises, and to brief (short-term) and time-limited therapy. Some clarification of the use of brief psychotherapy is indicated at this point since brief therapy has been somewhat loosely linked to the approach used in *crisis intervention*. Developmental, situational, and family crises can be chronic as well as acute, and they do not necessarily call for brief therapy, time-limited therapy, or crisis intervention techniques. And brief, focused, or time-limited therapy may be used to deal with other than crisis situations. Brief therapy may be used to treat mild reactive disorders as well as a variety of developmental problems, such as prolonged colic. Time-limited therapy is ordinarily associated with crisis intervention, which has a sound theoretical basis and which has been developed as a model of 1 form of brief therapy.

Many practitioners of crisis intervention (which became associated with the community mental health movement and to some seemed to repudiate psychoanalytic theory) are unaware that the theory of crisis intervention is based on Lindemann's observations of the reactions of relatives of people who died in the Cocoanut Grove fire in Boston in 1943.[148] Lindemann's attempts to help these families in their grieving process led to his awareness of the importance of helping families in a crisis situation. Lindemann observed that immediate intervention could help families who were having difficulty in grieving to begin this necessary adaptive process in a surprisingly short time and that many families could regain their equilibrium and function without further help, even though the grieving process (now a healthier one)

*They called their approach the Brief Evaluation and Treatment Service (BETS).

continued for months. He also found that immediate, brief intervention enabled some families to reach a more effective equilibrium and healthier coping styles. (An adaptation of Lindemann's approach that the physician can use to help parents mourn "adaptively" is discussed in Chapter 26.)

Caplan,[45] Parad,[182] Kaplan,[123] and others have further developed crisis theory, formulating a concept of crisis intervention to be used as the framework for a limited form of therapy for the resolution of other types of family crisis (e.g., the loss of a father's job or the birth of a premature infant). The approach suggested in these studies includes (1) identifying the crisis, (2) understanding its nature and its precipitants, (3) identifying the family member or members involved, (4) identifying the types of adaptive or maladaptive attempts to cope, (5) setting limits on therapeutic contacts (sometimes specific time limits), and (6) negotiating specific attainable goals (at the minimum, helping the family or the person regain the original equilibrium).

Such an approach calls for considerable training. The therapist must become skillful in rapidly assessing coping mechanisms and the degree of individual or family psychopathology, must learn to be direct and active in aiding problem-solving without becoming overly directive, must understand how to help an individual or a family terminate treatment, and must be able to evaluate, through follow-up, whether further treatment is required.

As Clifford, Tarnow, and others[52] have emphasized, when a child is involved in a family crisis, an assessment of his underlying developmental conflict (which may have precipitated the crisis) and the approach chosen to deal with the conflict are of vital importance.

The handling of psychiatric emergencies[40,129,161] lies at one end of a continuum of crises of varying intensity. Collier and Morrison[53] and Mattsson and his colleagues[161] have described a brief crisis-oriented treatment approach for the families of adolescents in a child emergency service who have attempted suicide. Morrison has pioneered in the development of an approach using a child psychiatry team in the emergency room, where crisis-oriented techniques can include the overnight stay of the parent and/or the child.[176]

The role the pediatrician can play in psychiatric emergencies* has been discussed in relation to pediatric wards by Mattsson and Naylor[162] and in regard to ambulatory situations by Haggerty.[98] Galdston and Hughes[82] have described the use of hospitalization as a form of crisis intervention, related to the evidence of diagnostic and therapeutic benefit of hospitalization for certain children who have mild-to-moderate emotional problems offered earlier by Solnit[218] and by Laybourne and Miller.[139]

As previously indicated, methods of psychiatric screening, involving the analysis of questionnaires by computer, did not seem to interest pediatricians in a clinic program or to result in the pediatricians' making appropriate interventions. But the response of mental health professionals in a pediatric setting to such psychiatric screening has been more positive. In a study of a program undertaken in a pediatric clinic of the Kaiser Permanente Foundation that used the services of psychiatric social workers, Tasen and his colleagues[226] have shown that, of the 70% of parents who indicated concern about their children's behavior or development on such questionnaires, the majority could be helped to deal satisfactorily with these concerns in 1 interview with a psychiatric social worker, who used reassurance, counseling, or (occasionally) crisis intervention techniques. About 15% of these families required referral to a mental health facility for more intensive treatment. These figures support the observation that parent concerns about the behavior of their children are often overlooked, and the findings parallel the results of the field survey methods of psychiatric screening that Hetznecker, Gardner, and their colleagues[109] developed for adults. Cooper[55] has shown, in a controlled study, that such brief interventions by mental health professionals in a pediatric setting can produce significantly positive results, and Chamberlain[48] (a behaviorally oriented pediatrician) has made effective use of such principles of primary prevention in a pediatric clinic.

In general, the child in longer-term psychotherapy derives support from a consistently understanding and accepting relationship with the therapist. (Varying degrees of educational guidance and emotional release are undoubtedly involved.) The child typically undergoes psychotherapy because an adult has decided he should. But some children may be brought to psychotherapy not only against their wishes but also without the benefit of their parents' support. The parents may be blind to their child's needs and seek psychiatric help only because they are pressured to do so by school or legal authorities. Thus some children undergoing psychotherapy may look on therapeutic change as a matter of their conforming to an inexorable demand or even an unwanted reality. On the other hand, as Allen and Axline have emphasized, children have in their favor active maturational and developmental forces, which in some respects make therapy with children more likely to be effective than therapy with adults.

The playroom is an important factor in the therapeutic technique. The various toys used are generally simple, and they are carefully selected to facilitate the child's communication of his fantasies and feelings. The approach at first derives from perception of the child's needs and it varies according to the therapist's individual style. The therapist may evoke the child's thoughts and elicit play activity in a more structured situation, or he may encourage the child to say whatever he wishes and to

---

*These include school phobia (discussed in Chapter 28) and other problems, some of which are only defined by the community as emergencies.

play freely. In general, the therapist creates an atmosphere of interest and trust in which he endeavors to get to know as much as possible about the child. He conveys to the child that he knows something about disturbed children and that he likes to help them. The therapist usually expresses warmth and even affection more openly and is more active with children than with adult patients. The therapist may engage in active play with dolls with a younger child, dart games with a school-age boy, and checkers with an early adolescent, talking with the child all the while. Or the therapist may observe the child's play and make comments about its meaning, adopting the role of a participating observer. Despite the relative permissiveness of the therapeutic situation, the therapist must set limits on the child's aggressive or destructive behavior. If the therapist does not, the child will feel guilty or he may fail to learn inner controls, as Jessner[120] has emphasized.

The therapist's role is a flexible one, and it may range from relative passivity to an active, intervening stance, depending on the child's needs at a particular time. Nonverbal communications, such as a child's facial expressions, gestures, posture, and motility in his play and productions, are important clues to the child's inner feelings. Children vary in their ability to verbalize spontaneously in the playroom, a fact that must be taken into account. Therapeutic interventions are considered along a continuum. At 1 end of the continuum are the questions the therapist asks to understand and clarify the child's problem. At the other end of the continuum are the therapist's confrontations and interpretations that reduce conflict and expand the patient's conscious awareness of himself. In addition, a patient may be offered new information, as well as advice, counsel, and direction designed to help him adopt a healthy course of action.

Parent Therapy

Therapy involving the parents of disturbed children has gone through a num-ber of phases. The early child psychoanalysts viewed the child's parents mainly as reporters of events at home and elsewhere, recognizing that the child's problems were largely rooted in those events. The analysis of the child's problems was counted on to desensitize him to family events that affected him adversely. In a later stage of the early child guidance movement, the parents were viewed as being in need of counseling about how to change their child's undesirable habits of behavior. That approach involved tandem therapy for the child and his parents. More recently, help for the child's parents has been a goal concomitant with psychotherapy for the child (but what help for parents means has not been defined explicitly).

In recent years, some workers (e.g., Ackerman[3]) have recommended several "in-between" techniques (in between advice or guidance and intensive psychotherapy) to deal with some of the unconscious components of the parent-child relationship. As Chethik[50] pointed out, there is surprisingly little in the psychiatric and psychologic literature about the in-between areas. Counseling has been advocated by Fraiberg,[74] Halpern and Kissel,[102] and others, "attitude therapy" was advocated by Levy,[145] a child-centered group guidance approach was described by Slavson,[215] and "parallel" group psychotherapy for parents of disturbed children has been discussed by Westman and his colleagues.[237]

In the child guidance movement, help was originally offered almost exclusively to parents. Such offerings tended to be designated as "casework,"[69] reflecting the case-oriented approach of early social welfare workers. Although the collaborative therapeutic approach is not emphasized in the literature, that approach involving both parents and children originated in the procedures developed by social workers later in the child guidance movement.

Dietz[59] has referred to "reciprocal interaction" in the parent-child relationship during psychotherapy, which seems to put parent therapy on a level with child therapy, even though the child is often presented as the disturbed member of the family and has often been referred to as the primary patient. The term reciprocal interaction seems to fit the mutually interactional or transactional concepts involved in disturbances already discussed, of parent-child relationships and family functioning.

In a collaborative or reciprocal approach to treatment, the therapist may accept the child's disturbed behavior as the problem initially if the parents cannot yet see themselves as also involved in the child's difficulties. In the case of young preschool-age children, it is not uncommon for the principal psychotherapeutic effort to be directed toward the parents, with limited direct involvement of the child. As the older preschool-age child becomes more capable of using play symbolically to deal with conflicts, he is usually more actively involved in the therapy. The school-age child, who is capable of both play and verbal interchanges, is usually treated directly, as is the largely verbal adolescent.

Parent therapy as it evolved from the social work approach has focused principally on the parent-child interaction and its vicissitudes. The parents rarely see themselves as patients initially, and elaborate reconstructions of their own early childhood experiences are ordinarily not appropriate. In this approach, the therapist deals with the parent's experiences or unconscious feelings only insofar as they shed light on the problem in the parent-child relationship. For example, a parent may unconsciously identify an active, vigorous child with a brother who had shown delinquent behavior and so tend to overcontrol the child to prevent his becoming like his brother. The child rebels against the overcontrol. A parent may identify a somewhat oppositional child with the "bad" part of himself or a parent may try to make up to a child for deprivations he himself experienced. Finzer[72] has developed the con-

cept of "localized neurotic interaction," in which a child in a particular developmental stage "reactivates" the conflicts his parent experienced when he was in that same developmental stage. The result may be that the parent unconsciously condones the child's antisocial behavior, or that he overcontrols the child, who, in rebellion, shows the same antisocial behavior the parent showed when he was a child. In such instances, a focal insight-promoting approach to therapy may help the parent to understand and alter his behavior while it helps the child to control his impulsive, rebellious, oppositional, or other behavior.

Different approaches may be called for in parent therapy. For example, a very dependent or seriously disturbed parent may need caring and concern before he can see his child as an individual;[126] an insight-promoting therapy approach can be initiated later. Support, counseling, guidance, or other techniques may be called for in some instances or may be offered intermittently during insight-promoting therapy.

If the relationship between a parent and a particular child is deeply symbiotic,* 2 therapists, working in tandem, may be needed to aid in the process of separation-individuation for both parent and child. Parents are often seen together in therapy, but if they begin to show deep anger or mistrust, they may have to be seen separately, sometimes with a third therapist added. Group therapy for fathers, mothers, or fathers and mothers[47,61,215] has been effective for parents who are not seriously disturbed. At times individual interviews may be needed to deal with increased anxiety or conflict or with other special problems. As the child improves with treatment and the parents' attitudes toward him change, the focus may shift to other important intrapsychic problems of 1 or both parents, who may then seek treatment for themselves. Sometimes a marital problem

---

*Tandem therapy may be necessary in other seriously disturbed parent-child relationships, following the collaborative approach between child and parent therapists.

is unveiled, and a change to marital therapy or counseling may be indicated.

In summary, "help" for parents has developed into a dynamic type of therapy that has special characteristics and challenges that make it quite different from (though reciprocally related to) individual psychotherapy for the child. The original team approach, developed in the early community child guidance clinics, called on the psychiatrist to evaluate and treat the child while the social worker helped the parents and the psychologist administered intelligence tests and personality tests. In the team approach now favored, the roles of the team members are much more flexible and overlap considerably. Psychologists and social workers are now trained to undertake therapy with children, while child psychiatrists and psychologists may treat parents. Workers from all 3 disciplines may provide family, group, or other forms of therapy, and child psychiatry nurses, still few in number, are beginning to do so too. Each discipline retains its uniqueness and has its particular value orientations. Thus the child psychiatrist offers medical diagnostic and drug therapy skills, the psychologist offers knowledge of testing and special understanding of research methods, the psychiatric social worker offers a unique grasp of the interaction of the family and the community, and the nurse offers sympathetic care. All these workers may be involved in research. Any one of these workers may be the administrative head of a program if a child psychiatrist is heavily involved in the program as a consultant or as a medical clinical director. If they are certified, all these workers may receive third-party reimbursement for the psychotherapeutic services they render under different local arrangements although as yet only psychiatrists and psychologists have national registers, which qualify them to receive reimbursement under federally sponsored programs.

Since the beginning of child therapy, gifted people from "nontraditional" backgrounds have become outstanding child therapists, among them such outstanding leaders as Anna Freud and Erik Erikson. I believe that there is a need for a new discipline—child therapy—that has a special curriculum, direct openings into the field, and a career ladder, somewhat like the new discipline of psychotherapy (with the degree Doctor of Mental Health) that has been developed recently by Wallerstein.

Treatment of the Poor and Ethnic Minorities

A number of myths about psychotherapy have persisted for many years. One of them is that mentally retarded children are untreatable. Another is that people who are poor are not good candidates for psychotherapy. That myth goes together with the myth that only a person who pays a fee has the proper motivation for psychotherapy.[147,149,227] McDonald and Adams[167] and Harrison and his colleagues[103] have indicated that the persistence of this myth is less a reflection on the poor than on a self-fulfilling prophecy of middle-class and upper-middle-class psychiatrists. Hollingshead and Redlich[111] and Harrison and his colleagues[104] have shown that many therapists in the past were trained to expect poor people and those with low-status jobs[115] to respond passively to treatment with drugs, electroshock, and environmental manipulation, offered only in crises, and not to respond to the various forms of psychotherapy. Adams as well as Pavenstedt[184] and Malone[153] are working to change such attitudes, using flexible approaches and "reaching out" through home visits. Studies have shown that patients who have lower socioeconomic backgrounds tend to drop out of treatment if they are assigned inexperienced residents who do not understand their problems.[22] Providing more experienced therapists and helping other therapists develop better insights into the problems of the poor can lead to fewer dropouts and greater success, as McKnight and his colleagues[169] have indicated.

More patients from ethnic minority groups have begun to seek psychotherapy recently, puncturing the myth that particular ethnic groups, often from backgrounds of poverty, cannot benefit from insight-promoting psychotherapy. Accordingly, problems in the relationships between therapists and patients of different ethnic backgrounds and other problems involved in offering help to minorities have begun to be explored.[4,20,42,93,209,233] Waite[231] and Jackson and her colleagues[116] have pointed out the pitfalls in such relationships. Those pitfalls, which arise from stereotyping and problems concerning attitudes of both groups, may include differences in socioeconomic background[51] and ethnic experiences and even language problems.[154] Calneck[43] has indicated that white racial prejudice can affect even the black therapist–black patient situations, because the black therapist must deal with his own feelings toward the white majority as well as his patient's problem. Much more understanding and study of such factors are needed if effective treatment is to be given in inpatient as well as outpatient settings.

Psychotherapy is generally indicated for children who have emotional and mental disorders that seem likely to impair maturation and development. In general, the contraindications to psychotherapy are difficult to delineate. Evidence that therapy will interfere with reparative forces, and may thus cause more difficulty than the original problem, may be sufficient reason to rule out the use of intensive or uncovering psychotherapy of any type. Instead, the development of a supportive relationship, suitable activities, or some other environmental measures may be helpful.

Family Therapy

In recent years Bell,[26] Ackerman,[2] Satir,[207] Haley,[100] Minuchin,[173] Howells,[114] and others[117] have attempted to shift the focus from the child as the primary patient to the family, which may present the child as a symptom of its pathologic functioning. As Zuk[244] has said, this approach explores the pathogenic relationships among family members and attempts to shift the balance so that new and healthier forms of relating become possible. In such situations, all or selected members of the family are treated simultaneously in a group. Family therapy has value in that it fosters real-life interactions and verbalizations and provides the opportunity to observe nonverbal interactions also. It may sometimes be more effective than tandem or other forms of therapy. Although there are different strategies for family therapy, as pointed out by Beels and Ferber,[23] a much more active, confrontational approach may be needed at times to keep feelings under reasonable control, and "side-taking" approaches designed to mobilize feelings have some real dangers. Very disturbed families may be seriously upset by the explosive force of the feelings thus mobilized. Thus there are some contraindications to family therapy as well as indications for it, as Wynne has emphasized.[242]

Although family therapy has been shown to be an effective type of treatment, it may not meet the family's expectations. Flexibility and a willingness to serve families on a level meaningful to them can fully engage some families in treatment who might otherwise refuse treatment or drop out of it.[205] Family therapy has been of value as a form of crisis intervention in emergencies involving suicide attempts and other problems in older children and adolescents seen in a child psychiatry emergency service.[161] Langsley and his colleagues[137,138,185] have shown that many adult patients can be kept out of the hospital by using appropriate methods of resolving family crises. Short-term approaches have evolved,[122] and family therapy has been carried on in the home.[24,81] But there is no need to see family therapy's primary approach to interpersonal forces as separate from, or opposed to, that of dynamic individual or child-parent psychotherapy, as some enthusiasts have urged. I believe that the family approach is often best used intermittently in the course of ongoing therapy with child and parents. It is axiomatic that the form of therapy should be fitted to the needs of the family, not the family to the therapy.

In one very real sense, as McDermott and Char[165] have emphasized, family therapy can be said to have raised serious problems. Ironically, its independent co-inventors, Bell[25] and Ackerman,[1] intended their techniques, which were new in the early 1950s, to benefit children in particular. Family therapy originally was designed to bridge the gap between adult and child mental health training and services and to improve the quality of mental health care services for families. But instead of becoming a synthesizing force, it has sometimes acted as a third major force, contributing to polarization, and it has undoubtedly resulted in less mental health care for children than before.

There are various reasons for these unfortunate developments. Child mental health professionals, who are usually brought up in the tradition of individual psychotherapy for the child and tandem therapy for the parents, have usually had little interest or training in family therapy, as McDermott and Char have pointed out. On the other hand family therapists, enthusiastic about their new therapeutic modality, have not grasped the importance of training in the understanding and treatment of children as individuals,[78] if they are to be viewed appropriately in the context of the family as a unit.

It was child mental health professionals who first recognized the significance of the influence of the environment on the child, with the relationships within the family being the most intimate and powerful forces. However, the development of family therapy coincided with the community mental health movement. With the gradual assumption by that movement of general systems theory as the basic conceptual scheme for family therapy, there arose the paradox of both an indirect and a direct ejection of the child from the family therapy process. As community mental health centers adopted the generic family approach as their basic therapeutic tool, the child began to be viewed as a miniature adult and no longer as an individual but merely as a part of the family system. Many new professionals were involved in this approach, which became oriented to action and immediate change, as opposed to observation and diagnostic formulation prior to therapeutic intervention.

In this phase, the child was viewed no longer as a patient, who was possibly suffering from an intrapsychic pathology that required specialized treatment. Generic family therapy was seen as capable of handling any symptoms or problems that children had. Although the stated goal of many family therapists was to help the child become an individual member of the family system,[208] the child's developmental level was rarely taken into account. A few family therapists, such as Bell,[26] Zilbach and her colleagues,[243] and Guttman[97] remained sufficiently child oriented to provide play materials for therapeutic purposes and continued to observe and interpret the play in the context of family interactions. But most family therapists had little understanding of child development, and they became frustrated with younger children who could not communicate easily on a verbal level. McDermott and Char, in their review of the literature, found that although many family therapists accepted the theory that the child's disorder was the family's presenting symptom, they began to exclude children from the therapy and to concentrate on the marital relationship as the real problem.

Family therapy was not a failure, as Ackerman later declared it to be,[3] nor was the community mental health movement a failure despite its problems. Through that movement, reach-out into the community was accomplished, and therapy was brought within the reach of more of the people who needed it, even though children did not receive their share. There are encouraging signs that family therapy is beginning to be seen as one approach in a continuum of necessary therapeutic services. Two of the manifestations of that change are the recent paper by Montalvo and Haley, "In Defense of Child Therapy,"[174] and Federal legislation that requires community health centers to include specialized children's services and personnel. Basic psychiatrists and, especially, child psychiatrists and other child mental health workers are beginning to be recognized as professionals who can contribute importantly to community mental health programs. Legislators are beginning to realize that follow-up services of various types are needed[183] for patients now being "deinstitutionalized" with the use of drugs and that more than family therapy is necessary to maintain them in the community.

Although the tensions between different schools of thought have not yet subsided, child psychiatrists are beginning to participate in family therapy programs, and leaders like Haley[99] are beginning to see the need for understanding the role of the child in the family approach. Adequate coverage for mental health services in a national health insurance program and Federal legislation for proportionate funding of services for different age groups, including the elderly, in community mental health centers would be 2 important steps toward a more balanced approach to family therapy.

A movement toward optimal treatment for the disturbed child is evidenced in the development of comprehensive community mental health centers for children, with outpatient, inpatient, and day treatment services for children and adolescents and the establishment of community consultation programs, especially for schools. Koret[130] has pioneered in this move, adding also a therapeutic nursery school and other

services. Although it has been traditional in the United States to provide separate services for children and youths with different categories of problems, N. Lourie[150] and others have recently called for a noncategorical approach to treatment programs. There is also a beginning movement away from institutional and toward community-based residential programs for disturbed children.[175]

Group Therapy

Group psychotherapy with children began in the early 1930s, when Slavson[214] and others[38] began to work with older school-age children in what they called activity group therapy. This approach laid the groundwork for further developments in the use of group psychotherapy with both younger children and adolescents. An analytic approach to group therapy for adolescents was later developed by Foulkes and Anthony.[73] Group therapy was later used effectively in treating disturbed hospitalized children and adolescents, and techniques were also developed for various settings, including correctional institutions, public schools, hospitals, residential treatment centers, and other specialty clinics. More recently, group therapy for children and adolescents has been an important part of community mental health programs.[49] Parents' groups,[237] mothers' groups,[61] fathers' groups,[47] and brief group approaches[66] have been valuable.

The child's age and developmental level influence the approach to group psychotherapy.[222] Play and activity must dominate in the various techniques used with younger children, while much verbalization and active discussion are encouraged in group activity with older children. With adolescents, interview groups, at times involving a more analytic approach,[33] have often been used. Psychodrama[140] and other adaptations of group therapy principles have also been used effectively.

Group psychotherapy seems to help children feel unconditionally accepted by the therapist and the other group members. Feelings are accepted, conflicts are aired, and insights can develop. Feelings of guilt, anxiety, inferiority, and insecurity find relief. Affection and aggression are manifested without danger of retaliation although within clearly established limits. The individual child is carried along by the momentum of the group, and may influence its development. Collaborative therapy with parents, individually or in groups, is necessary in most instances, and individual psychotherapy may have to be used in conjunction with the group approach for some individuals.[204] A new and very effective subdiscipline has recently developed in the field of social work—that of social group work. Social group workers offer activity group therapy for school-age children in pediatric hospital settings and interview group therapy for adolescents. They and other mental health professionals trained in this approach can offer valuable help to groups of disturbed children who suffer from many types of chronic physical illnesses or handicaps. They have also offered help to parents of such children in group discussions, with a pediatrician acting as co-leader. Sensitivity training and encounter groups grew out of this tradition. They can be most effective, but the training of the leader of such groups is most important. Acute psychotic episodes have been occasionally precipitated by overly intense T-group experiences.[118]

Therapeutic Nursery Schools

The therapeutic nursery school provides a special form of group therapy for disturbed, retarded, brain-damaged, or otherwise deviant preschool-age children. This form of therapy requires special training for the teachers working with such children, a high teacher-to-child ratio, and great flexibility in programming.[12] As Alpert[13] has shown, in addition to other types of therapy, a therapeutic nursery school can offer corrective or restitutional experiences for emotionally deprived children. Intensive therapy for preschool-age children with psychotic pictures can be offered in such a setting, as the work of Rank and her associates,[189] Staub, Mizner, and others has demonstrated.[223] Parent therapy, offered collaboratively for individuals, couples, or in groups as indicated, forms an important part of this approach. If they can remain in their homes, very seriously disturbed children may need long-term planning with follow-up care in a therapeutic program for older preschool-age children leading to day treatment. Ideally treatment at all stages is given in the same setting. Behavior therapy has been used successfully for less disturbed children in therapeutic nursery schools.[8]

A therapeutic nursery school can easily be added to an existing child guidance facility,[125] child development center, mental retardation program, or community mental health center. Some nursery school programs have been established in university medical centers and in community settings, but many more are needed, as are training programs for teachers of deviant children.[35]

Behavior Therapy

Behavior therapy is based on the presumption that all behavior, both normal and deviant, arises from what an individual has learned or not learned, and that it is possible to devise methods of learning, relearning, or unlearning which will produce healthier behavior. The focus of such learning theory is on overt behavior, rather than on the patient's thoughts and feelings, and the patient's symptoms are seen as maladaptive behavior or inappropriate habits, not as psychopathology. Pavlov's classic conditioning studies on animals,[95] which focused on the modification of a basic reflex, usually a reflex involving the autonomic nervous system, were later elaborated by Miller[172] and others into a motivational context involving approach-avoidance-conflict and other dimensions. Skinner's[221] studies of the effects of positive and negative reinforcement on naturally occurring behavior led to the concept of operant conditioning, according to which rewarded behaviors are learned and unrewarded or punished behaviors are extinguished. A broad review of the background and current status of behavior therapy has been offered by Urban and Ford.[228] Werry[236] has provided a helpful review of behavior therapy as it applies to children. Ross[203] has discussed behavior modification as it applies to theory, research, and therapy.

In both classical and operant conditioning, stimulus generalization can occur to other than the conditioning situations. The effect of a stimulus can be weakened if it is presented simultaneously with an antagonistic stimulus.

With their knowledge of the effects of stimuli and consequences for future behavioral responses, behavior therapists try to maximize the probability of occurrence and to strengthen healthy behavior at the expense of maladaptive alternatives. As Urban and Ford have pointed out, the choice of the technique to be used in treatment depends on the results of analysis of the behavior problem. If modification of the relationship between a response and the situation in which it occurs is indicated, therapy may involve:

1. *Desensitization*, in which the subject is exposed to the stimulus eliciting the response, with the intensity gradually increased until the inappropriate response is no longer elicited.
2. *Reciprocal inhibition*, which involves an effort to elicit, at a greater level of magnitude, another response, such as relaxation, which is incompatible with the initial response, such as inappropriate fear. A combination of the methods of desensitization and reciprocal inhibition

has been used to deal successfully with numerous phobias.

3. *Conditioned avoidance*, which involves the pairing of the situational stimuli that elicit the inappropriate response with aversive stimuli that elicit an unpleasant or uncomfortable reaction. This approach includes the administration of drugs such as Antabuse for patients with excessive alcohol intake.

If modification of the interrelationship between a response and its consequences is indicated, therapy may involve:

1. *Positive reinforcement*, in which efforts are made to increase the frequency of a desired response by systematically arranging for a positive, satisfying, and thus rewarding, experience whenever the desired response occurs. If the desired response does not occur in its final form initially, approximation, or shaping, techniques which reinforce only those responses that move in the direction of the final act can be used. Attention, praise,[142] and rewards (e.g., food and candy) can be used to reinforce socially effective behavior in children;[10] tokens, special privileges, and other rewards suitable for their age have been used successfully in the treatment of adolescents.[155]

2. *Negative reinforcement*, in which efforts are made to increase the probability of the desired response by providing an unpleasant or aversive stimulus beforehand and removing the stimulus as soon as the desired response occurs.

3. *Aversive conditioning*, which involves arranging for unpleasant consequences to occur after an undesirable response, thus reducing the likelihood of its recurrence. Aversive stimuli include electric shock[151] and various other forms of physical punishment. In a milder form, aversive conditioning has been used by Mowrer[177] and others in the treatment of enuritic children, with wetting leading to the sound of a bell and the awakening of the child.

4. *Extinction*, a technique that attempts to reduce the likelihood that an inappropriate response will occur by arranging, not for unpleasant consequences, but for no consequences at all. Extinction has also been used in combination with positive reinforcement: attention is withheld until appropriate behavior occurs and then that behavior is rewarded with attention and encouragement.

5. *Negative practice*, which involves the deliberate, frequent repetition of an undesired behaviour, has proved successful in eliminating some habitual maladaptive behaviours, including such disruptive activities as rocking back and forth in one's chair during classroom time.

Behavior therapy has been used to treat fears, phobias, tics, stuttering, enuresis, encopresis, anorexia nervosa, vomiting, sores produced by repeated scratching, photic and musicogenic seizures, and conversion and other neurotic symptoms in children. It has been used to diminish antisocial behavior of seriously disturbed adolescents on psychiatric wards, and in dealing with acting-out or delinquent children and adolescents in residential settings; it has also been used to encourage social interactions and speech patterns in chronically psychotic children and to diminish self-injurious behavior. Therefore the principles of behavior therapy should be familiar to all professionals who work with children.[34]

Certain qualifying statements must be made, however. Although behavior therapy has been shown to be effective in individual situations, the few follow-up studies available which compare the results of behavior therapy with the more traditional psychotherapeutic methods do not demonstrate any unequivocal superiority, as Werry has emphasized. The therapist, the therapeutic situation, and the relationship between the therapist and the patient are important variables. Patients may respond differently to different therapists who use similar methods,[216] and subjective responses are inevitably involved.

Children need to be motivated to participate in behaviour therapy, but that fact has often not been mentioned. Problems in motivating children and the number of experiments required in some conditioning or desensitization approaches may lengthen treatment significantly. Negative reinforcement has often been found to diminish the motivation of the patient to undergo treatment. Aversive conditioning, involving physical punishment, shock with a cattle prod, and similar techniques may have complex meanings to children beyond those intended by the therapist. The suppression of behavior induced during treatment may not continue outside the

setting in which the aversive stimulus is given; healthy behaviors may be inhibited also, and other unpredictable results may occur. Therapists administering such negative reinforcements must be not only well trained but also sensitive and in good command of their impulses, in order to prevent callousness or cruelty from creeping in. Simple punishment has been shown in the laboratory to be less effective than positive reinforcement.[228]

Positive reinforcement is a powerful tool in therapy, as well as in child rearing. Praise, attention, and encouragement may be more potent in shaping behavior with some children than concrete rewards. Extinction ("planned ignoring") also has a place, especially in combination with positive reinforcement. Punishment in the form of deprivation of privileges has some place in the treatment of seriously disturbed or deviant children, but, in my opinion, physical punishment rarely if ever does, even if it is administered by the peer group. Needless to say, the flagrant abuse of certain types of behavioral therapy as recently headlined in the press cannot be condoned. But their use without informed consent in the management of patients institutionalized following court procedures is difficult to monitor. Marmor[156] has pointed out that dynamic psychotherapy and behavior therapy have some elements in common. Both require the establishment of a close, positive, and confiding relationship, the arousal of expectations of help, offering the patient new information about his problem, a new way of explaining his symptoms and the approach to their relief, and the provision of success experiences. A study of two groups of patients, one treated by behavior therapy and the other by short-term dynamic psychotherapy, showed that patients in both groups placed a high value on trust, catharsis, insight, and the patient-therapist relationship, a finding that suggests that behavior therapy patients tend to place more emphasis than their therapists do on such subjective factors.[216] Recently, it has been demonstrated that an insight-promoting psychotherapeutic approach can be used in conjunction with behavior therapy.[156]

Behavior therapy is a new and complex field. It can help to some degree certain children who are not now helped, and it offers valuable implications for the treatment of children. Parents can be taught to use behavior techniques,[158] but some have difficulty applying them, and they should not be pressed to do so.[28] Behavior principles applied by other members of the patient's family, such as the planned ignoring of certain disturbed behavior by siblings, has been reported,[171] but here again, too much pressure can cause problems. The fact that relatively inexperienced personnel can be trained to undertake some behavior therapy under supervision has positive implications for the delivery of health services.*

Hypnosis

Hypnosis has been used primarily in adult therapy when blocks in psychotherapeutic treatment develop. It may also be used as the primary method of dealing suggestively with certain conversion symptoms.[37] The therapist should have training in the use of hypnosis, because the effectiveness of this type of therapy depends on how information elicited in the hypnotic state is used thereafter. The hypnotic trance, an altered state of consciousness, is not easy to define and is still only partially understood.[86,168] Recall by itself produces little, and it can be disturbing. Although hypnosis is not as dangerous as popular myths imply, occasional cases of unresolved hypnotic trances and rare episodes of posthypnotic depersonalization occurring in susceptible subjects have been reported. Although these reactions can

easily be dealt with by a skilled therapist,[57] hypnosis should be used cautiously, especially in treating adolescents and patients with hysterical personalities.

A vivid imagination and a susceptibility to suggestion are criteria that have been used to indicate that hypnosis can be successfully induced in adults. Experience indicates that 9 out of 10 people can be hypnotized to some degree and that about 2 out of 10 can reach deep trance states.[195] Most school-age children can be hypnotized readily, according to Wolberg[239] LaBaw,[133] and others. There does not appear to be a positive correlation between the depth of the trance state and the effectiveness of therapy, and it has been found that light trances are frequently helpful. Gardner[84] has used hypnosis in treating psychologic or mixed psychologic and physical symptoms in children. She reports that symptom removal of the psychologic component, if carried out gradually, does not ordinarily result in symptom substitution or other difficulties. She has also provided an extensive review of the literature on the use of hypnosis with children.

Hypnosis has been used to relieve pain during childbirth,[94] dental treatment,[212] and the setting of fractures. It has been used effectively in brain operations and other surgical procedures in which a general anesthetic may be contraindicated.[94] Skin rashes of psychologic origin and warts have been treated successfully with hypnosis, as have asthma and certain other symptoms of psychophysiologic origin. LaBaw has found hypnosis of great value for children with severe burns,[133] as have Bernstein[30] and others. LaBaw[136] also used hypnosis individually and in groups to treat hemophilia in children and adolescents, with a dramatic lessening in episodes of bleeding and hospitalization. Self-hypnosis can be taught to patients who have such disorders, and it can be useful also in habit control. LaBaw[135] has used hypnosis in children who have painful cancer and has

---

*The applications of behavior therapy to the treatment of specific problems of children and adolescents will be discussed in later chapters.

found suggestive therapy in lieu of terminal hospitalization of value for the patient, his family, and the attending physician.[134] Elements of insight-promoting psychotherapy and behavior therapy have been combined with hypnosis.[84]

Narcohypnosis (involving the use of sodium amytal) has been used to treat adults in much the same way as hypnosis has.[235,240] In my opinion, such therapy has no advantages and some dangers for children and adolescents.

Because of its wide applicability, child psychiatrists and child psychologists should have the opportunity to learn the use of hypnosis or "suggestive therapy"[133] with children, although, in the past, some therapists have been reluctant to do so.[85] Mental health professionals can then teach the approach to pediatricians, nurses, and other professionals.[85] In inducing hypnosis, most therapists (e.g., LaBaw[133]) after developing a relationship with the child and explaining the procedure, simply repeat monotonously repetitive suggestions, such as to relax, breathe deeply, close the eyes, and to feel sleepy. Some, like Gardner,[84] suggest that the child imagine himself in tranquil surroundings of a familiar type or imagine soothing situations. The use of elaborate gadgets is unnecessary and inappropriate.

Residential or Inpatient Treatment

Residential, or inpatient, treatment should be viewed as one point on a continuum of services necessary for children who suffer from serious emotional or mental disturbances. In the last 25 years or so, increasing attention has been focused on the need for specialized programs for such children. As a result, many treatment centers have been established that vary widely as to type and in their approach to administration, staffing, and programming.[199] Some facilities are under psychiatric direction and in a hospital[44]; others are run by a social or other community agency with psychiatric and other medical consultants.[15] Staff patterns range from psychiatric nurses and technicians in hospitals to highly trained child care workers in residential centers.[14] Some are "open," dealing only with children who will not run away; others are "closed," to make possible the treatment of potential runaways or adolescents who have suicidal, homicidal, or other serious antisocial tendencies. Some are "semi-open;" that is, they can be closed for individuals who move into an open program gradually as treatment progresses. A period of 1 to several years of residential treatment may be necessary for seriously disturbed or mentally ill children. Thus such programs are expensive, the more so since, if they are to be effective, a staff-patient ratio of about 2-to-1 is needed.

Inpatient treatment is indicated for a child whose symptoms are indicative of serious psychopathology that is supported or aggravated by his environment.[60,194] It may also be indicated for children whose symptoms are not amenable to the types of therapeutic intervention available in their locality and who are therefore not manageable in their home environment.[113] This is not to say that residential treatment should be regarded as a substitute for group foster homes, day treatment, or outpatient services, all of which should be coordinated with community mental health centers and other community programs.

Whatever the approach to treatment, the core of every residential or inpatient program includes (1) the separation of the child from his environment, (2) corrective emotional experiences in a therapeutic living situation, and (3) the opportunity for psychologic help. Therapy for parents and at times other family members is also necessary if the child is not to return to an unchanged family home environment.[164,186]

In recent years, hospitalization has been used more widely in diagnostic and short-term treatment units (where the child remains several weeks to several months).* Vasey and his colleagues[229] have found an inpatient program that combines diagnostic studies and planned living experiences[90] (milieu therapy[31,191]), integrated with formal treatment of the child and his family to be effective for school-age children. Preschool-age children should ordinarily be handled on an outpatient basis or in therapeutic nursery schools, but that approach may not be possible for occasionally wildly aggressive 4- or 5-year-old boys.[200] The short-term unit can function as a halfway house or as a clearinghouse, providing the opportunities for realistic long-term planning for the child and his family. The planning may involve (1) the child's return to the home with outpatient treatment, (2) day treatment of the child in a hospital setting, or (3) placement of the child in individual or group foster homes, cottage-type group-living settings, or institutions that have long-term residential treatment programs. Children can be handled on an emergency basis if necessary, or a planned admission can be arranged. Such a unit deserves a vital position in the umbrella of services within a large community; indeed, if the unit is to function, all of the other services described previously must be available. Short-term approaches are now being added to children's treatment programs at some residential treatment centers and state hospitals.

Seriously disturbed adolescents have often been treated in adult hospital settings, some of which have a separate integrated program of schooling and activities. Falstein,[68] Miller,[170] and others have used this approach. Barter and Langsley[21] have found that the attitudes of staff trained to work with adults can be a limiting factor in the management of adolescents.[87] A separate inpatient unit with specially trained staff for adolescents has definite advantages in a hospital setting for diagnostic and relative short-term treatment, as

*L. Bender was using such an approach in a city hospital more than 30 years ago.

Switzer and Hirschberg[60] and others[21] have concluded. Adolescent behavior may be better controlled on adult wards, but treatment proceeds more effectively if the adolescent learns to modulate or control his behavior[193] appropriately in a milieu that encourages a therapeutic relationship with the staff, involving the setting of appropriate limits[191] and rewards. Individual psychotherapy,[92,108] behavior therapy,[155] psychodrama,[140] and other treatment approaches can be integrated in such an environment. Drug therapy may be necessary initially, but the structure, relationships, and limits are often sufficient to provide a calming effect on seriously disturbed adolescents. Seclusion should be used as a therapeutic tool[88] for (for example) the adolescent who is out of control and who may hurt himself or someone else. Seclusion should never be used as a punishment for breaking the rules or other similar acts. A diagnostic and relatively short-term treatment setting for adolescents can function as a clearinghouse for long-term planning for the patient and his family, in the same manner described earlier. Planning for the treatment of seriously disturbed or psychotic deaf or blind children and adolescents leaves much to be desired. Mental hospitals need specially trained staff to deal with such physically handicapped patients, and schools for the deaf and blind need more mental health consultation.

In some instances, children and even adolescents have been committed to hospitals for diagnosis and treatment against their will and contrary to the wishes of the parents as well. The present trend is toward making all commitments voluntary, but involuntary commitments may have to be resorted to if the parents are unable to permit hospitalization of a child, particularly an adolescent, who is dangerous to himself or to others or if the patient is a seriously disturbed adolescent who runs away or who has committed an illegal act. A closed psychiatric treatment center for such adolescents can be helpful. Children or adolescents should not be simply locked up in a state hospital or other setting, however, as Hobbs[110] has emphasized. Active treatment, not custodial care, should be the goal of such programs. Young people and their parents should have the same right to legal review of their progress and eligibility for release as adults now enjoy (thanks to the efforts of Szasz and others that have led to the issuance of a position statement supporting such rights by the American Psychiatric Association[187]).

The effectiveness of residential treatment for disturbed children has sometimes been called into question. Evaluation of results is not easy, and improvement, especially in the case of psychotic children, is not easily related to specific types of treatment, as Davids and his colleagues[58] and others have emphasized. The fact that about 50% of seriously disturbed children require further treatment following their discharge from the hospital complicates the follow-up and evaluation of outcome. Nevertheless, questionnaire studies at the Bradley Home in Providence[58] and at the Brown Schools in Texas[46] indicated that about 75% of such children seen at these institutions showed significant improvement over admission status for at least several years after their discharge from these institutions and that about 50% seemed to have made a good adjustment. These results were similar to those reported by Levy[146] at the Menninger Clinic. Although these studies revealed that some patients showed no improvement and that some patients became worse after discharge, the data appear to support the conclusion that such programs are effective, especially considering the seriously disturbed nature of the patients in these settings. Although these are long-term programs, a recent survey by Marsden and McDermott[157] indicates that the length of stay in such settings has declined from about 3 years on the average to between 1 and 2 years. More re-

search in this difficult area is urgently needed.

Follow-up studies by Masterson[160] and Garber[83] of seriously disturbed adolescents treated on an inpatient basis are somewhat less optimistic, although the results were better than for a comparable group of adults and the average length of stay was shorter. Of the patients followed, 50% to 90% showed considerable improvement on discharge. However, they had trouble maintaining their gains, and they had many problems in social adjustment, although their work and family adjustments were good or fair. A review of follow-up studies by Gossett and his colleagues[91] confirmed these findings. Again, more outcome research is vital.

The work of Langsley and his colleagues[138] and others who used intervention in family crises (with appropriate follow-up) to keep large numbers of adult and older adolescent patients out of mental hospitals has pertinence for work with children and early adolescents, as does the use of emergency rooms for overnight stays.

Planning for after-care, or adequate follow-up treatment, should be emphasized in working with children and adolescents.[89] After-care planning should start before the child is admitted to an inpatient or residential setting; otherwise, agencies may not be in a position to assist when the time comes, and families may have difficulty accepting the returned child, who, as a consequence may be excluded from both his family and his community. After-care facilities should be as close to the child's home as possible, in order to facilitate contact between the parents and the agencies who may be working with them as well as with the child. A trend in the direction of de-institutionalization is underway, as is the development of community-based residential programs for disturbed children. To help in the patient's return to society, some residential programs have developed halfway houses or group foster homes of their own in the community.

Other approaches to treatment have been tried. One of them is the Five–Two Program at the Suffolk Center on Long Island.[234] The program involves an integrated treatment plan that combines short-term initial hospitalization with movement toward the child's attending a special school during the day and and undergoing behavior shaping by his parents at home at night and on weekends. As the patient improves, he makes increasing use of available community programs.

A most innovative approach has been developed by Hobbs[110] in Nashville, where the Project Re-Ed school provides educational therapy in a residential setting. Trained counselors live and work with the children on a 24-hour basis, combining therapeutic tutoring with a corrective living experience. Mental health and pediatric consultation is available. The results have been most impressive, and the length of stay at this facility is shorter than in the average residential psychiatric or hospital program. Although Project Re-Ed is an outstanding model, it is not a full substitute for an inpatient or residential treatment approach since the school does not take wildly agitated psychotic children or children who show severe acting-out behavior. The emphasis on the relationship between the counselor and the child bears some similarity to the approach of the European *educateurs*, practitioners of a new discipline, who work in and often manage residential settings for disturbed, retarded, homeless, or delinquent children.

Day Treatment (Partial Hospitalization)

In a day treatment program, the child spends the major part of the day in a therapeutic center and returns home in the evening and on weekends. Such a program is designed to serve children who require more therapeutic intervention than is offered by a child psychiatry clinic but who need not be removed from their homes for residential care. Many of these day treatment programs are connected with hospitals, schools, and other institutions as an extension of services already provided. They can fairly easily be added to an existing child guidance clinic or community mental health center that provides specialized children's services. Day treatment can help—and at less than half the cost—many children who were formerly treated in inpatient settings. Some day treatment programs are independent of other agencies or programs.

As in a residential program, the establishment of a therapeutic climate is necessary to aid rehabilitation and treatment in a day treatment program. Milieu therapy includes detailed planning to deal with such factors as the degree and form of structure, limits in the program, the individuality and consistency of experience to which the child is to be exposed, measures to reduce anxiety and provide satisfaction, the management of difficult behavior, and the apportionment of the therapeutic responsibility among various staff members.

Day treatment programs also vary in their emphasis on certain factors. Some centers use formal psychotherapy for the child and parents as the basic framework for the program,[32] while others view the opportunity for special education, the relationships with staff members, the part-time removal from a pathogenic home situation, or the opportunity for special education as the primary form of therapy.[70] Therapeutic methods may include group techniques usable in the classroom. Individual teachers may provide corrective emotional experiences, such as the use of "the life space" interview developed by Redl,[192] in which the teacher confronts the child with surface feelings, or the "stand-by" approach used by Blom and his colleagues[32] in the Day Care Center at the University of Colorado. In that approach events are handled as they occur. Since the school program takes up most of the child's day, in most day treatment centers today there is a close relationship between psychotherapy and special education (the psychoeducational approach). School is considered a vital therapeutic instrument, and so educational experiences are integrated into the total treatment plan. This coordination of education and therapy has the advantage of reinforcing therapeutic gains and self-esteem, fostering peer identification and offering opportunities to develop useful defenses against impulses and anxiety. Simultaneous treatment for the parent(s) aimed at altering unhealthy interactions with the child is indispensable. The parents may be seen in individual, group, or family therapy.

Day treatment is indicated for children who have emotional disorders that have seriously impaired their social and academic functioning. It is appropriate aftercare therapy for some chronically psychotic children, who can be placed in special group foster homes following inpatient treatment. On occasion, it can be used as a transition between hospitalization or residential treatment and complete return to the community. Although day treatment is often long-term, it can be useful on a short-term basis. It is contraindicated for children who are homicidal or suicidal, for children who run away repeatedly, or for children from disorganized homes. Day treatment for preschool-age children is relatively equivalent to that provided by some well-run therapeutic nursery schools.[79]

Camps for Disturbed Children

Beginning with the pioneering work of Redl[190] and Scheidlinger,[210] therapeutic summer camps for disturbed children have gradually become an established therapeutic modality. In addition to a well-planned therapeutic milieu balanced to fit the needs of the individual groups,[119] the various activities of camp life can help a child build his confidence around successful experiences at his own pace, and he can come to feel that he is a respected member of his peer group. Ongoing consultation and treatment are provided in helping to meet each child's individual needs. Parents are usually expected to participate in the camp experience, both in the treatment process and in some camp outings. Ordinary overnight camps and camps which emphasize survival have their merits, but they are too large and competitive for the disturbed child. Recently, therapeutic camping principles have been applied to the treatment of obese and diabetic children and adolescents. A camp experience alone cannot meet all the needs of a truly disturbed child; it must be coordinated carefully with ongoing treatment planning. Some residential treatment centers have set up their own summer therapeutic camps, to be used as the child's needs dictate.

Other Forms of Therapy

Music Therapy

Music has been shown by Heimlich,[105] Stein,[219] and others to be effective in communicating with children, in reducing anxiety, and in encouraging the expression of feeling individually or in groups. Heimlich has introduced a psychotherapeutic approach to music therapy for children and adolescents who have psychologic problems of even psychotic proportions, and Cooke[54] has used music creatively in a formal psychotherapeutic approach. Background music in low-stimulus study booths has been used by Scott[211] to diminish hyperactivity in children. Recently, Gerstein and others have combined music and dance therapy.

Art Therapy

Children's artistic productions have been used as media for the expression of feeling and symbolic fantasy in psychotherapy since the pioneering work of Klein and

Anna Freud. Naumberg[180] was one of the first to make a more systematic study of children's art work. More recently, Robbins and Sibley,[198] Kramer,[131] and others have developed art therapy programs for disturbed children and adolescents which foster the sublimation of emotional conflicts in a supportive context and a sense of creativity and identity. These programs also promote maturation in general.

Physical Methods of Therapy

Of the various physical methods of therapy for adults, insulin therapy, formerly used to treat psychotic adolescents, is no longer considered appropriate by child psychiatrists. For some years, Bender[27] and others used electroconvulsive therapy to treat psychotic children. Although this procedure did not cause brain damage, as Gurevitz[96] has demonstrated, it did not prove to be of therapeutic value, and was confusing to children. Its use has been virtually abandoned by child psychiatrists, although some psychiatrists still use it inappropriately. Some years ago, Schapire prohibited the use of electroconvulsive therapy in the treatment of patients under 18 years old in Colorado state hospital units without special review by 2 child psychiatrists and rigid precautions. The recent standards for psychiatric facilities serving children and adolescents have taken a similar stand.[220]

Today electroconvulsive therapy is of value primarily in the treatment of middle-aged depressed patients, especially men. It may be helpful to an occasional very depressed adolescent, but other methods of treatment, such as psychotherapy, drugs, and hospitalization are to be preferred. In my opinion, forms of sleep therapy, such as Dauerschlaf and electrosleep, should not be used for children.

Many physicians have believed that psychosurgery is a treatment of the past. However, a new wave of interest in psychosurgery seems to be rising.[36] In addition to lobotomy, cingulatomy, and other surgical procedures on adults (some with a diagnosis of neurosis), lobotomy and hypothalamotomy, and amygdalectomy have been used to control marked hyperactivity,[19] aggression,[206] and emotional instability in children.[179] I agree with Masserman[159] that the results of psychosurgical procedures are not fully predictable, even in adults, and that improvement is difficult to evaluate. A controlled study undertaken in 1959 by Smith and Kinder[217] showed marked definitive losses in psychologic performance in adult schizophrenics 8 years after operation. These results differed with the results of 3 previous studies, one involving the same patient, which showed no lasting impairment soon after the operation. Aldrich[6] long ago saw problems in social adjustment following lobotomy. Other methods of treatment are available for disorders in children and adolescents, and the developing brain needs no such insult. The American Orthopsychiatric Association issued a position statement in 1974[5] opposing the use of lobotomy in children and the use of surgical procedures involving the brain to deal with problems of drug addiction and crime. The association also recommended the appointment of a national commission to study current issues involving psychosurgical techniques in the United States and to develop guidelines and safeguards for selected and appropriate uses of such procedures.*

Other Services in the Community

Other community services which offer help to disturbed families include family and children's agencies (public, voluntary, and private) which provide therapy for a child and his parents or marital counseling for the parents. Some agencies offer home-

---

*Biofeedback approaches to the treatment of epilepsy, cardiac arrhythmias, and other disorders were referred to in Chapter 4. Megavitamin or so-called orthomolecular therapy will be discussed in Chapter 20.

maker services in order to keep a family from being broken up when the mother becomes ill[112,197] or to provide supportive rehabilitation of a disturbed parent who remains in the home.[7] Foster grandparents have been involved in the home treatment of disturbed children.[121] Trained neighborhood mental health workers are available in some out-reach programs, and trained volunteers are taking a more active role in community and hospital settings.[17,67,230] There are also agencies that specialize in marital counseling. Juvenile courts are becoming increasingly aware of psychosocial problems in the children referred to them, as are child welfare agencies, which offer aid to dependent children in broken or disadvantaged families, including adoption or placement in foster homes, or cottage-type group-living situations.

Bibliography

1. Ackerman, N: *Psychodynamics of Family Life.* New York, Basic Books, 1958.
2. Ackerman, N.W.: *Exploring the Base for Family Therapy.* New York, Family Service Association of America, 1961.
3. Ackerman, N.W.: The failure of family psychotherapy. In: *Expanding Theory and Practice in Family Therapy* (N.W. Ackerman, F.L. Beatman, and S.N. Sherman, Eds.). New York, Family Service Association of America, 1967.
4. Adams, P.L.: Dealing with racism in biracial psychiatry. J. Am. Acad. Child Psychiatry, 9:33, 1970.
5. Alder, J.: Psychosurgery: Ethical issues and a proposal for control. Am. J. Orthopsychiatry, 44:661, 1974.
6. Aldrich, C.K.: Problems of social adjustment following lobotomy. Am. J. Psychiatry, 107:459, 1950.
7. Aldrich, C.K.: Homemaker service in psychiatric rehabilitation. Am. J. Psychiatry, 114:993, 1958.
8. Allan, K.E., et al.: Effects of social reinforcement on isolated behavior of a nursery school child. Child Dev., 35:511, 1964.
9. Allen, F.H.: *Psychotherapy with Children.* New York, Norton, 1942.
10. Allen, R.P., et al.: Behavior therapy for socially ineffective children. J. Am. Acad. Child Psychiatry, 15:500, 1976.
11. Alpern, E.: Short clinical services for children in child guidance clinic. Am. J. Orthopsychiatry, 26:314, 1956.
12. Alpert, A.: The treatment of emotionally disturbed children in a therapeutic nursery. Am. J. Orthopsychiatry, 25:826, 1955.
13. Alpert, A.: A special therapeutic technique for prelatency children with a history of deficiency in maternal care. Am. J. Orthopsychiatry, 33:161, 1963.
14. Alt, H.: Responsibilities and qualifications of the child care worker. Am. J. Orthopsychiatry, 23:670, 1953.
15. Alt, H.: *Residential Treatment for the Disturbed Child.* New York, International Universities Press, 1960.
16. Anthony, E.J.: Behavior disorders of childhood. In: *Carmichael's Manual of Child Psychology*, 3rd Ed. Vol. 2 (P. Mussen, Ed.). New York: Wiley, 1970.
17. Arffa, M.S.: High school and college student volunteers in community and psychiatric settings: A bibliography with selected annotations. Supplementary Mailing from Mental Hospital Service, American Psychiatric Association, April, 1966.
18. Axline, V.M.: *Play Therapy.* New York, Ballantine Books, 1969.
19. Balasubramaniam, V., Kanaka, T., and Ramamurthi, B.: Surgical treatment for hyperkinetic and behavior disorders. Int. Surg., 54:18, 1970.
20. Barter, E.R., and Barter, J.T.: Urban indians and mental health problems. Psychiatr. Ann., 4:36, 1974.
21. Barter, J.T., and Langsley, D.G.: The advantages of a separate unit for adolescents. Hosp. & Community Psychiatry, 19:241, 1968.
22. Baum, O.E., et al.: Psychotherapy, dropouts, and lower socioeconomic status. Am. J. Orthopsychiatry, 36:629, 1966.
23. Beels, C.C., and Ferber, A.: Family therapy: A view. Family Process., 8:280, 1969.
24. Behrens, M.L., and Ackerman, N.W.: The home visit as an aid in family diagnosis and therapy. Soc. Casework, 1:11, 1956.
25. Bell, J.E.: Family group therapy: A method for the psychological treatment of older children, adolescents and their families. Public Health Monograph No. 64, Washington, Government Printing Office, 1961.
26. Bell, J.E.: Family group therapy—A new treatment method for children. Family Process, 6:254, 1967.
27. Bender, L.: One hundred cases of childhood schizophrenia treated with electric shock. Trans. Am. Neurol. Assoc., 72:165, 1947.
28. Berkowitz, B., and Graziano, A.: Training parents as behavior therapists: A review. Behav. Res. Ther., 10:297, 1972.
29. Bernstein, I.: Indications and goals of child analysis compared with child psychotherapy. J. Am. Psychoanal. Assoc., 5:158, 1957.
30. Bernstein, N.: *Emotional Care of the Facially Burned and Disfigured.* New York, Little, 1976.
31. Bettelheim, B., and Sylvester, E.: A therapeutic milieu. Am. J. Orthopsychiatry, 18:191, 1948.
32. Blom, G.E., et al.: A psychoeducational approach to day care treatment. J. Am. Acad. Child Psychiatry, 11:492, 1972.
33. Boulanger, J.B.: Group psychoanalytic therapy

in child psychiatry. Can. Psychiatr. Assoc., 6:272, 1961.

34. Brady, J.P.: Behavior therapy. In: *Comprehensive Textbook of Psychiatry*, 2nd Ed., Vol. 2 (A.M. Freedman, H.I. Kaplan, and B.J. Sadock, Eds.). Baltimore, Williams & Wilkins, 1976.
35. Braun, S.J., and Lasher, M.G.: *Preparing Teachers to Work with Disturbed Preschoolers*. Cambridge, Mass., Nimrod Press, 1970.
36. Breggin, P.: The return of lobotomy and psychosurgery. U.S. Congressional Record, 118:E3380–E3386, 1972.
37. Brenman, M., and Gill, M.M.: *Hypnotherapy*. New York, International Universities Press, 1960.
38. Bronner, A.: Group therapy and private practice. Am. J. Psychother., 8:54, 1954.
39. Bruch, H.: Brief psychotherapy in a pediatric clinic. Q. J. Child Behav., 1:2, 1949.
40. Burks, H.L., and Hockstra, M.: Psychiatric emergencies in children. Am. J. Orthopsychiatry, 34:134, 1964.
41. Buxbaum, E.: Technique of child therapy: A critical evaluation. Psychoanal. Study Child, 9:297, 1954.
42. Callan, J.P.: Meeting mental health needs of Puerto Rican families. Hosp. Community Psychiatry, 24:330, 1973.
43. Calneck, M.: Racial factors in the counter transference: The black therapist and the black client. Am. J. Orthopsychiatry, 40:39, 1970.
44. Cameron, K.: A psychiatric in-patient department for children. J. Ment. Sci., 95:560, 1949.
45. Caplan, G.: *Principles of Preventive Psychiatry*. New York, Basic Books, 1964.
46. Carr, R.: A Follow-up Study on Children Discharged From the Oaks. *The Oaks Newsletter*, 1:1, 1972.
47. Chalpin, G.: The father's group: An effective therapy medium for involving fathers in a child psychiatric clinic treatment room. J. Acad. Child Psychiatry, 5:125, 1966.
48. Chamberlain, R.W.: Approaches to child rearing: Early recognition and modification of vicious cycle parent-child relationships. Clin. Pediatr., 6:469, 1967.
49. Chance, E.: Group psychotherapy in community mental health programs. Am. J. Orthopsychiatry, 37:920, 1967.
50. Chethik, M.: Work with parents: Treatment of the parent-child relationship. J. Am. Acad. Child Psychiatry, 15:453, 1976.
51. Christmas, J.: Group rehabilitative approaches in socially and economically disadvantaged communities. In: *Progress in Group and Family Therapy* (C. Sager and H. Kaplan, Eds.). New York, Brunner/Mazel, 1972.
52. Clifford, G., et al.: Unpublished material.
53. Collier, J.G., and Morrison, G.C.: Family treatment approaches to suicidal children and adolescents. J. Am. Acad. Child Psychiatry, 8:140, 1969.
54. Cooke, R.: Personal communication.
55. Cooper, M.M.: Evaluation of the mother's advisory service. Monogr. Soc. Res. Child Dev., 12:1, 1947.

56. Coppolillo, H.P.: A technical consideration in child analysis and child therapy. J. Am. Acad. Child. Psychiatry, 8:411, 1969.
56a. Cummings, N., and Follette, W.: Psychiatric services and medical utilization in a prepaid health plan setting. II. Med Care, 6:31, 1968.
57. Danto, B.L.: Management of unresolved hypnotic trances as forms of psychiatric emergencies. Am. J. Psychiatry, 124:1, 1967.
58. Davids, A., Ryan, R., and Salvatore, P.D.: Effectiveness of residential treatment for psychotic and other disturbed children. Am. J. Orthopsychiatry, 38:469, 1968.
58a. Deuhrssen, Von, A., and Jorswieck, E.: An empirical-statistical investigation into the efficacy of psychoanalytic therapy. Nervenarzt, 36:166, 1965.
59. Dietz, C.R., and Costell, M.E.: Reciprocal interaction in the parent-child relationship during psychotherapy. Am. J. Orthopsychiatry, 26:376, 1956.
60. Disturbed Children. Menninger Clinic, Children's Division. San Francisco, Jossey-Bass, 1969.
61. Durkin, H.E.: *Group Psychotherapy for Mothers*. Springfield, Ill., Thomas, 1969.
62. Eisenberg, L.: Treatment for disturbed children: A follow-up study. In: *Mental Health Program Reports*. Public Health Service Publication No. 1568, Bethesda, Md., 1968.
63. Eisenberg, L., Conners, K.C., and Lawrence, S.: A controlled study of the differential applications of out-patient psychiatric treatment for children. Jap. J. Child Psychiatry, 6:125, 1965.
64. Eissler, K.R.: Notes on problems of technique in the psychoanalytic treatment of adolescents. In: *The Psychoanalytic Study of the Child*, Vol. 13. New York: International Universities Press, 1958.
65. Egan, M.H., and Robinson, K.: Home treatment: An addition to our continuum of therapy. Curr. Psychiatr. Ther., 7:24, 1968.
66. Epstein, N.: Brief group therapy in a child guidance clinic. Soc. Work, 3:33, 1970.
67. Ewalt, P.I.: *Mental Health Volunteers: The Expanding Role of the Volunteers in Hospital and Community Mental Health Services*. Springfield, Ill., Thomas, 1967.
68. Falstein, E.: Personal communication.
69. Feldman, Y.: A casework approach toward understanding the parents of emotionally disturbed children. Soc. Work, 3:23, 1958.
70. Fenichel, C., Freedman, A.M., and Klapper, Z.: Day school treatment. Am. J. Orthopsychiatry, 30:130, 1960.
71. Finzer, W.F., and Kirkpatrick, S.: Unpublished material.
72. Finzer, W.F., and Kisley, A.J.: Localized neurotic interaction. J. Am. Acad. Child Psychiatry, 3:265, 1964.
73. Foulkes, S.H., and Anthony, E.J.: *Group Psychotherapy: The Psychoanalytic Approach*. New York, Penguin Books, 1957.
74. Fraiberg, S.: Counselling for the parents of the very young child. Soc. Casework, 35:47, 1954.
75. Frank, J.D.: Problems of controls in psychotherapy as exemplified by the psychotherapy re-

search project of the Phipps psychiatric clinic. In: *Research in Psychotherapy* (E.A. Rubinstein and M.B. Parloff, Eds.). Washington, D.C., American Psychological Association, 1959.

76. Frank, J.D.: Psychotherapy: The restoration of morale. Am. J. Psychiatry, 131:271, 1974.

77. Freud, A.: *The Psychoanalytical Treatment of Children*. London, Imago, 1946.

78. Freud, A.: The child as a person in his own right. Psychoanal. Study Child, 27:621, 1972.

79. Frommer, E.A.: A day hospital for disturbed children under five. Lancet, 1:377, 1967.

80. Freeman, R.D.: The home visit in child psychiatry: Its usefulness in diagnosis and training. J. Am. Acad. Child Psychiatry, 6:276, 1967.

81. Friedman, A.S.: Family therapy as conducted in the home. Fam. Process, 1:132, 1962.

82. Galdston, R., and Hughes, M.C.: Pediatric hospitalization as crisis intervention. Am. J. Psychiatry, 129:97, 1972.

83. Garber, B., Ed.: *Follow-up Study of Hospitalized Adolescents*. New York, Brunner/Mazel, 1972.

84. Gardner, G.G.: Hypnosis with children. Int. J. Clin. Exp. Hypn., 22:20, 1974.

85. Gardner, G.G.: Attitudes of child health professionals toward hypnosis: Implications for training. Int. J. Clin. Exp. Hypn., 24:63, 1976.

86. Gill, M.M., and Brenman, M.: *Hypnosis and Related States*. New York, International Universities Press, 1960.

87. Glasser, B., Hartman E., and Avery, N.: Attitudes toward adolescents on adult wards of a mental hospital. Am. J. Psychiatry, 124:317, 1967.

88. Glynn, E.: The therapeutic use of seclusion on an adolescent ward. J. Hillside Hosp., 6:156, 1957.

89. Glynn, E.: An after care program for adolescents. J. Hillside Hosp., 9:61, 1960.

90. Goldsmith, J.M., Schulman, R., and Grossbard, H.: Integrating clinical processes with planned living experiences. Am. J. Orthopsychiatry, 24:281, 1954.

91. Gossett, J.T., et al.: Follow-up of adolescents treated in a psychiatric hospital. I. A review of studies. Am. J. Orthopsychiatry, 43:602, 1973.

92. Greaves, D.C., and Regan, P.F.: Psychotherapy of adolescents at intensive hospital treatment level. In: *Psychotherapy of the Adolescent* (B.H. Balser, Ed.). New York, International Universities Press, 1957.

93. Green, J.M., Trankina, F.J., and Chavez, N.: Therapeutic intervention with Mexican-American children. Psychiatr. Ann., 6:68, 1976.

94. Group for the Advancement of Psychiatry: *Medical Uses of Hypnosis*. Symposium No. 8. New York, Group for the Advancement of Psychiatry, 1962.

95. Group for the Advancement of Psychiatry: *Pavlovian Conditioning and American Psychiatry*. Symposium No. 9. New York, Group for the Advancement of Psychiatry, 1964.

96. Gurevitz, S., and Helme, W.H.: Effects of electroconvulsive therapy on personality and intellectual functioning of the schizophrenic child. Dig. Neurol. Psychiatry, 3:11, 1955.

97. Guttman, H.A.: The child's participation in conjoint family therapy. J. Am. Acad. Child Psychiatry, 15:490, 1976.

98. Haggerty, R.J.: Family crises: The role of the family in health and illness. In: *Ambulatory Pediatrics* (M. Green and R. Haggerty, Eds.). Philadelphia, Saunders, 1968.

99. Haley, J.: Beginning and experienced family therapists. In: *The Book of Family Therapy*. (A. Ferber, M. Mendelsohn and A. Napier, Eds.). New York, Science House, 1972.

100. Haley, J., and Hoffman, L.: *Techniques of Family Therapy*. New York, Basic Books, 1967.

101. Hallowitz, D., and Cutter, A.V.: A collaborative diagnostic and treatment process with parents. Soc. Work, 6:2, 1961.

102. Halpern, W.I., and Kissel, S.: *Human Resources for Troubled Children*. New York, Wiley-Interscience, 1976.

103. Harrison, S.I., et al.: Social class and mental illness in children: Choice of treatment. Arch. Gen. Psychiatry, 13:411, 1965.

104. Harrison, S.I., et al.: Social status and child psychiatric practice: The influence of the clinician's socioeconomic origin. Am. J. Psychiatry, 127:652, 1970.

105. Heimlich, E.P.: The specialized use of music as a mode of communication in the treatment of disturbed children. J. Am. Acad. Child Psychiatry, 4:86, 1965.

106. Heinecke, C.M.: Frequency of psychotherapeutic session as a factor affecting outcome: Analysis of clinical rating and test results. J. Abnorm. Psychol., 74:553, 1969.

107. Heinecke, C.M., and Goldman, A.: Research on psychotherapy with children: A review and suggestions for further study. Am. J. Orthopsychiatry, 30:483, 1960.

108. Henrickson, W.J., Holmes, D.J., and Waggoner, R.W.: Psychotherapy with hospitalized adolescents. Am. J. Psychiatry, 116:527, 1959.

109. Hetznecker, W., et al.: Field survey methods in psychiatry: A symptom check list, mental status, and clinical status scales for evaluation of psychiatric impairment. Arch. Gen. Psychiatry, 15:427, 1968.

110. Hobbs, N.: Project Re-Ed: *New Concepts for Helping Emotionally Disturbed Children*. Nashville, Tenn., George Peabody College, 1969.

111. Hollingshead, A., and Redlich, F.: *Social Class and Mental Illness: A Community Study*. New York, Wiley, 1958.

112. Homemaker Service in Public Welfare: The North Carolina Experience. Bureau of Family Services. Washington, Government Printing Office, 1965.

113. Howells, J.G.: Child-parent separation as a therapeutic procedure. Am. J. Psychiatry, 119:922, 1963.

114. Howells, J.G.: *Theory and Practice of Family Psychiatry*. New York, Brunner/Mazel, 1976.

115. Hunt, R.G.: Occupational status and the disposition of cases in a child guidance clinic. Int. J. Soc. Psychiatr., 8:199, 1962.

116. Jackson, A.M., Berkowitz, H., and Farley, G.K.: Race as a variable affecting the treatment in-

volvement of children. J. Am. Acad. Child Psychiatry, *13*:20, 1974.

117. Jackson, D.D., and Weakland, J.H.: Conjoint family therapy. Some considerations on theory, technique, and results. Psychiatry, *24* (Suppl.):30, 1961.

118. Jaffee, S.L., and Scherl, D.J.: Acute psychosis precipitated by T-group experiences. Arch. Gen. Psychiatry, *21*:443, 1969.

119. Jensen, S.E., McCreary, J.A., and Brown, J.S.: Disturbed children in a camp milieu. Can. Psychiatr. Assoc. J., *13*:371, 1968.

120. Jessner, L.: Discipline as a problem in psychotherapy with children. Nerv. Child., *9*:147, 1951.

121. Johnston, R.: Foster grandparents for emotionally disturbed children. Children, *14*:46, 1967.

122. Kaffman, M.: Short term family therapy. Family Process, *4*:241, 1965.

123. Kaplan, D.: Study and treatment of an acute emotional disorder. Am. J. Orthopsychiatr., *35*:1, 1965.

124. Karasu, T.B.: Psychotherapies: An overview. Am. J. Psychiatry, *134*:851, 1977.

125. Katan, A.: The nursery school as a diagnostic help to the child guidance clinic. Psychoanal. Study Child, *14*:250, 1959.

126. Kaufman, I.: Maximizing the strengths of parents with severe ego defects. Soc. Casework, *36*:443, 1955.

127. Kellner, R.: The evidence in favor of psychotherapy. Br. J. Med. Psychol., *40*:341, 1967.

128. Klein, M.: *The Psychoanalysis of Children.* London, Hogarth Press, 1937.

129. Kliman, G.: *Psychological Emergencies of Childhood.* New York, Grune & Stratton, 1968.

130. Koret, S.: The children's community mental health center emerges. Child. Psychiatry Hum. Dev., *3*:243, 1973.

131. Kramer, E.: *Art As Therapy with Children.* New York, Schocken Books, 1971.

132. Kramer, S., and Settlage, C.F.: On the concepts and technique of child analysis. J. Am. Acad. Child Psychiatry, *1*:509, 1962.

133. LaBaw, W.L.: Assisting adults and children with remedial uses of their trance capability: A frequent imperative for health professionals. Behav. Neuropsychiatry, *1*:24, 1969.

134. LaBaw, W.L.: Terminal hypnosis in lieu of terminal hospitalization. Gerontol. Clin., *11*:312, 1969.

135. LaBaw, W.L., et al.: The use of self-hypnosis by children with cancer. Am. J. Clin. Hypn., *17*:233, 1975.

136. LaBaw, W.L.: Regular Use of Suggestibility by Pediatric Bleeders. Haematologia, *4*:419, 1970.

137. Langsley, D.G., and Kaplan, D.M.: *The Treatment of Families in Crisis.* New York, Grune & Stratton, 1968.

138. Langsley, D., et al.: Follow-up evaluation of family crisis therapy. Am. J. Orthopsychiatry, *39*:753, 1969.

139. Laybourne, P.C., and Miller, H.C.: Pediatric hospitalization of psychiatric patients: Diagnostic and therapeutic implications. Am. J. Orthopsychiatry, *32*:596, 1962.

140. Lebovici, S.: Psychodrama as applied to adolescents. J. Child Psychol. Psychiatry, *1*:298, 1961.

141. Leventhal, T., and Weinberger, G.: Evaluation of a large scale brief therapy program for children. Am. J. Orthopsychiatry, *45*:119, 1975.

142. Levin, G.R., and Simmons, J.J.: Response to praise by emotionally disturbed boys. Psychol. Rep., *11*:539, 1962.

143. Levitt, E.E.: The results of psychotherapy with children: An evaluation. J. Consult. Psychol., *21*:189, 1957.

144. Levitt, E.E.: Psychotherapy with children: A further evaluation. Behav. Res. Ther., *1*:45, 1963.

145. Levy, D.M.: Attitude therapy. Am. J. Orthopsychiatry, *7*:103, 1937.

146. Levy, E.Z.: Long-term follow-up of former inpatients at the children's hospital of the Menninger clinic. Am. J. Psychiatry, *125*:1633, 1969.

147. Lievano, J.: Observations about payment of psychotherapy fees. Psychiatry. Q., *41*:324, 1967.

148. Lindemann, E.G.: Symptomatology and management of acute grief. Am. J. Psychiatry, *101*:141, 1944.

149. Lorand, S., and Consolo, W.A.: Therapeutic results in psychoanalytic treatment without fee. Int. J. Psychoanal., *39*:59, 1938.

150. Lourie, N.V., and Lourie, B.P.: A noncategorical approach to treatment: Programs for children and youth. Am. J. Orthopsychiatry, *40*:684, 1970.

151. Lovaas, O.I., Schaffer, B., and Simmons, J.Q.: Building social behavior in autistic children by use of electric shock. J. Exper. Res. Personal., *1*:99, 1965.

152. Luborsky, L., Singer, B., and Luborsky, L.: Comparative studies of psychotherapies. Arch. Gen. Psychiatry, *32*:995, 1975.

153. Malone, C.H.: Child psychiatry services for low socioeconomic families. J. Am. Acad. Child. Psychiatry, *6*:332, 1967.

154. Marcos, L.R., and Alpert, M.: Strategies and risks in psychotherapy with bilingual patients: The phenomenon of language independence. Am. J. Psychiatry, *133*:1275, 1976.

155. Marks, I.M.: The current status of behavioral psychotherapy: Theory and practice. Am. J. Psychiatry, *133*:253, 1976.

156. Marmor, J.: Dynamic psychotherapy and behavior therapy. Arch. Gen. Psychiatry, *24*:22, 1971.

157. Marsden, G., McDermott, J.F., and Miner, D.: Residential treatment of children: A survey of institutions and characteristics. J. Am. Acad. J. Psychiatry, *9*:333, 1970.

158. Mash, E.J., Hardy, L.C., and Hamerlynck, L.A., Eds.: *Behavior Modification Approaches to Parenting.* New York, Brunner/Mazel, 1976.

159. Masserman, J.H.: *Psychoanalysis and Human Values.* New York, Grune & Stratton, 1960.

160. Masterson, J.F.: Prognosis in adolescent disorders. Am. J. Psychiatry, *114*:12, 1958.

161. Mattsson, A., Hawkins, J., and Seese, L.: Child psychiatric emergencies: Clinical characteristics and follow-up results. Arch. Gen. Psychiatry, *17*:584, 1967.

162. Mattsson, A., and Naylor, K.A.: Psychiatric emergencies on the pediatric ward: Clinical char-

acteristics and suggestions for management. In: *Emergencies in Child Psychiatry* (G.C. Morrison, Ed.). Springfield, Ill., Thomas, 1975.

163. Mattsson, A., Seese, L.R., and Hawkins, J.W.: Suicidal behavior as a child psychiatric emergency: Clinical characteristics and follow-up results. Arch. Gen. Psychiatry, 20:100, 1969.

164. Maxwell, A.: The interrelated movement of parent and child in resident treatment. Q. J. Child Behav., 2:185, 1950.

165. McDermott, J.F., Jr., and Char, W.F.: The undeclared war between child and family therapy. J. Am. Acad. Child Psychiatry, 13:483, 1974.

166. McDermott, J.F., et al.: Social class and mental illness in children: observations of blue collar families. Am. J. Orthopsychiatry, 35:500, 1965.

167. McDonald, N.F., and Adams, P.L.: The psychotherapeutic workability of the poor. J. Am. Acad. Child Psychiatry, 6:663, 1967.

168. McGlashan, T.H., Evans, F.J., and Orne, M.T.: The nature of hypnotic analgesia and placebo response to experimental pain. Psychosom. Med., 31:227, 1969.

169. McKnight, J.A., et al.: Unpublished material.

170. Miller, D.H.: The treatment of adolescents in an adult hospital. Bull. Menninger Clin., 21:189, 1957.

171. Miller, N.B., and Cantwell, D.P.: Siblings as therapists: A behavioral approach. Am. J. Psychiatry, 133:447, 1976.

172. Miller, N.E.: Learning of visceral and glandular responses. Science, 163:434, 1969.

173. Minuchin, S.: Conflict-resolution family therapy. Psychiatry, 28:278, 1965.

174. Montalvo, B., and Haley, J.: In defense of child therapy. Fam. Process, 12:227, 1973.

175. Montanari, A.J.: A community-based residential program for disturbed children. Hosp. and Community Psychiatry, April, 1963.

176. Morrison, G.C., Ed.: *Emergencies in Child Psychiatry: Emotional Crises of Children, Youth, and Their Families.* Springfield, Ill., Thomas, 1975.

177. Mowrer, O.H.: *Learning Theory and Personality Dynamics.* New York, Ronald Press, 1950.

178. Naftulin, D., Donnelly, F., and Wolkon, G.: Four therapeutic approaches to the same patient. Am. J. Psychother., 29:66, 1975.

179. Narabayashi, H., et al.: Stereotactic amygdalotomy for behavior disorders. Arch. Neurol., 9:1, 1963.

180. Naumberg, M.: *An Introduction to Art Therapy: Studies of the "Free" Art Expression of Behavior Problem Children and Adolescents as a Means of Diagnosis and Therapy.* New York, Teachers College Press, 1973.

181. Noshpitz, J.D.: The therapeutic aspect of residential treatment. J. Phila. Assoc. Psychoanal., 10:71, 1976.

182. Parad, H.J.: *Crisis Intervention: Selected Readings.* New York, Family Service Association of America, 1965.

183. Paul, J.L., Stedman, D.J., and Neufeld, G.R., Eds.: *Deinstitutionalization: Program and policy development.* Washington, D.C., National Institute of Mental Health, 1972.

184. Pavenstedt, E., et al.: *The Drifters: Children of Disorganized Lower-Class Families.* Boston, Little, Brown, 1967.

185. Pittman, F., et al.: Family therapy as an alternative to psychiatric hospitalization. Report No. 20. Washington, D.C.: American Psychiatric Association, 1966.

186. Polskin, S.R.: Working with parents of mentally ill children in residential care. Soc. Work, 6:4, 1961.

187. Position statement by board of trustees, American Psychiatric Association, on involuntary hospitalization of the mentally ill. Am. J. Psychiatry, 128:11, 1972.

188. Proskauer, S.: Focussed time-limited psychotherapy with children. J. Am. Acad. Child Psychiatry, 10:619, 1971.

189. Rank, B., et al.: A special adaptation of the psychoanalytic approach to the treatment of children with atypical ego development. Am. J. Orthopsychiatry, 16:391, 1946.

190. Redl, F.: Psychopathologic risks of camp life. Nerv. Child, 6:139, 1947.

191. Redl, F.: The concept of a therapeutic milieu. Am. J. Orthopsychiatry, 29:721, 1959.

192. Redl, F.: Strategy and techniques of the life-space interview. Am. J. Orthopsychiatry, 29:1, 1959.

193. Redl, F., and Wineman, D.: *Controls from Within: Techniques for the Treatment of the Aggressive Child.* Glencoe, Ill., Free Press, 1952.

194. Reid, J.H., and Hagan, H.R.: *Residential Treatment of Emotionally Disturbed Children.* New York, Child Welfare League of America, 1952.

195. *Report on Medical Use of Hypnosis.* (American Medical Association Council on Mental Health.) JAMA, 168:1053, 1958.

196. Rexford, E.: Child psychiatry and child analysis in the United States today. J. Am. Acad. Child Psychiatry, 1:365, 1962.

197. Rice, E.P.: Homemakers Service in Maternal and Child Health Programs. Department of Health, Education, and Welfare. (Health Services and Mental Health Administration, Maternal and Child Health Service), 1965.

198. Robbins, A., and Sibley, L.B.: *Creative Art Therapy.* New York, Brunner/Mazel, 1976.

199. Robinson, J.M., et al., Eds.: *The Psychiatric Inpatient Treatment of Children.* Washington, D.C., American Psychiatric Association, 1958.

200. Robinson, J.F.: Psychiatric inpatient care of the younger patient. Ment. Hosp., January, 1965.

201. Rosenfeld, E., Frankel, N., and Esman, A.H.: A model of criteria for evaluating progress in children undergoing psychotherapy. Am. J. Acad. Child Psychiatry, 8:193, 1969.

202. Rosenthal, A., and Levine, S.: Brief psychotherapy with children: A preliminary report. Am. J. Psychiatry, 127:646, 1970.

203. Ross, A.O.: *Psychological Disorders of Children: A Behavioral Approach to Theory, Research, and Therapy.* New York, State University at Stonybrook, 1974.

204. Sager, C.J.: Concurrent individual and group analytic psychotherapy. Am. J. Orthopsychiatry, 30:225, 1960.

205. Sager, C.J., et al.: Selection and engagement of patients in family therapy. Am. J. Orthopsychiatry, *38*:15, 1968.
206. Sano, K., et al.: Posteromedial hypothalamotomy in treatment of aggressive behavior. Confin. Neurol., *27*:164, 1969.
207. Satir, V.: Family systems and approaches to family therapy. J. Fort. Logan Ment. Health Cent., *4*:81, 1967.
208. Satir, V.: Including the children in the family group. In: *Conjoint Family Therapy*, Rev. Ed. Palo Alto, Calif., Science and Behavior Books, 1967.
209. Schacter, J.S., and Butts, H.: Transference and counter transference in interracial analyses. J. Am. Psychoanal. Assoc., *16*:792, 1968.
210. Scheidlinger, S., and Scheidlinger, L.: The treatment potentialities of the summer camp for children with personality disturbances. Nerv. Child, *6*:232, 1947.
211. Scott, J.T.: The use of music to reduce hyperactivity in children. Am. J. Orthopsychiatry, *40*:677, 1970.
212. Shaw, S.J.: *Clinical Applications of Hypnosis in Dentistry.* Philadelphia, Saunders, 1958.
213. Shulman, J.L.: One visit psychotherapy with children. Prog. Psychother., *5*:86, 1960.
214. Slavson, S.R.: *Analytic Group Psychotherapy with Children, Adolescents and Adults.* New York, Columbia University Press, 1950.
215. Slavson, S.R.: *Child-Centered Group Guidance of Parents.* New York, International Universities Press, 1958.
216. Sloane, R.B., et al.: Patient's attitudes towards behavior therapy and psychotherapy. Am. J. Psychiatry, *134*:134, 1977.
217. Smith, A., and Kinder, E.F.: Changes in psychological test performances of brain-operated schizophrenics after 8 years. Science, *129*:149, 1959.
218. Solnit, A.J.: Hospitalization: An aid to physical and psychological health in childhood. Am. J. Dis. Child., *99*:155, 1960.
219. Stein, J.: Music therapy treatment techniques. Am. J. Orthopsychiatry, *33*:521, 1963.
220. *Standards for Psychiatric Facilities Serving Children and Adolescents.* Washington, D.C., American Psychiatric Association, 1971.
221. Skinner, B.F.: *Science and Human Behavior.* New York, Macmillan, 1953.
222. Slavson, S.R.: Differential methods of group therapy in relation to age levels. Nerv. Child, *4*:196, 1945.
223. Staub, E., et al.: Unpublished material.
224. Strupp, H.: Specific vs. nonspecific factors in psychotherapy and the problem of control. Arch. Gen. Psychiatry, *23*:393, 1970.
225. Strupp, H.H., and Bergin, H.E.: Research in Individual Psychotherapy: A Bibliography. Department of Health, Education, and Welfare (Pub. Health Service. National Institute of Mental Health, 1969.)
226. Tasen, W.M., Dasteel, J.C., and Goldenberg, E.B.: Psychiatric screening and brief intervention in a pediatric program utilizing allied health personnel. Am. J. Orthopsychiatry, *44*:568, 1974.
227. Terestman, N., Miller, J.D., and Weber, J.J.: Blue collar patients at a psychoanalytic clinic. Am. J. Psychiatry, *131*:261, 1974.
228. Urban, H.B., and Ford, D.H.: Behavior Therapy. In: *Comprehensive Textbook of Psychiatry* (A. Freedman and H.Kaplan, Eds.). Philadelphia, Saunders, 1967.
229. Vasey, I., et al.: Unpublished material.
230. *Volunteer Services in Mental Health: An Annotated Bibliography.* National Institute of Mental Health, National Clearing House for Mental Health Information. Publication No. 1002. Washington, Government Printing Office, 1978.
231. Waite, R.: The negro patient and clinical theory. J. Consult. Clin. Psychol., *32*:427, 1968.
232. Waldfogel, S., Tessman, E., and Hahn, P.B.: A program for early intervention in school phobia. Am. J. Orthopsychiatry, *29*:324, 1959.
233. Warren, R.C., et al.: Differential attitudes of black and white patients toward treatment in a child guidance clinic. Am. J. Orthopsychiatry, *43*:384, 1973.
234. Weber, G.H., and Haberlein, B.J.: *Residential Treatment of Emotionally Disturbed Children.* New York, Behavioral Publications, 1972.
235. Weinstein, E.A., and Malitz, S.: Changes in symbolic expression with amytal sodium. Am. J. Psychiatry, *111*:198, 1954.
236. Werry, J., and Wollerstein, J.P.: Behavior therapy with children. A broad overview. J. Am. Acad. Child. Psychiatry, *6*:346, 1967.
237. Westman, J.C., et al.: Parallel group psychotherapy with the parents of emotionally disturbed children. Int. J. Group Psychother., *13*:52, 1963.
238. Witmer, H.: A comparison of treatment results in various types of child guidance clinics. Am. J. Orthopsychiatry, *5*:351, 1935.
239. Wolberg, L.R.: *Medical Hypnosis.* New York, Grune & Stratton, 1948.
240. Wolf, S., and Ripley, H.S.: Studies on the action of intravenously administered sodium amytal. Am. J. Med. Sci., *215*:56, 1948.
241. Wolman, B.B.: *Handbook of Child Psychoanalysis: Research, Theory, and Practice.* New York, Van Nostrand Reinhold, 1972.
242. Wynne, L.: Some indications and contraindications for exploratory family therapy. In: *Intensive Family Therapy* (I. Boszormenyi-Nagy and J.L. Framo, Eds.). New York, Harper & Row, Hoeber Medical Division, 1965.
243. Zillbach, J.J., Bergel, E., and Gass, C.: The role of the child in family therapy. In: *Progress in Group and Family Therapy.* New York, Brunner/Mazel, 1972.
244. Zuk, G.H.: The side-taking function in family therapy. Am. J. Orthopsychiatry, *37*:553, 1967.

General References

Ackerman, U.W.: Family psychotherapy and family psychoanalysis: The implications of difference. Fam. Process, May, 1962.

Adams, P.L.: *A Primer of Child Psychotherapy*. Boston, Little, Brown, 1974.

Ambrose, G.: Hypnotherapy for children. In: *Hypnosis in Modern Medicine* (J.M. Schneck, Ed.). Springfield, Ill., Thomas, 1962.

Atcheson, J.D., Alderton, H.R., and Harvey, R.: The development and organization of a children's psychiatric hospital. Can. Med. Assoc. J., *25*:158, 1964.

Augenbraun, B., Reid, H., and Friedman, D.: Brief interventions as a preventive force in disorders of early childhood. Am. J. Orthopsychiatry, *37*:697, 1967.

Barten, H.H., and Barten, S.S., Eds.: *Children and Their Parents in Brief Therapy*. New York, Behavioral Publications, 1973.

Becket, P.G.S.: *Adolescents Out of Step: Their Treatment in a Psychiatric Hospital*. Detroit, Wayne State University Press, 1965.

Berlin, I.N.: Crisis intervention and short-term therapy: Approach in a child psychiatric clinic. J. Am. Acad. Child Psychiatry, *9*:595, 1970.

Bettelheim, B.: *Love is Not Enough: The Treatment of Emotionally Disturbed Children*. Glencoe, Ill., Free Press, 1950.

Bettelheim, B.: *Truants from Life: The Rehabilitation of Emotionally Disturbed Children*. Glencoe, Ill., Free Press, 1955.

Blom, G.E., and Finzer, W.F.: The development of specific treatment approaches to the emotionally disturbed children: Psychiatric inpatient and day care treatment. Am. J. Med. Sci., *243*:112, 1962.

Boszormenyi-Nagy, I., and Framo, J.L., Eds.: *Intensive Family Therapy: Theoretical and Practical Aspects*. New York, Harper & Row, Hoeber Medical Division, 1965.

Bowen, M.: Family psychotherapy. Amer. J. Orthopsychiatry, *31*:40, 1961.

Bruch, H.: *Learning Psychotherapy: Rationale and Ground Rules*. Cambridge, Mass., Harvard University Press, 1975.

Caplan, G. Ed.: *Prevention of Mental Disorders in Children*. New York, Basic Books, 1961.

Cooper, S.: New trends in work with parents: Progress or change? Soc. Casework, *42*:342, 1961.

Cutter, A.V., and Hallowitz, D.: Different approaches to treatment of the child and the parents. Am. J. Orthopsychiatry, *32*:152, 1962.

d'Amato, G.: *Residential Treatment for Child Mental Health*. Springfield, Ill., Thomas, 1969.

Drechsler, R.J., and Shapiro, M.J.: A procedure for direct observation of family interaction in a child guidance clinic. Psychiatry, *24*:163–170, 1961.

Durkin, H.E.: The group therapy movement. Psychiatr. Ann., *2*:14, 1972.

Eysenck, H.J.: Learning theory and behavior theory. J. Ment. Sci., *105*:61, 1959.

Fielding, J.M.: A technique for measuring outcome in group psychotherapy. Br. J. Med. Psychol., *48*:189, 1975.

Fleck, S.: Psychotherapy of families of hospitalized patients. In: *Current Psychiatric Therapies* (J. Masserman, Ed.). 3rd Ed. New York, Grune & Stratton, 1963.

Furman, R.A., and Katan, A.: *The Therapeutic Nursery School: A Contribution to the Study and Treatment of Emotional Disturbances in Young Children*. New York, International Universities Press, 1969.

Geleerd, E.R.: *The Child Analyst at Work*. New York, International Universities Press, 1967.

Ginott, H.G.: *Group Psychotherapy with Children: The Theory and Practice of Play-Therapy*. New York, McGraw-Hill, 1961.

Gottschalk, L.A., Fox, R.A., and Bates, D.E.: A study of prediction and outcome in a mental health crisis clinic. Am. J. Psychiatry, *130*:1107, 1973.

Grob, M., and Singer, J.: *Adolescent Patients in Transition: Impact and Outcome of Psychiatric Hospitalization*. New York, Human Services Press, 1974.

Group for the Advancement of Psychiatry: *The Field of Family Therapy*. Report No. 78. New York, Group for the Advancement of Psychiatry, 1970.

Hammer, M., and Kaplan, A.M.: *The Practice of Psychotherapy with Children*. Homewood, Ill., Dorsey Press, 1967.

Hayworth, M.R., Ed.: *Child Psychotherapy: Theory and Practice*. New York, Basic Books, 1967.

Heinecke, C.M.: Aiding "at risk" children through psychoanalytic social work with parents. Am. J. Orthopsychiatry, *46*:89, 1976.

Holmes, D.: *The Adolescent in Psychotherapy*. Boston, Little, Brown, 1964.

Klein, D., and Lindemann, E.: Preventive intervention in individual and family crisis situations. In: *Prevention of Mental Disorders* (G. Caplan, Ed.). New York, Basic Books, 1961.

Konopka, G.: The role of the group in residential treatment. Am. J. Orthopsychiatry, *25*:679, 1955.

Krug, O.: The application of principles of child psychotherapy in residential treatment. Am. J. Psychiatry, *108*:695, 1952.

Kubie, L.S.: Some theoretical principles underlying the relationship between individual and group psychotherapy. Int. J. Group Psychother., *8*:1, 1958.

LaVietes, R.L.: Crisis intervention for ghetto children: Contraindications and alternative considerations. Am. J. Orthopsychiatry, *44*:720, 1974.

LaVietes, R., et al.: Day treatment center and school: Seven years experience. Am. J. Orthopsychiatry, *35*:160, 1965.

Lippman, H.S.: *Treatment of the Child in Emotional Conflict*, 2nd Ed. New York, McGraw-Hill, 1962.

Mattsson, A.: Emergencies in child psychiatry. JAMA, *202*:538, 1967.

McDermott, J.F., Fraiberg, S., and Harrison, S.J.: Residential treatment of children: The utilization of transference behavior. J. Am. Acad. Child Psychiatry, *7*:169, 1968.

Minuchin, S.: *Families and Family Therapy*. Cambridge, Mass., Harvard University Press, 1974.

Moustakas, C.E.: *Children in Play Therapy*. New York, Jason Aronson, 1973.

Noshpitz, J.D.: Notes on the theory of residential treatment. J. Am. Acad. Child Psychiatry, *1*:284, 1962.

Pearson, G.H.J.: *Handbook of Child Psychoanalysis*. New York, Basic Books, 1968.

Pittinger, R.E., and Martineau, F.: Some notes on the authority structure and the responsibility of adolescents in the George Junior Republic. J. Nerv. and Ment. Dis., *133*:339, 1961.

Residential Treatment of Emotionally Disturbed Children: Annotated Bibliography. New York, Child Welfare League of America, 1952.

Rosen, V.H.: Changes in family equilibrium through psychoanalytic treatment. In: *Neurotic Interaction in Marriage.* (V.W. Eisenstein, Ed.). New York, Basic Books, 1956.

Schaefer, C., Ed.: *Therapeutic Uses of Child's Play.* New York, Jason Aronson, 1975.

Slavson, S.R.: *An Introduction to Group Therapy.* Cambridge, Mass., The Commonwealth Fund, 1943.

Slavson, S.R., and Schiffer, M.: *Group Psychotherapies for Children: A Textbook.* New York, International Universities Press, 1975.

Swanson, F.L.: *Psychotherapists and Children: A Procedural Guide.* New York, Pitman, 1970.

Sutton, H.A.: "Some nursing aspects of a children's psychiatric ward." Am. J. Orthopsychiatry, *17*:675, 1947.

Trieshman, A.E., et al.: *The Other 23 Hours: Child Care Work with Emotionally Disturbed Children in a Therapeutic Milieu.* New York, Aldine, 1969.

Waldfogel, S., and Gardner, E.G.: Intervention in crises as a method of primary prevention. In: *Prevention of Mental Disorders in Children.* (G. Caplan, Ed.). New York, Basic Books, 1961.

Weinrab, J. Ed.: *Recent Developments in Psychoanalytic Child Therapy.* New York, International Universities Press, 1960.

Witmer, H.L., Ed.: *Psychiatric Interviews with Children.* Cambridge, Harvard University Press, 1946.

Wolpe, J.: *The Practice of Behavior Therapy,* 2nd Ed. New York, Pergamon Press, 1973.

Yalom, I.D.: *The Theory and Practice of Group Psychotherapy,* 2nd Ed. New York, Basic Books, 1975.

12

The Psychotherapeutic Aspects of the Role of the Pediatrician

> *Some patients, though conscious that their condition is perilous, recover their health simply through their contentment with the goodness of the physician.*
> *(Hippocrates)*

The Doctor-Patient Relationship

Most of the complaints about medical care and the frequent failure of patients to follow medical advice stem from a perceived lack of warmth and humanity in the doctor-patient relationship. Contacts with physicians in hospitals and clinics tend to reinforce these perceptions. As Korsch[33] has indicated, the doctor-patient relationship is too important to be left to chance or intuition alone; it must be studied and taught as a part of the art of medicine, known to family physicians in the past but unfortunately neglected today.

Szasz and Hollender[53] have usefully conceptualized 3 models of the doctor-patient relationship. They are (1) the model of *activity-passivity*, in which the physician is active and the patient is more or less completely passive, (2) the model of *guidance-*

cooperation, in which the patient obediently cooperates with the physician, (3) the model of *mutual participation*, an adult relationship in which the physician helps the patient to help himself.

Any one of these models can be appropriate, depending on the individual situation. Sometimes the doctor-patient relationship passes through all 3 phases. For example, if the physician is called on to treat a late adolescent in a diabetic coma, an active and authoritative approach to immediate diagnosis and treatment is vital, and can be most reassuring to the parents and the patient as he recovers from the coma. Later, as the patient begins to learn how to control his diabetes, the guidance of the physician and his associates becomes paramount, and the mutual participation phase gradually evolves. There are, of course, certain inherent dangers in the first

2 models. The activity-passivity model gratifies the needs of certain physicians for mastery and a feeling of superiority, and these physicians may not treat the patient or parent with dignity and respect. The guidance-cooperation model permits the physician to feel he is "competent" and "right" in his actions, but he may be tempted to go beyond this and "play God," or attempt to mold the patient into an image of himself.

Since their contacts in medical school were largely with bedridden patients, the mutual participation model is the hardest model for many physicians to use effectively. Although it is the most appropriate model for use in supportive psychotherapy with parents and children who have psychosocial components to their problems, many pediatricians feel uncomfortable with the mutual participation model. They tend to feel that it is not sufficiently active; they may feel guilty about charging parents for "talking," without offering a prescription or other traditional therapeutic measures which involve doing something "to" or "for" the patient. The fact that the parents or the child may feel helped or relieved as a result of a therapeutic relationship that permits mutual participation is not always easy for physicians to comprehend. This model involves much active empathy with the patient's or parent's feelings. It has a "partnership" element which helps the patient get to know himself more fully and to change his functioning or behavior where indicated.

The activity-passivity model may be used most effectively, with some very dependent or needy parents, whereas anxious, tense, or immature parents may benefit most from the guidance-cooperation approach. The physician must know himself and his feelings intimately if he is to employ these approaches flexibly, especially if he feels it appropriate to help parents gradually move toward the mutual participation model.

The guidance-cooperation model may be used effectively with many older children and adolescents. However, it should be used cautiously with adolescents. Some very sick, dependent, or regressed children and adolescents may require the activity-passivity approach, although they should be encouraged at least to move toward the guidance-cooperation model. Some adolescents almost demand, and can use effectively, the mutual participation model of the doctor-patient relationship.

In the doctor-patient relationship, whatever its nature, attention should be paid to attitudes and feelings which are transferred onto the physician from past experiences with key figures. Ordinarily such feelings are not dealt with directly in a supportive approach, but awareness of their origin, (gathered from his knowledge of the family history and current observations) will help the pediatrician avoid reacting as if such transference feelings were directed toward him personally. Occasionally it may be necessary to confront the child or his parent with the fact that such attitudes or feelings of mistrust or anger, for example, do in fact derive from earlier experiences, such as desertion or deprivation. In addition, the physician must look into himself if certain types of behavior by children or parents repeatedly anger or frustrate him. Such feelings may be influenced at least in part by his own past experiences and represent a type of countertransference which may not be appropriate to the current situations.

The transference relationship is often seen most clearly in the physician's relationship with the child, who tends to expect the doctor to react to him as his parents have in the past. Fearful parents may react as they used to react to their own parents. Thus, as Coddington[14] has pointed out, the physician taking care of children often finds himself in the unique position of being symbolically a surrogate parent for child and parent simultaneously. Some parents may seek fatherly advice; an anxious mother may unconsciously reenact a relationship with a seductive father by behaving seductively toward the physician. In addition to transference and countertransference phenomena, the physician must recognize that current feelings or conflicts may be displaced onto him. The child may show anxiety, reflecting the parents' irrational fears about his condition; or a wife may show mistrust derived from her feelings about a husband with whom she is having serious marital conflict.

The Diagnostic-Evaluative-Treatment Process

As indicated in Chapter 9, diagnosis and treatment, though usually considered separate processes, actually cannot be easily separated, particularly in regard to the psychosocial aspects of the child's or adolescent's problem as it relates to his family. Change and improvement can occur during the process of diagnosis and evaluation. The step toward requesting help for any problem, particularly a problem that has significant psychosocial aspects, is most important. Indeed, as Senn[50] has emphasized, the approach to management of psychosocial problems may be said to be set in motion even before the family is seen, during the period when the decision to call or visit the doctor is made by the parents. If the parents perceive the need and can bring themselves to ask for help for a child who has a school problem, the effectiveness of the evaluation-treatment approach will be enhanced considerably. This is in contrast to the situation in which the parents, out of guilt or apprehension, need to deny the implications of the problem, and must be urged or otherwise motivated to seek help. As Finzer[18] has indicated, during an evaluation interview with father, mother, and son about a school problem, a father may be surprised to learn that quarrels between him and his wife have upset his son considerably and have interfered with his son's school work. The fath-

er's recognition of the situation and his subsequent attempts to change his interactions with his wife can bring therapeutic change in the evaluation phase.

Setting the Stage

In considering the approach to the "helping process," it is useful to regard the initial interviews as exercises in communication between the parents and the physician and between the child and the physician. The process of encouraging positive and mutual communication begins with the secretary or nurse who handles the first request for an appointment. A warm and friendly response tends to make the parents feel that help will be forthcoming, even if it will be some time before the doctor can see them. A cold response or an implication that the doctor is very busy, even though an appointment is made, can make the parent feel "one down" even before the doctor-patient relationship has started.

In the first contact, the physician's manner and manifest attitudes as a person as well as a physician are of fundamental importance. A study by Korsch and her colleagues[33] showed that parents who perceived the pediatrician as friendly, concerned, and sympathetic were significantly more satisfied after the visit than were the parents who perceived the physician as "businesslike." Other positive factors include such things as a pleasant waiting room and an appointment system which makes only a relatively short wait necessary. (Some loyal parents wait patiently for long periods of time; anxious, tense, angry, or guilty parents do not wait comfortably; and parents from minority groups may misinterpret long waits as evidence of discrimination.)

The interview should be conducted in quiet surroundings, and it should be as free as possible from interruptions or other pressures on the physician. Most patients do not like to be seated across a desk from the physician; a desk so placed is a barrier, and it makes the physician seem more distant. Putting the chair or chairs at the corner of the desk, diagonally facing the physician, eliminates the barrier, and makes the patient feel closer to the physician and more important to him.

As numerous studies attest, the use of medical jargon by the physician is all too often a barrier to communication. Such terms as sphincter, edema, peristalsis, or work-up come easily to the physician; a few parents or patients may be impressed by the physician's erudition, but most feel confused, put off, or put down. And terms such as appendectomy that are understandable to parents may be incomprehensible or frightening to children.

Communication is only rarely completely "logical." The feelings of the parent and the nonverbal communication of the physician who (for example) glances impatiently at his watch may interfere significantly with the logical interchange of ideas. A perfunctory, impersonal "checklist" approach bespeaks disinterest, while an overly vigorous "checking-up" approach may seem like an interrogation to the parent or patient.

As Korsch's study also emphasized, parent or patient satisfaction is more related to effective communication than to the length of time in the interview. Five or 10 minutes can be as effective and satisfying as 45 minutes, whether the complaint is serious or minor. This finding was supported in the study by Finklestein and Walker[17] of the effectiveness of the communication to the parents concerning a diagnosis of congenital heart disease, referred to in Chapter 7.

Gaps in Communication

The expectations of the doctor and of the parents in their first contact are identical: the diagnosis and treatment of the child patient. At a minimum, the parents expect a competent evaluation of the child's problem and adequate communication to them of its cause, treatment, and prognosis. As mentioned earlier, parents also expect the doctor to be friendly, concerned, and sympathetic. The physician for his part expects the parents to fully communicate their concerns, to provide the details of the history of the child's condition, and to accept his diagnosis and cooperate with his recommendations. As discussed in Chapter 7, "roadblocks" or "filters" in the communication process may lead to unfulfilled expectations on both sides.

The Interviewing Process: Exploration and Evaluation

The best approach to interviewing from the evaluation (information-getting) point of view involves active listening by the interviewer (something more than "hearing"), warmth, acceptance, openmindedness, a willingness to understand (nonjudgmental), patience, freedom from distraction, concentration, and alertness to verbal or behavioral cues. Asking open-ended questions ("What is your main worry?", "What troubles you most?", or "What is really worrying you?") can assist in the active listening process and in the clarification of the parent's concern. Understanding or "accepting" responses, with a sympathetic rejoinder—"Yes, I see," "That must be difficult," "You're concerned about what might happen,"—or supplying a word during an emotional block can offer the parent positive reinforcement that will encourage revelation of concerns or feelings more effectively than will evaluative responses or probing. Hostile responses on the interviewer's part may occur; these are always occasions for self-examination since they indicate that countertransference feelings, misunderstanding, overidentification with the child, or other problems are arising.

As Garrett[23] has suggested, the interviewer must look for clues which may indicate basic underlying problems. He makes hypotheses and tests them out by further questions in that area, although he does not usually reveal the hypotheses or his interpretations to the patient or parent. Questions such as, "What was going on about the time Johnny got sick," and "You must have had some feelings about the way the teacher handled the situation" may lead to important revelations, perhaps a family problem related to the child's illness or about a battle between parent and teacher over a child's behavior in school.

In Levy's[37] Attitude Study Project, certain key questions were developed in order to put the parent at ease and draw her out. "Tell me about it," "Tell me more about it," or "How do you feel about it" can encourage a mother to talk about highly charged topics freely and in a relaxed way. In a series of "quickies and openers" the question "Do you get any help in the care of the children?" yields a surprisingly emotional and revealing response from many mothers. "Who's the chief critic in your family?" or "How do you manage?" are also markedly effective in revealing family dynamics. In asking about sibling rivalry, the question, "How did he take the baby's coming?" is much more productive than "Did he show any jealousy?" which leads most parents to deny any such behavior. "When did he discover that part of his anatomy?" was found to be much more effective in bringing out data and feelings about masturbation than "Does he masturbate?" The physician should ask questions which avoid putting answers into the parent's mouth: "What about play?", "How about school?", "What does his father like to do with him?" are significant examples. (Similar principles of interviewing are discussed in "Health Supervision of Young Children," a monograph prepared by the American Public Health Association[25a].)

The physician can use "generalized" responses to help parents deal with their self-blame or other feelings.* The comments "It's pretty hard for parents not to be afraid they haven't done everything possible to prevent their child from getting sick" and "Most parents tend to blame themselves for having done something or not having done everything when their child gets sick" usually result in self-revelation, whereas "Did you blame yourself?" is usually answered by a socially acceptable "No."

A technique developed by Rogers[46] is readily adaptable to pediatric interviewing. Reflecting feelings by repeating emotion-laden words or phrases, often with some clarification, is most effective in helping parents explore further their feelings or conflicts. "You feel that you can't get through to your daughter?" can open up an important block to understanding of a child by a parent. Selecting the emotionally charged word in a sentence and repeating it is effective; (e.g., "angry?", "confused?"). Levy's technique of "restatement" is similar: "Your husband's ideas of discipline seem crude to you" can help open up an area of conflict between wife and husband. "You don't see eye-to-eye about handling him" can help open up a marital problem involving a battle between the parents about the handling of the child.

In his Attitude Study Project Levy also offers techniques designed to assess the parent's capacities and needs. "What do you think?" "What would you like to do?" "How do you explain that?" "Why do you think he does it?" All these questions may elicit valuable information about the parent's beliefs, degree of understanding, emotional strengths, and openness to help. "What are your thoughts about feeding the baby?" can be of predictive value regarding the mother's attitude to breast or bottle feeding. "How do you feel about toilet training?" can offer valuable information about the parent's needs and attitudes that will influence the use of anticipatory guidance and pediatric counseling.

*This represents "incision and drainage of guilt," referred to earlier.

Pacing the Interview

As Levy points out, in the process of learning how to let "the mother talk," inexperienced interviewers may become concerned that once the "floodgates" are open, the interview will get out of hand. If a parent wanders too far from the central topic, the interviewer can interrupt and set the interview back on the track. He can pick up a key phrase, ("You were saying that your son. . . " or "I'm getting a little lost; let's go back to. . . ") and guide the interview to where he feels it will be most profitable. If the parent is still talking vigorously when it is time to terminate the interview, the physician can say something like, "I'm sorry, but it's time for us to stop today; we'll continue next time" or "Let's make another appointment so that we can talk more about these things." Occasionally a parent or an adolescent patient will pour out so much self-revelatory material that, he or she may be reluctant to return to talk further, fearing that the interviewer cannot possibly see him as a "good" or adequate parent or person. If the interviewer senses that this is occurring, he can intervene by saying, "I'm very much interested in your feelings, and we'll talk more about them. I'd like now to go back to. . . " and return to a more factual or less emotionally charged point.

If the parent or parents make partial, irrelevant, or inaccurate responses, the interviewer can say, "I'm sorry, but I don't quite understand" or, "I don't quite see the connection between what you're saying and what we were talking about." This may help the parent to elaborate on a partial or inaccurate response, to explain what is only apparently an irrelevant response, or to return to the flow of the interview. Nonresponses or silence generally reflect a feeling of dissatisfaction or of being misunderstood. The interviewer can say something like, "I have a feeling that we're not communicating" or "It seems to be hard for you to talk about this," which generally will elicit a response with which he can deal.

In all approaches, the interviewer's tone and manner are vitally important. As indicated earlier, interest, acceptance, and a non-critical attitude on the part of the interviewer are far more important than any specific technique he may use.

The Interviewing Process: Interpretation

Once evaluation is completed, interpreting the findings for the parents and the child is vitally important if the treatment phase is to proceed effectively. (Some general principles involved in the implementation of the results of the clinical evaluation were discussed in Chapter 10.) In a broader sense, all parents require a full explanation of the cause of their child's illness and relief of any feelings of self-blame they may have. Balint[7] has called attention to the needs of parents for a "name" for their child's illness, however vague the name may be. All parents also need some discussion of appropriate treatment measures and of prognosis although a discussion may be difficult if no active treatment can be undertaken or if it is impossible to give the prognosis. A specific prognosis should *never* be given (e.g., "6 months to live" or "this will take 3 months to clear up") since if the physician is wrong, the parents may be very resentful, and no physician can be that accurate. If he has doubts, he should admit honestly his inability to predict and should help the parents to live with ambiguity.

The importance of phrasing explanations in everyday language has been emphasized, as has giving the parents the opportunity to ask questions once an explanation is given. If no questions are forthcoming, the physician can say, "You probably have some questions" which both implies the existence of questions and gives the parents permission to ask them. It has been demonstrated that the more completely the parents or patient understands the medical situation, the more likely it is that the follow-through will be successful, especially if the relationship with the physician is positive and continuing.

The Interviewing Process: Treatment

As mentioned earlier, evaluation, interpretation, and treatment overlap, and some therapeutic benefit may well come from the evaluation approach. An example is the development of a feeling of emotional support on the part of the parent or patient as the result of his perception that the interviewer is interested in and cares about what has happened or is happening to him. Also, considerable ventilation of feelings as well as constructive clarification of the medical situation or of the patient's main worry may have taken place during the evaluation interview.

Supportive Psychotherapy

The supportive psychotherapeutic approach that can be usefully employed by the pediatrician can be contrasted with the intensive psychotherapeutic approach of the mental health professional in terms of an analogy between supportive medical treatment and the operative interference of the surgeon.

The supportive psychotherapeutic approach has as its goals:

1. Helping the parent, patient, or family to regain an adaptive equilibrium and previous level of functioning, if mild decompensation has occurred in the face of stressful events.
2. Helping the parent, patient, or family to maintain an adaptive equilibrium, when this is fragile or shaky.
3. Helping the parent, patient, or family to move toward a healthier adaptive equilibrium, when this is possible without requiring sweeping personality changes.
4. Helping the parent, patient, or family resolve a crisis situation.

Some overlapping of course exists between the supportive approach and the intensive psychotherapeutic approaches. In general, however, the more intensive approach involves active, probing, interpretative, and other insight-promoting techniques, with the goal being the uncovering of unconscious conflicts that must be dealt with in order to achieve a significant change in personality or family functioning. (Vigorous probing and deep interpretations can cause much anxiety or other harmful responses if used unwisely. Interpretations are two-edged weapons, like ACTH, and are used sparingly by the most skillful psychotherapists.) The goals of supportive psychotherapy are generally relieving symptoms, mobilizing strengths, and dealing with conscious and usually current conflicts.

The techniques recommended for the nonpsychiatric physician in the approach to supportive psychotherapy have generally been those crystallized long ago by Levine[35] for work with adults and by Levy[36] for children and parents. They have also been discussed by Bruch[11] in relation to brief psychotherapy in a pediatric clinic and more recently by Coddington[14] in relation to pediatric practice. Discussions of supportive therapy by psychologically sophisticated pediatricians for adolescents have been offered by Gallagher,[20] Wessel,[57] and, more recently, Fine.[16] A cluster of these techniques, which really belong under the category of *counseling*, a type of supportive psychotherapy, include guidance and advice, persuasion, reassurance, ventilation of feelings, confession, sympathy and encouragement, and suggestion, all of which should be offered in a generally accepting, noncritical, empathetic, and supportive context.

All the techniques just listed are important and can be helpful. However, as Senn[50] pointed out, in his classic paper "The Psychotherapeutic Role of the Pediatrician," it is neither necessary nor desirable in every case to do more than offer the patient an opportunity to establish a relationship; whatever is of therapeutic value will often flow out of such a positive relationship developed at the outset. Indeed, without such a relationship ("therapeutic alliance")[29] that involves empathy and acceptance of the patient's feelings by the physician and trust and expectation of help on the part of the patient, no techniques will be effective.

The concept of psychotherapy as a process based on a relationship (as described by Senn for the pediatrician) originated in earlier developments, particularly in psychoanalytic psychology, and it has been adapted to other types of psychotherapy. In discussing this topic, a discussion of the psychotherapeutic process in terms of phases may be helpful. The following list is adapted from some ideas of Gardner,[21] with some influence from Rogers.[46]

1. *Establishment of a relationship.* With patients or parents who have milder problems and considerable strengths, the establishment of a relationship itself may result in the ability to cope with problems, the amelioration of symptoms, the alleviation of discomfort, or the reestablishment of a personal or an interpersonal adaptive equilibrium.

2. *Exploration.* Exploration in the direction of clarifying anxieties and fears, or in areas of largely conscious individual emotional conflicts or interpersonal conflict, can lead toward the identification of the focal problem or problem area.

3. *Confrontation.* Confronting the patient or parent with recurrent themes of thought and feeling or nonverbal behavior relating to the focal problem may involve such approaches as pointing out particular behavior or highlighting inconsistencies in thought or feeling.

4. *Interpretation.* Interpretation of the sources of anxieties, conflicts, and defenses, which are often related to experiences in early childhood or other experiences and to current precipitating events, involves helping the patient or his parents achieve insight into the causes of his problems and into methods of dealing with them adaptively.

5. *Integration.* Integration or working through (over) all the foregoing, until the insights achieved can be applied to current situations in such a way as to permit the individual to cope with stresses, resolve problems, or change un-

healthy reactions or behavior in the direction of a balanced adaptive equilibrium.

From this model, it can readily be seen that a positive answer can be given to Seitz's[49] question ("Can the general practitioner do psychotherapy?") and that the pediatrician or family physician can learn with training to offer supportive psychotherapy by working within the first 3 phases of the total psychotherapeutic process, largely employing the mutual participation model. (Nurses and health associates can also learn this approach with training).

As indicated earlier, the establishment of a positive relationship and the emotional support thereby provided may in itself suffice to help the parent or patient suffering from a mild disorder regain an adaptive equilibrium, with a return of coping capacities and the alleviation of distress or symptoms. This process, which has been termed "relationship therapy," may involve some discussion of the child's problems with the parent and may result in some ventilation of feelings and the development of spontaneous insights at the conscious level.

With preschool-age and younger school-age children, improvement may occur with very little verbal interchange between the child and the physician.[62] The child's play may express nonverbally themes that are symbolic of problems[51,61] and may involve considerable release[36] of feelings in the process. Within the framework of an accepting, supportive relationship with an empathic adult, the expressive use of toys can help the child move toward self-realization, mastery, and maturity, as Allen[1] has demonstrated and Axline[6] has confirmed more recently in her nondirective approach to play therapy. Although a rather permissive approach supports free play, appropriate limits must be set,[28] as indicated in Chapter 8. (In general, it is best not to take notes during therapy with children and adolescents.)

Exploration of anxieties, fears, and conflicts, leading to identification of focal problem areas, may be necessary in more complicated situations. With parents and older children and adolescents, this process involves more initial activity on the physician's part, using some of the interviewing techniques of drawing-out and clarification discussed earlier in this chapter and elsewhere. Verbal interchange is more actively involved with children, although methods of exploration through play are important for most older children and some younger adolescents.[8,15] Considerable ventilation of feelings, sometimes amounting to a revelation of disturbing feelings about particular events or situations, may take place in this phase. The development of spontaneous insights by the child or his parents and improvement without full identification of problem areas may occur in this phase at times.

Confrontation of recurrent emotional themes or nonverbal behavior, identification of behavioral inconsistencies, and problem areas may be direct or tentative, as the situation demands, but the confrontation should be *gentle* and nonthreatening. During this phase, while avoiding deep probing or interpretation of the parents' or patient's unconscious thoughts or emotional conflicts,[62] the physician may be able to verbalize certain feelings or thoughts for them, such as guilt or anger, that are obviously near to consciousness. This approach may touch off spontaneous insights which can illuminate the connections between events and feelings. The parents may be able to perceive the child's feelings and behavior more clearly and to become aware of the problems raised by their attitudes toward him or their handling of him. The older child or adolescent may be helped to understand his misconceptions about his parents' feelings or the contributions of his own behavior to the problem. Both parents and child may see more clearly how the problem began, and they may begin to talk together, in or out of treatment, about how it can be resolved.

This approach to supportive psycho-therapy, which largely involves the model of mutual participation in the treatment situation, is not inconsistent with elements of the other 2 models at certain points. Obviously, the physician must be more active in the phases of exploration and confrontation (if these phases are necessary), and he may offer guidance, advice, reassurance, or information at appropriate times. Of course confrontation may involve elements of implied interpretation; and some superficial interpretations, best offered in the form of questions, may indeed be appropriate at times. Also, the physician may have to help the parents integrate or work through feelings or conflicts already recognized, particularly those related to a serious illness in their child.

If the parent seems to be working out a solution to a problem or, when questioned, makes an intuitively constructive response to a situation, the physician can use positive reinforcement, involving encouragement and praise. For certain parents or children, he may need to use suggestion, persuasion, reeducation, or other methods of supporting constructive actions, without undue pressure. (The judicious use of elements of behavior therapy has been discussed in Chapter 11.)

After 1 or 2 long interviews initially, 20-to-30-minute interviews with parents and child, individually or together, will usually suffice for the supportive psychotherapeutic approach described. Longer interviews may be needed occasionally in a crisis situation. Physicians should not be reluctant to make a reasonable charge for their time. If the fee is discussed in advance, most parents are glad to pay for their help. Setting aside a special afternoon or evening for more complicated situations usually permits the physician to integrate them into his busy schedule.

The Interviewing Process: Termination

In a supportive psychotherapeutic approach of the type described, the goals of treatment are limited to those discussed earlier. With preschool-age children who have mild reactive disorders, several interviews will often suffice to help the parents achieve more consistent discipline, recognize and handle sibling rivalry, or deal with a feeding, sleeping, or toilet-training problem. A school phobia in a 6- or 7-year-old child, involving a developmental crisis, may respond to "first aid" measures offered in a few interviews, coupled with appropriate contacts with the school. School-age children with more chronic problems, such as enuresis, may have to be followed for some months. In the case of mild adolescent developmental or situational crises, a few interviews suffice to deal with the immediate problem.

In all cases, the door should be left open for return visits, and, in many instances, a follow-up appointment should be scheduled after the immediate problem has been resolved. Follow-up care is especially important for adolescents, who may have a continuing need for "someone to talk to" but may have difficulty verbalizing such a need. It is important (and not always easy), especially with adolescents, to be able to "let go" when appropriate, even though not every problem may be completely resolved. As Allen[1] has pointed out, the physician should watch for signs of a pushing for independence on the part of parents as well as in adolescents and older children, and he should give them a choice about "tapering off." Of course, in a supportive approach, in some cases the physician may have to settle for intermittent contacts over months or even years.

Case Examples of Supportive Psychotherapy by Pediatricians

Case Example. (Improvement during the diagnostic-evaluation process). A 3-year-old girl was brought to the pediatrician by her mother. The girl's history indicated that for the past 2 months she had refused to talk or to play spontaneously, sitting quietly most of the time and occasionally whispering to herself. She also clung constantly to her mother. When her mother was asked about the events surrounding the onset of the child's behavior, she recalled that it coincided with the birth of her second child, a boy, although she had not previously made this connection herself (nor had her husband). The girl's birth and developmental histories indicated no problems, and the results of the physical examination were within normal limits. The physician was unable to talk directly with the girl. He suggested a return visit a few days later to explore the problem further.

On the second visit, in the presence of the mother (since the girl could not separate from her), the physician set up on a small table a play situation involving a girl doll and a baby doll. The girl simply sat quietly in front of the table until the physician asked in a whisper how the girl doll felt about having a baby brother. Without answering, the girl pushed the baby off the table and then laughed spontaneously. The mother, who seemed to understand the meaning of this behavior, held out her arms to the little girl, who rushed over to her, saying, "Mommy, Mommy!" The mother then said spontaneously that she realized she had been preoccupied with the new baby, who had been fussy and slept poorly at first (though less so lately). Her husband had been away on several business trips, and the mother had not really discussed the problem with him. She had not mentioned the baby's fussiness previously to the physician, feeling ashamed of it and hoping it would disappear.

The mother broke down and cried, saying the girl's problem was her fault. The physician let her cry and then said simply that such problems were not really anyone's fault. The mother said she would spend more time with the girl and would encourage her husband to do so also. The physician supported her determination; he suggested that a brief "time alone" daily with the girl was more important than the length of time involved. When the girl and her mother returned home, the girl talked freely with her mother. On a follow-up visit 2 weeks later, the mother said there had been no further problems.

Comment. In this case, the focal problem presented itself during the diagnostic-evaluative process, during the taking of the history and a brief diagnostic play interview with the little girl. The positive effects of expression of feelings in play were clearly evident. In the supportive context of the interview, the mother easily understood the situation without its being clarified, and she was able to ventilate her feelings of self-blame spontaneously. The physician was wise to let her cry, and, in effect, he gave her absolution from her guilt. He then positively reinforced her plan to deal with the focal problem, using a bit of explanation in the process. Obviously, this mother, although anxious about her handling of the new baby and experiencing a temporary loss of support from her husband, had considerable strength as a parent and a person. The parent's relationship with the girl had clearly been a positive one prior to the birth of the new baby, and the temporary absence of the father may have played a role in the girl's reactive process of withdrawal mixed with only mild depression.

Case Example. (Brief supportive psychotherapy with a preschool-age child). A 4-year-old boy, an only child, was referred to a physician because of "hyperactivity." His mother brought him to the physician's office; she said that the father would not come because he did not believe there was a problem. During the history, it became clear that the mother really meant that the child's behavior was aggressive rather than hyperactive although he had been an active child since birth. His aggressiveness involved provoking fights with other children in the nursery school he attended, and he refused to obey the teachers at times. At home, he exhibited only temper tantrums, and he suffered frequent nightmares. His mother said that his father had been very strict with the boy since he had begun to move around and explore things in his second year. She felt the boy was afraid of his father, who had spanked him when he showed oppositional or negativistic behavior. She said the boy always did what she asked, and she felt she had no problems with him. The boy's birth and developmental history were otherwise unremarkable, as were the results of the physical examination.

The physician scheduled a return interview to explore the problem further. In a play interview, after a brief conversation about school, (the boy said school was "nice"), the boy began to talk of monsters, who could hurt people, and at first he showed no provocative or aggressive behavior. He played with dart guns, first shooting at a target but gradually directing his shots toward the physician. When the physician said that shooting at people was against the rules in the office, the boy promptly returned to the target. The rest of the time he spent with a doll family, which comprised a mother and father who were always "arguing" and a boy who was afraid to go out of the house.

The physician felt that he needed more in-formation and, with the mother's permission, called the head of the nursery school. She told the physician that the boy had been somewhat aggressive toward other children and provocative toward the teachers when he entered the school in the fall. Firm limits were set on his aggression and his provocative behavior was purposely ignored. These techniques helped the child control his behavior although he was occasionally somewhat demanding and unaccountably fearful. The head of the nursery school had told the boy's mother of his aggressive behavior in the fall and had suggested that the mother talk with their physician. But the mother had come to the scheduled spring conference without having done so.

The physician was puzzled, and he told the mother that he needed to talk to the father in order to understand the situation more fully. Although the mother had predicted the father would not come in, the father readily agreed to do so when the physician called him. The father indicated that he had been quite strict with the boy in his early years, because he had felt the mother set no limits and that the boy needed some discipline. He said that in the last year he had yielded to the mother's pleas and had no longer been strict with the boy. He now felt that the mother let the boy do whatever he wanted and that his temper tantrums occurred when he occasionally intervened out of frustration at the boy's demands on the mother. He also said that he and his wife had had frequent arguments over the years.

When the physician saw the parents together, the physician commented that apparently the parents didn't see "eye-to-eye" about discipline. An argument ensued, with the mother's insisting she had to protect the boy from the father and the father insisting that he was no longer overly strict and that the mother let the boy have his will. Both parents had been ashamed to bring the boy in when the teacher suggested it. The mother had brought him in only after a particularly bitter argument with the father. The physician said that he felt the boy was confused by the parents' inability to agree on such matters but that the school report indicated he was not seriously disturbed and had responded to limits. The parents asked if they had "damaged" their child by their arguments, and the physician said that he did not regard such problems as anyone's fault. He said that in his interview with the boy, the boy seemed to be "inviting limits" by his testing-out behavior and really was afraid of losing control of his aggressive feelings. The physician suggested a brief series of play interviews with the child and tandem interviews with the parents in order to help everyone to understand and work together.

In a series of 5 half-hour bi-weekly interviews with the child, the boy again seemed to be inviting limits, at first principally in regard to the dart gun play. He quickly responded to the limits the physician set, and much of his play thereafter was with the doll family. The parent dolls still "argued" at first. The boy shot them both "dead" with the dart gun, although they were quickly resurrected and soon stopped arguing. The boy doll was no longer afraid to go out of the house, saying he knew "what to do" now. His parents indicated that his nightmares had ceased. He was reported to need less attention at school, to be less fearful, and to show more positive behavior and an increased capacity for cooperative play.

During the same period, the physician saw the parents separately from the child for 5 half-hour interviews. The physician confined his nonjudgmental approach largely to asking "drawing-out" questions, with some reflection of feelings and clarification of conflicts or misunderstandings between the parents. After several visits, the mother spontaneously revealed that her fear of masculine aggressive behavior in general had led her to be afraid to provoke her own boy with discipline and controls, and she saw a connection between her fears and her response in childhood and adolescence to an extremely stern father. She also acknowledged she had failed to see the change in her husband's behavior. During the same time, father came to realize that he had been overly strict at first because he felt that his own father had been too lenient with him. He also came to feel he had been wrong in generally withdrawing and letting the mother handle the discipline herself. Both parents talked about their inconclusive arguments, and they were able to see spontaneously how their son must have been troubled and confused over "what to do." At this point, the physician suggested that, since they now understood the sources of their differences and could see the boy needed and even wanted limits, the parents work together to find limits they could agree upon. He helped them to begin this, and their arguments at home ceased. They returned once several months later to discuss some minor points. Two years later, having moved to another city, the parents wrote to the physician, saying gratefully that the boy was well adjusted and doing well in school, and that they were much happier in their marriage.

Comment. In this instance, the presenting problem did not turn out to be the focal prob-

lem. The boy's hyperactivity turned out to be aggressive behavior, but even that problem existed more in the eyes of the beholder—the mother—than in fact. When the physician invited the father to come in, he realized that the focal problem was an interpersonal one—the inability of the parents to agree on limits on behavior for their boy.

In this case, the physician had to use an active approach, calling the father,* in order to build a relationship with all 3 members of the family. Also, it was necessary for the physician to use confrontation with the parents regarding their differences and the child's confusion (and to minimize self-blame in the process) before clarification could take place. (Such a variation in the usual stages is occasionally necessary.) The physician offered a diagnostic formulation of the focal problem, with some explanation of the child's behavior, and he set up a brief supportive psychotherapeutic approach for the parents and the child. With his help, the parents were able to clarify their misunderstandings and disagreements, which stemmed in part from their own past experiences, and to achieve spontaneous insights that made change possible. The child mainly used expression of feeling, without interpretation, to achieve exploration and clarification in his play, and he benefited from his parents' progress. The physician wisely set limits in the therapeutic process, a necessary procedure in a number of cases.[55]

Case Example. (Longer-term supportive psychotherapy with a school-age child). A 9-year-old boy was referred to a pediatrician who had a special interest in psychosocial problems. The boy had repeated asthmatic attacks, which had begun about 2 years before. The attacks were mild at first and occurred about once a month. Gradually they had become more severe though the frequency remained the same. The boy had been treated by a family practitioner, who had tried the usual medical approach without much benefit and who had referred the boy to an allergist for desensitization, again without significant benefit over a year and a half. Within the past year, the attacks had been severe enough to require that the boy be hospitalized 10 times. Each time, an extremely rapid remission had occurred, before any special change in the medical regimen could be effected. The fam-

---

*As mentioned in the initial interview the mother indicated that her husband would refuse to come to an interview, although he readily agreed to come in when the physician called him. This is frequently the case. Also, in middle-class families, the mother is likely to be the parent who takes the child to the doctor, but in some ethnic groups taking the child to the doctor is seen to be the father's responsibility.

ily practitioner suspected that the boy's asthma had a psychologic component, and so he referred the child to the pediatrician.

During the history, which was given by both parents, the pediatrician asked what had been going on in the family when the boy's asthma began. The mother recalled that she had been quite ill at that time, with influenza complicated by pneumonia and had been hospitalized for more than 2 weeks. The parents did not know what underlay the monthly occurrence of the boy's asthmatic attacks. They had become aware, however, that most attacks began with mild wheezing and that the boy then became quite frightened and his fear seemed to intensify the attacks.

The boy's birth and developmental history were normal, except that the parents remarked that the boy was "almost too good" and was rather dependent on them, especially on the mother. At school, the boy got top grades, but he had no real friends. The physical examination revealed that he had only mild pulmonary wheezing at the moment. He seemed quite concerned about his bodily functioning, particularly that of his lungs, and he asked the pediatrician rather sophisticated questions.

The family survey indicated that a grandparent and a sibling on the mother's side had asthma. The parents had a younger daughter, aged 8. The family was quite close and was extremely interested in music. The father, who was in his 40s, was a successful professional man. He played the piano. The mother, who was also in her 40s, worked part-time. She played the viola. The boy played the flute, and the sister played the violin. Both children were remarkably talented musically, as were the parents, and the family's favorite activity was playing together. The parents had extremely high expectations of the children, particularly in regard to music, and the children spent many hours practicing. They had very little time for or interest in social activities with their peers.

In an interview with the child alone, the boy sat and talked like a small adult. He ignored the puppets[9] and the other play materials. He gave only brief replies to questions, and the replies were revealing only in that they confirmed his social isolation. He liked school, but his only real interest was practicing the flute and playing quartets with the family. He wanted to be a professional flutist, probably a soloist, when he grew up. He was not sure he wanted to be married or have children. He gave 3 wishes: (1) to be a good boy, (2) not to want sundaes—the sugar was bad for his teeth, and (3) to be a famous flutist when he grew up because his

parents wanted him to. He did not respond to a suggestion that he make up a story,[22] and he said he would not draw a picture because he was not talented in drawing and it would not be perfect. His only mention of his asthma was in reply to a question. He said it worried him because it interfered with his flute playing and schoolwork. The physician agreed that that was a problem.

The pediatrician talked with the parents and said that he agreed that the boy's fear was involved in the asthma, and that emotional tension could aggravate the asthma. He dealt reassuringly with the mother's expressed guilt about the tendency toward asthma that was present in her side of the family. He said he thought the sources of the boy's fear were in the back of his mind, where he could not get at them, despite his obvious high intelligence, and that a combination of talks and play therapy, probably for several months, could be of help. He also said that he would need their help regularly in thinking out loud about ways to help the boy help himself. He later told the boy that there was a way to help with his worries over the asthma, and that it involved regular talks and some play. He told the boy that his parents would meet with him, the pediatrician, to try to help too but that the details of the things he and the boy talked about would be between themselves.

The pediatrician arranged for half-hour weekly sessions with the boy on an afternoon set aside for this purpose. He saw the parents separately for a half hour every 2 weeks, spending 5 minutes or so after the boy's interview with the parent who brought the boy (usually the mother) to learn of current developments. For 2 months, the boy remained the little adult of the first session. He talked only in response to questions and then briefly, with little self-revelation and continued denial of the degree and intensity of his fear. He seemed to like coming, however, and he began to thank the pediatrician at the end of each session. He admitted on one occasion that he loved sundaes, but that he had no hope of getting one because of his parents' beliefs. Immediately after the diagnostic evaluation the pediatrician changed the boy's medication slightly, and his monthly attacks became a little less severe, requiring brief hospitalization for only one out of 2 attacks.

During this period of slowly building a relationship with the boy, the pediatrician, receiving a growing trust from the parents, was able to explore much more actively with them than with the boy. He learned that the boy had been extremely fearful that his mother would die when she was hospitalized 2 years before and that his attacks began while she was in the hospital. It became clear that the boy had been very dependent on his mother since his sister's birth (when he was a little over a year old). He had clung so closely to her then that he interfered with her care of the baby, making her both sorry for him and somewhat angry at him. Although he had come to be able to function independently as he developed, he still was markedly attached to his mother.

As the talks continued, it was noted that his asthma attacks seemed to correlate with his mother's menstrual periods, at which times she regularly developed severe, sometimes migrainous headaches, and she usually took to her bed for a few hours or even a day. At these times, the boy would seem to fear that his mother would die, and he would again cling to her. He would begin to wheeze and then, expressing fears of his own death, would have a full-blown asthmatic attack. The parents had been concerned about his dependent tendencies in infancy; they were concerned again at these monthly intervals that the boy would return to his clinging and fail to return to his high level of educational and musical attainment. After each such episode, the parents would urge the boy to get back to school and to his music practice as soon as possible.

During the third month, the boy noticed a small rubber ball on the toy shelf in the pediatrician's office. He bounced it idly and somewhat awkwardly; he soon missed catching it, and it rolled toward the pediatrician's chair. The pediatrician picked up the ball and tossed it back to the boy, who caught it and returned the toss. Thus began a regular game of catch, which took up each session and became more and more vigorous as the boy tossed the ball harder and harder, sometimes saying, "Take that, you old devil." While throwing the ball, he began to talk a little more spontaneously, about his subjects at school, and he once mentioned that he had had a dream about his almost falling over a precipice, but being saved. He could not elaborate or make any association to the dream,[39] saying only, "I forget." The pediatrician offered the thought that the boy had a pretty good "forgetter," but the boy only smiled in response. He told the pediatrician that his birthday was to come the next month, and when the pediatrician said he would like to give him a present,[34] (he had told the parents that this was his practice), the boy said he would like a sundae.[25] The pediatrician said he would have to talk that over with his parents. During this month, the boy's asthmatic attack was much milder.

When the pediatrician next talked with the parents, he told them of the boy's request. During this month, they had begun to become aware both of their own fears of the boy's dependency and of their high expectations of him. (The pediatrician had helped stimulate this spontaneous insight when the mother complained of the boy's fears about her death and his. The father then said that the mother was afraid the boy would die in an asthmatic attack, and even he had also been afraid at times. The pediatrician then used a mild confrontation, saying it seemed a little inconsistent that the parents felt the boy's fears were unreasonable and yet could experience fear themselves. He also said that although the boy's fears were somewhat excessive, all children and even adults have fears.) The parents responded by recognizing that they had expected a lot of the boy in regard to his performance as well as fears. Thus when he mentioned the boy's birthday request, the parents were ready to agree with him that a sundae on a special occasion was a reasonable request from a child and that a little sugar occasionally would probably not damage the boy's teeth.

This episode appeared to be a turning point. The boy began to throw the ball even harder, talked more freely about his heavy schedule of practice and schoolwork, and also asked his parents if he could go out for the baseball team. The parents said yes, and they continued to reexamine their high expectations, coming to feel that the boy was practicing too much to allow him enough social and other activity. The boy played baseball and began to engage in other age-appropriate activities. During the fourth and fifth months, the boy's asthmatic attacks stopped completely. The parents extended their reconsiderations to their daughter, who eagerly moved out socially. After a mutually arranged tapering off of appointments during the sixth month, the parents and the child felt ready to terminate their visits. They continued their muscial activities but on a much more relaxed and limited basis, and the parents went out more socially. A year later, the boy was still free of asthma, and he and the family had continued their freer though still constructive adaptive balance.

Comment. In this case, the therapy moved more classically through the stages of the supportive therapeutic process. The process took longer (about 6 months, with the interviews diminishing in frequency during the last month) because the boy's personality tendencies and the family's life-style were much more longstanding than would have been the case with a preschool-age child. The focal problem, which related to the imbalance between the boy's un-satisfied dependency needs and the parents' high expectations, thus took longer to work through toward parental understanding and the development of true independence on the boy's part.

The boy's anger toward his parents, which probably intensified, through guilt, his fears of his mother's and his own death, was never ver-balized directly. However, the intensity of the ball-throwing activity, which involved some displacement, certainly resulted in a great ven-tilation of feeling, and the boy did talk some-what complainingly about his heavy schedule. The single dream related to the boy's being saved from danger was not interpreted, but it probably indicated his unconscious awareness that the relationship with the physician was helping him. (The psychophysiologic relation-ships between asthma, which in this case was probably of milder nature, and the psychosocial factors involved are discussed more fully in Chapter 21.)

Finally, the boy and his parents certainly had more psychosocial strengths than many people, possibly because of their close family relation-ships, temperamental qualities, and other fac-tors.

Case Example. (Supportive psychotherapy with an adolescent). A 15-year-old girl was re-ferred by her father to a pediatrician because she had exhibited withdrawal and social isola-tion at home and at school for the past year and a half, with brief angry outbursts toward her parents at times and a gradual decline in her grades in school. Her mother had recently achieved success as a professional entertainer, and for the past 2 years she had been away on trips much of the time. Her father (who gave the history) was the owner of a small business, and he often worked until late at night. The girl's birth history and developmental survey gave little hint of abnormality although she was said to have been a stubborn child since in-fancy.[12] The results of the physical examination were within normal limits although the girl's pubertal development was a little delayed.

The father, a rather quiet man, was genuinely concerned about the girl, but he had delayed doing anything about her problems, because he and the girl's mother thought she would grow out of her social, emotional, and academic prob-lems. A week before, the girl had had a verbal outburst, during which she accused her parents of not caring for her. The outburst had led the father to bring the girl to the pediatrician. He talked on the telephone with the mother, who was away on a trip, and she agreed somewhat

reluctantly to the visit. The father, who was in his early 50s, was considerably older than the mother. He had 2 children by a previous mar-riage. They were married and lived at a consid-erable distance. Thus the 15-year-old daughter was the only child in the home.

In an interview, the girl was almost com-pletely silent. In response to a question, re-garding difficulties with her school work, she said only, "Yes," but would not elaborate or talk about any of her problems with her peers or her parents. The pediatrician said he realized she did not want to talk about her problems at this point but that she might like doing so later. He waited a short time, but, since no response was forthcoming, he began to ask her a few questions about her future aspirations. She an-swered only, "I don't know" to questions about career possibilities, and said, "No" to questions about her wishes for marriage and children. There was an angry tone to her voice and a somewhat depressed expression on her face, and the pediatrician could feel in himself an answering sense of anger and frustration. He was tempted to respond with silence, but he realized that the girl might misinterpret this as disinterest or hostility on his part, and he con-tinued to be reasonably active.

Resorting to a superficial interpretation, he offered the thought that the girl might feel an-gry about his asking questions. He received the monosyllabic reply, "No." The thought that she might wish that her father had not brought her in received the answer, "I don't care." At this point, the pediatrician, sensing that her replies to these interpretations indicated that she was not totally negative about seeing him, sug-gested that they make another appointment in which they could talk further about her "school problems," in order to find a way to secure some help. The girl replied, "If you want to," and left silently, with an appointment to return in 2 weeks. (The pediatrician felt that a 1-week return appointment might make her feel locked into a relationship with him which she was not ready to accept.)[63]

In a talk with the father, the pediatrician said that it had been difficult for the girl to talk al-though he had the intuitive feeling that she would not totally resist help. He said further that he did not know the reasons for her with-drawal, occasional angry outbursts, or academic difficulties, but that he suspected they had something to do with her feelings about herself in her adolescent phase of development.

Although in the early part of his interview with the girl, the pediatrician had considered suggesting it might be easier for her to talk with a woman, her responses to his interpretations and her acquiescence to a return appointment for further exploration made him feel that the girl could eventually develop a positive relationship with a man.[41] He therefore told the father that he would set up a series of interviews every 2 weeks and would try to help the girl to work out her problems. If he failed to be able to do so after a reasonable time, he would suggest referring her to a mental health professional. This seemed agreeable to the father, as did the suggestion that every 3 to 4 weeks he and the physician meet to keep up on developments in the girl's life and other matters.

The girl came a few minutes early for her next appointment. She was dropped off and later picked up by her father's sister, with whom she had a somewhat detached relationship. Her silent behavior continued throughout half-hour interviews, with the pediatrician continuing to ask questions and to offer occasional speculative interpretations. For example, when he had asked how things had been since their first contact, the girl had replied, "Oh," and shrugged. When later he offered the thought that she might be wishing to be somewhere else, she replied tonelessly, "Where?" The pediatrician was somewhat flustered at this response, because he knew she had withdrawn from friendships and activities. He said he meant she might not wish to be here, and might not like his asking questions. The girl simply shrugged her shoulders again. At the end of the interview, she said "So long" in a more pleasant tone than she had yet employed. However, the general pattern continued over the next four biweekly visits. At one point, the pediatrician told the girl that she did not have to come if she did not want to. She answered, "Oh, my father would make me come."

During this period the pediatrician had 2 interviews with the father. He learned that the father believed the girl's problems stemmed from her mother's frequent and long absences, because both phenomena had begun about the same time and because the girl seemed angry and had more frequent angry outbursts when her mother returned from a trip. These outbursts seemed related to the fact that the girl spent most of her time at home in her room, with the door closed, and the mother, feeling shut out, wanted her to keep her door open. The father admitted he felt the same way. Recently, he said the outbursts had centered around the controversial door, with the girl shouting at both parents, "You don't understand me"— and slamming the door. The father also expressed some guilt about his frequent

late working hours, and he realized that the girl was alone much of the time.

After the father's second visit, the mother called and asked to see the pediatrician. She said she had been talking with her husband about their daughter, and she expressed some guilt about the effect her many trips had on the girl. She expressed some blame toward the father, however, and said that his late working hours had helped her return to her previous career, with much greater success, in an attempt to find a meaningful life for herself.

Beginning with the fifth visit, the girl began to say, "Hello" in a pleasant tone when she arrived for the interview. Though still generally silent, she spontaneously mentioned in the sixth interview having had a test at school and said she did not like the teacher. In the eighth interview, she said that her parents wanted her to keep her door open and that she wanted to keep it closed. This had been her only mention of problems at home.

During this period, the pediatrician arranged to see both parents together. They indicated they had been talking together about their daughter for the past few weeks, the first time they had done so in the last year and a half. They said that at first each had blamed the other for neglect. Both could now see that each was partly responsible. The mother said the real problem was in their marriage, and the father agreed, saying they needed some help to make it work. The pediatrician supported this idea, but he said that kind of help was not within his competence. He added that he could refer them to a marriage counselor, an offer they accepted.

Both parents then asked if their preoccupations with their work had affected their daughter. The pediatrician asked what they thought, and they indicated they felt she had been affected, which made help for the marriage, with continuing help for their daughter, all the more urgent. They reported that while she had been seeing the pediatrician, she had become much less withdrawn from them and from her former friends, had had almost no verbal outbursts and was doing much better in school.

The pediatrician saw the girl 4 more times. Her silent behavior gradually lessened, and she seemed much happier. She told the pediatrician she was glad her parents were getting help, and she admitted that she had blamed herself for their problems, feeling she was not worth their spending time with her. She spoke of her previous behavior as her "bad side," and she said the "good side" was now back, making her feel worthwhile. She decided she did not need further help, and she said that her parents were already happier and spending more time at home.

Comment. In this case, the power of an accepting, nonjudgmental, and empathic relationship is clearly demonstrated, despite the special problem presented by the silent adolescent. The fact that the girl came each time and gave a few clues to her wish for help (e.g., resisting an opportunity to stop coming), indicated that a relationship was developing. The pediatrician's patience, self-control, and continuing interest in the girl were essential to the development of the relationship. Exploration produced only the symbolism of the door, but the girl was improving rapidly outside the interview setting (at first without the pediatrician's knowledge).

Despite the deterioration of their marriage, the parents possessed considerable strengths. Their reopening of communication and their spontaneous insights into the focal problem—the marriage—together with their developing awareness of their need for help, undoubtedly was also a factor in the girl's rapid improvement, as well as in her opening up in the office in the last phase of treatment.

Parent Therapy: Treatment of the Parent-Child Relationship

A number of terms have been used in discussing work with parents. Arnold[3] has recently defined the term parent guidance as "the offering to parents of information, clarification, advice, support, counsel, directives, supportive psychotherapy, or other interaction with a professional helper, with the intention of indirectly helping the child." The following discussion concentrates on the principles of supportive psychotherapy for parents, with "stages" similar to those with children. For convenience the generic term parent therapy is used although a number of the other techniques of guidance summarized by Arnold may be involved in the process.

In supportive psychotherapy with parents, the focus should be kept on the interaction between the parents and the child.[13,24,56] As demonstrated in several of the preceding cases, in which parent therapy as well as child therapy is demon-

strated, the physician may need to keep the focus entirely on the child initially, because many parents are not ready to look at their interactions with their children until later in the treatment process. The physician should go into the parent's own problems as little as possible. Exploration of the parents' past should be held to that needed to illuminate the parents' problems in handling the child if that can be done without much probing.

Asking the parent to talk a little about his own growing up may bring to light a problem the parent had at the same developmental stage, perhaps one from which he is trying to protect his child. A parent may reveal that her boy reminds him of her brother, who was always bossy or demanding. Certain parents may recognize that they identify the child with a parent who deserted them, or with their own "bad" side. Other types of parent-child interactions or family transactions, such as those in which the child is scapegoated or acts out the unconscious feelings of the parent generally involve more seriously disturbed families and require referral to a mental health professional or facility. The ubiquitous influence of self-blame or guilt is demonstrated in most of the preceding case examples.

In supportive therapy with parents, the rule is that the physician avoid deep interpretation and rely on the relationship, exploration with clarification, and confrontation. But the physician may combine gentle confrontation with superficial interpretation, usually offered as a question or speculatively. For example, a parent who reveals that he had a deprived childhood, might be told, "You seem to be determined that your girl's life will be different from yours, and so it's hard to tell her she can't have anything. Maybe that's connected with her tantrums, when you feel so helpless."

If parents from ethnic minority backgrounds seem mistrustful, the white middle-class physician is wise to acknowledge his awareness that they might have difficulty in trusting someone from his background. Bringing such a problem out in the open generally helps the parents or patient to feel more comfortable. (The successful treatment of persons in limited economic circumstances with the use of low fees or no fees has been discussed elsewhere, as has the possibility that middle-class therapists[43] might be biased about the treatment outcomes of these patients.)

One of the pitfalls in parent therapy of a supportive (or insight-promoting) nature is overidentification with the child. It is easy for the physician to feel anger at parents who do not seem to understand their child. The anger may be inevitable, but it must be kept under control. Another pitfall is taking at face value the picture one parent gives of the other parent. (The other parent is usually much different than described.) Seeing both parents together initially will avoid this pitfall. The physician should see each parent if at all possible, even if they are divorced and must be seen separately. Also, male physicians must avoid overidentification with the father-husband; the reverse caution is important for female physicians.

Occasionally, a parent's own problems may become so manifest during parent therapy (or even during the diagnostic-evaluative process) that the focus must be shifted from the parent-child interaction to the parent as a patient. Generally this shift calls for referral of the parent to a mental health professional or facility. Psychiatric consultation may be helpful in making such a decision, or the parent himself may recognize such a need. Also, a couple may be helped to see (or may themselves come to see) the need for referral for marital therapy or counseling. Regardless of the situation, if the physician continues supportive therapy with the child, he should either maintain direct contact with the parents, using a reporting type of relationship combined with more superficial counseling, or make sure, in contacts with the mental

health professional, that they combine such an approach with individual treatment, if they wish to do so.

In recent years, as described by Townsend,[54] a part-time social worker has been included in the group practices of some pediatricians. The social worker acts as a consultant or works therapeutically with parents in the various approaches just described. Other pediatric groups have included psychologists, social workers, and nurses with special training.[60]

With mildly disturbed preschool-age children, parent therapy alone, without direct therapy for the child, may be possible in some instances.[19] An approach of this kind has been carefully evaluated and successfully demonstrated by Heinecke.[26]

Case Example (Parent therapy with a preschool-age child). A 4-year-old Chicano girl was brought by her foster mother, (who also was Chicano) to an Anglo female pediatrician because the child had a 2-year history of "unmanageable" behavior. She made constant demands, had frequent tantrums, and made angry statements, such as "You don't love me!" The family, including 2 older children, had been treated for years in a neighborhood health center. However, the mother, whose husband had died of a "heart attack" $2^{1}/_{2}$ years before, felt that she was not getting enough help at the center with this child, and she had asked to be referred to a private "children's specialist." She could not pay the pediatrician's usual fee for an office visit, and so a lower fee was arranged.

On the first visit, the mother indicated that she had taken the girl as a foster child several months after her husband's death, feeling that she "had to do something." At first, the child had been responsive and generally obedient, but after several months, her tantrums, demands, and related behavior had begun. The foster mother knew little of the child's previous history, except that she was the child of a young Chicano couple who had been killed in an automobile accident. The couple had broken away from their own parents, who lived in another city and who did not want to take the child. Since the foster mother had handled successfully several foster babies in brief placement some years before, she was given the little girl when she applied to Social Services.

The results of the girl's physical examination were normal. In a brief play interview that involved doll play, the girl played the role of a mother; she disciplined a "bad girl" by slapping her repeatedly. The pediatrician suggested a return visit to allow further exploration of the child's problems.

The mother did not come to the return visit. After a few days, the pediatrician called her to arrange for another appointment and discovered that her telephone had been disconnected temporarily. The pediatrician made a home visit. She was received somewhat distantly by the foster mother. The pediatrician inquired about the child, and said she hoped to see her again. At first, the foster mother said that she had not been feeling well and that she had been unable to bring the girl in for the return appointment. After a time, the mother seemed to warm up to the pediatrician, and she talked more freely of some of her economic and other problems. The pediatrician then said she wondered if the foster mother might have some trouble trusting Anglos. The foster mother said that she did have trouble, but then, to the surprise of the pediatrician, she said that she also had problems relating to some of the Chicano staff at the neighborhood health center. When the pediatrician asked about it, the foster mother cried openly. The pediatrician let her cry for a few minutes, simply saying, "You are upset about something." The foster mother gained control of her feelings and then said, "You don't know what it's like not to belong to anybody."The pediatrician said she would like to know, and the foster mother then poured out her own story.

She herself had been a foster child. She had been placed at 3 years of age with an Anglo family, when her mother died and her father had disappeared. She said she had been treated as a black sheep in her foster family, and she had felt she was punished unfairly compared to the family's own children. She also said that she realized her background had something to do with her difficulties with her foster child. She was planning to remarry a Chicano man, who had said he would join her in adopting the child. However, she felt her problems with the child were coming between her remarriage, which she wanted, and the adoption, about which she had mixed feelings.

The pediatrician said she could understand that the foster mother felt torn in this situation, and she suggested that they continue talks for a while at her office. The foster mother readily agreed, and arrived early for the next appointment 5 days later. She seemed eager to talk but said she did not know where to start. The pediatrician reminded her that she had said she thought her own experience as a foster child

had something to do with her difficulties with the little girl. The foster mother seemed relieved, and she said that she recalled her own unhappy childhood so clearly that she found it hard to deny her foster child anything or to punish her. She said that if the girl were her own child, she would have slapped her or punished her in some other way, such as shaming her; her older children were well controlled.

The pediatrician said that she could understand her feelings but that perhaps she really wanted to punish the child sometimes, even though she could not bring herself to do so. The foster mother agreed but said that her angry feelings at such times made her feel that she would be letting the child down by punishing her. The pediatrician said that children need limits and even occasional punishment; and sometimes they invite the setting of limits by testing the parent (by misbehaving). She also said she did not feel that such an approach would be letting the child down, but she did not press the point.

At the next interview, a week later, the foster mother said she had been thinking about their last talk. She had come to feel that perhaps she was letting the little girl down by not setting limits or punishing her. The problem now was that she did not know what to do. If she gave in to her angry feelings, she might really hurt the child. Also, she said, she still felt guilty at times for even thinking of punishment. The little girl had been abandoned by her Chicano grandparents (as she herself felt she had been abandoned by her Chicano parents). She added that these experiences must have something to do with her difficulty in accepting help from the Chicano staff at the health center. With her mistrust of Anglos (related to her experience with her Anglo foster parents and later contacts with other Anglos) and her feelings that Chicanos would let you down (even her husband had died and left her) she did not feel fully comfortable with either ethnic group.

The pediatrician said, "I guess that's why you said you didn't belong to anybody." The foster mother agreed, and also said that if she did use punishment, she didn't know whether to use Chicano methods (e.g., a light slap or shaming) or Anglo methods (e.g. hard spanking). An appointment was made to talk further in a week.

During the next interview, the foster mother said that she had tried Chicano methods of disciplining the little girl and that she was surprised to see how positively the child responded. In the final interview, a week later, the foster mother indicated that she now "felt more like a Chicano" and that things were going very well with the child. She was proceeding with her plans to adopt the child and to marry the Chicano man. She said she felt she no longer needed special help and would return to the neighborhood health center for follow-up care. The door was left open for her to return to the pediatrician if she felt the need to do so.

Comment. The establishment of a relationship was complicated by a minority mother's mistrust of an Anglo. The pediatrician sensed the mistrust and realized that the broken appointment[2] was especially significant. Her reaching out with a home visit and her bringing up the subject of "ethnic" mistrust helped cement the relationship and allowed exploration to proceed. Exploration brought forth the focal problem—the foster mother's identification with the girl to the point that she was unable to set limits for or punish the girl.

The discipline problem was compounded by the fact that the foster mother was caught between 2 cultures. The pediatrician helped the foster mother face this conscious conflict with her gentle confrontation about a statement she had made—that she belonged to nobody. The confrontation combined with the pediatrician's acceptance and warmth (the fact that the pediatrician was a woman may have helped), seemed to help resolve the woman's identity conflict. In accepting her own ethnic identity, the foster mother, who must have had much emotional strength, could find culturally acceptable methods of disciplining the child, who desperately wanted disciplining.

Family Approaches

As I mentioned before, I believe that intensive family therapy requires training and experience beyond that of the family physician or health associate. However, some pediatricians who, like David Friedman, have special expertise in the psychosocial aspects of pediatrics, have described an approach involving psychotherapeutic consultation with families by social workers[5] operating in a pediatric setting. Friedman's approach involved a maximum of 3 interviews with each family following an evaluation and a "firm referral" by the pediatrician, with a follow-up interview 6 to 9 months later. The families studied each had a preschool-age child who had sleep and feeding disturbances, excessive crying, and gastrointestinal disturbances. The family interviews involved meeting with the child, both parents, and the therapist in a room in which the child was free to move around and to make use of various play materials. In the cases described, the room was the pediatrician's office, which emphasized the service as part of pediatric practice. The parents were encouraged to talk about family problems and their feelings about themselves and their child. The preschool-age children generally demonstrated their feelings through play with toys and interaction with the adults. The families selected for this approach were largely families that seemed to have considerable strength and families whose symptom-producing behavior did not seem rooted in profoundly unconscious conflicts.

The principles of supportive psychotherapy were drawn on: rapid development of a relationship with the child and his parents, considerable exploration, and gentle confrontation of actual behavior as seen in the family interview. The goals of this brief approach were to identify the focal problem quickly, and to help the families develop a conscious awareness of explicit behavior and insight into implicit conflicts and motivation. Although some superficial interpretations of the ramifications of actual behavior in symptom formation were employed, the goal was to help the families use this understanding, combined with spontaneous insights, and thus become able to control behavior and to learn more effective modes of interaction (integration of insights). In the interviews, the therapist sometimes gave examples of behavior that was more appropriate to the particular family.

In some instances, the child's symptom disappeared during the interviews and the children were still symptom free a year later. Most of the families responded positively and considered the interviews helpful. In a few families, conflicts were found to be deeper and the children much more severely disturbed than they had seemed earlier. These patients were referred to a child psychiatrist.

I believe that this approach can be used successfully by a physician, nurse, or health associate who is interested and can avail himself of the services of social workers or other mental health professionals trained to work with children and families along these lines. The pediatrician can sit in on interviews at first, operate as a co-leader later, and finally carry the treatment out on his own.

Group Discussions

In their private practice, a few pediatricians have used group discussions with parents of the type described by Wishik.[59] It is usually mothers who are involved although fathers occasionally participated. Wishik[58] and others[10] have described a similar approach to child health conferences. This approach has also been found helpful by Kirschner[30] in maternity programs; in dealing with the parents of ill and handicapped children by Korsch, Fraad and Barnett,[32] and others,[40,44] and with mothers of newborns on maternity services.[32] Parent Effectiveness Training, a specially structured approach, is also usually taught in groups.

Group discussions of these types are usually led by pediatricians, nurses, or (more recently) pediatric health associates. In a recent helpful review, Arnold and his colleagues,[4] have described group therapy and group guidance or discussion as being at opposite ends of a continuum, with some overlapping in the middle. (Group therapy was discussed in Chapter 11.) Discussion groups are often open ended, and involve short, inconsistent, or no commitment of time from the members. The format is well structured, and some content is offered initially by the leader. During the discussion, the leader provides information and advice and the participants exchange information advice with each other. Suppor-

tive and anxiety-reduction techniques are relied on, and the focus is generally on the child's behavior, with some consideration of the effectiveness of the parents' reaction to and interaction with the child.

As Arnold and his colleagues have pointed out, much empathic peer support is generated in such groups, which facilitates a healthy ventilation of feelings. Vicarious learning, mutual help, and mutual imitation and identification among the participants and with the leader are importantly involved, and contributing to the discussion fosters the development of self-esteem and adequacy, as well as hope and expectation. "Blessings by comparison" (i.e., learning that other parents have had similar problems) and "blessings by contrast" (i.e., learning that others have had more severe problems) are additional spin-offs from such discussions.

The leader must maintain some control over the discussion. If it drifts too much, he should bring it back to a focus related to its goals. The leader must occasionally intervene gently but firmly (a sense of humor often helps) if the discussion becomes too heated or if one member consistently attacks another. Occasionally a question raised by a group member is so intimate or self-revealing that the leader is wise not to pursue it in the group. Otherwise, the person involved may feel too uneasy to return to the group. Such a parent may need a personal interview and possibly referral for mental health consultation or treatment.

Discussion groups have been valuable in helping adolescents who have a chronic illness, handicap, or other problem. The formation of groups of people who have common disorders has been found helpful. Groups involving both parents and children have occasionally been successful, but they can easily become difficult to manage.

If the physician, nurse, or health associate has not had experience in leading group discussion, the addition of a co-leader, perhaps a social worker can be most helpful. In fact, the co-leader system has certain advantages, as when the leader cannot attend a session. Weekly group meetings lasting 60 to 90 minutes (occasionally longer) seem to be most effective.

Special Problems

The angry or "irate" parent presents a special challenge to the physician. Most pediatricians find it difficult to deal with this type of situation, and, as Schulman[48] has pointed out, tend to avoid such contacts whenever possible or to become upset, anxious, or angry if forced to face them. Schulman's suggestions for the "management of the irate parent" are pertinent and positive. As a first principle, he recommends carrying out the interview in a private office without the child present. If the parent resists a private interview and persists in talking in the presence of others, the pediatrician should firmly but kindly insist that the discussion take place in his office. If this invitation is ignored, he should issue a second invitation and walk toward his office as if expecting the parent to follow, (the parent usually does).

Once in a private spot, the physician should encourage the parent to talk, being careful not to take the outburst as a personal attack. Usually the anger is a result of the anxiety of the parents about the child's illness, of guilt projected onto the doctor or the hospital staff, or of poor or faulty communication. The physician must control his temper, even if he is slightly at fault, and he should avoid interrupting the parent's flow of feelings by defensive responses. Reflection of feelings and understanding responses, regardless of whether the physician agrees or disagrees with what is being said, will help the parents to talk out their anger. Even if the parents pause momentarily, the physician should invite further comments. When their anger is drained, he should indicate his honest concern about their problem and promise to look into the situation and to institute any

necessary or constructive changes. If he has made an error, as occasionally happens, he should acknowledge it and offer a plan for rectification. Usually this approach, plus arrangements for further communication, will be sufficient. Self-blame or other feelings on the parents' part that may emerge during the interview can be dealt with later.

In managing patients or parents with massive denial of the serious implications of a catastrophic illness, chronic handicap, or potentially fatal illness, the physician as a general principle should avoid tackling the denial in a frontal attack in order to help in "facing reality." This will only increase the denial. An "around end" approach that deals with self-blame or other feelings, using "incision and drainage of guilt" or some other supportive technique, combined with patience, is the approach of choice. The use of supportive psychotherapeutic principles will help many parents with mild-to-moderate overprotective, overcontrolling, rejecting or similar tendencies, but some parents may have to be referred for psychiatric consultation or for treatment by mental health professionals. Parents who are overly dependent on the physician can be encouraged to use a "telephone lifeline" to the physician or nurse.[52] Such freely available support, combined with praise for successes, usually leads to greater independence rather than dependence. If referral of the child or his parents to mental health resources seems indicated to the physician, but referral is refused, "incision and drainage of guilt" may be helpful. If not, a supportive approach, involving an accepting relationship and counseling, plus limited further exploration or confrontation, will often ultimately lead to acceptance of referral.

Crisis Intervention

Some psychiatric emergencies (e.g., incipient psychotic episodes, suicide attempts by seriously disturbed adolescents, homicidal, assaultive, or destructive behavior, certain psychotic-like responses to the abuse of drugs, and violent fights between parents and children) require the services of child psychiatrists or other child mental health professionals. However, as Mattsson and his colleagues[42] have shown, next to violent conflicts between parents and children, the most common factors precipitating an emergency are exacerbation of a chronic physical illness, a physical injury, and surgery. (Psychiatric emergencies, along with crisis theory and the approach to crisis intervention, were discussed in general in Chapter 11. Drug therapy, when a part of the treatment approach to crises or emergencies, is discussed in Chapter 13.)

Family crisis situations, which may be urgent but not emergencies, are often first encountered by physicians, nurses, and health associates. Consequently, they should be familiar with the principles of crisis intervention: the rapid identification and assessment of the focal problem in the crisis, the setting of reasonable but limited goals, the offering of brief interventions as appropriate and in a direct and authoritative (but not authoritarian) manner, the prompt referral of the person in crisis to the appropriate professional person or agency when more skilled mental health treatment is called for, and if intervention is undertaken, arranging for its termination and disposition. Crises may arise as a result of a family's disorganized, depressed, or otherwise disturbed response to the loss of the father's job, a death in the family, the unexpected birth of a premature or a defective infant, the diagnosis of a fatal illness in a child, or the sudden exacerbation of a chronic illness.

In managing crisis situations, the physician draws on the principles of supportive psychotherapy. Moreover, if he had not known the parents and child previously, he must quickly establish a working relationship or therapeutic alliance with them. He must also use active exploration and confrontation in a rapid and direct manner. He may have to use incision and drainage of guilt, and if the family is in a state of shock, he may have to think out loud the thoughts and feelings he senses they are having. In some cases, he may be wise to urgently recommend a consultation with a child psychiatrist,[47] who, in turn, should respond promptly. Once the family grasps the fact that the physician can help them to cope with the situation, the physician can arrange for follow-up care as indicated, by himself or by appropriate community agencies or professionals. Occasionally, as Lindemann[31] has pointed out, crisis intervention may be both immediately therapeutic and prevent more serious disorders. Also, it may help to promote a new psychologic or interpersonal equilibrium at a more adaptive level and prevent future crises as well.[45]

Case Example. A pediatrician was called in the evening by the mother of a $2^{1}/_{2}$-year-old girl he had seen in his practice. She said the little girl was in a panic, screaming uncontrollably and running agitatedly around the room. This behavior had built up gradually since the day before, and the child had had nightmares the last 2 nights. The mother and father were at a loss to explain or cope with the situation. The pediatrician told the parents to bring the girl to the emergency room of the local children's hospital, and he met them there. He found the parents to be agitated also, and he could not get a coherent history because of their fear that something was terribly wrong. He had difficulty in examining the child because of her screaming and hyperactivity, but he found no serious physical abnormalities. In her screaming, he could only make out the single word, "Mommy."

At this point, the pediatrician called a child psychiatrist, who had done consultations for him before and said he wondered whether the child was psychotic. The psychiatrist went quickly to the emergency room, and he found the situation as the pediatrician had described it. At first he could make no more headway with the child or parents than the pediatrician had, though he thought the little girl was in a panic state and was probably not psychotic. He did manage to calm the mother somewhat, but he could get no history of a precipitating event.

Still puzzled, the psychiatrist happened to

notice that the mother had one foot in a cast, and he asked what had happened. The mother replied that she had broken several bones in her foot some weeks before in an automobile accident. She had had the cast removed 2 days before, and the little girl while bouncing up and down on her mother's lap, had somehow fallen off onto the foot. The foot was rebroken, and the cast had been replaced by the mother's orthopedist the same day. She had not scolded the child, and she had not thought to mention the incident to the pediatrician or the psychiatrist.

The psychiatrist then said he might have the answer to the problem, and he spoke directly to the little girl, who, the mother had said, ordinarily talked reasonably well for her age. He told her that she had not meant to hurt Mommy's foot and that she was not a bad girl. The child suddenly looked directly at the psychiatrist, stopped screaming, and said clearly "Mommy's foot; bad girl." The psychiatrist repeated, "Not bad girl." The mother echoed this response, and the little girl, still hyperactive, ran over to the mother, clinging to her and sobbing (rather than screaming).

It was now well after midnight, and the parents and child (not to mention the physicians) were exhausted by the evening's experience. The psychiatrist recommended that the girl (who was calming down) and her mother be admitted for an overnight stay in the hospital. He suggested a mild dose of chloral hydrate for the girl and some sedation for the mother as well as for the father, who was advised by the pediatrician to go home and get some rest.

The pediatrician came to the hospital in the morning, and he found the girl and her mother much better and calmer. The event was discussed, and the little girl said, "Not bad girl." The mother expressed some guilt that she had not connected the two events, but she responded to the pediatrician's reassurance and support. The girl remained mildly hyperactive and clung to her mother for several days, but then she resumed her normal behavior.

Case Example. An 11-year-old black boy was brought to a pediatrician because he exhibited sudden withdrawal, involving virtually complete immobilization and inability to function, over the preceding week or so. The history taken from the boy's parents indicated that the boy had been previously well adjusted, had good social relationships, and performed excellently in school. No physical abnormalities were found. The boy's grandfather, who had lived in the boy's home and to whom the boy was closely attached, had died about 10 days before of sudden "heart failure." The parents had apparently been grieving appropriately, but the boy had shown no grief (which puzzled the parents) and had not wished to attend the funeral. In essence, he had not talked about the grandfather since his death. During the history and physical examination, the boy had been completely silent, and he did not respond to questions.

The pediatrician finally said to the boy in the presence of the parents, "I wonder if you're thinking about your grandfather and wishing he were alive. Maybe you're blaming yourself." The boy suddenly broke into tears and then said, "It was my fault. I didn't get him the drink." The pediatrician gave the boy his handkerchief. After the boy had sobbed bitterly for a few moments, the pediatrician put his arm around him, and said in a sympathetic tone, "Tell me about it."

The boy, still sobbing occasionally, told the pediatrician that he had been in his grandfather's room, when the grandfather suddenly began to breathe heavily and choked out the words, "Get me some water." The boy ran to do this, but when he returned the grandfather was dead. The parents had not known of this incident, and the father quickly said, "It wasn't your fault; he's had heart trouble for years, and we knew it was bound to come. You just happened to be there." The pediatrician and the mother reinforced this explanation, and the boy seemed immensely relieved, hugging his mother and crying quietly. The pediatrician said that he thought the boy would be all right, and he suggested that the family return in a week. During that time, the boy seemed sad at times, and he cried at times, but he was able to talk about his grandfather and to function in the home, returning to school at the end of the week. On a return visit 1 month later, he had returned to his previous adjustment although he said that he still felt sad at times about his grandfather's death.

Case Example. A 16-year-old white boy was brought to a pediatrician by his mother because he had had explosive vomiting and diarrhea intermittently for the past few days. He had some fever at first, and his mother kept him in bed but did not call the doctor. When the boy's fever subsided but his symptoms continued (though less severely), the mother became worried and brought the boy in for an examination. The history indicated no developmental or previous medical abnormalities, except occasional mild diarrhea over the past 2 years, and the results of the physical examination were normal, except for some borborygmi.

The pediatrician talked with the mother alone

for a few minutes. He discovered that the parents had been divorced years before and that the father had severed all contact with the family. The boy had missed his father, and often argued with the mother, at first blaming her for the divorce. She had been working since the divorce, but she had lost her job the week before and had had to go on welfare.

The pediatrician then talked with the boy, who said that he and his mother did argue sometimes but that he no longer blamed her for the divorce. He was worried that she had lost her job, and he said that having her home made him think of his father and miss him more. When he talked with the mother and boy together, the pediatrician said that the boy's symptoms must have started with the flu but that emotional tension could aggravate such symptoms, which he thought would subside soon. With the boy's permission, he told the mother that her presence at home the past week aroused memories in the boy of his father and that such feelings could produce sadness and some emotional tension. Both the mother and boy seemed satisfied with this explanation. The mother said she did not think their arguing was a serious problem, and the boy agreed. No return appointment was made but the pediatrician said they could return any time they wanted.

A week later, the boy called the pediatrician and said he was still having some diarrhea occasionally. The pediatrician saw the boy and found no abnormalities on examination. The boy talked again about missing his father and mentioned things they did together. This time, the pediatrician sensed that the boy needed to talk further and that he seemed reluctant to leave. After talking with the mother by telephone, the pediatrician set up biweekly half-hour interviews with the boy. The boy responded eagerly in the interviews, and he talked of many things, including his interests in mechanical things. His diarrhea subsided in several weeks. In the third interview, he complained of some numbness in his little finger. The pediatrician, after again examining the boy, suspected the numbness was an unconscious conversion mechanism. He told the boy that he thought it was a lingering manifestation of emotional tension and that it would probably go away soon with their talks. He said, however, that the boy did not have to have any symptoms to continue the talks.

By the next interview, the numbness had subsided. At the following interview, the boy said, "I feel better now that I have someone to talk to." Their biweekly talks continued for several months, (the mother had long since found another job), when the boy said he thought he no longer needed to come regularly but would appreciate it if he could come in and talk if he needed to. With this arrangement, the boy made an appointment every three to four months, "to bring the pediatrician up-to-date on developments." The arrangement continued until the boy graduated from high school and went to college in another state. For the next several years, he occasionally wrote the pediatrician, who replied promptly.

It is hoped that this chapter demonstrates clearly that pediatricians, family physicians, nurses, and health associates can be trained to use supportive psychotherapy in its various forms with children and parents, if they are interested (and many are not). There will of course be occasional failures, as there are in intensive insight-promoting psychotherapy carried out by mental health professionals with more seriously disturbed children and parents. Nevertheless, I believe that the principles of supportive psychotherapy should be offered in pediatric residencies (as they have been by the author and his colleagues, Eckhardt, Rabin, and Sakamoto, as well as by some others) and in the training programs of the other disciplines, as well as in continuing education programs, on a part-time basis, for pediatricians and for people in other disciplines. (Parents and children will usually accept a gradual movement from a guidance or counseling posture to a supportive psychotherapeutic approach. They may have difficulty, even if the physician is fully trained to do so, in accepting a change in the physician's role to that of an intensive insight-promoting psychotherapist, as Menahem et al.[43a] have pointed out.)

Bibliography

1. Allen, F.: *Psychotherapy for Children*. New York, Norton, 1942.
2. Alpert, J.J.: Broken appointments. Pediatrics, 34:127, 1964.
3. Arnold, L.E., Ed.: *Helping Parents Help Their Children*. New York, Brunner/Mazel, 1978.
4. Arnold, L.E., Rowe, M., and Tolbert, H.A.: Par-

ents' groups. In: *Helping Parents Help Their Children* (L.E. Arnold, Ed.). New York, Brunner/Mazel, 1978.

5. Augenbraun, B., Reid, H.L., and Friedman, D.B.: Brief intervention as a preventive force in disorders of early childhood. In: *Children and Their Parents in Brief Therapy* (H.H. Barten and S.S. Barten, Eds.). New York, Behavioral Publications, 1973.

6. Axline, V.M.: *Play Therapy*, Rev. Ed. New York, Ballantine Books, 1969.

7. Balint, M.: *The Doctor, His Patient, and the Illness*, 2nd Ed. New York, Pitman, 1964.

8. Beiser, H.R.: Play equipment for diagnosis and therapy. Am. J. Orthopsychiatry, 25:761, 1955.

9. Bender, L., and Woltman, A.: The use of puppet shows as a psychotherapeutic method for behavior problems in children. Am. J. Orthopsychiatry, 6:341, 1936.

10. Bleiberg, N., and Forrest, S.: Group discussions with mothers in the child health conference. Pediatrics, 24:118, 1959.

11. Bruch, H.: Brief psychotherapy in a pediatric clinic. Q. J. Child. Behav., 1:2, 1949.

12. Chess, S., and Thomas, A.: Temperamental individuality from childhood to adolescence. J. Am. Acad. Child Psychiatry, 16:5, 1975.

13. Chethik, M.: Work with parents: Treatment of the parent-child relationship. J. Am. Acad. Child Psychiatry, 15:453, 1976.

14. Coddington, R.D.: The use of brief psychotherapy in a pediatric practice. J. Pediatr., 60:259, 1962.

15. Durfie, M.B.: The use of office equipment in play therapy. Am. J. Orthopsychiatry, 12:495, 1942.

16. Fine, L.L.: *After All We've Done for Them: Understanding Adolescent Behavior*. Englewood Cliffs, N.J., Prentice-Hall, 1977.

17. Finkelstein, M., and Walker, C.: Unpublished material.

18. Finzer, W.: Unpublished material.

19. Furman, E.: Treatment of under-fives by way of their parents. Psychoanal. Study Child, 12:250, 1937.

20. Gallagher, J.R., and Harris, H.I.: *Emotional Problems of Adolescents*, 3rd Ed. New York, Oxford University Press, 1976.

21. Gardner, George: Unpublished material.

22. Gardner, R.A.: *Therapeutic Communication with Children: The Mutual Story-Telling Technique*. New York, Science House, 1971.

23. Garrett, A.: *Interviewing: Its Principles and Methods*. New York, Family Welfare Association of America, 1942.

24. Halpern, W.I., and Kissel, S.: Parent counselling. In: *Human Resources for Troubled Children* (W.I. Halpern, Ed.). New York, Wiley, 1976.

25. Haworth, M.R., and Keller, M.J.: The use of food in the diagnosis and therapy of emotionally disturbed children. J. Am. Acad. Child Psychiatry, 1:548, 1962.

25a. Health Supervision of Young Children: A Guide for Practising Physicians and Child Health Conference Personnel. New York, American Public Health Association, 1955.

26. Heinecke, C.M.: Aiding "at risk" children through

psychoanalytic social work with parents. Am. J. Orthopsychiatry, 46:89, 1976.

27. Jessner, L.: Some aspects of permissiveness in psychotherapy of children. Child Dev., 21:13, 1950.

28. Jessner, L., and Kaplan, S.: "Discipline" as a problem in psychotherapy with children. Nervous Child., 9:147, 1951.

29. Keith, C.R.: The therapeutic alliance in child psychiatry. J. Am. Acad. Child. Psychiatry, 7:31, 1968.

30. Kirchner, A.: Parents' classes in a maternity program. Am. J. Public Health, 43:896, 1953.

31. Klein, D.C., and Lindemann, E.: Preventive intervention in individual and family crisis situations. In: *Prevention of Emotional Disorders in Childhood*. (G. Caplan, Ed.). New York, Basic Books.

32. Korsch, B., Fraad, L., and Barnett, H.L.: Pediatric discussions with parent groups. J. Pediatr., 44:269, 1954.

33. Korsch, B.M.: Practical techniques of observing, interviewing, and advising parents in pediatric practice as demonstrated in an attitude study project. Pediatrics, 18:467, 1956.

34. Levin, S., and Werner, H.: The significance of giving gifts to children in therapy. J. Am. Acad. Child Psychiatry, 5:630, 1966.

35. Levine, M.: *Psychotherapy in Medical Practice*. New York, Macmillan, 1942.

36. Levy, D.M.: Trends in therapy: Release therapy. Am. J. Orthopsychiatry, 9:713, 1939.

37. Levy, D.M.: Observations of attitudes and behavior in the child health center. Am. J. Public Health, 41:182, 1951.

38. Levy, D.M.: Advice and reassurance. Am. J. Public Health, 44:1113, 1954.

39. Lippman, H.S.: Dreams in psychiatric work with children. Psychoanal. Study Child, 1:123, 1945.

40. Luzzati, L., and Dittmann, B.: Group discussions with parents of ill children. Pediatrics, 13:269, 1954.

41. Mattsson, A.: The male therapist and the female adolescent patient. J. Am. Acad. Child Psychiatry, 9:707, 1970.

42. Mattsson, A., Hawkins, J.W., and Seese, L.R.: Child psychiatric emergencies: Clinical characteristics and follow-up results. Arch. Gen. Psychiatry, 17:584, 1967.

43. McDermott, J.F., et al.: Social class and child psychiatric practice: The clinician's evaluation of the outcome of therapy. Am. J. Psychiatry, 126:951, 1970.

43a. Menahem, S., Lipton, G.F., and Caplan, G.: The psychologically oriented pediatrician and the provision of psychoanalytic psychotherapy. Child Psychiatry Hum. Dev., 12:67, 1981.

44. Milliken, S.: Group discussion of parents of handicapped children from the health education viewpoint. Am. J. Public Health, 43:900, 1953.

45. Paul, L.: Crisis intervention. Ment. Hygiene, 50:141, 1966.

46. Rogers, Carl R.: *Counselling and Psychotherapy*. New York, Houghton Mifflin, 1939.

47. Schowalter, J.E., and Solnit, A.J.: Child psychiatry consultation in a general hospital emergency room. J. Am. Acad. Child Psychiatry, 5:534, 1966.

48. Schulman, J.L.: The management of the irate parent. J. Pediatr., *77*:338, 1970.
49. Seitz, P.F.D.: Can the general practitioner do psychotherapy? Gen. Pract., *11*:126, 1959.
50. Senn, J.J.E.: The psychotherapeutic role of the pediatrician. Pediatrics, 2:147, 1948.
51. Smolen, E.N.: Nonverbal aspects of therapy with children. In: *Child Psychotherapy: Practice and Theory* (M.R. Haworth, Ed.). New York, Basic Books, 1964.
52. Strain, J., and Miller, D.: The preparation, utilization, and evaluation of a registered nurse trained to give telephone advice in a private pediatric office. Telephone advice by nurse in private pediatrician's office. Pediatrics, *47*:1051, 1971.
53. Szasz, T., and Hollender, M.: A contribution to the philosophy of medicine: The basic models of the doctor-patient relationship. Arch. Intern. Med., *97*:585, 1956.
54. Townsend, E.H.: The social worker in pediatric practice: An experiment. Am. J. Dis. Child, *107*:77, 1964.
55. Wenar, C.: The therapeutic value of setting limits with inhibited children. J. Nerv. Ment. Dis., *125*:390, 1957.
56. Werkman, S.: The involvement of parents in adolescent emotional difficulties. In: *Adolescence: Special Cases and Special Problems*, Rev. Ed. (R. Steimal, Ed.). Washington, D.C., Catholic University Press, 1968.
57. Wessel, M.A., and LaCamera, R.E.: The pediatrician and the adolescent: An extraordinary opportunity to be helpful. Clin. Pediatr., *6*:227, 1967.
58. Wishik, S.M.: Parents' group discussions in a child health conference. Am. J. Public Health, *43*:888, 1953.
59. Wishik, S.M.: Contributor's section: Pediatrics and society. Pediatrics, 24:117, 1959.
60. Wiskingrad, L., Schulkuff, J.T., and Slavsky, A.: The role of a social worker in a private practice of pediatrics. Pediatrics, 32:1, 1963.
61. Woltmann, A.G.: Diagnostic and therapeutic considerations of nonverbal projective activities with children. In: *Child Psychotherapy: Practice and Theory* (M.R. Haworth, Ed.). New York, Basic Books, 1964.
62. Zulliger, H.: Child psychotherapy without interpretation of unconscious content. Bull. Menninger Clin., *17*:180, 1953.
63. Zwick, P.A.: Gauging dosage and distance in psychotherapy with adolescents. Am. J. Orthopsychiatry, *30*:645, 1960.

General References

Abel, T.M., and Mitraux, R.: *Culture and Psychotherapy*. New Haven, Conn., College & University Press, 1974.
Adams, P.L.: *A Primer of Child Psychotherapy*. Boston, Little, Brown, 1974.
Anthony, J.: Communicating therapeutically with the child. J. Am. Acad. Child Psychiatry, 3:106, 1964.

Balser, B.H., Ed.: *Psychotherapy of the Adolescent*. New York, International Universities Press, 1936.
Barten, H.H., and Barten, S.S., Ed.: *Children and Their Parents in Brief Psychotherapy*. New York, Behavioral Publications, 1973.
Blos, P.: *On Adolescence*. Glencoe, Ill., Free Press, 1959.
Blos, P.: *The Young Adolescent*. New York, Free Press, 1972.
Caplan, G., and Lebovici, S.: *Adolescence: Perspectives*. New York, Basic Books, 1969.
Conger, J.J.: *Adolescence and Youth: Psychological Development in a Changing World*, 2nd Ed. New York, Harper & Row, 1977.
Cooper, S., and Wanerman, L.: *Children in Treatment: A Primer for Beginning Psychotherapists*. New York, Brunner/Mazel, 1977.
Deutsch, H.: *Selected problems of adolescence: With special emphasis on group formation*. Psychoanal. Study Child., *3*:63, 1967.
Douvan, E., and Gold, M.: Model patterns in American adolescence. In: *Review of Child Development Research*. New York, Russell Sage Foundation, 1966.
Eisenberg, L., and Gruenberg, E.M.: The current status of secondary prevention in child psychiatry. Am. J. Orthopsychiatry, *31*:355, 1961.
Erikson, E.H.: The problem of ego identity. J. Am. Psychoanal. Assoc., *4*:56, 1956.
Erikson, E.H.: *Identity and the life cycle*. Psychol. Issues, *1*:1, 1959.
Erikson, E.H.: *Identity, Youth, and Crisis*. New York, Norton, 1968.
Fraiberg, S.: Some considerations in the introduction to therapy in puberty. In: Psychoanal. Study Child, 10:264, 1955.
Frank, J.D.: The dynamics of the psychotherapeutic relationship: Determinants and effects of the therapist's influence. Psychiatry, 22:17, 1959.
Frank, J.: *Persuasion and Healing*, Rev. Ed. Baltimore, Johns Hopkins University Press, 1973.
Freud, A.: *The Ego and the Mechanisms of Defense*. New York, International Universities Press, 1946.
Fromm-Reichmann, F.: *Principles of Intensive Psychotherapy*. Chicago, University of Chicago Press, 1950.
Gallagher, J.R., and Harris, H.I.: *Emotional Problems of Adolescents*, 3rd Ed. New York, Oxford University Press, 1976.
Gardner, G.: Psychiatric problems of adolescence. In: *American Handbook of Psychiatry* (S. Arieti, Ed.). New York, Basic Books, 1959.
Gardner, R.A.: *Psychotherapeutic Approaches to the Resistant Child*. New York, Jason Aronson, 1975.
Group for the Advancement of Psychiatry: *Normal Adolescence: Its Dynamics and Impact*. Report No. 68. New York, Group for the Advancement of Psychiatry, 1968.
Halpern, W.J., and Kissel, S.: *Human Resources for Troubled Children*. New York, Wiley, 1976.
Hammer, M., and Kaplan, A.M.: *The Practice of Psychotherapy with Children*. Homewood, Ill., Dorsey Press, 1967.
Harrison, S.I., and Carek, D.J.: *A Guide to Psychotherapy*. Boston, Little, Brown, 1966.

Haworth, M.R., Ed.: *Child Psychotherapy: Practice and Theory.* New York, Basic Books, 1964.

Heald, F.P., Dangela, M., and Brunschuyler, P.: Physiology of adolescence. N. Engl. J. Med., *268*:192, 1963.

Holmes, D.J.: *The Adolescent in Psychotherapy.* Boston, Little, Brown, 1964.

Jersild, A.: *The Psychology of Adolescence,* 2nd Ed. New York, Macmillan, 1963.

Josselyn, J.: *The Adolescent and His World.* New York, Family Service Association of America, 1952.

Josselyn, I.M.: Psychotherapy of adolescents at the level of private practice. In: *Psychotherapy of the Adolescent* (B.H. Balser, Ed.). New York, International Universities Press, 1957.

Josselyn, I.M.: *Adolescence: Report of the Joint Commission on Mental Health of Children.* New York, Harper & Row, 1971.

Lippman, H.: *Treatment of the Child in Emotional Conflict.* 2nd Ed. New York, Blakiston, 1962.

Marcus, D., et al.: A clinical approach to the understanding of normal and pathologic adolescence. Arch. Gen. Psychiatr., *15*:569, 1966.

Masterson, J.E., Jr.: Psychotherapy of the adolescent: A comparison with psychotherapy of the adult. J. Nerv. Ment. Dis., *127*:511, 1958.

Meeks, J.E.: Children who cheat at games. J. Am. Acad. Child Psychiatry, *9*:157, 1970.

Meeks, J.E.: The fragile alliance: An orientation to the outpatient psychotherapy of the adolescent. Baltimore, Williams & Wilkins, 1971.

Moustakas, C., Ed.: *The Child's Discovery of Himself.* New York, Ballantine Books, 1972.

Moustakas, C., and Shalock, H.D.: An analysis of therapist-child interaction in play therapy. Child Dev., *26*:143, 1955.

Offer, D., and Offer, J.B.: *The Psychological World of the Teenager.* New York, Basic Books, 1969.

Piaget, J., and Inhelder, G.: *The Growth of Logical Thinking from Childhood to Adolescence.* New York, Basic Books, 1958.

Psychiatric Approaches to Adolescence. Sixth International Congress of the International Association for Child Psychiatry and Allied Professions. Edinburgh, 1966.

Salzman, L.: Truth, honesty, and the therapeutic process. Am. J. Psychiatry, *130*:1280, 1973.

Schaefer, C., Ed.: *Therapeutic Use of Child's Play.* New York, Jason Aronson, 1976.

Schonfeld, W.A.: General practitioner's role in management of personality problems of adolescents. JAMA, *147*:1424, 1951.

Solnit, A.J.: The vicissitudes of ego development in adolescence. Panel report. J. Am. Psychoanal. Assoc., *7*:523, 1959.

Strupp, H.H.: *Psychotherapists in Action.* New York, Grune & Stratton, 1960.

Swanson, F.L.: *Psychotherapists and Children: A Procedure Guide.* New York, Pitman, 1970.

Tanner, J.M.: *Growth at Adolescence,* 2nd Ed. Philadephia, Blackwell Scientific Publications, 1961.

Timmons, F.R.: Brief psychotherapy in an adolescent medical clinic: A case example. J. Pediatr. Psychol., *2*:138, 1977.

Walz, G.R., and Benjamin, L.: *Transcultural Counseling: Needs, Programs, and Techniques,* Vol. 7. New York, Human Sciences Press, 1978.

Witmer, H.L., Ed.: *Psychiatric Interviews with Children.* New York, The Commonwealth Fund, 1946.

13
Psychopharmacologic Treatment

Raze out the written troubles of the brain
And with some sweet oblivious antidote
Cleanse the stuffed bosom of that perilous stuff
Which weighs upon the heart.
(William Shakespeare)

Psychopharmacologic drugs have a definite though limited place in the treatment of psychosocial disorders in children and adolescents. After widespread overuse (and overly rigid opposition in some quarters), the approach to the clinical use of such drugs in child psychiatry and pediatrics is gradually becoming more balanced and thoughtful. Eisenberg[17] has remarked that the certainty of convictions held in this area has tended to vary inversely with the depth of the base of knowledge. The paucity of well-designed and well-controlled studies that use homogeneous samples of adequate size has been pointed out by Sprague and Werry[47] in a critical review of research in child psychopharmacology and by Freeman[26] in a thorough and incisive review of psychopharmacology as it relates to retarded children. Cogent and balanced reviews of the use of drugs in children and adolescents have been provided by Eisenberg[16] and Werry[51] and in excellent books that were edited recently by Wiener[53] and Werry.[52]

Recent years have seen considerable improvement in research methodology in this field. The investigations of Eisenberg and his associates[19] and of others[9,10] have provided sound models for the approach to studies of drugs used for children and adolescents. Although more is known about the effectiveness, side-effects, and toxicity of some of these drugs, the mode of action of most such drugs is still not fully understood, and their use is still largely empirical. No drug can replace the interpersonal relationship between the child, his parents, and the physician, and medication should never be the sole component of treatment.

In general, psychotropic drugs seem to be less effective in the treatment of children and adolescents than adults. This may be due to the fact that metabolic factors operate differently at different levels of de-

235

velopment, to the greater complexity of the physician-patient-parent relationship when the patient is a child, or to other factors. The information available on the long-term effects of psychotropic drugs on children and adolescents is limited. As Campbell[7] has pointed out, however, studies show some effects on the endocrine and the central nervous systems of adults, which indicates that further investigations in the childhood age range are urgently needed. Eisenberg[17] has cogently discussed the ethical issues involved in drug therapy with children, including problems related to the "control" of behavior, questions about "normality" and its influence by chemicals, and the increasingly recognized long-term side-effects of drug therapy on growth and development.

The available evidence indicates that drug therapy can be effective in reducing anxiety and hyperactivity and the consequent diminution of impulsiveness and irritability can result in lessened anxiety, an improved attention span, and some increase in cognitive effectiveness. Drug therapy can, within limits, increase the spontaneous activity and responsiveness of patients suffering from apathy and withdrawal. As a result of diminution in anxiety and disorganized behavior, some severely disturbed or psychotic children can be helped to participate in group activities or special classes. They may also become more amenable to psychotherapy.

As the foregoing discussion implies, the term "psychotherapeutic drug" is a misnomer. More correctly, the effects of psychotropic drugs upon certain symptoms may help seriously disturbed children become more amenable to psychotherapy. There is no evidence that any drug can improve intellectual functioning by direct action on the central nervous system. Drug therapy can modify responses to current experience, but it cannot by itself undo previously learned behavior or alter fixed personality traits or neurotic patterns.

A major factor in a child's response to drug therapy is the psychologic effect of administering medication. It is clear that a drug can influence a child either directly, by way of his own expectations, or indirectly, through changes in parental attitudes of behaviour, usually in anticipation of a change in the child, or in both ways. In addition, the confidence of the physician administering the drug may influence the expectations of child and parents. Kraft[34] has observed that the basic pharmacodynamic actions of a drug may be enhanced or diminished, depending upon the attitude of the child, his parents, and, at times, other helping figures, such as teachers. Beecher[4] has demonstrated that about one-third of the pharmacotherapeutic effectiveness of any drug results from the placebo effect, which derives from psychologic anticipation. The placebo effect can be enhanced if a positive doctor-patient-parent relationship is present. The placebo effect can be diminished, and the drug may even be ineffective if the relationship is mistrusting or negative or if the physician prescribes the drug out of exasperation or other negative feelings. Stress in the patient's life may also influence both the action of the drug and its placebo effect, as Beecher[5] has shown. When prescribing drugs, the physician should inform parents and older children and adolescents not only of the expected therapeutic effects, but also of the limitations of drug treatment, as well as possible adverse effects.

Basic Principles of Drug Treatment

The principles discussed under this heading are adapted from Eisenberg's cogent discussion.[16]

Many clinicians agree that it is difficult to use formal diagnostic categories as a guide in prescribing psychotropic medication. On the other hand, both Conners[10] and Werry[49] believe that the use of diagnostic systems is important to compare categories and for other research implications. In prescribing drugs, the tendency is to try to alleviate certain target symptoms, such as a high anxiety level, marked hyperactivity, and disruptive or disorganized behavior. Most psychiatrists agree that a careful clinical evaluation, including a review of the history of the child's symptoms and prior development and an assessment of the past and present adaptive functioning of the child and his parents, should be undertaken before medication is prescribed. In brief, drug treatment should be only part of a comprehensive treatment plan which is based on the strengths, weaknesses, feelings, and needs of the child and his parents. With mild to moderately anxious children, it is better not to start with a drug, since many will respond to supportive psychotherapeutic measures alone.[20]

Although some severely disturbed or psychotic children who show intense anxiety and disorganized behavior may be helped by major tranquilizers, others who show withdrawn or isolated behavior may not benefit. Children who have chronic personality disorders are generally not helped by drugs. However, stimulant drugs may help some older children and adolescents who have aggressive and impulsive behavior patterns if they are being treated in residential settings.[21]

As Eisenberg and his colleagues[20] have shown, most children who have psychoneurotic problems respond better to psychotherapy than to drugs. But some children who have marked phobias or overwhelming anxiety may exhibit more spontaneous behavior and improved adaptive functioning if tranquilizers are combined with psychotherapy in the initial approach. Mental retardation and intellectual limitations due to cerebral lesions in chronic brain syndromes are not modifiable by any drug, but stimulant drugs may help to control the hyperactivity and distractibility which can occur with these conditions. The use of drugs to treat reactive disorders is indicated only rarely, unless a panic state

supervenes or sedation is needed to alleviate acute and intense anxiety in response to stress.

Appropriate drugs should be chosen according to firm indication and should be used with discrimination.

Major tranquilizers, while appropriate for the treatment of moderate-to-severe clinical pictures in children who show marked anxiety, are not indicated in the treatment of milder anxiety or fearfulness because of the possibility of toxicity. Nor are they usually appropriate for hyperactive children. An abnormal electroencephalogram (EEG) in a disturbed child is not in itself indicative of a need for anticonvulsant or tranquilizing drugs; psychosocial study of the child in the family is called for, as the EEG findings may be of no clinical significance. No more than one tranquilizing drug should be prescribed at a time; a recent review of the literature shows that there is no advantage in using drugs in combinations,[25] and some harm may accrue from polypharmacy. (If a referred child is taking several drugs and seems lethargic, it is my usual practice to hospitalize him and to remove him from all medication in order to achieve a baseline for observation. Care should be taken to avoid "iatrogenic" drug interactions, which are difficult to predict, as well as possible potentiation of drug effects by patent medicines, particularly cold remedies.

Tranquilizing drugs are usually contraindicated in cases of even mild delirium, as their side-effects may increase confusion and disorientation. A sedative, such as chloral hydrate, may be prescribed if necessary. In my opinion, tranquilizing drugs are also contraindicated in treating children—especially adolescents—who have incipient or borderline psychotic pictures. The side-effects of tranquilizers (e.g., drowsiness or blurred vision) may increase the patient's feelings of depersonalization or confusion about his body image or identity. Tranquilizing drugs have been known occasionally to precipitate psychoses in such situations. Even in less precarious situations, the effect of drugs on the child's psyche and various physiologic systems should be considered. In some cases, a child's self-image may be adversely affected by the need to take drugs, and this may be an overriding consideration even though certain symptoms would be improved with the use of medication.

In my opinion, tranquilizing drugs are still prescribed too frequently by some physicians, although less so than in the past. Mastery of some fears or anxiety, with other types of supportive help when indicated, may even be necessary to help spur development in children. Because of the possibility of suicide attempts or drug habituation, adolescents should be given small amounts of any drug prescribed. Ordinarily, only enough medication should be prescribed to last until the next visit, which should be scheduled within 3 to 7 days. A seriously disturbed adolescent who comes from a disorganized family may have to be hospitalized in order to initiate medication.

The physician who prescribes drugs should have a thorough knowledge of their pharmacologic properties, particularly of their side-effects and toxic manifestations.

The severity of the child's disorder and the potential for improvement must justify the possible impact of side-effects or toxicity. The development of seizures or extrapyramidal symptoms in a frightened child in an anxious family has negative implications for all concerned, and the psychologic consequences may be far reaching. The dosage must be carefully regulated to avoid impairing a child's intellectual alertness and acuity.

Some tranquilizers are contraindicated for children because of their propensity for producing toxic manifestations more often in young persons than in adults. A history of previous hypersensitivity is also a contraindication to the use of certain drugs. Special screening of drugs used to treat disturbed children is vital, because a drug's action may be unpredictable owing to the child's immaturity or level of development. In the case of teenage pregnancy, the physician should be aware of the possibility of toxic effects on the newborn (e.g., extrapyramidal symptoms and jaundice) if the child's mother has taken phenothiazines.[32] The NIMH Pediatric Psychopharmacological package[41] outlines formal methods for the careful medical surveillance of psychopharmacologic treatment of children, including the screening of all body systems, especially the nervous system, checking and plotting height and weight curves, and considering the necessity for blood tests. In all cases, expected benefits must outweigh possible disadvantages.

The dosage must be individualized for each patient.

Although the standard dosage of tranquilizers for children may be expressed in body weight (mg/kg/day) or in relation to body surface, the dosage may have to be varied to achieve therapeutic effectiveness. Generally, it is best to prescribe the lowest possible dose that will produce a beneficial response, since toxicity occurs with high doses more often in children than in adults. As a rule of thumb, Werry[51] recommends beginning with half the minimum recommended dose; recent studies have shown that the usual recommended dose is often too high for children. Individualization, with careful monitoring, is necessary, however, since undertreatment or overtreatment may occur because of metabolic uniqueness. Certain drugs, such as stimulants, can be used in higher doses in children than adults, but important individual differences still occur. Since psychotropic drugs are generally long-acting, the dosage should not be increased more often than at weekly intervals.

A well-tested and familiar drug should generally be used rather than a new or unfamiliar one.

In the rush to find new and more effective drugs, many drugs on the market have not been sufficiently tested, particularly for their side-effects and toxicity in children. Past experience has proved that a drug's toxicity may not be manifested until it has been in general use for some time. The physician is therefore well advised to familiarize himself with 1 or 2 drugs in each category and to use as few as possible.

Drugs should be used sparingly and no longer than necessary.

Since symptom control is the goal of drug therapy, drug therapy should be discontinued as soon as possible. Campbell[7] has advised that the use of major tranquilizers in treating acutely psychotic children be limited to 4 to 6 weeks. A hyperactive child on stimulant medication should have a drug-free trial after several months. Lowering the dosage periodically will permit termination of drug therapy if symptoms do not recur.

Since drug therapy affects symptoms only, the physician must continue to seek and treat the basic causative factors that underlie the symptoms.

Contrary to the view of some physicians, the relief of symptoms may be a vital component of the total treatment plan, and its importance should not be underrated. Mastery of certain troubling symptoms may provide a significant impetus to the development of some children. However, the physician should not permit his concerns about the basic underlying physical, psychologic, or social factors to be lulled by symptomatic relief alone. If he does, he is not fulfilling his professional obligations to the child and his family.

Types of Drugs

Psychoactive agents may be classified in 1 of 5 major categories: (1) tranquilizers, (2) hypnotics and sedatives, (3) stimulants, (4) antidepressants, and (5) hallucinogens or psychotomimetics. On the basis of their chemical structure and potency, the tranquilizers may be further identified as major and minor. Their site of action is poorly understood, but they are believed to be most active at the subcortical level.

Major Tranquilizers

The major tranquilizers are used primarily to treat hospitalized or severely disturbed or psychotic children; they have a calming effect on agitated, impulsive, or excited patients, without significant clouding of consciousness, paradoxic excitement, or depressive effect. They may facilitate social adjustment and reduce or help control delusions and hallucinations and thus increase the patient's ability to communicate. The major tranquilizers may be helpful in treating severely disturbed children in other diagnostic categories.* Low dosages of these drugs should be employed initially, with the dosage increased at intervals of about 7 days until a satisfactory response is obtained, or until side-effects or evidence of toxicity is seen. The dosage can then be reduced or the medication terminated. In acute disturbances, an initial parenteral dose may be given (although parenteral administration should be avoided in children if possible). The major tranquilizers are powerful drugs that apparently act through a depressant effect[51]; they should therefore be used only when there are definite indications for their use—and then with due caution. Ordinarily they should not be used to alleviate anxiety of the type seen in psychoneurotic disorders, reactive disorders, or milder problems.

Phenothiazine Derivatives. The phenothiazines are the most potent of the tranquilizers, and they have received the most extensive clinical use since the discovery of chlorpromazine in the 1940s. Within this group, there are 3 major subgroups, which are discussed in the following paragraphs.**

Dimethylaminopropyl (Aliphatic) Series.

---

*Thus the term "antipsychotic" is not appropriate.
**Some of the early phenothiazines have been withdrawn from the market.

This group includes chlorpromazine (Thorazine), promazine (Sparine), and triflupromazine (Vesprin). *Chlorpromazine* has relatively low toxicity and a fairly good safety margin of therapeutic activity over toxicity. Controlled studies[7,22] have demonstrated that chlorpromazine has a useful though limited effect on severely disturbed or psychotic children (including some with mental retardation), particularly if intense anxiety, agitation, or psychomotor excitement is present. Chlorpromazine has some sedative effects, however, and high doses can impair learning and performance. Common side-effects include anticholinergic responses (e.g., dryness of the mouth, blurred vision, difficult micturition, constipation, and gastric upset), skin changes (e.g., dermatitis, photosensitivity, and, if treatment is long continued, pigmentation), extrapyramidal syndromes (e.g., Parkinsonism, dystonias, choreiform movements, tremors, rigidity, and akathisia), nausea and vomiting, and drowsiness.[15] Endocrine abnormalities and unexplained bodily temperature changes also occur although they are less common. Electrocardiographic changes have also been described. In one study,[42] a group of children and adolescents treated with phenothiazines and haloperidol on a long-term basis developed tardive dyskinesia, often presenting as choreoathetotic movements of the lips and tongue, when the drugs were withdrawn. In about 50% of these patients the involuntary movements subsided spontaneously, while the other patients required medication with another tranquilizer, which raised the possibility that these side-effects were irreversible. Werry[51] and others believe that tardive dyskinesia as a side-effect of phenothiazine medication is the result of postsynaptic sensitization to dopamine, whose transmission is blocked by these drugs.

Potentially serious toxic effects of these drugs include blood dyscrasias (agranulocytosis; aplastic anemia), seizures, cholangiolitic jaundice and (rarely) sympatholytic responses involving marked hypotension, tachycardia, and a shock-like state (at times accompanying parenteral administration of high doses). Regular blood studies should be routine when these drugs are given. Sudden death, involving cardiovascular collapse associated with arrhythmias and/or marked hypotension, has been reported (rarely) in adult patients taking high doses of certain phenothiazines.[35] The relationship is as yet unclear.

Toxicity or troublesome side-effects can ordinarily be managed by decreasing the dose or by changing to another drug. Extrapyramidal signs can usually be relieved by the oral administration of antiparkinsonism drugs, such as biperidon (Akineton) or benztropine (Cogentin). Diphenhydramine (Benadryl) given intravenously over 5 minutes (2 mg/kg) seems to be the best antidote for severe dystonia and rigidity and for marked nausea and vomiting,[29] and it may be helpful in cases of accidental ingestion.[14]

Promazine does not seem to be as effective as chlorpromazine, and a higher incidence of seizures has been reported.

Triflupromazine seems to be no more effective than promazine, and a fairly high incidence of troublesome side-effects has been reported.

Piperazine Series. This group includes trifluoperazine (Stelazine), fluphenazine (Prolixin), prochlorperazine (Compazine), and perphenazine (Trilafon). *Trifluoperazine* has been reported to have a somewhat stimulating or "activating" effect on withdrawn, apathetic patients. No controlled studies have as yet established this fact, however, and side-effects, including marked extrapyramidal symptoms, seem to be more frequent with trifluoperazine than with chlorpromazine. *Fluphenazine* can be administered in much smaller doses than chlorpromazine, but questions regarding its effectiveness have been raised in 1 controlled study, and a high incidence of side-effects has been reported. The effectiveness of *perphenazine* has also been questioned in 2 controlled investigations, and the incidence of side-effects, including serious extrapyramidal syndromes, is quite high in children. Similar questions have been raised regarding *prochlorperazine*. Acetophenazine and other drugs in the piperazine series seem to have no advantages over chlorpromazine. Tardive dyskinesia seems to be an even more common and distressing syndrome resulting from prolonged use of the piperazines than the phenothiazines, and recent reports[8,39] raise the possibility that tardive dyskinesia is life threatening.

Piperidine Series. Thioridazine (Mellaril) is the principal drug in the piperidine group. It has fewer side-effects than most drugs in the aliphatic and piperazine subgroups, with the incidence of extra pyramidal effects especially low. However, cardiac irregularities have occurred in the treatment of adults. Several controlled studies have indicated that disturbed and stereotyped behavior in mentally retarded children and adolescents is especially responsive to thioridazine, and the drug is reported to have some antidepressant effects in seriously disturbed adolescents. Administration on a once-a-day basis is possible, and the presence of a convulsive disorder is not a contraindication for its use. The fact that thioridazine is not available in a palatable liquid form limits its usefulness for children.

The *thioxanthenes* are related to the phenothiazines. One drug in the thioxanthene group, *chlorprothixene* (Taractan), has been said to be effective in treating disturbed children, but the only controlled study reported to date casts doubts on its effectiveness. Its side-effects and contraindications are about the same as for the phenothiazines. It is approved only for patients over 6 years old.

In summary, the safest and most effective drug in the aliphatic series of phenothiazines is chlorpromazine (Thorazine). No drug in the piperazine series is superior to chlorpromazine, and trifluoperazine (Stelazine), perphenazine (Trilafon), and fluphenazine (Compazine) are not safe for children, because of the frequency of painful torticollis, trismus, and violent extrapyramidal side-effects. In the piperidine series, thioridazine (Mellaril) is an effective drug, and it has fewer side-effects than chlorpromazine. The phenothiazines potentiate the effects of barbiturates, and, as with other tranquilizing drugs, their activity is potentiated by alcohol and certain other drugs.

Rauwolfia Alkaloids. The rauwolfia alkaloids seem to be less reliable in their effects than the phenothiazines. Reserpine, which is thought to act by reducing serotonin levels, was formerly used to treat psychotic and markedly disorganized children, but its use is now largely confined to the treatment of hypertension. Lethargy, nasal congestion, gastric hypersecretion, diarrhea, and other disturbing side-effects are frequently encountered in children when these drugs are prescribed in adequate doses.

Butyrophenones. Although the butyrophenones are unrelated to the phenothiazines, their pharmacologic action is similar. Haloperidol (Haldol) may have a specifically beneficial effect on severe tic syndromes in some cases, especially maladie de tics (Gilles de la Tourette's) syndrome. However, the safety and effectiveness of this drug have not been established for children, and it is not approved for use in patients under 12 years old. (The drug has been used to treat psychotic adult patients.) Reported side-effects include a high incidence of extrapyramidal syndromes, as well as laryngospasm, bronchospasm, and hypotension. Bronchopneumonia and liver damage have been reported as possible toxic effects; and shock-like states, associated with respiratory depression and hypotension, have been described following the administration of haloperidol in large doses. Tardive dyskinesia is at least as common in patients treated with drugs in this group as with the piperazines. Death has occasionally occurred in adults receiving haloperidol although the relationship is not clear. In my opinion haloperidol is not a safe drug, even for adolescents.*

Minor (or Mild) Tranquilizers

Because of their beneficial effects on milder psychological disorders, the minor tranquilizers are frequently used for the outpatient treatment of children. Occasionally these drugs are helpful with more seriously disturbed children if their behavior patterns are reasonably malleable, but they are not adequate substitutes for the major tranquilizers.

Diphenylmethanes. Several drugs in the diphenylmethane group have antihistaminic as well as tranquilizing effects. Toxicity is not common, although the usual precautions should be taken. *Diphenhydramine* (Benadryl) has been used extensively as an antianxiety agent as well as a sedative and an antiemetic. Side-effects, which are generally mild, include dryness of the mouth, dizziness, drowsiness, and, occasionally, overexcitation. In one controlled study diphenhydramine has been reported to be effective in treating somewhat anxious children and children who have sleep disorders. Its effectiveness is reported to be greatest in younger children, with a fall off at puberty, although some pediatricians have used it successfully with adolescents. The taste of Benadryl is not unpleasant, and it is available in elixir form.

Hydroxyzine (Atarax, Vistaril) has been used to control mild anxiety states, night terrors, and reactions to somatic difficulties. Various studies, mostly uncontrolled, suggest that hydroxyzine is less potent than diphenhydramine but that its side-effects are about the same. The same seems to be true of *azacyclonol* (Frenquel). The dosage of drugs in this group cannot be increased significantly because of their atropine-like side-effects.

---

*In some severe cases of Gilles de la Tourette's syndrome, the possible benefits *may* outweigh the disadvantages, if the drug is used cautiously.

Propanediols. *Meprobamate* (Equanil, Miltown) and *mephenesin* (Tolserol) have only limited tranquilizing effects on children, and their use may give rise to drowsiness, rashes, hypotension, and other undesirable side-effects. Habituation and withdrawal effects have been reported in adults. Acute toxicity has resulted from accidental ingestion of large amounts. Because of their muscle-relaxing qualities, these drugs have been most useful in treating children who have cerebral palsy and related disorders.

Benzodiazepines. *Chlordiazepoxide* (Librium) and *diazepam* (Valium) are apparently effective in reducing anxiety in adults and in animals, but not enough is known about their effectiveness in children. In a controlled study, Librium was found to stimulate hyperactivity in disturbed and retarded children. Its side-effects include drowsiness, ataxia, overexcitation, hypersensitivity, and jaundice. Diazepam has been claimed to have potent muscle relaxant properties, and it may be useful in treating spastic conditions and as an anticonvulsant in status epilepticus.

Hypnotics and Sedatives

These drugs seem to act more at the cortical level than do the tranquilizing drugs. *Barbiturates* have been found of little value in treating moderately or severely disturbed children, but they are sometimes useful in treating acutely agitated children. Except for the use of phenobarbital in treating children who have convulsive disorders, prolonged administration of barbiturates is unwise, because of the confusion, anxiety, disorientation, and increased agitation they frequently produce. Even in short-term usage, barbiturates may paradoxically stimulate preschool-age children or children with hyperactivity resulting from anxiety or brain damage. *Chloral hydrate* continues to be one of the most effective sedatives for children and adolescents. It is an extremely safe drug, and the best drug for delirium if a sedative is required. Although *paraldehyde* is equally potent and even safer, its odor as it is excreted through the lungs creates problems with children. A mild tranquilizer, such as Benadryl, has been used for sedative effects in children. The other nonbarbiturate sedatives, such as *glutethimide* (Doriden) and *ethchlorvynol* (Placidyl), have no place in the treatment of children.

Stimulants

Drugs in this group include *amphetamine* (Benzedrine), *dextroamphetamine* (Dexedrine), and *methamphetamine* (Methedrine), all of which are sympathomimetic amines with adrenergic effects. Amphetamine was first used by Bradley[6] in 1937. Controlled studies by Eisenberg,[18] Conners,[12] and their colleagues have documented that dextroamphetamine has the paradoxical effect of quieting or inhibiting the behavior of truly hyperactive children (i.e., children who are markedly hyperactive at home, at school, and in other social situations). The source of these effects is unclear. Other studies have shown dextroamphetamine to be superior to chlorpromazine in reducing hyperactivity in nonneurotic children. (Thioridazine has been shown to be effective also, but it should be reserved for psychotic or other seriously disturbed children who are hyperactive and whom stimulants may affect adversely.) There seems to be little difference between the dextro and levo rotatory isomers of amphetamine.[2]

Conners and his colleagues[13] have demonstrated the positive effects of dextroamphetamine on perception, learning, and achievement in certain hyperactive children with nonneurotic learning disorders. Other investigators, though reporting a reduction in hyperactivity, have reported no effect on attention and learning in mentally retarded children. The amphetamines do not seem to be effective antidepressants in children, and a "let-down" effect has been noted following their use for this purpose.

For reasons that are not clear, they do not stimulate seizure activity and so can be used with anticonvulsants for hyperactive children who have convulsive disorders, although they should not be used concomitantly with tranquilizers. The inhibiting effect of the amphetamines is said to diminish at puberty, when they may act as a true stimulant. Individual differences in response patterns have been observed in adolescents and young adults, however.

Although the statement has been made that stimulant drugs can be of value in determining the etiology of hyperactivity, there is no solid evidence to support the claim. Fish[23] in offering evidence to explode the "one drug, one child" myth has pointed out that hyperactivity may be seen in children in different diagnostic categories and that some may be helped by amphetamines and some (e.g., psychotic children) may be made worse. Children with brain damage who exhibit hyperactivity (many do not) may respond positively as may children whose hyperactivity stems primarily from anxiety or from a masking of depression.

The side-effects of the amphetamines include irritability, tearfulness, insomnia, anorexia, and stomachaches, as well as adrenergic effects. Occasionally overquieting effects, with marked inhibition, tearfulness, and even depression may occur. Dyskinetic syndromes have been rarely reported;[38] ordinarily they can be controlled by lowering the dosage. Overdoses can result in toxic psychosis,[51] with hallucinations and other symptoms. Although Beck and his colleagues[3] and other groups have followed some hyperactive patients into adolescence and found no apparent effects on growth or habituation stemming from prolonged use of amphetamines, Safer and his colleagues[43] have reported long-term effects involving weight loss and inhibition of growth. Grinspoon[28] has noted some risk of habituation in adolescents.

Methylphenidate (Ritalin) acts as a central nervous stimulant also, although it has a different chemical structure and so does not produce the adrenergic effects of the amphetamines. In a controlled study, Conners and Eisenberg[11] have shown methylphenidate to be effective in treating hyperactive nonneurotic children, and also have reported some improvement in learning. The side-effects of methylphenidate include anorexia, insomnia, and occasional overexcitation. Hallucinosis has been reported from overdoses.[37]

Deanol acetamidolbenzoate (Deaner) has been said to produce results similar to the amphetamines without adrenergic effects. However, recent controlled investigations have raised considerable doubt about its effectiveness in children.

In prescribing amphetamines for truly hyperactive school-age children, one can start with 5 mg of dexedrine and give it in the morning (to avoid insomnia). The drug should be given 30 minutes before breakfast; a positive effect may occur by breakfast. Half a tablet (2.5 mg) may produce good results in preschool-age children. If no improvement occurs in 2 to 3 days, the dosage can be increased by 5 mg every several days, (in divided doses, one in the morning and one in the early afternoon) until improvement occurs or until side-effects, such as anorexia or difficulty in falling asleep, ensue. If no noticeable improvement has occurred after 2 weeks, dexedrine should be discontinued, and methylphenidate can be tried, starting with a 10 mg dose. The Council on Child Health of the Academy of Pediatrics[1] has concluded that the dosage for school children may be increased to a maximum of 80 mg per day (2 mg/kg) for methylphenidate and about 40 mg per day for dextroamphetamine. An occasional child who does not respond to either of these drugs may respond to amphetamine. Werry,[51] on the other hand, believes that dosage at this level should be regarded as exceptional rather than average. In his opinion, most children will respond to lower doses and

the higher doses could have an adverse effect on growth and weight.

Antidepressants

Drugs classified as antidepressants include the monoamine oxidase inhibitors and the iminodibenzyl (tricyclic) derivatives. The monoamine oxidase inhibitors are thought to exert an effect on the metabolism of serotonin and norepinephrine. Initially these drugs were greeted with enthusiasm, but now they seem to have little place in the treatment of children. The types of depressions said to be treated successfully in adults do not occur often in childhood and adolescence. In addition, adverse side effects and toxicity are a serious problem. Serious effects involving hypertension may occur with the ingestion of cheese, alcohol, and other foods and from sympathomimetic amines in patent medicine and other preparations. *Iproniazide* (Marsalid), which has produced liver intoxication and other markedly adverse effects in adults, is now banned in the United States. Isocarboxazid (Marplan) also has produced adverse side-effects, including cardiac dysrhythmias, hypotension, and disturbances in a number of physiologic systems.

Several of these agents have been used to treat disorders other than depression. *Nialamide* (Niamid) and *phenelzine* (Nardil) have been administered to autistic and seriously withdrawn adolescents. They were reported to show an increased awareness of their surroundings as a consequence. The results seem equivocal, however, and adverse effects remain a problem.

Drugs in the iminodibenzl group have been reported to alleviate depression in adolescents, and some controlled studies[51] support the conclusion that *imipramine* (Tofranil) has this beneficial effect. The effects of this drug on children's moods and behavior is still under investigation by the Food and Drug Administration, however, and its use for patients under 12 years old is not approved. Imipramine has also been reported to be effective in the symptomatic treatment of enuresis in a number of uncontrolled and in some controlled studies, although positive effects were not demonstrated in some other controlled studies. It has also been used to treat hyperactivity and school phobia,[27] but the studies that were done had some methodologic problems, and the adverse effects of the drug were significant.

The side-effects of imipramine include dryness of the mouth, dizziness, lethargy, sweating, increased heart rate and blood pressure, nausea, insomnia, constipation, disturbance of appetite, agitation, and tremors. Winsberg and his colleagues[54] have reported serious toxic reactions in children, including electrocardiographic abnormalities, with sufficient prolongation of the PR interval to produce continuing first-degree atrioventricular block in some patients. In another study, a child who developed hypotension after being treated with imipramine for enuresis also showed a first-degree atrioventricular block. Seizures in previously seizure-free children have been reported,[40] and Saraf and his colleagues[44] reported the sudden death of a child who had received an unusually large single dose of imipramine at bedtime (14.7 mg/kg) for school phobia.

Because of these findings and other considerations, the Food and Drug Administration[31] has recommended that in further investigations of imipramine the dosage be limited to a maximum of $2\frac{1}{4}$ mg per kg of body weight per day, and that regular electrocardiographic monitoring be instituted when doses approach this limit. Werry[51] recommends a maximum total daily dose of 100 mg except under unusual circumstances.

Amitryptyline (Elavil) is closely related to imipramine. It has been said to be effective in the treatment of enuresis and hyperactivity. Its side-effects include convulsions, overexcitement, and hypotension. *Protriptyline* (Aventyl) has also been used to treat enuresis, but its side-effects have been found to be more intense than those of imipramine and amytryptyline.

Clearly, the iminodibenzyl compounds are potent drugs, and they have been used in many studies. But they have dangerously adverse side-effects, particularly imipramine, and if they are prescribed at all for children, they should be used with great caution and in low dosages. In my opinion, the risks do not outweigh the benefits. They are not generally helpful in alleviating depression in children, and they are only occasionally of benefit in the treatment of depression in adolescents.[51]

Hallucinogens (Psychotomimetics)

The hallucinogenic drugs, which include lysergic acid diethylamide (LSD–25), mescaline, and psylocybin, have been mainly used in research studies on adults. LSD–25 has been used in the treatment of seriously withdrawn and chronically psychotic children, but the results of the treatment are not clear-cut. The safety of these drugs for children is not certain, and their use is not recommended.[7,46]

Other Drugs

Lithium carbonate has been used to treat adults who have manic-depressive (affective) psychotic disorders. Such disorders do not seem to occur in any explicit form in children, and they occur only rarely in adolescents. The drug has some adverse side-effects, and it has been used only investigationally in the treatment of adolescents. *Anticonvulsants,* such as Dilantin, have been used to treat children who have behavior disorders without seizures, particularly when their EEGs are abnormal. However, several studies indicate that these drugs have no positive effects and their adverse effects can be serious. According to reviews by Campbell[7] and Sprague and Werry,[46] *hormones, glutamic acids,* and *megavitamins* do not benefit children who have psychotic disorders. The removal of certain foods and additives from the diet of hyperactive children, as recommended by Feingold,[24] has only recently received careful study. In a double-blind crossover study of school-age children, Harley and his colleagues[30] have found no support for the Feingold hypothesis, and Werry[50] believes that the cumbersome diet may carry a slight risk in inadequately supervised cases in which nutrition may already be a problem.

Summary

Many sophisticated clinicians now agree that the psychoactive drugs that have been carefully studied and proved useful, and at the same time have no significantly harmful side-effects, are relatively small in number. In my opinion, thioridazine (Mellaril) is the safest drug to administer to children who have markedly agitated, disorganized, or severely disturbed (sometimes psychotic) behavior patterns. If thioridazine is ineffective chlorpromazine (Thorazine) can be used. Children who are hyperactive, impulsive, and (sometimes) aggressive respond best to dextroamphetamine (Dexedrine) or methylphenidate (Ritalin), as part of a program of treatment and educational measures. Certain other target symptoms, (e.g., maladie des tics and enuresis) may be helped by drugs such as haloperidol and imipramine, but not without risk. With proper precautions, adolescents who are seriously depressed can be treated with imipramine (Tofranil) in conjunction with psychotherapy or other treatment. Markedly anxious but nonpsychotic children may respond best to diphenhydramine (Benadryl) as a part of the total treatment plan. When sedation is indicated for children, it is best achieved with chloral hydrate or Benadryl, whereas paraldehyde is a useful drug for sedating adolescents.

Ordinarily it is best to defer the use of psychoactive drugs until clinical evaluation of the child and parents has been completed and a diagnostic formulation and total treatment plan achieved. The supportive effect of such an approach, particularly if it is carried out in a hospital setting, sometimes results in clinical improvement that might otherwise be attributed to the effects of drugs.[48] When required, liquid forms of medication are generally preferable to crushed tablets for children. In *emergency or crisis situations*, involving panic states, agitated behavior, disorganized thinking, sweeping regression or "frozen" withdrawal in children or adolescents, immediate use of medication may be necessary. Medication can be withheld later in order to gauge the child's ability to cope, as Fish[22] has suggested. In brief, significant symptomatic improvement in the shortest period of time with a minimum of side-effects is the goal of such treatment. As Smith[45] has indicated, however, some transient side-effects may be permissible in order to prevent further decompensation of the child's adaptive balance and his psychologic support systems. Higher dosages than would be acceptable in a routine approach therefore may be used initially, sometimes to the point of significant side-effects. However, a balance between symptomatic relief and minimal side-effects should be sought that does not result in impairment of the child's functioning. Of course, the possible side-effects must be fully discussed with the parents and older children if outpatient management is undertaken.

Even in crisis situations in which some side-effects may be acceptable, the least toxic drug possible should always be used. Some investigators, such as Lourie,[36] recommend a major tranquilizer, such as one of the phenothiazines, to treat adolescents who have acute anxiety states or acute psychotic states accompanied by disorganized thought patterns or depression. Some (e.g. Fish[23]) feel that reduction of anxiety or hyperactivity in children and young adolescents can usually be achieved with the use of a minor tranquilizer, most often diphenhydramine, which can be given intramuscularly if necessary. In the opinion of Kavanaugh and Mattsson[33] the use of major tranquilizers in crisis situations should be reserved for patients whose acute personality disorganization poses serious management problems and for whom the less potent minor tranquilizers have not been rapidly effective. I subscribe to their view, as well to their belief that the stimulant drugs have little place in crisis situations involving children showing hyperactivity, because of limited time for diagnostic evaluation.

If a major tranquilizer is used, it should be given in adequate dosage. A major portion of the 24-hour dose should be administered at bedtime in order to take advantage of the sedative effects and to minimize the possibility of drowsiness during waking hours. Kavanaugh and Mattsson have found that chlorpromazine is usually the most quickly effective of the major tranquilizers. This drug can be given rectally or intramuscularly if indicated; intravenous administration is not recommended. Thioridazine may also be effective; it is available in liquid form. It is not recommended for children under 2 years old. Imipramine may be used with appropriate precautions to treat acutely depressed adolescents, although thioridazine, which has some antidepressant effect, may be safer. If major tranquilizers are administered parenterally, careful observation for symptoms of hypotension, dystonia, and other potentially serious side-effects should be maintained for at least 1 hour following administration, and antidotes such as Benadryl and Cogentin should be readily available. If medication is prescribed, particularly if it is to be administered by injection, both the parents and the child should be prepared in advance, in accordance with the principles outlined in Chapter 7. Particular care should be taken that medication not be interpreted by younger children

as punishment or by older children and adolescents as an attempt at control or domination on the part of the physician or parents.

Bibliography

1. American Academy of Pediatrics, Council on child health: Medication for hyperkinetic children. Pediatrics, 53:560, 1975.
2. Arnold, L., et al.: Levoamphetamine vs. dextroamphetamine in minimal brain dysfunction. Arch. Gen. Psychiatry, 33:292, 1976.
3. Beck, L., et al.: Childhood chemotherapy and later drug abuse and growth curve: A follow-up study of 30 adolescents. Am. J. Psychiatry, 132:436, 1975.
4. Beecher, H.K.: Measurement of Subjective Responses: Quantitative Effects of Drugs. New York, Oxford University Press, 1959.
5. Beecher, H.K.: Increased stress and effectiveness of placebos and "active drugs." Science, 132:91, 1960.
6. Bradley, C.: The behavior of children receiving benzadrine. Am. J. Psychiatry, 94:577, 1937.
7. Campbell, M.: Psychopharmacology in childhood psychoses. Int. J. Ment. Health, 4:238, 1975.
8. Casey, D.E., and Rabins, P.: Tardive dyskinesia as a life-threatening illness. Am J. Psychiatry, 135:486, 1978.
9. Conners, C.K.: Psychopharmacology of psychopathology in childhood. In: Psychopathological Disorders of Childhood (H. Quay, and J. Werry, Eds.). New York, Wiley, 1972.
10. Conners, C.K.: Methodological considerations in drug research with children. In: Psychopharmacology in Childhood and Adolescence. (J.M. Wiener, Ed.). New York, Basic Books, 1977.
11. Conners, C.K., and Eisenberg, L.: The effects of methylphenidate on symptomatology and learning in disturbed children. Am. J. Psychiatry, 120:458, 1963.
12. Conners, C.K., Eisenberg, L., and Barcai, A.: The effect of dextroamphetamine on children. Arch. Gen. Psychiatry, 17:478, 1967.
13. Conners, C.K., et al.: Dextroamphetamine sulfate in children with learning disorders: Effects on perception, learning, and achievement. Arch. Gen. Psychiatry, 21:182, 1969.
14. Davis, J.M., et al.: Overdosage of psychotropic drugs: A review. I. Dis. Nerv. Syst., 29:157, 1968.
14a. Davis, J.M., et al.: Overdosage of psychotropic drugs: A Review. II. Dis. Nerv. Syst., 29:246, 1968.
15. DiMascio, A., Soltys, J.J., and Shader, R.I.: Psychotropic drug side effects in children. In: Psychotropic Drug Side Effects, Clinical and Theoretical Perspectives. (R.I. Shader and A. DiMascio, Eds.). Baltimore, Williams & Wilkins, 1970.
16. Eisenberg, L.: The role of drugs in treating disturbed children. Children, 11:167, 1964.
17. Eisenberg, L.: Principles of drug therapy in child psychiatry with special reference to stimulant drugs. Am. J. Orthopsychiatry, 41:371, 1971.

18. Eisenberg, L.: The clinical use of stimulant drugs in children. Pediatrics, 49:709, 1972.
19. Eisenberg, L., Connors, C.K., and Sharpe, L.: A controlled study of the differential application of outpatient psychiatric treatment of children. Jap. J. Child Psychiatry, 6:125, 1965.
20. Eisenberg, L., et al.: The effectiveness of psychotherapy alone or in conjunction with perphenazine or placebo in the treatment of neurotic and hyperkinetic children. Am. J. Psychiatry, 117:1088, 1961.
21. Eisenberg, L., et al.: A psychopharmacologic experiment in a training school for delinquent boys: Methods, problems, findings. Am. J. Orthopsychiatry, 33:431, 1963.
22. Fish, B.: Drug use in psychiatric disorders of children. Am. J. Psychiatry, 124: (Suppl.) 31, 1968.
23. Fish, B.: The "one child, one drug" myth of stimulants in hyperkinesis: Importance of diagnostic categories in evaluating treatments. Arch. Gen. Psychiatry, 25:193, 1971.
24. Feingold, B.: Why Your Child Is Hyperactive. New York, Random House, 1975.
25. Freeman, H.: The therapeutic value of combinations of psychotropic drugs: A review. Psychopharmacol. Bull., 4:1, 1967.
26. Freeman, R.D.: Psychopharmacology and the retarded child. In: Psychiatric Approaches to Mental Retardation. (F.J. Menascolino, Ed.). New York, Basic Books, 1970.
27. Gittelman-Klein, R., and Klein, D.F.: Controlled imipramine treatment of school phobia. Arch. Gen. Psychiatry, 25:204, 1971.
28. Grinspoon, L., and Bakalar, J.B.: The amphetamines: Medical uses and health hazards. Psychiatr. Ann., 7:81, 1977.
29. Gupta, J.M., and Lovejoy, F.H.,Jr.: Phenothiazine toxicity may be relieved by diphenhydramine. Pediatrics, 39:771, 1967.
30. Harley, J.P., et al.: Hyperkinesis and food additives: Testing the Feingold hypothesis. Pediatrics, 61:818, 1978.
31. Hayes, T., Panitch, M., and Barker, E.: Imipramine dosage in children. Am. J. Psychiatry, 132:546, 1975.
32. Hill, R.M., Desmond, M.M., and Kay, J.L.: Extrapyramidal dysfunction in an infant of a schizophrenic mother. J. Pediatr., 69:589, 1963.
33. Kavanaugh, J.C., and Mattsson, A.: Drug therapy in child psychiatric emergencies. In: Emergencies in Child Psychiatry (G.C. Morrison, Ed.). Springfield, Ill., Thomas, 1975.
34. Kraft, I.A.: The use of psychoactive drugs in the outpatient treatment of psychiatric disorders of children. Am. J. Psychiatry, 124:95, 1968.
35. Leestma, J.E.: Sudden death and phenothiazines: A current controversy. Arch. Gen. Psychiatry, 18:137, 1968.
36. Lourie, R.S.: Psychoactive drugs in pediatrics. Pediatrics, 34:691, 1964.
37. Lucas, A.R., and Weiss, M.: Methylphenidate hallucinosis. JAMA, 217:1079, 1971.
38. Mattson, R.H., and Calverley, J.R.: Dextroamphetamine sulfate-induced dyskinesis. JAMA, 204:400, 1968.

39. Mehta, D., Mallya, A., and Volavka, J.: Mortality of patients with tardive dyskinesia. Am. J. Psychiatry, 135:371, 1978.
40. Petti, T.A., and Campbell, M.: Imipramine and seizures. Am. J. Psychiatry, 132:538, 1975.
41. Pharmacotherapy of Children: Pediatric psychopharmacological packages. In: Psychopharmacological Bulletin Special Issue. Washington, D.C., National Institute of Mental Health, 1973.
42. Polizos, P., et al.: Neurological consequences of psychotropic drug withdrawal in schizophrenic children. Autism Childhood Schiz., 3:247, 1973.
43. Safer, D., Allen, R., and Barr, E.: Depression of growth in hyperactive children on stimulant drugs. N. Engl. J. Med., 287:217, 1972.
44. Saraf, K.R., et al.: Imipramine side effects in children. Psychopharmacologia, 37:265, 1974.
45. Smith, W.F., Jr.: Determinants influencing the use of psychoactive drugs in the management of psychiatric emergencies in children and adolescents. In: Emergencies in Child Psychiatry (G.C. Morrison, Ed.). Springfield, Ill., Thomas, 1975.
46. Sprague, R., and Werry, J.: Methodology of psychopharmacological studies with the retarded. In: International Review of Research in Mental Retardation (N.R. Ellis, Ed.). New York, Academic Press, 1971.
47. Sprague, R.L., and Werry, J.: Psychotropic drugs in handicapped children. In: Second Review of Special Education (L. Mann, and D. Sabatino, Eds.). Philadelphia, Journal of Special Education Press, 1974.
48. Vasey, I., and Prugh, D.G.: Unpublished material.
49. Werry, J.S.: Diagnosis for psychopharmacological studies in children. In: Psychopharmacological Bulletin Special Issue: Pharmacotherapy of Children. Washington, D.C., National Institute of Mental Health, 1973.
50. Werry, J.: Diet and Hyperactivity. Med. J. Aust., 2:281, 1976.
51. Werry, J.S.: The use of psychotropic drugs in children. J. Am. Acad. Child. Psychiatry, 16:446, 1977.
52. Werry, J.S., Ed.: Pediatric Psychopharmacology. New York, Brunner/Mazel, 1978.
53. Wiener, J.M., Ed.: Psychopharmacology in Childhood and Adolescence. New York, Basic Books, 1977.
54. Winsberg, B.G., et al.: Imipramine and electrocardiographic abnormalities in hyperactive children. Am. J. Psychiatry, 132:542, 1975.

General References

Beecher, H.K.: The powerful placebo. JAMA, 159:1602, 1955.
Boatman, J.J., and Berlin, I.N.: Some implications of incidental experiences with psychopharmacologic drugs in a children's psychotherapeutic program. J. Am. Acad. Child Psychiatry, 1:431, 1962.
Cytryn, L., Gilbert, A., and Eisenberg, L.: The effectiveness of tranquilizing drugs plus supportive psychotherapy in treating behavior disorders of

children: A double-blind study of eighty out-patients. Am. J. Orthopsychiatry, *30*:113, 1960.

Fisher, S., Ed.: *Child Research in Psychopharmacology.* Springfield, Ill., Thomas, 1959.

Gerard, R.W.: Drugs for the soul: The rise of psychopharmacology. Science, *125: 201, 1957.*

Heninger, G., DiMascio, A., and Klerman, G.L.: Personality factors in variability of response to phenothiazines. Am. J. Psychiatry, *121*:1091, 1965.

Lucas, A.R.: Psychopharmacologic treatment. In: *The Psychiatric Disorders of Childhood* (C.R. Shaw, Ed.). New York, Appleton-Century-Crofts, 1966.

Malitz, S., and Kanzler, M.: Are antidepressants better than placebo? Am. J. Psychiatry, *127*:41, 1971.

Naditch, M.P., Alker, P.C., and Joffe, P.: Individual differences and setting as determinants of acute adverse reactions to psychoactive drugs. J. Nerv. Ment. Dis., *161*:326, 1975.

Oettinger, L., Jr.: The use of deanol in the treatment of disorders of behavior in children. J. Pediatr., *53*:671, 1958.

Prugh, D.G., and Kisley, A.: Psychopharmacologic agents. (Appendix D.) In: *The Mental Health of Children: Services, Research, and Manpower* (Reports of Task Forces IV and V and Report of the Committee on Clinical Issues by the Joint Commission on Mental Health of Children.) New York, Harper & Row, 1973.

Stone, W.N., et al.: Impact of the psychosocial factors on the conduct of combined drug and psychotherapy research. Br. J. Psychiatry, *127*:432, 1975.

Werry, J.S., and Sprague, R.L.: Psychopharmacology. In: *Mental Retardation*, Vol. 4. (J. Wortis, Ed.). New York, Grune & Stratton, 1972.

14
Principles of Diagnosis and Classification

Physicians think they do a lot for a patient when
they give his disease a name.
(Immanuel Kant)

The classification of individual personality pictures is necessary and helpful, but it is arbitrary and artificial in many respects. The marked discrepancies in approaches to the classification of psychopathologic disorders in children and adolescents and the disparities among the terms used to refer to those disorders underscore the need for a classification that is separate from that of adults and that uses reasonably explicit and clearly defined categories that can be employed by clinicians from varying theoretical or experiential backgrounds. Although as Hobbs[25] has pointed out, there are dangers in making loose diagnoses or "labeling," categories are needed to facilitate communication in practice, teaching, and research.

The current official psychiatric classification of children's disorders ("Behavioral Disorders of Childhood and Adolescence") appears in the 1969 revision of the AMA *Standard Nomenclature of Diseases and Oper-*ations. (It is also published in the second (1969) edition of the *Diagnostic and Statistical Manual of Mental Disorders*—DSM II).[1] This is an improvement over the previous psychiatric classification (DSM–I) in that it at least has a separate section on children's disorders (the DSM–I did not). However, the children's section has been widely criticized by child psychiatrists and other child mental health professionals[15,18,20,41,55] as being a typology, not a classification, composed mainly of symptom complexes or partial symptom responses. That limitation and the fact that child mental health professionals use a variety of diagnostic terms make it difficult to collect epidemiologic data on mental and emotional disorders in childhood and adolescents.

The available data,[3,5,10,31,50,52,61] which have been well summarized by Anthony,[2] support the view of Buckle and Lebovici[11] that all children sometimes show signs of disturbed behavior (e.g., breath holding, nail biting, and excessive fearfulness). I agree with Anthony that the dividing line between normal behavior and disordered behavior is not a fixed one, and that it fluctuates in different social and cultural settings, with "sensitive" periods at different levels of the child's development. In 1970, the Joint Commission on Mental Health of Children[12] estimated that 8% to 12% of the children and adolescents in the United States (between 2 and 3 million) needed professional help for emotional and mental disorders. It was estimated also that only about 10% of these young people were receiving diagnostic evaluation and about 10% of those evaluated would receive the treatment they needed. In 1962, the President's Commission on Mental Retardation[43] had estimated that 3% of the children and adolescents in the United States were mentally retarded. There is probably some overlapping in these figures, as there is with the estimate that 10% to 15% or more[56] of children in the United States have learning problems. In the 1979 report of the President's Commission on Mental Health,[44] the estimates of emotional and mental disorders were even higher, particularly among impoverished and minority families. (The estimates took into account the high-risk factors mentioned in Chapter 2.)

A classification of psychopathologic disorders of childhood and adolescence has been proposed in recent years by the Committee on Child Psychiatry of the Group for Advancement of Psychiatry (GAP).[23] The classification is based upon a conceptual framework embracing 3 basic propositions: (1) the psychosomatic concept, (2) the developmental concept, and (3) the psychosocial concept. That conceptual framework is in basic harmony with the concepts of health and disease, adaptation, and the interrelationships among physiologic, psychologic, and social levels of organization and development of the human personality discussed earlier in this book.

The psychosomatic concept underlies the unity of response of the human organism. Psychopathologic syndromes represent only one type of response, at the psychologic level, when adaptation breaks down, with other levels also involved. The developmental concept underscores the fact that classification is relative, depending upon the child's developmental stage and the dimension of development that is involved. The psychosocial concept supports the conclusion that the clinician must regard the family rather than the individual as the essential unit for the study and treatment of health and disease. All three propositions support the concept of multiple etiologic factors of predisposing, contributory, precipitating, and perpetuating nature, as suggested by the unitary theory of health and disease mentioned earlier.

As the GAP Report indicated, the ideal classification would permit a synthesis of the clinical picture, the psychodynamic and psychosocial factors, considerations about the developmental level of origin of conflicts,* the major etiologic forces, a concise prognosis, and the appropriate method of treatment. But although the present knowledge of parent-child relationships and family patterns of interaction is growing, it is still too limited to permit classification on these grounds. Because internal (intrinsic or innate) and external (experiential or acquired) etiologic factors are involved in all disease pictures, classification of psychopathologic disorders on the basis of etiology is difficult (although an international committee of the World Health Organization has begun an attempt to do so.[51]) For example, the death of a parent during a child's early years bears a significant relationship to such adult disorders

---

*Freud used the term genetic-dynamic to refer to the developmental level of origin of emotional conflicts. But Freud's term is easily confused with hereditary origins, and it is mentioned here only because the reader may encounter it in some psychoanalytic publications. Engel coined the term "genic" to clarify the difference. I will use the term developmental level of origin, because I think it is clearer.

as psychoneurosis, schizophrenia, delinquency, depression, and alcoholism, as various studies[10] have demonstrated. Yet many times the death of a parent is not associated with these disorders; multiple etiologic factors, including unresolved grief, are undoubtedly involved.

In regard to prognosis, there are other problems. Different disorders often arise at different levels of development. The available longitudinal studies,[17,29,38,46,47,58] although they support the concept that, without help, children who have many or severe problems do not "grow out of them," leave unanswered some questions about the relationship of certain early disorders to later ones. As Rutter[49] has pointed out in a recent review, some disorders (e.g., delinquency and antisocial behavior) have their roots in early childhood and if they are not treated they often continue into adult life. Other disorders, such as psychoneurotic disorders, seem to be different in important ways from the adult form, and they may not continue into adult life. Similar symptoms at a particular developmental stage (e.g., adolescence) may be associated with different degrees of disorder in adaptation.

That there are sex differences in the incidence of reported symptom patterns from early childhood is evident from the literature.[8,32,60] In his wide-ranging review of disorders in behavior, Anthony[2] estimates that in Western countries boys are referred for help for social or emotional disorders more than 10 times as often as girls are. These disorders include aggressive behavior and delinquency in general, stuttering, reading difficulties and school failure, and speech, hearing, and eye problems. There appears to be a sex difference in the peak ages of referrals. Boys begin to peak when they are 9 to 10 years old, and they reach their peak at 14 to 15 years old. Girls begin to peak when they are 14 to 15 years old, and they reach their peak at 15 to 17 years old. It is well known that infant mortality and morbidity are higher for boys than for girls.

Referrals of nonwhite children occur less often in childhood but rise sharply during adolescence.

Anthony concludes that many sex differences probably are a result largely of the cultural factors that determine the sex roles. He believes that the differences between boys and girls in regard to physical aggressiveness, which are apparent at least in the early preschool-age period, may be related to physical or hormonal factors or to a difference in how boys and girls respond to challenge (as Murphy[39] has suggested) but that social and cultural factors are certainly importantly involved also. In a recent study,[48] parents were found to have perceptions of their child's "maleness" or "femaleness" within the first 24 hours of the child's birth, which suggests that sextyping and sex-role socialization of the child begin at his birth.

The sex roles of women and the family roles of men have been changing significantly,[6,26] and with the help of Horney[28] and other women psychoanalysts and psychologists, views on feminine psychology have undergone major changes. These observers see feminine psychology much differently than did Helena Deutsch[13] and other earlier writers.

For various reasons, attempts to balance these factors must be reserved for the diagnostic formulation. At present, only the clinical-descriptive aspects can be dealt with in a classification that is susceptible to the use of statistical methods and that can be used by people from different schools of thought.

The GAP (Group for Advancement of Psychiatry) Classification

The GAP classification involves a set of operational definitions of clinical categories. It is based on a conceptual framework with which it was hoped that clinicians from varying backgrounds might agree. Besides the psychosomatic, developmental, and psychosocial points of view mentioned, the GAP classification considers contributions from psychoanalysis, as well as from learning theory, neurophysiology, child development, social science, and ethology. The GAP classification is descriptive, not explanatory, although some inferences about etiology are inevitably present in the operational definitions of some of the categories. The schema enables multiple classifications to be made where appropriate and thus permits a more total personality diagnosis to be made. For example, a more total personality diagnosis of a psychoneurotic or personality disorder may be added to a "part" diagnosis of (for example) psychophysiologic disorder, brain syndrome, or mental retardation. The GAP classification includes an extensive list of symptoms that permits symptoms to be reported independently or in association with diagnosis, and it permits the diagnosis of "normality" ("healthy responses") to be made. It also offers a concept of "developmental deviations" appropriate to childhood and familiar to child clinicians, as well as definitions specific to childhood in regard to other categories, and a glossary of terms.

The GAP classification was presented simply as a point of departure for clinicians who work with children to use, criticize, and modify, since there was no available classification of child psychopathologic disorders on which clinicians agree, in spite of over 20 attempts in this country and Europe. The GAP classification has generally been well received, but it has not been universally approved. Its conceptual approach and its theoretical framework have been critized by some.[18,20,22,53] But Ashburner,[3] in Australia, feels that its conceptual approach is coherent and that the system can readily be understood by clinicians from different schools of thought. Criticisms of its failure to employ criteria for disorders in psychosocial functioning that may not correspond with clinical diagnosis have

been rightly made. The author, who was chairman of the GAP committee when it formulated its classification, later offered to the Joint Commission on Mental Health of Children a proposed classification based on levels of psychosocial function and dysfunction[41] that involved a developmental framework and that correlated with the GAP nomenclature. This was developed in order to try to meet the above criticism and to encourage its usage and modification by others, including those who are not mental health professionals. The classification also involved the concept of a "grid,"[22] composed of community agencies and professionals necessary for the diagnosis and treatment of disorders at different developmental levels and of differing degrees of limitations in functioning.

Since its appearance, the GAP classification has been widely used by individual professionals and in children's psychiatric facilities in the United States and elsewhere. As an alternative to the AMA Standard Nomenclature, it has been recommended for use in at least 2 major textbooks,[21,54] and it has been translated into several languages. Although it deals with social class and ethnic[14] factors to only a limited extent, its use in an urban child psychiatry service has been supported by Bemporad and his colleagues,[9] as well as others. Loof[34] has found at least parts of the classification helpful in dealing with the problems of rural children in Appalachia. Ashburner[3] and others have made specific suggestions about how the GAP classification might be modified or adapted to the Standard Nomenclature or the International Classifications of Diseases (ICD–8)[59] to permit a more effective and appropriate classification of psychopathologic disorders in childhood and adolescence. Ashburner's recommendations about how to integrate the GAP classification into Section 5 of the ICD–8 have been accepted by the National Health and Medical Research Council of Australia,[40] and the GAP classification is used officially by the Child Psychiatry Society of Australia and New Zealand.

The applicability of the GAP classification to different settings and in different countries has been demonstrated, and the classification may properly be thought of as at least having international implications for child mental health professionals. In my view and that of Jordan and Schmitt, (cited in Chapter 9), the diagnoses based on the GAP classification can also be used by pediatricians and other health care personnel, sometimes with consultative aid, in evaluating and planning the treatment of children and adolescents who have various types of psychosocial disorders. Since its conceptual framework is based on a developmental and adaptational model, it fits well with broader theoretical approaches, such as Erikson's (see Chapter 5), and it does not suffer from the narrower "disease-oriented" limitations of the traditional "medical" model. (All categories in the GAP classification are referred to as disorders.)

The discussion which follows in Chapters 15 to 23 draws heavily on the work of the GAP committee, using operational definitions drawn up by them, with some modifications.

The proposed major categories and subcategories are arranged rather arbitrarily in a hierarchy that ranges roughly from healthy responses, through milder to more severe psychologic disorders, to syndromes in which somatic factors may predominate. The placing of the healthier (or the less disturbed) groups at the top of the hierarchy reflects the committee's general optimism about prognosis in childhood disorders, with significant exceptions. The following is a list of the major categories and the proposed subcategories.

1. Healthy Responses
   a. Developmental crises
   b. Situational crises
   c. Other responses
2. Reactive disorders
3. Developmental deviations
   a. Deviations in maturational patterns
   b. Deviations in specific dimensions of development
      (1) Motor
      (2) Sensory
      (3) Speech
      (4) Cognitive functions
      (5) Social development
      (6) Psychosexual
      (7) Affective
      (8) Integrative
   c. Other developmental deviations
4. Psychoneurotic disorders
   a. Anxiety type
   b. Phobic type
   c. Conversion type
   d. Dissociative type
   e. Obsessive-compulsive type
   f. Depressive type
   g. Other psychoneurotic disorders
5. Personality disorders
   a. Compulsive personality
   b. Hysterical
   c. Anxious
   d. Overly dependent
   e. Oppositional
   f. Overly inhibited
   g. Overly independent
   h. Isolated
   i. Mistrustful
   j. Tension-discharge disorders
      (1) Impulse ridden personality
      (2) Neurotic personality disorder
   k. Sociosyntonic personality disorder
   l. Sexual deviation
   m. Other personality disorders
6. Psychotic disorders
   a. Psychoses of infancy and early childhood
      (1) Early infantile autism
      (2) Interactional psychotic disorder
      (3) Other
   b. Psychoses of later childhood
      (1) Schizophreniform psychotic disorder
      (2) Other
   c. Psychoses of adolescence
      (1) Acute confusional state
      (2) Schizophrenic disorder, adult type
      (3) Other
7. Psychophysiologic disorders
   a. Skin
   b. Musculoskeletal
   c. Respiratory
   d. Cardiovascular
   e. Hemic and lymphatic
   f. Gastrointestinal
   g. Genitourinary

h. Endocrine
i. Of the nervous system
j. Of the organs of special sense
k. Other psychophysiologic disorders
8. Brain syndromes
   a. Acute
   b. Chronic
9. Mental retardation
10. Other disorders

Modifying statements may be added to the major categories, as in the Standard Nomenclature. The modifying statements would incorporate the dimension of acuteness or chronicity (with acuteness distinguished from reversibility), degree of severity (mild, moderate, or severe), and the manifest nature of individual symptoms. Although certain disorders, such as psychoneuroses, personality disorders, and particular types of psychotic disorders, are viewed as occurring only after a particular point in development, the broad age range and the developmental level can be specified in each instance (infancy, early childhood, later childhood, or adolescence).

Although there is not a published study that is based on the results of systematic concomitant use of the GAP nomenclature and DSM II, one study by Bemporad and his colleagues[9] compared the GAP classification with the previous version of the Standard Nomenclature (DSM I) and concluded that the GAP classification differentiated diagnostic categories more effectively. Others have had the impression that the GAP classification is more reliable and is more readily susceptible to statistical treatment than is the current version of the Standard Nomenclature.[4,19] Various investigators, such as Finch,[18] Fish,[20] Harrison,[24] Rexford,[45] and Engel,[16] have approved the use of the category "healthy responses," (formerly unclassifiable*) and of the category "developmental deviations" (also formerly unclassifiable) as a primary diagnosis or in combination with an accompanying personality diagnosis. They also expressed

the opinion that including childhood variants of some adult personality disorders in the classification allowed the diagnosis of less severe and as yet unsolidified personality disorders. These include the term "isolated" rather than "schizoid" and "mistrustful" rather than "paranoid." In addition, it has been felt that the inclusion of new subcategories of personality disorders (e.g., overly dependent, oppositional, and overly inhibited) permitted clinicians to describe more specifically the types of personality problems actually encountered in children.

For the sake of clarity, several examples of the nomenclature which can be used in actual classification and diagnosis are given in the following pages; these examples draw on the principal categories and the subcategories, as well as on the symptom list. (The symptom list is organized around (1) disturbances related to bodily functions, (2) disturbances related to cognitive functions, (3) disturbances in affective behavior, (4) disturbances related to development, (5) disturbances in social behavior, and (6) disturbances in integrative behavior.)

1. Healthy response of early childhood—developmental crisis type, acute, mild, manifested by separation anxiety and clinging behavior.
2. Reactive disorder of early childhood—acute, moderate, manifested by regressive encopresis, thumb sucking, and withdrawn behavior.
3. Developmental deviation of later childhood—delayed maturational pattern type, chronic, moderate, manifested by impulsive behavior, low frustration tolerance, continued enuresis, reading disability, and persistence of prelogical thought processes.
4. Psychoneurotic disorder of later childhood—phobic type, acute, severe, manifested by fear of school,** separation anxiety, and morning nausea.

---

*Under the DSM-II, to diagnose health clinicians have had to choose the category "no disease" or the category "no diagnosis".

**School phobia, a syndrome, may be part of a phobic psychoneurotic disorder, or, in children just entering school, a manifestation of a marked developmental crisis over separation-individuation. It may be also part of a reactive disorder to a chronic physical illness, or it may even be one of a constellation of symptoms in a psychotic disorder. Other syndromes may also fall into different diagnostic categories.

5. Personality disorder of later childhood—compulsive type, chronic, moderate, manifested by ritualistic behavior, counting compulsions, and obsessive rumination.

6. Psychotic disorder of later childhood—schizophreniform type, chronic, severe, manifested by autistic behavior, associative (thought) disorder, resistance to change, whirling, echolalia, ritualistic behavior, and panic states.

7. Psychophysiologic skin disorder of early adolescence—chronic, moderate, manifested by neurodermatitis, marked scratching, and inhibited behavior.

8. Personality disorder of middle adolescence—overly inhibited type, chronic, severe, manifested by withdrawn behavior, learning inhibition, and hesitant speech.

The principles involved in making diagnostic formulations, a prognostic statement, and a treatment plan, were discussed in Chapter 9. The diagnostic categories and subcategories are discussed in greater detail in Chapters 15 to 23. (In this approach, enuresis and hyperactivity are treated as symptoms. Enuresis may be a continuing feature of a developmental deviation, a symptom of a regressive nature in a reactive disorder, a conversion symptom as part of a psychoneurotic disorder, or one of a constellation of symptoms in a psychotic disorder. Hyperactivity may be part of a developmental deviation, a symptom of anxiety in a reactive disorder, a manifestation of diffuse brain damage, or part of a psychotic disorder. Encopresis and other symptoms are treated similarly.)

Although the GAP classification is widely used in child mental health facilities,[9,19,37,42] it has not yet been accepted by the American Psychiatric Association and the American Medical Association. Official data are still reported in the form of DSM-II,[1] which has been adapted to the Psychiatric Section of the ICD-8. (The GAP classification can be similarly adapted, as Ashburner[3] has shown.) North Carolina, on the recommendation of Behar,[7] has officially adopted the GAP classification, and has arranged with Blue Cross and CHAMPUS to accept it. (The GAP section on mental retardation

recommends the use of the currently accepted classification of mental retardation offered by the American Association on Mental Deficiency.[36])

In 1974 a task force on the classification of emotionally disturbed children was set up; it was composed of Prugh, Engel, and Morse.[42] The classification was part of a project on classification of children that was led by Hobbs[25] and underwritten by the Department of Health, Education, and Welfare. The task force recommended the GAP classification as a workable system for child mental health clinicians and other health professionals that transcends the traditional "medical" model but can be integrated into the "official" classification systems used nationally and internationally. Since the GAP classification has no inherent pejorative or "professional" implications, it could be meshed with a classification based on levels of psychosocial functioning that is similar to the one contemplated in North Carolina. Such an approach could be used by other than mental health clinicians, thus offering the possibility of correlation between categories of functioning and appropriate types of intervention and support systems.

As the task force pointed out, the definitions of levels of psychosocial functioning could be translated into a list of the fundamental mental and emotional needs of healthy and disordered children at different levels of development, with important implications for prevention and treatment. Categorical terms will still need to be used for clinical, research, and epidemiologic purposes, but, as Lourie[35] has pointed out, those terms need not dictate treatment patterns, which has often happened in the United States, sometimes with political implications.

A committee of the American Psychiatric Association has revised DSM-II. The revision is referred to as DSM-III. The DSM-III adopts primarily a descriptive approach and, in its early drafts, did away with the distinction between neurotic and psychotic disorders (an important distinction in the view of Kubie[30] and Hollender[27]). Recently, DSM-III has been officially adopted by the American Psychiatric Association.

The DSM-III does have a separate section on the classification of disorders of children and adolescents. This retains a few features from DSM-II, such as conduct disorders, and adds a few drawn from the GAP classification, such as oppositional disorders and some "specific" developmental disorders; it offers several new features, such as attention deficit disorder, with or without hyperactivity. The DSM-III uses a multiaxial approach (proposed originally by the child psychiatry group of the World Health Organization[51]); this permits the estimation of the severity of psychosocial stressors and the level of adaptive functions (the latter somewhat like the approach recommended earlier by Prugh[41]). As a result of pressure from many psychiatrists, the distinction between neurotic and psychotic disorders was retained, although some terms for neurotic disorders were changed. Differential diagnoses are appropriately included. In my opinion, however, the DSM-III often regards symptoms as disorders, and, as discussed by Spitzer and his colleagues,[33] it changes entirely (and inappropriately, in the view of Prugh and others) the approach to psychophysiologic disorders. The writer, though not unbiased regarding the GAP classification, still feels it is the best teaching framework for health care personnel.

Bibliography

1. American Psychiatric Association: *Diagnostic and Statistical Manual of Mental Disorders*, 2nd Ed. Washington, D.C., 1969.
2. Anthony, E.J.: Behavior disorders of childhood. In: *Carmichael's Manual of Child Psychology*, 3rd Ed., Vol. 2 (P. Mussen, Ed.). New York, Wiley, 1970.
3. Ashburner, J.V.: Some problems of classification with particular reference to child psychiatry. Aust. N.Z. J. Psychiatry, 2:244, 1968.
4. Bahn, A.: Personal communication, 1968.
5. Bahn, A.K., Chandler, C.A., and Eisenberg, L.: Diagnostic characteristics related to services in psychiatric clinics for children. Milbank Mem. Fund Q., 1962.
6. Bardwick, J.M.: *Psychology of Women: A Study of Biocultural Conflicts.* New York, Norton, 1970.
7. Behar, L., and Early, B.: A review of several diagnostic classification systems in child mental health. Unpublished material.
8. Beller, E.K., and Neubauer, P.B.: Sex differences and symptom patterns in early childhood. J. Am. Acad. Child Psychiatry, 2:417, 1963.
9. Bemporad, J.R., Pfeiffer, C.M., and Bloom, W.: Twelve months' experience with the GAP classification of childhood disorders. Am. J. Psychiatry, 127:658, 1970.
10. Birtchnell, J.: Early parent death and mental illness. Br. J. Psychiatry, 116:281, 1970.
11. Buckle, D., and Lebovici, S.: *Child Guidance Centers.* Geneva, World Health Organization, 1960.
12. *Crisis for the 70's: Report of the Joint Commission on Mental Health of Children.* New York, Harper & Row, 1970.
13. Deutsch, H.: *The Psychology of Women*, Vols. 1,2. New York, Grune & Stratton, 1945.
14. Deutsch, M., Katz, I., and Jensen, A.: *Social Class, Race, and Psychological Development.* New York, Holt, Rinehart, & Winston, 1968.
15. Engel, M.: Dilemmas of classification and diagnosis. J. Spec. Ed., 3:231, 1969.
16. Engel, M.: *Psychopathology in Childhood: Social, Diagnostic, and Therapeutic Aspects.* New York, Harcourt, Brace, Jovanovich, 1972.
17. Escalona, S., and Heiden, G.M.: Prediction and outcome: A study in child development. In: *Culture and Mental Health* (M.H. Opler, Ed.). New York, Macmillan, 1959.
18. Finch, S.M.: Nomenclature for children's mental disorders needs improvement. Int. J. Psychiatry, 7:414, 1969.
19. Finzer, W.F., and Wagonfeld, S.: Personal communication, 1969.
20. Fish, B.: Limitations of the new nomenclature for children's disorders. Int. J. Psychiatry, 7:393, 1969.
21. Freedman, A.M., and Kaplan, H.I.: *Comprehensive Textbook of Psychiatry*, 2nd Ed. Baltimore, Williams & Wilkins, 1967.
22. Group for the Advancement of Psychiatry: *Critique of Joint Commission Report.* New York, Group for the Advancement of Psychiatry, 1972.
23. Group for the Advancement of Psychiatry: *Psychopathological Disorders in Childhood: Theoretical Considerations and a Proposed Classification*, Vol. 6. Report No. 62. New York, Group for the Advancement of Psychiatry, 1966.
24. Harrison, S.: Review of "psychopathological disorders in childhood: theoretical considerations and a proposed classification." Am. Assoc. Psychiatr. Serv. Child., 14: No. 4, 9, 1967.
25. Hobbs, N., Ed.: *Issues in the Classification of Children: A Sourcebook on Categories, Labels, and Their Consequences.* San Francisco, Jossey-Bass, 1974.
26. Hoffman, L.W.: Changes in family roles, socialization, and sex differences. J. Am. Psychol. Assoc., 32:644, 1977.
27. Hollender, M.H., and Szasz, T.X.: Normality, neurosis, and psychosis. Some observations on

the concepts of mental health and mental illness. J. Nerv. Ment. Dis., 125:599, 1957.

28. Horney, K.: *Feminine Psychology*. New York, Norton, 1973.
29. Kagan, J., and Moss, H.A.: *Birth to Maturity: A Study in Psychological Development*. New York, Wiley, 1962.
30. Kubie, L.S.: The fundamental nature of the distinction between normality and neurosis. Psychoanal. Q., 23:187, 1954.
31. Lapouse, R., and Monk, M.: An epidemiologic study of behavior characteristics in children. Am. J. Public Health, 48:1134, 1958.
32. Lee, P.C., and Stewart, R.: Sex Differences: Cultural and Developmental Dimensions. New York, Urizen Books, 1976.
33. Lipp, M.R., Looney, J.G., and Spitzer, R.L.: Classifying psychophysiologic disorders: A new idea. Psychosom. Med., 39:285, 1977.
34. Loof, D.H.: *Appalachia's Children*. Lexington, Ky., University of Kentucky Press, 1971.
35. Lourie, N.V., and Lourie, B.P.: A noncategorical approach to treatment programs for children and youth. Am. J. Orthopsychiatry, 40:684, 1970.
36. *Manual on Terminology and Classification in Mental Retardation*. H. Grossman, Ed. Washington, D.C., American Association on Mental Deficiency, 1977.
37. May, J.G.: Nosology and diagnosis in child psychiatry. In: *Basic Handbook of Child Psychiatry* (J. Noshpitz, et al., Eds.). New York, Basic Books, 1980.
38. McFarlane, J.W., Allen, L., and Honzik, M.P.: *A Developmental Study of the Behavior Problems of Normal Children*. Berkeley, University of California Press, 1954.
39. Murphy, L.: *Vulnerability, Coping, and Growth: From Infancy to Adolescence*. New Haven, Connecticut, Yale University Press, 1976.
40. National Health and Medical Research Council. *Glossary of Mental Disorders*. Canberra, Australia, 1967.
41. Prugh, D.G.: Psychosocial disorders in childhood and adolescence: Theoretical considerations and an attempt at classification. Report of the Joint Commission on Mental Health of Children. In: *The Mental Health of Children: Services, Research, and Manpower: Report of the Committee on Clinical Issues of the Joint Commission on Mental Health of Children*. (Appendix B.) New York, Harper & Row, 1973.
42. Prugh, D.G., Engel, M., and Morse, W.: Emotional disturbance in children: Report of the Task Force. In: *Issues in the Classification of Children*, Vol. 1, (N. Hobbs, Ed.). New York, Jossey-Bass, 1974.
43. *Report of the President's Panel on Mental Retardation*. Washington, Government Printing Office, 1962.
44. Report to the President from President's Commission on Mental Health. Washington, D.C., Government Printing Office, 1979.
45. Rexford, E.: Personal communication.
46. Robins, L.: *Deviant Children Grown Up*. Baltimore, Williams & Wilkins, 1966.
47. Robins, L.N., and O'Neal, P.: The marital history of former problem children. Social Problems, 5:347, 1958.
48. Rubin, J.Z., Provenzano, F.J., and Luria, Z.: The

eye of the beholder: Parents' views on sex of newborns. Am. J. Orthopsychiatry, 44:512, 1974.
49. Rutter, M.L.: Relationships between child and adult psychiatric disorders: Some research considerations. In: *Annual Progress in Child Psychiatry and Child Development*. New York, Brunner/Mazel, 1973.
50. Rutter, M., Tizard, J., and Whitmore, K.: *Education, Health, and Behavior*. London, Longmans, 1970.
51. Rutter, M., et al.: A tri-axial classification of mental disorders in childhood: An international study. J. Child Psychol. Psychiatry, 10:41, 1969.
52. Ryle, A., Pond, D., and Hamilton, M.: The prevalence and patterns of psychologic disturbance in children of primary age. J. Child Psychol. Psychiatry, 6:101, 1965.
53. Santostefano, S.: Beyond nosology: Diagnosis from the viewpoint of development. In: *Perspectives in Child Psychopathology* (H.E. Rie, Ed.). Chicago, Aldine Atherton, 1971.
54. Shaw, C.R., and Lucas, A.R.: *The Psychiatric Disorders of Childhood*, 2nd Ed. New York, Appleton-Century-Crofts, 1970.
55. Silver, L.B.: DSM-II and child and adolescent psychopathology. Am. J. Psychiatr., 125:161, 1969.
56. Stringer, L., and Glidewell, I.C.: *Final Report for Early Detection of Emotional Illness in School Children*. Washington, D.C., National Institute of Mental Health, 1967.
57. Thomas, A., Chess, S., and Birch, H.G.: *Temperament and Behavior Disorders in Children*. New York, New York University Press, 1968.
58. Thomas, A., and Chess, S.: Evolution of behavior disorders into adolescence. Am. J. Psychiatry, 133:539, 1976.
59. U.S. Department of Health, Education, and Welfare: *International Classification of Diseases* (ICD-8). (Adapted for use in the United States) Washington, Government Printing Office, 1969.
60. Wolff, S.: Behavioral characteristics of primary school children referred to a psychiatric clinic in childhood. Br. J. Psychiatry, 113:885, 1967.
61. Wolff, S.: *Children Under Stress*. London, Allen Lane, 1969.

General References

Anthony, E.J.: Taxonomy is not one man's business. Int. J. Psychiatry, 3:173, 1967.
Bazelon, D.F.: Mental disorders: The need for a unified approach. Am. J. Orthopsychiatry, 34:39, 1964.
Benjamin, J.D.: The innate and the experiential in child development: In: *Childhood Psychopathology* (S.I. Harrison, & J.F. McDermott, Eds.). New York, International Universities Press, 1972.
Calobrisi, D.: Classification of children's mental disorders. Am. J. Psychiatry, 125:1457, 1969.
Dohrenwend, B.F., and Dohrenwend, B.: *Social Status and Psychological Disorder: A Causal Inquiry*. New York, Wiley, 1969.
Eisenberg, L.: The Role of Classification in Child Psychiatry. Int. J. Psychiatry, 3:179, 1967.
French, A.P.: *Disturbed Children and Their Families: Innovations in Evaluation and Treatment*. New York, Human Sciences Press, 1977.
Freud, A.: *Normality and Pathology in Childhood: Assessment of Development*. New York, International Universities Press, 1965.
Hammer, M., Salsinger, K., and Sutton, D., Eds.:

Psychopathology: Contributions from the Biological, Behavioral and Social Sciences. New York, Wiley, 1973.

Harrison, S.J., and McDermott, J.F., Eds.: *Childhood Psychopathology.* New York, International Universities Press, 1972.

Hobbs, N.: *Issues in the Classification of Children,* Vol. 2. New York, Jossey-Bass, 1974.

Hoch, P., and Zubin, J., Eds.: *Psychopathology of Childhood.* New York, Grune & Stratton, 1955.

Jenkins, R.L., and Cole, J.O., Eds.: *Diagnostic Classification in Child Psychiatry,* Washington, D.C., American Psychiatric Association, 1964.

Kessler, J.W.: *Psychopathology of the Child.* Englewood Cliffs, N.J., Prentice-Hall, 1966.

Kessler, J.W.: Nosology in child psychopathology. In: *Perspectives in Child Psychopathology* (H.E. Rie, Ed.). Chicago, Aldone & Atherton, 1971.

Linn, N.W., et al.: A social dysfunction rating scale. J. Psychiatr. Res., 6:299, 1969.

Quay, H., and Werry, J., Eds.: *Psychopathological Disorders of Childhood.* New York, Wiley, 1972.

Rie, H.E., Ed.: *Perspectives in Child Psychopathology.* Chicago, Aldine-Atherton, 1971.

Robins, L.M., and O'Neal, P.L.: The strategy of follow-up studies with special reference to children. In: *Modern Perspectives in International Child Psychiatry* (J. G. Howells, Ed.). Edinburgh, Oliver & Boyd, 1969.

Rutter, M.: Classification and categorization in child psychiatry. J. Child Psychol. and Psychiatry, 6:71, 1965.

Schopler, E., and Reichler, R., Eds.: *Psychopathology and Child Development: Research and Treatment.* New York, Plenum Press, 1976.

Steinhauer, P., and Rae-Grant, Q.: *Psychological Problems of the Child and His Family.* Toronto, Macmillan of Canada, 1977.

Wolman, B.B.: *Manual of Child Psychopathology.* New York, McGraw-Hill, 1972.

15
Healthy Responses

The growth of flesh is but a blister;
childhood is health.
(George Herbert)

Although the definition of normality in development has a certain relativity, in regard to individual variations in behavior[9,17] and in different cultural[2] and historical[1] settings, a positive assessment of healthy behavioral responses can be made[3,5,10,13] clinically. The general path of development of the normal personality[7,8,17] was discussed in Chapter 5, as was the fact that almost all children have some problems in development at some time.

A basic consideration in assessing healthy behavior in a child is its age- or stage-appropriateness. The balance of progressive and regressive forces is important, as is the evaluation of the "smoothness of development."[5] The child's intellectual, social, and emotional functioning should be considered,[11] as should his overall adaptive capacity, including the balance of his vulnerability and strengths, the flexibility of his patterns of response, and the effectiveness of coping mechanisms.[10] Those factors must be evaluated in accordance with the child's basic endowment (his genetic and constitutional capacities), with the nature of the stresses in his family and social settings, and with other factors.[12] Among the types of healthy responses are developmental crises and situational crises.[5]

Developmental Crises

The diagnostic features of a developmental crisis are:

1. The crisis is usually brief, and transient, and its behavioral manifestations are mild to moderate in degree.

2. The crisis is obviously related to a particular developmental stage, and it involves healthy attempts by the child to resolve appropriate psychosocial tasks.

3. Examination of the child and the child's history show him to be normal except for the behavioral manifestations of the developmental crisis.

General Considerations

Developmental crises are related to the child's attempt to resolve such psychosocial tasks as the establishment of trust, autonomy, initiative, industry, and identity. Examples are the "stranger"[15] and "separation" anxieties[16] characteristic of the second half of the child's first year. These anxieties are related to the infant's capacity to distinguish first between his mother and other people, and shortly after that to differentiate between his mother and himself, thus perceiving and comprehending her absence. A push toward and an attempt to consolidate autonomy is associated with oppositional behavior or normally negativistic behavior in the second and third years of life. The irrational fears[6] or normal phobias of the older preschool-age child are largely a result of his attempts to deal with the issues of initiative and sexual differentiation. The school-age child's pseudocompulsive or ritualistic behavior represent efforts to contain and to consolidate his push toward accomplishment and industry. The pseudoindependent, sometimes oppositional, and often inconsistent behavior of the adolescent is related to a developmental crisis in his search for his identity.

Developmental crises are fundamentally related to maturational forces within the child although these of course interact with the behavior of the child's parents and other forces external to him.

Clinical Findings

The history shows the child's adjustment in previous stages to have been within normal limits. Ordinarily there are no relevant physical findings, although a concurrent physical illness can intensify a developmental crisis as a result of increased regression or dependence. Anxiety, oppositional behavior, or other manifestations are more marked when the basic developmental conflict is most intense; for example, when the infant or young child is separated from the parent or the parents impose discipline on an adolescent. Family functioning and parent-child relationships seem generally healthy.

Treatment and Prognosis

Although most developmental crises resolve spontaneously, a supportive counseling of the child and his parents by the physician may help the child master the developmental crisis more quickly and comfortably and begin to move to his next developmental stage. "Anticipatory guidance" often helps parents understand the behavioral characteristics of a coming developmental crisis (e.g., separation anxiety or normally negativistic behavior). Some parents may otherwise interpret such behavior as abnormal, or they may handle the child overpermissively or overpunitively.

A developmental crisis that is handled ineffectively may build up into a reactive disorder or, later, may crystallize into a structured psychoneurotic or personality disorder. If a developmental crisis occurs early or late, it may represent a developmental deviation.

Case Example. For several months a 20-month-old girl, an only child, had become more physically active and exploratory in her behavior, requiring more careful supervision by her parents. Although she still became anxious and clung tightly, crying, to the mother when the parents had to leave her with a sitter, she showed signs of increasing oppositional behavior at other times. She would often resist vigorously attempts to control her behavior, and, when she was asked to do things, she regularly replied with a strong, no. (Although she spoke a number of words, she had not yet learned to say yes.) Occasionally, she had a brief temper tantrum when her wishes were frustrated. Her parents were troubled by her behavior, but they were able to avoid pitched battles and to maintain reasonably firm limits about important matters. The child's behavior continued unabated for about 4 months, and then gradually (24 to 30 months) became much more muted. She still tolerated frustration poorly at times, and she had brief bursts of strongly oppositional behavior until she was about 3 years old.

Comment. The girl's behavior shows a normal push toward autonomy during the toddler phase. Her parents understood the developmental significance of her oppositional behavior and her "normal negativism." They were able to meet her conflicting needs for support and limits, thus helping her to resolve the developmental crisis in favor of realistic steps toward beginning independence and impulse control.

Situational Crises

The diagnostic features of a situational crisis are:

1. The crisis is usually relatively brief and transient.

2. The crisis is obviously related to situations in the child's family or environment that are acutely stressful for the child.

3. The child's behavior seems to be a normal response to the crisis, not deeply disturbed behavior.

4. Examination of the child and the child's history show him to be normal except for his response to the crisis situation.

General Considerations

Situational crises are related to the child's attempt to adapt to stressful circumstances (e.g., an acute minor illness, the short-term hospitalization of a preschool child, or other environmental shifts, with the alterations in interpersonal relations that may be involved. A response to a family crisis or to the illness or death of a parent are other examples. The child's behavioral response is considered to be age appropriate and adaptive, as in the "work of mourning" characteristic of a healthy grief reaction. (Grief reactions are discussed more fully in Chapters 26 and 28). Absence of grief is a matter of concern. Often it occurs because parents have difficulty in permitting or supporting the child's grief responses, which may upset them.

Clinical Findings

The child's history shows that his adjustment before the situational crisis was within normal limits. Ordinarily there are no relevant physical findings, but a concurrent physical illness can intensify the behavioral manifestations, which may resemble those in developmental crises. Sadness and occasional crying, associated with talking about a dead or absent[14] parent, are characteristic of grief reactions in children, and some temporary depression may occur, along with guilt and misinterpretation of events. Depressive equivalents may be manifested by a temporary loss of appetite, sleep disturbances, or underactivity or overactivity, particularly in younger children. Regression is also characteristic of situational crises, sometimes with a temporary abandonment of speech by infants or a loss of bowel and bladder control in toddlers. Physiologic concomitants of anxiety are common (e.g., the elevated blood pressure or tachycardia seen almost routinely on a child's admission to the hospital), and they may lead to diagnostic confusion with heart disease or thyrotoxicosis.

Treatment and Prognosis

Situational crises are self-limited although they may last for weeks or several months (e.g., in a grief response). Supportive counseling by the physician may help the child to mourn,[4] to cope with environmental or interpersonal stresses, and to resolve the crisis, with appropriate understanding and management by the child's parents or other adults. Anticipatory guidance (e.g., about stage-appropriate responses to illness or hospitalization) may help greatly. Preventive measures (e.g., preparing the child and his parents for hospitalization or the availability of facilities for overnight stay by a parent) can also help greatly.

If the stressful circumstances are too intense or prolonged, if the child's adaptive capacity is weakened by a concurrent physical illness or other contributory factors, or if the parents or other care-taking adults are unable to respond adequately to the child's emotional needs, the behavioral manifestations may fail to resolve or they may be intensified. Thus, they may lead to reactive disorders or to other, more structured psychopathologic disorders. Psychiatric consultation may be helpful in evaluating the degree of psychopathology.

Case Example. A 3½-year-old boy experienced the birth of a sister. He had been prepared for the birth, and he had talked a good deal about his "baby sister" and how he would play with her. When the baby came home from the hospital, however, he seemed interested in her only briefly. For the next few days, he repeatedly tried to get the mother's attention when she was with the baby, he became more dependent and fearful, and he began to suck his thumb. Although he had been dry at night for over 6 months, he wet the bed regularly for about 10 days. On several occasions, he told his father that he wished the baby would "go back where she came from." After 2 weeks, he began to seem less jealous and less demanding, especially after his mother began to spend some time alone with him each day. In about 3 weeks, he seemed to have generally returned to his previous level of adjustment. He showed more interest in the baby, but he still was jealous and demanding occasionally, especially when he was tired.

Comment. The boy showed some immediate jealousy and mild regression, which are normal responses to the birth of a sibling. His capacity to cope with the situation was helped by his ability to talk about his feelings and by his mother's recognition of his needs.

Bibliography

1. Aries, P.: *Centuries of Childhood.* New York, Knopf, 1962.
2. Eisenberg, F.: The human nature of human nature. Science, 76:123, 1972.
3. Freud, A.: *Normality and Pathology in Childhood: Assessments of Development.* New York, International Universities Press, 1965.
4. Friedman, S.B.: Management of death in a parent or sibling. In: *Ambulatory Pediatrics* (M. Green and R. Haggerty, Eds.). Philadelphia, Saunders, 1968.
5. Group for the Advancement of Psychiatry: *Psychopathological Disorders in Childhood: Theoretical Considerations and a Proposed Classification.* Report No. 62. New York, Group for the Advancement of Psychiatry, 1966.
6. Jersild, A.T.: *Child Psychology,* 3rd Ed. New York, Prentice-Hall, 1947.
7. Kagan, J., and Moss, H.: *Birth to Maturity: A Study in Psychological Development.* New York, Wiley, 1961.
8. McFarlane, J.W., Allen, L., and Honzik, M.P.: *A Developmental Study of the Behavioral Problems of Normal Children.* Berkeley, University of California Press, 1954.
9. Murphy, L.B.: *The Widening World of Childhood.* New York, Basic Books, 1962.
10. Murphy, L.B.: *Vulnerability, Coping, and Growth: From Infancy to Adolescence.* New Haven, Conn., Yale University Press, 1976.
11. Prugh, D.G.: Psychosocial disorders in childhood and adolescence: Theoretical considerations and an attempt at classification. Report of the Joint Commission on Mental Health of Children. In: *The Mental Health of Children: Services, Research and Manpower. Report of Committee on Clinical Issues of the Joint Commission on Mental Health of Children.* (Appendix B.) New York, Harper & Row, 1973.
12. Prugh, D.G., Engel, M., and Morse, W.: Emotional disturbance in children: Report of the Task Force. In: *Issues in the Classification of Children,* Vol. 1. (N. Hobbs, Ed.). New York, Jossey-Bass, 1974.
13. Stuart, H.C., and Prugh, D.G.: *The Healthy Child: His Physical, Psychological and Social Development.* Cambridge, Mass., Harvard University Press, 1960.
14. Sugar, M.: Children of divorce. Pediatrics, 46:588, 1970.
15. Tennes, K.H., and Lample, E.E.: Stranger and separation anxiety in infancy. J. Nerv. Ment. Dis., 139:247, 1964.
16. Tennes, K.H., and Lample, E.E.: Some aspects of mother-child relationship pertaining to infantile-separation anxiety. J. Nerv. Ment. Dis., 143:426, 1966.
17. Thomas, A., et al.: *Behavioral Individuality in Early Childhood.* New York, New York University Press, 1963.

General References

Allen, F.H.: *Positive Aspects of Child Psychiatry.* New York, Norton, 1963.
Ausubel, D.P.: *Theory and Problems of Adolescent Development.* New York, Grune & Stratton, 1954.
Ausubel, D.P.: *Theory and Problems of Child Development.* New York, Grune & Stratton, 1958.
Bowlby, J.: Grief and mourning in infancy and early childhood. Psychoanal. Study Child, 15:9, 1960.
Burks, H.L., and Harrison, S.J.: Aggressive behavior as a means of avoiding a depression. Am. J. Orthopsychiatry, 32:416, 1962.
Chess, S.: Psychiatric disorders of childhood. I. Healthy responses, developmental disturbances, and stress or reactive disorders. In: *Comprehensive Textbook of Psychiatry* (A.M. Friedman and H. Kaplan, Eds.). Baltimore, Williams and Wilkins, 1967.
Douvan, E., and Gold, M.: Modal patterns in American adolescence. In: *Review of Child Development Research,* Vol. 2 (L.W. Hoffman, and M.L. Hoffman, Eds.). New York, Russell Sage Foundation, 1966.
Erikson, E.H.: *Identity and the Life Cycle.* New York, International Universities Press, 1959.

Erikson, E.H.: *Childhood and Society*, 2nd Ed. New York, Norton, 1963.

Erikson, E.H.: *Identity: Youth and Crisis*. New York, Norton, 1968.

Harper, P.A.: *Preventive Pediatrics: Child Health and Development*. New York, Appleton-Century-Crofts, 1962.

Hartmann, H.: *Ego Psychology and the Problem of Adaptation (1939)*. New York, International Universities Press, 1958.

Illingworth, R.: *The Development of the Infant and Young Child, Normal and Abnormal*, 34th Ed. Baltimore, Williams & Wilkins, 1966.

Josselyn, I.M.: *Psychosocial Development of Children*. New York, Family Service Association of America, 1948.

LaPouse, R., and Monk, M.A.: An epidemiologic study of behavior characteristics in children. Am. J. Public. Health, *48*:1134, 1958.

Lewis, M.: *Clinical Aspects of Child Development*. Philadelphia, Lea & Febiger, 1971.

Lidz, T.: *The Person: His and Her Development Throughout the Life Cycle*. 2nd Ed. New York, Basic Books, 1968.

Richmond, J.B., and Lustman, S.L.: Total health: A conceptual visual aid. J. Med. Ed., *29*:23, 1954.

Senn, M.J.E., and Solnit, A.J.: *Problems in Child Behavior and Development*. Philadelphia, Lea & Febiger, 1968.

Spock, B.: *Baby and Child Care*, Rev. Ed. New York, Pocket Books, 1957.

Steinhauer, P.D., and Rae-Grant, Q.: *Psychological Problems of the Child and His Family*. Toronto, Macmillan of Canada, 1977.

Thomas, A., Chess, S., and Birch, H.G.: *Temperament and Behavior Disorders in Children*. New York, New York University Press, 1968.

Westley, W.: Emotionally healthy adolescents and their family backgrounds. In: *The Family in Contemporary Society* (L. Gladstone, Ed.). New York, International Universities Press, 1958.

Witmer, H., Kotinsky, R., Eds.: *Personality in the Making*. New York, Harper, 1952.

III

Specific Clinical Considerations: The Diagnosis, Treatment, and Management of Disorders of Development and Adaptation in Children and Adolescents

In children may be observed the traces and seeds of what will one day be settled psychological habits.
(Aristotle)

16

Reactive Disorders

*Children are not simply micro-adults, but have
their own specific problems.*
(Bela Schick)

The diagnostic features of a reactive disorder are:

1. The behavior and/or the symptoms appear in reaction to an event, a set of events, or a situation.
2. The behavioral disturbance is of pathologic degree.
3. The disorder is usually temporary, responding well to treatment, but it may become chronic or it may develop into more severe psychopathologic pictures.
4. The disorder usually occurs in pre-school-age and early school-age children although it may occur in older children or adolescents.
5. Except for the reactive disorder, the child is ordinarily normal in regard to his examination and history. He may have had previous difficulties in adaptation in his family, or he may have an acute physical illness that has caused the reactive disorder.

General Considerations

A reactive disorder can be regarded as a manifestation of a predominantly conscious conflict between the child's drives, impulses, or needs and his social environment and not as an unconscious, internalized process. A great variety of events or situations, often those involving family crises (e.g., illness, accident, or hospitalization, the loss of a parent; marked changes in the attitudes and/or behavior of others, particularly parents; school pressures; or premature, excessive, or inappropriate stimulation) may precipitate or perpetuate a reactive disorder. A disturbing situation that has arisen suddenly and unexpectedly may have a profound effect on the child, particularly on the young child. A disturbing situation that has evolved gradually may allow the child time for mastery.

The diagnosis should be based on a careful examination of the child in his social environment, using positive criteria and avoiding methods of exclusion. It should be demonstrated that a specific event, set of events, and/or situation exists that is emotionally traumatic for the particular child and that acts as a precipitant. A simple coincidence in time may suggest the

267

cause but does not prove it. Positive psychologic evidence such as that just described must be obtained to make the diagnosis. In making the diagnosis, the physician should emphasize the effect of the stress on the child's adaptive balance and the child's reaction to the stress, rather than the degree of stress. Some situations (e.g., the death of a child's parent or the divorce of his parents) are considered potentially traumatic for all children. (See Chapter 2 for a fuller discussion of stressful stimuli and their effects. The management of parent loss by death, divorce, or desertion is dealt with in Chapter 28.) But even a mild stressful stimulus may produce a reactive disorder in a particular child. The child's response depends on what the stress means to the child and to his parents, the nature of the child's experiences, his basic endowment, including his temperament, his developmental level, and his adaptive capacity. A situation that would have little effect on an older child may have a marked effect on an infant. The child's response may depend on his having reached a particular level of development.

Reactive disorders can occur in children of any age, but they are more likely to occur in infants and preschool-age children. Among their other differences and special vulnerabilities, younger children do not yet have the capacity to repress strong feelings, to internalize conflict, and to develop a structured psychopathologic response, which are ways of coping with emotional stress. Although accurate figures on incidence and prevalence are not yet available, particularly for younger children, statistics from the Biometrics Branch of the National Institute of Mental Health[1] support the impression that situational-reactive disorders are the most common ones seen in children and adolescents.

Clinical Findings

The nature of the reaction depends on the child's stage of development, his past experience, his basic endowment, his available defenses and coping devices, his adaptive capacity, his family's response, and other factors. The reaction may take the form of regression, a temporary arrest in development, or a variety of psychologic or behavioral symptoms. Often a part of the clinical picture may represent attempts to cope or to maintain his adaptive balance by, for example, aggressive or regressive behavior to ward off a depression.[3] Part may be evidence of adaptive failure (e.g., by marked withdrawal and difficulty in functioning). The child may show physiologic concomitants of anxiety or other emotions. In a child who is psychologically and physiologically predisposed, a psychophysiologic disorder, such as a peptic ulcer or ulcerative colitis, may be precipitated during the reactive disorder.

The infant who does not have adequate mothering may show apathy, marked depression,[14] eating and sleeping disturbances,[6,12,13] or failure to thrive.[2] The young child may show separation anxiety,[16] withdrawal, thumb sucking, manipulation of parts of his body, or rocking.[5] Some children may try to coerce, punish, or otherwise manipulate people by aggressive behavior, passive resistance, or oppositional or negativistic behavior.[8] Pica,[9,10,17] rumination,[15] and trichotillomania[4] may also represent reactions to emotional deprivation. Marked fears, panic states (see Chapter 12 for an example of an acute and severe reactive disorder involving a panic state in a preschool child and treated by crisis intervention), excessive day-dreaming, preoccupation with fantasy, or other psychologic responses may occur, especially in young children. Regression to infantile patterns, (e.g., wetting and soiling[11]) is also common. Overt depression may occur, with suicidal manifestations in adolescents or depressive equivalents in children and adolescents. The depressive equivalents may be eating or sleep disturbances, apathy, or an increase or a decrease in activity patterns. (These disorders and others that are strongly affected by developmental factors, are discussed more fully in Chapter 28.)

Occasionally, a child identifies with a seriously disturbed or psychotic parent and shows behavior or symptoms that are similar to his parent's, but not psychosis. Such a *folie á deux* may be a reactive disorder on the part of the child; or it may have progressed to a chronic personality disorder or some other structured psychopathologic disorder.

The category of reactive disorders includes a number of entities that are variously referred to in the literature (e.g., conduct disturbances, behavior disorders, neurotic traits, habit disturbances, anaclitic depressions, situational disorders, and stress reactions).

Treatment and Prognosis

Some mild reactive disorders may resolve fairly quickly if the parents or other adult figures (e.g., teachers) are able to understand their nature and origins, offer emotional support to the child, and deal constructively with the environmental situation. Other reactive disorders require supportive psychotherapy by the physician for the child and his parents. If long continued, some other reactive disorders may require referral and intensive psychotherapy for the child and his parents. Behavior therapy, especially desensitization, has helped relieve marked fears and other symptoms of reactive disorders. Adverse reactions by an older child to hospitalization may be largely prevented by preparing him (and his parents) for the experience, and the reactions of preschool children may be abated by permitting unrestricted visiting or overnight stay by the mother. In the hospital, "replacement therapy"—the use of parent-substitutes—may help a child overcome rumination or other feeding disturbances, failure to thrive, or other reactions to emotional deprivation.

Follow-up is essential, and some children may have to be referred to a specialist. Anticipatory guidance may help prevent developmental or situational crises from becoming pathologic reactive disorders. The use of homemakers (e.g., to help a sick mother in a single-parent family) may prevent a child's being put in a foster home. Foster grandparents can be sent into homes to help parents deal with acutely disturbed children.[7]

The prognosis for response to supportive treatment is ordinarily good. But sometimes the child can become chronically incapacitated. A reactive disorder in an infant that temporarily arrests his development may become a developmental deviation. A structured psychoneurotic disorder may arise from a reactive disorder. A psychiatric consultation may help decide whether the child needs intensive psychotherapy.

In certain cases, a reactive disorder may be superimposed on a structured psychoneurotic disorder that has fixed patterns or even on a chronic, moderate psychosis. Supportive, often brief treatment may help a child who has a chronic obsessive-compulsive personality disorder deal with the situation to which he is reacting and to return to his previous level of compensation. The prognosis otherwise may depend on the response to treatment of the underlying psychopathologic disorder.

Case Example. A boy who was 3 years and 10 months old, an only child, had shown isolated, withdrawn, and stereotyped behavior, bedwetting, nightmares (several times a week), and somewhat unclear speech since he was $2^1/_2$ years old. The boy's psychomotor development had apparently been normal up to that time, and he had been able to speak clearly in short sentences. When he was $2^1/_2$ years old, his mother had infectious hepatitis, associated with rather marked depression, and she was unable to care for the boy for at least 6 months. During this period, the father cared for the boy with the help of a series of housekeepers. The mother had to be hospitalized for several weeks early in her illness, and before she left for the hospital, the boy screamed and clung desperately to her. At first, he seemed depressed and inconsolable in her absence. Gradually, he became withdrawn and isolated, and he showed little reaction when the mother returned home. He had sleep disturbances, markedly regressed behavior, including an almost complete loss of speech for a period of several months and a temporary loss of bowel control, which he had just attained. From that time up to the present, his withdrawn and isolated behavior had continued. It was associated with many bedtime rituals, frequent nightmares, and unclear speech.

When he was observed during 2 play interviews, the boy was at first withdrawn and aloof, and he played alone in a stereotyped fashion. His speech was infantile; he had much difficulty pronouncing consonants in particular. Toward the end of the first interview, he began to include the examiner in his play. In the second interview, he was able to relate to the examiner more comfortably and with increasing warmth, talking a little more intelligibly about his frightening dreams about monsters "taking her away." Physical examination was within normal limits, and he had no history of birth injury or significant illness.

The mother seemed still to be depressed and to be worried about her health. She herself had been an only child. She had been very dependent on her mother and rather distant from her father. She had become pregnant after 6 years of marriage and 3 miscarriages. She said that she had felt "incomplete" without a baby to care for. Up to the point of her illness, she had been somewhat anxious about and overprotective of the boy (e.g., she found it difficult to leave him with sitters), and he had been quite dependent on her. On her recovery from the hepatitis, she had still felt depressed. She was disturbed by the boy's withdrawn behavior, and she made occasional desperate attempts to "get through to him," feeling helpless and guilty when she failed to do so. The father was a driving, dominating person, who directed his wife's care of the household. He had been constantly dissatisfied with his son, even from infancy, because of his failure to "take things like a man."

Comment. Although there had been problems in the parent-child relationships in this family before the mother became ill, the boy's reaction to the temporary loss of his mother appeared to be the central factor in the rather sudden onset of his disturbed behavior. His previous overdependence on the mother (a response to her anxious, overprotective, and overvaluing approach as well as the father's criticism of him and inability to relate warmly to him), were fac-

tors that made him both especially vulnerable to the loss of the mother and angry at her for her apparent desertion of him (as he misperceived the consequences of her illness). The disorder in behavior was of sufficient intensity and duration, with evidence of failure to cope, to permit its categorization as a reactive disorder which would not resolve spontaneously, and required the help of a mental health professional. After a curbstone consultation at a hospital with a child psychiatrist, the family was referred to a clinical psychologist, who carried on intensive, insight-promoting play therapy for the boy and therapy for the parents for nearly a year, to help them resolve their problems successfully. The father later sought therapy for himself.

Bibliography

1. Bahn, A.K., Chandler, C.A., and Eisenberg, L.: Diagnostic characteristics related to services in psychiatric clinics for children. Milbank Mem. Fund Q., *40*:1, No. 3, 1962.
2. Bullard, D., et al.: Failure to thrive in the "neglected" child. Am. J. Orthopsychiatry, *37*:680, 1967.
3. Burks, H.L., and Harrison, S.J.: Aggressive behavior as a means of avoiding a depression. Am. J. Orthopsychiatry, *32*:416, 1962.
4. Delgardo, R.A., and Mannino, F.V.: Some observations on trichotillomania in children. J. Am. Acad. Child Psychiatry, 8:229, 1969.
5. Evans, J.: Rocking at Night. J. Child Psychol. Psychiatr. Other Discip., 2:71, 1961.
6. Hirschberg, J.C.: Parental anxieties accompanying sleep disturbance in young children. Bull. Menninger Clin., 21:129, 1957.
7. Johnson, R.: Foster grandparents for emotionally disturbed children. Children, 14:46, 1967.
8. Levy, D.M.: Oppositional syndromes and oppositional behavior. In: *Childhood Psychopathology* (S.I. Harrison and J.F. McDermott, Eds.). New York, International Universities Press, 1972.
9. Millican, F.K., et al.: Study of an oral fixation: Pica. J. Am. Acad. Child. Psychiatry, 7:79, 1968.
10. Millican, F.K., and Lourie, R.S.: The child with pica and his family. In: *The Child in His Family.* (E.J. Anthony and C. Koupernik, Eds.). New York, Wiley, 1970.
11. Prugh, D.G., et al.: A study of the emotional reactions of children and families to hospitalization and illness. Am. J. Orthopsychiatry, 23:70, 1953.
12. Sperling, M.: Etiology and treatment of sleep disturbance in children. Psychoanal. Q., 6:79, 1958.
13. Sperling, M.: Pavor nocturnus. J. Am. Psychoanal. Assoc., 6:79, 1958.
14. Spitz, R.A., and Wolf, K.: Anaclitic Depression. Psychoanal. Study Child., 2:313, 1946.
15. Stein, M.L., Rausen, A.R., and Blau, A.: Psy-

chotherapy of an infant with rumination. JAMA,
171:2309, 1959.
16. Tennes, K.H., and Lampl, E.E.: Defensive reactions to infantile separation anxiety. J. Am. Psychoanal. Assoc., *17*:1142, 1969.
17. Wortis, H., et al.: Children who eat noxious substances. Am. Acad. Child Psychiatry, *1*:536, 1962.

General References

Chess, S.: Psychiatric disorders of childhood. I. Healthy responses, developmental disturbances, and stress or reactive disorders. In: *Comprehensive Textbook of Psychiatry* (A.M. Freedman and H. Kaplan, Eds.). Baltimore, Williams & Wilkins, 1967.

Kaplan, D.M.: A concept of acute situational disorders. Soc. Work, *7*:15, 1962.

Kaplan, D.M.: Study and treatment of an acute emotional disorder. Am. J. Orthopsychiatry, *35*:69, 1965.

Sullivan, A.W.: Psychologic aspects of pediatric practice: Acute psychiatric illness in children. N. Y. State J. Med., *58*:1665, 1958.

17
Developmental Deviations

He who watches a thing grow
has the best view of it.
(Heraclitus)

The diagnostic features of a developmental deviation are:

1. The deviation occurs as a characteristic of a child's development over a period of months or years.
2. The deviation may involve a single aspect of development (e.g., motor or sensory), or it may be characterized by a lag, an unevenness, or a precocity in patterns of maturation.

General Considerations

Developmental deviations are deviations in personality development that are outside the range of normal variation because they occur to a degree, in a sequence, or at a time not appropriate to the child's age or stage of development. A developmental crisis that appears very early or very late may represent a developmental deviation.

Biologic (hereditary, constitutional, temperamental, and maturational) factors seem to contribute importantly to developmental deviations.[2] A developmental deviation may be modified or intensified by the child's experience. This may arise from a family's interactions,[5] emotional deprivation,[3] environmental influences,[4] and other factors. An unresolved reactive disorder that occurred when the child was an infant may be a predisposing factor. Chess and her colleagues[5] and others think that hyperactivity may often derive from the child's temperamental patterns (a high activity level[1] and related characteristics) that emerge early in his life and remain stable throughout his childhood. Such a developmental deviation may become intensified and progress to a clinical behavior disorder if the child's parents are unable to cope with such patterns. A mild deviation in a child who lives in a family that has a marital or other type of conflict may become a marked one because of the disturbed interactions between the parents and the child. Deviations that are predominantly physical (e.g., precocious puberty, delayed menstruation, or delayed growth) can be regarded as primary deviations, and the child's reaction to the physical deviation—whether a healthy response, a reactive disorder, or some other response—can be regarded as secondary. (As discussed in Chapter 21, delayed menstruation or growth may at times be influenced by psychophysiologic factors.)

Clinical Findings

Some developmental deviations seem to involve almost the whole maturational timetable, while others apply only to individual aspects of development. Children who have deviations in a single dimension (e.g., a motor or a sensory deviation) may later develop an associated personality disorder or other total personality disturbance. In such instances the personality disturbance is the primary diagnosis, and the developmental deviation is the secondary diagnosis.

Deviations in Maturational Patterns

Deviations in maturational patterns include broad or almost total lags, marked unevenness, or precocities in maturation in a number of dimensions. They include also deviations in a child's capacity for controlling or integrating such bodily functions as speech, sleeping, and bladder and bowel functions.

Deviations in Specific Dimensions of Development

Deviations in Motor Development. Deviations in motor development include long-standing deviations in activity levels (hyperactivity or hypoactivity) and psychomotor capacities, deviations in handedness, coordination, and other largely motor capacities (at times associated with perceptual problems). Brain damage or other factors do not seem to be involved in such deviations. Some hyperkinetic chil-

dren who do not have brain damage would be considered in this category. Disorders in which anxiety produces the hyperactivity are considered reactive disorders or total personality disorders, and the hyperactivity is considered a symptom.

Deviations in Sensory Development. Deviations in sensory development include difficulties in monitoring stimuli that range from tactile stimuli to social stimuli. Children who have such difficulties may overreact to ordinary sensory input by becoming easily overstimulated, or they may show underreactive or uneven responses. Their responses to stimuli may range from problems in falling asleep to regressive, exhibitionistic, or apathetic behavior, and the problems may be specified as individual symptoms.

Deviations in Speech Development. Deviations in speech development include significant delays or lags in the development of speech that are not associated with deafness, oppositional behavior, elective mutism, brain damage, or early childhood psychosis. Included in the category are certain children who have disorders of articulation, rhythm, phonation, or comprehension of speech, usually of a persistently infantile type and without physical abnormalities, as well as some children who have a marked precocity in the development of speech. Not included are the normal repetition of words by a healthy early preschool-age child and stuttering, where it is considered a conversion reaction.

Deviations in Cognitive Functions. Deviations in cognitive functions include developmental lags or other deviations in the child's capacity for symbolic or abstract thinking or in his perceptual-motor capacities which may affect his ability to read and write and to work arithmetic problems. Some children may show persistent prelogical thought processes or delays in the repression of primitive fantasies and other deviations in cerebral integration that are unrelated to brain damage. Some children who are referred to as "late bloomers," some children who are "pseudo-retarded," and some who were formerly called "borderline retarded" (i.e., who are at the lower end of the normal distribution curve of intellectual potential) are considered to have deviations in cognitive functions, as are children who are precocious in regard to their intellectual development.

Deviations in Social Development. Deviations in social development include delayed, precocious, or uneven patterns of social capacities or relationships that have not become true personality disorders. A child's delayed capacity to separate from his parents, dependence, marked shyness, oppositional behavior, inhibitions, and immaturely aggressive behavior are examples.

Deviations in Psychosexual Development. Deviations in psychosexual development include significant deviations in the onset of sexual curiosity, markedly precocious or delayed heterosexual interests, or the persistence of infantile autoerotic patterns. Deviations in heterosexual identifications, such as those seen in passive, feminine boys or somewhat masculine girls who do not show actual sexual inversion or perversion, are also included. Such children who have those deviations may show an internalized conflict but no psychoneurosis or personality disorder. Passive, feminine boys especially have learning inhibitions, which are regarded as a symptom.

Deviations in Affective (Emotional) Development. Deviations in emotional development include emotional lability inappropriate to the child's level of development, an overcontrol of emotions inappropriate to his level of development, apathetic or mildly depressed tendencies, and other emotional patterns but no structured psychoneurotic reactions or personality disorders. Included in the category are "cyclic" behavior patterns that resemble hypomania and euphoria that alternate with diminished activity and a somewhat depressed state.

Deviations in Integrative Development.

Deviations in integrative development include deviations in the child's ability to tolerate frustration or control his impulses. Also included are certain overactive or uneven defense mechanisms (e.g., projection or denial) in the absence of personality disorder or psychosis.

Treatment and Prognosis

A developmental deviation is not necessarily fixed. The passage of time, advances in maturity, or help from parents or some other external figures can lead to its diminution or disappearance. But depending on how the child is handled later or on other factors, the deviation may presage the development of a more structured disorder. The distinction can be made only by further evaluations.

In many instances, formal treatment is not necessary. The physician's explanation to the parents that the deviation is largely biologic and that it will improve with the child's development may relieve the parents' confusion, anxiety, or conflict between themselves or with the child. Counseling the parents about managing a poorly coordinated or a socially immature child may be important, however. It may include recommendations for motor training or for putting the child in a nursery school. Other therapeutic measures may be indicated; for example, supportive psychotherapy for a child who has developed an emotional or behavior disorder or a sweeping lag in maturation that may have been intensified by family problems, with supportive psychotherapy for the child's parents. Therapy with one of the stimulant drugs (along with other measures) may be indicated for a child who is markedly hyperactive. Speech therapy may be indicated for a child who has a lag in speech development, or remedial tutoring may be indicated for a child who has a cognitive lag. If a serious personality or psychoneurotic disorder is superimposed on or has evolved out of a developmental deviation, more intensive psychotherapy may be indicated.

Preventive steps can be undertaken if lags in the cognitive development or the speech development of late preschool-age children are discovered early. Physicians, nurses, other health personnel, and educators must work together in screening for those lags and in taking preventive measures.

Case Example. An 8-year-old boy about to enter the third grade was brought to a pediatrician by his parents, both professional people, because he had difficulties in school and gross problems in motor coordination. He had been teased for his poor coordination by the other children in his class. In the history, the developmental survey indicated that he had no other problems than the motor clumsiness and poor coordination and their social consequences. The motor problems had been present since the boy was an infant, and the parents and the boy's pediatrician in another city had been inclined to disregard them, because neither parent was well coordinated. The boy was anxious about his performance in school, especially about his handwriting, which was hard for him, and led him to perform below the level the teachers felt his intellectual capacities indicated. This and the teasing had led the school personnel to suggest that the boy be examined by a physician.

The boy's medical survey showed no significant illnesses in the child or his family. The family's survey showed that the parents had been somewhat protective of the boy, who was an only child, particularly because of his poor coordination (of which, however, they were careful not to be critical). Their relationship with the boy seemed otherwise to be warm and positive.

The results of the boy's physical and neurologic examinations were within normal limits, except for his marked difficulty in coordination and his rather small size. In a play interview, the boy talked freely about his feelings of inferiority in regard to his poor coordination and the teasing of other children. He mentioned also his anxiety about his handwriting, which led him not to try at times. He refused to draw a picture, write, or read a second-grade paragraph. He "would do terrible." His 3 wishes and other fantasy material centered on his hopes for help with his problems. He set up a family doll play situation in which a boy was "'sad," and his parents could not help him. The boy doll also resented his parents' not letting him

try certain things because they thought he would fail.

After the pediatrician talked by telephone with the school principal and the boy's teacher, who confirmed and elaborated on the parents' and the boy's stories, the pediatrician decided that a psychologic consultation was indicated. He referred the boy for testing to a child clinical psychologist whose consultation services he had used regularly. He asked the psychologist to analyze the boy's abilities, including any perceptual-motor difficulties. He prepared the boy for the tests, saying that they were not like school tests and that he could not fail them. The psychologist administered the Wechsler Intelligence Scale for Children (WISC), the Bender-Gestalt Test, and other tests. She found that the boy had a Verbal I.Q. of 154, a Performance I.Q. of 74, and a Full-Scale I.Q. of just over 100. The low Performance I.Q. was explained entirely by the boy's motor incoordination. The WISC and the other tests indicated the boy had no perceptual problems. Parts of the projective tests, such as the Children's Apperception Test (CAT), indicated that the boy had feelings of sadness, loneliness, and hopelessness, though not true depression, together with anxiety about his performance, and some resentment toward his parents. The psychologist felt that those feelings could have intensified the boy's motor incoordination.

The pediatrician interpreted the psychologist's report first for the parents, then for the boy separately, and then for all three of them together. He told the parents that the boy had very high or superior intelligence, and that his motor difficulties represented a developmental lag that had constitutional and temperamental bases, and that was compounded by the boy's worries about himself. He said there was no evidence of brain damage (the parents had feared that) and that the boy could be helped. The pediatrician arranged for the boy to see a teacher who specialized in motor training (and who was recommended by the psychologist), and he set up a short series of supportive psychotherapeutic interviews with the child and parents, seeing them in tandem. He saw the boy alone weekly and the parents together biweekly, both in half-hour interviews. He also talked again with the boy's teacher, telling her his general opinion of the boy and his problems, based on his impressions and the psychologist's testing. The teacher had felt the boy's basic intelligence was above average, but she was surprised to learn about his high Verbal I.Q., and she seemed reassured and supportive of the pediatrician's plan.

Over a 10-week period, the boy responded well, talking more about and playing out his original feelings and then gradually becoming more confident and less anxious and less resentful of his parents. The parents gradually came to understand the boy's feelings more fully, realizing spontaneously their overprotective tendencies, and expressing some guilt about them and about possible hereditary influences (guilt the pediatrician was able to relieve). The boy liked the motor training, which centered on simple and gentle games with balls and other objects, and his motor coordination in school began to improve. At the end of 10 weeks, the parents felt they could handle the situation. The boy seemed to feel so too, and the last family interview showed a warmer interaction and a mutual understanding between parents and child. The motor training was continued for several months, with the door left open for the family to return to the pediatrician at any time.

A follow-up interview held 6 months later indicated that the boy was performing much closer to his intellectual level, that he was much better adjusted in school, that his motor performance in writing and in general was much better, and that the teasing had subsided. The parents supported the boy's wish to learn to ride a bicycle (which they had discouraged); they felt the family was much happier, and they were thinking of having another child. Follow-up testing by the psychologist 9 months later indicated that the boy's Verbal I.Q. was about the same, but that his Performance I.Q. had risen to low average.

Bibliography

1. Fries, M., and Woolf, P.: Some hypotheses on the role of congenital activity type in personality development. Psychoanal. Study Child, 8:94, 1954.
2. Group for the Advancement of Psychiatry: *Psychopathological Disorders in Childhood: Theoretical Considerations and a Proposed Classification*, Vol. 6. Report No. 62. New York, Group for the Advancement of Psychiatry, 1966.
3. Lax, R.F.: Infantile deprivation and arrested ego development. Psychoanal. Q., 27:501, 1958.
4. Malone, C.: Developmental deviations considered in the light of environmental factors. In: *The Drifters* (E. Pavenstedt, Ed.). Boston, Little, Brown, 1967.
5. Thomas, A., Chess, S., and Birch, H.G.: *Temperament and Behavior Disorders in Children*. New York, New York University Press, 1968.

General References

Chess, S.: Psychiatric disorders of childhood. I. Healthy responses, developmental disturbances, and stress or reactive disorders. In: *Comprehensive Textbook of Psychiatry* (A.M. Freedman and H. Kaplan, Eds.). Baltimore, Williams & Wilkins, 1967.
Escalona, S.K.: *The Roots of Individuality*. Chicago, Aldine, 1968.
Thomas, A., et al.: *Behavioral Individuality in Early Childhood*. New York, New York University Press, 1963.

18
Psychoneurotic Disorders

A child's feelings are none the less acute for
being in part unwarranted.
(Andre Maurois)

The diagnostic features of a psychoneurotic disorder are:
1. It is ordinarily chronic and structured and it pervades the child's personality.
2. It is characterized by psychologic symptoms (free-floating anxiety, obsessive thoughts, phobias) that can cripple the child seriously.
3. It is not usually seen in flagrant form before the early school-age period.
4. The child does not show a gross disturbance in reality testing despite the seeming irrationality of his fears or other symptoms.

General Considerations

Psychoneurotic disorders are based on a person's unconscious conflicts over the handling of his sexual and aggressive impulses which, though repressed from the person's consciousness, are active and unresolved. The unconscious conflicts are usually derived from earlier conscious conflicts between the child and persons important to him, such as his parents and siblings, and they occur as the young child struggles to master himself and his environment. Thus psychoneurotic disorders have their genesis in the preschool years, when the child is involved in individuation, early sex identification, and social integration. But they do not usually become manifest until the early school-age period, when the child is able to repress and internalize his emotional conflicts, with the help of his developing conscience (or superego), newly developed psychologic defenses, and the now developed mechanism of symptom formation.

If early conflicts between the child and his parents are not resolved, the child tends to internalize and render unconscious his conflicting emotions. His conflict may thus become chronic and self-perpetuating—a kind of self-reinforcing and reverberating feedback system. The child's unconscious conflict, together with the psychologic defenses he uses maladaptively, becomes an integral part of his personality, with limited potentiality for change. The model is that of a psychoneurosis and it is a definitive example of a "structured" psychopathology.[46]

A conflict a person is unable to resolve but tries to handle neurotically by too strenuous repression characteristically arouses anxiety. The anxiety is perceived by the conscious portion of the person's personality, and it may produce an unconscious association of ideas, emotion, and events. The anxiety, acting as a "danger signal" to the ego, ordinarily sets into operation certain defensive mechanisms that intensify the repression, and leads to the formation of psychologic symptoms that deal with the conflict symbolically, thus achieving a partial—and unhealthy—solution. The symptom (e.g., an obsessive doubt) is at times recognized by the child as something foreign and painful ("ego-alien") over which he has no control. The recognition occurs less consistently in children, particularly in the early stages of the symptom, than in adults. Patients who develop manifest psychoneurotic disorders in adolescence or adult life have been shown to have had mothers who died before the patients were 5 years old significantly more often than had the general population.[8] The finding is not specific to a psychoneurotic patient, however; it is true also of adult patients who have other disorders.

Clinical Findings

During the preschool-age period, various symptomatic reactions may occur, and they may fluctuate and change. Individual neurotic symptoms of a symbolic nature, (e.g., obsessions or phobias[91]) may occasionally occur in children as young as 3 or 4 years old, although structured psychoneurotic disorders are rare at that age. Precursors of the neurosis may be unresolved developmental or situational crises, which may become intensified in the face of unhealthy reactions or conflicts in the parents;[27] psychoneurotic disorders may appear later. A reactive disorder may be followed by internalization of the conflict and the development of a structured psychoneurosis if precipitating external events (usually multiple) occur and intensify the original conflict and, in time, change the person's adaptive equilibrium. Occasionally, the precipitating situation may be so overwhelming that a "traumatic neurosis" may crystalize from a latent or subclinical neurotic disorder.[3] It is hard to understand why one child develops a psychoneurotic disorder and another child develops another type of disorder in the presence of similar conflicts and to understand what determines the type of neurotic symptom that appears in the child.[46] Innate differences in the capacity for repression of feelings or in cognitive styles may be involved, as Witkin[104] has pointed out, as may family patterns or predispositions.

Children who have true psychoneurotic disorders may show disturbances in behavior in addition to symbolic symptoms. Although the children are not usually openly aggressive (they often fear loss of control of their aggressive impulses), aggressive behavior related to fears of harm or attack may occur. Hyperactivity, usually intermittent, may also occur in such children, particularly those who have psychoneurotic disorders of the anxiety type. Psychoneurotic disorders in children seem to be more common in middle-class families.[43] The children are usually members of intact families, and they are frequently referred for medical examination. The differential diagnosis includes reactive disorders, developmental deviations, healthy developmental crises, and some disorders that are predominantly physical—for example thyrotoxicosis and certain paralyses—whose symptoms may resemble those of psychoneurotic disorders of the anxiety and conversion types, respectively. (The prognosis and management are discussed later.)

Mixed psychoneurotic disorders, which are common in children, should be diagnosed according to their predominant feature, with a qualifying statement about the trends of another subtype. Individual symptoms can be further described, as in other types of disorders.

Psychoneurotic Disorders of the Anxiety Type

The anxiety arising from the unconscious internalized conflict appears to break through into awareness as an intense and diffuse feeling of apprehension or of impending disaster, in contrast to normal apprehensions, conscious fears of objective dangers, or content-specific phobias. The anxiety is ordinarily free floating, without the appearance of stable defense mechanisms or symbolic symptom formation in its early stages, and it may arise in a variety of situations. The physiologic concomitants of anxiety (e.g., flushed face, rapid pulse, moist palms, palpitations, dizziness, disturbances in respiration, and gastrointestinal disorders, such as diarrhea and urinary frequency or urgency) are often present in varying degrees. But unlike psychophysiologic disorders, anxiety disorders do not lead to structural changes in the organ systems involved. Anxiety may be chronic or it may occur in attacks, often in response to upsetting experiences. The attacks may last a few minutes or for hours, and they may occur several times a week or even several times a day.[3,9,57]

In children, anxiety neuroses are not apt to remain diffuse; they often develop into one of the more crystalized "symptom" neuroses.[46] Anxiety neuroses must be distinguished from acute panic states, which are frequently reactive disorders of anxious children in hypochondriacal families or, in adolescents, acute confusional states.

Case Example. An 8-year-old boy was brought to a pediatrician because he had episodes of trembling of his whole body, especially of his hands. The episodes occurred almost daily, and they lasted several minutes. The episodes had begun when the boy was about 7 years old, and they occurred at home and in school. During the episodes, the boy was virtually immobilized, and he emitted a soft, groaning sound. After an episode, he would often say that he felt dizzy, that his heart was pounding, and that his stomach felt funny. Neither the boy nor his parents could identify any precipitating factor; his history indicated only that he had been somewhat fearful and dependent during the preschool-age period. (He did well academically in his present school.)

During a visit to the pediatrician's office, the boy had an episode of trembling when the physician asked him about school. The boy's palms were moist and cold (which made hyperthyroidism unlikely). The boy was given a complete work-up; it ruled out cardiac abnormalities, petit mal, hyperthyroidism, and other disorders. The physician told the parents that emotional tension could cause such episodes, and he arranged for a consultation with a child psychiatrist.

The consultation revealed both that the boy felt "something terrible" might happen during the episodes of trembling and that the episodes occurred at times when the boy felt he might not perform well or might do "something wrong." It was learned also that he was the first-born child, that he had a younger sister, and that his father, who had worked hard and had become outstandingly successful in his profession, had very high standards of achievement for the boy. The mother, on the other hand, was very protective of the boy, especially when the father was away on a trip (as he often was). A diagnosis of psychoneurotic disorder of the anxiety type was made, and psychotherapy was recommended for the boy and his parents, a recommendation that the pediatrician supported. The boy underwent psychotherapy for 15 months. During that time, he gradually became symptom free and confident. The boy's parents were gradually able to reconcile their conflicts about handling the boy.

Psychoneurotic Disorders of the Phobic Type

In psychoneurotic disorders of the phobic type, the child has unconsciously displaced the content of his original conflict onto an object or a situation in the external environment that has symbolic significance for him. The fears generated by the unconscious internal conflict break through into his consciousness, but they are distorted and irrational. Thus the child avoids those objects and situations that revive or intensify his displaced conflict, and he frequently projects his unacceptable feelings onto the external feared object or situation. He may show a conscious fear of animals, school, dirt, disease, high places, elevators, or of dying. Some of the reversible physiologic concomitants that were described in relation to anxiety neuroses may also be seen.[3,21,46,61]

Developmental crises involving separation anxiety (with the child's concern for the whereabouts of his mother) should be differentiated from phobic disorders (e.g., psychoneurotic school phobias), which have internalized and structured characters. The mild fears[50,58] and transient phobias[3] of the healthy preschool-age child (which are somewhat different in girls and in boys), and the fears of specifically stressful experiences that characterize reactive disorders[74] (as in the young child who, after having been hospitalized, fears people in white coats) should also be differentiated from neurotic phobic disorders. In making the diagnosis, the specific character of the phobic manifestations (e.g., fear of animals or fear of dirt) can be listed as an individual symptom.

The school phobia syndrome[88] may have a classic psychoneurotic phobic structure. Or it may represent (1) a prolongation of separation anxiety as part of a developmental crisis in children beginning school, (2) a reactive disorder with phobic mechanisms, arising from a family illness or other crisis or a move to a new school in the early school-age period, (3) intensification of a chronic personality disorder of anxious or phobic nature, or (4) a manifestation of a borderline or incipient psychotic state.[88,102] (School phobia is discussed more fully in Chapter 28.)

Case Example. A 10-year-old boy had had strong fears of animals since he was about 4 years old. These fears had gradually become worse, and they focused on dogs. The boy had to be taken to and from school by one of his parents (usually his mother), and he was unable to participate in outdoor recess because of his fears. (He performed well enough in the classroom.) The school psychologist had tried desensitizing behavior therapy without success. The boy was finally referred to a pediatrician by the school because he was absent from school more and more. His parents said that the boy was now often completely unable to leave the house, even in their company, because of his paralyzing fear that he might meet a dog. The boy's history indicated that he had been frightened by a dog when he was about 2 years old although his fear did not become marked until 2 years later and did not focus on dogs until he was about 6 years old. The boy's mother also had some fears about animals. His father, a perennially unsuccessful man who drank heavily, had for a long time tended to ridicule his wife's fears. He had also punished the boy physically in an effort to eradicate his fears, but to no avail.

The boy was referred to a child psychiatrist. During the consultation, it was apparent that the boy could not discuss his fears easily. He did draw a picture of a tiny barking dog that was confronted by a fierce "father" dog. The drawing led the psychiatrist to infer that the boy was unconsciously displacing his fear of the father onto large dogs and projecting his own ineffectual anger toward the father onto dogs— all the while fearing retaliation. Psychotherapy helped the boy uncover and come to grips with his fears. His mother was able to help him in his efforts to become independent of her. His father, who was at first unable to become involved, later was able to accept referral for treatment of his problems. His treatment was moderately successful.

Psychoneurotic Disorders of the Conversion Type

In psychoneurotic disorders of the conversion type, the original conflict seems to have been dealt with unconsciously (after having been repressed) through a "conversion" centrally into a somatic dysfunction that involves a disturbance in the functioning of bodily structures or organs supplied by the voluntary portion of the central nervous system. Such dysfunctions thus ordinarily involve the striated musculature and the somatosensory apparatus.[46] Conversion disorders may produce disturbances in motor function (e.g., paralysis or motor tics), disturbances in sensory perception (e.g., blindness or deafness), disturbances in awareness (e.g., conversion syncope, which often involves "gradual" faints, with no vasomotor changes and partial consciousness) or conversion seizures, which usually involve thrashing movements that do not have tonic-clonic components and with memory for events. Marked psychologic invalidism associated with intense weakness, bizarre paralyses, conversion seizures, or other symptoms may be disturbances in the total body image of seriously disturbed adolescents. Conversion disorders may also produce disturbances of the upper and lower ends of the gastrointestinal tract (e.g., certain types of vomiting[49] or encopresis), disturbances of the voluntary components of respiration (e.g., hyperventilation or coughing or barking tics), and disturbances of the genitourinary organs (e.g., certain types of enuresis or bladder atony). In all the structures mentioned, voluntary innervation is at least partly involved. Pain of conversion origin is common; for example, abdominal pain in children who have school phobia and chest pain in adolescents who fear heart disease.

The exact neurophysiologic mechanisms of the conversion phenomena are not known.[80] Presumably some change in the electrochemical activity of the cerebral cortex takes place in response to psychologic or interpersonal stressful stimuli, as a result of which the individual muscular components or the particular organ of special sense acts "as if" its function were suspended, blocked, or altered. Certain EEG changes have been reported to occur when such a symptom disappears, but the EEG changes are nonspecific and are not indicative of a structural change in the cerebral cortex. Local structural changes are not demonstrable in the body parts involved. Distortions in the perception of pain, touch, and other senses may occur in reverse, as if such stimuli were perceived centrally without the existence of specific sources in the local sites affected. Secondary changes in structure can of course occur; for example, contractures in long-standing conversion paralysis or changes in calcium metabolism and excretion in a person who is bedridden.

In conversion disorders, the symptom seems to symbolize the conflict. A partial solution results—at the cost of illness and suffering but with unconscious secondary gain accruing from increased dependence or from other sources. The anxiety aroused by the conflict appears to be "bound" to the symptom, and the person feels little conscious concern (the classic *la belle indifference* that was described in the early literature on hysteria). The unconscious psychologic determinants of the symptom may vary.

1. The symptom may be a translation into *body or "organ" language* of an unacceptable wish and the defense against it (unconsciously, "I wish to see; I should not see; therefore I cannot see").

2. The symptom may take the form of *identification* with an important figure, usually a parent who has suffered from a particular symptom that the child now experiences in a distorted fashion.

3. The symptom may be a *revival of a "memory trace"* of a previous physical experience, generally a painful physical sensation or a sexually overexciting contact.

4. The symptom may be a *punishment for an unacceptable wish or impulse* directed against a person the child loves, with the child himself suffering "magically" what he wished on that person.[78]

Some cases may involve combinations of these factors. Engel[31] has recently emphasized the central importance of the memory trace of some type of bodily experience.

The disturbance in function or sensation does not follow anatomical lines of distribution; it conforms to the child's unconscious need and his naive concepts of his body. Paralyses or sensory disturbances may be totally one sided, most frequently on the left side.[37] Transient conversion symptoms, such as weakness of a limb or abdominal pain, may occur in reaction to specific situational stresses in children, including convalescence from physical illness,[14] and during developmental and situational crises in adolescents. They do not have the character of fixed conversion disorders.[34,35] As indicated earlier, conversion mechanisms are often mixed with psychophysiologic disorders and reactions to physical illness. In older adolescents and adults, conversion disorders frequently occur in hysterical personalities, most common in women, but also in men. They may appear in other personality pictures, however, particularly during childhood.

Conversion disorders in childhood and adolescence have been extensively reviewed by Engel[31] and others.[77] Loof's[62] studies have suggested that conversion disorders occur more commonly in families that do not speak freely about their emotions and in which sexual conflicts are predominant. Cultural factors[107] seem to be related to incidence; in the United States, conversion disorders seem to occur more often in isolated rural subcultures, where repressive attitudes and superstition and belief in magic may be more common. Epidemics of paralyses[53] and "benign myalgia"[69,70] have been described in a number of countries, formerly in association with fears of a polio epidemic. According to Halliday,[47] the *grande hysterie* described by Charcot (which is associated with major, often multiple, and often recurrent conversion symptoms in patients who have hysterical personality disorders) seems to occur less often in recent years. The decrease is possibly related to the less repressive attitudes toward sexuality that exist today. But *grande hysterie* can still occur, as the following case examples show.

Case Example. A 14-year-old girl was admitted to the pediatric ward because she had anorexia accompanied by ketosis, as well as seizure-like episodes that involved opisthotonic postures associated with marked arching of the back and pelvic writhings but without loss of consciousness. Apparently she had been bedridden at home for almost 2 years. The girl's legs were weak, so much so that she fell if she was made to stand. In the hospital, she quickly began to eat and drink, and her ketosis subsided. A physical examination showed that she had no physical abnormalities, and that her EEG was normal. The girl had been born out of wedlock, and her mother was living in the girl's home (although the girl's maternal grandmother gave the history).

A consultation with a child psychiatrist indicated that the weakness of the girl's legs had come on gradually, beginning about 2 years before. At that time, the rural school the girl attended had collaborated with the local health department in waging an immunization campaign, and somehow the girl had been given her first multiple immunizations without her grandmother's consent. (The grandmother was a large, strong woman who dominated the girl and her mother.) The grandmother insisted that the girl had developed "polio" from the injection, although the girl had had only a mild febrile response to the injection and had not had a polio shot. The grandmother believed that the girl's legs were paralyzed, and she kept her in bed, saying that she would devote her life to caring for the girl. Although the girl (and her mother) had given in to the grandmother's dictates, the anorexia and the conversion seizures that the girl had developed over the last few months apparently were related to her unconscious conflicts between her need to be cared for and her resentment about being controlled. (When the girl was 10 years old, she had observed a relative having a seizure. The girl's seizures seemed to be related to her identification with the relative.) The weakness of the girl's legs seemed to symbolize her inability to "stand on her own feet" in regard to her submission to her grandmother and to her inability to express her anger. Psychologic tests showed that the girl's I.Q. was in the range of 60 to 70.

At first, the girl was treated supportively on the pediatric ward by the psychiatrist. She responded in a month by becoming able to stand alone. It was difficult for the psychiatrist to see the grandmother regularly. One day, the grandmother came to the hospital and took the girl home, saying that she "could care for her better than any doctor or nurse." The psychiatrist let the grandmother take the girl home (because he knew the strength of the symbiotic bond between the girl and her grandmother), but he encouraged her to bring the girl back to the hospital if the symptoms recurred. The symptoms recurred in several weeks, and the grandmother brought the girl back to the hospital. She repeated the taking home and bringing back

2 more times. By that time, the psychiatrist had been able to develop a relationship with the grandmother. She had told him that she had a stomach ulcer, and he had made arrangements for her to be treated by an internist. A social worker also had become involved in the grandmother's case, and reluctantly the grandmother had become dependent on her.

The girl allowed herself to be "taught to walk again." As soon as the girl was well enough—and as soon as the grandmother allowed it—the girl was transferred to a psychiatric adolescent unit, where she remained for 14 months. She underwent individual therapy and milieu therapy, and she became able to function independently. Her I.Q. rose into the 90s. The grandmother, whose life was now more satisfying to her, continued to permit the girl to progress. The girl was followed supportively at gradually longer intervals for several years. When she was 18, she married and left home. She later gave birth to a normal infant, and she seemed to be raising the child in a healthy manner. The girl's mother remained a shadow of the grandmother (the grandmother had relinquished control of her granddaughter but now controlled her daughter). The grandmother died a few years later, and the girl's mother became more independent.

Case Example. An 11-year-old Chicano girl from a small, rural town was admitted to the pediatric ward because she was paralyzed from the neck down. The paralysis had come on over a period of a week, approximately 4 weeks before. The girl had no history of fever or other symptoms. The paralysis was associated with insensitivity to touch and pain, and the symptoms did not follow anatomical lines of distribution. The girl could swallow, and although she was sad, she did not seem seriously depressed or anxious. An extensive work-up showed that she had no physical abnormalities. The referring health professional mentioned that a hex cult was rumored to be operating in the girl's school. He said that the girl's aunt and uncle (with whom the girl lived) and the girl herself had told a social worker that a hex could not possibly be involved in the paralysis.

The girl, who was in a respirator, was interviewed by a child psychiatrist in a group conference in the pediatric ward. When it was suggested to her that some people in such a situation might think a hex or witchcraft was involved, the girl replied that she did not think so, but her mother did. The psychiatrist called a consulting *curandera*, a folk healer, who had recently joined the staff of a community mental health center. The *curandera* came to the hospital

to interview the girl and her parents. The parents told the *curandera* that they believed (and that the girl did too) that a hex had been placed on their child. The psychiatrist thought that the girl had a major conversion disorder expressed in ethnic terms, and he felt that the *curandera* should be allowed to try to help the girl. A psychologist agreed with the diagnosis, but he felt that hypnosis was the approach of choice. A hypnotic interview was held, but it produced no change in the girl's condition.

The *curandera* treated the girl in 2 private sessions. She first explained to the girl that power came through her from God and that she could dispense her power through a ceremonial necklace she possessed. In the first session, the *curandera* touched each part of the girl's upper trunk with the necklace, and functioning was restored to that part of the girl's body. The next day, the *curandera* repeated the same procedure on the girl's lower trunk, with similar results. The *curandera* then recommended that the girl have some follow-up physiotherapy.

The girl's family gave the *curandera* some information that they had not given the staff. They told her that they had considered turning over the girl to the care of another member of the family, a more distant relative. That possibility had so angered a member of the community in which the family lived that he put a hex on the family. The girl's possible loss of her home had apparently thrown her into a serious emotional conflict. Also, she had overheard a violent argument between her aunt and uncle. The argument, the threatened loss of her home, and the fear of the hex had precipitated the girl's paralysis.

The *curandera* explained the paralysis in ethnic terms—as the girl's response to the danger of death from the hex—and she based her cure on that interpretation. The psychiatrist explained the paralysis in traditional psychiatric terms—as a symbol of the girl's complete helplessness and her need for care. The girl seemed also to derive secondary gain from the paralysis in that the paralysis made it impossible for her aunt and uncle to turn her over to someone else's care.

The *curandera* visited the girl's family in their home. She recommended to them that they keep the girl, and she referred them for marital therapy to the local mental health clinic, which had Chicano professionals on its staff. Two years later, the girl was still symptom free, she had adjusted well at home, and she performed well at school.

When conversion disorders occur in a person who does not have a hysterical personality, the appropriate personality diagnosis should also be specified. Conversion disorders must be distinguished principally from the symptoms of predominantly physical illness and from psychophysiologic disorders; these disorders are sometimes mixed, (e.g., in Sydenham's chorea and epileptic seizures), and multiple diagnoses should be made as needed. Ruling out physical illness is not sufficient to make a diagnosis of a conversion disorder. Positive signs of psychosocial disturbance must be demonstrated in conversion disorders and in certain other psychoneurotic disorders. As indicated earlier, positive psychologic data must be demonstrated: (1) a chronic, unresolved, unconscious and internalized emotional conflict in the child in the family setting, (2) relevant stressful and precipitating circumstances, (3) symbolic psychologic determinants of the symptom, and (4) unconscious secondary gain, with partial resolution of the conflict or other perpetuating forces. A study of the psychosocial factors should accompany an investigation of the physical factors, and it should not be left until the end of an exhaustive (and exhausting) set of laboratory studies. Early psychiatric consultation may help make the diagnosis. When the diagnosis is made, the child's symptoms should be accepted as real (as they are psychologically), and not as "in his head" or "put on."

True malingering is rare in children and adolescents. As Engel[32] has pointed out, such patients need to be nurtured or to suffer. Many of them are accident prone, and submit readily to painful procedures. Prazar and Friedman[77] believe that the phenomenon may be associated with patients in institutions in which advantages may accrue to the state of being ill or threats may be circumvented. Such terms as Münchausen's syndrome are more nearly epithets than clinical diagnoses; there are adult pathologic liars, but, in my view, these are sick individuals.

Specific Conversion Disorders

Certain conversion disorders, such as conversion deafness, trismus,[95] and paraplegia, occur rarely in children, although aphonia[7] and blindness[105] are not uncommon in children.[105] Some conversion disorders, such as the hyperventilation syndrome,[33,40] occur more often, particularly in adolescents. The hyperventilation syndrome involves initial conversion mechanisms but the hyperventilation may trigger off psychophysiologic sequelae. Patients often report "black-outs" or other types of "spells" and sensations of shortness of breath, choking, or smothering (rather than tingling and numbness of the extremities, overbreathing, lightheadedness, or generalized weakness). The patient is usually unaware of the anxiety that has resulted in the hyperventilation, which can lead to tetany or syncope. If the physician suspects the child has the hyperventilation syndrome, he should ask the child to hyperventilate for several minutes to help make the diagnosis. Having the child rebreathe into a bag and reassuring him often brings him immediate relief. But the conflicts that underlie the symptom must be investigated. In milder cases, counseling of the child and his parents may suffice. In some cases, however, the hyperventilation is only one of several symptoms of the child's emotional disturbance, and more intensive psychotherapy is usually indicated.

Fainting. *Conversion syncope* is usually but not always seen in patients who have hysterical personality disorders. It usually occurs in older school-age and adolescent girls who have conflicts, particularly about their sexuality, although boys may also exhibit it. The differential diagnoses include vasodepressor syncope, syncope associated with epilepsy or hyperventilation, and (occasionally) syncope related to such physical causes as cardiac abnormalities, anemia, and paroxysms of coughing.[30] Attacks of conversion syncope may be sudden and dramatic, but often the person simply slumps over or even faints while sitting, without showing the prodromal signs of anxiety or vasomotor changes that occur in vasodepressor syncope, and without injury (though the attack is "real" psychologically). Consciousness is usually only partly lost, with considerable variations in its level. The eyes may be open, fluttering, or held tightly closed. Bizarre movements are often seen, with various sounds emitted at times. The attack may last for a few seconds or for hours.

Conversion syncope is usually precipitated by disturbing events, sometimes related to sexual issues,[43,44] or by situations in which the patient might be expected to do or say something troubling to her. The attack thus seems to symbolize an unconscious blocking out of conflict-producing sights or situations although the posture or movements of the patient during the faint may be provocative in sexual or other ways. Psychiatric consultation is usually indicated, and intensive psychotherapy is often needed to deal with the unconscious underlying conflicts as well as with the family situation.

Vasodepressor syncope, the most common type of fainting, may occur in school-age children, but it usually occurs in adolescents. The attack of syncope may occur in response to frightening or disturbing situations, such as venipuncture and the sight of blood or in anticipation of pain from other sources.[30] Usually the patient is standing when the attack begins, although the syncope occasionally occurs when the patient is sitting or even lying down. Fatigue (particularly when the person has been standing still for a long time), hot or humid surroundings, or prolonged periods without food may be precipitants or contributory factors. Lightheadedness, weakness, dizziness, pallor, numbness, nausea, excessive salivation, feelings of warmth, sweating, blurring of vision, and yawning or sighing may be prodromal symptoms. The symptoms may disappear spontaneously, or the person may faint suddenly.

The person loses consciousness completely, and the fall may be painful; consciousness is usually regained in a few seconds or at most several minutes. If unconsciousness persists for more than half a minute or so, clonic movements may appear.

Many children have a single attack of syncope under the circumstances described. Recurrent attacks may be aborted by putting the child's head low or by other methods, including avoiding situations that are likely to precipitate an attack. Children who have frequent attacks of syncope are often anxious and somewhat inhibited, and they tend to fear punishment or damage to the integrity of their body, carrying over from the preschool period. I have seen several adolescents in whom the visible prodromal symptoms of vasodepressor syncope seemed to activate conversion mechanisms and to change the type of attack.

Carotid sinus syncope, which results from a hyperactive carotid sinus reflex, is relatively rare in children. It also may sometimes be associated with anxiety. Attacks of syncope may occasionally occur as a result of paroxysmal tachycardia, which may be touched off by emotional crises in anxious children who have a biologic predisposition.[30]

Tics. Tics usually first occur in the school-age period.[3,46] Tics are abrupt, stereotyped involuntary movements of particular muscle groups. Eye blinking, nose twitching, facial grimaces, and movements of the neck or head are types of tics. Like nail biting, tics are habit disturbances, and they affect nearly 50% of children during the school-age period. They are more common in boys, and they are usually mild and transient, lasting a few weeks or several months in emotionally healthy children. They may originate in purposive movements, such as blinking because of eyestrain or twitching because of nasal irritation. In tense, over-conscientious, and restless children who often are under undue pressure from their parents, tics may change from one to another type. In disturbed children who have conflicts with their parents, tics are sometimes more constant and are pathologic. They then assume the characteristics and symbolic meanings of conversion symptoms; for example, they may represent an unconsciously aggressive gesture or self-punishment through identification with a fantasied figure who is being choked or attacked.

Other types of tics are respiratory tics—coughing,[10,54] sniffling, clearing the throat, inspiratory stridor, or hiccoughing, often occurring in a child who had a respiratory infection during a conflict. In more seriously disturbed children, barking tics[11] may occur. They may symbolize the child's identification with a feared or a loved animal.

Tics have been said to be difficult to treat, although some tics (e.g., the respiratory tics) have responded to counseling or brief psychotherapy. Recovery probably depends on the degree of the child's personality disturbance and his family's pathology.[3,39,66] Most children who have 1 or 2 conversion tics do well.[66,97] Tics appear within children who have different personality pictures, however, including obsessive-compulsive, overly inhibited personality disorders, in which conflicts over the handling of aggressive impulses are paramount. A few tics are associated with hysterical personality disorders; some occur in children whose disorders border on psychoses. A psychiatric consultation may be most helpful for children who have long-standing and multiple tics, and long-term intensive psychotherapy is indicated for children who are more severely disturbed and for their families.

Maladie des Tics. The rare syndrome of maladie des tics (often called *Gilles de la Tourette's* syndrome, after the clinician who described it in the late 1800s) includes a number of severe tics that involve sudden involuntary movements of different parts of the body. The disorder typically begins before the child is 10 years old, but it may occur from the preschool years up to late adolescence. Eye blinking, facial twitching, and neck movements usually occur first. Explosive but initially transient movements of the shoulders, chest, and upper extremities appear later. As the disorder progresses, the tics occur more frequently, and they gradually spread to the trunk and lower extremities. Occasionally, complex involuntary movements may involve the entire body, including sudden and impulsive acts of kicking, jumping, wringing the hands, protrusion of the tongue, and slapping the face. At some point, vocal tics appear—inarticulate sounds, such as clearing the throat and grunting, barking, or quacking noises, or sudden vocalizations that have no apparent meaning. In about 50% of the cases, the final symptom is the explosive utterance of obscenities (coprolalia). In some patients, imitative speech (echolalia) and imitative movements may appear. Rarely, vocal tics or coprolalia may be the earliest symptom of the disorder.

The symptoms generally are intensified by fatigue, excitement, anger, or stressful situations, and they improve with relaxation, fever, and drowsiness to the point of disappearing during sleep. The disorder is usually progressive, but periods of waxing and waning can occur, as can spontaneous remissions. In the past, the prognosis was said to be poor, and mental deterioration or psychosis was believed to occur in the final phase in most cases (although little systematic follow-up data were available). That view has changed, and Mahler,[67] Eisenberg and Kanner,[29] Lucas[63,64] and others[16] recently have reported gradual amelioration of symptoms in late adolescence and early adulthood.

As Woodrow[106] and Kelman[52] have indicated in recent reviews, the views about the etiology of *maladie des tics* have varied. They range from early views of the disorder as hereditary (there is little evidence that it is), to more recent attempts to understand the etiology by investigating the psychodynamic or somatic factors. The personality characteristics and intrafamilial dynamics of the patients described in the literature vary somewhat.[3,5,28] Some patients have been described as extroverted and gregarious; more often they have been described as having obsessive-compulsive personality traits, being perfectionistic, conforming, and anxious, and having much difficulty controlling their aggressive impulses and in expressing their feelings of anger. Some patients have been described as schizophrenic.

Probably patients fall along a continuum in regard to the severity of their personality disturbance, and show some variations in the nature of their personality disturbance. (For that reason I prefer the designation of "multiple tics," with much variation in the severity of the tics and the personality disturbance.) In my experience with 5 patients of school age, 3 patients had obsessive-compulsive personality disorders, 1 patient was overly inhibited, and 1 patient had a neurotic personality disorder and some oppositional tendencies and some mild acting out of aggressive impulses. One of the obsessive-compulsive patients had some defects in reality testing and a clinical picture that bordered on psychosis.

A number of investigators have viewed the tics as the person's symbolic expressions of anger he considers unacceptable, with displacement onto obscene language and dissociation from responsibility as the result of the involuntary nature of the symptoms. That view seems to fit with the finding in some studies of family psychopathology that at least 1 parent is usually domineering, controlling, rigid, demanding, and punitive. My experience supports those findings, but the samples in most investigations are so small that the formulations cannot be considered definitive.

Recently, in an uncontrolled study Shapiro and his colleagues[89] found evidence of physical abnormalities. Such abnormalities have generally included nonspecific EEG abnormalities, soft neurologic signs, per-

ceptual-motor difficulties as shown by the Bender Gestalt Test, and discrepancies between the child's Verbal I.Q. and his Performance I.Q. (noted also by Lucas[63,64]). As indicated in Chapter 22, other investigators find such evidence of brain damage equivocal at best, especially in children. As Eisenberg and his colleagues[29] have pointed out, the minimal changes in the size and density of small cells in the corpus stratum that were seen in 1 autopsy by Balthasar, a pathologist, were not seen by other pathologists, and the findings were not replicated by Balthasar himself in another autopsy on a patient who had had maladie des tics. Only 1 other autopsy has been carried out on a patient who had maladie des tics (and without microscopic examination). Finally, it is difficult to conceptualize the type of lesion in the brain that produces the striking clinical picture of maladie des tics. It is of course possible that in certain cases mild cerebral dysfunction could be mixed with psychodynamic factors. Lake and his colleagues[56] found no abnormalities in catecholamine metabolism. (Other studies of serotonin and dopamine metabolism are currently being carried on.) As Brun and Shapiro[15] have pointed out, the differential diagnoses should include toxic disorders, vascular accidents, dystonia musculorum deformans, the choreas, postencephalitic disorders, and various rare disorders (e.g., Wilson's disease and the "bobble-head doll syndrome" described by Nellhaus[73]).

A plethora of physical, environmental, and other psychologic approaches to the treatment of maladie des tics has produced generally equivocal results. Mahler[65] and others have reported definitive cases in which improvement or remission occurred after different types of psychotherapy were used. I have successfully treated 2 such patients, but the follow-up of these patients, like the other follow-ups that have been reported, was limited. Eisenberg, Ascher, and Kanner[29] reported on a similarly treated case in 1959, and at that time they favored trying a completely psychiatric management of patients who had maladie des tics. Since then, several patients have been treated successfully with behavioral therapy,[20] and Lucas[63,64] and others[89] found haloperidol to have a relatively specific effect on the tics that were motor and vocal.

In a large scale follow-up of mostly adult patients who were treated with haloperidol, Lucas,[63,64] and Shapiro and his colleagues[89] found convincing evidence for its effectiveness in children. But they also found that its effectiveness was severely hampered by side-effects that often forced patients to compromise between maximum relief of symptoms and minimal discomfort—or forced them to discontinue the drug and live with their symptoms. I feel that haloperidol, which is not approved for children, is dangerous for adolescents, and that it should be used in conjunction with intensive psychotherapy in only the severest cases. In my experience, residential or inpatient treatment can be valuable for severely disturbed children who have maladie des tics. If haloperidol is used, it seems safest to begin to use it (with other treatment measures) in a hospital setting.

Urinary Retention. Another conversion syndrome is urinary retention, often with marked atony of the bladder. It occurs principally in adolescent girls and women, who often have hysterical personality disorders. Brief psychotherapy can help relieve the symptom (which usually is related to sexual conflicts) although long-term therapy is generally indicated.[19,99]

Astasia-Abasia. A rare conversion syndrome in children is astasia-abasia,[4] a condition in which the patient can move his legs normally in bed but has trouble putting them on the floor. He shows a variety of uncoordinated and dysrhythmic movements when he attempts to get out of bed. The syndrome may also be seen in patients who have hysterical personality disorders, often those who have psychologic invalidism. I have seen several milder cases in older school-age girls and boys who have

conflicts about convalescence. Counseling those children and their parents was effective although intensive long-term psychotherapy is usually employed.

Camptocormia. Another rare conversion syndrome in adults is camptocormia,[6,85] (the bent back syndrome), which involves a flexion deformity of the vertebral column. I have seen several mild cases in adolescents, who seemed to have conflicts about looking up and "bearing up" that responded to psychotherapy. One school-age child showed what seemed to be a combination of astasia-abasia and camptocormia in a stressful situation that involved an ambiguous diagnosis of a physical illness. The psychodynamics were not completely clear, but the symptoms cleared with support and when the diagnosis was clarified. (Although the final diagnosis was that of a more serious illness, it relieved the boy of certain pressures within the family.)

Psychoneurotic Disorders of the Dissociative Type

Psychoneurotic disorders of the dissociative type are based on neurotic conflicts that lead to some temporary general disorganization of the personality, with repressed impulses or affects giving rise to anxiety. The results are aimless motor discharge or "freezing," fugue states, catalepsy, cataplexy, transient catatonic states without underlying psychosis, and other pictures. In adolescents particularly, the self-representation of the personality may be disturbed; and depersonalization, dissociated personality, or multiple personalities, and amnesia may occur. Disturbances in consciousness may occur, and hypnogogic and hypnopompic or so-called twilight states, marked somnambulism (often associated with sleep-talking), and pseudo-delirious and stuporous states may result.[3]

These disorders, like conversion disorders, often occur in hysterical personalities. But they may also appear in association with other psychopathologic disorders and (rarely) isolated symptoms of some of these disorders may occur transiently in healthy people as the result of an acute physical illness or overwhelmingly stressful situations. Other total personality diagnoses should thus be mentioned when it is appropriate to do so. The diagnosis should indicate the symptoms, and the disorders should be differentiated from panic states (usually marked reactive disorders), acute brain syndromes, psychotic disorders, and epileptic equivalents (in which episodic EEG abnormalities occur).

Psychoneurotic Disorders of the Obsessive-Compulsive Type

In psychoneurotic disorders of the obsessive-compulsive type, the anxiety aroused by the unconscious conflict seems to be counteracted by the occurrence of thoughts (obsessions) or impulses to act (compulsions), or mixtures of both, that are isolated from the original unacceptable impulse. The child frequently recognizes his ideas or behavior as being unreasonable, but he is nevertheless compelled to repeat his compulsions or suffer his obsessive thoughts, and sometimes he becomes incapacitated. Often the behavior is the opposite of the unconscious wish (reaction formation). An example is excessive orderliness and washing compulsions that overlie impulses to soil or to mess. Counting and touching rituals frequently occur, and the child shows marked anxiety if someone tries to interfere with the ritual.[46,51,81,90]

In Adams' recent studies,[1,2] the onset of obsessive-compulsive symptoms, at times associated with tics, took place in children 6 to 7 years old or (occasionally) older. A few children were said to have shown the symptoms in the preschool-age period. Three quarters of the patients were boys. Children who have the disorder are said to be of high intelligence and to show precocious ego development,[72] although ob-

sessional pictures have been reported in retarded children. Adams said that the children were characteristically very verbal and underactive physically, were excessively concerned with social conformity, had a rigid sense of right and wrong, tended to label rather than think, and communicated very little feeling. The children's inability to express even appropriate anger and their difficulty in controlling aggressive impulses seemed to reflect their central unconscious conflicts, and fears of insanity often represent fears that they would lose control of their feelings and their world. Adams' study of the children's parents indicated that the parent had very similar obsessive-compulsive styles and that they were also highly verbal and usually underactive physically. The mothers were generally the dominant persons in the families, which tended to derogate maleness. The parents valued social conventions, rectitude, and cleanliness highly, and they had a tendency to hoard. They tended also to live rather isolated, withdrawn lives, and had trouble making warm friendships. Adams commented on their conventional but hollow lives and pointed out that many of the parents were tired of their empty conformity. The possibility of some biologic predisposition and hereditary influence in obsessive behavior has long been considered, but the facts are not clear.[42]

These disorders must be distinguished from normal compulsive-like ritualistic behavior, such as the bedtime rituals of young children and the pseudo-compulsions and rituals of the early school-age child. They must also be distinguished from the obsessive tendencies in some psychotic children.[26] The specific symptom patterns can be listed in the diagnosis.

Psychoneurotic Disorders of the Depressive Type

As indicated earlier, depression in children and adolescents up to 16 or 17 years old or older may be manifested somewhat differently from depression in adults.[36,60,92,96] In infants depressive equivalents are often manifested by fussing, eating and sleeping disturbances, head banging, and bed rocking although a depression may be overt, such as the so-called anaclitic depression,[94] a reactive disorder caused by a loss of maternal emotional support. Older infants and young children may show withdrawal,[79] apathy, regression, hyperactivity or hypoactivity, insomnia, weight loss, vomiting, diarrhea, or constipation. Chronic depression in emotionally deprived infants and young children can lead to permanent emotional and intellectual impairment, failure to thrive, increased susceptibility to physical illness, and even death.[93] The school-age child may show such depressive equivalents as significant behavioral disturbance, involving temper tantrums, negativism, truancy, running away from home, accident-proneness, and acting-out behavior of an aggressive nature, which may help the child ward off more serious depression.[17] Depression may also be manifested by school phobia, learning difficulties, speech problems, irritability, abdominal pain, enuresis, hyperventilation, physical complaints, or a tendency to fatigue easily.[82] In adolescents, boredom, failing in school, dropping out of school, or delinquent behavior may also occur.[96] Psychophysiologic disorders may be precipitated in children and adolescents by depression or feelings of hopelessness and "giving-up," and depression may exacerbate an underlying psychotic process. Physical illness may precipitate depression at any age. Psychomotor retardation is ordinarily less marked in children (except young infants) than in adults, as are the other biologic signs of depression.

Recent studies by Poznanski and Zrull[76] and others[48,68,86] have drawn attention to the fact that overt and directly observable depression, based on internalized neurotic conflict, is more common in childhood than was formerly believed. The children studied were described as sad, unhappy, or openly depressed, showing low self-esteem and a negative self-image, difficulties in handling aggression, withdrawal, and excessive crying. The children expressed feelings of inadequacy, had difficulty in sleeping, and were excessively concerned about dying. Their families had considerable pathology. The parents showed a high incidence of depression, difficulties in handling aggression, and often overt rejection of their children. A follow-up of the children into adolescence and young adulthood[75] showed that they had the same degree of psychopathology, and neurotic conflicts but not psychoses. Fifty percent of the group were still depressed, mostly those who had lost a father through divorce (and who had never seen him again). Some who had been openly depressed as children but not when they were older had lost a parent through death. Those whom the follow-up showed to be still depresssed generally had had no parent at all to whom they could relate. They still had poor peer and heterosexual relationships and their performance in school was below their capacities. They had become more passive and overtly dependent. Thus the loss of a parent seemed to be an important factor in chronic depression, a conclusion reached in another study also.[18] On follow-up their disorders thus resemble adult depressive pictures more closely (in adult depressive disorders, parental loss in childhood is very high[8]). Apparently most of the young people either had not received treatment or had not followed through on it.

More recently, Cytryn and McKnew[24] proposed the following classification, or typology, of childhood depression: acute depression, chronic depression, and masked depression. In their study, *acute depression* was manifested by openly depressed feelings and some depressive equivalents that were always related to the sudden loss of an important family member (not always a parent), through divorce, a move, or the withdrawal of that person because of other preoccupations (without the substitute of another appropriate figure). The parents of the children studied did not have overt clinical depression.[71] All the children who had *chronic depression* had at least 1 parent who had clinical depression; and that group also had many instances of frequent separations, some evidence of depreciation and rejection, with fewer instances of loss of involvement.[71] Among the children who had *masked depression,* a term first used by Glaser,[41] a condition characterized only by depressive equivalents, there had often been an acute loss or a loss of involvement and almost always depreciation and rejection, but few instances of depression in their parents.

Thus a child who has an acute or a chronic depression may be aware of his depressed feelings, even if he also has some depressive equivalents. In masked depression, which may be acute or chronic, any of the physiologic, psychologic, or behavioral equivalents just discussed may be present without the child's being aware of his depressed feelings. Many adolescents, particularly those from the ghettos or barrios who feel frustrated or alienated, may manifest chronic depression by acting-out behavior that is associated with anger or rage. Why some children do not become depressed or why some develop other disorders in situations similar to those just described is not clear. (Mourning of course is more effective in healthier families, as indicated in Chapter 6.) The question of a genetic[87] or biochemical[103] predisposition to depression in adults has been raised recently, but convincing evidence of such a predisposition in children and adolescents is lacking.[23,25]

Acute depression may accompany grief or bereavement. If the child is permitted to grieve and if the "work of mourning" is accomplished, the prognosis is usually good. Acute depression may continue as part of a reactive disorder, or, in a young child, the associated conflicts may be internalized, and a chronic psychoneurotic

depressive disorder may develop. Depressions of psychotic proportions do not seem to occur in childhood, although a few adolescents exhibit them. Depressions should also be distinguished from fleeting feelings of depression in healthy children who undergo developmental or situational crises and from the cyclical behavioral and mood swings that occasionally occur in children who have developmental deviations. Suicide threats or suicide attempts may be made by older children or adolescents who have any of the disorders discussed.[45]

Treatment and Prognosis of Psychoneurotic Disorders

Even though the child may have internalized and repressed earlier conflicts, he is still in the process of development. Changes in his disorder may still occur, leading to the prevalence of symptomatology at certain stages or to changes in his symptoms. Some mild psychoneurotic disorders may resolve spontaneously as the child reworks the conflicts at a higher level of maturation, and accomplishes the developmental tasks he had been unable to master. The parent or the whole family may develop, giving the child greater emotional support; or changes may occur in the family's adaptive equilibrium that diminish the child's conflicts and release him from his developmental impasse.

Even moderate psychoneurotic disorders seem to be self limited, over a period of several years. Robins[83] has shown in a long-term follow-up study that most children who have diagnosed psychoneurotic disorders do not have them as adults. However, more severe disorders that are not treated, may continue for many years, as Waldron[100] has shown. Rutter[84] indicated that the sex incidence changes; psychoneurotic disorders are more common in males during childhood and in females during adulthood. Sampling problems in clinical studies and the use of different nomenclatures make research in such behavioral areas difficult. There are as yet no adequate incidence and prevalence data about emotional and mental disorders in childhood.

Despite the self-perpetuating character of established psychoneurotic disorders, the response to treatment is generally good in childhood, especially in regard to anxiety, phobic, conversion, and depressive types. These types usually respond well to intensive psychotherapy for the child and his parents that is continued for a year or more. Marked obsessive-compulsive,[42] severely phobic, and dissociative types may be treated successfully, but they are more recalcitrant and difficult and often require several years of psychotherapy. Such phobic and obsessive disorders may respond better to child analysis than to psychotherapy.[12,13] Hypnosis or hypnotherapy may be effective in the moderate forms[38] or to relieve symptoms.[55] Mild tranquilizers, such as Benadryl, may help to control free-floating anxiety (see Chap. 13). But such drugs ordinarily have limited value for children. Eisenberg and his colleagues have found psychotherapy more effective than drugs for these disorders. Severely depressed adolescents may respond to antidepressants, but they must be used with due caution. Behavior therapy can be of value in less severe psychoneurotic disorders (e.g., certain phobias,[59] obsessive-compulsive disorders,[101] and conversion symptoms), and it has been used successfully to treat urinary retention that is a conversion syndrome.[22] Hospitalization of children with psychoneurotic disorders is rarely indicated, except at times for diagnostic evaluation, for children who have attempted suicide, and for severely disturbed adolescents who have severe depressions or marked conversion disorders.

Children who have early or mild psychoneurotic disorders—and their parents—may be treated with supportive psychotherapy by the pediatrician. He often makes the diagnosis, using psychiatric consultations when indicated. As Friedman[34] has shown, abdominal pain may be especially responsive to supportive psychotherapy. (The "first-aid" management of school phobia and the management of depressed or otherwise troubled children who make suicidal threats or attempts are discussed in Chapter 28.) For children who have milder conversion disorders, particularly while they are convalescing from a physical illness, the positive use of suggestion, combined with supportive measures, (e.g., arranging for a nurse to "teach" a child who has a leg weakness to walk again) or hypnotic suggestive therapy[55] may help the child return to functioning in several weeks. But the family's problems should not be overlooked. The more severe psychoneurotic disorders, even those that respond to the approaches described, may recur if the underlying conflicts are not resolved by intensive psychotherapy.

Bibliography

1. Adams, P.L.: Family characteristics of obsessive children. Am. J. Psychiatry, *128*:1414, 1972.
2. Adams, P.L.: *Obsessive Children: A Sociopsychiatric Study.* New York, Brunner/Mazel, 1973.
3. Anthony, J.E.: Neurotic Disorders. In: *Comprehensive Textbook of Psychiatry*, 2nd Ed. (A.M. Freedman, H.I. Kaplan, and B.J. Saddock, Eds.). 2: Baltimore, Williams & Wilkins, 1975.
4. Asch, S.S. and Sabbath, J.C.: Astasia abasia—two cases. J. Hillside Hosp., *3*:32, 1954.
5. Ascher, E.: Psychodynamic considerations in Gille de la Tourette's disease (maladie des tics). Am. J. Psychiatry, *105*:267, 1948.
6. Ballenger, J.C.: A case of camptocormia occurring in psychotherapy. J. Nerv. Ment. Dis., *162*:291, 1976.
7. Bangs, J.L. and Freidinger, A.: Diagnosis and treatment of a case of hysterical aphonia in a thirteen-year-old. J. Speech. Hear. Dis., *15*:316, 1950.
8. Barry, H., Jr., and Lindemann, E.: Critical ages for maternal bereavement in psychoneuroses. Psychosom. Med., *22*:166, 1960.
9. Bergman, P.: Neurotic anxieties in children and their prevention. Nerv. Child., *5*:37, 1946.
10. Berman, B.A.: Habit of cough in adolescent children. Ann. Allerg., *24*:43, 1966.

11. Bernstein, L.: A respiratory tic: The barking cough of puberty. Laryngoscope, 73:315, 1963.
12. Bornstein, B.: Phobia in a six-year-old boy. Psychoanal. Study Child, 34:181, 1949.
13. Bornstein, B.: Fragment of an analysis of an obsessive child: The first six months of analysis. Psychoanal. Study Child, 8:313, 1953.
14. Brazelton, T.B.: The pediatrician and hysteria in childhood. Nerv. Child, 10:306, 1953.
15. Brun, R.D., and Shapiro, A.K.: Differential diagnosis of Gilles de la Tourette syndrome. J. Nerv. Ment. Dis., 155:328, 1972.
16. Brun, R.D., et al.: A follow-up of 78 patients with Gilles de la Tourette's syndrome. Am. J. Psychiatry, 133:944, 1976.
17. Burks, H.L. and Harrison, S.I.: Aggressive behavior as a means of avoiding depression. Am. J. Psychiatry, 32:416, 1962.
18. Caplan, M. and Douglas, V.: Incidence of parental loss in children with depressed mood. J. Child Psychol. Psychiatry, 10:225, 1969.
19. Chapman, A.H.: Psychogenic urinary retention in women: Report of a case. Psychosom. Med., 21:119, 1959.
20. Clark, D.F.: Behavior therapy of Gilles de la Tourette's syndrome. Br. J. Psychiatry, 112:395, 1966.
21. Colm, H.N.: Phobias in children. Psychoanal. Rev., 46:65, 1959.
22. Cooper, A.J.: Conditioning therapy in hysterical retention of urine. Br. J. Psychiatry, 111:575, 1965.
23. Cytryn, L., Logue, M. and Desai, R.B.: Biochemical correlates of affective disorders in children. Arch. Gen. Psychiatry, 31:659, 1974.
24. Cytryn, L. and McKnew, D.H.: Proposed classification of childhood depression. Am. J. Psychiatry, 129:149, 1972.
25. DeLeon-Jones, F., et al.: Diagnostic subgroups of affective disorders and their urinary excretion of catecholamine metabolites. Am. J. Psychiatry, 132:1141, 1975.
26. Despert, J.L.: Differential diagnosis between obsessive-compulsive neurosis and schizophrenia in children. In: Psychopathology of Children (P. Hoch and J. Zubin, Eds.). New York, Grune & Stratton, 1953.
27. Downs, J. and Simon, K.: Psychoneurotic patients and their families. Psychosom. Med., 15:463, 1953.
28. Dunlap, J.R.: A case of Gilles de la Tourette's disease (maladie des tics): A study of intrafamily dynamics. J. Nerv. Ment. Dis., 130:340, 1960.
29. Eisenberg, L., Ascher, E. and Kanner, L.: A clinical study of Gille de la Tourette's disease (maladie des tics) in children. Am. J. Psychiatry, 115:715, 1959.
30. Engel, G.L.: Syncope. Springfield, Ill., Thomas, 1962.
31. Engel, G.L.: A reconsideration of the role of conversion in somatic disease. Compr. Psychiatr., 9:316, 1968.
32. Engel, G.L.: Conversion symptoms. In: Signs and Symptoms: Applied Physiology and Clinical Interpretation (C.M. MacBryde and R.S. Blacklow, Eds.). Philadelphia, Lippincott, 1970.
33. Enger, N.B. and Walker, P.A.: Hyperventilation syndrome in childhood: A review of 44 cases. J. Pediatr., 70:521, 1967.
34. Friedman, R.: Some characteristics of children with "psychogenic pain": Observations on prognosis and management. Clin. Pediatr., 11:331, 1972.
35. Friedman, S.: Conversion symptoms in adolescents. Pediatr. Clin. North Am., 20:873, 1973.
36. Frommer, E.A.: Depressive illness in childhood. Br. J. Psychiatry, 2:117, 1968.
37. Galin, D., Dismond, R., and Braff, D.: Lateralization of conversion symptoms: More frequent on the left. Am. J. Psychiatry, 134:578, 1977.
38. Gardner, G.G.: Hypnosis with children. Int. J. Clin. Exp. Hypn., 22:20, 1974.
39. Gerard, M.W.: The psychogenic tic in ego development. Psychoanal. Study Child, 2:133, 1946.
40. Gillespie, J.B.: The hyperventilation syndrome in childhood. Arch. Pediatr., 71:197, 1954.
41. Glaser, K.: Masked depression in childhood and adolescents. Am. J. Psychother., 21:565, 1967.
42. Goodwin, D.W., et al.: Follow-up studies in obsessional neurosis. Arch. Gen. Psychiatry, 20:182, 1969.
43. Green, A.W.: The middle class male child and neurosis. In: Social Perspectives on Behavior (H.D. Steinard, R.A. Cloward, Eds.). Glencoe, Ill., Free Press, 1958.
44. Green, M.: Fainting. In: Ambulatory Pediatrics (M. Green and R.J. Haggerty, Eds.). Philadelphia, Saunders, 1968.
45. Greer, S.: The relationship between parental loss and attempted suicide: A control study. Br. J. Psychiatry, 110:698, 1964.
46. Group for the Advancement of Psychiatry: Theoretical Considerations and a Proposed Classification of Psychopathological Disorders in Childhood. New York, Group for the Advancement of Psychiatry, 1966.
47. Halliday, J.L.: Psychosocial Medicine: A Study of the Sick Society. New York, Norton, 1948.
48. Harrower, M.R.: Neurotic depression in a child. In: Case Histories in Clinical and Abnormal Psychology (A. Burton and R.E. Harris, Eds.). New York, Harper, 1947.
49. Hill, O.W.: Psychogenic vomiting and hypokalemia. Gut, 8:98, 1967.
50. Jersild, A.T., and Howes, F.B.: Children's Fears. New York, Bureau of Public Teachers College, Columbia University, 1935.
51. Judd, L.L.: Obsessive compulsive neurosis in children. Arch. Gen. Psychiatry, 12:136, 1965.
52. Kelman, D.H.: Gilles de la Tourette's disease in children: A review of the literature. J. Child Psychol. Psychiatry, 6:219, 1965.
53. Knight, J.A., et al.: Epidemic hysteria: A field study. Am. J. Public Health, 55:858, 1965.
54. Kravitz, H., et al.: Psychogenic cough tic in children and adolescents. Clin. Pediatr., 8:580, 1969.
55. LaBaw, W.L.: Assisting adults and children with remedial uses of their trance capability. Behav. Neuropsychiatr., 1:24, 1969.
56. Lake, C.R., et al.: Catecholamine metabolism in

Gilles de la Tourette's syndrome. Am. J. Psychiatry, *134*:257, 1977.

57. Langford, W.S.: Anxiety states in children. Am. J. Orthopsychiatry, *7*:40, 1937.

58. Lapouse, R. and Monk, M.A.: Fears and worries in a representative sample of children. Am. J. Orthopsychiatry, *29*:803, 1959.

59. Lazarus, A.A.: The elimination of children's phobias by deconditioning. In: *Behavior Therapy and the Neuroses: Readings in Modern Methods of Treatment Derived from Learning Theory* (H.J. Eysenck, Ed.). New York, Macmillan, 1960.

60. Lesse, S.: The mutivariant masks of depression. Am. J. Psychiatry, *124*:35, 1968.

61. Lippman, H.S.: The phobic child and other related anxiety states. In: *The Practice of Psychotherapy with Children* (M. Hammer and A.N. Kaplan, Eds.). Homewood, Ill., Dorsey Press, 1967.

62. Loof, D.H.: Psychophysiological and conversion reactions in children: Selective incidence in verbal and nonverbal families. J. Am. Acad. Child Psychiatry, *9*:318, 1970.

63. Lucas, A.R.: Gilles de la Tourette's disease: An overview. N.Y. State J. Med., *70*:2197, 1970.

64. Lucas, A.R., Kauffman, P.E., and Morris, E.M.: Gilles de la Tourette's disease: A clinical study of fifteen cases. J. Am. Acad. Child Psychiatry, *6*:700, 1967.

65. Mahler, M.S.: A psychoanalytic evaluation of tics in the psychopathology of children. Psychoanal. Study Child, *3/4*:279, 1949.

66. Mahler, M.S., Luke, J.A. and Daltroff, W.: Clinical and follow-up study of the tic syndrome in children. Am. J. Orthopsychiatry, *15*:631, 1945.

67. Mahler, M.S., and Rangell, L.: A psychosomatic study of maladie des tics (Gilles de la Tourette's disease). Psychiatr. Q., *17*:579, 1943.

68. Malmquist, C.P.: Depression in childhood and adolescence. N. Engl. J. Med., *284*:955, 1971.

69. McEvedy, C.P. and Beard, A.W.: Concept of benign myalgic encephalomyelitis. Br. Med. J., *1*:11, 1970.

70. McEvedy, C.P., and Beard, A.W.: Royal free epidemic of 1955: A reconsideration. Br. Med. J., *1*:7, 1970.

71. McKnew, D.H. and Cytryn, L.: Historical background in children with affective disorders. Am. J. Psychiatry, *130*:1278, 1973.

72. Nagera, H.: *Obsessional Neuroses: Developmental Psychopathology.* New York, Jason Aronson, 1976.

73. Nellhaus, G.: The bobble-head doll syndrome: A "tic" with a neuropathologic basis. Pediatrics, *40*:250, 1967.

74. Poznanski, E.O.: Children with excessive fears. Am. J. Orthopsychiatry, *43*:428, 1973.

75. Poznanski, E.O., Krahenbugl, V. and Zrull, J.P.: Childhood depression: A longitudinal perspective. J. Am. Acad. Child Psychiatry, *15*:491, 1976.

76. Poznanski, E. and Zrull, J.P.: Childhood depression: Clinical characteristics of overtly depressed children. Arch. Gen. Psychiatry, *23*:8, 1970.

77. Prazar, G. and Friedman, S.B.: Conversion reactions. In: *Principles of Pediatrics: Health Care of the Young.* (R.A. Hoekleman et al., Eds.). New York, McGraw-Hill, 1978.

78. Prugh, D.G.: Toward an understanding of psychosomatic concepts in relation to childhood. In: *Modern Perspectives in Child Development.* (A.J. Solnit and S.A. Provence, Eds.). New York, International University Press, 1963.

79. Putnam, M.C., Rank, B. and Kaplan, S.: Notes on John J.: A case of primal depression in an infant. Psychoanal. Study Child, *6*:38, 1951.

80. Rangell, L.: The nature of conversion. J. Am. Psychoanal. Assoc., *7*:362, 1959.

81. Regner, E.G.: Obsessive-compulsive neuroses in children. Acta Psychiatr. Neurol. Scand., *34*:110, 1959.

82. Rie, H.E.: Depression in childhood: A survey of some pertinent contributions. J. Am. Acad. Child Psychiatry, *5*:653, 1966.

83. Robins, L.: *Deviant Children Grown Up.* Baltimore, Williams & Wilkins, 1966.

84. Rutter, M.: Relationships between child and adult psychiatric disorders. In: *Annual Progress in Child Psychiatry and Child Development* (S. Chess and A. Thomas, Eds.). New York, Brunner/Mazel, 1973.

85. Sandler, S.A.: Camptocormia or the functional bent back. Psychosom. Med., *9*:197, 1947.

86. Sandler, J. and Joffe, W.G.: Notes on childhood depression. Int. J. Psychoanal., *46*:88, 1965.

87. Schildkraut, J.J.: Biogenic amine metabolism in depression illness: Basic and clinical studies. In: *Recent Advances in the Psychobiology of Depression Illness.* (T. Williams, M. Katz, and J. Shield, Jr., Eds.). Washington, D.C.: Department of Health, Education, and Welfare. Washington, Government Printing Office, 1972.

88. Schmitt, B.D.: School phobia—the great imitator: A pediatrician's viewpoint. Pediatrics, *48*:433, 1971.

89. Shapiro, A.K., et al.: Tourette's syndrome: Summary of data on 34 patients. Psychosom. Med., *35*:420, 1973.

90. Silverman, J.S.: Obsessional disorders in childhood and adolescence. Am. J. Psychother. (Suppl.), *26*:362, 1972.

91. Sperling, M.: Animal phobias in a two year old child. In: *The Psychoanalytic Study of the Child*, Vol. 7. New York, International Universities Press, 1952.

92. Sperling, M.: Equivalents of depression in children. J. Hillside Hosp., *8*:138, 1959.

93. Spitz, R.A.: Hospitalism: An inquiry into the genesis of psychiatric conditions in early childhood. Psychoanal. Study Child, *1*:53, 1945.

94. Spitz, R.A. and Wolff, K.M.: Anaclitic depression. Psychoanal. Study Child, *2*:313, 1946.

95. Stolzenberg, J.: Case report on periodic hysterical trismus in oral surgery. Med Pathol., *6*:453, 1953.

96. Toolan, J.M.: Depression in children and adolescents. Am. J. Orthopsychiatry, *36*:404, 1966.

97. Torup, E.: A follow-up study of children with tics. Acta Pediatr., *51*:261, 1962.

98. Udell, B. and Hornstra, R.K.: A comparative study of neurotics seen in a community mental health center and in private practice. Hosp. Community Psychiatry, *27*:269, 1976.

99. Wahl, C.W. and Golden, J.S.: Psychogenic urinary retention. Psychosom. Med., 25:543, 1963.

100. Waldron, S., Jr.: The significance of childhood neurosis for adult mental health: A follow-up study. Am. J. Psychiatry, 133:533, 1976.

101. Weiner, I.B.: Behavior therapy in obsessive-compulsive neurosis: Treatment of an adolescent boy. Psychother. Theory, Res. Pract., 4:27, 1969.

102. Williams, H.R. and Prugh, D.G.: School phobia. In: *Ambulatory Pediatrics* (M. Green & R.J. Haggerty, Eds.). Philadelphia, Saunders, 1968.

103. Williams, T.A., Katz, M.M., and Shield, J.A., Jr., Eds.: Recent Advances in the Psychobiology of the Depressive Illnesses. Department of Health, Education and Welfare Publication (HSM) 70-9053 Washington, Government Printing Office, 1972.

104. Witkin, H.A., et al.: *Psychological Differentiation: Studies of Development.* New York, John Wiley & Sons, 1962.

105. Wolff, E. and Fachman, G.S.: Hysterical blindness in children. Am. J. Dis. Child, 55:743, 1938.

106. Woodrow, K.M.: Gilles de la Tourette's disease—A review. Am. J. Psychiatry, 131:1000, 1974.

107. Ziegler, F.J. and Imboden, J.B.: Comtemporary conversion reactions. Arch. Gen. Psychiatry, 6:259, 1962.

General References

Anthony, E.J. and Benedek, T., Eds.: *Depression and Human Existence.* Boston, Little, Brown, 1975.

Anthony, E.J. and Gilpin, D.C.: *Three Clinical Faces of Childhood.* New York, Spectrum, 1976.

Benedek, T.: Toward the biology of the depressive constellation. J. Am. Psychoanal. Assoc., 4:389, 1956.

Bennet, I.: *Delinquent and Neurotic Children: A Comparative Study.* New York, Basic Books, 1960.

Bergman, P.: Neurotic anxieties in children and their prevention. Nerv. Child, 5:37, 1946.

Bibring, E.: The mechanism of depression. In: *Affective Disorders.* (P. Greenacre, Ed.). New York, International Universities Press, 1953.

Borland, L.R.: Hysterical symptoms as a factor in oral diagnosis. *Oral Surg.* Oral Med. Oral Pathol., 6:444, 1953.

Bowlby, J.: Pathological mourning and childhood mourning. J. Am. Psychoanal. Assoc., 11:500, 1963.

Chodoff, P. and Lyons, H.: Hysteria, the hysterical personality and "hysterical" conversion. Am. J. Psychiatry, 114:734, 1958.

English, O.S. and Pearson, G.H.J.: *Emotional Problems of Living: Avoiding the Neurotic Pattern.* New York, Norton, 1945.

Fenichel, O.: *The Psychoanalytic Theory of Neurosis.* New York, Norton, 1945.

Freud, A.: Problems of infantile neurosis. Psychoanal. Study Child, 9:9, 1954.

Freud, A.: *Normality and Pathology in Childhood.* London, Hogarth Press, 1966.

Freud, S.: *Mourning and Melancholia Collected Papiers,* Vol. 4 (J. Riviere, trans.). London, Hogarth Press, 1917.

Freud, S.: Analysis of a phobia in a five-year-old boy. In: *Standard Edition,* Vol. 5. London, Hogarth Press, 1955.

Hollender, M.H. and Szasz, T.S.: Normality, neurosis and psychosis: Some observations on the concepts of mental health and mental illness. J. Nerv. Ment. Dis., 125:599, 1957.

Kolansky, H.: Clinical problems of the prelatency and latency child: Treatment of a three-year-old girl's severe infantile neurosis: Stammering and insect phobia. Psychoanal. Study Child, 15:261, 1960.

Kubie, L.S.: The fundamental nature of the distinction between normality and neurosis. Psychoanal. Q., 23:187, 1954.

Marks, I.M., et al.: Obsessive compulsive neurosis in identical twins. Br. J. Psychiatry, 115:991, 1969.

Parker, N.: Close identification in twins discordant for obsessional neurosis. Br. J. Psychiatry, 110:496, 1964.

Rachman, S. and Costello, C.M.: The aetiology and treatment of children's phobias: A review. Am. J. Psychiatry, 118:97, 1961.

Rock, N.: Conversion reactions in childhood: A clinical study of childhood neuroses. J. Am. Acad. Child Psychiatry, 10:65, 1961.

Sperling, M.: *The Major Neuroses and Behavior Disorders in Children.* New York, Jason Aronson, 1975.

Sperling, M.: The neurotic child and his mother: A psychoanalytic study. Am. J. Orthopsychiatry, 21:351, 1951.

19
Personality Disorders

*The childhood shows the man
as morning shows the day.*
(John Milton)

The diagnostic features of a personality disorder are:

1. The disorder is ordinarily chronic and structured and it pervades the child's personality.
2. The disorder is characterized by chronic or fixed pathologic or maladaptive personality traits or patterns, derived from the child's responses to earlier conflicts, that have become deeply ingrained in his personality structure.
3. The disorder is not commonly seen in flagrant form before the late school-age period.

General Considerations

In personality disorders, chronic pathologic behavioral or psychologic trends are present, with the quality of traits characteristic of the personality. For reasons that are not clear, symptom formation of a psychoneurotic nature is rarely seen, even though earlier neurotically repressed conflicts may have led to the patterns of response that have crystalized into the personality or behavioral traits manifested.[41] In most but not all such disorders, the child does not perceive these trends or traits as sources of intrapsychic distress or anxiety, and so they can be said to be "ego-syntonic."

Since such personality traits are not clearly or consistently present in most children until at least the later school-age period, when the child's personality structure has crystalized and his personality traits begin to "calcify," personality disorders are not commonly fully developed before that period.[41] Nevertheless, the developmental experiences and the constitutional and other factors that contribute to the genesis of personality disorders often are present during infancy and early childhood, and premonitory patterns are often seen. Most personality disorders seem to involve strong fixations in the child's early psychosexual and psychosocial development that are related to his earlier conflicts about dependency, autonomy, aggressive impulses, and sexual differentiation. Young children who develop chronic illnesses or handicaps often have associated personality disorders, as may children who have psychophysiologic disorders.

In discussing personality disorders, the concept of a continuum is useful.[41] At one end of the continuum are people who have relatively well-organized personalities and (for example) "constructive" compulsive traits or somewhat overdependent traits that are mild-to-moderate exaggerations of healthy personality traits. These people may blend into their environment and may pass unnoticed unless their network of interpersonal relationships changes suddenly or radically. At the other end of the continuum are people who have markedly impulsive, sometimes poorly organized personalities and who come into dramatic conflict with society because of their sexual or social behavior. Marked regression may be present in some of these disorders without evidence of true psychosis. In some severe forms, however, signs of an underlying thought disorder (a borderline psychotic picture) may be present, and a psychotic disorder may occasionally supervene. In milder forms, the child may decompensate in the face of external stresses, and neurotic symptom formation may be superimposed on the basic personality picture. A reactive disorder may also occur in a child who has a chronic personality disorder.

In diagnosing a personality disorder, the physician should consider the total personality picture and not a single symptom or behavioral characteristic, such as hyperactivity, aggressive behavior, enuresis, or shyness. Addiction to drugs, alcohol, or other substances, (e.g., glue), is ordinarily considered a single symptom. Mixed personality disorders often occur. They should be diagnosed according to the predominant set of personality patterns, and a

statement should be made about any trends or features of another type.

Clinical Findings

The subtypes of personality disorders that are discussed in the following paragraphs are based on the GAP nomenclature.[41] They are somewhat different from those in the Standard Nomenclature. The differences arise in part from the shifting nature of childhood disturbances (which may change significantly during adolescence) and in part from certain conceptual considerations.

Obsessive-Compulsive Personality Disorder

Children who have obsessive-compulsive personality disorders show chronic and excessive concern about orderliness, cleanliness, and conformity that is related to their continuing conflicts at the psychosocial level of the establishment of autonomy versus shame or doubt. Their personalities are ordinarily relatively rigid and inflexible, and they have trouble relaxing. When their patterns of behavior are disrupted, these children may be aware of some tension or anxiety, but they usually perceive their environment or other people as being responsible for their distress.[41] They may have some obsessive thoughts and compulsive rituals, but during increased conflict and anxiety they rarely decompensate to the point where these thoughts and rituals are crippling. Ordinarily these children perform well, and they often show a kind of pseudo-maturity in the presence of adults, who may consider this to be healthy childhood behavior. These children often have problems in socializing with their peers, and those who have more severe disorders may need intensive psychotherapy or psychoanalysis. An obsessive-compulsive personality disorder often occurs in firstborn children (often boys) who are trying to meet their parents high expectations of them. Their parents also often have obsessive tendencies.[1,2,22]

Hysterical Personality Disorders

Children and adolescents (mostly girls[41,87] but some boys[12,62]) who have hysterical personality disorders tend to be overdramatic, flamboyant, labile, excitable, oversuggestible, coy, provocative, and at times seductive.[53,79] They often seem to be overly dependent on their environment to establish their independent identities, and they may have a pseudo-social poise. Despite their often misleading overt heterosexual behavior, they give evidence of unusual repression of sexual impulses and seem to have trouble establishing their sexual identities and sexual relationships. (They have conflict about psychosocial issues of initiative versus guilt in the oedipal phase of their psychosexual development). They may have an unconscious masochistic need to suffer that arises from guilt about their sexual impulses, and at times their aggressive impulses. Symptom formation of a conversion or a dissociated type often occurs at times of increased conflict, as may visual or aural wish-fulfilling hallucinations. (But these phenomena appear rarely in people who have milder hysterical personality disorders.[23]) In more severe cases, a variety of shifting symptoms may occur, as may psychologic invalidism that reflects a deep disturbance in body-image formation.

People who have hysterical personalities are often very manipulative or demanding in a passive-aggressive way, indicating that fixation of their conflicts that occurred at very early stages of their personality development (related to psychosocial issues of trust and autonomy[63]) underlie their hysterical trends (which derive from a higher level of pseudo-sexual nature). They may use suicidal threats to manipulate others. Occasionally they make serious suicidal attempts, however, and that possibility should be kept in mind.

The developmental histories and family backgrounds of people who have hysterical personalities are revealing.[6] Such disorders appear to occur more often in woman relatives of women patients, indicating that identification may play a part.[100] As Celani[21] has indicated in a recent review, the mothers of girls who have hysterical personalities seem to be women who are envious of their husbands and competitive with them and who have conflicts about being mothers. They have trouble giving emotionally on a daily basis, but they can be "motherly" when their children are sick or hurt. Their children thus receive attention mainly when they are frail, ill, or disabled. These children seem to turn to their fathers as substitute mothers. The fathers have been described as superficially charming and somewhat seductive men, who often have difficulty in forming close relationships. The girls seem to use their charm and seductive behavior to attract their fathers. A reciprocally seductive relationship develops that intensifies the covert strife between the parents.

Such a triangular relationship is of course familiar, and it is only an exaggeration of the normal. What leads to the development of the life-long patterns of the hysterical personality is less clear. In some cases, the girl may actually have been seduced by her father or another close male relative—or the girl actually believes this to be so. (But seduction and incest in themselves do not produce hysterical personalities.) Both parents may unconsciously select a child to play such a role, or other as yet unknown predisposing factors may be involved.

In the view of Berblinger[12] and others, the girl continues in adolescence and adulthood to communicate frailty, weakness, and helplessness to men (hysterical males communicate the same message to women[11]) in a manner that attracts the interest and attention of men. Ironically, the girl's seductiveness and superficial warmth permit the avoidance of feelings of closeness at a deeper level, with resultant vulnerability to rejection. The girl's basic unfulfilled need to have supportive, maternal gratifications from men seems to combine with her guilt about her former close relationship with the father and her rivalry with her mother to make her relationships with men basically asexual ones. If the man responds to the sexual implications the female is usually outraged at his advances. (Most such women are frigid even when they marry.) Essentially the patient needs constantly to test men and to control them because she has an unconscious fear of being rejected. She is dependent on the responses of men, but she gets little deep emotional satisfaction, even when she finds a man who is strong, protective, and nurturing but who does not make sexual demands. Intensive long-term psychotherapy for the young person and her parents can be most effective.[24,53,79]

Case Example. A 14-year-old girl was admitted to the pediatric ward because she had a severe respiratory infection. As her infection responded to medical treatment, the girl, who was attractive and well-developed, began to act seductively toward the male staff, touching them frequently, sitting on their laps, and making sexually provocative remarks, upsetting the staff in the process. When the girl began talking about having had intercourse with a number of boys and men, it was decided to discuss her case at a psychosomatic conference in the pediatric department. In an interview before the interdisciplinary staff, the girl said laughingly that she could make her father do whatever she wanted, and she exhibited coy behavior toward the psychiatrist holding the conference. She recounted a dream she had about being "attacked" by a monster (male). These and other features led the physician to make a diagnosis of a hysterical personality disorder and to observe that the girl was really frightened of sexual intercourse and probably was a virgin. The house staff were skeptical, and they arranged for a gynecological consultation. The gynecologist said that the girl's hymen was intact and that she had the most virginal introitus he had ever seen. The girl later admitted her fears, and psychotherapy was arranged for her and her parents, who had been concerned about her seductive behavior.

Certain hysterical personality disorders that occur occasionally in older children and adolescents partake of the quality of a psychosis. The Ganser syndrome[4,38,74,98] is one of the so-called hysterical psychoses,[51] that may also have elements of a dissociative disorder (see Chap. 18). The Ganser syndrome may be precipitated by situations in which the patient wishes to escape from responsibility. The patient is able to give "approximate answers" to questions he is asked, which indicates that he has a basic contact with reality and a basic understanding, but his responses are distorted. As in other "hysterical psychoses," the patient's naive concept of what "craziness" may be like lends to his absurd behavior, in this case, his approximate answers. Persons with such disorders are not malingering. Some of them are more seriously disturbed than is the usual person who has a hysterical personality,[98] and they have a history of problems in personality functioning.

Anxious Personality Disorder

Children who have anxious personality disorders are chronically tense and apprehensive about new situations, often because of the extraordinarily vivid fantasies they have.[59] They usually perceive their environment as threatening, however, and are not aware of and do not show crippling anxiety, as do children who have anxiety neurosis.[41] They do not have marked inhibitions or constriction of the total personality, and they are often able to cope with new situations despite their initial anxiety, unlike children with developmental deviations who do not have stage-appropriate coping behaviors available. Supportive psychotherapy by the pediatrician may suffice for those who have milder clinical pictures although some children may require more intensive treatment by a mental health professional. Mild tranquilizers, such as Benadryl, may be palliative but they are usually not helpful on a long-term basis.

Overly Dependent Personality Disorder

Children who have overly dependent personality disorders are chronically helpless, clinging, and overdependent, and they have trouble achieving autonomy and initiative. They may be markedly demanding in a passive-aggressive way. Often their parents have been overprotective.[60] The child's temperament, development, and experience may also be involved.[83,91] Counseling and supportive psychotherapy may help, but intensive psychotherapy for the child and his parents may be necessary. Some children who would formerly have been classified as passive-aggressive, passive-dependent, immature, or unstable personalities would be included in this category.

Oppositional Personality Disorder

Children who have oppositional personality disorders express their aggressiveness by oppositional patterns of passive nature. Their behavior may have some actively aggressive aspects, however. They may seem to be conforming, but they continually provoke others. Their negativism, stubbornness, dawdling, and other measures show their covert underlying aggressiveness. These children may also show passive-dependent or demanding trends.[61] If these trends affect their learning, the children may have trouble learning because of emotional blocking out, "failing to hear," or passively resisting external pressure.[4] In a sense, these children may insist on their autonomy by oppositional adaptive maneuvers, which fail to achieve that goal. Children who have oppositional personality disorders formerly had to be classified as having passive-aggressive personalities. They should be differentiated from children who have developmental deviations and from children who have tension-discharge disorders, who act out their feelings aggressively. Oppositional personality disorders usually arise from struggles for control between the older infant and his parents, but the child's temperament (his degree of stubbornness) is probably also involved. Intensive psychotherapy is often necessary in the more severe cases.

Overly Inhibited Personality Disorder

Children who have overly inhibited personality disorders show superficial passivity, often with extreme ("pathologic") shyness, inhibition of motor action or initiative, and marked constriction of their personality functions, including at times diminished speech. They are to be differentiated from children who have so-called schizoid (isolated) personalities by the fact that they seem to wish for warm and meaningful relationships but cannot achieve them. They are often less inhibited in the home than at school or in other social settings. Some conscious anxiety may be evident, but the "frozen," inhibited quality is usually paramount.[41] Some negativism and other oppositional features are often part of the picture although they do not seem to predominate. These children show considerable self-doubt and lack of achievement of autonomy and initiative.

Although their inhibitions, which are related primarily to their unconscious fears of losing control of their aggressive or sexual impulses, render these children somewhat dependent on others to "get going," they are not usually overly dependent in many other respects, and they may be able to function independently in situations in which they feel comfortable. Their inhibitions often affect their academic learning. They may have trouble assimilating knowledge as well as in putting it to use, because they fear aggression or competition and because of their constricted, unspontaneous personalities. (Learning problems are discussed more fully in Chapter 28.) Although most of these children need intensive treatment, follow-up studies[67,73] indicate that even without long-term treatment, the majority become reasonably well-adjusted, although quiet and retiring, adults. Some seem to be only marginally adjusted, but the incidence of schizophrenia in late adolescence or adult life is extremely low.

Children who have elective mutism often fall into this group, although a few may have psychoneurotic school phobias, obsessive-compulsive personality disorders, or even psychotic disorders. Most children who have elective mutism have at least adequate intelligence. They often had mild speech difficulties when they were younger or problems in communication within their families. Some of their parents had conflicts about talking, particularly about family secrets. Although the term "refusal to talk" (in school)[101] has been used to describe the behavior of these children, most of these children have not refused to talk but are afraid[46] or too inhibited[19] to speak outside the home, and they are often relieved when treatment frees them to speak.

Elective mutism occurs more often in girls than in boys. As Pustrom and Speers[80] and others have indicated, the child often has an ambivalent and overly dependent (hostile-dependent) relationship with the mother, and the father is distant and passive. The mother's unconscious need to keep the child involved with her may be her way of dealing with her marital problems. The child's inability to talk outside her home usually involves much repressed anger—the hostile side of her relationship with her mother. When the parents have a conflict about talking, the child may be acting out their conflict. A study[17] of children in immigrant families in Canada indicated that the hostile-dependent relationship between a mother and her child was furthered by the mother's tendency to remain isolated and indifferent to the need to learn the language of the country. The child's mutism fed into the mother's dream of returning to her native land. Although some children respond to intensive short-term psychotherapy,[101] many require long-term help,[5] and some are exceedingly difficult to treat.[26]

Case Example. A 10-year-old girl had been shy and quiet at school since she began kindergarten although she was more talkative and active at home. This pattern became more marked each year. At the beginning of the fifth grade, she spoke in school only in whispers, and she gradually stopped speaking at all in class, although her written work remained excellent. She occasionally spoke on the playground, and she engaged in appropriate play with some evident pleasure. On the WISC, which was given by the school psychologist, the girl had a Performance I.Q. that was high average, but her Verbal I.Q. was untestable. She made no verbal responses to parts of several projective tests. Her pediatrician found no physical abnormalities of her speaking parts or her central nervous system. In talking with her parents, however, he discovered that the parents had had increasing difficulty in communicating for the past few years because they had marital problems.

Overly Independent Personality Disorder

Children who have overly independent personality disorders show chronically ebullient and active, (but not usually hyperactive) behavior. They seem to rush toward independence, and they have trouble accepting teaching or the setting of limits. Their behavior may be pseudo-precocious or pseudo-adult, and they are ordinarily not aggressive in a destructive or an antisocial sense.[41]

Although these children may show negativism, they generally have positive attitudes. They are impatient to grow up and they may be overly responsible. Many tend to strongly deny their feelings of helplessness and their dependency. Some may overcompensate for a fantasied defect or cover up their fears of being harmed or their anxiety that has arisen from sexual conflicts. When they are physically ill, they drive themselves too soon into overambitious activity, or they may have other difficulties in convalescence (because of the increased dependency needs—and the gratification of those needs—that convalescence brings). For some, a chronic illness or a handicap may help cause the disorder. Those who have milder cases may respond to supportive therapy, but some require long-term intensive treatment. Therapy is a must for their parents also.

Isolated Personality Disorder

Children who have isolated personality disorders tend to be distant, detached, cold, or withdrawn toward their family and friends. Often they are isolated and seclusive or "isolating". They have trouble competing and in expressing even their healthy aggressive feelings although some may have occasional and unpredictable outbursts of bizarre aggressive or sadistic behavior.[41]

These children appear to differ quantitatively and qualitatively from children who have overly inhibited personalities. They have a restricted capacity for emotional experiences unlike inhibited children, who have a capacity for emotional experiences but have trouble expressing their feelings. They may show shyness, oversensibility, inhibition, and passivity and oppositional behavior, but their inability to form warm relationships is predominant. They also seem introverted and withdrawn and too satisfied with their isolation. They have a rich fantasy life, and they are preoccupied with their daydreams and autistic reveries, unlike children who have inhibited personalities, who maintain relationships despite their difficulty in expressing their feelings.

Isolated children are often able to achieve success in certain areas of functioning, particularly intellectual areas, although many show mild deviations in their thinking or concept formation (but not true thought disorders). They are generally pliant and unobtrusive socially, but they may have occasional outbursts of aggressive, even homicidal behavior or of other kinds of negative behavior that seem to be unrelated to external stimuli. They tend to show increased withdrawal and detachment in adolescence, but only a small percentage seem to be preschizophrenic (at least on the basis of clinical impression[3]), and they do not seem to have latent schizophrenia. For that reason the term schizoid personality, formerly used to describe what seemed to be latent or preschizophrenic tendencies, seems inappropriate, and the term isolated personality seems appropriate. A constitutional tendency would seem to be present, and the child's early experience may play a significant role. Bowlby[16] used the term "affectionless character" to describe some older children and adolescents who had had marked emotional deprivation in their early childhood. Some of these people may fit the isolated personality category although others may belong in the tension-discharge category. Treatment is difficult and protracted, and it may have to be given in a hospital or a residential setting.

Mistrustful Personality Disorder

Mistrustful personality disorder is rare in childhood. It occurs occasionally in late preadolescence or early adolescence. The children may have features of the isolated personality disorder, but their condition is characterized by suspiciousness (beyond the adolescent norm), intense mistrust of others, fears that they will be harmed, and marked rigidity of thinking. Those characteristics are often related to emotional deprivation in their early years. The disorder does not ordinarily progress to an actual paranoid state, as seen in adults,[41] and for that reason, the term mistrustful personality seems to be preferable to the term paranoid personality. If the adult type occurs in late adolescence (it occasionally does,[47]) the term paranoid personality can be applied to it. The patients can be treated successfully although involving the parents, who may themselves show mistrustful or paranoid patterns,[50] may be difficult.

Tension-Discharge Disorder

Children who have tension-discharge disorders show chronic patterns of aggressive and sexual behavior that conflict with society's norms. They have difficulty "storing" tension, and they discharge it by "acting." They act out their feelings or impulses toward people or society in an antisocial or destructive way, rather than inhibit or repress them and develop other psychologic defenses or symptoms. The terms antisocial personality, psychopathic personality, impulsive character, sociopathic personality, dissocial personality, affectionless character, acting-out personality, neurotic character disorder, primary behavior disorder, neurotic behavior disorder, conduct disorder, and unsocialized aggressive reaction have been used by different investigators to describe the different people and behaviors that fit the tension-discharge category. The large number of terms suggests that the category has several subcategories. Temperament undoubtedly figures in the tension-discharge disorders,[99] but the studies of Rexford[84] and others[16] support the idea that familial and social factors are the most important ones.

Impulse-ridden Personality Disorder. Children who have impulse-ridden personality disorders have shallow relationships with adults and other children and have a very low tolerance of frustration. They have great difficulty controlling their aggressive and sexual impulses, which they often act on immediately, without regard for the consequences. These children have little anxiety, internalized conflict, or guilt; their conflicts remain largely external—between society and their impulses. Some internalized conflict may be present, and some overlap exists in children who have neurotic personality disorders. In some, psychoneurotic symptoms are present.[78] Their basic inability to control their impulses seems to be reinforced by a defect in conscience (superego) formation; they are unable to store tension and to postpone gratifications. They usually have primitive defense mechanisms; they strongly deny their dependency or other needs, and they project their hostile feelings onto adults or society while rationalizing their own behavior.[41]

Children who have tension-discharge disorders often were seriously deprived emotionally as infants and young children and had frequent and prolonged separations from their mothers or suffered the loss of a parent. A large number of them come from lower socioeconomic groups, although they may be from any level of society. Many had parents and grandparents who exhibited antisocial behavior. Those adults were poor and some of them were victims of racism. A constitutional tendency toward motor discharge of tension may be present. A number of these children have abnormally dysrhythmic EEG tracings,[54] but usually no true epileptic patterns. In some there is a high correlation of enuresis since infancy and fire-setting.[68] Stealing, fire-setting, vandalism, destruction, aggressive attack, and other antisocial acts may frequently occur, and their behavior may sometimes change from one form to another or to several others. Drug addiction is not infrequent in older children and adolescents. Although these children have poor judgment and a poor concept of time, they usually are of adequate intelligence and their reality testing in certain areas is quite good.[81]

Children who have chronic brain damage but have not been emotionally deprived may show a somewhat similar picture in regard to impulse control and judgment. But they usually are able to form relationships, and they may show marked guilt and evidence of true conscience formation.

Neurotic Personality Disorders. Children who have neurotic personality disorders may show behavior superficially similar to that seen in the impulse-ridden personality disorders as they act out or discharge tension that arises from conflict. They seem, however, to have reached a higher level of personality development, which indicates a strong influence from earlier repressed neurotic conflicts. Their behavior often becomes repetitive and their acts have unconscious symbolic significance rather than show a predominance of discharge phenomena. They often have associated psychoneurotic symptoms.[41] Evidence of conscience formation is manifested by their conflict, which is accompanied by apparent anxiety and guilt. The guilt sometimes leads them unconsciously to invite limits or punishment (by allowing themselves to be caught stealing or otherwise "tempting" an adult to control them). In the absence of exacerbations of conflict, they seem to be able to control their impulses to some extent. Their antisocial behavior, when it occurs, is either predominantly a reaction to the intensification of conflicts[52] rather than the sudden discharge of tension in response to frustration that occurs in the impulse-ridden disorders, or the result of their limitations in ego controls that sometimes occurs in certain brain-damaged children. Their relationships with others are warmer and more meaningful although often very ambivalent. Marital discord, overpunitiveness or overpermissiveness, and inconsistency about setting limits are common in their families.[95]

Some overlapping with the impulse-ridden disorders of course exists. During middle or late adolescence, many of these children have been described as neurotic characters or neurotic criminals. Hysterical or other personality trends may be mixed with their tension-discharge problems.

Sociosyntonic Personality Disorder

There are two subtypes of sociosyntonic personality disorder and they overlap somewhat. Children who have one subtype show aggressive, destructive behavior or antisocial personality trends which, though deviant by society's standards, may be consonant with the standards of the child's neighborhood group, gang—or even of his family.[41] These children should be distinguished from children who have developmental or situational crises of later childhood or adolescence, from children who have reactive disorders, and from children who have other psychopathologic disorders. Some of these children may become impulse ridden or may develop neurotic personality disorders although not as a rule.

The other subtype includes personality pictures that derive from cultures other than the majority group. The subtype includes children who live in isolated rural settings who may have repeated hallucinatory experiences, as do others in their subculture, as well as members of groups who practice magic (e.g., voodoo). If these manifestations or others (e.g., social inhibition when in strange groups), occur only occasionally and are not combined with other personality characteristics and patterns of thought and perception strongly deviant from the predominant societal patterns, such children may be said to have reactive disorders or developmental deviations—or even to show healthy responses.

Sexual Deviation

A child should be classified as having a sexual deviation only when a sexual deviation is regarded as the major personality disturbance and is chronic and pervasive enough to dominate his orientation toward social life. Confusion, disturbance, or deviation in heterosexual identifications and sexually deviant behavior of course may occur in a variety of childhood and adolescent pictures. They should be classified under such headings as developmental deviations, psychoneuroses, and psychoses. Many healthy boys and girls have transient homosexual experiences in late preadolescence and early adolescence; and effeminate behavior in school-age boys or masculine behavior in school-age girls does not necessarily mean that those children will become homosexuals. Homosexual behavior occurs transiently in correctional institutions and residential treatment settings.[48] It is often related to status and to other social considerations. Historical and cultural factors have undoubtedly affected the prevalence of homosexual behavior in certain societies (e.g., in ancient Greece).

When actual inversion of the child's heterosexual identification occurs on a relatively fixed basis in middle or late adolescence and when homosexual or other sexually deviant behavior continues steadily, the child's basic personality picture should be carefully considered to establish the primary diagnosis. Such trends can change somewhat in adolescence and early adult life, and latent homosexual or other tendencies be present without overt manifestations throughout life. A significant number of adults can function bisexually.

The concept of sexual deviation or perversion is being reexamined. A recent survey conducted by a task force on homosexuality set up by the National Institute of Mental Health (NIMH) estimated that between 3 to 4 million Americans are predominantly homosexual. The development of the Gay Liberation movement and the report of a recent controlled psychological study which indicated that well-adjusted homosexuals cannot be distinguished from equally well-adjusted heterosexuals, would seem to support Freud's idea that homosexuality should not be considered a mental illness, a vice, or a degradation. The NIMH task force recommended that a national center be set up to study sexual behavior, to do more epidemiologic and other studies, and to consider legal changes to remove penalties for sexual acts in private among consenting adults. Such steps have already been taken in England, where the Parliament adopted the recommendations of the Wolfenden

Report, and those steps have been recommended by the Ninth International Congress on Criminal Law and by the American Law Institute. Discrimination against homosexuals in employment practices has already been declared unconstitutional by the U.S. Supreme Court, a step that should gradually eliminate blackmailing and other kinds of harassment of homosexuals. The American Psychiatric Association, under much pressure from the Gay Liberation movement and after much conflicting discussion[45,64,94] recently recommended that homosexuality not be considered a psychopathologic disorder. As several authorities have pointed out, however, legal changes or classification changes alone will not change immediately the social attitudes toward homosexuality in the United States, which are different from those of most European countries and numerous past civilizations, as well as most primitive societies. In most societies, homosexual behavior is not accepted if it involves the seduction of a minor, force or violence, or public solicitation or exhibition. The approach in the United States to the regulation of sexual behavior has involved threats to the homosexual individual (e.g., the invasion of his privacy) as well as the use of informers and entrapment although that approach is changing. Deisher and his colleagues[25] have pointed up the problems in identifying and rehabilitating young male prostitutes and has called for pediatricians, child psychiatrists, and other professionals to become leaders in developing a clinical approach to homosexuality that is based on humanistic traditions.

Although the concept of sexual perversion is rightfully being reexamined, many psychiatrists still consider homosexuality a gender identity disorder. A biologic predisposition or vulnerability to homosexuality may exist (the evidence is conflicting[35,37]), but in people studied by psychiatrists, the principal causative factors in homosexuality seem to be acquired and to be rooted in the homosexual's early family and child-rearing experiences.[14,44] Until recently, most psychotherapists, following Freud's view, felt that attempts to help a homosexual person become heterosexual were futile; they felt that the most they could offer was to help the person who had a conflict about being homosexual live more comfortably with his homosexuality. Since the early 1960s, there have been reports of increasing success in reversing homosexuality, as Hadden[44] has noted. The methods used are intensive psychotherapy, psychoanalysis, and behavior therapy.[15,29] Thus although a person should not have to suffer in society because he is homosexual, if he wants to change, his chances of being able to change seem to be getting better.

Although feminine behavior in boys and masculine behavior in girls does not necessarily predispose them to homosexuality, recent reports have indicated that boys who show excessive feminine behavior do not necessarily become more masculine in time.[7,102] Indeed, as Newman[76] has pointed out, recent evidence indicates that those boys are at high risk for adult gender identity disorders, including homosexuality, transsexualism, and transvestism. As Green[39] has pointed out, "tomboyism" in girls is much more common than "sissiness" in boys, is more readily tolerated by our society, and more often changes to more conventional feminine behavior in adolescence. But one study has suggested that tomboyism may be associated with later feminine homosexual orientation.[89]

Extremely feminine boys commonly engage in cross-dressing, feminine mannerisms, and feminine fantasy play and have feminine mannerisms from the preschool period. During the school-age period, they are teased and rejected by their male peers. The boys' mothers and sometimes the other female members of their families have tolerated and even encourage the boy's fem-

inine behavior from an early age.[32]* The mother often keeps the boy close to her and insulated from the masculine world. She needs his dependence on her and his companionship for unconscious reasons that are related to her own family background and usually to an unsatisfying marital relationship or sometimes because she lacks and needs a male figure. The father usually resents and avoids his son, and he often joins with the mother in rationalizations about the boy's feminine behavior. Fear of losing the son's companionship often makes the mother reluctant to undertake treatment.

Newman[75] defines certain "major criteria" (first-category behaviors) which, he believes, call for treatment as a type of primary prevention of transsexualism and other gender disorders. These behaviors include, besides cross-dressing and assuming feminine roles in fantasy games or play (and resisting masculine roles), the verbal expression of wishes to become a girl or grow up to be a woman, and an exaggeratedly feminine manner, gait, and way of speaking. Newman thinks that such behaviors as a dislike of rough and competitive boys' games, a dislike of mechanical toys, enjoying girls as playmates, being graceful in body movements and gestures (as opposed to imitation of feminine behavior), a preference for artistic or sedentary activities, and being teased as a "sissy" by other boys are "minor criteria." They may occur with the major criteria, but if they occur alone, the gender pathology is probably not serious enough to produce later significant disorders. Indeed, Newman believes that some boys who have

---

*The studies of Money[71,72] have indicated that the gender role begins to be established by the latter part of the child's second year of life. Another study[88] suggests that sex-typing and sex-role socialization may begin at birth. These findings point up how important it is to decide, as soon as possible after birth, whether an infant who has ambiguous external genitalia should be raised as a boy or a girl. The decision is based on the results of the physical examination, laboratory studies, and other methods (even laparotomy in true hermaphroditism).[69]

such minor criteria may grow up to be creative adults.

Newman and his colleagues have found that psychotherapy for extremely feminine boys that was begun when the boys were 5 to 12 years old usually helped them. The treatment consisted of 1 or 2 individual play therapy sessions a week with a male therapist for several years, combined with counseling or parent therapy. In a series of 5 boys, all 5 became more masculine and more aggressive, and they discontinued their specifically feminine behaviors, such as cross-dressing. Newman discussed whether in the light of the changing attitudes toward homosexuality, transsexualism, and transvestism, such boys should be treated. He thinks that treatment can at least help the boy have a happier childhood, and that the prevention of an adult gender disorder is a related goal of treatment. Other treatment approaches that have produced similar results are psychoanalysis[90] and behavior therapies[9] that reinforce masculine behavior.

Over the past 25 years, much has been written about the treatment of transsexuals. Adults and adolescents, often males, who are convinced that their true (inner) gender is different from their "external" gender and who have a history in childhood of cross-dressing and an expressed wish to be a person of the opposite sex, as well as other signs of a core gender disorder, including occasional autocastration,[43] have been described clearly by Stoller,[92,93] Green and Money,[40] and others. Surgical treatment of those people was formerly viewed with some skepticism.[58] But recently Newman and Stoller[77] have suggested that the pendulum may have swung too far in the other direction. They and others[56] have cautioned that a number of patients presenting as transsexuals may not really have serious gender disorders. Some of these patients seem to have seized on the idea of sex reassignment as a sort of magical solution to a crisis, or they may even be attempting to ward off a psychotic

episode. Benjamin[10] has warned about the possibility of iatrogenic influence upon the request for sex reassignment. Although transsexuals have been reported to have a high incidence of intermittent depression preoperatively and a nearly 20% suicide attempt rate,[96] another study[49] showed a 16% postoperative suicide attempt rate, a finding that raises questions about the patients' postoperative adjustments.

There have been occasional reports that apparently transsexual adolescents and adults have responded to psychotherapy[33] or behavior therapy,[8,82] although most true transsexuals are said to be unresponsive.[77] Kirkpatrick and Friedman[56] believe that consulting psychiatrists should consider the patient's total personality rather than focus on the genuineness of the perceived gender disorder and that psychotherapy should be offered whatever the decision about the genuineness of the disorder.

Clinical studies have indicated that other sexual deviations that involve exhibitionism[66] and pedophilia[70] in adults are based on a developmental psychopathology, at times a serious one. Early childhood experiences, usually ones that involve an overcontrolling or overprotective mother and an absent or distant father, appear to render boys who are potentially exhibitionists inordinately eager to please and likely to have continuing conflicts about expressing and inhibiting their hostility, especially their hostility toward women. The exhibitionism thus may be simultaneously an unconscious retaliation, a declaration of masculinity, a covert solicitation, and a refuge from insecurity and a sense of failure. In certain instances, the unconscious hostility may be directed toward a child, perhaps one who represents the exhibitionist's sibling or some other developmental figure important to him. A few exhibitionists who have extremely strong conflicts may under certain circumstances become violent or psychotic, engaging in sexual molestation, rape, or even murder. (These topics are discussed more fully in Chapter 28).

If sexual deviation is considered the primary diagnosis, other trends in the child's personality should also be listed (e.g., overdependence and isolation). The type of sexually deviant behavior can be specified (e.g., voyeuristic behavior, exhibitionistic behavior, or panic reaction in a homosexual adolescent boy).

Treatment and Prognosis

The prognosis for these generally deep-rooted and ingrained disorders in personality functioning varies considerably from disorder to disorder and according to their severity. People who have mild obsessive-compulsive, anxious, hysterical, or overly dependent disorders may blend with their environment, and they may not even be regarded as significantly disturbed. A certain degree of compulsiveness is an asset in certain types of jobs. Some hysterical trends may be an asset to entertainers or people in other fields that call for a certain amount of exhibitionism. But more severe degrees of those disorders may be more crippling, and even moderate oppositional and overly independent disorders can interfere with a person's academic or social functioning.

Older children and adolescents who have moderate-to-severe isolated or mistrustful personality disorders, especially boys, often come in conflict with the law, through bizarre outbreaks of sadistic behavior in the former and aggressive behavior designed to ward off feared attacks in the latter. Those who have sociosyntonic personality disorders may adjust well as long as they remain in their own subculture (e.g., a gang in a disadvantaged neighborhood) where their behavior is adaptive. But if they join the army (for example), their values and behavior and those of the majority group or social institution will conflict seriously.

Children who have tension-discharge disorders are often regarded by society as being delinquent. (Delinquency is a category that includes many other clinical entities, and it will be discussed later.) Children who have impulse-ridden personalities have the poorest prognosis, since they tend to fight off or run away from treatment by representatives of the society they distrust, and some of them become criminals as adults. In a long-term follow-up, Robins[86] has concluded that about 50% of these disorders do carry over into adult life, especially if the child's parents have shown antisocial behavior. But some of these disorders "burn out," and the people have become more sociable and organized in their behavior by the time they are 25 to 30 years old. Children who have neurotic personality disorders—and who often are unconsciously asking to be controlled— ordinarily have a better outlook.

Mild-to-moderate obsessive, hysterical, anxious, overly dependent or independent, oppositional, and overly inhibited disorders can be treated on an ambulatory basis. Some early school-age children who have milder forms of these disorders can be treated successfully along with their parents, by supportive therapy by the pediatrician, by counseling about how they can become more independent, diminish their inhibitions, improve their self-control, and deal with their parents' overly high aspirations for them. Often teachers, social workers, and consulting psychiatrists can help.

Children who have moderate-to-severe disorders are best treated by intensive psychotherapy, usually on an outpatient basis, unless their disorders interfere seriously with their functioning. Some overly inhibited children who have elective mutism can respond to a short-term therapy that focuses on the mutism. Others will resist such an approach and will respond only to a long-term therapy that involves a trusting relationship. Such children are difficult to treat and are a source of frustration for the therapist. They may speak to him only toward the end of treatment or they may never speak to him, even though they gradually have come to talk to everyone not involved in their therapy. A few children must be hospitalized briefly to get their treatment started. Day hospital programs, that have a psychoeducational approach or a special class in school may be of great value if the child has associated learning difficulties.

Children and adolescents who have the more severe disorders respond best to long-term residential therapy. Some who have learning difficulties respond best to residential educational therapy. Tranquilizers are rarely very helpful, unless the child has considerable anxiety.

Children who have moderate-to-severe isolated or mistrustful personality disorders generally require intensive residential therapy—in a hospital, a cottage-type group-living setting, or a group foster home. (The mental health treatment facilities must be adequate.) Children who have neurotic personality disorders require formal psychotherapy, which may be carried out on an ambulatory basis. Many of these children require residential therapy. They need therapeutic controls to keep them out of the courts. Some of the children just described and some children who have sociosyntonic personality disorders who have become involved in delinquent acts may respond to therapy in a treatment-oriented correctional institution for "predelinquents." There they can be offered warmth, structure, consistent limits, and positive relationships with well-trained staff who have access to mental health consultation. Tranquilizers or other drugs usually help these children very little.

Older children and adolescents who have tension-discharge disorders of the impulse-ridden type and who often have had much emotional deprivation in their early years, can often be treated only in a "closed" residential setting. Consistent, firm control of their acting-out behavior, combined with the staff's warm personal

interest and individual therapy and milieu therapy, can help these children internalize their conflicts with the world, mobilize their guilt, build up their internal controls. Redl[81] has shown that surprisingly good results can be achieved if treatment is begun by early adolescence and is continued for several years. Tranquilizers rarely help although amphetamines may help with hyperactivity and impulsivity.

Children who have true sexual deviations can often be treated successfully by intensive psychotherapy or behavior therapy on an ambulatory basis during adolescence. If they are not treated until they become adults (when their patterns are fixed and they are poorly motivated to change), the results of even psychoanalysis may be limited. However, even adult sexual offenders can be treated fairly effectively if the court orders them to be put in a closed psychiatric hospital, where they can undergo intensive individual and group therapy. Such an approach in a special unit for sex offenders at Atascadero in California has shown surprisingly low recidivism rates. Some adolescents who have various types of personality pictures and who have become addicted to drugs or alcohol may not respond to community programs or outpatient therapy, and inpatient treatment may be necessary.

Some patients who have extremely severe personality disturbances have been termed borderline personalities because they exhibit clinical pictures which "border" on psychosis. Borderline personalities in adults have been much discussed by Kernberg[55] and others,[18,57] and they were the subject of an excellent review recently by Gunderson and Singer.[42] They have been described in children by Anna Freud[34] and others[36,97] and in adolescents by Masterson,[65] but the most intensive and incisive long-term study of borderline personalities in children and adolescents was carried out by Ekstein and his colleagues.[27,28] The young people studied showed marked defects in ego functioning[13,31] and difficulties in distinguishing fantasy from reality, and in social relations. Some might have progressed to the point where they developed shaky neurotic or personality disorders (e.g., hysterical, obsessive-compulsive, neurotic personality, or mixed disorders and hypochondriacal tendencies[85]) but with a tendency toward sweeping regression and often an underlying disorder in thinking that involved psychotic mechanisms. Others may have shown developmental failure and exhibited intense narcissism or demanding behavior, deep ambivalence toward and difficulty in trusting other persons, primitive defense mechanisms, such as heavy denial or projection, bursts of primitive rage or acting-out behavior,[20] and distortions in reality testing which are exacerbated in the face of increased anxiety.[30]

If the clinical picture has the coloration of a personality disorder, personality disorder can be the primary diagnosis, with specific descriptions of his other difficulties (e.g., in reality testing). Other disorders might be called severe developmental deviations in cognitive, social, and other areas, or mild psychotic disorders.

Such children may make borderline adjustments for many years, may drift in and out of reality, or may decompensate into a brief psychotic episode periodically. They are difficult to treat. At least several years of intensive psychotherapy is required for them and for their deeply disturbed families. For those whose main difficulty is fluctuating drifts away from reality, outpatient therapy may be effective. For some who have arrested development, the treatment must begin in a hospital or residential setting, and periodic readmissions are often required. Treatment must be very supportive initially, (often for many months). Some therapists have emphasized the need to give the child a great deal emotionally and to permit him to regress, with limits put on his aggression or manipulative demands, of course. When a trusting relationship has been developed between the

child and his therapist, limits can gradually be set on the satisfaction of the child's dependency needs, and the therapy can move toward an insight-promoting approach. Not all therapists can tolerate such a complicated and often demanding relationship over such a lengthy period of time, but if this can be done, the patient's response over a period of years can be remarkable.

Bibliography

1. Adams, P.L.: Family characteristics of obsessive children. Am. J. Psychiatry, 128:1414, 1972.
2. Adams, P.L.: Obsessive Children: A Socio-Psychiatric Study. New York, Brunner/Mazel, 1973.
3. Anthony, E.J.: Developmental Antecedents of Schizophrenia. In: Transmission of Schizophrenia (S. Katz and D. Rosenthal, Eds.). London, Pergamon Press, 1968.
4. Anthony, E.J.: Neurotic disorders. In: Comprehensive Textbook of Psychiatry, 2nd Ed., Vol. 2. (A. Freedman, H. Kaplan, and B. Saddock, Eds.). Baltimore, Williams & Wilkins, 1975.
5. Anthony, E.J., and Gilpin, D.C.: Three Clinical Faces of Childhood. New York, Spectrum, 1976.
6. Arkonac, O., and Guze, S.B.: Family background of hysteria. N. Engl. J. Med., 268:239, 1963.
7. Bakwin, H.: Deviant gender-role behavior in children; Relation to homosexuality. Pediatrics, 41:620, 1968.
8. Barlow, D.H., Reynolds, E.J., and Agras, W.S.: Gender identity change in a transsexual. Arch. Gen. Psychiatry, 28:569, 1974.
9. Bates, J.E., et al.: Intervention with families of gender-disturbed boys. Am. J. Orthopsychiatry, 45:150, 1975.
10. Benjamin, H.: The Transsexual Phenomenon. New York, Julian Press, 1966.
11. Berblinger, K.W.: The quiet hysteric and his captive respondent. Dis. Nerv. Syst., 21:386, 1960.
12. Berblinger, K.W.: The hysterical personality. Am. J. Psychiatry, 132:741, 1975.
13. Beres, D.: Ego disturbances associated with early deprivation. J. Am. Acad. Child Psychiatry, 4:188, 1965.
14. Bieber, I., et al.: Homosexuality: A Psychoanalytic Study. New York, Basic Books, 1962.
15. Birk, L., et al.: Avoidance conditioning for homosexuality. Arch. Gen. Psychiatry, 25:314, 1971.
16. Bowlby, J.: Maternal Care and Mental Health. Bull. WHO, 3:355, 1951.
17. Bradley, S., and Solomon, S.: Elective mutism in immigrant families. J. Am. Acad. Child Psychiatry, 15:510, 1976.
18. Brody, E.B.: Borderline state, character disorder and psychotic manifestations: Some conceptual formulations. Psychiatry, 23:75, 1960.

19. Browne, E., Wilson, V., and Laybourne, P.: Diagnosis and treatment of elective mutism in children. J. Am. Acad. Child. Psychiatry, 2:605, 1963.

20. Cain, A.C.: On the meaning of "playing crazy" in borderline children. Psychiatry, 27:278, 1964.

21. Celani, D.: An interpersonal approach to hysteria. Am. J. Psychiatry, 133:1414, 1976.

22. Chethik, M.: The therapy of an obsessive-compulsive boy: Some treatment considerations. J. Am. Acad. Child. Psychiatry, 8:465, 1969.

23. Chodoff, P., and Lyons, H.: Hysteria, the hysterical personality, and "hysterical" conversion. Am. J. Psychiatry, 114:734, 1958.

24. Dawes, L.G.: The psychoanalysis of a case of "grand hysteria of Charcot" in a girl of fifteen. Nerv. Child, 10:272, 1954.

25. Deisher, R.W., Eisner, V., and Sulzbacher, S.J.: The young male prostitute. Pediatrics, 43:936, 1969.

26. Elson, A., et al.: Follow-up study of childhood elective mutism. Arch. Gen. Psychiatry, 13:182, 1965.

27. Ekstein, R.: *Children of Time and Space, of Action and Impulse.* New York, Appleton-Century-Crofts, 1966.

28. Ekstein, R., and Wallerstein, R.: Observations on the psychology of borderline and psychotic children. Psychoanal. Study Child, 9:344, 1954.

29. Ellis, A.: *Homosexuality—Its Causes and Cure.* Secaucus, N.J., Lyle Stuart, 1965.

30. Engel, M.: On the psychological testing of borderline children. Arch. Gen. Psychiatry, 8:426, 1963.

31. Erikson, E.H.: The problem of ego identity. J. Am. Psychoanal. Assoc., 4:56, 1956.

32. Fischoff, J.: Preoedipal influences in a boy's determination to be "feminine" during the oedipal period. J. Am. Acad. Child. Psychiatry, 3:273, 1964.

33. Forrester, B.M., and Swiller, H.: Transsexualism: Review of syndrome and presentation of possible successful therapeutic approach. Int. J. Group Psychother., 22:343, 1972.

34. Freud, A.: The assessment of borderline cases. In: *The Writings of Anna Freud,* Vol. 5. New York, International Universities Press, 1956.

35. Friedman, R.C., et al.: Hormones and sexual orientation in men. Am. J. Psychiatry, 134:571, 1977.

36. Frijling-Schreuder, E.C.M.: Borderline states in children. Psychoanal. Study Child, 24:307, 1969.

37. Gartrell, N.K., Loriaux, D.L., and Chase, T.U.: Plasma testosterone in homosexual and heterosexual women. Am. J. Psychiatry, 135:1117, 1977.

38. Goldin, S., and MacDonald, J.E.: The Ganser state. J. Ment. Sci., 101:267, 1955.

39. Green, R.: Childhood cross-gender behavior and subsequent sexual preference. Am. J. Psychiatry, 136:106, 1979.

40. Green, R., and Money, J.: *Transsexualism and Sex Reassignment.* Baltimore, Johns Hopkins Press, 1969.

41. Group for Advancement of Psychiatry: *Psychopathological Disorders of Childhood: Theoretical Considerations and a Proposed Classification.* Report No.

62. New York, Group for Advancement of Psychiatry, 1966.

42. Gunderson, J.G., and Singer, M.T.: Defining borderline patients: An overview. Am. J. Psychiatry, 132:1, 1975.

43. Haberman, M.A., and Michael, R.P.: Autocastration in transsexualism. Am. J. Psychiatry, 136:347, 1979.

44. Hadden, S.B.: Treatment of homosexuality by individual and group psychotherapy. Am. J. Psychiatry, 114:810, 1958.

45. Hadden, S.B.: Homosexuality: Its questioned classification. Psychiatr. Ann., 6:62, 1976.

46. Halpern, W.I., Hammond, J., and Cohen, R.: A therapeutic approach to speech phobia: Elective mutism reexamined. J. Am. Acad. Child. Psychiatry, 10:94, 1971.

47. Harrison, S.I., and Hess, J.H.: Paranoid Reactions in Children. J. Am. Acad. Child Psychiatry, 5:105, 1966.

48. Harrison, S.I., and Klapman, H.J.: Relationships between social forces and homosexual behavior observed in a children's psychiatric hospital. J. Am. Acad. Child Psychiatry, 5:105, 1966.

49. Hastings, D.W.: Post-surgical adjustment of male transsexual patients. Clin. Plast. Surg., 1:335, 1974.

50. Hitson, H.M., and Funkenstein, D.H.: Family patterns and paranoidal personality structure in Boston and Burma. Int. J. Social Psychiatry, 5:182, 1959.

51. Hollender, M.H.: Hysterical psychosis. Am. J. Psychiatry, 120:1066, 1964.

52. Johnson, A., and Szurek, S.: The genesis of antisocial acting-out in children and adults. Psychoanal. Q., 21:323, 1952.

53. Kaufman, I.: Conversion hysteria in latency. J. Child Psychiatry, 1:385, 1962.

54. Kennard, M.: The electroencephalogram and disorders of behavior. J. Nerv. Ment. Dis., 124:103, 1956.

55. Kernberg, O.: Borderline personality disorganization. J. Am. Psychoanal. Assoc., 15:641, 1967.

56. Kirkpatrick, M., and Friedmann, C.T.H.: Treatment of requests for sex-change surgery with psychotherapy. Am. J. Psychiatry, 133:1194, 1976.

57. Knight, R.P.: Borderline States. Bull. Menninger Clin., 17:1, 1953.

58. Kubie, L.S.: Critical issues raised by operations for gender transformation. J. Nerv. Ment. Dis., 147:431, 1968.

59. Langford, W.S.: Anxiety states in children. Am. J. Orthopsychiatry, 7:40, 1937.

60. Levy, D.M.: *Maternal Overprotection.* New York, Columbia University Press, 1943.

61. Levy, D.: Oppositional syndromes and oppositional behavior. In: *Childhood Psychopathology* (S. Harrison, & J. McDermott, Eds.). New York, International Universities Press, 1972.

62. Linsada, P.V., Peele, R., and Pittard, E.A.: The hysterical personality in men. Am. J. Psychiatry, 131:518, 1974.

63. Marmor, J.: Orality in the hysterical personality. J. Am. Psychoanal. Assoc., 1:656, 1953.

64. Marmor, J.: Sexual behavior. Psychiatric Ann., *1*:45, 1971.

65. Masterson, J.F.: *Treatment of the Borderline Adolescent: A Developmental Approach.* New York, Wiley, 1972.

66. McDonald, J.M.: *Indecent Exposure.* Springfield, Ill., Thomas, 1973.

67. Michael, C.M., Morris, D.P., and Soroker, E.: Follow-up studies of shy, withdrawn children. II. Relative incidence of schizophrenia. Am. J. Orthopsychiatry, *27*:331, 1957.

68. Michaels, J.J.: *Disorders of Character.* Springfield, Ill., Thomas, 1955.

69. Migeon, C.J.: Ambiguity of the external genitalia in the newborn. In: *Principles of Pediatrics: Health Care of the Young* (R.A. Hackelman et al., Eds.). New York, McGraw-Hill, 1978.

70. Mohr, J.W., Turner, R.E., Turner, M.B.: *Pedophilia and Exhibitionism: A Handbook.* Toronto, University of Toronto Press, 1964.

71. Money, J.: Psychologic evaluation of the child with intersex problems. Pediatrics, *36*:51, 1965.

72. Money, J., Hampson, J.G., and Hampson, J.L.: Imprinting and the establishment of gender-role. Arch. Neurol. Psychiatry, *77*:333, 1957.

73. Morris, D.P., Soroker, E., and Burruss, G.: Follow-up studies of shy, withdrawn children. I. Evaluation of later adjustment. Am. J. Orthopsychiatry, *24*:743, 1954.

74. Nardi, T.J., and DiScipio, W.J.: The Ganser syndrome in an adolescent Hispanic-black female. Am. J. Psychiatry, *134*:453, 1977.

75. Newman, L.E.: Transsexualism in Adolescence: Problems in Evaluation and Treatment. Arch. Gen. Psychiatry, *23*:112, 1970.

76. Newman, L.E.: Treatment for the parents of feminine boys. Am. J. Psychiatry, *133*:683, 1976.

77. Newman, L.E., and Stoller, R.J.: Nontranssexual men who seek sex reassignment. Am. J. Psychiatry, *131*:437, 1974.

78. Noshpitz, J.D., and Spielman, P.: Diagnostic study of the differential characteristics of hyperaggressive children. Am. J. Orthopsychiatry, *31*:111, 1961.

79. Proctor, J.T.: Hysteria in childhood. Am. J. Orthopsychiatry, *28*:394, 1958.

80. Pustrom, E., and Speers, R.W.: Elective mutism in children. J. Am. Acad. Child Psychiatry, *3*:287, 1964.

81. Redl, F.: *The Aggressive Child.* Glencoe, Ill., Free Press, 1957.

82. Rekers, G.A., and Lovaas, O.I.: Behavioral treatment of a "transsexual" preadolescent boy. J. Abnorm. Child Psychol., *2*:99, 1974.

83. Rexford, E.: A developmental concept of overdependency in young children. Child. Dev., *25*:125, 1954.

84. Rexford, E.: A developmental concept of the problems of acting out. J. Am. Acad. Child. Psychiatry, *2*:6, 1963.

85. Richards, E.L.: Following the hypochondriacal child for a decade. J. Pediatr., *16*:337, 1948.

86. Robins, L.: *Deviant Children Grown Up.* Baltimore, Williams & Wilkins, 1966.

87. Robins, E., and O'Neal, P.: Clinical features of hysteria in children with a note on prognosis: A two to seventeen year follow-up study of forty-one patients. Nerv. Child., *10*:246, 1953.

88. Rubin, J.Z., Provenanzo, F.J., and Luria, Z.: The eye of the beholder: Parents' views on sex of newborns. Am. J. Orthopsychiatry, *44*:512, 1974.

89. Saghir, M., and Robins, E.: *Male and Female Homosexuality.* Baltimore, Williams and Wilkins, 1973.

90. Sperling, M.: The analysis of a boy with transvestite tendencies. Psychoanal. Study Child., *19*:470, 1964.

91. Stendler, C.B.: Possible causes of overdependency in young children. Child Dev., *25*:125, 1954.

92. Stoller, R.J.: Male childhood transsexualism. J. Am. Acad. Child. Psychiatry, *7*:193, 1968.

93. Stoller, R.J.: *Sex and Gender: On the Development of Masculinity and Femininity.* New York, Science House, 1968.

94. Stoller, R.J., et al.: A symposium: Should homosexuality be in the APA Nomenclature? Am. J. Psychiatry, *130*:1207, 1973.

95. Van Amerongen, S.T.: Permission, promotion, and provocation of antisocial behavior. J. Am. Acad. Child. Psychiatry, *2*:99, 1963.

96. Walinder, J.: *Transsexualism.* Stockholm, Scandinavian University Books, 1967.

97. Weil, A.P.: Certain severe disturbances of ego development in childhood. Psychoanal. Study Child., *8*:271, 1953.

98. Weiner, H., and Braiman, A.: The Ganser syndrome: A review and addition of some unusual cases. Am. J. Psychiatry, *3*:767, 1955.

99. Weinreb, J., and Counts, R.M.: Impulsivity in adolescents and its therapeutic management. Arch. Gen. Psychiatry, *2*:548, 1960.

100. Woerner, P.J., and Guze, S.B.: A family and marital study of hysteria. Br. J. Psychiatry, *114*:161, 1968.

101. Wright, H.L.: A clinical study of children who refuse to talk in school. J. Am. Acad. Child Psychiatry, *7*:603, 1968.

102. Zuger, B.: Effeminate behavior present in boys from early childhood. I. The clinical syndrome and follow-up studies. J. Pediatr., *69*:1098, 1966.

General References

Abraham, K.: Contributions to the theory of the anal character. In: *Selected Papers.* London, Hogarth Press, 1942.

Bakwin, H., and Bakwin, R.M.: *Behavior Disorders in Children,* 4th Ed. Philadelphia, Saunders, 1972.

Brown, W., and Pisetsky, J.E.: Sociopsychologic factors in hysterical paraplegia. J. Nerv. Ment. Dis., *119*:283, 1954.

Buxbaum, E.: *Troubled Children in a Troubled World.* New York, International Universities Press, 1970.

Clausen, J.A.: Family structure, socialization, and personality. In: *Review of Child Development Re-*

search (M. Hoffman and I. Hoffman, Eds.). New York, Russell Sage Foundation, 1966.

Creak, M.: Hysteria in childhood. Acta Paedopsychiatr., *36*:269, 1969.

Engle, M.: On the psychological testing of borderline children. Arch. Gen. Psychiatry, *8*:426, 1963.

Franz, A.: The Neurotic Character. Int. J. Psychoanal., *11*:292, 1930.

Green, R.: *Sexuality Identity Conflict in Children and Adults*. New York, Basic Books, 1974.

Horton, P.C.: The psychological treatment of personality disorder. Am. J. Psychiatry, *133*:262, 1966.

Ingram, I.M.: The obsessional personality and obsessional illness. Am. J. Psychiatry, *117*:1016, 1961.

King, C.H.: Counter-transference and counter-experience in the treatment of violence-prone youth. Am. J. Orthopsychiatry, *46*:43, 1976.

Makkay, E.S., and Schwabb, E.H.: Some problems in the differential diagnosis of antisocial character disorders in early latency. J. Am. Acad. Child Psychiatry, *1*:414, 1962.

Mead, M.: The implications of culture change for personality development. In: *Personal Character and Cultural Milieu*, 3rd Ed. (D.G. Haring, Ed.). Syracuse, Syracuse University Press, 1956.

Money, J., and Ehrhardt, A.: *Man and Woman: Boy and Girl*. Baltimore, Johns Hopkins Press, 1973.

Redl, F.: *The Aggressive Child*. Glencoe, Ill., Free Press, 1957.

Rexford, E.N., Schliefer, M., and Van Amerongen, S.T.: A follow-up study of 57 antisocial young children. Ment. Hyg., *40*:196, 1956.

Saghir, M.T., and Robbins, E.: *Male and Female Homosexuality: A Comprehensive Investigation*. Baltimore, Williams and Wilkins, 1973.

Solnit, A.J.: Bisexuality gone awry—The child is father to the man. Pediatrics, *43*:913, 1969.

Stoller, R.J.: Overview: The impact of new advances in sex research on psychoanalytic theory. Am. J. Psychiatry, *130*:241, 1973.

Teicher, J.D.: Personality disorders. In: *Comprehensive Textbook of Psychiatry*, 2nd Ed., Vol. 2. (A.M. Freedman, H. Kaplan, and B. Saddock, Eds.). Baltimore, Williams & Wilkins, 1975.

20
Psychotic Disorders

The mind is its own place and itself can
make a Heaven of Hell, a Hell of Heaven.
(John Milton)

The diagnostic features of psychotic disorders are:

1. The onset may be sudden or gradual and there are differences in the clinical picture that are related to the child's developmental level.
2. The essential features are (a) a failure to develop an awareness of reality or a withdrawal from reality, with a preoccupation with one's fantasy life, (b) a failure to develop an emotional relatedness to human figures (or a retreat from such relatedness), (c) an inability to express emotions appropriately or to use speech communicatively, and (d) bizarre, stereotyped, or otherwise seriously inappropriate behavior.
3. Hallucinations and delusions, as well as other classic signs of adult psychoses rarely occur until the late school-age or the early adolescent period.
4. Obsessive, compulsive, phobic, conversion, and other psychologic or behavioral symptoms may occur. The symptoms are markedly intense and tenacious, and the child usually is not aware that the symptoms are illogical or inappropriate.

General Considerations

A psychotic disorder in a child is a basic and sweeping disorder in the child's personality functioning and extreme distortion in his ego development. The distortion is revealed in disturbances of the ego functions that subserve thought, the expression of emotions, perception, motility, speech, and individuation. Associated disorders in the child's relatedness to his parents or to other adults and in reality testing are also present to a significant degree. Some manifestations of psychotic behavior seem to represent the child's efforts to make restitution or to compensate for the psychotic process.[71]

The criteria for diagnosis of psychotic

disorder are different at different developmental levels. The earliest behavioral manifestations in infancy and very early childhood are severe disturbances in the child's achievement of attachment to his mother, in beginning the process of individuation, and in his relatedness to other persons. In the preschool-age and early school-age periods, a failure to integrate functions, a disintegration of the personality, a regression, or an arrest in development may occur, along with the child's failure to relate to people or to test reality in various regards. In later childhood and adolescence, severe disturbances may occur in the child's social relationships, sense of identity, thought processes (with looseness of associations or a breakthrough of primitive, prelogical, or magical thinking) and in other areas related to his ego functioning.

Children who have psychoses of the types just discussed do not ordinarily show signs of brain damage, true aphasia,[33] or other neurologic disorders.[180] They usually have a history of disturbed family functioning. For example, his mother may have trouble relating to him, because she is depressed about a family crisis or as the result of an underlying deep-seated personality disorder. Marital problems are often present, with absence of emotional support by the father. A number of investigators have described pathologic relationships, attitudes, or conflicts on the part of one or (often) both parents that involve the patient particularly. Several controlled studies[9,62] have shown significant differences in child-rearing attitudes, parent-child relationships, and family styles of interaction and communication and perceptions of the external world between the parents of so-called schizophrenic children and the parents of normal or psychoneurotic children. Several studies involving adults have demonstrated a significantly higher incidence of parent loss by death or separation during childhood among schizophrenic patients than in the general population.[77]

The findings just listed are pertinent and significant, but most of them are not specific to psychoses in children. They occur also in families that produce disturbed but not necessarily psychotic children.[37] As mentioned earlier, a history of parent loss in childhood is found also in patients who have psychoneurotic disorders, especially depressive types, and delinquent behavior. In my opinion, there is no such thing as a "schizophrenogenic mother." Disturbances in parent-child relationships and distortions in the family's interaction can be found in association with other disorders. Most clinicians think that children who develop psychotic disorders have a biologic predisposition or special vulnerability to psychosis. Evidence for truly hereditary factors is not impressive in those psychoses which develop in infancy and early childhood, although the interaction of experience and genetic mechanisms seems to play a causative role in psychoses that appear in late adolescents and adults.

Some innate or constitutional aberration in the child's threshold of response to sensory stimuli or in his levels of arousal have been postulated by some for children who have the psychoses of early childhood. That aberration may affect and may be affected by disturbances in the early emotional relationship of the mother and her infant,[66] which in turn may be affected by problems in the family's equilibrium and functioning. In studies of identical twins who were discordant for schizophrenia, differences in the twin's size, behavior, and maturation that were present at birth often led parents to suspect that there was some abnormality in the twin who later became schizophrenic or to perceive and handle that child differently.[157] Although the child's premorbid personality did not seem to be the so-called schizoid personality, a greater submissiveness and sensitivity were among the personality traits described in the schizophrenic twins.[156] In a long-term follow-up study of children who were seen in a child guidance clinic, those who developed schizophrenia in adult life were noted to have shown in childhood more symptoms of all kinds, and in particular more aggressive behavior, than did a "no-disease" group.[126] But these and other childhood behavioral characteristics described in other studies[3] are not predictive of adult schizophrenia.

Children who have chronic brain syndromes or mental retardation may also show evidence of psychotic disorders superimposed on their underlying difficulty, which may render some children more vulnerable to psychosis, especially if their environmental circumstances are adverse. For these children the appropriate primary diagnosis should be given, with the psychotic reaction given as a secondary diagnosis. If the child's intellectual development is seriously blunted or invaded by the psychotic process, it may be exceedingly difficult to estimate his inherent capacities or to rule out interwoven diffuse brain damage or mental retardation. A trial of therapy may be needed before the child is able to undergo formal psychologic testing.

This category does not include children who have disorders often referred to as borderline personalities, children who are borderline psychotic, children who show "circumscribed interest;" children who have latent psychosis, or children who are pseudoneurotic. Some children are categorized as having severe personality disorders, with continuing mild or intermittent thought disorders. These disorders are probably best classified under the predominant personality heading in the chapter on personality disorders (Chap. 19), with a qualifying statement about a disturbance in cognitive functioning and some difficulty in reality testing. A few late preschool-age or early school-age children who have marked developmental lags in their cognitive functioning or in their capacity for repression, and persistent prelogical or magical thinking, seem to have a severe

enough superimposed disturbance in their psychosocial functioning to be regarded as borderline psychotic. These children are probably best classified as having developmental deviations, with a statement made regarding the degree of their disturbance in ego functioning (see Chap. 17). The same would hold for children who show the so-called prepsychotic picture and have evidence of impending disorganization and decompensation in ego functioning, often associated with marked hypochondriacal concerns[101] (unless they show further changes permitting a more definitive diagnosis). Such considerations reflect the view that not all thought disorders are psychoses and that not all psychoses are schizophrenia.

In childhood, psychotic disorders are characterized by marked, pervasive deviations from the behavior that is expected for the child's age. Psychotic disorder is often revealed by severe and continued impairment of the child's emotional relationships with persons, disturbances in communication that are associated with irrelevant or diminished speech or failure in speech development, disturbances in sensory perception, bizarre or stereotyped behavior and motility patterns, outbursts of intense and unpredictable anxiety or panic, disturbances in the child's self-concept or the absence of a sense of personal identity, and blunted, uneven, or fragmented intellectual development. In some cases, however, the child's intellectual performance may be adequate or better than adequate, with the psychotic disorder confined to other aspects of the child's personality functioning.

The following special categories of psychotic disorders are recognized as characteristic of childhood. They are discussed in the order of their chronologic appearance since classification is based heavily on developmental considerations. Some psychotic disorders in later childhood and adolescence have some of the features of psychotic disorders in adulthood, but differences related to developmental factors are seen at all levels. Some workers (e.g., Eaton and Menolascino[47]) believe that the process that produces the clinical picture, whether it reduces or interferes with integrated personality functioning, is the same at all developmental levels and that the clinical subgroups are related to the child's stage of development at the onset of his psychotic disorder, the response of the child's environment, and other factors. Some, like Rutter,[145] feel the processes are different in different disorders. Whatever the cause, parents have great difficulty in coping with the psychotic child[113] and his treatment,[164] and his siblings may also be affected.[74]

Psychotic Disorders of Infancy and Early Childhood

Primary Early Infantile Autism

Primary infantile autism must be distinguished from the secondary form, in which the autism, or self-referent behavior, follows brain damage or mental retardation. Early infantile autism, (a term first used by Kanner in 1944[85,86]) appears to have its onset during the child's first few months or first year of life. The infant fails to develop an attachment to his mother. He remains aloof, showing little or no awareness of other people, with absence or avoidance of eye contact, fails to smile, and is very much preoccupied with inanimate objects. The infant thus fails to move out of the "normal autistic"[111] phase of early infancy and, having failed to develop attachment, does not develop stranger anxiety or separation anxiety.

The child's speech development is ordinarily delayed or absent. When the child does begin to speak, he does not use speech appropriately or to communicate. Often he has a mechanical tone, reverses pronouns, shows echolalia, and uses neologisms.[150]

He shows a strong need for the maintenance of "sameness" and tends to resist change, responding with marked outbursts of temper or acute and intense anxiety when his routines are altered. Extreme aloneness and preoccupation with the preservation of sameness are considered by Kanner and Eisenberg to be the hallmarks of the condition.[51] The child's sleeping and feeding problems are often severe. Stereotyped motor patterns often occur. They are often bizarre or primitive, and they often involve whirling, rocking, or other movements. Hand flapping, toe walking, and sudden lunging or darting movements also occur often. The child may fail to react to verbal sounds, but he may be hyperresponsive to the sound of a vacuum cleaner or a barking dog, or he may show outbursts of anxiety that are apparently related to internal stimuli. His intellectual development occasionally is normal or advanced. More often it is restricted and uneven, and he may function at a retarded level. It is possible that the remarkable calendar calculation[78] and other isolated feats performed by apparently retarded persons—so called idiots savants—may represent a peak of uneven intellectual development in certain autistic children. In general, the child's development is uneven.[87]

The differential diagnoses must include brain damage, such as that caused by congenital rubella or cerebral lipoidosis, mental retardation from a variety of causes, sensory defects, such as complete or partial blindness or deafness, developmental aphasia, epilepsy, environmental deprivation or hospitalism, and anaclitic depression.[122] Emotional shock from a seriously traumatic event, such as an accident or a burn, may produce a withdrawn, autistic-like state in certain older infants and very young children. Children who have mental retardation and chronic brain damage may show autistic phenomena, such as disturbances in speech and communication, a preoccupation with inanimate objects, and stereotyped or rhythmic movements. They do not ordinarily show the extreme aloneness and preservation of sameness as do children who have early infantile autism. A few such children do show associated brain damage; some have been said to develop such signs at a later point. Children who have early infantile autism later develop seizures somewhat more frequently than do healthy children.[145]

Theories about the etiology of early infantile autism are legion, and research has blossomed recently. In a recent critical review, Ornitz and Ritvo[128] found little evidence that prenatal and perinatal or hereditary factors played a part. No chromosomal abnormalities have been found in children who have early infantile autism;[84] the results of their neurologic examinations are generally unremarkable and the results of their EEG studies are inconclusive (including evoked auditory responses and state of arousal). One study that investigated the possible presence of slow-acting viruses demonstrated no abnormalities in cerebrospinal immunoglobulins.[178] Metabolic,[34] biochemical,[34,179] and hematologic studies have turned up some apparent abnormalities, but attempts to replicate those findings have not had conclusive results, as Ornitz and Ritvo report. Neurophysiologic research has been limited because of difficulties in obtaining the cooperation of patients who have early infantile autism, although neurochemical studies have shown promise.[35] Ornitz and Ritvo[127] have demonstrated certain differences in the perceptual processes and vestibular functions of autistic children, and they are continuing their research in this important area. The special problems in diagnosis are being attacked with the use of behavior-rating scales.[32,61]

Although some studies have shown no differences in the families of autistic children from normal subjects, some investigators (e.g., Rank,[134] Despert,[42] and Reiser[136]) have reported disturbances in family dynamics at an early period in children who had similar disorders that may be significant. Bettelheim[14] has reported the same finding on a retrospective basis. Clinical observations[37] support the idea that having a child with early infantile autism was extremely difficult, even anguishing for the parents, but most of the cases observed involved older children. Other clinical data offered by Call,[20,22] admittedly retrospective, support the impression that besides the infants' problems in attaching to their mothers, the mothers often have trouble feeling warm toward the infants because of serious conflicts during the pregnancy, marital problems, depression, or deep personality problems. Kanner had the impression originally that the parents' unemotionality contributed to infantile autism,[87] although that impression has not been fully substantiated. Eisenberg[50] has described the fathers (as well as the mothers) of such children as having serious personality difficulties which markedly impaired the normal fulfillment of their paternal role.

Although the focus of many investigators has shifted to the child's inherent difficulties in relating, which involves sensory-integrative or other problems, some investigators, including Call and Prugh, believe that the problems come from both the child's and the parents' sides. One theory is that infants who have early infantile autism have unusual constitutional characteristics that involve differences in their levels of sensory responsiveness to stimulation[13] or in their arousal[81] mechanisms. Some infants may have high thresholds of response and thus would require considerable stimulation, which might not be supplied by a depressed or withdrawn parent. Some infants may have low thresholds of response and thus would easily be overstimulated by an anxious or conflicted parent. Sander's[148] work showing that infant caretaker's activities can affect the newborn infant's biologic rhythms and other physiologic functions may be pertinent to the situation of infants who have some constitutional vulnerability of these or other types. Thus such problems might arise in the context of such a negative feedback system between infant and parent, as others, around feeding and sleeping, are now believed to occur. Such an interactional theory is not (indeed, no theory is) fully explanatory, but it may be closer to the truth than the theories which center the problem in either the infant or the parent alone.

Interactional Psychotic Disorder

This category includes children who have so-called symbiotic psychosis, which was first described by Mahler.[109] But it also includes other disorders that have somewhat different features, while symbiotic parent-child relationships may be seen in disorders other than psychoses.[71] Children who have symbiotic psychotic disorders seem from their histories to have developed adequately for the first year or 2 of life, with awareness of and attachment to their mothers appearing during their first year. Subsequently the child may show unusual dependence on his mother in the form of an intensification and prolongation of the attachment. Thus the child does not achieve separation and individuation. That failure seems to be at least partly the result of the unconscious need of the child's parent, usually his mother, to bind the child to her in an intense symbiotic or interdependent phase of ego development. She does so to satisfy vicariously her own emotional needs that arise from inadequate gratification in her marriage, other family problems, or a marked personality disturbance of her own.

In the child's second to fourth or fifth year, the onset of the psychotic disorder occurs, ordinarily in relation to some shift in the balance within the parent-child relationship (e.g., the birth of a sibling and the preoccupation of the mother with the baby, depression in or withdrawal by the mother, or a severe family crisis). The young child, who is overdependent on the now disrupted symbiotic interaction, often rather suddenly shows intense separation anxiety and clinging and regressive manifestations in an apparent attempt to restore the symbiotic relationship. When the attempt is unsuccessful, the child seems to retreat to a defensive autistic posture, as Mahler terms it.[110] The picture is one of gradual withdrawal, emotional aloofness, the appearance of autistic behavior, and a distorted perception of reality. The picture may resemble that of early infantile autism, and the diagnosis can only be made by examining the child's history. Occasionally the father or some other family member becomes the symbiotic partner, perhaps because of a shift in parental or familial roles. Again the question of some constitutional predisposition on the child's part remains unanswered. In twins, alternating psychotic pictures that begin in early childhood[82] are also seen occasionally, as are other interactional patterns.

Other Psychotic Disorders of Early Childhood

This category includes disorders whose pictures do not conform closely to those of early infantile autism or interactional psychosis although they may show some features of each disorder. The category includes some children who have "atypical" or fragmented ego development, which was first described by Rank.[134] These children exhibit some autistic behavior and emotional aloofness, but they may also show some strengths in adaptive behavior and assets in personality development.[136,137]

The differential diagnoses of psychotic disorders in early childhood include developmental lags in cognitive functioning, acute brain syndromes in which some similar behavior may be seen, marked depression and apathy, identification with a psychotic parent or other adult, and intense anxiety and inhibition that leads to the picture of the "frozen" child, who has action paralysis.

Psychotic Disorders of Later Childhood

Schizophreniform Psychotic Disorder

This disorder, which was originally called "schizophrenic-like" by Lourie, Pacella, and Piotrowski,[105] is usually seen in children 6 to 12 or 13 years old, most often in the early school-age period or just before. The disorder is more common in boys than in girls, and its severity is often underestimated in the early stages, attention being focussed on the child's minor and apparently physical complaints. Children whose disorders fit in this category have been most frequently designated as having "childhood schizophrenia," following the lead of Potter,[133] and Bender.[10] Definitions of the disorder and attitudes toward the children who have it vary.[40,65] Many of these children are seen in the disorder's chronic phase, long after its onset. The term schizophreniform, which is used in the GAP nomenclature,[71] has the advantage of indicating the parallels between this disorder and the adult form of schizophrenia while emphasizing the developmental differences, as well as suggesting that children who have the disorder do not necessarily develop the later adult disorder.

The onset is usually gradual, with dependent and clinging behavior usually noted from the time the child begins school. Often neurotic symptoms, such as conversion headaches and abdominal pains, are present and are associated with a low tolerance for frustration, hypochondriacal tendencies, and intense temper outbursts. By the child's third or fourth school year or sometimes earlier, the psychotic process becomes manifest, with marked anxiety, especially over separation from his mother,

difficulty in relating to his peers, gradual withdrawal from teachers, marked preoccupation with fantasy, bizarre or disruptive behavior, gross disturbances in reality testing, persecutory fantasies that have the characteristics of poorly organized delusions, and hallucinatory experiences, especially visual hallucinations at night but occasionally auditory hallucinations as well.[41] The hallucinations usually are macabre, bizarre, or strangely vague, in contrast to the transparent, comprehensible, largely auditory[100] and usually wishfulfilling hallucinations in hysterical disorders. Looseness of associations may be followed by a true thinking disorder, with distorted symbolization, condensation of several thoughts into one, and other manifestations of a breakthrough of prelogical thought processes. In the early stages, these patients seem to be able to relate fairly well to a helping adult; disturbances in thinking and reality testing can fairly readily be brought under control with the use of the adult as a kind of auxiliary ego.

A recent study of Jordan and Prugh[83] of 22 cases generally confirmed the GAP description. It included 6 additional cases in which more acute and sudden eruptions of the psychotic process occurred, accompanied by sweeping anxiety, uncontrollable obsessions, rituals, or phobias, and marked withdrawal leading to distorted reality testing, delusional thinking, and withdrawn or bizarre behavior. "Catastrophic reactions" of this type have been described following severe bodily injury although they may be precipitated by family crisis or other traumatic experiences. Children who have the schizophreniform disorder have usually been markedly overdependent during the preschool-age period, and they do not seem to have accomplished successfully the separation-individuation process necessary for school adjustment.

The families of the children in Jordan's and Prugh's study were generally quite disturbed, with only a few reasonably stable homes and a good deal of distortion of reality, as in other studies.[16,65] In 50% of the cases, the fathers had left their families and a number of parents were alcoholic, and 3 mothers were psychotic. The siblings generally were mildly to moderately disturbed, although only 1 was regarded as psychotic. The mothers generally were markedly overprotective and overindulgent, tending to keep the patients close to them at home.

In many of these children, regression is ordinarily not as marked as in adults. True hallucinations are not commonly recognized until the child is 8 or 9 years old, (partly because in the early school-age child, the presence of fantasy, some persistence of magical thinking, and an evolving though uneven mastery of difficulties makes it difficult to be certain about such phenomena). Bizarre behavior and stereotyped motor patterns, such as whirling, are frequently present. Some children show sudden and wild outbursts of aggressive, violent, or self-mutilating behavior,[70] inappropriate mood swings, and suicidal threats and attempts. Ideas of reference ("People can read my mind with that machine"), dissociative phenomena, somatic delusions ("My arms are falling off"), catatonic behavior, paranoid thinking, and other manifestations seen in adults may occur. If the psychotic process has progressed to the point where intellectual deterioration is a prominent feature, the child's intellectual capacities may be difficult to determine.[38] Christ[31] has found a Piagetian framework helpful in the cognitive assessment of psychotic children. Crystalization of the disorder into definite subtypes, as in adults, does not seem to occur in schizophreniform psychosis during this age period.

From the interpersonal approach, Garmezy and his colleagues[62] have described differences from normal controls in child-rearing attitudes in parents of schizophrenic patients. Kaufman and his colleagues[92] have identified characteristic types of defense in parents of schizophrenic children. Szurek and his colleagues[162,181] see various types of family psychopathology. Others, such as Bateson and his colleagues,[7,167] see more specific pathologic interactions, such as the double bind, or, with Lidz and his group,[102] disturbances in family role functioning and the "transmission of irrationality." Wynne and his colleagues see a "lack of communicative clarity"[177] and a "pseudo-mutuality" of relatedness,[176] while Goldfarb and his colleagues see "parental perplexity" and problems in cohesion in the patients' families.[9,65]

The differential diagnosis should include severe panic states (reactive disorders) in which thinking can become temporarily disorganized by anxiety, severe obsessive-compulsive disorders,[43] and marked developmental lags in cognitive functioning or repressive capacities, in which prelogical thinking may persist beyond the preschool-age period. Children who have delusions or (more often) visual hallucinations associated with an acute brain syndrome or delirium usually show a rather quick subsidence of symptoms from such a psychotic episode once the underlying disturbance is corrected. Children who have chronic brain syndromes show definitive signs of neurologic damage and are usually able to relate positively to others and to test basic reality. Heller's syndrome, a rare type of degenerative encephalopathy,[112] may involve dementia, which is usually readily distinguishable. But it too may have a number of causal factors in a psychotic picture, as Chmiel and Mattsson[30] have indicated. Differentiating the disorder from mental retardation in the preschool-age period may require psychotherapy, as Loomis and his colleagues have indicated.[151] These investigators used both standardized play observations and tests in their study.

There are 2 main theories of the cause of psychosis during childhood. One theory is that psychosis in childhood is the result of

factors that derive from atypical development and organization of the central nervous system,[11] perhaps related to some form
of brain dysfunction.[5] The other theory is
that psychosis in childhood is principally
the result of disturbed family relationships
and disordered parent-child relationships
in particular.

Some evidence for brain dysfunction or
neurointegrative deficiencies has been ad-
duced by Gittelman and Birch,[64] Pollack,[131]
and others.[165] Goldfarb[65] has maintained
that some children diagnosed as schizophrenic are neurologically impaired, with
their behavior resulting in a pathogenic effect on the family. Some criteria for the
presence of brain damage have been somewhat loose in some studies. As in early
childhood psychoses, genetic factors do not
appear to be significantly involved in cases
appearing in the school-age range.

The truth probably lies somewhere between the 2 theories just described. For one
thing, there are undoubtedly problems in
sampling. Some cases apparently do involve some brain dysfunction, and brain
damaged and mentally retarded children
may be liable to develop a picture resembling that of schizophreniform psychosis
(although many do not). The child's family
problems play an important part, but they
do not explain the whole picture. Undoubtedly, the child has some type of vulnerability[47] to the disorder. Mednick[119] believes that the child may have a physiologic
predisposition; that is, certain components
of the child's autonomic nervous system
may be unusually responsive to mild stress
and thus vulnerable to learned avoidance
thinking or a thinking disorder. Much more
systematic research on the behavioral level
and metabolic levels are needed to arrive
at a full answer to this important question.
With others,[58] I favor an interactional point
of view.

Manic-depressive psychotic disorder is
virtually nonexistent in childhood, although it does occur (rarely) in the late
school-age period.[4] Paranoid psychotic dis-

orders also do not occur in the school-age
period. (As mentioned in Chapter 19, paranoid reactions and personality patterns are
occasionally seen in early adolescence.)

Psychotic Disorders of Adolescence

Acute Confusional State

During late adolescence and the post-
adolescent period, a particular type of psychotic disorder may occur. It is related to
the developmental problems of the stage,
and it was first described by Carlson.[27] The
onset of the disorder is often rather abrupt,
with acute and intense anxiety, depressive
trends, confusion in thinking, and feelings
of depersonalization ("I don't feel like myself"), among other manifestations. The
person's disturbances in the development
of a sense of identity are apparent, but he
usually lacks evidence of a true thought
disorder or a marked breakdown in reality
testing. The young person often has a capacity for meaningful emotional relationships despite the disorder, and he shows
(unevenly) the presence of varying adaptive capacities.

The differential diagnosis includes adult-
type schizophrenic disorders, acute panic
states (usually a reactive disorder, although occasionally one involving latent
homosexual trends), acute brain syndromes, and the feelings of anxiety,
depression, confused thinking or of depersonalization which occur at times in
normal adolescents who are under stress.
Admixtures of hysterical and other psychoneurotic symptoms may be present.
They can be classified as secondary personality disorders under their appropriate
categories or they can be regarded as symptoms. The outlook for immediate recovery
is generally good, but later a deep-seated
personality disorder may be seen to underlie the psychotic picture; or it may be

related to an acutely decompensating personality disorder. When such prior personality trends can be seen clearly, the personality disorder can be specified as the primary diagnosis, and the acute confusional state can be classified as the secondary diagnosis.

Schizophrenic Disorders of the Adult Type

These disorders, which begin to resemble adult schizrenia, involve a breakdown in reality testing, thought disorders, hallucinations or delusions, limited socialization, and, at times, a breakdown in impulse controls.[104,171] Some differences that are related to the child's developmental level may be present, often making diagnosis difficult. Although many cases are undifferentiated and are often acute and subside rapidly, subtypes of a simple, catatonic, paranoid, or hebephrenic nature may be seen on a more chronic or recurrent basis, as in adults. The distinction between process and reactive forms of schizophrenia begins to be helpful diagnostically in late adolescence.[46,88] The process form reaches back in years, involves serious difficulties or adjustment, and has a gradual or insidious onset. The reactive form appears more suddenly and in response to precipitating stress.

Other Psychoses of Adolescence

This general category should be reserved for disorders which do not fit the categories in adolescence already discussed. This category may include reactive psychoses[166] or sweeping regressive pictures of a psychotic degree,[149] related to situational stresses, with mild thought disorders that do not have true schizophrenic coloration. Transient catatonic states[98] or marked dissociative states may also be seen, at times with strong hysterical, obsessive, or phobic features. Some people in whom these states occur may have severe underlying personality disorders, which can be specified.

Manic-depressive psychotic disorder was not included as a major category in the GAP nomenclature. Harms[73] (in 1952) and Campbell[24] (in 1959) had written about children who had cyclical patterns of elation and sadness; the diagnostic criteria those investigators used were considered not clear, and such cases were included in the category of developmental deviations. At the time the GAP report was published, Anthony, a member of the GAP committee, had done the only current review and case study. He concluded that manic-depressive disorders were not encountered before 11 years of age and only rarely in adolescence[3] (in which case the adult diagnosis could be used). Anthony found only 1 case in which the disorder continued into adult life. Since 1966, when the GAP report was published, manic-depressive disorders have been described as occurring occasionally in early adolescence[28] and slightly more often in later adolescence.[54,56,175] The diagnostic criteria have been modified somewhat from the strict ones of Anthony. I am somewhat skeptical of the rare reports of manic-depressive pictures,[2] manic[168] and hypomanic behavior[118] and psychotic-like depression[169] as well as of the results of the uncontrolled studies of the responses to lithium of disturbed children who have manic-depressive parents[2,45] who responded favorably to lithium.

In adults, bipolar affective disorders, in which both manic and depressive episodes occur, and unipolar disorders, in which mania does not appear, have been described. The trend is less clear in adolescents.

So-called hysterical psychoses, the Ganser syndrome, and related disorders were discussed in Chapter 19.

Treatment and Prognosis

As implied, the presence or absence of a psychotic disorder alone is not necessarily related to the long-term outlook in childhood or adolescence, nor, as indicated earlier, to the level of psychosocial functioning in any exact sense. This is particularly true for school-age children with schizophreniform psychotic disorder. They usually respond to outpatient psychotherapy that involves tandem therapy for their parents. Their symptoms subside and they seem to achieve greater independence and social relatedness if they are treated for a year or more within 2 years after the onset of the disorder. If they are not treated within 2 years, as Jordan and Prugh[83] have emphasized, a chronic, gradually deteriorating state that resembles what many have called childhood schizophrenia or psychosis may supervene. It is much more difficult to treat. Such children may lose their capacity to relate to adults; their I.Q.s may drop 10 to 30 points, and the children may be excluded from school or referred for residential care. If the onset is acute, psychiatric hospitalization on a relatively short-term basis (several weeks to several months), and milieu therapy and tandem psychotherapy for the child and his parents can help the child recompensate and may enable him to return home for outpatient or day treatment, as Vasey and his colleagues[163] have demonstrated.

Children who have psychotic disorders of early childhood have a more guarded prognosis and a more limited outlook. Follow-up studies by Eisenberg and Kanner[48,51] and by Rutter[146,147] in Britain of children who had early infantile autism indicated that by adolescence more than two-thirds were making poor social adjustments. Those who had not acquired speech by the time they were 5 years old or who had low I.Q.s often required long-term institutional care. About one-third improved, some of them becoming self-supporting. Although many did not receive adequate treatment, very few become classic adult schizophrenics. With the greater availability of more modern and intensive treatment, more of these children might have improved, as Rutter

has indicated (in my experience, even children who do not speak until they are 5 years old may respond). Weiner[172] has summarized the results of available studies of the outcome of actual treatment of children with early infantile autism by stating that substantial improvement can be expected in 25% of cases, with 50% probably requiring residential placement by the end of adolescence.[48]

More than 50% of a group of very young children with "atypical development" (infantile psychosis) who were followed up by Brown and Reiser[17,18,138] after long-term psychoanalytically oriented therapy in a therapeutic nursery school showed capacities for functioning in society by adolescence. (Some of these children may have had early infantile autism.) Detailed follow-up data, although limited, are available. Children who have symbiotic psychotic pictures also apparently have a somewhat better prognosis than do those who have early infantile autism. In the experience of Staub and her colleagues[158] 6 out of 9 preschool-age children showed marked improvement, to the point where they could function adequately socially and educationally, following therapy for child and parents combined with a therapeutic nursery school program and later day treatment. Further systematic follow-up studies of early childhood psychosis are badly needed.

Although in general, the earlier the onset the more guarded the prognosis, in my opinion, the somewhat pessimistic, rather static attitudes of some clinicians toward psychotic disorders in these age groups are not appropriate. One reason for the pessimism has been the tendency of many investigators to regard all cases in a particular category as a unit. Kanner[86] and Eisenberg[51] emphasized long ago that there were different degrees of early infantile autism, and Szurek and his colleagues[162] applied the concept of a gradient to the severity of childhood psychoses, with cases ranging from less severe to more severe.

Havelkova[75] has reported on patients who had very mild cases of early childhood psychosis that improved spontaneously. He observed also that among patients who had milder cases and who were treated, those who were treated earlier had a better outcome than those who were treated later. I have seen 4 cases of mild early infantile autism; 1 of the children progressed to apparent normality in 2 years without treatment (the child's parents refused treatment). Some parental counseling was given, and the child was placed in a nursery school.

Case Study. J. was 30 months old when she was referred to the child psychiatry clinic for evaluation of generalized but uneven developmental delays (most notably in language, where her developmental age was 12 to 14 months). "Unusual behaviors" were also manifest, including head banging, a relative disinterest in people, including her mother, minimal eye contact, and at times a lack of response to sounds, despite having normal hearing.

J. was described as having been a quiet, independent baby who seemed to prefer lying in bed to being held. She never displayed stranger or separation anxiety, and she did not walk alone until she was 18 months old. When she was 26 months old, she had virtually no language. When J. was 3 months old, her mother began to work part-time, and when J. was 6 months old, her mother was working full-time, leaving J. with a number of different baby-sitters. J.'s parents gave a history of long-standing marital discord which amounted to virtual chaos within the family.

During the initial evaluation sessions, J. displayed no language, and she was largely emotionally detached. She did display 3 distinctly positive prognostic signs. In the first session, she spontaneously climbed into the evaluator's lap, and she had momentary eye contact with him. By the third play session she was able to actively engage and utilize the evaluator's help in mastering tasks, and was clearly disturbed by being left alone in the playroom. In addition, she spontaneously raised a telephone receiver to her ear and babbled into the mouthpiece.

In the 9 months following the evaluation, J. attended a toddler's day care program 2 to 4 hours per day 3 to 5 days per week, and she was seen fairly regularly (1 hour per week) in individual play therapy. During the same time, the turmoil in her family increased, and attempts at engaging her parents in psychotherapy were only minimally successful. Despite these difficulties, J. developed a clear attachment to her therapist, as manifested by her greeting him with a smile and open arms and by intermittently sharing her play with him. By the end of the 9-month period, she had a 15-word vocabulary and could count to 5.

Call[21] has made a plea for the prevention of autism in infancy. He has reported several cases in which early intervention and, in 1 case, counselling of a mother of a very young infant in a well-child clinic seemed to be successful.

Treatment methods differ somewhat, depending on the child's age and developmental level, as well as on his clinical picture. I believe that every child who has an early childhood psychosis deserves an initial trial of therapy on an ambulatory basis, beginning as early in the preschool-age period as possible. As has been indicated, some surprisingly good results may be achieved, even in early infantile autism. At the very least, the initial treatment on an ambulatory basis with the child and parents may pinpoint the child's basic intellectual endowment. Or it may help the parents to accept long-term placement or other steps if these become clearly necessary after at least a year of treatment. Whatever the etiologic factors, parents of these children need compassion as well as much support and relief from guilt.

In the treatment of these young children, play therapy and tandem therapy for the parents may be combined with the contributions of a therapeutic nursery school, as Rank and her colleagues,[134,135] and Staub and his colleagues[158] have indicated. Operant conditioning, particularly that involving positive reinforcement or rewards (praise, affection, candy, or food) for bits of healthy behavior, has been reported[123] to help these children develop some speech and achieve some degree of socialization or to help them control self-mutilating behavior. Aversive behavior therapy involving electric shock has also been used,[107] but it can confuse the child and its benefits are limited. In the "symbiotic" psychosis, the child should not be placed in a nursery school until the child and his parents are ready to separate without marked anxiety, as Mahler[108] has indicated. Family conjoint therapy seems to have limited value, and it may be contraindicated in the early stages of treatment. Psychoactive drugs have limited value in very young children unless the children are sweepingly anxious, hyperactive, or destructive.[26] Home training programs implemented by competent people who visit the parents and help them to train children toward self-help and socialization can be of real value. The National Society for Autistic Children, based in Albany, New York, offers parents information and group support.

The treatment of such children must extend over a number of years, and it must be closely coordinated with educational and other programs. An outpatient clinic that functions in collaboration with a therapeutic nursery school and a day treatment program can facilitate the child's entry into public school, as Halpern and Gold[72] have demonstrated. They use structured language training as the educational core. Of a group of 15 children who had features resembling those of early infantile autism (including several children who had brain damage) who were handled by such an approach, 11 were in public school, (3 were in regular classes and the other 8 were in special or modified classes) at the time of a 4-year follow-up. The other 4 children were in residential treatment facilities. Although 9 had no useful speech and 6 had only the most rudimentary speech when they entered the preschool program, all had useful speech at the time of the follow-up. Even in the severest cases, in which long-term residential treatment is indicated and children of school age often have no speech, Bettleheim[15] has reported a "good" outcome in 42% of 40 patients, a "fair" outcome in 38%, and a "poor" outcome in 20%.

School-age children who have chronic psychotic pictures that often resemble those of schizophreniform disorders that were not treated early have been treated in a variety of ways. Psychoanalytically oriented outpatient psychotherapy has been used by Ekstein,[53] Kaufman and his colleagues,[90] Escalona,[55] and others,[55,60] and psychoanalysis has been used,[63] as has individual psychotherapy for a blind psychotic child.[159] Group therapy of psychotic children has also been found helpful.[155] Behavior therapy has been found valuable in reinforcing speech development and social behavior and in dealing with particular symptoms[79,106] although in the opinion of Prugh and others, ideally it should be used in conjunction with dynamic psychotherapy.

Contemporary treatment approaches emphasize the need for parent therapy as well (as Szurek and Berlin,[161] Kaufman and his colleagues,[91,93] and others[36,53,129,153] have indicated), including group therapy where appropriate.[124,130] In addition to music and art therapy, various types of body stimulation have been employed.[79]

Psychoactive drugs have been used in superabundance for children with these disorders. As indicated in Chapter 13, I believe that most such drugs are not helpful to children and may be harmful. They should only be used as adjuncts in a comprehensive treatment approach. Of the major tranquilizers, chlorpromazine (thorazine) and Mellaril can be used safely for school children or adolescents to control bursts of panic or hyperactivity or aggressive behavior that often is based on fear of attack and to control certain other symptoms, but how much they affect the psychotic process itself is unclear. Campbell[25] has found thiothixene (Navane), a thioxanthene, to be a safer and more effective antipsychotic drug than are the phenothiazines. She feels the hypnotics, sedatives, stimulants, and antidepressant drugs essentially have no place in the treatment of the psychotic child and that some may be harmful. She also believes that before a child is given a major tranquilizer, Benadryl, a safer drug, should be tried in individualized doses. The use of the hallucinogen LSD–25 by Bender and her colleagues[12] and by others[154] has little to recommend it and has some dangers.[59] Lithium can be effective in the occasional manic-depressive adolescent,[25] but because of its possible toxic effects, it is inappropriate for hyperactive and aggressive children.

Megavitamin treatment has been advocated by Rimland[140] for chronically psychotic disorders (and by others for various learning disabilities). A task force of the American Psychiatric Association[121] thoroughly evaluated the available reports and concluded that megavitamin therapy does not meet the criteria for scientific validity and that well-controlled trials of nicotinic acid therapy with adult schizophrenic patients have shown such therapy to have no value. The Committee on Nutrition of the American Academy of Pediatrics agreed.[1] It saw no value in and some possibly harmful physical effects from the use of megavitamin therapy for learning disorders. As indicated earlier, electroshock therapy has no place in the treatment of children.

Some children who have chronic psychotic disorders respond well to a day program. The program may be (1) a day treatment program, with an educational approach combined with psychotherapy for children and parents,[68] (2) a day school program with therapeutic aspects[57] or (3) a day activity and education program, with parents enlisted as co-therapists.[152] Other children of school-age require treatment in hospital or residential settings.

Psychiatric hospitalization may be used briefly or episodically,[94] or it may involve long-term therapeutic use of the planned milieu, combined with the various treatment modalities, as Szurek and Berlin[161] and Brunstetter[19] have stressed. Although children's programs in state hospitals have been much maligned as being custodial, if the staff is adequate and if cottage-type units are available, those programs can provide effective long-term treatment, as Williams[173] has demonstrated. Residential treatment centers put special emphasis on the milieu approach and the living in of the child care staff, along with various forms of treatment. Outstanding programs have been offered at the Orthogenic School, in Chicago,[15] the Menninger Clinic, in Topeka,[52] Bellefaire, in Cleveland,[116] the Jewish Board of Guardians, in New York, and the Residential Treatment Center, in Rochester, New York, among others.

In all such out-of-home placements, therapy for parents and other family members is vital (even if the therapy must be carried out at a distance) to prevent the child or adolescent patient from being extruded from his family.[164] It is also difficult for the patient to return home to a family that has not changed. There is a trend toward deinstitutionalization, which is healthy, but an effective monitoring system must be established if the trend is to be effective. Some children, especially those who have serious medical or drug problems and psychosis, a marked suicidal potential, run-away tendencies, and other problems require care for a period in closed hospital units, and others need residential treatment for several years. When appropriate (either at the outset or when the child has reached the point of maximal benefit in a hospital or residential setting), placement of the child as near home as possible in either a small cottage-type group residential setting that has a specially trained staff or in a "professional" group foster home is undoubtedly best. But those facilities should have an adequate treatment staff or associated treatment facilities. Many group homes do not. Some children cannot go home again, because the family has dissolved or cannot handle them, and they may have to remain in treatment-oriented group living settings for many years.[99]

Although there are a number of treatment modalities for the school-age psychotic child and his family, it is not easy to evaluate the outcomes of those treatments. Except for a few, the samples have been small, and differences in terms, criteria for diagnosis, and etiological concepts render conclusions difficult. To date, no major attempt has been made to compare the effectiveness of different types of treatment. Most of the available follow-up studies have involved some form of ambulatory or residential psychotherapy, sometimes with other forms of therapy.

As mentioned, the prognosis for the child who has acute schizophreniform psychotic disorder is good.[83] Of 22 children studied on an outpatient basis, 10 received a year or more of weekly individual psychotherapy, with tandem therapy for their parents, mostly their mothers. Within 2 years after the onset of their disorder, 3 children received several months of treatment only, for a variety of reasons related to the treatment plan. Nine patients received no therapy, either because their families had moved, the child showed a mild, temporary improvement, or the parents refused therapy (only 6 of these 9 could be followed). Of the 10 who received appropriate therapy, 9 showed marked improvement in their functioning. Their reality testing returned, any delusional fantasies and hallucinations they had disappeared, and they exhibited greater independence from their mothers and teachers as well as an ability to relate (superficially) to their peers. About 1 year after termination of their treatment, they were known to have maintained their improvement; they were living at home and attending school. Phenothiazines were given to 5 patients, with little or uncertain effect. The tenth patient showed mild improvement only. The 3 patients who broke off treatment showed mild improvement, but they generally relapsed, and 2 were admitted to a state hospital. Five of the 6 patients who received no treatment and who could be followed were eventually put in residential facilities or a

state hospital. The sixth patient remained at home but was chronically psychotic.

The outcome studies of the treatment of chronically psychotic patients involve largely residential treatment settings. Davids and his colleagues[39] reported that about one-third of the group treated had made a good school adjustment and about 50% made a good overall adjustment. But about 40% of the rest had to be put in institutions. (This figure actually amounts to 8% to 9% of the total treated.) Weiner[171] has summarized the available data on the outcome of chronically ill patients treated in residential settings by such workers as Goldfarb,[67,69] Szurek and Berlin,[162] and Kemph,[95] as well as studies that included outpatients.[49,75] He stated that about one-third make a moderately good adjustment during adolescence, and another one-third make a marginal adjustment outside an institution, and the remaining one-third require more or less permanent residential care. Goldfarb[67] found more improvement in patients who did not have brain damage and a worse result for those who had, as did Eaton and Menascolino[47] and Rutter.[144] Havelkova's[75] study indicated that the earlier the treatment the better the results, while Kemph found the best improvement in those treated most intensively. In a comparison of residential and day care treatment programs, both Kemph's and Goldfarb's studies showed that children who were treated intensively improved more than children who were not treated intensively.

The treatment and prognosis of psychotic disorders in the school-age group have been discussed in some detail to emphasize the importance of early recognition and referral for treatment of children who have schizophreniform disorders. Although the children who were treated early (reported by Jordan and Prugh) are a small group, and are possibly a skewed sample, their prognosis seems to be dramatically better than the prognosis of children who were not treated early and who seem to develop chronic psychotic disorders. In my opinion, pediatricians, family physicians, educators, and other professionals who detect and refer such children soon after the onset of the psychotic process can make an important contribution to secondary prevention.

Psychotic disorders that occur during adolescence vary widely in prognosis and response to treatment. Again the etiologic concepts vary widely, and they influence attitudes toward treatment. In addition, some investigators consider most psychotic disorders in adolescence schizophrenic (and some consider them manic-depressive), while others see acute confusional states and acutely regressive, transiently catatonic, or other psychotic disorders that appear to be reactive to situational and interpersonal stresses as psychodynamic responses (often of people who have been previously disturbed).

Although systematic follow-up data are limited, it seems that the reactive pictures, including acute confusional states, have generally good prognoses, and usually they respond well to psychotherapy,[80] and some therapy for the parents, (which often is not given). Brief (occasionally longer) periods of hospitalization may be needed. The structure, external controls, and individual and milieu therapy offered in a hospital can produce remarkable personality reorganization and adaptive advances.[23,98] Psychoactive drugs seem to be more effective in adolescents than in children when they are used as adjuncts to psychotherapeutic measures on an outpatient basis (with the cautions described in Chapter 13).

As indicated earlier, in adolescence a type of schizophrenia closer to that seen in adults begins to occur. In addition to interpersonal problems within the adolescent's family, hereditary factors begin to be involved, as in adult schizophrenia, a point that was clarified recently by Kety and his colleagues[97] and Helgason,[76] among others. Biochemical aberrations in the functioning of brain biogenic amines have been described in adults[96] although some workers, such as Ban,[6] question whether the biochemical changes are caused by disordered psychopathological processes or are the result of those processes. Kety believes that genetic factors represent only the potential for development of schizophrenia, which is brought out if pathologic and environmental force interact. The contribution of hereditary factors seems to be much smaller than was believed some years ago.

The prognosis for and response to treatment of schizophrenia in adolescents has been reported by Masterson,[114] and others[132] to be considerably less favorable than in adults. (In the past, about one-third of adults suffered a single episode, one-third had periodic recurrences, and one-third became chronic patients.) Masterson[115] and others[120,125] point out the difficulty in differentiating borderline disorders, depression, and other clinical pictures from schizophrenia. The distinction made by Easson[46] of the difference in prognosis of process and reactive forms is also pertinent; the reactive form shows an early response to treatment. Along with Symonds and Herman[160] and Weiner[170] I am somewhat more optimistic about the response of the individual schizophrenic adolescent to adequate treatment although I recognize that there is a group who have serious predisposing factors and continuing problems and whose prognosis is more guarded.

The therapeutic approach[89] used with adolescent schizophrenic patients has included individual psychotherapy, with therapy for the parents, group therapy, family therapy, drug therapy, hospital or residential treatment, and day treatment.[103] Major tranquilizers have been widely used, particularly in hospital settings, and indeed they have seemed to have considerable value. Some have come to regard the use of tranquilizers as the therapy of choice for schizophrenic patients. (Virtually all child psychiatrists think that electroconvulsive therapy and psychosurgery have no place in the treatment of schizophrenic adolescents.) But a recent report by Carpenter and his colleagues[29] has indicated that adult schizophrenic patients treated in a hospital setting by individual and group psychotherapy and milieu therapy showed outcomes at a 1-year follow-up that were similar to those of a a group treated with phenothiazines. (But methodologic differences may be involved.) The study does not indicate that drugs should not be used but it does call for a more balanced reappraisal of therapeutic approaches, with more systematic research in the comparison of the effectiveness of different treatment modalities.

In regard to the manic-depressive disorders that occasionally occur in adolescents, a genetic causative factor may be involved, as demonstrated in the bipolar type of manic-depressive disorders in adults,[174] although there are too few cases reported to permit a conclusion. Evidence that genetic factors contibute to the unipolar type of depressive disorder in adults is still suggestive only,[44] and it is not yet clear if this type of depressive disorder occurs in adolescents. A recent small-scale controlled study by Robbins and his colleagues[142] has suggested that the children of manic-depressive mothers are at risk for affective disorders. Biochemical investigations in adults have implicated a derangement of neuroendocrine mechanisms that apparently involve an unexplained disturbance in the metabolism of catecholamines and other biogenic amines.[139]

Psychosocial investigations indicate that losses of key figures, whether actual or symbolic, play a large part in the onset of both bipolar[141] and unipolar[117] depressive disorders, with the manic state, when it occurs, somehow acting as an emergency defense reaction[8] to deal with the underlying depression. Much further research is needed, but again the etiologic concepts of an interaction among genetic, biochemical,

developmental and psychosocial factors seem most appropriate.

Lithium carbonate can be used as part of a comprehensive treatment program for a truly manic-depressive adolescent,[24,141] but because of possible toxic effects it is inappropriate for hyperactive or aggressive children. Electroconvulsive therapy has helped occasionally in very seriously depressed adolescents, but it should be undertaken only after consultation with 2 qualified child psychiatrists.

Bibliography

1. American Academy of Pediatrics, Committee on Nutrition: Megavitamin therapy for childhood psychoses and learning disabilities. Pediatrics, 58:910, 1976.
2. Annell, A.L.: Lithium in the treatment of children and adolescents. Acta Psychiatr. Scand. (Suppl)., 207:19, 1969.
3. Anthony, E.J.: Developmental antecedents of schizophrenia. In: *Transmission of Schizophrenia.* (S. Katz and D. Rosenthal, Eds.). London, Pergamon Press, 1968.
4. Anthony, J., and Scott, P.: On manic-depressive psychosis in childhood. J. Child. Psychol. Psychiatry, 1:53, 1960.
5. Bakwin, H., and Bakwin, R.M.: Schizophrenia in childhood. Pediatr. Clin. North Am., August, 1958.
6. Ban, T.R.: *Recent Advances in the Biology of Schizophrenia.* Springfield, Ill., Thomas, 1973.
7. Bateson, G., et al.: Toward a theory of schizophrenia. Behav. Sci., 1:251, 1956.
8. Bateman, J.F., et al.: The manic state as an emergency defense reaction. J. Nerv. Ment. Dis., 119:349, 1954.
9. Behrens, M.L., and Goldfarb, W.: A study of patterns of interaction of families of schizophrenic children in residential treatment. Am. J. Orthopsychiatry, 28:300, 1958.
10. Bender, L.: Schizophrenia in childhood: Its recognition, description, and treatment. Am. J. Orthopsychiatry, 26:499, 1956.
11. Bender, L.: Childhood schizophrenia: A review. Int. J. Psychiatry, 5:211, 1968.
12. Bender, L., Goldschmidt, L., and Sankar, D.: Treatment of autistic schizophrenic children with LSD-25 and UML-491. In: *Recent Advances in Biological Psychiatry* (J. Wortis, Ed.). New York, Plenum Press, 1963.
13. Bergman, P., and Escalona, S.: Unusual sensitivities in very young children. Psychoanal. Study Child, 314:33, 1948.
14. Bettelheim, B.: *The Empty Fortress: Infantile Au-*

tism and the Birth of the Self. New York, Macmillan, 1967.

15. Bettelheim, B.: *A Home for the Heart.* New York, Knopf, 1974.
16. Block, J., et al.: A study of the parents of schizophrenic and neurotic children. Psychiatry, *21*:387, 1958.
17. Brown, J.: Follow-up of children with atypical development (infantile psychosis). Am. J. Orthopsychiatry, *33*:855, 1963.
18. Brown, J.L.: Adolescent development of children with infantile psychosis. Semin. Psychiatry, *1*:79, 1969.
19. Brunstetter, R.W.: Milieu treatment for psychotic children. In: *Clinical Studies in Childhood Psychoses* (S. Zurek and I. Berlin, Eds.). New York, Brunner/Mazel, 1973.
20. Call, J.D.: Interlocking affective freeze between an autistic child and his "as-if" mother. J. Am. Acad. Child. Psychiatry, *2*:319, 1963.
21. Call, J.S.: Prevention of autism in a young infant in a well-child conference. J. Am. Acad. Child Psychiatry, *2*:451, 1963.
22. Call, J.D.: A quiet crisis. In: *Emergencies in Child Psychiatry* (G.C. Morrison, Ed.). Springfield, Ill., Thomas, 1975.
23. Cameron, K.: Inpatient therapy of psychotic adolescents. Br. J. Med. Psychol., *23*:107, 1950.
24. Campbell, J.D.: Manic-depressive psychoses in children. JAMA, *158*:154, 1959.
25. Campbell, M.: Biological intervention in psychoses of childhood. J. Autism Child. Schizophr., *3*:347, 1973.
26. Campbell, M.: Pharmacotherapy in early infantile autism. Biol. Psychiatry, *10*:399, 1975.
27. Carlson, H.B.: Characteristics of an acute confusional state in college students. Amer. J. Psychiatry, *114*:900, 1958.
28. Carlson, G.A., and Strober, M.: Manic-depressive illness in early adolescence: A study of clinical and diagnostic characteristics in six cases. J. Am. Acad. Child Psychiatry, *17*:138, 1978.
29. Carpenter, W.T., Jr., McGlasham, T.H., and Strauss, J.S.: The treatment of acute schizophrenia without drugs: An investigation of some current assumptions. Am. J. Psychiatry, *134*:14, 1977.
30. Chmiel, A.J., and Mattsson, A.: Heller's syndrome: A form of childhood psychosis of multicausal origin. J. Am. Acad. Child Psychiatry, *14*:337, 1975.
31. Christ, A.E.: Cognitive assessment of the psychotic child: A Piagetian framework. J. Am. Acad. Child Psychiatry, *16*:227, 1977.
32. Cohen, D.J., et al.: Agreement in diagnosis: Clinical assessment and behavior rating scales for pervasively disturbed children. J. Am. Acad. Child Psychiatry, *17*:589, 1978.
33. Cohen, D.J., Carparulo, B., and Shaywitz, B.: Primary childhood aphasia and childhood autism. J. Am. Acad. Child Psychiatry, *15*:604, 1976.
34. Cohen, D.C., et al.: Biogenic amines in autistic and atypical children: Cerebrospinal fluid measures of homovanillic acid and 5-hydroxyin-

doleacetic acid. Arch. Gen. Psychiatry, *31*:845, 1974.
35. Cohen, D.J., and Young, J.G.: Neurochemistry and child psychiatry. J. Am. Acad. Child Psychiatry, *16*:353, 1977.
36. Cooper, B., and Ekstein, R.: Casework with psychotic children and their parents: Fusion, separation, individuation. Reiss-Davis Clin. Bull., *6*:122, 1969.
37. Creak, M., and Ini, S.: Families of psychotic children. J. Child Psychol. Psychiatry, *1*:156, 1960.
38. Davids, A.: Intelligence in childhood schizophrenics, other emotionally disturbed children and their mothers. J. Consult. Psychol., *22*:159, 1958.
39. Davids, A., Ryan, R., and Salvatore, P.D.: Effectiveness of residential treatment for psychotic and other disturbed children. Am. J. Orthopsychiatry, *38*:469, 1968.
40. Des Lauriers, A.M.: The schizophrenic child. Arch. Gen. Psychiatry, *16*:194, 1967.
41. Despert, J.L.: Delusional and hallucinatory experiences in children. Am. J. Psychiatry, *104*:528, 1948.
42. Despert, J.L.: Some considerations relating to the genesis of autistic behavior in children. Am. J. Orthopsychiatry, *21*:335, 1951.
43. Despert, J.L.: Differential diagnosis between obsessive-compulsive neurosis and schizophrenia in children. In: *Psychopathology of Childhood* (P. Hoch and J. Zubin Eds.). New York, Grune & Stratton, 1953.
44. Dorzab, J., et al.: Depressive disease: Familial psychiatric illness. Am. J. Psychiatry, *127*:1128, 1971.
45. Dyson, W.L., and Barcai, A.: Treatment of children of lithium-responding parents. Curr. Ther. Res., *12*:286, 1970.
46. Easson, W.M.: The psychotic adolescent. In: *The Severely Disturbed Adolescent.* New York, International Universities Press, 1969.
47. Eaton, L., and Menolascino, F.J.: Psychotic reactions of childhood: A follow-up study. Am. J. Orthopsychiatry, *37*:521, 1967.
48. Eisenberg, L.: The autistic child in adolescence. Am. J. Psychiatry, *112*:607, 1956.
49. Eisenberg, L.: The course of childhood schizophrenia. Arch. Neurol. Psychiatry, *78*:69, 1957.
50. Eisenberg, L.: The fathers of autistic children. Am. J. Orthopsychiatry, *27*:715, 1957.
51. Eisenberg, L., and Kanner, L.: Early infantile autism, 1943–55. Am. J. Orthopsychiatry, *26*:556, 1956.
52. Ekstein, R.: *Children of Time and Space, of Action and Impulse.* New York, Appleton-Century-Croft, 1966.
53. Ekstein, R., Friedman, S., and Caruth, E.: The psychoanalytic treatment of childhood schizophrenia. In: *Manual of Child Psychopathology* (B. Wolman, Ed.). New York, McGraw-Hill, 1972.
54. Engstrom, F.W., Robbins, D.R., and May, J.G.: Manic-depressive illness in adolescence: A case report. J. Am. Acad. Child Psychiatry, *17*:514, 1978.
55. Escalona, S.: Some considerations regarding

psychotherapy with psychotic children. In: *Child Psychotherapy* (M.R. Hayworth, Ed.). New York, Basic Books, 1964.

56. Feinstein, S.C., and Despert, E.A.: Juvenile manic-depressive illness: Clinical and therapeutic considerations. J. Am. Acad. Child Psychiatry, *12*:123, 1973.

57. Fenichel, C., Freedman, A.M., and Klapper, Z.: A day school for schizophrenic children. Am. J. Orthopsychiatry, *30*:130, 1960.

58. Fessil, W.J.: Interaction of multiple determinants of schizophrenia. Arch. Gen. Psychiatry, *11*:1, 1964.

59. Fink, M.: Prolonged adverse reactions to LSD in psychotic subjects. Arch. Gen. Psychiatry, *15*:450, 1966.

60. Ford, E.S.C., Robles, C., and Harlow, R.G.: Psychotherapy with child psychotics. Report of two cases. Am. J. Psychother., *14*:705, 1960.

61. Freeman, B.J., et al.: The behavior observation scale for autism: Initial methodology, data analysis, and preliminary findings on 89 children. J. Am. Acad. Child Psychiatry, *17*:576, 1978.

62. Garmezy, N., Stockner, C., and Clarke, A.R.: Child-rearing attitudes of mothers and fathers as reported by schizophrenic and normal control patients. Am. Psychol., *14*:333, 1959.

63. Geleerd, E.R.: The psychoanalysis of a psychotic child. Psychoanal. Study Child, *3/4*:311, 1949.

64. Gittelman, M., and Birch, H.G.: Childhood schizophrenia: Intellect, neurological status, perinatal risk, prognosis, and family prognosis. Arch. Gen. Psychiatry, *17*:16, 1967.

65. Goldfarb, W.: *Childhood Schizophrenia.* Cambridge, Mass., Harvard University Press, 1961.

66. Goldfarb, W.: The mutual impact of mother and child in childhood schizophrenia. Am. J. Orthopsychiatry, *31*:738, 1961.

67. Goldfarb, W.: A follow-up investigation of schizophrenic children treated in residence. J. Jewish Board Guard, *1*:5, 1970.

68. Goldfarb, W., Goldfarb, N., and Potlack, R.C.: Treatment of childhood schizophrenia: A three year comparison of day and residential treatment of schizophrenic children. Arch. Gen. Psychiatry, *14*:119, 1966.

69. Goldfarb, W., et al.: *Psychotic Children Grown Up: A Prospective Follow-up Study in Adolescence and Adulthood.* New York, Human Sciences Press, 1978.

70. Green, A.H.: Self-mutilation in schizophrenic children. Arch. Gen. Psychiatry, *17*:234, 1967.

71. Group for the Advancement of Psychiatry: *Theoretical Consideration and a Proposed Classification of Psychopathological Disorders of Childhood.* New York, Group for the Advancement of Psychiatry, 1966.

72. Halpern, W., and Gold, J.: The schooling of autistic children: Preliminary findings. Am. J. Orthopsychiatry, *40*:665, 1970.

73. Harms, E.: Differential pattern of manic-depressive disease in childhood. Nerv. Child, *9*:326, 1952.

74. Havelkova, M.: Abnormalities in siblings of schizophrenic children. Can. Psychiatr. Assoc. J., *12*:363, 1967.

75. Havelkova, M.: Follow-up study of 71 children diagnosed psychotic in preschool age. Am. J. Orthopsychiatry, *38*:846, 1968.

76. Helgason, T.: Epidemiology of mental disorders in Iceland. Acta Psychiatr. Neurol. Scand. (Suppl.), *40*:173, 1964.

77. Hilgard, J.R., and Newman, M.F.: Evidence for functional genesis in mental illness. J. Nerv. Ment. Dis., *132*:3, 1961.

78. Hill, A.L.: An investigation of calendar calibration by an idiot savant. Am. J. Psychiatry, *132*:557, 1975.

79. Hingtgen, J.N., and Bryson, C.Q.: Recent developments in the study of early childhood psychoses: Infantile autism, childhood schizophrenia, and related disorders. In: *Annual Progresss in Child Psychiatry and Child Development.* New York, Brunner/Mazel, 1973.

80. Holmes, D.J.: *The Adolescent in Psychotherapy.* Boston, Little, Brown, 1964.

81. Hutt, C., et al.: Arousal and childhood autism. Nature, *204*:908, 1964.

82. Jacobs, E.G., and Meanikoff, A.M.: Alternating psychoses in twins: Report of cases. Am. J. Psychiatry, *117*:791, 1961.

83. Jordan, K., and Prugh, D.G.: Schizophreniform psychosis of childhood. Am. J. Psychiatry, *128*:323, 1971.

84. Judd, L.L., and Mandell, A.J.: Chromosome studies in early infantile autism. Arch. Gen. Psychiatry, *18*:450, 1968.

85. Kanner, L.: Autistic disturbance of affective contact. Nerv. Child., *2*:217, 1943.

86. Kanner, L.: Early infantile autism. J. Pediatr., *25*:211, 1944.

87. Kanner, L., and Lesser, L.J.: Early infantile autism. Pediatr. Clin. North Am., Aug., 711, 1958.

88. Kantor, R.E., and Herron, W.G.: *Reactive and Process Schizophrenia.* Palo Alto, Calif., Science and Behavior Books, 1966.

89. Katz, P.: Therapy of Adolescent Schizophrenia. Am. J. Psychiatry, *127*:132, 1978.

90. Kaufman, J., et al.: Adaptation of treatment techniques to a new classification of schizophrenic children. J. Am. Acad. Child. Psychiatry, *2*:460, 1963.

91. Kaufman, I., et al.: Treatment implications of a new classification of parents of schizophrenic children. Am. J. Psychiatry, *116*:920, 1960.

92. Kaufman, I., et al.: Four types of defense in mothers and fathers of schizophrenic children. Am. J. Orthopsychiatry, *29*:460, 1959.

93. Kaufman, I., et al.: Childhood schizophrenia: Treatment of children and parents. Am. J. Orthopsychiatry, *27*:683, 1957.

94. Kemph, J.P.: Brief hospitalization in the treatment of the psychotic child. Psychiatr. Digest, *27*:35, 1966.

95. Kemph, J.: Follow-up of psychotic children treated in residential treatment centers. In: *Annual Progress in Child Psychiatry and Child Development.* (S. Chess and A. Thomas, Eds.). New York, Brunner/Mazel, 1973.

96. Kety, S.S.: Current biochemical approaches to schizophrenia. N. Engl. J. Med., *276*:1271, 1967.

97. Kety, S.S., et al.: Mental illness in the biological and adoptive families of adopted schizophrenics. Am. J. Psychiatry, *128*:302, 1971.

98. Kurland, L., and Teicher, J.D.: Treatment of adolescent catatonia. Calif. Med., *99*:312, 1963.

99. Lamb, H.R.: The state hospital: Facility of last resort. Am. J. Psychiatry, *134*:1151, 1977.

100. Levin, M.: Auditory hallucinations in "non-psychotic" children. Am. J. Psychiatry, *88*:1119, 1932.

101. Levy, D.M.: Body interest in children and hypochrondriasis. Am. J. Psychiatry, *12*:295, 1932.

102. Lidz, T.: The intrafamilial environment of the psychiatric patient. VII. Transmission of irrationality. Arch. Neurol. Psychiatry, *58*:521, 1958.

103. Linnihan, P.C.: Adolescent day treatment: Community alternative to institutionalizatin of the emotionally disturbed adolescent. Am. J. Orthopsychiatry, *47*:679, 1977.

104. Loeb, L.: Adolescent schizophrenia. In: *The Schizophrenic Syndrome* (L. Bellak and L. Loeb, Eds.). New York, Grune & Stratton, 1969.

105. Lourie, R.S., Pacella, B.L., and Piotrowski, Z.A.: Studies on the prognosis in schizophrenia-like psychoses in children. Am. J. Psychiatry, *99*:542, 1943.

106. Lovaas, O.I.: A behavior therapy approach to the treatment of childhood schizophrenia. In: *Minnesota Symposium on Child Psychiatry.* (J. Hill, Ed.). Minneapolis, University of Minnesota Press, 1967.

107. Lovaas, O.I., Schaffer, B., and Simmons, J.Q.: Building social behavior in autistic children by use of electric shock. J. Exp. Res. Personal., *1*:99, 1965.

108. Mahler, M.S.: Personal communication.

109. Mahler, M.S.: On child psychosis and schizophrenia: Autistic and symbiotic infantile psychosis. Psychoanal. Study Child, *7*:286, 1952.

110. Mahler, M.S.: On early infantile psychosis. The symbiotic and autistic syndromes. J. Am. Acad. Child Psychiatry, *4*:554, 1965.

111. Mahler, M.S., and Furer, M.: Certain aspects of the separation-individuation phase. Psychoanal. Q., *32*:1, 1963.

112. Malamud, N.: Heller's disease and childhood schizophrenia. Am. J. Psychiatry, *116*:215, 1959.

113. Marcus, L.M.: Patterns of coping in families of psychotic children. Am. J. Orthopsychiatry, *47*:388, 1977.

114. Masterson, J.F.: Prognosis in adolescent disorders: Schizophrenia. J. Nerv. Ment. Dis., *124*:219, 1956.

115. Masterson, J.F.: *The Psychiatric Dilemma of Adolescents.* Boston, Little, Brown, 1967.

116. Mayer, M.F., and Blum, A. Eds.: *Healing Through Living.* Springfield, Ill., Thomas, 1971.

117. McKnew, D.H., and Cytryn, L.: Historical background in children with affective disorders. Am. J. Psychiatry, *130*:1278, 1973.

118. McKnew, D.H.,Jr., Cytryn, L., and White, I.: Clinical and biochemical correlates of hypomania in a child. J. Am. Acad. Child Psychiatry, *13*:576, 1974.

119. Mednick, S., and Schulsinger, F.: Factors related to breakdown in children at high risk for schizophrenia. In: *Life History Research in Psychopathology* (M. Rolf, and D. Ricks, Eds.), Minneapolis, University of Minnesota Press, 1970.

120. Meeks, J.E.: *The Fragile Alliance.* Baltimore, Williams & Wilkins, 1971.

121. *Megavitamin and Orthomolecular Therapy in Psychiatry.* Task Force Report No. 7. Washington, D.C., American Psychiatric Association, 1973.

122. Menolascino, F.J.: Autistic reactions in early childhood: Differential diagnostic considerations. J. Child. Psychol. Psychiatry, *6*:203, 1965.

123. Metz, J.R.: Conditioning generalized imitation in autistic children. J. Exp. Child Psychol., *4*:389, 1965.

124. Moe, M., Waal, N., and Urdahl, B.: Group psychotherapy with parents of psychotic and neurotic children. Acta Psychother. Psychosom., *8*:134, 1956.

125. Neubauer, P., and Steinert, J.: Schizophrenia in adolescence. Nerv. Child, *10*:129, 1954.

126. O'Neal, P., and Robins, L.N.: Childhood patterns predictive of adult schizophrenia: A thirty year follow-up study. Am. J. Psychiatry, *115*:385, 1959.

127. Ornitz, E., and Ritvo, E.: Perceptual inconstancy in early infantile autism. Arch. Gen. Psychiatry, *18*:76, 1968.

128. Ornitz, E.M., and Ritvo, E.R.: The syndrome of autism: A critical review. Am. J. Psychiatry, *133*:609, 1976.

129. Pavenstedt, E., and Anderson, I.: Complementary treatment of mother and child with atypical development. Am. J. Orthopsychiatry, *22*:607, 1952.

130. Peck, H.B., Rabinovitch, R.D., and Cramer, J.B.: A treatment program for parents of schizophrenic children. Am. J. Orthopsychiatry, *19*:592, 1949.

131. Pollack, M.: Brain damage, mental retardation, and childhood schizophrenia. Am. J. Psychiatry, *115*:422, 1958.

132. Pollack, M., Levenstein, S., and Klein, D.F.: A three year post-hospital follow-up of adolescent and adult schizophrenia. Am. J. Orthopsychiatry, *38*:94, 1968.

133. Potter,, H.W.: Schizophrenia in Children. Am. J. Psychiatry, *12*:1253, 1933.

134. Rank, B.: Adaptation of the psychoanalytic technique for the treatment of young children with atypical development. Am. J. Orthopsychiatry, *19*:130, 1949.

135. Rank, B.: Intensive study and treatment of preschool children who show marked personality deviations or "atypical development" and their parents. In: *Emotional Problems of Early Childhood* (G. Caplan, Ed.). New York, Basic Books, 1955.

136. Reiser, D.E.: Psychosis of infancy and early childhood, as manifested by children with atypical development. I. N. Engl. J. Med., *269*:790, 1963.

137. Reiser, D.E.: Psychosis of infancy and early childhood as manifested by children with atyp-

ical development. II. N. Engl. J. Med., *269*:844, 1963.

138. Reiser, D., and Brown, J.: Patterns of later development in children with infantile psychosis. J. Am. Acad. Child Psychiatry, *3*:650, 1964.

139. Ridges, A.P.: Biochemistry of depression: A review. J. Int. Med. Res., *3*:42, 1975.

140. Rimland, B.: High-dosage levels of certain vitamins in the treatment of children with severe mental disorders. In: *Orthomolecular Psychiatry* (D. Hawkins and L. Pauling, Eds.). San Francisco, Freeman, 1973.

141. Robbins, D.R., Engstrom, F.K., and May, J.G.: The treatment of an adolescent: A multiple systems approach, with a review of the literature. Unpublished material.

142. Robbins, D.R., et al.: Psychological characteristics of children of manic-depressive mothers. (Paper presented at the Annual Meeting of the American Academy of Child Psychiatry.) Houston, Texas, October, 1977.

143. Rose, J.A.: The prevention of mothering breakdown associated with physical abnormalities of the infant. In: *Prevention of Mental Disorders in Children* (G. Caplan, Ed.). New York, Basic Books, 1961.

144. Rutter, M.: The influence of organic and emotional factors on the origins, nature, and outcome of childhood psychosis. Dev. Med. Child Neurol., *7*:518, 1965.

145. Rutter, M.: Infantile autism and other childhood psychoses. In: *Child Psychiatry: Modern Approaches* (M. Rutter and L. Hersov, Eds.). London, Blackwell Scientific Publications, 1976.

146. Rutter, M., Greenfield, D., and Lockyer, L.: A 5–15 year follow-up study of infantile psychosis. II. Social and behavioral outcome. Br. J. Psychiatry, *113*:504, 1967.

147. Rutter, M., Greenfield, D., and Lockyer, L.: A 5 to 15 year follow-up study of infantile psychosis. In: *Annual Progress in Child Psychiatry and Child Development* (S. Chess and A. Thomas, Eds.). New York, Yearbook, 1968.

148. Sander, L., Julia, J.L., Steckler, G., and Burns, P.: Continuous 24-hour interactional monitoring in infants reared in two caretaking environments. Psychosom. Med., *34*:114, 1972.

149. Sands, B.E.: The psychoses of adolescence. J. Ment. Sci., *102*:308, 1956.

150. Savage, V.A.: Childhood autism: A review of the literature with particular reference to the speech and language of the autistic child. Br. J. Disord. Commun., April, 1968.

151. Schachter, F.F., Meyer, L.R., and Loomis, E.A., Jr.: Childhood schizophrenia and mental retardation: Differential diagnosis after one year of psychotherapy. Am. J. Orthopsychiatry, *32*:584, 1962.

152. Schopler, E., and Reichler, R.J.: A program for psychotic children: The child research project, Chapel Hill, North Carolina. Hosp. Comm. Psychiatry, *23*:307, 1972.

153. Shapiro, M.J., and Shugart, G.: Ego therapy with parents of the psychotic child. Am. J. Orthopsychiatry, *28*:786, 1958.

154. Simmons, J.Q.: Modification of autistic behavior with LSD-25. Am. J. Psychiatry, *123*:1201, 1966.

155. Speers, R.W., and Lansing, C.: *Group Therapy in Childhood Psychosis*. Chapel Hill, University of North Carolina Press, 1965.

156. Stabenau, J.R.: Heredity and environment in schizophrenia: The contribution of twin studies. Arch. Gen. Psychiatry, *18*:458, 1968.

157. Stabenau, J.R., and Pollin, W.: Early characteristics of monozygotic twins discordant for schizophrenia. Arch. Gen. Psychiatry, *17*:723, 1967.

158. Staub, E., Mizner, J., Roberts, M., and Prugh, D.G.: Unpublished material.

159. Stewart, R.H., and Sardo, R.: The psychotherapy of a blind schizophrenic child. J. Am. Acad. Child Psychiatry, *4*:123, 1965.

160. Symonds, A., and Herman, M.: The patterns of schizophrenia in adolescence. Psychiatr. Q., *31*:521, 1957.

161. Szurek, S., and Berlin, I.: Elements of psychotherapeutics with the schizophrenic child and his parents. Psychiatry, *19*:1, 1956.

162. Szurek, S.A., and Berlin, I., Eds.: *Clinical Studies in Childhood Psychoses: 25 Years in Collaborative Treatment*. New York, Brunner/Mazel, 1973.

163. Vasey, I., et al.: Unpublished material.

164. Veiga, M.: The missing child: Family reactions to hospitalization of children with mental disorders. J. Am. Acad. Child Psychiatry, *2*:413, 1963.

165. Walker, H.A., and Birch, H.G.: Neurointegrative deficiencies in schizophrenic children. J. Nerv. Ment. Dis., *151*:104, 1970.

166. Warren, W., and Cameron, K.: Reactive psychosis in adolescents. J. Ment. Sci., *96*:448, 1950.

167. Weakland, J.H.: The "double-bind" theory of schizophrenia and three-party interaction. In: *The Etiology of Schizophrenia*. (D. Jackson, Ed.). New York, Basic Books, 1960.

168. Weinberg, W., and Brumback, R.: Mania in children. Case studies and literature review. Am. J. Dis. Child, *130*:380, 1976.

169. Weinberg, W., et al.: Depression in children referred to an educational diagnostic center. J. Pediatr., *83*:1065, 1973.

170. Weiner, J.B.: *Psychological Disturbance in Adolescence*. New York, Wiley-Interscience, 1970.

171. Weiner, J.B.: Schizophrenia. In: *Psychological Disturbances in Adolescents*. New York, Wiley-Interscience, 1970.

172. Weiner, J.B.: Childhood psychosis. In: *Principles of Pediatrics: Health Care of the Young* (R.A. Hoekelman, et al., Eds.). Baltimore, Williams & Wilkins, 1978.

173. Williams, J.: Unpublished material.

174. Winokur, G.: Genetic and methodological considerations in manic depressive disease. Br. J. Psychiatry, *117*:267, 1970.

175. Winokur, G., Clayton, P.J., and Reich, T.: *Manic-Depressive Illness*. St. Louis, Mosby, 1969.

176. Wynne, L., et al.: Pseudo-mutuality in the family relations of schizophrenics. Psychiatry, *21*:205, 1958.

177. Wynne, L., and Singer, M.: Communication styles in parents of normals, neurotics, and

schizophrenics. In: *Family Structure, Dynamics and Therapy* (I.M. Cohen, Ed.). Psychiatric Research Report No. 20. Washington, D.C., American Psychiatric Association, 1966.

178. Young, J.G., et al.: Childhood autism: Cerebrospinal fluid examination and immunoglobulin levels. J. Am. Acad. Child Psychiatry, 16:174, 1977.

179. Young, J.G., et al.: Decreased urinary free cate-cholamines in childhood autism. J. Am. Acad. Child Psychiatry, 17:589, 1979.

180. Zimet, C.N., and Fishman, D.B.: Psychological deficit in schizophrenia and brain damage. Ann. Rev. Psychol., 21:113, 1976.

181. Zurek, S.A., and Berlin, I.N.: *Clinical Studies in Childhood Psychoses.* New York, Brunner/Mazel, 1973.

21
Psychophysiologic Disorders

*A physician is obligated to consider more than a
diseased organ, more even than the whole
man. . . he must view the man in his world.*
(Harvey Cushing)

*Anger is my meat; I shall sup upon myself and
so shall starve with feeding.*
(William Shakespeare)

The diagnostic features of psychophysiologic disorders are:

1. The disorders involve organs or organ systems which are innervated by the autonomic nervous system, in contrast to conversion disorders, which involve the striated musculature and somatosensory apparatus, and which have voluntary innervation.

2. In the disorders biological predisposing factors seem to be involved with probably latent biochemical defects. Psychologic and social factors are predisposing, contributing, precipitating, and perpetuating factors.

3. The disorders do not alleviate anxiety, in contrast to conversion disorders, in which anxiety is repressed and seems to be "bound" to the symbolic symptom.

4. The disorders may be mild or severe, transient, or chronic. Probably a continuum exists, with the disorders ranging from those that involve a milder biologic predisposition and a greater psychologic influence for their appearance and perpetuation to those that involve a heavier biologic predisposition and a lesser psychologic influence.

General Considerations

In the Standard Nomenclature, the term psychophysiologic disorders is used in preference to the term psychosomatic disorders, because the latter term refers to an approach to the field of medicine as a whole rather than to a certain specified condition. The term psychophysiologic disorder is also preferred to the term somatization reactions, which implies that the disorders referred to are simply other forms of psychoneurotic disorders that involve bodily organs. (In DMS III, published since this book went to press, the term psychophysiologic disorder has been changed to "psychological factors affecting physical condition.")

The term psychophysiologic disorders (or vegetative disorders) refers to disorders in which there is a significant interaction between physiologic and psychologic components in the clinical picture, with varying degrees of weighting of each component. Psychophysiologic disorders may be precipitated and perpetuated by psychologic or social stressful stimuli. Such disorders ordinarily involve the organ systems that are innervated by the autonomic (involuntary) part of the central nervous system. The symptoms of disturbed functioning at the vegetative level are regarded as pathophysiologic rather than as having psychologic symbolic significance, as in conversion disorders, which involve structures innervated by the voluntary portion of the central nervous system. Some overlapping occurs, as discussed in Chapter 4. In psychophysiologic disorders structural changes occur and may continue to a point that may be irreversible and even life threatening. The psychophysiologic disorders seem not to be simple physiologic concomitants of emotions, as may be true in psychoneurotic disorders of the anxiety type, reactive disorders, or other pictures, including healthy responses. Biologic predisposing factors of a genetic or inborn nature, developmental psychosocial determinants that have a limited specificity, and current precipitating events of individually stressful significance seem to be among the multiple etiologic factors in these disor-

ders. The psychophysiologic interrelationships involved in these disorders are discussed in general in Chapter 3. A more specific discussion of these relationships follows. What is discussed may not apply to all such disorders. (Recent studies have demonstrated that there are subtypes of essential hypertension and peptic ulcer, among others.[259])

Although conflict situations of particular types may be consistently involved in the predisposition toward and precipitation of psychophysiologic disorders, no type-specific personality, parent-child relationship, or family pattern has as yet been associated with the individual psychophysiologic disorders. Many similar psychologic or psychosocial characteristics may be found in children who have other disorders but not psychophysiologic disturbances. Psychophysiologic disorders may also involve more than 1 organ system in sequence, and occasionally more than 1 disorder occurs simultaneously. Psychologic factors may play a minor role in some disorders that involve a heavier biologic predisposition, while in other disorders such factors may play a major role, with somatic factors less prominent, supporting the idea of a continuum. Certain psychophysiologic disorders are associated with chronic and/or severe personality disorders of varying types, some that even border on psychosis, while others may occur in conjunction with milder personality disorders or reactive disorders. Most cases reported have been studied in hospital settings, where patients tend to have more serious physical and psychologic disorders. Milder cases in patients who show less severe disturbances in personality functioning are often encountered in ambulatory pediatric practice. Developmental considerations are involved, as in the more global, undifferentiated responses of young infants, the rise in incidence of a number of disorders in children in the school-age period, and the stormier course of some disorders (e.g., diabetes) during adolescence. In some psychophysiologic disorders, racial and ethnic differences (e.g., in hypertension[102]) as well as sex differences (e.g., in peptic ulcer[164]), along with other factors, have been described.

A secondary diagnosis of the type of personality picture seen with the psychophysiologic disorder should be specified. If conversion mechanisms in structures that are fully or partly voluntarily innervated are admixed with psychophysiological mechanisms (e.g., in the vomiting that may occur in adolescents who have anorexia nervosa), that fact can be added as a separate diagnosis, and the particular symptoms can be specified. Responses to predominantly acute or chronic somatic illnesses should be considered a secondary diagnosis. Reactive disorders are frequently though not exclusively seen in reactions to acute illness; and a variety of personality disorders, from overly dependent to overly independent disorders, or other disorders are associated with chronic illness (see Chap. 25).

Clinical Findings

In the following discussion of disorders of particular organ systems that may be involved in psychophysiologic disorders, some disorders that occur only in children are mentioned, as well as disorders that may occur in both children and adults. (A fuller discussion of the psychophysiologic interconnecting mechanisms and relevant theoretical considerations is found in Chapter 3.)

Psychophysiologic Skin Disorders

The category psychophysiologic skin disorders includes certain cases of psoriasis, neurodermatitis, seborrheic dermatitis, urticaria, angioneurotic edema, alopecia areata and alopecia totalis, acne, and certain cases of atopic eczema.

Atopic eczema may occur in an infantile form as well as in a later, more chronic form.[14] It usually occurs in children in families who have an allergic diathesis.[73,118] Children affected by chronic atopic eczema are generally rigid and tense, and sometimes they are compulsive. They have a tendency to repress strong emotions, particularly resentment toward overcontrolling parents who may have offered their children inadequate contact comforts in infancy.[168]

Exacerbations of the disorder are often related to conflicts in the parent-child relationship.[16] During adolescence exacerbations are usually related to increased conflicts about independence and sexuality. Many people who have atopic eczema become overly inhibited, have strongly narcissistic concerns about their bodies, have unconscious exhibitionistic trends (that are covered up by the skin lesions) and find unconscious pleasure, (akin to sexual pleasure) and satisfy their self-punishing needs by persistent and harmful scratching.[270] In *psoriasis*, although a different biologic predisposing factor must be involved, somewhat similar relationships between stressful life events and the severity of the psoriasis have been demonstrated.[89,270] *Neurodermatitis* that does not have an allergic component often begins with pruritus that is related to emotional conflicts.[156] Scratching intensifies the lesions. These disorders can be helped by intensive psychotherapy in conjunction with dermatologic measures. Reinforcement procedures have also been tried with benefit in severe scratching.[3]

Recurrent *urticaria* appears to be closely related to dermatographia. The skin's reactivity is often constitutionally derived, and it is frequently associated with positive scratch tests.[103] The clinical manifestations may be brought out by emotionally traumatic experiences[88a] or intensified by conflicts about sexuality and independence.[270] Children who have recurrent urticaria are often shy and easily embarrassed and they blush readily. They are also often passive, immature, withdrawn, or inhibited children who have feelings of inadequacy and unconscious exhibitionistic trends and who are overdependent on their mothers. In younger children, urticaria may be brought on by overexertion or overexcitement. *Angioneurotic edema*[173] may be seen in anxious infants or young children. A supportive psychotherapeutic approach based on helping the parents and child with their underlying conflicts is often effective in treating these conditions. Tranquilizers have been used, but the intensity and danger of their side-effects makes them of dubious value.

Alopecia areata[159] can occur in relation to emotionally traumatic events, (e.g., actual or symbolic losses), as may *alopecia totalis*.[123] Psychotherapy may be helpful in alopecia areata, but it is not often helpful in alopecia totalis, and cosmetic measures are important.

Severe *acne* may be deeply troubling to adolescents, and it may continue into early adult life. People who have marked and chronic acne are often shy and inhibited, and they have conflicts about their sexuality and about growing up.[185] Stressful life events can exacerbate the acne. The increased production of skin-surface free fatty acids, with secondary infection, may play a role.[129] These factors are often combined with an adolescent's resistance to skin care, which is related to oppositional behavior or a negative identity. Psychotherapy and dermatologic measures are most helpful.

Besides its basic functions (e.g., protection and secretion), the skin is an organ of emotional expression, as indicated by blushing, pallor, and other phenomena. As an organ of emotional expression, the skin receives central representation as a part of the body image. Thus certain conversion phenomena may somehow take place in the skin[221] (as in the somatosensory apparatus), even though no voluntary innervation is involved. Hypnotic suggestion has long been known to produce blisters (from a "suggested burn") and other changes in the skin. Some cases of dermatitis thus seem to involve conversion mechanisms,[9] at times with psychophysiologic components. This observation may also help to explain the effects of suggestion[252] on certain types of *warts* (e.g., verruca vulgaris), in the etiology of which a virus is known to be involved. Psychosocial factors may also be involved in certain cases of recurrent herpes simplex.[18]

Psychophysiologic Musculoskeletal Disorders

This category includes certain cases of rheumatoid arthritis, tension headaches, and myalgias such as backache.[112]

Juvenile Rheumatoid Arthritis. Children who have juvenile rheumatoid arthritis often have conflicts about their aggression and dependence and are intensely close to and dependent on their mothers.[23,38] The arthritis itself may be a type of autoimmune response; the psychophysiologic interrelationships are not fully understood.[163] Exacerbations of the disorder may be clinically related to shifts in the family's interpersonal balance.[147] Such a shift often involves situations in which the child fears loss of a key relationship, together with angry feelings that he is afraid to express. Muscle tension related to inner conflicts may help to intensify the inflammation around the joints involved.[163] Psychotherapeutic measures designed to help the child deal with these feelings and to help the parents understand the child's conflicts, as well as their own, may add to the effectiveness of medical treatment.

Tension Headaches. Tension headaches involve a tightening of the scalp and neck muscles that is related to emotional conflicts in tense, often compulsive, people.[76,274] Psychotherapeutic intervention can be most effective.[95] New biofeedback techniques have helped reduce symptoms in adults.[29] (Headaches are discussed more fully in Chapter 18).

Psychophysiologic Respiratory Disorders

This category includes certain cases of bronchial asthma, allergic rhinitis, and chronic sinusitis.[110] Breath holding spells often begin voluntarily. Hyperventilation syndromes and sighing respirations usually involve conversion mechanisms admixed with anxiety.[58] These phenomena are discussed elsewhere in the book.

Bronchial Asthma. Bronchial asthma occurs twice as often in boys as in girls. The basic defect appears to be an altered state of the host which is reflected in the labile bronchial tree ("twitchy lung"). In children who have a hereditary predisposition to asthma, attacks may be triggered by fears of separation or threatened alienation from the parent, open conflict between child and parent, marital battles, and other conflict situations.[144,183] Coughing spells can be consciously and unconsciously motivated, and not infrequently they trigger an asthma attack. Involuntary psychophysiologic mechanisms (which may involve conditioned vagal responses that produce reflex bronchoconstriction and increased bronchial mucus) overlap with symbolic or voluntary components in triggering attacks. Other trigger mechanisms include intrinsic factors (e.g., exercise and drug sensitivity) and extrinsic factors (e.g., allergic, infectious, and irritant substances), which may be combined with and augmented by psychosocial factors.[214]

During an attack, the parent may fear that the child will die from suffocation. The fear frequently results in overanxious and overprotective parental behavior that leads to overdependent child behavior[268] or other behavior patterns reflecting internalized fear or panic. Certain parents may show resentment or ambivalence toward the asthma or to the child, who may then feel rejected. The child may respond to such parental feelings by denying his illness or with oppositional or manipulative behavior. Struggles for control can develop, with the child manipulating the parent by hyperventilating or coughing to trigger an attack of asthma, which may then become involuntary. Problems of childhood omnipotence are severe in some families of children with asthma.[183]

In a study by Block and her colleagues,[22] children who scored low on a scale measuring allergic potential (APS) showed greater psychopathology and more conflicts in their family and parent-child relationships than did those who had a higher allergic potential. Psychologic differences between "rapidly remitting" and "steroid-dependent" groups of children have been demonstrated by Purcell.[195] These studies, though useful, need to be replicated with the use of current pulmonary physiologic measurement techniques. More recent studies have documented the effects of suggestion on pulmonary functions measured by total body plethysmography and wedge spirometry.[214]

The attitudes of the primary physician can significantly affect the outcome of the treatment of asthma. For less seriously disturbed children, he can offer supportive psychotherapy along with appropriate medical measures. Anticipatory guidance is often helpful, particularly in regard to disciplinary methods to be used with children who have asthma. The parents should be encouraged to have time away from their child. The major psychologic issues to be dealt with are the child's separation anxiety, his guilt, and his anger toward his parents and the health professionals. Psychologic support must be offered to the parents, especially the mother, to help them with their feelings of guilt and resentment and with their feelings of inadequacy about helping their child. Intensive psychotherapy for the child and parents may be necessary.[183,238] It is most effective if serious structural change has not occurred. Hypnosis has helped certain patients abort asthma attacks and has helped them to realize that they have some control over the onset and the degree of severity of an attack. Behavior modification programs also seem to be helpful.[169] Group therapy for parents of asthmatic children has been effective in reducing the parents' guilt and anxiety. Self-care clubs have been established to offer children considerable emotional support.[214]

Long-term hospitalization or residential placement should be reserved for children who have severe and protracted asthma or children who would find frequent hospitalizations too disruptive to their development.[214] The change in the child's social environment[126] and the use of related medical and psychologic approaches to treatment can help the child develop new adaptive skills, as well as help him to separate asthma from family conflicts. Parental visiting and work with the family, perhaps through an agency in the parents' home town, can help bring about family change.[165] "Parentectomy" alone not only may make some very dependent children worse but also increases the feelings of guilt in parents who already feel that they may have caused their child's asthma. Recreational group programs in summer camps are another way to promote healthy separation and to foster development. They have been helpful when they are combined with individual support for the child and his family.

The dangers of overmedication and the possibility of psychologic dependence on nebulizers and steroids are all-important considerations in the medical management of asthma.[247] Incipient changes in the child's body image and a lag in his growth that is caused by prolonged steroid therapy must also be considered.[176]

Case Example. Steve was a 15-year-old boy, who was brought to the pediatric outpatient clinic by his mother because he had "severe asthma." Steve's mother indicated that his asthma had been mild and occasional until about 10 months earlier. Since that time, she said, Steve had been so incapacitated by his asthma that he could no longer attend school. His mother said that Steve's father had had asthma as a child. When the pediatric resident asked

where the father was, the mother said that he had died about a year ago. Steve's history was otherwise unrevealing. His physical examination showed that he had only mild wheezing and had no clubbing of his fingers or other signs. A psychiatric consultation was requested.

Steve's mother was interviewed by herself. When she was asked about her husband's death, she broke down and cried, expressing both sorrow and bitterness toward her husband, who had been killed in an auto accident while he was intoxicated. She said that she had had to go to work a month after her husband's death. The boy had complained of asthma at the time of his father's death, but the mother was too depressed and preoccupied to pay any attention to him. She said in the interview that she felt guilty about that. She had not become aware of the boy's missing school frequently until recently, when the school had contacted her.

In an interview with the boy, he too cried openly and said that he had been unable to go to school because of his feelings of helplessness and abandonment by his father. He was afraid that his mother was not interested in him because of her preoccupation with her work. She left for work before the boy had to leave for school, and many times he stayed home, lying on the couch in a depressed state, watching television. The boy said that his asthma had bothered him a little, but that really he had just "given up."

In talking with the pediatric resident, the psychiatric consultant recommended the positive use of pediatric hospitalization, with support for the mother and patient, gradual mobilization of the boy, who seemed to be "at a crossroads," from which he could take the road toward emotional invalidism. He was admitted to the hospital, in spite of his mild asthma, and a special program was planned for him. The pediatric resident saw the boy daily, and a social worker saw his mother. The resident developed a supportive relationship with the boy, who quickly became less depressed, and talked about his wish to become a doctor or an x-ray technician. On the second day, he went to school for an hour. His attendance was stepped up gradually to three hours, with an increasing program of recreational activities, into which he entered with increasing enthusiasm.

The boy was discharged after 10 days. He was to return to school on a half-time basis for a week and then was to return to school full-time. The mother was less depressed, bitter, and guilty, and she planned to change her time of work so that she could see the boy off to school. They made an appointment with the pediatric resident to return in 2 weeks. At that time, the boy was eager to return to school full-time, and he and his mother seemed much closer, having talked together a good deal.

The pediatric resident saw the family at 2 week intervals for about 2 months, and then, at the boy's request, tapered off the relationship, increasing the interval to 1 month, then 2 months. At the end of 6 months, at the last visit the boy was told he could come back if he wanted to discuss any problems. The resident had seen the boy first for 15 minutes each time and then the mother for 5 to 7 minutes afterward. He had advised the mother to gradually give the boy greater privileges. The boy took them eagerly. When his case was presented at a grand rounds a year after admission, the boy had "moved out" socially at school, had a girlfriend, and was doing better academically than he had before his father's death. Both he and the mother seemed to have completed their mourning over the father's death, and the mother had become involved in social activities that she found satisfying.

Allergic Rhinitis. Allergic rhinitis in adolescents and adults has been shown by Holmes and his colleagues[111] (in randomly chosen sensitive subjects) to become exacerbated in settings of increased emotional conflict. Supportive psychotherapeutic measures may make medical measures more effective in reducing nasal hyperemia, hypersecretion, and other symptoms.[40,110,197] (Most allergic syndromes are affected to some degree by psychosocial factors.[103])

Psychophysiologic Cardiovascular Disorders

Psychophysiologic cardiovascular disorders, which may overlap somewhat with respiratory disorders, include certain cardiac arrhythmias (e.g., paroxysmal supraventricular tachycardia), essential hypertension, certain cases of hypotension, vasodepressor syncope, migraine, and certain types of peripheral vascular spasm (e.g., Raynaud's disease).

Some children show intense autonomic responses to emotional conflicts or stressful situations, which may trigger off attacks of *paroxysmal supraventricular tachycardia* that

are followed by attacks of syncope.[63,205] An increase in catecholamines seems to be involved (as may be the case in certain other cardiac arrhythmias[196]). Supportive psychotherapy may help reduce conflicts or stress, and, if appropriate medical treatment is also given, may help to prevent such attacks. Modification of arrhythmias by conditioning has been said to show promise.[91]

Children who have *essential hypertension* have not been extensively studied from a psychophysiologic point of view. It is now recognized, however, that essential hypertension occurs fairly commonly during childhood and adolescence.[157] Adults who have essential hypertension have shown significant conflicts in dealing with their feelings of anger and their conflicts about dependence.[177,272] Differences in heart rate, blood pressure, and the incidence of hypertension have been shown to vary in different ethnic and socioeconomic groups.[74,102,217,218]

Studies have shown that in both normotensive and hypertensive subjects increased catecholamine levels and peripheral resistance, as well as renal artery constriction,[181,224] accompanied rises in blood pressure[149] when those subjects discussed "conflictual" topics. Hypertensive subjects showed a much more intense and prolonged response. The intensification of conflicts in patients who have benign hypertension has been seen to precipitate malignant hypertensive changes.[200] Psychophysiologic vasoconstrictive responses to chronic emotional conflict have been presumed, though not proven, to lead to structural changes in the kidney and vascular bed, although cholesterol and other factors are also certainly involved. In an experimental study by Henry,[106] mice that had had deficient early experiences that were subjected to situations involving social disorder showed an increase in catecholamine-synthesizing enzymes and eventually showed a sustained increase in both blood pressure and arteriosclerotic degeneration of the vascular bed.

The relationship of such responses to the renin-angiotension-aldosterone system is not yet clear.[261] Adrenergic stimulation appears to release renin under certain circumstances, and to be related to the production of angiotensin.[258] In a recent study, an acceleration in cardiac rate that was produced by operant conditioning seemed to be associated with an increase in renin activity,[276] and in anther study[36] plasma renin secretion seemed to be increased in healthy subjects when they felt anxious.

Findings of the type just described suggest that it is possible that emotional stimuli could affect both renal vascular flow and the various systems involved in the maintenance of blood pressure in susceptible people. Hypertension is significantly more common in the parents of hypertensive children.[200] Hyperresponsivity to cold pressor tests is seen in some infants, and young adults who develop hypertension show a premorbid tendency to marked fluctuations in blood pressure. Some biologic predisposition thus is probably involved. Much research remains to be done in this area, and different mechanisms may be involved in different subtypes of hypertension.[261]

Medical treatment should be combined with supportive psychotherapeutic measures. It is possible that such an approach may help prevent mildly hypertensive children from developing serious hypertension, with all its complications. Biofeedback[225] may help reduce blood pressure in hypertensive adults although its effectiveness recently has been called into question.[107a] Training in yoga[45] and transcendental meditation and other relaxation techniques has had some definite results, and those techniques seem to be more promising than is biofeedback.

Children who have chronic or recurrent *orthostatic hypotension* seem to be tense, anxious, and emotionally restricted.[6] Constitutionally labile autonomic responses also seem to be involved. A supportive psychotherapeutic approach combined with parent counseling can be helpful. At times, the child may need to be referred for intensive psychotherapy.

Similar autonomic mechanisms seem to be active in children or adolescents who have *vasodepressor syncope*, which involves sudden relaxation of the visceral nervous system with associated bradycardia and a fall in blood pressure.[56] Vasodepressor syncope may be brought on by a sudden fright while one is standing or sitting, by the pain of a venipuncture, by anticipation of pain, or by a threat[228] from other sources. The child does not lose consciousness completely, but he may be dizzy or weak or he may faint. Children who repeatedly have vasodepressor syncope are usually anxious and somewhat inhibited. They also tend to fear punishment or mutilation. Psychotherapeutic measures and desensitization techniques can be effective. *Carotid sinus syncope*, which results from a hyperactive carotid sinus reflex, is uncommon in children. It is usually associated with anxiety states. (Syncope is discussed more fully in Chapter 18.)

The types of syncope just discussed must be distinguished from conversion syncope,[211] which often occurs in children (usually girls) who have hysterical personalities. In conversion syncope, vascular changes do not occur, and the degree of the child's loss of consciousness varies. Other conversion symptoms often occur. Conversion syncope is of central origin, and it seems symbolically to be an unconscious attempt to block out a conflict-producing situation. None of the types of syncope discussed appear to bear any relationship to epilepsy, and all of them are fairly easily distinguished from the Stokes-Adams syndrome.[95a]

Migraine begins to appear during the school-age period. (Headaches of any type occur infrequently in preschool-age children, who localize pain poorly.) There seems to be some relationship between migraine and idiopathic epilepsy.[113] Both disorders occur in families and at times in the same person. Attacks of migraine are paroxysmal, sometimes periodic, and often hemicranial. They are associated with focal EEG changes, transient reflex changes, and other reflex localized neurologic disturbances, which are related to first vasoconstriction and then vasodilation of the cerebral blood vessels, phenomena that are mediated through the autonomic nervous system.[100]

It is often difficult to determine whether an aura has preceded the child's migraine attack. Nausea and vomiting may be more predominant symptoms than headache. Juvenile migraine may present as a confusional state[55] or with perceptual abnormalities and distortion in the child's time sense and body image.[84] Such symptoms may lead to a mistaken diagnosis of psychosis, drug-ingestion, or other clinical conditions. Emotional crises or overfatigue often precipitate an attack.[113] Migraine patients tend to be overcompliant, rigid, and perfectionistic and to have trouble handling their feelings of anger.[132,273] Their parents are often tense and overcontrolling, and the patient may have a special conflict-producing role in the family.[161] Migraine headaches should be distinguished particularly from tension headaches and conversion headaches. Conversion headaches are often based on the child's unconscious identification with the parent of the same sex, who also has headaches. Medical measures and supportive psychotherapy of the child and counseling of the parents can be of help. Intensive psychotherapy is often necessary.[237] Ergotamine tartrate should be used cautiously in children, because its side effects (e.g., numbness of the extremities) may be quite distressing, and it may produce nausea and vomiting. Biofeedback techniques[216] have been helpful in reducing symptoms in adults, as have hypnosis and other relaxation approaches.

Raynaud's disease has not been well studied in children. In adults who have Raynaud's disease, stressful circumstances have been shown to be associated with a rapid fall in skin temperature, which is followed by severe pain in the cyanosed fingers.[90] The disorder responds well to psychotherapy if no irreversible tissue pathology has occurred.[166]

Coronary heart disease and myocardial infarction, which appear to have psychophysiologic components in adults[37,77,213] rarely occur in childhood.[172] (Some discussion of such cardiovascular disorders is included in Chapter 4.)

Psychophysiologic Hemic and Lymphatic Disorders

Numerous physiologic concomitants of anxiety or responses to stress are encountered in relation to this system. These include changes in the blood levels of leukocytes, lymphocytes, eosinophils, and glutathione values, and changes in relative blood viscosity, clotting time, hematocrit, and sedimentation rates.[53,175] The changes ordinarily are reversible, and they present principally diagnostic problems. (Changes of this nature are discussed more fully in Chapter 3.) Chronic or recurrent states of leukocytosis may occur, however, as may "stress" ("benign") polycythemia,[160] which involves a decrease in plasma volume with a normal red cell volume. Evidence exists that "spontaneous" bleeding that is unrelated to injury may occur in response to emotional stress in children who have hemophilia.[158] The exact mechanisms are not known. Transient rash and hematuria have been reported to occur in relation to exercise and emotion. In addition, chronic, recurrent purpura has been described as occurring in situations that involve emotional conflict or other stressful stimuli. Such patients often show evidence of hysterical personalities, but what mechanisms are involved in the purpuric response is not clear.[2,142]

Psychophysiologic Gastrointestinal Disorders

Psychophysiologic gastrointestinal disorders include a wide variety of disorders since the gastrointestinal tract is so responsive to emotional stimuli. Nonaganglionic megacolon, peptic ulcer, ulcerative colitis, the irritable bowel syndrome, certain types of recurrent abdominal pain, cyclic vomiting, cardiospasm, so-called "idiopathic" celiac disease, regional enteritis, obesity, and anorexia nervosa are the major psychophysiologic gastrointestinal disorders. Pylorospasm, persistent colic, psuedo-peptic ulcer syndrome,[256] some cases of gastritis, certain types of constipation and diarrhea, certain disorders in salivation, and some types of periodontal disease[188] may involve psychophysiologic factors to some degree.

Nonaganglionic megacolon of psychophysiologic origin* has its origin in the infant's withholding of the stool during coercive toilet training.[182,206] Autonomic imbalance seems to contribute to the enlargement of the colon, and some constitutional factor may be involved in the predisposition to this disorder. In its treatment, initial cleaning out of the bowel with oil-retention or other types of enemas and an attempt to regularize evacuation of the bowels may be helpful, but psychotherapeutic measures are usually also necessary.[32]

Peptic ulcer and *ulcerative colitis* begin to appear with some frequency in the school-age period. Both conditions have been reported to occur at birth and in the neonatal period. These early cases, however, probably represent a response by pituitary-adrenal mechanisms to stress or medication, perhaps related to the higher gastric acidity and the higher level of adrenocortical steroids which occur during the first few hours and days of life. Both disorders may of course later occur as complications of ad-

*I prefer the term psychophysiologic (nonaganglionic) megacolon to "psychogenic megacolon" because the disorder involves more than conversion factors.

renal steroid or ACTH therapy. Acute "stress" ulcers with massive bleeding may occur in response to intense physical exertion associated with emotional tension.[226]

In school-age children and adolescents, the symptoms of peptic ulcer are different from those in adults. A preponderance of duodenal ulcers is seen, and boys are predominantly affected. The abdominal pain is not well localized, and the symptoms are not as clearly related to meals. Nausea and vomiting are more common. Anorexia, headaches, and early morning pain are often seen. Acute peptic ulcers, sometimes healing spontaneously, probably occur more often in children than has been believed, and they are more common in children than in adults. There is a high incidence of peptic ulcer in the child's family.[164]

Changes in the child's emotional state can produce, through cerebral cortical-hypothalamic interconnections and vagal stimulation, changes in his gastric and duodenal motility and secretion and mucosal engorgement. These changes may lead to minute petechial hemorrhages and small ulcerations.[271] The mechanisms which produce chronic discrete ulcers are not clearly understood. There seems to be a diminution in the mucosal protective mechanisms which may be a result of food stasis that is secondary to an increase in circulating adrenal cortical steroids or ACTH and an increase in gastric acidity.[167] Septic, traumatic processes or certain hormonal mechanisms may also be involved. Most people who develop peptic ulcers show an apparent biologic predisposition. The presence of high serum pepsinogen levels and high levels of conflict about dependence have made it possible to predict what young adults would develop peptic ulcers later when they were in a stressful situation.[260] Children and adults who develop peptic ulcers have difficulty in handling their feelings of anger. They are generally tense and overcompliant and often passive and dependent. At the same time, they are often demanding of affection.

Their mothers are usually dominant and overprotective, but they may be cold in their handling of their children. Their fathers often are distant and passive, though occasionally rigid and punitive.[39,249] The ulcer frequently develops in a setting of divorce, the death of a loved one, an intensified marital conflict, or other situations that involve actual, threatened, or symbolic loss.[109] Some overlapping exists with the school phobia picture, with which an acute peptic ulcer may occasionally coexist.

Children who have peptic ulcer often respond readily to bland diets, antacids, and antispasmodics.[164,186] Such a medical regimen should be combined with a supportive psychotherapeutic approach. Intensive psychotherapy for the child and his parents may be necessary, especially if pain is a prominent symptom.[249] Surgery is rarely indicated, but it may be life saving when the occasional complications of perforation or massive bleeding occur.

Ulcerative Colitis. Ulcerative colitis is a potentially severe, even life-threatening disorder. Children who have ulcerative colitis are generally overdependent, passive, inhibited, and show some compulsive tendencies.[5,148,193] In some cases, they show considerable manipulation of their parents in regard to the illness. Some children show only mild-to-moderate reactive disorders, some show disorders of psychotic or borderline psychotic proportions, and some show chronic personality disorders. Often there is a core of depression. Within broad limits, the more seriously disturbed children show stormier courses of illness.[174,193]

As Engel[56a] has shown in adults, the initial onset of ulcerative colitis in childhood often involves bleeding rather than diarrhea.[193] Precipitation of a fulminating type of onset of colitis usually takes place in a situation involving actual or threatened loss of emotional support from a key figure, usually a parent.[133] On the other hand, the insidious type of onset is usually associated with stressful forces, which gradually build up to significant levels. An acute mild onset may also occur, with bleeding for only a few days or weeks.[193] An apparently permanent remission will often occur in these less disturbed children with lesser biologic predisposition.

The mother is usually the dominant person in the family and the fathers are passive and retiring. The family characteristically exhibits problems in communication, especially of negative feelings.

The nonspecific inflammatory response usually begins in the lower colon, and it may progress upward, even into the terminal ileum.[47] The probable predisposing factors include familial patterns of autonomic response to stress that involve the lower gastrointestinal tract in "bowel-oriented" families, and possible conditioning of the defecation reflex to emotional conflict during coercive toilet training.[193] Overprotection and domination in the child's early life by his mother lead the child to become overdependent as well as resentful.

Emotional conflict has been shown to produce changes in motility, secretion, and vascularity in the colon of normal people, leading to petechial hemorrhages and minute ulcerations.[88] Some unidentified biologic predisposing factor (possibly one related to an abnormality in the inflammatory process) seems to produce the abnormal mucosal response of bleeding in patients who develop ulcerative colitis. Autoimmunization may be involved in some of the other manifestations, such as arthritis, reinforcing the impression that the process is often a systemic one rather than one involving only the bowel.

Treatment of this potentially life-threatening illness should always include both medical and psychotherapeutic measures. Several studies[133,193] have demonstrated the contribution of psychotherapy to physiologic improvement, but other studies[5] suggest that only psychologic improvement occurs. The psychotherapeutic approach should ordinarily be limited to supportive measures in the early phases. Exacerbations can be produced by premature emotional insights in the more fragile, overly dependent patient. Later more insight-producing psychotherapeutic approaches can be valuable. Sperling[239] has employed psychoanalysis successfully.

In the case of the child who feels depressed or hopeless and who is not responding to steroid therapy but is too ill for surgery, psychotherapy may be life saving.[193] Children who have milder physical and psychologic disorders often respond readily to a supportive approach that permits them some regression. They rapidly become dependent on the pediatrician, often with prompt cessation of their symptoms. The more seriously disturbed, overdependent, or manipulative children require more intensive psychotherapy. It includes extensive work with the parents, who tend to respond overanxiously to the child's fears or demands. Marital conflicts are common. As Finch and his colleagues[148] have demonstrated, cooperation of the physician, nurse, psychiatrist, social worker, and surgeon is especially important. The pediatrician should be the captain of the team.

Good follow-up care is essential. Ulcerative colitis may be of a remitting, chronic intermittent, or chronic continuous type.[47] Sigmoidoscopy can be a stressful experience for children, and it has been associated with exacerbations of the colitis. It should ordinarily not be done more than once every 6 months (preferably once a year), and it may be done under general anesthesia if the child is especially anxious. A significant percentage of children who had an early onset and chronic continuous courses of ulcerative colitis may later develop bowel carcinoma, even after many years of remission. However, if the symptoms of ulcerative colitis are under control, surgery to prevent carcinoma does not seem to be warranted. If a significant response to combined medical and psychologic measures does not appear within 2 years, or if "silent" progression of struc-tural bowel changes occurs despite psychologic improvement, surgery should be considered.[193]

In addition to the other indications for surgery, a long-continued delay in the adolescent growth spurt (beyond 15 years) should lead to consideration of surgical procedures.[13] But even after colectomy or colostomy, psychotherapeutic measures should be continued. Surgery may result in a striking physical improvement, but psychosocial disorders, overdependency, manipulative behavior, or school phobia may continue. The child and his parents, who often have compulsive trends, frequently have a great deal of unrecognized difficulty in adjusting to a colostomy. Recurrence of the colitis in ileostomy stumps, breakdowns in incisions, anxiety over colostomy bags, and other postoperative complications are frequent.[193] Ileostomy clubs can offer valuable group support to older adolescents.

Case Example. A 3 ½-year-old girl developed an acute fulminating form of ulcerative colitis. She did not respond to steroid therapy and other medical measures, and she was considered too ill for surgery. A therapist tried to undertake supportive therapy with her. The girl remained withdrawn and aloof, however, clinging to her mother during visits and developing several bloody stools when the mother tried to leave. Her illness had begun the day after her mother had returned home after having had a baby.

On her return home, the mother had given the little girl 2 goldfish, 1 of whom died when the girl "accidentally" dropped them on the floor in her room. Knowing that, the therapist set up a doll family scene and had a little girl doll expressing her dislike of the mother's new baby. When the baby doll accidentally fell off the table, the little girl smiled. The therapist then made the little girl doll repeatedly kick the baby doll off the table, and the patient responded with laughter. Thus a relationship between the therapist and the little girl was begun. In several days, and after repeated doll play, the little girl began to talk and engage in the play. She showed first rapid subsidence and then complete remission of her symptoms within several weeks. Follow-up therapy with the child and her parents was carried on, and the girl remained symptom free until she was 6 $\frac{1}{2}$ years old, when she developed diabetes.

Older children and adolescents who have chronic nonspecific diarrhea ("spastic colitis," "mucous colitis," *"irritable bowel" syndrome*) have many of the same psychosocial conflicts in their family backgrounds as do patients who have ulcerative colitis. They are generally less disturbed, however.[190,264] Bowel response to vagal stimulation caused by intensified emotional conflict seems to be even more active in patients who have chronic nonspecific diarrhea than in patients who have ulcerative colitis.[48] They also have strong family tendencies toward their condition, in conjunction with frequently coercive bowel training and other predisposing factors.[194] But they seem to have no biologic predisposition toward abnormal tissue response and mucosal bleeding; and combined medical and supportive psychotherapeutic measures by the pediatrician in conjunction with the social worker and consulting psychiatrist seem to help them more than such measures help children who have ulcerative colitis. Intensive psychotherapy for child and parents may be necessary.[190,235,264]

Recurrent Abdominal Pain. Recurrent abdominal pain is common; it occurs in about 10% of boys and 13% of girls. Although some do show 14 and 6 per second positive spikes on the EEG, these signs are not diagnostic. They occur in many normal children in the early school-age period who have no associated symptoms.[162] So-called abdominal migraine or abdominal epilepsy, which involves paroxysmal attacks in association with EEG changes and which is followed by sleep, is very rare in children.[52] More than 90% of children who have recurrent abdominal pain show no physical basis for the pain.[4] Localization of pain is poor in school-age children, and most symptoms are epigastric or periumbilical. School phobic manifestations are present in some children, as are other symptoms, such as headaches, dizziness, sleep disturbances, diarrhea, and vomiting. The re-

current episodes of pain are usually related to some emotional crisis in tense, timid, apprehensive, inhibited, and often overly conscientious children. The children usually have been overprotected by their parents.[94] Abdominal pain, headache, or "nervous tension" is frequently present in 1 of the parents or in another close family member. There seems to be no relationship between the ingestion of milk and recurrent abdominal pain. Some children show disturbances in colonic motility and changes in secretion and engorgement but no bleeding.[244] These responses seem to be oversensitive autonomic responses that have constitutional and often familial bases. Or conversion mechanisms may be involved in the child's pain, which is based on his identification with a family member or which has other determinants. A supportive approach by the pediatrician is often helpful, with reassurance to the patient and his parents about the absence of serious physical causes.[94] The possibility of a school adjustment problem may be discussed with the child's teacher. Drugs are of little help, except for their possible placebo effects. Intensive psychotherapy for child and his parents may be necessary.

Cyclic Vomiting. Cyclic vomiting seems to have no relationship to epilepsy. (Some authors use the term recurrent vomiting for the cyclic vomiting syndrome, which can often be handled initially in a pediatric hospital setting, with psychiatric consultation.) It occurs usually in tense, anxious, easily overstimulated, and overdependent children. The parents have often been overanxious and overprotective, and their children may respond by being demanding or manipulative.[7] In certain cases, a symbiotic relationship between the child and his mother has been described, together with a failure of the child to achieve separation and individuation.[199] Episodes of vomiting may be touched off by infections, frightening new situations, marital discords, or other family crises.[17] Headache, abdominal pain, and some fever are often associated with the vomiting. A familial tendency is common, and the vomiting and other symptoms have continued into adult life in a number of people who received no psychologic treatment.[101] Although conversion mechanisms may contribute to the vomiting, an overactive gag reflex and the physiologic concomitants of anxiety seem to be involved in many cases, and a constitutional predisposition to a particular pattern of autonomic response to stressful stimuli may be involved.[66] The dehydration and metabolic disturbances caused by the vomiting can be serious, even life threatening, and they may arouse great anxiety and guilt in the child's parents.[116] Thorazine and other antiemetics have been helpful in aborting an attack

Psychotherapeutic intervention for the child and his parents is usually necessary,[135] and inpatient psychiatric help may be required.[46]

Cardiospasm. Cardiospasm has been described in adults,[64,269] but the condition is rare in children.[151] Changes in smooth muscle functioning that involve the lower two-thirds of the esophagus[64] may affect the efficacy of the involuntary components of the act of swallowing as a result of emotional influences. The reflex activity of the cardiac sphincter of the stomach is related coordinatively to the swallowing movements of the mouth and esophagus.[262] The exact psychophysiologic mechanisms that produce the cardiospasm, however, are not clear.[151] I have treated one patient, an anxious, tense early adolescent boy who had an overprotective mother and whose father was absent. With intensive psychotherapy, the symptoms disappeared, and a year later, at a follow-up visit, improvement was shown to have been maintained.

Idiopathic Celiac Disease. So-called idiopathic celiac disease characteristically has its onset in an infant 6 to 18 months old; the initial signs are a disturbance in appetite, failure to gain weight, irritable behavior, and diarrhea alternating with constipation. These signs are followed by the gradual appearance of large, foul, pale stools, striking fluctuations in weight, abdominal distention, increasing wasting and retardation in growth, marked muscular weakness, anorexia or capricious appetite, evidence of severe depression, and other features. Intestinal malabsorption is present, together with a pattern of abnormal gastrointestinal motility and histologic abnormalities of the mucosa of the jejunum. Clinical evidence of vitamin and mineral deficiencies (and anemia) and secondary infection may be associated with the chronic picture. With modern methods of treatment, these latter problems can be dealt with successfully, thus doing away with the high mortality formerly observed. Other causes of the celiac syndrome (e.g., infection, obstruction, infestation, and malrotation of the intestines) must of course be ruled out. Celiac disease in children and nontropical sprue in adults appear to be different phases of the same syndrome although the adult form is ordinarily not as severe.[187]

Recent investigations have indicated that people who have celiac disease have trouble metabolizing the gliadin fraction of wheat gluten in particular, which seems to be an enzymatic defect and not a true allergy. The disorder has a familial character, supporting the impression that genetic factors operate in the defect; a latent form is often found in relatives who do not show the characteristic clinical picture.[191] A gluten-free diet has in many instances produced gradual remission. The disorder seems to be less common today than formerly.

A consistent though nonspecific personality picture of an anxious, rigid, moderately compulsive nature has been noted among the mothers of children who have celiac disease; their fathers are often rather distant and passive. A basic disturbance in the mother-child relationship is ordinarily present, beginning in struggles for control over feeding in early infancy. It is usually related to family or marital problems centered on the pregnancy, delivery, or neo-natal period for the particular child.[187] The mother's (occasionally the father's) anx-iously controlling approach may be inten-sified by her feelings of fear and guilt about her child's disorder. Children and adoles-cents who have celiac disease are fre-quently overdependent and outwardly passive and inhibited, they have marked difficulties in handling angry or resentful feelings, and they often show some pas-sive-aggressive or negativistic behavior.[33] They generally find it hard to separate from the significant parent. Having a chronic ill-ness or frequent exacerbations of that ill-ness undoubtedly contributes to the pic-ture although adults who have nontropical sprue often show similar personality char-acteristics, even those who have no early history of celiac disease.[191]

In many instances, the onset of celiac disease is related to precipitating events that most often involve an actual, a threat-ened, or a fantasied loss of dependent grat-ifications from the mother or another key nurturing person.[33,187] Depression in the mother that is related to marital problems or intercurrent circumstances has appeared prior to the onset of the child's disease, leading the mother to handle the infant more anxiously and often to withdraw emotionally from him, occasionally to the point of neglect.[154] An "answering" depression may occur in the infant. It is associated with regression in the child's be-havior and disturbance in his feeding and bowel habits, with a chronologic relation-ship to the onset of the prodromal symp-toms of celiac disease. At times, such in-terpersonal events are combined with a respiratory infection or some other physi-cal illness in the child.

Exacerbations of celiac disease in older children and adults have been noted to oc-cur in relation to emotional conflict, par-ticularly a conflict about dependency or ac-tual or symbolic separation from supportive figures that is associated with feelings of helplessness.[33,191] Such exacerbations may

be influenced also by depression or other emotions, leading to a conscious or an un-conscious giving up of a gluten-free diet. Resolution of the conflicts can be associ-ated with an apparently spontaneous re-mission of the symptoms. When gluten is present in the diet, steatorrhea may occur with exacerbations that are related to emo-tional conflict. When gluten is absent from the diet, only diarrhea may occur.[92] Gluten ingested in the absence of emotional con-flict may not cause symptoms. Apparently the presence of gluten in the diet is a "nec-essary but not sufficient" condition for the appearance of steatorrhea; emotional con-flict, or, at times, an intercurrent infection may also be required.

Physiologic studies have indicated that the absorption defect in celiac disease may be reversed temporarily by parasympa-thomimetic or sympathetic-blocking drugs, as well as by the administration of corti-sone.[187] These and other studies seem to suggest that the autonomic nervous sys-tem and the neuroendocrine system play a part in absorption defects, both systems being capable of influencing bowel activity and perhaps the development of the his-tologic changes. Emotional influences on absorption may be transmitted through both systems with the mediation of the hy-pothalamic-pituitary-adrenal cortical axis. Psychophysiologic influences on the me-tabolism of gluten are not known.

A number of remedies for celiac disease have been recommended over the years, but many of them have been used suc-cessfully only by their originators. Before the use of gluten-free diets, diets that con-tained only simple carbohydrates and low fat were used with considerable success, and, more recently, cortisone was noted to produce remissions in many patients who had celiac disease and nontropical sprue. A psychotherapeutic approach involving supportive work with the mother, and sometimes hospitalization of the infant (who is assigned 1 nurse to feed and care for him) has also proved effective in some cases within a short time, without any change in the diet and without any other kind of treatment.[187] Supportive psychotherapeutic measures used to treat exacerbations of nontropical sprue in adults have had the same effects.[191] Thus the most essential ingredient in the favorable response even to gluten-free diets seems to be a positive doctor-patient-parent relationship, one involving confidence and a supportive psychotherapeutic effect. Besides the use of dietary measures and the correction of metabolic abnormalities or deficiency states, psychiatric consultation may be indicated and, sometimes, the use of more intensive psychotherapy for the patient and his family. Since the underlying defect in metabolism remains after remission, often because of persistent histologic changes in the intestinal mucosa, a continuing relationship with the physician can help prevent exacerbations related to emotional conflict or other factors.

Early studies of children who had *regional enteritis* showed principally the psychologic effects of a chronic illness.[128] More recent investigations have indicated that children who have regional enteritis have many of the psychosocial characteristics of children who have ulcerative colitis.[204] However, children who have regional enteritis are generally less disturbed than are the children who have ulcerative colitis. Both disorders tend to respond to similar treatment.[150,204,236] But surgery is rarely indicated for regional enteritis, and it may only compound the difficulties encountered in the course of the disorder. It is possible that, for undetermined reasons, the predominant involvement of the ileum rather than the colon is responsible for the differences in the pathophysiologic and clinical pictures of the two disorders.[87]

Obesity. Obesity in children is becoming more common in the United States, possibly because of increased affluence and overeating.[189] Although endocrine factors or pituitary lesions had been thought to be prominently involved in many cases of obesity, it appears now that such factors are only rarely influential. As Bruch[26] has shown, most cases of obesity result from an excess of intake over output of calories, as a result of overeating that is usually associated with inactivity. Obesity tends to occur in families who tend to overeating. Increased appetite, a psychological phenomenon, can far outreach physiologic hunger.

Metabolic or other biologic predisposing factors may also play a part. The hypothalamic regulation of eating (the "glucostatic mechanism") may be influenced by the amount of fat in the body, whether as circulating metabolites or in fat deposits. The level of free fatty acids in the blood can apparently be affected by autonomic stimulation, while steroid mechanisms may influence the storage of fat. Thus, the "dynamics of fat metabolism" may possibly respond to changes in "psychologic dynamics" in situations of conflict, through neuroendocrine interrelationships in people who have a biologic predisposition to obesity.[191] Some people seem to be constitutionally predisposed to obesity. Obesity has been shown to occur often in persons from the lower socioeconomic groups,[245] with some ethnic variations.[121]

Bruch[26] has shown that from the psychosocial point of view, markedly obese children and adolescents have one of two major types of obesity: the reactive type of obesity or the developmental type of obesity. The *reactive* type of obesity is related to overeating and underactivity in response to an emotionally traumatic experience, such as the death of a parent or sibling, the break-up of a family through divorce, or school failure. Children who have the reactive type of obesity tend to use food as a substitute for basic emotional gratifications lost through the traumatic experience. Rather sudden gains of 40 to 50 pounds have been observed in children and adolescents who have had such traumatic experiences.[189] The gain is sometimes reversed when parent-substitute relationships have been established or when the conflict has been resolved. In the reactive type of obesity, supportive psychotherapeutic measures by the pediatrician, with occasional psychiatric consultation, are often helpful. However, children who come from more disturbed families may require intensive outpatient individual or family psychotherapy to relieve the more persistent psychosocial problems.

The *developmental* type of obesity usually has its origins in strong familial tendencies toward overeating and obesity. It represents a disturbed way of life ("family frame") that involves the patient and his whole family. The mother, who often was emotionally deprived as a child, usually dominates and overprotects her child. The child's father is ordinarily passive and retiring. But both parents may unconsciously use 1 particular child to satisfy vicariously their own emotional needs or compensatory tendencies. Often the child is overvalued by the parents, sometimes because another child has died. Overfeeding may also represent the parents' attempt to deal with guilt. Or, as Bruch[28] has indicated, the mother may be able to respond to her infant's show of discomfort only by feeding him. She sets up a pattern that the child later internalizes. The child is often large at birth, becomes obese in early infancy because he is overfed, and continues to be markedly obese. After his early demanding behavior has subsided, the child usually becomes passive and oversubmissive, overdependent, and immature. The child is often taller than average, and he actually has an increased lean body mass, in contrast to the child who has the reactive type of obesity, whose fat alone accounts for his gain in weight.[189]

Obese children often have feelings of helplessness and despair and a tendency to withdraw from social interaction that is associated with their tendency to overeat. As Hamburger[99] has indicated, these children may unconsciously use eating to deal with their anxiety or tension or to ward off depression or feelings of hostility. Eating or chewing may acquire unconscious symbolic significance as a conversion symptom, or patterns of "addiction" to food may result. Although obesity is a social handicap, some children or adolescents hide behind their "wall of weight" and ward off their sexual conflicts with the feeling that they are ugly or unattractive.[26] The result is a disturbance in their body image, and a lack of awareness of satiety. In the Pickwickian syndrome,[30] alveolar hypoventilation, compensatory polycythemia, and drowsiness are associated with marked obesity. A too-rapid loss of weight may produce a "dieting depression" or even a psychotic picture in some markedly obese and seriously disturbed adolescents.[191]

Children and adolescents from the families described may be very hard to treat. The parents or the patient may not be able to see the child's obesity as a serious problem. If the patient and his parents can be helped to take positive steps, the physician must choose carefully between individual psychotherapy, group therapy, and family therapy. Long-term psychiatric hospitalization or residential treatment may be necessary.

For patients who are severely depressed, diets and anorectic drugs are ordinarily of little use by themselves. The parents of these children are unable to help the children remain motivated to lose weight, and they may even unconsciously sabotage the treatment. The anorectic drug approach used alone may have more complications than benefits. The central nervous system stimulants may become habit forming, and they should not be used with children and adolescents.

Surgery to reduce intestinal absorption in very obese persons has not been carefully evaluated clinically by an interdisciplinary approach. Some patients seem to respond to such surgery without showing signs of psychotic or other decompensation, but paradoxical psychologic difficulties may be encountered.[34]

Some seriously disturbed obese persons are probably better off psychologically without marked weight reduction but rather aim to achieve and maintain a "preferred weight." A supportive relationship with the physician may be the most important factor. Weight Watchers techniques, which include the use of group support, have been more successful in helping markedly obese persons than have most other techniques. Behavior modification techniques have also been shown to be valuable.[180]

In her recent approach, Bruch[28] has concentrated on helping the adolescent who has the developmental type of obesity to achieve an identity separate from his parents' and a heightened awareness of his own concerns and needs. Weight reduction is a secondary goal. Bruch feels that prevention can be achieved by helping mothers who habitually overfeed their infants develop a better way to respond to the child's needs.

Obesity that appears during adolescence generally has a better prognosis than obesity that has been present since the child's early life. Obesity that appears during adolescence is usually reactive obesity. But the obese adolescent has serious secondary conflicts related to society's approving attitude toward slimness and its critical attitude toward obesity. These attitudes are partly justified medically since obese adults have a greater incidence of hypertension, diabetes, and heart disease. If the adolescent has a positive motivation to lose weight, the pediatrician can take a supportive approach with him, in combination with counseling the child's parents and the judicious use of diets and mild exercise.[189] Overstrenuous dieting or overly strong pressure on the child to diet or to exercise should be avoided. Summer "diet camp" programs can give some obese adolescents significant help. These programs provide adequate social satisfactions as well as group discussions or individual therapy. Some obese adolescents show particular

difficulties in resolving problems about their sexual identity. Their problems often reflect their parents' unresolved sexual problems. Their parents often have marital conflicts. Zakus and Solomon[277] have shown that such adolescents may respond to more intensive psychotherapy, with additional help offered to their parents in alleviating their overconcern and overcontrolling tendencies.

Case Example. A 14-year-old boy, an only child, was admitted to a pediatric ward weighing 422 pounds. Physical examination showed no other abnormalities; he was not above the height normal for his age, but his bones were quite large. The boy's mother had overfed him since his infancy, and she had centered her life on him since her divorce during his second year of life. She herself was not seriously obese, but she had developed an incisional hernia the size of a basketball from a laparotomy some years before, which she had refused to have repaired. She had resisted previous attempts to help the boy lose weight, and the school principal was able to persuade the mother to bring the boy to the hospital only by declaring him a fire hazard because he nearly blocked most doors.

Although the boy seemed motivated to lose weight, his mother could not accept the recommendation of the child psychiatry consultant that the boy be transferred to the adolescent psychiatry unit for intensive treatment. The boy was followed in the pediatric clinic on a diet, the mother unconsciously discouraged the dieting, however, giving Metrecal to the boy after meals. The child psychiatry consultant made it a point to be in the pediatric clinic at the time of the mother's visits to her boy, and he gradually developed a supportive relationship with the mother as well as the boy.

After about a year, the mother decided to have her hernia repaired, and the consultant helped her contact the surgical services to arrange this. After her recovery, the mother wrote to the consultant, asking him to have her son admitted to the adolescent psychiatric unit. Over 10 months, with intensive individual psychotherapy and milieu therapy for the boy, with tandem help for the mother, the boy's weight dropped dramatically (he would chew ice cubes at times when he felt hungry, crunching them angrily). He became more sociable, did better academically, and became interested in athletics. The boy's weight leveled off, and the psychiatric staff felt it was wise to settle for a happy, outgoing 285 pounder, already showing progress in football, then to try for more weight loss. On his return home, the mother at first offered him excess amounts of food; he refused it, however, and 1 year later his weight was still around 287 pounds.

Anorexia Nervosa. Anorexia nervosa is observed most frequently during adolescence or postadolescence. It may, however, appear during the late school-age or prepubertal periods. It should be differentiated from anorexia as a symptom of depression or other disorders. In true anorexia nervosa, the conflict about eating becomes internalized and chronic.[232] Loss of psychologic appetite, denial of physical hunger, aversion to food, severe weight loss, hypoproteinemia (at times with edema), emaciation and pallor, amenorrhea, an increase in body hair, a lowered body temperature, pulse rate, and blood pressure, flat or occasionally diabetic blood sugar levels, dryness of the skin and brittleness of the nails, and intolerance to cold may occur singly or in combination and in varying degrees of severity. The patient often remains active, often to a striking degree and even in the face of marked loss of body weight (denial of emaciation), and some patients may even exercise to lose weight. Patients often appear preoccupied or irritable, and they have difficulty talking about their feelings. Some of the symptoms appear to be the result of a psychophysiologic disturbance involving the pituitary-hypothalamic axis. Other symptoms, such as amenorrhea, may be the result of starvation (although menstruation may not return until long after a normal body weight is achieved[20]). Although "pituitary cachexia" or hypopituitarism must be ruled out, its occurrence is rare.

Anorexia nervosa occurs predominantly in girls, but it may occasionally be seen in boys.[61] It often begins in relation to a strenuous attempt at dieting; the diet is then continued until it cannot be controlled. The mother (occasionally the father) has usually been strongly overcontrolling toward the patient, and there is an ambivalent and hostile-dependent relationship between the mother and the daughter. The patient often has a history of early feeding problems. The parents may value slimness and physical attractiveness; and the girl's relationship with her father may have an overtly seductive quality. Not infrequently the parents and some late adolescent patients have jobs that involve the preparation of food. Those jobs may provide a compensatory sublimation for a few early or mild chronic cases.

Preadolescent patients are often overconscientious, energetic, and highly achieving persons. They remain strongly dependent on their parents, but they unconsciously resent their parents' control. Problems in emancipation from their parents, which reflect their underlying difficulties in separation-individuation, are also usually involved.[28] Food intake then becomes something over which the patients can have control. Many girls have been chubby or obese or have had fears of becoming fat. Alternating periods of obesity and anorexia[15] have been described in certain of these girls, as have periods of bulimia followed by self-induced vomiting. During puberty, these patients have significant difficulties in their heterosexual relationships, and they often avoid dating or other types of social interaction by engaging in many kinds of activities, including sports, or by isolating themselves socially. The onset of anorexia nervosa may be related to the menarche or to traumatic experiences, often sexual ones.

Diagnostically, there are three main groups of patients[138] and the groups overlap somewhat: (1) patients who have psychoneurotic disorders who have mixed hysterical and phobic trends and for whom eating appears to have strong sexual implications that are derived from their earlier unresolved conflicts. Those patients attach highly symbolic meanings to their weight and body contours, and they often have associated unconscious fears or fantasies about pregnancy, (2) patients who have obsessive-compulsive personality disorders and rigid, overconscientious, driving, and sometimes secretive personality trends and who develop fears of contamination of or dirt in their food, and (3) patients who have schizophrenic or borderline psychotic states, in which the thought disorder and the massive projection involved often leads to fears of poisoning. Self-destructive or unconsciously suicidal implications of the failure to eat may be involved in the inability to eat in all 3 groups. A small group of patients show a severe reactive disorder with strong depressive trends that is superimposed on an overly dependent or other mild personality disorder. Underlying the personality disturbance is often a distorted self-image with a failure to be in touch with body sensations or functions.[28]

The largest group of patients are those in whom the symptoms begin around puberty. These patients are more often involved in developmental crises, and they tend to exhibit reactive disorders or hysterical psychoneurotic pictures with phobic trends. They are less disturbed, and if they are treated, usually their prognosis is good. Those who show obsessive-compulsive personality disorders are more rigid and difficult to treat. Those who develop this syndrome in late adolescence or just after adolescence tend to be of the schizophrenic or borderline psychotic type, and their prognosis is much more guarded. If the person's weight loss is 50% of her original body weight, serious physical debility or even death may occur.[20]

Hospitalization had been almost universally employed in the past.[21,79] Recently a number of patients have been treated successfully on an outpatient basis,[203] sometimes following brief hospitalization, with a combined medical and psychological approach. Patients who are in the less disturbed, mildly psychoneurotic or reactive group can benefit from a supportive psychotherapeutic approach by a pediatrician, with the judicious use of psychiatric consultation and help for the parents to avoid battles over food. Intensive psychotherapy for the patient and her parents may be necessary for the patient who is more severely neurotic,[27] however, and family therapy may be especially effective in these patients.[141] Behavior therapy that gives positive rewards for weight gain has helped some of these patients;[19] follow-up care is important, and work with parents is essential if behavioral methods are used. For patients who have a more rigid, obsessive-compulsive personality disorder, treatment by a psychiatrist or psychologist working closely with the pediatrician can often be effective.[83] Individual outpatient psychotherapy can be combined with family therapy.[141] If necessary, a pediatric adolescent inpatient ward can serve as a temporary adjunct to outpatient treatment.[79]

Seriously disturbed patients who have schizophrenic, borderline, and severe reactive disorders, particularly those who are extremely manipulative and controlling toward their parents, can be treated most successfully by psychiatric hospitalization or residential treatment.[146,203] In such a setting, the patient can be permitted to prepare her own food on the ward, which may help her deal with her fears about the food she is given. The patient should not be pressured to eat although the seriousness of her problem should be pointed out to her and to her parents. Bruch[28] has pointed out that the primary psychotherapeutic challenge is to help the patient in her desperate struggle to gain a separate and self-respecting identity. A healthier identity can permit her to give up her rigid regulation of her food intake and her low body weight, made necessary by her need to achieve and maintain her shaky and unhealthy type of control and identity. (Intensive follow-up is necessary, since seriously disturbed adolescents who appear to recover from anorexia nervosa may develop other types of self-destructive behavior.[246])

If the patient's body weight falls near 50% of its original level, combined medical and psychiatric treatment, using tube feeding if necessary, should be employed. The patient can be helped to accept the tube feedings if she is told they are needed to protect her from doing herself harm from her diet. Patients usually respond favorably when the doctor "takes over" responsibility for their welfare during this critical time.

Case Example. A 13-year-old girl was admitted to the hospital because of her gradual loss of weight (almost 30 pounds) over the past year. She had begun to diet around menarche although she had not been obese. As she put it, she could not stop dieting, and she added an exercise program, running as much as 5 miles a day (she continued this regimen in the hospital, running "laps" around the ward). Psychiatric consultation showed her to be a girl who had a moderately severe obsessive-compulsive personality disorder, who came from a home where the parents had experienced severe marital conflict for many years, with the father often turning to the girl, the oldest of 3 children, for solace and support. The girl developed a positive relationship with a male pediatric resident, and she had long talks with him about her returning wish to be "pretty" and regain weight. Since the parents lived across the state, a plan was worked out for the girl to stay in a nearby group home, and the resident continued to follow her case twice a week, with supervision from the child psychiatry consultant. Her parents were referred to a marital counseling agency in their home town.

The girl gradually gave up her exercise program and she stopped dieting although it took some months for her to regain her weight. After nearly a year, the parants' marriage had improved markedly, and the girl returned home, with no reappearance of her symptoms. She continued to return once a month for supportive contacts with the resident over the next school year; her obsessive-compulsive tendencies remained, but these were much milder and they even helped her in her school work. Finally, she decided that she could get along on her own, and she terminated the contacts with the resident. For another year, however, she wrote monthly letters to the resident, who had gone into practice, and she seemed to maintain her gains.

Psychophysiologic Genitourinary Disorders

The category psychophysiologic genitourinary disorders includes certain types of menstrual disturbances (e.g., dysmennorhea, amenorrhea, and premenstrual tension), certain types of functional uterine bleeding, certain types of polyuria and dysuria, certain types of urinary retention or "vesical paralysis," some cases of urinary frequency and urgency, certain types of urethral and vaginal discharges, and some cases of persistent glycosuria without diabetes. Disturbances in the sexual functioning of the genital organs in older adolescents (e.g., vaginismus, frigidity, impotence, frequent erections, dyspareunia, and priapism) often involve conversion disorders of the voluntarily innervated musculature. Certain cases of these disturbances, however, may have psychophysiologic components.

Menstrual disturbances are common in early adolescence. Irregularity is usually the rule in the first year or so after menarche, and menorrhagia, metrorrhagia, and temporary amenorrhea are not uncommon. These disturbances may be intensified or perpetuated by emotional "shock" and emotional conflicts, as can functional bleeding[105] and amenorrhea[57] in late adolescents and adult women. Although the hypothalamic-pituitary-ovarian axis seems to be involved, the exact psychophysiologic interrelationships are still unclear.[98,223]

Dysmenorrhea, which usually occurs only after ovulation begins, occurs in as many as 12% of high-school girls in the United States, and it causes much absence from school.[51] Its incidence may be influenced by the attitudes of secrecy, misunderstanding, inconvenience, and disgust toward menstruation which still are widespread.[104,265] Long-standing and severe dysmenorrhea usually indicates that the girl is having trouble accepting the feminine role and in assuming the responsibilities of womanhood.[78,108] The psychophysiologic mechanisms in dysmenorrhea are not fully understood.

Premenstrual tension, which is characterized by fatigue, irritability, anxiety, and mild depression, is frequent in adolescent girls.[230] It is somehow associated with the hormonal, electrolyte, and other physiologic changes that precede menstruation.[119] Although subjective effects have been reported, the menstrual cycle seems to have no objective effects on the cognitive and perceptual-motor performances of emotionally healthy females.[231] However, 2 studies[44,251] have indicated that women who are menstruating or who are about to menstruate tend to bring their young children to the hospital more often for minor illnesses than do "intermenstrual" women, suggesting that a woman's menstrual status may affect the way she responds emotionally to illness in her children.

Sterility in late adolescent girls and adult women may have a psychophysiologic basis, related to expulsive contractions of the uterus arising from anxiety over sexual activity.[10] Anovulation, tubal spasm, and changes in cervical mucus may also be involved.[215] *Habitual abortion* occurs in young women who have significant conflicts about sexuality and motherhood[96,122] and in whom "uterine dynamics" (strong contractions) seem to parallel psychodynamics.[153] Although the psychophysiologic mechanisms are not as yet completely understood, emotional stress apparently can result in an increase in posterior pituitary hormones, with oxytocin accounting for the augmented uterine activity.[152] Vandenbergh and Taylor[253] have shown that emotional illness is much higher in women with habitual abortion after suture of the incompetent cervical os unless psychotherapy is offered concurrently.

In many menstrual disorders, discussion of attitudes, fears, or conflicts in the context of a supportive relationship with the pediatrician or pediatric gynecologist, together with counseling for the parents, will bring relief.[131] Some adolescent girls who have marked premenstrual tension and severe dysmenorrhea or persistent amenorrhea without other causes have marked personality problems. These patients often respond to intensive psychotherapy combined with counseling of their parents. Married adolescent females who are sterile or who have habitual abortions can benefit from psychotherapy, and/or marital therapy.[219] Cain[31] has described the reactions of children in disturbed families to the mother's miscarriage; their reactions may include anger and guilt.

Infertility in late adolescent and adult males may stem from impotence and problems in ejaculation.[178] In addition, there is some evidence that emotional stress leads to oligospermia.[24] The hypothalamic-pituitary axis, which regulates gonadotropin excretion, is presumably involved although the psychophysiologic interrelationships are not fully understood. Supportive psychologic measures may be helpful.

Disorders of urination are not uncommon, especially in adolescents. Enuresis, like encopresis, ordinarily involves conversion, regressive, or other mechanisms, and it is not considered a true psychophysiologic disorder. Urinary retention occurs most often in adolescent females although it may occur in males. The unconscious equation of genital and urinary functioning is characteristic, with conflicts about sexuality that derive from experiences in childhood. Identification with relatives who have urinary disorders may also be involved, as may an earlier disorder of the genitourinary system or accidents that involve the pelvis and affect urinary functioning.[255] The patient may be unable to void for days or weeks. Catheterization removes the urine, but it does not cure the retention problem. Urethral spasm is ordinarily present, and bladder hypofunction, sometimes amounting to vesical paralysis, may be associated with a conversion mechanism that involves the external bladder sphincter. Measurement of bladder pressure in an experimental interview that involved exposure to stressful topics has shown that hypofunction occurred in some patients in relation to emotional conflict.[207] Such studies have shown that other patients exhibit hyperfunctioning related to urinary frequency in the same situations. Supportive therapy may be helpful in some cases of urinary retention. In other cases, more intensive psychotherapy may be required. That is also true for some cases of urinary frequency, particularly if they are associated with symptoms of urgency or with "stress incontinence."[1]

Polyuria may result from an increased water intake that has a symbolic meaning, as in some cases of "psychogenic" polydipsia.[136] Supportive psychotherapy may be helpful.

Psychophysiological Endocrine Disorders

This category includes certain cases of hyperinsulinism, as well as diabetes, thyrotoxicosis, growth failure, pseudocyesis, and, in adolescent and adult females, certain disorders in lactation.

Hyperinsulinism[184] and cases of "idiopathic" hypoglycemia[41] related to emotional tension have been reported in adolescents. The psychophysiologic mechanisms, which presumably involve increased vagal activity, and the predisposing factors are not clearly understood. Unrecognized depression may be more important than the physiologic manifestations in certain cases.[69] Psychiatric consultation can be helpful, and formal psychotherapy may be necessary.

Diabetes. Diabetes is known to involve a hereditary predisposition and to be significantly influenced by psychophysiologic mechanisms. Metabolic changes undoubtedly antedate the onset of the manifest clinical disorder, as suggested by the high percentage of women (particularly obese women) who give birth to babies who weigh more than 11 pounds, and who later develop diabetes. Prediabetic people often have elevated oral glucose tolerance curves without other signs or symptoms.[97] In a controlled study, adolescent diabetics had a significantly higher incidence of parental loss and severe family disturbance before

the onset of diabetes than did a comparable group of adolescents who had blood dyscrasias.[241] A number of studies have indicated that diabetes is often triggered by increased conflict, most often a conflict involving a real or threatened loss of a key figure or relationship.[97,140] Exacerbations, including diabetic coma in children and adolescents, are frequently triggered off by family crises or other stressful stimuli. In such exacerbations, an initial fall in blood sugar often occurs, and it is associated with an increase in blood and urine ketone bodies and a diuresis that precede the actual rise in blood sugar, ketones, and free fatty acid levels and the appearance of the other phenomena that lead to coma.[107a]

In childhood diabetes, particularly during adolescence, the onset is often more abrupt and the course stormier than it is in the adult form.[62] Unlike some other psychophysiologic disorders, diabetes is a permanent handicap, and children and parents must be able to mourn effectively the loss of certain expectations (and to mourn them again at each level of the child's development). The mourning is necessary even though the child has no visible signs of disability and the resultant immediate changes in his life-style may not be great.

Adolescents may feel socially isolated because of their diabetes,[248] and they may worry about marriage and the effect of their illness on their children.[243] Different styles of coping with the impact of the disorder occur.[250] Some adolescents may try to control their diet rigidly, and they take the insulin carefully. Others may deny that they have diabetes, and they refuse to take the insulin and thus precipitate hypoglycemia and insulin reactions. If those conditions are severe and occur often, they can produce brain damage[80] and have deleterious effects on the adolescents' academic and social functioning.

There is no personality picture specific to diabetes. However, some retrospective observations have suggested that adolescents who develop diabetes were more demanding as infants and young children about feeding (perhaps because of premonitory metabolic changes).[241] Some patients are over-anxious and dependent, while others are overly independent (pseudo-independent). Younger children may misinterpret diabetes and its treatment as punishment. Their parents' reactions may range from overprotection and overanxiety to rigidity and (occasionally) rejection. Struggles for control between parents and child may result in the child's stealing food or overeating. In a number of healthier families,[240] however, the parents have no serious difficulty in accepting the child's illness, and no significant personality disturbance appears in the child.

The use of a "flexible"diet, one that includes appropriate snacks that are "covered" by adequate amounts of insulin and that forbids only concentrated sweets and second helpings of some desserts, seems to help make life more normal for children and adolescents who have diabetes.[71] There is some controversy about whether or not such flexibility affects the incidence of diabetic complications in adult life. One problem is that good criteria regarding the control of diabetes are lacking. A flexible diet may also help to avoid daily battles over food, the child's stealing and hoarding food, and related problems. A few adolescents, however, seem to want some external controls, and they may do better with the structure a basic diet offers, with permission to deviate somewhat from the diet on special occasions. The substitution of oral insulin preparations for injected insulin in patients who have mild diabetes has no place in the treatment of juvenile diabetes although it may have some research value.

Counseling within a supporting relationship with the pediatrician will often suffice for many children and parents. Chase and his colleagues[35] have written a booklet for children who have diabetes and for their parents. Group discussions have been helpful with older children and adolescents, and special summer camp programs have helped children develop self-care.[257] Disturbed adolescents who use their diabetes to control or rebel against their parents or who exhibit unconsciously self-destructive behavior by overeating or refusing to take insulin require a more intensive psychotherapeutic approach. This approach must involve the close cooperation of the psychiatrist, the social worker, and the pediatrician. Inpatient pediatric or psychiatric settings may be needed for these adolescents. There is suggestive evidence that beta-adrenergic blocking drugs may help prevent emotionally induced exacerbations, particularly in certain subtypes of diabetes. Their use, however, is still in the experimental stage.

Anxious parents who have intense guilt, particularly those who blame their heredity for their child's diabetes, may have great difficulty in injecting insulin into ("hurting") their young child. Parents who are overprotective may not be able to let the child learn to take his own insulin when he is ready to do so. Early education about the disease, combined with counseling and support, including group discussions, has helped many parents. Some parents need more intensive psychotherapy. Family therapy has been indicated and helpful in some difficult situations, particularly those involving adolescents who have so-called "brittle" diabetes.

Thyrotoxicosis. Children and adolescents who have thyrotoxicosis often experience the onset of the disorder in the context of gradually intensifying stressful circumstances or under conditions of a real or threatened loss of an important emotional relationship.[140] They seem to have particular difficulty handling their dependency needs. Some patients have overt tendencies toward dependency, while others attempt to deny and cover up such tendencies with a pseudo-independent facade. Some patients are chronically depressed. Unplanned pregnancies, marital conflicts, overcontrolling parents, maternal deprivation, and broken homes are frequent in the histories of these patients.[25] In adult studies, those who had higher levels of tension that involved motor, autonomic, and verbal activity showed higher serum iodine levels (but within the normal range) than did those who had lower serum iodine levels.[68] The decay of radioactive iodine has been shown to be increased in stressful interviews, and it has been possible to predict the rate of decay on the basis of the subject's personality configuration, which was derived from a cluster of personality traits.[50] A longitudinal study of thyroid "hot spots" (areas which are hyperavid for radioactive iodine) in euthyroid people has indicated that their personalities were similar to those of people who developed thyrotoxicosis. In contrast to a normal control group, the subject group showed a waxing and waning of hot-spot activity in a predictable direction as a concomitant consequence of life stress.[254] Various data suggest that hot spots can progress into nodular and diffuse hyperthyroidism under conditions of prolonged or severe stress. Through limbic-hypothalamic interconnections, stressful experiences result in an increase in anterior pituitary thyrotropic hormone, which brings about an increased thyroid secretion. Since an increased rate of decay of radioactive iodine has been found in people who have a family history of thyrotoxicosis,[50] there must be a relationship among thyroid functioning, stress, and a constitutional factor.

The effectiveness and ease of medical treatment of thyrotoxicosis in childhood usually makes formal psychotherapy unnecessary for the disorder itself. Successful treatment of adults by psychotherapy alone has been reported by Cope and his colleagues.[42] However, problems about dependency ordinarily continue, and psychotherapy may be indicated for the child and his parents. Lability of mood and occasionally intense projection may require at least brief psychotherapeutic intervention. Since surgery carries some risks, brief psychotherapy may help an essentially disturbed child to respond to medical measures or may prepare him for surgery.

Growth Failure. Growth failure in its various forms seems to involve certain psychophysiologic effects on endocrine functioning. These effects have not been fully clarified, however, and much overlapping with nutritional and other factors exists. Growth failure that occurs in situations involving psychosocial disruption has long been recognized by pediatricians. "Environmental deprivation," "maternal deprivation," and "sensory deprivation" have been used as descriptive terms,[67] as have "deprivation dwarfism" and "masked emotional deprivation" (which may be involved in the production of a variety of other disorders than growth failure), as Prugh and Harlow[192] have indicated. "Failure to thrive," which refers to a syndrome that arises from environmental stress and without relevant somatic etiologic factors, is a more broadly applicable term, and it is now generally accepted as differentiating the syndrome from other forms of growth failure.

As Barbero and his colleagues[8] have pointed out, the weight of infants and very young children who fail to thrive characteristically is below the third percentile on standard scales. Although weight-growth failure is often present, a delay in height gain is less common than is a delay in weight gain. A delay in the child's psychomotor development is often present although the child may not show significant lags in reaching his developmental milestones. In a few cases, only a developmental delay is present, without evidence of weight-growth failure. Apathy or, at times, extreme irritability may be present. Withdrawn behavior may predominate, or warding-off behavior involving the hands may be present.

Other symptoms (e.g., physical weakness, distended abdomen, vomiting, diarrhea, anemia, or recurrent respiratory infections) may be associated with a failure to thrive. These symptoms call for careful physical and laboratory studies, but they are generally secondary to the basic problem of deprivation.[137,179] In some cases, failure to thrive may be associated with a primary somatic disorder. The somatic disorder may not be sufficient to account for the growth failure, or it may have brought about family responses leading to failure to thrive.

In most instances, weight gain, acceleration in development, disappearance of associated symptoms, and behavioral improvement occur in several weeks when the child has been hospitalized for diagnostic study. The most important factor in the recovery seems to be an environment that provides adequate care and nurturing, with the use of parent-substitute relationships from foster grandmothers or other staff members ("replacement therapy") and work with the parents.

Reinhart and his colleagues[60] studied 40 families of infants and young children who had been hospitalized for failure to thrive. Most of the families were from lower socioeconomic groups. They had both rural and urban backgrounds, they tended to be isolated socially, and one-third of the fathers were absent from the home. Three groups were delineated, each comprising about one-third of the total. In the first group, adequate living conditions and good physical care of the child were noted. All the mothers were described as extremely depressed; they verbalized fears their children would die, or they perceived their children as retarded. All the mothers made efforts to feed and cuddle their babies although in a strained, unsure manner. All the mothers had had a severe loss (e.g., the death of a parent) within 4 months before their child's hospitalization, and they traced the breakdown in mothering to the loss. The mothers visited their children daily, accepted help in feeding and handling their children, and could express feelings of depression and ambivalence. The mothers were most responsive to follow-up contacts, and they showed improvement in nurturing their children and in their family's functioning. Long-term follow-up evaluation indicated that the children had maintained and extended their initial gains in weight, height, and development, and that they continued to thrive.

The families in the second group showed some similarities to those in the first group. They seemed to have fewer strengths, however, and to be unable to cope with crises and longstanding problems. Most were in the lowest socioeconomic group. Their living conditions were deprived, and the children had received poor physical care. The children in this group were often the youngest members of a large family. Most of the mothers showed severe depression that usually was compounded by marked or chronic medical problems, and they had marital difficulties. The mothers themselves had received poor mothering, they had experienced chronic economic and cultural deprivation, and they seemed helpless and uncertain about caring for their children. They perceived their children as being very ill or retarded. Most of these mothers were unable to relate easily to the hospital staff, and they needed much help with their economic and other needs. Although all the children improved dramatically in the hospital, most of the children did not maintain the improvement despite the valiant efforts of the staff to help the families. Improvement occurred only when there were occasional dramatic changes in the family's functioning, when a mother left an alcoholic, abusing husband, or when different parenting figures were involved. For the families who could not mobilize sufficient strengths, even when they had continued help, removal of the child from the home was seriously considered. In these families, the child's failure to thrive seemed to be not simply a product of a disturbed parent-child relationship but rather the result of severe socioeconomic deprivation that had its roots in the backgrounds of both parents.

In the third group, the families' living conditions were adequate, and the physical care of children had been generally good. All the mothers displayed overt and extreme anger and hostility, as well as antagonism and provocative behavior toward the hospital staff. They were overtly angry and often quite punitive toward their children, perceiving them as "bad" rather than ill or retarded. They seemed to identify the child with their own "bad" side and to project their anger onto the hospital staff. They denied guilt about or responsibility for their children's problems. These mothers seemed to have had poor mothering themselves, and they also seemed to have had difficulty in establishing meaningful relationships. They could not accept help from the hospital staff, and they generally rejected follow-up contacts. In some of these families, the other children showed failure to thrive and there was considerable evidence of physical abuse.* The children who remained in their homes showed continued retardation in growth and social functioning. Immediate removal of the child from the home was generally indicated because of gross family pathology.[198] When the children were removed, they improved dramatically.

Other studies[82] have agreed with the frequent need for foster home placement in certain families of children who fail to thrive and whose prognosis is guarded.* But there also seem to be some indications for treatment in the home.[82,137] In either case, good follow-up care must be given.[54] Even when the child's physical response is good, emotional, behavioral, and educational problems[115] are often present and continuing intellectual retardation has been reported. A nonjudgmental approach to the parents by the hospital's staff is important to help foster a therapeutic alliance. Guilt about the child's improvement in the hands of other people is common in the parents, and those feelings must be recognized and dealt with positively. Although failure to thrive often occurs in families from lower socioeconomic groups, it may occur at any socioeconomic level and it may overlap somewhat with battering and other types of child abuse.

Some investigators believe that the cause of the failure to thrive is related to nutritional deficiencies. In some cases, that may be true, or a lack of appetite may be a partial mechanism. But the disturbed parent-child relationship and the parents' inability to provide adequate warmth, nurturing, and appropriate stimulation seems to be basic to most cases.[267]

In some instances (e.g., older children who show the "deprivation dwarfism" picture described by Silver[227]) the child has a voracious appetite. In those instances, the child's growth hormone levels are low, normal, or borderline. Silver thinks that a functional insufficiency in the effects of growth hormone is the psychophysiologic mechanism. In another study,[130] 50% of the children who had "deprivation dwarfism" showed elevated cortisol secretion rates compared with those in the control group, who showed growth failure from other causes. Increased biologic activity of cortisol, resulting from stimulation of pituitary-adrenal cortical functioning by emotional stress, could produce a relative undernutrition in the child[179] despite his voracious appetite. Further studies are needed, but the psychophysiologic effects of chronic emotional conflict on endocrine functioning and interrelationships seem to be importantly involved. Constitutional factors may help determine whether weight-growth failure or developmental delay may predominate. Whether (as certain data suggest[212]) delayed puberty or delayed growth in adolescence may result from psychophysiologic influences remains to be more fully investigated.

---

*As indicated in Chapter 28, there is some overlap between failure to thrive and physical child abuse, and some workers suggest that these may occur along a continuum.[127]

Pseudocyesis. Pseudocyesis may occur in adolescents. It has also been reported in school-age girls (the youngest was 6 years old).[222] The enlargement of the abdomen that occurs may involve conversion mechanisms although increases in fatty tissue, gas, or fecal material have also been thought to be involved.[75] The physiologic changes of pregnancy which appear in most women who have pseudocyesis, (even the improvement of diabetic symptoms) seem to derive from psychophysiologic influences on endocrine functions.[93] Psychic factors seem to act on the hypothalamic-pituitary axis, causing a shift in the levels of various hormones.[242] Evidence of increased corpus luteum activity has been reported in some cases.[220] A full understanding of the psychophysiologic interrelationships has not been reached.

Although pseudocyesis often occurs in females who have hysterical personality disorders, it may sometimes occur early in the marriage in some young women who have milder developmental conflicts about their feminine identity and the assumption of the responsibilities of motherhood.[170] Women who have pseudocyesis generally have a conscious wish for a baby but often have unconscious fears or negative feelings about motherhood. In some more disturbed adolescent girls who have repressed knowledge of sexual matters because of serious conflicts, pseudocyesis may appear after the first experience of kissing or petting or with any genital contact.[124] Psychiatric consultation is indicated. Although a supportive, reality-oriented approach may suffice to bring about cessation of the symptoms of pregnancy, intensive psychotherapy and/or marital therapy may be needed to deal with the underlying personality problems.

Disorders in Lactation. This group includes cessation of milk flow related to acute emotional stress or intensified conflict.[171] A central inhibition of oxytocin has been demonstrated in such cases, presumably through hypothalamic-posterior pi-tuitary interconnections.[43] Supportive psychotherapy may lead to conflict resolution and the return of lactation.

Psychophysiologic Nervous System Disorders

These disorders include idiopathic epilepsy (petit mal, psychomotor equivalents, and grand mal), narcolepsy, motion sickness, some recurrent fevers of psychophysiologic origin, and hyperactivity. Psychophysiologic factors may be involved in certain types of dizziness, vertigo, and sleep disturbance.

Children who have so-called *idiopathic epilepsy* often have personality disturbances before the onset of epilepsy. The onset of the epilepsy itself frequently produces psychic trauma, and the disorder still carries stigma. Parents are often understandably anxious about the child's safety during a seizure, and often they are unrealistically restrictive about the child's activity. They tend to blame themselves for the hereditary factor. However, heredity is not as significant as many people believe. At least 10% of the general population—and many more, especially during the critical period of neural integration (3 to 9 years of age)—have abnormal EEG records but do not develop seizures.[162] Parents often unconsciously equate the child's seizure with death or "craziness," and they may fear what he will do during a seizure.

Children who have idiopathic epilepsy often have feelings of inferiority, of shyness, and of being different. Many epileptic children show inhibition of their aggression associated with an increase in seizure activity.[86] However, some may show irritability, temper outbursts, or aggressive behavior, particularly before a seizure. Children tend to have fears of death just before a seizure, and they may fear they have said or done something "bad" during the amnesic period afterward. They are often afraid to ask what happened. There is no type-specific epileptic personality. Most of the disturbances in behavior are the result of the reaction of the child and his parents to the illness.

With proper seizure control, few children who have the idiopathic type of epilepsy "deteriorate," intellectually or otherwise. The impression that such deterioration occurred came from the earlier tendency to include in this group children who have "symptomatic" epilepsy and who show brain damage due to trauma or disease and those who have reversible depression of mental activity caused by sedative drugs. The lack of educational and social opportunities for epileptic children, who formerly were kept out of school or away from normal social interaction, also contributed to the impression that they had deteriorated. Children who have febrile seizures in the preschool-age period are slightly more likely to later develop idiopathic epilepsy than are children who do not have febrile seizures. The former group may have a lowered convulsive threshold because of hereditary or other reasons.

Seizures occur more often during periods of emotional conflict or crisis within the family, sometimes with a build-up of tension. They are often precipitated initially in such a context.[86] Experimental studies of adolescents and adults have demonstrated paroxysmal changes in EEG activity[125] and the triggering of actual seizures[11] in response to the experiencing of different emotional states. Such emotional factors, involving hypothalamic-cortical interconnections, are regarded by some as the most common triggering factors. Fatigue, low blood sugar, head trauma, and other factors may also precipitate seizures in people who have a lowered threshold for convulsions.

The influences just mentioned are especially prominent in children who have *petit mal* epilepsy. Petit mal seizures involve brief "absences," and at times they are associated with minor motor or vegetative phenomena. Petit mal seizures occur most commonly during the school-age pe-

riod. Frequent seizures may interfere with school performance. Continuous seizures (petit mal status epilepticus) may be confused with functional psychosis.[263] With adequate medical treatment the prognosis is usually good, and petit mal epilepsy usually disappears by late adolescence. Children who have petit mal epilepsy are often inhibited emotionally, and they show considerable guilt and conflict about their feelings of anger.

Scolding, anxiety, upsetting sights, or unacceptable anger may all trigger petit mal attacks;[234] or the child may have attacks only in the presence of a parent with whom he is in conflict. Some adolescents can inhibit seizures, but the mechanism is poorly understood. Various types of sensory stimulation, often associated originally with a disturbing experience, may also serve to precipitate attacks (that have auditory, musicogenic,[70] television-like photosensitivity,[210] or "flicker fusion" effects). Some disturbed children when confronted by conflict situations may even touch off such attacks themselves by moving their fingers rapidly in front of their eyes or in other ways.[210] At times they use such attacks in a manipulative fashion.[139]

Psychomotor equivalents are encountered in school-age children. They may involve episodes of bizarre, automatic, or stereotyped movements that are associated with autonomic disturbances emanating from a temporal lobe focus. Some clouding of consciousness and partial or complete amnesia may occur. Chewing and smacking movements, incoherent or irrelevant speech, outbursts of rage, and confused or somnambulism-like states may appear suddenly, and last for a few minutes or for several hours. Such episodes often appear in relation to some emotional crisis.[209] At times, the content of the seizures may have psychodynamic significance[59] although the behavior is not organized or purposeful.

Other symptoms (e.g., headache, abdominal pain, and burst of destructive behavior) have been said to represent latent epilepsy or seizure equivalents. Attacks of paroxysmal pain, usually periumbilical in location and colicky in nature, have been described. They are associated with ictal discharge on the EEG, and they are often followed by sleep. Those attacks have been referred to as abdominal epilepsy or as abdominal migraine. Such attacks are quite rare, however,[52] and they should be differentiated from the recurrent abdominal pain mentioned earlier, as well as other types of pain. Headaches associated with ictal discharges are extremely rare. Ictal behavior disturbances are even rarer if they exist at all. (Children who have epilepsy may of course exhibit associated reactive, neurotic, or other disorders.) The tendency to make a diagnosis of "epileptic equivalent" on the basis of exaggerated fears, repeated tantrums, aggressive behavior, marked withdrawal, running away from home, or sleepwalking, combined with poorly defined abnormalities on the EEG, is far too widespread. Most of the children suspected of having epileptic equivalents show disturbances in behavior related to conflicts within the family, and "treatment of the EEG" with anticonvulsant medication is not indicated.

Grand mal seizures may also be precipitated by emotional conflicts, as well as by sensory stimulation, hyperventilation, lowered blood sugar levels, head trauma, or other stimuli. Voluntary arrest of grand mal seizures by changes in mental or physical activity has been reported in adolescents and adults, who often have had an aura.[143] Grand mal seizures must be differentiated from "hysterical" or conversion seizures that involve symbolic psychologic conversion mechanisms. Conversion symptoms are often admixed with those deriving from the epilepsy, and conversion "seizures" may continue after the epilepsy is controlled.

In treating these disorders, the pediatrician can help parents, through counseling and support, to see their child's illness more realistically and to deal with their guilt as well as with their fears of the child's death, mental illness, or retardation. He can help them to keep their anxiety from overrestricting the child (beyond such prohibitions as not to climb high trees and not to swim alone), and he can help the parents and child avoid oppositional struggles about drug therapy or other "control issues." Group discussions with parents[11a] and with children[49] have been helpful. Through a supportive relationship, the physician or health associate can help the child deal with his fears or social difficulties and can offer greater understanding of the child's problems to parents, teachers, or other adult figures.[143] The prognosis for response to treatment is good, as is the child's chance to live an independent, constructive life with few restrictions.

A few parents openly reject or stigmatize the child because of guilt or other feelings. In such a situation, early referral for psychiatric help is indicated. For more seriously disturbed children, psychotherapy for the child and his parents can help them deal with basic emotional conflicts.[86,234] It can help decrease the anxiety involved in emotional trigger mechanisms, and it can render drug therapy more effective. Family therapy has been reported to be beneficial.[139] A few children may require psychiatric hospitalization or residential treatment. Hypnosis has been reported to be effective in some children who have petit mal epilepsy.[81] Conditioning techniques have had some success on patients whose seizures had photosensitivity[210] and musicogenic components.[70]

If possible, the goal of therapy should be complete control of seizures. The threat of another seizure is devastating to some children and their parents. Nevertheless, care should be taken to avoid using too many or too high dosages of antiepileptic drugs, which may make the child "dopey" or even mildly delirious. In addition, the use of phenobarbital can result in paradoxic stimulation with resultant hyperactivity. This paradoxic effect is seen more frequently in preschool-age children. As in other psychophysiologic disorders or in any chronic illness, complete relief from symptoms may pose a problem in readaptation for children in families in which the child's invalidism has become a significant feature in the family's equilibrium.[65]

A variety of symptomatic pictures have frequently been thought to bear some relationship to idiopathic epilepsy. The association of epilepsy with migraine has already been mentioned, as has the lack of its association with syncope, recurrent abdominal pain, and cyclic vomiting. Narcolepsy is another disorder mentioned in this connection.

Narcolepsy is a syndrome characterized by paroxysmal and recurrent attacks of irresistible sleep, often precipitated by a sudden change in the person's emotional state that is related to a conflict situation.[134] Narcolepsy is uncommon in childhood, and it is said to occur more frequently in boys than in girls.[275] The attacks of overpowering sleep may come on suddenly during various activities. There may be one or two or many attacks a day. They may be associated with cataplexy[229] (sudden attacks of muscle weakness without loss of consciousness) and hypnagogic hallucinations, between waking and sleeping. The sleep during attacks is light, and the patient is easily awakened. Nocturnal sleep is usually normal.

Although some unknown biologic predisposing factor may be involved, the major factors seem to be psychopathologic,[11] often related to conflicts about independence or the handling of feelings of anger. The EEG recordings show signs of only light sleep during attacks and are otherwise normal. Although the course is generally chronic, spontaneous improvement may occur. Narcolepsy is to be differentiated from the Pickwickian syndrome,[30] in which sudden attacks of somnolence occur in markedly obese children and from so-called hysterical trance or dissociative states. Narcolepsy appears to bear no relationship to epilepsy. Stimulants, such as methylphenidate or the amphetamines, may be of some help in treatment, but intensive psychotherapy is often needed to deal with the patient's underlying conflicts.[155]

Motion sickness (including car sickness from riding in trains and elevators and on swings) is more common in children than in adults. Seasickness and sickness from riding in airplanes are less common. Vestibular irritation, autonomic responses, and psychologic factors are all probably involved to different degrees in different children. Motion sickness usually improves markedly by adolescence.[6] Tense, apprehensive children, or children who have psychoneurotic phobic pictures are most affected, and family arguments during driving are often a factor. Dramamine usually is of value in treatment, but psychotherapy may be necessary for phobic children.[202]

Fever of psychophysiologic origin may occur in certain children who show excitement[201] or continued emotional tension[85] in the absence of physical overactivity. Such fever may occur on a chronic low-grade basis in infants with "hospitalism"[266] or in school-age children who are chronically anxious. In the latter instance, the child's parents, especially his mother, are often overanxious, and they continue to take the child's temperature daily, long after a mild respiratory or other infection has subsided. The fever (generally under 101° F) usually disappears when the temperature taking stops. The physician should discuss the parents' fears, which may be related to guilt or other feelings rather than offer them blanket reassurance about the child's health. After the discussion, discharge from the hospital of an infant who has such a fever, but no other signs of physical illness usually brings his temperature down to normal.

Hyperactivity occurs in many children who have no signs of brain damage. (Brain damage and management of hyperactivity are discussed more fully in Chapters 22 and 28.) Anxious children who are active from birth may show hyperactivity associated with impulsivity and distractibility in response to anxiety they feel because of their parents' overrestrictiveness or other family tensions. Such hyperactivity may represent an intensification of a developmental deviation or a reactive disorder. Stimulants may help, as with hyperactive children who have brain damage, if the child is hyperactive at home as well as at school. Other psychologic measures should always be employed, however, and psychotherapy may be necessary, particularly for children who show hyperactivity only outside the home, perhaps in response to competition and other sources of anxiety.

Psychophysiologic Disorders of the Organs of Special Sense

These disorders include glaucoma (certain cases), keratitis, blepharospasm, Meniere's syndrome,[72] and certain types of tinnitus and hyperacusis. Most of the research that has indicated that psychophysiologic components precipitate or intensify these disorders has been done on adults.[40,219] In patients who have glaucoma (it is rare in children) an increased severity of eye symptoms and an elevation of intraocular pressure coincided with the accentuation of previous frustration or with threats to security.[278] In one study, these findings were replicable in interviews,[208] and in another study, hypnosis produced a significant lowering of intraocular pressure.[12] Other research has indicated that there is no specific glaucoma personality.

Treatment and Prognosis

When possible, prognosis and treatment were mentioned in the discussion of the specific syndromes. Many interacting factors are involved, including the nature and

degree of the patient's biologic predisposition, the severity of his personality disturbance and family disruption, the extent that psychosocial factors help perpetuate the disorder, and its response to psychotherapeutic treatment and medical treatment. In some disorders (e.g., failure to thrive in infancy), only treatment of the basic emotional deprivation, with replacement measures offered by parent substitutes, together with help for the parents, will bring about an improvement.[145] In disorders that have milder psychologic components (e.g., some cases of asthma), medical measures taken in the context of a supportive relationship with the physician or health associate will suffice.

Therapeutic Approach

The treatment of these disorders should be based on an adequate diagnostic evaluation and a weighting of the physical and psychologic factors. In potentially serious or life-threatening disorders, (e.g., ulcerative colitis and diabetes), psychotherapeutic measures should never be undertaken without concomitant medical treatment and follow-up care. In some milder disturbances, the pediatrician may use a supportive psychotherapeutic approach with child and parents, using child psychiatric consultation initially and as needed. If the patient is hospitalized, seeing the patient for brief periods at the beginning and/or the end of the day may be more effective than seeing him an hour or 2 a week. The patient is encouraged to be dependent on the pediatrician initially, with later gradual "weaning." If the psychophysiologic disorder continues, it becomes a chronic illness, and has the effect of a chronic illness on the child's growth and personality development and on his family as well. Again, the pediatrician sees some children and families in ambulatory practice who are able to cope surprisingly well with these disorders. Long-term follow-up may be indicated for some children, particularly those who have ulcerative colitis, who may have later exacerbations when they begin high school or go away to college, or make other major changes.

The Use of Psychotherapy

In more seriously disturbed children, intensive psychotherapy for the child and his parents may have to be carried out by a child psychiatrist or other mental health professional. In most such children, especially those who have ulcerative colitis and asthma, more supportive psychologic measures should be taken at the beginning, to avoid stirring up intense feelings that might lead to an exacerbation.[193] Later, a more intensive, insight-promoting approach may be employed as indicated,[120] including child analysis in some cases.[233] Formal psychotherapy, along with appropriate medical measures, has been reported to be effective in such disorders as asthma and other allergic problems, ulcerative colitis, anorexia nervosa, migraine headaches, and skin disorders. The efficacy of psychotherapy in other disorders, such as peptic ulcer, seems to vary. In hypertension, rheumatoid arthritis, and hyperthyroidism, the results are more difficult to evaluate.[34a] However, a supportive psychotherapeutic approach with children and parents should be considered part of a comprehensive therapeutic approach for all such disorders.

Collaboration and Coordination in the Approach to Treatment

In treating children with these disorders, the pediatrician must observe certain basic principles. *Continuity* of the relationship between the child and his parents and a single physician (and nurse or other professional when the child is in the hospital) is vital. *Communication* among professionals is needed to bring about good *collaboration* among the disciplines and consistency in management. *Consultation*

with child psychiatrists, psychologists, social workers, surgeons, and other specialists must be freely available and appropriately employed. Finally, *coordination* of all such activities must be effected if a unified plan of therapy that has a balance of physical, psychological, and social measures is to be evolved.

In many cases, the pediatrician is best equipped to coordinate a team approach to the management and treatment of children with these disorders. Coordination is easier to accomplish in the hospital, where professionals and nonprofessionals (e.g., foster grandparents or other parent substitutes) are freely available, and where a weekly or semiweekly ward management conference can help in observing the principles mentioned. A team approach can also be used by the pediatrician in private practice, with the help of social workers, nurses, medical aides (and other members of the newly evolving health team), and psychiatric, psychologic, and other consultants.

In some instances, the child who has a psychophysiologic disorder may be so disturbed that he may need psychiatric hospitalization. In such a case, the psychiatrist may act as the coordinator, drawing on the contributions of the pediatrician and other consultants regarding the medical or surgical aspects of treatment.

In all such efforts, close and cooperative contact with the parents should be maintained, in the context of a therapeutic alliance with the professional personnel involved. Also, competition for the exclusive care of the child by any one service or profession must be avoided if the child is to be treated as a human being and as a member of a family that needs help.

Suggested References

1. Aboulker, P., and Chertok, L.: Emotional factors in stress incontinence. Psychosom. Med., 24:507, 1962.
2. Agle, D.P., Ratnoff, O.D., and Wasman, M.:

Conversion reactions in autoerythrocyte sensitization. Arch. Gen. Psychiatry, *20*:438, 1969.

3. Allen, K.E., and Harris, F.R.: Elimination of a child's excessive scratching by training the mother in reinforcement procedure. Beh. Res. Ther., *4*:79, 1966.

4. Apley, J.: The child with recurrent abdominal pain. Pediatr. Clin. North Am., *14*:63, 1967.

5. Arajarvi, T., Pentti, R., and Aukee, M.: Ulcerative colitis in children: A clinical, psychological, and social follow-up study, Am. Pediatr. Fenn., *7*:259, 1962.

6. Bakwin, H., and Bakwin, R.M.: *Clinical Management of Behavior Disorders in Children,* 2nd Ed., Philadelphia, Saunders, 1958.

7. Barbero, G.J.: Cyclic vomiting. Pediatrics, *25*:740, 1960.

8. Barbero, G.J., and Shaheen, E.: Environmental failure to thrive: A clinical view. J. Pediatr., *71*:639, 1967.

9. Barchilon, J., and Engel, G.L.: Dermatitis: An hysterical conversion symptom in a young woman: psychosomatic conference. Psychosom. Med., *14*:295, 1952.

10. Bardwick, J.M., and Behrman, S.J.: Investigation into the effects of anxiety, sexual arousal, and menstrual cycle phase on uterine contractions. Psychosom. Med., *29*:468, 1967.

11. Barker, W.: Studies in epilepsy: Personality patterns, situational stress, and the symptoms of narcolepsy. Psychosom. Med., *10*:193, 1948.

11a.Baus, G., Letson, L., and Russell, E.: Group sessions for parents of children with epilepsy. J. Pediatr., *52*:270, 1958.

12. Berger, A.S., and Simel, P.J.: Effect of hypnosis on intraocular pressure in normal and glaucomatous subjects. Psychosom Med., *20*:321, 1958.

13. Berger, M., Gribetz, D., and Korelitz, B.I.: Growth retardation in children with ulcerative colitis: The effect of medical and surgical therapy. Pediatrics, *55*:459, 1975.

14. Bergman, R., and Aldrich, C.K.: The natural history of infantile eczema. Psychosom. Med., *25*:495, 1963.

15. Berlin, I.N., et al.: Adolescent alteration of anorexia and obesity. Am. J. Orthopsychiatry, *31*:228, 1957.

16. Berlin, I.N., and Szurek, S.A., Eds.: Psychosomatic disorders in childhood: An overview. In: *Psychosomatic Disorders and Mental Retardation in Children. The Langley Porter Child Psychiaty Series,* Vol. 3. (S.A. Szurek and I.N. Berlin, Eds.). Palo Alto, Calif., Science and Behavior Books, 1968.

17. Berlin, I.N., et al.: Intractable episodic vomiting in a 3 year old child. Psychiatr. Q., *31*:1, 1957.

18. Blank, H. and Brody, M.W.: Recurrent herpes simplex: A psychiatric and laboratory study. Psychosom. Med., *12*:254, 1950.

19. Blinder, B.J., Freeman, D.M.A., and Stunkard, A.J.: Behavior therapy of anorexia nervosa. Am. J. Psychiatry, *126*:1093, 1970.

20. Bliss, E.L., and Branch, C.H.: *Anorexia Nervosa.* New York, Hoeber, 1960.

21. Blitzer, J.R., Rollins, N., and Blackwell, A.: Children who starve themselves: Anorexia nervosa. Psychosom. Med., *23*:369, 1961.

22. Block, J., et al.: Interaction between allergic potential and psychopathology in childhood asthma. Psychosom. Med., *26*:307, 1964.

23. Blom, G., and Nicholos, G.: Emotional factors in children with rheumatoid arthritis. Am. J. Orthopsychiatry, *24*:588, 1954.

24. Bos, C., and Cleghorn, R.A.: Psychogenic Sterility. Fertil. Steril., *9*:84, 1956.

25. Boswell, J.: Hyperthyroid children: Individual and family dynamics, A study of 12 cases. J. Am. Acad. Child. Psychiatry, *6*:64, 1967.

26. Bruch, H.: *The Importance of Overweight.* New York, Norton, 1957.

27. Bruch, H.: Psychotherapy in primary anorexia nervosa. J. Nerv. Ment. Dis., *150*:51, 1970.

28. Bruch, H.: *Eating Disorders: Obesity, Anorexia Nervosa, and the Person Within.* New York, Basic Books, 1973.

29. Budzynski, T.H., Stoyva, J.M., and Adler, C.S.: Feedback-induced muscle relaxation: Application to tension headache. Behav. Ther. Exp. Psychiatry, *1*:205, 1970.

30. Burwell, C.S., et al.: Extreme obesity associated with alveolar hypoventilation—A pickwickian syndrome. Am. J. Med., *21*:819, 1956.

31. Cain, A.C., et al.: Children's disturbed reactions to their mother's miscarriage. Psychosom. Med., *26*:58, 1964.

32. Call, J.D., et al.: Psychogenic megacolon in 3 preschool boys: A study of etiology through collaborative treatment of child and parents. Am. J. Orthopsychiatry, *33*:923, 1963.

33. Campagne, W.V.L.: Ein Enquite Bij Coeliakpatienten, Luctor Emergo, Leiden, Drukkerij, 1960.

34. Castelnuovo-Tedesco, P., and Schnabel, D.: Studies of super-obesity. II. Psychiatric appraisal of jejuno-ileal bypass surgery. Am. J. Psychiatry, *133*:26, 1976.

34a.Chalke, F.C.R.: Effect of psychotherapy for psychosomatic disorders. Psychosomatics, *6*:125, 1965.

35. Chase, H.P., et al.: *Understanding Juvenile Diabetes: A Manual for Children with Diabetes and Their Parents.* 3rd Ed. Fort Collins, Colo., The Old Army Press, 1977.

36. Clamage, D.M., Vander, A.J., and Mouro, D.R.: Psychosoial stimuli and human plasma renin activity. Psychosom. Med., *39*:393, 1977.

37. Cleveland, S.E., and Johnson, D.L.: Personality patterns in young males with coronary disease. Psychosom. Med., *24*:600, 1962.

38. Cleveland, S.E., Reitmann, E.E., and Brewer, E.J.: Psychological factors in juvenile rheumatoid arthritis. Arthritis Rheum., *8*:1152, 1965.

39. Coddington, R.D.: Peptic ulcers in children. Psychosomatics, *9*:38, 1968.

40. Coleman, D.: Psychosomatic aspects of disease of the ear, nose and throat. Laryngoscope, *59*:709, 1949.

41. Conn, J.W., and Seltzer, H.S.: Spontaneous hypoglycemia. Am. J. Med., *19*:460, 1955.

42. Cope, O.: *Man, Mind, and Medicine.* Philadelphia, Lippincott, 1967.

43. Cross, B.A.: Neurohumoral mechanisms in emotional imbalance of milk ejection. J. Endocrinol., *12:*29, 1955.

44. Dalton, K.: Children's hospital admissions and mother's menstruation. Brittania Med. Journal, 2:27, 1970.

45. Datey, K.K., et al.: Shavasan: A yogic exercise in the management of hypertension. Angiology, 20:325, 1969.

46. Davenport, C.W., et al.: Cyclic vomiting. J. Am. Acad. Child. Psychol., *11:*66, 1972.

47. Davidson, M., Bloom, A.A., and Kugler, M.M.: Chronic ulcerative colitis of childhood: An evaluative review. J. Pediatr., *67:*47, 1965.

48. Davidson, M., and Wasserman, R.: The irritable colon of childhood (chronic nonspecific diarrhea syndrome). J. Pediatr., *69:*1027, 1966.

49. Defries, Z., and Browder, S.: Group therapy with epileptic children and their mothers. Bull. N.Y. Acad. Med., *28:*235, 1952.

50. Dongier, M., et al.: Psychophysiological studies in thyroid function. Psychosom. Med., *18:*310, 1956.

51. Doster, M.E., et al.: Data on incidence and degree of dysmenorrhea. American J. Public Health, *51:*1845, 1961.

52. Douglas, E.F., and White, P.T.: Abdominal epilepsy: A reappraisal. J. Pediatr., *78:*59, 1971.

53. Dreyfus, F.: Coagulation time of blood, level of blood eosinophils, and thrombocytes under emotional stress. Psychosom. Med., *1:*252, 1956.

54. Elmer, E., Gregg, G.S., and Ellison, P.: Late results of failure to thrive syndrome. Clin. Pediatrics, *8:*584, 1969.

55. Emery, E.S.: Acute confusional state in children with migraine. Pediatrics, *68:*110, 1977.

56. Engel, G.L.: *Fainting: Physiological and Psychological Considerations,* 2nd Ed. Springfield, Ill., Thomas, 1962.

56a.Engel, G.L.: Psychological aspects of gastrointestinal disorders. *American Handbook of Psychiatry,* Vol. 4 (S. Arieti, Ed.). New York, Basic Books, 1976.

57. Engels, W.D., Pattee, C.J., and Wittkower, E.D.: Emotional settings of functional amenorrhea. Psychosom. Med., *26:*682, 1964.

58. Enzer, N.B., and Walker, P.A.: Hyperventilation syndrome in childhood. J. Pediatr., *70:*521, 1967.

59. Epstein, A.W., and Ervin, F.: Psychodynamic significance of seizure content in psychomotor epilepsy. Psychosom. Med., *18:*43, 1956.

60. Evans, S.L., Rheinhart, J.B., and Succop, R.A.: Failure to thrive: A study of 45 children and their families. J. Am. Acad. Child. Psychiatry, *11:*440, 1972.

61. Falstein, E.I., Feinstein, S.C., and Judas, I.: Anorexia nervosa in the male child. Am. J. Orthopsychiatry, *26:*751, 1956.

62. Falstein, E.I., and Judas, I.: Juvenile diabetes and its psychiatric implications. Am. J. Orthopsychiatry, *25:*330, 1955.

63. Falstein, E.J., and Rosenblum, A.H.: Juvenile paroxysmal supraventricular tachycardia: Psychosomatic and psychodynamic aspects. J. Am. Acad. Child Psychiatry, *1:*246, 1962.

64. Faulkner, W.B.: Severe aesophageal spasm. Psychosom. Med., *2:*139, 1940.

65. Ferguson, S.M., and Rayport, M.: The adjustment to living without epilepsy. J. Nerv. Ment. Dis., *140:*26, 1965.

66. Ferholt, J., and Provence, S.: Diagnosis and treatment of an infant with psychophysiological vomiting. Psychoanal. Study Child., *31:*439, 1976.

67. Fischoff, J., Whitten, C.F., and Pettit, M.G.: A psychiatric study of mothers and infants with growth failure secondary to maternal deprivation. J. Pediatr., *79:*209, 1971.

68. Flagg, G.W., et al.: A psychophysiological investigation of hyperthyroidism. Psychosom. Med., *27:*497, 1965.

69. Ford, C.V., Bray, G.A., and Swerdloff, R.S.: A psychiatric study of patients referred with a diagnosis of hypoglycemia. Am. J. Psychiatry, *133:*290, 1976.

70. Forster, F.M., et al.: Modification of musicogenic epilepsy by extinction technique. Proc. 8th Int. Congr. Neurol., *4:*269, 1965.

71. Forsyth, C.C., and Payne, W.W.: Free diets in the treatment of diabetic children. Arch. Dis. Child., *31:*245, 1956.

72. Fowler, E.P., and Zeckel, A.: Psychosomatic aspects of Meniere's disease. J. Am. Med. Assoc., *148:*1265, 1952.

73. Freeman, E.H., et al.: Psychological variables in allergic disorders: A review. Psychosom. Med., *26:*543, 1964.

74. Freis, E.D.: Age, race, sex, and other indices of risks in hypertension. Am. J. Med., *55:*275, 1973.

75. Fried, P., et al.: Pseudocyesis: A psychosomatic study in gynecology. JAMA, *145:*1329, 1951.

76. Friedman, A., and Harms, E.: *Headaches in Children.* Springfield, Ill., Thomas, 1967.

77. Friedman, M., and Roseman, R.H.: Type A behavior pattern: Its association with coronary heart disease. Ann. Clin. Res., *3:*300, 1971.

78. Frisk, M., Widholm, O., and Hortling, H.: Dysmenorrhea—psyche and soma in teenagers. Acta Obstet. Gynecol. Scand., *44:*339, 1965.

79. Galdston, R.: Mind Over Matter: Observations on 50 patients hospitalized with anorexia nervosa. J. Am. Acad. Child Psychiatry, *13:*246, 1974.

80. Garder, L.J., and Reyersback, G.C.: Brain damage in juvenile diabetic patients associated with insulin hypoglycemia. Pediatrics, *7:*210, 1951.

81. Gardner, G.G.: Use of hypnosis for psychogenic epilepsy in a child. Am. J. Hypn., *15:*166, 1973.

82. Glaser, H.H., et al.: Physical and psychological development of children with early failure to thrive. J. Pediatrics., *73:*690, 1968.

83. Goetz, P.L., Succop, R.A., Reinhart, J.B.: Anorexia nervosa in children: A follow-up study. Am. J. Orthopsychiatry, *47:*597, 1977.

84. Golden, G.S.: The Alice in Wonderland syndrome in juvenile migraine. Pediatrics, *63:*517, 1979.

85. Goodell, H., Graham, D.T., and Wolff, H.G.: Changes in body heat regulation associated with varying life situations and emotional states. In: *Life Stress and Bodily Disease.* (H.G. Wolff, S.G.

Wolf, and C.C. Hare, Eds.). Baltimore, Williams and Wilkins, 1950.

86. Gottschalk, L.A.: Effects of intensive psychotherapy on epileptic children. Arch. Neurol. Psychiatry, 70:361, 1953.

87. Grace, W.J.: Life stress and regional enteritis. Gastroenterology, 23:542, 1953.

88. Grace, W.J., Wolf, S., and Wolff, H.G.: *The Human Colon*. New York, Hoeber, 1951.

88a. Graham, D.T.: The Pathogenesis of Hives: Experimental study of life situations, emotions, and cutaneous vascular reactions. In: *Life Stress and Bodily Disease*. (H.G. Wolff, S.G. Wolf, and C.G. Hare, Eds.). Baltimore, Williams and Wilkins, 1950.

89. Graham, D.T.: The relation of psoriasis to attitudes and to vascular reactions of the human skin. J. Invest. Dermatol., 22:379, 1954.

90. Graham, D.T.: Cutaneous vascular reactions in Raynaud's disease and in states of hostility, anxiety, and depression. Psychosom. Med., 17:200, 1955.

91. Graham, D.T.: Conditioned modification of arrhythmias. In: *New Applications of Conditioning to Medical Practice*. Madison, University of Wisconsin Press, 1972.

92. Grant, J.: Unpublished material.

93. Greaves, D.C., Green, P.E., and West, L.J.: Psychodynamic and psychophysiological aspects of pseudocyesis. Psychosom. Med., 22:24, 1960.

94. Green, M.: Psychogenic recurrent abdominal pain: Diagnosis and treatment. Pediatrics, 40:84, 1967.

95. Green, M.: Headaches. In: *Ambulatory Pediatrics*. (M. Green and R. Haggerty, Eds.). Philadelphia, Saunders, 1968.

95a. Green, M.: Fainting. In: *Ambulatory Pediatrics*. (M. Green and R. Haggerty, Eds.). Philadelphia, Saunders, 1968.

96. Grimm, E.: Psychological investigations of habitual abortion. Psychosom. Med., 24:369, 1962.

97. Ham, G.C., Alexander, F., and Carmichael, H.T.: A psychosomatic theory of thyrotoxicosis. Psychosom. Med., 13:18, 1951.

98. Hamburg, D.A., Moos, R.H., and Yalom, J.D.: Studies of distress in the menstrual cycle and the postpartum period. *Endocrinol. Human Behavior* (R. Michael, Ed.). London, Oxford University Press, 1968.

99. Hamburger, W.W.: Psychological aspects of obesity. Bull. N.Y. Acad. Med., 33:771, 1957.

100. Hamburger, W.W., Reiser, M., and Plunkett, J.: Electroencephalographic and psychological studies of a case of migraine with severe preheadache phenomena with concomitant cerebral vasospasm and focal hypertensive encephalopathy. Psychosom. Med., 15:337, 1953.

101. Hammond, J.: The late sequelae of recurrent vomiting of childhood. Dev. Med. Child Neurol., 16:15, 1974.

102. Harburg, E.: Socio-ecological stress, suppressed hostility, skin color, and black-white male blood pressure: Detroit. Psychosom. Med., 35:276, 1973.

103. Harms, E., Ed.: *Somatic and Psychiatric Aspects of Childhood Allergies*, Vol. I. (International Series of Monographs on Child Psychiatry.) Macmillan, New York, 1963.

104. Heald, F.P., et al.: Dysmenorrhea in adolescence. Pediatrics, 20:121, 1957.

105. Heiman, M.: The role of stress situations and psychological factors in functional uterine bleeding. J. Mt. Sinai Hosp., 23:755, 1956.

106. Henry, J.P., Meehan, J.P., and Stephens, P.: The use of psychosocial stimulation to induce prolonged systolic hypertension in mice. Psychosom. Med., 29:408, 1967.

107. Henry, J.P.: Relaxation methods and the control of blood pressure. Psychosom. Med., 40:273, 1978.

107a. Hinkle, L.E., and Wolf, S.: A summary of experimental evidence relating life stress to diabetes mellitus. J. Mt. Sinai Hosp., 19:537, 1952.

108. Hirt, M., et al.: The relationship beween dysmenorrhea and selected personality variables. Psychosomatics, 8:350, 1967.

109. Hollender, M.H., Soults, F.B., and Ringold, A.L.: Emotional antecedents of bleeding from peptic ulcer. Psychiatr. Med., 2:199, 1971.

110. Holmes, T.H., et al.: *The Nose: An Experimental Study of Reactions Within the Nose in Human Subjects During Varying Life Experiences*. Springfield, Ill., Thomas, 1949.

111. Holmes, T.H., Treuting, T., and Wolff, H.G.: Life situations, emotions, and nasal disease: Evidence on summative effects exhibited in patients with hay fever. Psychosom. Med., 13:71, 1951.

112. Holmes, T.H., and Wolff, H.G.: Life situations, emotions and backache. Psychosom. Med., 14:18, 1952.

113. Holquin, J., and Fenichel, G.: Migraine. J. Pediatr., 70:290, 1962.

114. Hoyt, C.S., and Stickler, G.G.: A study of 44 children with the syndrome of recurrent (cyclic) vomiting. Pediatrics, 25:775, 1960.

115. Hutton, I.N., and Oates, R.K.: Nonorganic failure to thrive: A long term follow-up. Pediatrics, 59:73, 1977.

116. Illingworth, R.S.: Practical observations and reflections. II. Vomiting without organic cause. Clin. Pediatr., 4:865, 1965.

117. Illingworth, R.S., and Holt, K.S.: Transient rash and hematuria after exercise and emotion. Arch. Dis. Child., 32:254, 1957.

118. Jacobs, M.A., et al.: Interaction of psychologic and biologic predisposing factors in allergic disorders. Psychosom. Med., 29:572, 1967.

119. Janowsky, D.S., Berens, S.C., and Davis, J.M.: Correlations between mood, weight, and electrolytes during the menstrual cycle: A renin-angiotensin-aldosterone hypothesis of premenstrual tension. Psychosom. Med., 35:143, 1973.

120. Jessner, L.: Psychotherapy of children with psychosomatic disorders. In: *The Practice of Psychotherapy with Children* (M. Hammer and A.M. Kaplan, Eds.). Homewood, Ill., Dorsey Press, 1967.

121. Kahn, E.J.: Obesity in children: Identification of a group at high risk in a New York ghetto. J. Pediatr., 77:771, 1970.

122. Kaij, L., et al.: Psychiatric aspects of spontaneous abortion. II. The importance of bereavement, attachment, and neurosis in early life. J. Psychosom. Res., 13:53, 1969.

123. Kaplan, H., and Reisch, M.: Universal alopecia: A psychosomatic appraisal. N.Y. State J. Med., 52:1144, 1952.

124. Kaplan, A.J., and Schopbach, R.R.: Pseudocyesis: A psychiatric study. Arch. Neurol. Psychiatry, 65:121, 1951.

125. Kemph, J.P., and Feldman, B.H.: A case study of some emotional factors affecting paroxysmal cerebral activity during interviews. J. Am. Acad. Child Psychiatry, 7:663, 1968.

126. Kluger, J.M.: Childhood asthma and the social milieu. J. Am. Acad. Child Psychiatry, 8:353, 1969.

127. Koel, B.S.: Failure to thrive and fatal injury as a continuum. Am. J. Dis. Child., 118:565, 1969.

128. Kraft, I.A., and Ardali, C.: A psychiatric study of children with diagnosis of regional ileitis. South. Med. J., 57:799, 1964.

129. Kraus, S.J.: Stress, acne, skin surface free fatty acids. Psychosom. Med., 32:503, 1970.

130. Krieger, I., and Good, M.H.: Adrenalcortical and thyroid function in the deprivation syndrome: Comparison with growth failure due to undernutrition, congenital heart disease or prenatal influences. Am. J. Dis. Child., 120:95, 1970.

131. Kroger, W.S., and Freed, S.C.: *Psychosomatic Gynecology*. Hollywood, Calif., Wilshire, 1962.

132. Krupp, G.R., and Friedman, A.P.: Migraine in children: A report of fifty children. Am. J. Dis. Child., 85:146, 1953.

133. Langford, W.S.: The psychological aspects of ulcerative colitis. Clin. Proc. Child. Hosp. Wash., D.C., 20:89, 1964.

134. Langworthy, O.R., and Betz, B.J.: Narcolepsy as a type of response to emotional conflicts. Psychosom. Med., 6:211, 1944.

135. Laybourne, P.C.: Psychogenic vomiting in children. Am. J. Dis. Child., 86:726, 1953.

136. Leiken, S.J., and Caplan, H.: Psychogenic polydipsia. Am. J. Psychiatry, 123:1563, 1967.

137. Leonard, M.F., Rymes, J.P., and Solnit, A.J.: Failure to thrive in infants: A family problem. Am. J. Dis. Child., 111:600, 1966.

138. Lesser, L.J., et al.: Anorexia nervosa in children. Am. J. Orthopsychiatry, 30:572, 1960.

139. Libo, S.S., Palmer, C., and Archibald, D.: Family group therapy for children with self-induced seizures. Am. J. Orthopsychiatry, 41:506, 1971.

140. Lidz, T., and Whitehorn, J.C.: Life situations, emotions, and Graves' disease. Psychosom. Med., 12:184, 1950.

141. Liebman, R., Minuchin, S., and Baker, L.: The role of the family in the treatment of anorexia nervosa. J. Am. Acad. Child. Psychiatry, 13:264, 1974.

142. Lindahl, M.W.: Psychogenic purpura: Report of a case. Psychosom. Med., 39:358, 1977.

143. Livingston, S.: The social management of the epileptic child and his parents. J. Pediatr., 51:137, 1957.

144. Long, R.T., et al.: The psychosomatic study of allergic and emotional factors in children with asthma. Am. J. Psychiatry, 115:114, 1958.

145. Lourie, R.S.: Experience with therapy of psychosomatic problems in infants. In: *Psychopathology in Childhood* (T. Hock & J. Zubin, Eds.). New York, Grune & Stratton, 1955.

146. Lucas, A.R., Duncan, J.W., and Piens, V.: The treatment of anorexia nervosa. Am. J. Psychiatry, 133:1034, 1976.

147. McAnarney, E.G., et al.: Psychological problems of children with chronic juvenile arthritis. Pediatrics, 53:523, 1974.

148. McDermott, J.F., and Finch, S.M.: Ulcerative colitis in children: Reassessment of a dilemma. J. Am. Acad. Child. Psychiatry, 6:512, 1967.

149. McKegney, F.P., and Williams, R.B.: Psychological aspects of hypertension. II. The differential influence of interview variables on blood pressure. Am. J. Psychiatry, 123:1539, 1967.

150. McKegney, F.P., et al.: A psychosomatic comparison of patients with ulcerative colitis and Crohn's disease. Psychosom. Med., 32:153, 1970.

151. McMahon, J.M., et al.: The psychosomatic aspects of cardiospasm. Ann. Int. Med., 34:608, 1951.

152. Malmquist, A., et al.: Psychiatric aspects of spontaneous abortion. I. A matched control study of women with living children. J. Psychosom. Res., 13:45, 1969.

153. Mann, E.C.: Habitual abortion. Am. J. Obstet. Gynecol., 77:706, 1959.

154. Manson, G.: Neglected children and the celiac syndrome. J. Iowa Med. Soc., 54:228, 1964.

155. Markowitz, I.: Psychotherapy of narcolepsy in an adolescent boy: Case presentation. Psychiatr. Q., 31:41, 1957.

156. Marmor, J., et al.: The mother-child relationship in the genesis of neurodermatitis. Arch. Dermatol., 74:599, 1956.

157. Masland, R.P., Heald, F.P., and Goodale, W.T.: Hypertensive vascular disease in adolescence. N. Engl. J. Med., 255:894, 1956.

158. Mattsson, A., Gross, S., and Hall, T.W.: Psychoendocrine study of adaptation in young hemophiliacs. Psychosom. Med., 33:215, 1971.

159. Mehlman, R.D., and Griesemer, R.D.: Alopecia areata in the very young. Am. J. Psychiatry, 125:605, 1968.

160. Mendels, J.: Stress polycythemia. Am. J. Psychiatry, 123:1570, 1967.

161. Menkes, M.M.: Personality characteristics and family roles of children with migraine. Pediatrics, 53:560, 1974.

162. Metcalf, D.R., and Jordan, K.: EEG ontogenesis in normal children. In: *Drugs, Development and Cerebral Function* (W.L. Smith Ed.). Springfield, Ill., Thomas, 1971.

163. Meyerowitz, S.: The continuing investigation of psychosocial variables in rheumatoid arthritis. In: *Modern Trends in Rheumatology*. (A.G.S. Hill, Ed.). London, Butterworth, 1971.

164. Millar, T.P.: Peptic ulcers in children. In: *Modern Perspectives in International Child Psychiatry*. (J.G. Howells, Ed.). Edinburgh, Oliver and Boyd, 1969.

165. Miller, H., and Baruch, D.W.: Psychotherapy of parents of allergic children. Ann. Allergy, *18*:990, 1960.

166. Millet, J.A.P., Lief, H., and Mittelmann, B.: Raynaud's disease: Psychogenic factors and psychotherapy. Psychosom. Med., *15*:61, 1953.

167. Mirsky, I.A.: Physiologic, psychologic, and social determinants in the etiology of duodenal ulcer. Am. J. Dig. Dis., *3*:285, 1958.

168. Mohr, G.J., et al.: Studies of eczema and asthma in the preschool child. J. Am. Acad. Child Psychiatry, *2*:271, 1963.

169. Moore, N.: Behavior therapy in bronchial asthma: A controlled study. J. Psychosom. Res., *9*:257, 1965.

170. Moulton, R.: The psychosomatic implications of pseudocyesis. Psychosom. Med., *4*:376, 1942.

171. Newton, N., and Newton, M.: Psychological aspects of lactation. N. Engl. J. Med., *277*:1179, 1969.

172. Nora, J.J., and Nora, A.H.: The pediatric roots of coronary heart disease. Chest., *68*:714, 1975.

173. Obermayer, M.E.: *Psychocutaneous Medicine.* Springfield, Ill., Thomas, 1955.

174. O'Connor, J.: Prognostic implications of psychiatric diagnosis in ulcerative colitis. Psychosom. Med., *28*:375, 1966.

175. Ogston, D., MacDonald, G.A., and Fullerton, H.W.: The influence of anxiety in tests of blood coaguality and fibrinolytic activity. Lancet, 2:521, 1962.

176. Orbach, C., and Tallent, N.: Modification of perceived body and of body concepts. Arch. Gen. Psychiatry, *12*:126, 1965.

177. Ostfeld, N.M., and Lebowits, B.Z.: Personality factors and pressor mechanisms in renal and essential hypertension. Arch. Intern. Med., *104*:43, 1959.

178. Palti, Z.: Psychogenic male infertility. Psychosom. Med., *31*:326, 1969.

179. Patton, R.G., and Gardner, L.L.: *Growth Failure in Maternal Deprivation.* Springfield, Ill., Thomas, 1963.

180. Penick, S.B., et al.: Behavior modification in the treatment of obesity. Psychosom. Med., *33*:49, 1971.

181. Pfeiffer, J.B., and Wolff, H.G.: Studies in renal circulation during periods of life stress and accompanying emotional reactions in subjects with and without essential hypertension: Observations on the role of neural activity in regulation of renal blood flow. J. Clin. Invest., *29*:1227, 1950.

182. Pinkerton, P.: Psychogenic megacolon in children: The implications of bowel negativism. Arch. Dis. Child., *33*:371, 1958.

183. Pinkerton, P., and Weaver, C.M.: Childhood asthma. In: *Modern Trends in Psychosomatic Medicine.* (O.M. Hill, Ed.). London, Butterworth, 1970.

184. Portis S.A.: Life situations, emotions, and hyperinsulinism. In: *Life Stress and Bodily Disease,* Vol. 29. (H.G. Wolff, and C.G. Hare, Eds.) Baltimore, Williams & Wilkins, 1950.

185. Powers, D.: Emotional implications of acne. N.Y. State J. Med., *57*:751, 1957.

186. Prouty, M.: Peptic ulcers in childhood. Pediatr. Digest, *9*:35, 1967.

187. Prugh, D.G.: A preliminary report on the role of emotional factors in idiopathic celiac disease. Psychosom. Med., *13*:200, 1951.

188. Prugh, D.G.: Psychological and psychophysiological aspects of oral activities in childhood. Pediatr. Clin. North Am., *3*:1049, 1956.

189. Prugh, D.G.: Some psychological problems concerned with the problem of overnutrition. Am. J. Clin. Nutr., *9*:538, 1961.

190. Prugh, D.G.: Natural history of children with chronic diarrhea. In: *Psychosomatic Aspects of Gastrointestinal Illness in Childhood.* (Report of the 44th Ross Conference on Pediatric Research.) Columbus, Ohio, Ross Laboratories, 1963.

191. Prugh, D.G.: Psychophysiological aspects of inborn errors of metabolism. In: *The Psychological Basis of Medical Practice.* (H.I. Lief, V.F. Lief, and N.R. Lief, Eds.). New York, Harper & Row (Hoeber), 1963.

192. Prugh, D.G., and Harlow, R.G.: Masked deprivation in infants and young children. In: *Deprivation of Maternal Care: A Reassessment of Its Effects.* Public Health Papers No. 14. Geneva, World Health Organization, 1962.

193. Prugh, D.G., and Jordan, K.: The management of ulcerative colitis in childhood. In: *Modern Perspectives in International Child Psychiatry.* (J.G. Howells, Ed.). London, Oliver and Boyd, 1969.

194. Prugh, D.G., and Schwachman, H.: Observations on "unexplained" chronic diarrhea in early childhood. Society transactions. Am. J. Dis. Child., *90*:496, 1955.

195. Purcell, K.: Critical appraisal of psychosomatic studies of asthma. N. Y. State J. Med., *65*:2103, 1965.

196. Rahe, R.H., and Christ, A.E.: An unusual cardiac (ventricular) arrhythmia in a child: Psychiatric and psychophysiological aspects. Psychosom. Med., *28*:181, 1966.

197. Rees, L.: Physiogenic and psychogenic factors in vasomotor rhinitis. J. Psychosom. Res., *8*:101, 1964.

198. Reinhart, J.B., and Drosh, A.L.: Psychosocial dwarfism: Environmentally induced recovery. Psychosom. Med., *31*:165, 1969.

199. Reinhart, J.B., Evans, S.L., and McFadden, D.J.: Cyclic vomiting in children: Seen through the psychiatrist's eye. Pediatrics, *59*:371, 1977.

200. Reiser, M.F., Ferris, E.B., and Levine, M.: Cardiovascular Disorders, Heart Disease, and Hypertension. In: *Recent Developments in Psychosomatic Medicine.* (E.D. Wittkower, and R.A. Cleghorn, Eds.). Philadelphia, Lippincott, 1957.

201. Renbourn, E.T.: Body temperature and pulse rate in boys and young men prior to sporting contests, a study of emotional hyperthemia: With a review of the literature. J. Psychosom. Res., *4*:149, 1960.

202. Reinhart, R.F.: Motion sickness: A psychophysiological gastrointestinal reaction. Aerosp. Med., *30*:802, 1959.

203. Reinhart, J.B., Kenna, M.D., and Succop, R.A.:

Anorexia nervosa in children: Outpatient management. J. Am. Acad. Child Psychiatry, *11*:114, 1972.

204. Reinhart, J.B., and Succop, R.A.: Regional enteritis in pediatric patients: Psychiatric aspects. J. Am. Acad. Child Psychiatry, *7*:252, 1968.

205. Richmond, J.B.: Discussion of juvenile paroxysmal supraventricular tachycardia: Psychosomatic and psychodynamic aspects. J. Am. Acad. Child Psychiatry, *1*:265, 1962.

206. Richmond, J.B., Eddy, E.J., and Garrard, S.D.: The syndrome of fecal soiling and megacolon. Am. J. Orthopsychiatry, *24*:391, 1954.

207. Ripley, H.S., et al.: Disturbances of bladder function associated with emotional states. J. Am. Med. Assoc., *141*:1139, 1949.

208. Ripley, H.S., and Wolff, H.G.: Life situations, emotions, and glaucoma. Psychosom. Med., *12*:215, 1950.

209. Robertiello, R.C.: Psychomotor epilepsy in children. Dis. Nerv. Syst., *14*:337, 1953.

210. Robertson, E.: Photogenic epilepsy: Self-precipitated attacks. Brain, *77*:232, 1964.

211. Romano, J., and Engel, G.L.: Studies of syncope. III. Differentiation between vasodepressor and hysterical fainting. Psychosom. Med., *7*:3, 1945.

212. Rosenbaum, M.: The role of psychological factors in delayed growth in adolescence: A case report. Am. J. Orthopsychiatry, *29*:762, 1959.

213. Rosenman, R.H., et al.: Clinically unrecognized myocardial infarction in the Western Collaborative Group Study. Am. J. Cardiol., *19*:776, 1967.

214. Sadler, J.E.: The long-term hospitalization of asthmatic children. Pediatr. Clin. North Am., *22*:173, 1975.

215. Sandler, B.: Emotional stress and infertility. J. Psychosom. Res., *12*:51, 1968.

216. Sargent, J.D., Green, E.E., and Walter, E.D.: Preliminary report on the use of autogenic feedback training in the treatment of migraine and tension headaches. Psychosom. Med., *35*:129, 1973.

217. Schachter, J., et al.: Phasic heart rate responses: Different patterns in black and white newborns. Psychosom. Med., *37*:326, 1975.

218. Schachter, J., Lachin, J.M., and Wimberly, F.C.: Newborn heart rate and blood pressure: Relation to race and to socioeconomic class. Psychosom. Med., *38*:390, 1976.

219. Schlaegel, T.F., and Hoyt, M.: *Psychosomatic Ophthalmology*. Baltimore, Williams & Wilkins, 1957.

220. Schwartz, N.B., and Rothchild, I.: Changes in pituitary LH concentration during pseudopregnancy in the rat. Proc. Soc. Exper. Biol. Med., *116*:107, 1964.

221. Seitz, P.F.D.: Psychological aspects of skin diseases. In: *Recent Developments in Psychosomatic Medicine*. (E. Wittkower, and R. Cleghorn, Eds.). Philadelphia, Lippincott, 1957.

222. Selzer, A.G.: Pseudocyesis in a 6 year old girl. J. Am. Acad. Child Psychiatry, *7*:693, 1968.

223. Shanan, J., et al.: Active coping behavior, anxiety, and cortical steroid excretion in the prediction of transient amenorrhea. Behav. Sci., *10*:461, 1965.

224. Shapiro, A.P.: Psychophysiologic mechanisms in hypertensive vascular disease. Ann. Intern. Med., *53*:64, 1960.

225. Shapiro, D., et al.: Effects of feedback and reinforcement on the control of human systolic blood pressure. Science, *63*:588, 1969.

226. Shenkin, H.A., and Feldman, W.: Elevated cortisol levels in patients with G. I. bleeding of stress origin. J. Clin. Endocrinol. Metab., *28*:15, 1968.

227. Silver, H.K., and Finklestein, M.: Deprivation dwarfism. J. Pediatr., *70*:317, 1967.

228. Sledge, W.H.: Antecedent psychological factors in the onset of vasovagal syncope. Psychosom. Med., *40*:568, 1978.

229. Smit, C.M., and Hamilton, J.: Psychological factors in the narcolepsy-cataplexy syndrome. Psychosom. Med., *21*:40, 1959.

230. Smith, S.L., and Sander, C.: Food cravings, depression, and premenstrual problems. Psychosom. Med., *31*:281, 1969.

231. Sommer, B.: The effect of menstruation on cognitive and perceptual-motor behavior: A review. Psychosom. Med., *35*:515, 1973.

232. Sours, J.A.: Clinical studies of the anorexia nervosa syndrome. N. Y. State J. Med., *68*:1363, 1968.

233. Sperling, M.: Problems in analysis of children with psychosomatic disorders. Q. J. Child Behav., *1*:12, 1949.

234. Sperling, M.: Psychodynamics and treatment of petit mal in children. Int. J. Psychoanal., *34*:248, 1953.

235. Sperling, M.: Observations from the treatment of children suffering from nonbloody diarrhea or mucous colitis. J. Hillside Hosp., *4*:25, 1955.

236. Sperling, M.: The psychoanalytic treatment of a case of chronic regional ileitis. Int. J. Psychoanal., *4*:612, 1960.

237. Sperling, M.: Further contributions to the psychoanalytic study of migraine and psychogenic headaches. Int. J. Psychoanal., *45*:549, 1964.

238. Sperling, M.: Asthma in children: An evaluation of concepts and therapies. J. Am. Acad. Child. Psychiatry, *7*:44, 1968.

239. Sperling, M.: Ulcerative colitis in children: Current views and therapies. J. Am. Acad. Child. Psychiatry, *8*:336, 1969.

240. Starr, P.H.: Psychosomatic consideration of diabetes in childhood. J. Nerv. Ment. Dis., *121*:493, 1955.

241. Stein, S.P., and Charles, E.: Emotional factors in juvenile diabetes mellitus: A study of early life experiences of adolescent diabetics. Am. J. Psychiatry, *128*:56, 1971.

242. Steinberg, A., et al.: Psychoendocrine relationship in pseudocyesis. Psychosom. Med., *8*:176, 1946.

243. Sterky, G.: Family background and state of mental health in a group of diabetic school children. Acta Paediatr., *52*:377, 1963.

244. Stone, R.T., and Barbero, G.J.: Recurrent abdominal pain in childhood. Pediatrics, *45*:732, 1970.

245. Stunkard, A., et al.: Influence of social class on obesity and thinness in children. JAMA, *221*:579, 1972.
246. Sturzenberger, S., et al.: A follow-up study of adolescent psychiatric inpatients with anorexia nervosa. I. The assessment of outcome. J. Am. Acad. Child Psychiatry, *16*:703, 1977.
247. Sulz, H.A., et al.: Asthma and eczema. In: *Long-term Childhood Illness*. Pittsburgh, University of Pittsburgh Press, 1972.
248. Swift, C.R., Seidman, F., and Stein, H.: Adjustment problems in juvenile diabetics. Psychosom. Med., *29*:555, 1967.
249. Taboroff, L.H., and Brown, W.H.: A study of the personality patterns of children and adolescents with the peptic ulcer syndrome. Am. J. Orthopsychiatry, *24*:602, 1954.
250. Tietz, W., and Vidman, T.: The impact of coping styles on the control of juvenile diabetes. Psychiatr. Med., *3*:67, 1972.
251. Tuch, R.H.: The relationship between a mother's menstrual status and her response to illness in her child. Psychosom. Med., *37*:388, 1975.
252. Ulman, M., and Dudek, S.: On the psyche and warts. II. Hypnotic suggestion and warts. Psychosom. Med., *20*:68, 1960.
253. Vandenburgh, R.L., Taylor, E.S., and Drose, V.D.: Emotional illness in habitual aborters following suturing of the incompetent cervical os. Psychosom. Med., *28*:257, 1966.
254. Voth, H.M., et al.: Thyroid hot spots: Their relationship to life stress. Psychosom. Med., *32*:561, 1970.
255. Wahl, C.W., and Golden, J.S.: Psychogenic urinary retention. Report of 6 cases. Psychosom. Med., *25*:543, 1963.
256. Warson, S.R., Turkel, S., and Schiels, H.S.: Pseudopeptic ulcer syndromes in children. J. Pediatr., *35*:215, 1949.
257. Weil, W.B., et al.: Social patterns and diabetic glycosuria. Am. J. Dis. Child., *113*:464, 1967.
258. Weiner, H.: Essential hypertension and psychosomatic research. Psychosom. Med., *38*:1, 1976.
259. Weiner, H.: The heterogeneity of psychosomatic disease. Psychosom. Med., *38*:371, 1976.
260. Weiner, H., et al.: Etiology of duodenal ulcer. I. Relation of specific psychological characteristics to rate of gastric secretion (pepsinogen). Psychosom. Med., *19*:1, 1957.
261. Weiner, H., et al.: Cardiovascular responses and their psychological correlates. Psychosom. Med., *24*:477, 1962.
262. Weiss, E.: Cardiospasm, A psychosomatic disorder. Psychosom. Med., *6*:58, 1944.
263. Weissberg, M.: A case of petit mal status: A diagnostic dilemma. Am. J. Psychiatry, *132*:1200, 1975.
264. Wender, E.H., et al.: Behavioral characteristics of children with chronic nonspecific diarrhea. Am. J. Psychiatry, *133*:20, 1976.
265. Whisnaut, L., and Zegans, L.: A study of attitudes toward menarche in white middle-class American adolescent girls. Am. J. Psychiatry, *132*:809, 1975.
266. White, K.L., and Long, W.N.: The incidence of psychogenic fever in a university hospital. J. Chron. Dis., *8*:567, 1958.
267. Whitten, C.F., Pettit, M.G., and Fischoff, J.: Evidence that growth failure from maternal deprivation is secondary to undereating. J. Am. Med. Assoc., *209*:1675, 1969.
268. Williams, J.S.: Aspects of dependence-independence conflict in children with asthma. J. Child. Psychol. Psychiatry, *16*:199, 1975.
269. Winkelstein, A.: Some general observations on cardiospasm. Med.Clin. North Am., *28*:589, 1944.
270. Wittkower, E.D., and Russell, B.: *Emotional Factors and Skin Diseases*. New York, Hoeber, 1963.
271. Wolf, S., and Wolff, H.G.: *Human Gastric Function*. New York, Oxford University Press, 1947.
272. Wolf, S., et al.: *Life Stress and Essential Hypertension*. Baltimore, Williams & Wilkins, 1955.
273. Wolff, H.G.: Personality features and reactions of subjects with migraine. Arch. Neurol. Psychiatry, *36*:895, 1937.
274. Wolff, H.G.: *Headache and Other Head Pain*. New York, Oxford University Press, 1963.
275. Yoss, R.E., and Daly, D.D.: Narcolepsy in children. Pediatrics, *25*:1025, 1960.
276. Young, L.D., Langord, H.G., and Blanchard, E.G.: Effect of operant conditioning of heart rate on plasma renin activity. Psychosom. Med., *38*:278, 1976.
277. Zakus, G., and Solomon, M.: The family situations of obese adolescent girls. Adolescence, *8*:33, 1973.
278. Zimet, C.N., and Berger, A.S.: Emotional factors in primary glaucoma: An evaluation of psychological test data. Psychosom. Med., *22*:391, 1960.

General References

Amsterdam, Elsevier, Physiology, Emotion, and Psychosomatic Illness. Ciba Foundation Symposium, 1972.
Anthony, E.J., and Koupernik, C., Eds.: *The Child in His Family*. New York, Wiley, 1970.
Chalke, F.C.R.: Effect of psychotherapy for psychosomatic disorders. Psychosomatics, *6*:125, 1965.
Costell, R.M., and Liederman, P.H.: Psychophysiological concomitants of social stress: The effects of conformity pressure. Psychosom. Med., *30*:298, 1968.
Dubos, R.: *Man, Medicine, and Environment*. New York, American Library, 1968.
Engel, G.L.: A unified concept of health and disease. Perspect. Biol. Med., *3*:459, 1960.
Engel, G.L.: *Psychological Development in Health and Disease*. Philadelphia, Saunders, 1962.
Engel, G.L.: Psychological aspects of gastrointestinal disorders. *American Handbook of Psychiatry*, Vol. 4 (S. Arieti, Ed.). New York, Basic Books, 1976.
Engel, G.L.: The need for a new medical model: A challenge for biomedicine. Science, *196*:129, 1977.
Finch, S.M.: Psychophysiological disorders in children. In: *Comprehensive Textbook of Psychiatry* (A.M. Freedman, H.I. Vaplan, and B.J. Saddock, Eds.). Baltimore, Williams & Wilkins, 1975.

Group for the Advancement of Psychiatry: *Psychopathological Disorders in Childhood: Theoretical Considerations and a Proposed Classification.* Report No. 62. New York, Group for the Advancement of Psychiatry, 1966.

Hill, O., Ed.: *Modern Trends in Psychosomatic Medicine.* London, Butterworth, 1970.

Jores, A., and Freyburger, H., Eds.: *Advances in Psychosomatic Medicine: Symposium of the Fourth European Conference on Psychosomatic Research.* New York, Brunner, 1961.

Lipowski, J.J.: Psychosomatic medicine in the seventies: An overview. Am. J. Psychiatry, *134:*233, 1977.

Lipowski, J.J., Lipsilt, D.R., and Whybrow, P.C., Eds.: *Psychosomatic Medicine: Current Trends and Clinical Applications.* New York, Oxford University Press, 1977.

Lipton, E.L., Steinschneider, A., and Rochmond, J.B.: Psychophysiological disorders in children. In: *Review of Child Development Research,* Vol. 2 (M. Hoffman and L. Hoffman, Eds.). New York, Russell Sage Foundation, 1966.

Loof, D.H.: Psychophysiologic and conversion reactions in children: Selective incidence in verbal and nonverbal families. J. Am. Acad. Child Psychiatry, *9:*318, 1970.

Mason, J.W.: Over-all hormonal balance as a key to endocrine organization. Psychosom. Med., *30:*791, 1968.

Mattsson, A.: Long-term physical illness in childhood: A challenge to psychosocial adaptation. Pediatrics, *50:*801, 1972.

Mirsky, I.A.: The psychosomatic approach to the etiology of clinical disorders. Psychosom. Med., *19:*424, 1957.

Prugh, D.G.: Psychological and psychophysiological aspects of oral activities in childhood. Pediatr. Clin. North Am., 3:1049, 1956.

Prugh, D.G.: Toward the understanding of the psychosomatic aspects of illness in childhood. In: *Modern Perspectives in Child Development* (A. Solnit and S. Provence, Eds.). New York, International Universities Press, 1963.

Reiser, M.F.: Changing theoretical concepts in psychosomatic medicine. In: *American Handbook of Psychiatry,* Vol. 4 (S. Arieti, Ed.). New York, Basic Books, 1976.

Schottstaedt, W.W.: *Psychophysiologic Approach in Medical Practice.* Chicago, Year Book, 1960.

Sperling, M.: Psychosomatic Disorders. In: *Adolescents* (S. Lorand and H.J. Schneer, Eds.). New York, Hoeber, 1961.

Sperling, M.: Transference neurosis in patients with psychosomatic disorders. Psychoanal. Q., *36:*342, 1967.

Sperling, M.: *Psychosomatic Disorders of Childhood.* New York, Jason Aronson, 1978.

Venables, P.H., and Christie, M.J.: *Research in Psychophysiology.* New York, Wiley, 1975.

Weiner, H.: *Psychobiology and Human Disease.* New York, Elsevier, 1977.

Witthower, E.D., and Warner, H., Eds.: *Psychosomatic Medicine: Its Clinical Applications.* New York, Harper & Row, 1977.

Witthower, E.D., Peterfly, G., and Pinter E.J.: Psychosomatic aspects of endocrinologic disorders. Postgrad. Med., 47:146, 1970.

Wolf, S.: *Children Under Stress.* London, Allen Lane, 1969.

22
Brain Syndromes

In bodily diseases, a wandering mind
is often found.
(Lucretius)

The diagnostic features of brain syndromes are:

1. They are characterized by impairment of orientation, judgment, discrimination, learning, memory, and other cognitive functions, as well as by emotional lability.

2. They are associated with evidence of cerebral dysfunction, including (a) abnormal neurologic findings, (b) a definitely abnormal EEG, (c) perceptual-motor disturbances as shown by psychologic tests, and (d) a clear history of an insult to the central nervous system. All 4 of these criteria should be present to establish the diagnosis.

3. They are admixed with psychologic disturbances that either preceded or are secondary to the brain damage. There is no "pure" cerebral dysfunction without associated psychologic reactions.

General Considerations

Brain syndromes are basically caused by localized or diffuse damage to brain tissue, particularly that of the cerebral cortex, from any cause. Associated with the basic syndrome, in children as in adults, may be other personality disturbances, such as psychotic manifestations, neurotic manifestations, or disturbances in behavior. These associated disturbances are not necessarily related to the degree of the brain tissue dysfunction or to the degree of brain damage. They are determined by the child's predisposing personality patterns, current emotional conflicts, level of development, and interpersonal relationships in his family, as well as by the nature of the precipitating brain disorder and its meaning to the child and his parents.[42]

As in adults, these associated disturbances in children are often looked on as having been released by the brain disorder or as having been superimposed on it or intertwined with it. In infants and young children, however, later personality development may be influenced by such disturbances, whose manifestations may be quite different from those in older children

377

and adults. The young child appears to be able, to a great extent, to compensate during his later development for insults to the central nervous system, as certain case examples and the results of the Apgar test[26,84] suggest. Certain functions the child developed most recently may be most vulnerable to such insults, whereas functions he developed earlier may be less affected. On the other hand, functions he has not yet developed may be interfered with, particularly those related to the cognitive aspects of learning and the development of impulse controls. It is thus much harder in children than in adults to correlate the severity of cognitive difficulty with the severity of the brain damage. The child's premorbid personality characteristics, temperamental patterns, and environmental factors are also involved in varied responses that can occur even to similar brain injuries. Artificial separations into totally "organic" and totally "functional" problems are particularly inappropriate, conceptually and clinically, as indicated earlier in a more general sense.

Children who have localized rather than diffuse lesions of the brain may react to them in various ways, depending only in part on what brain functions are interfered with. These children can often compensate to a considerable degree during the course of their development. Within broad limits, the reactions of the child's parents and other members of his family, together with other factors in his environment, seem to be the most influential determinants of how the child handles the defect.[35]

To quote the Standard Nomenclature, "The brain syndromes of diffuse nature are separated, with much overlap, into acute and chronic, with regard to differences in prognosis, treatment, and in the course of illness. The terms acute and chronic refer primarily to the degree of reversibility of brain pathology and the accompanying brain syndrome, and not to the etiology or even necessarily the onset or duration of the initial illness or insult to the central nervous system. Since the same etiology may produce either temporary or permanent damage, a brain disorder which appears reversible, hence acute, at its beginning, may prove later to have left permanent damage and a persistent brain syndrome, which will then be diagnosed as chronic." These observations apply to children as well as adults. Since the physical aspects of brain syndromes have been discussed in detail in several excellent textbooks on pediatric neurology, emphasis will be laid in this chapter on the psychologic and social ramifications of brain damage in children.

Clinical Findings

Acute Brain Syndromes

This category includes those types of acute brain disorders that are associated with intracranial infection of bacterial or viral origin, systemic infection with high fever, drug or poison (including alcohol) intoxication, trauma (including burns), circulatory disturbances, certain types of convulsive disorder, cardiorespiratory and metabolic disorders, as in renal insufficiency, and certain disorders of unknown etiology, such as multiple sclerosis.

The principal manifestation of an acute brain syndrome in children, as in adults, is delirium, a toxic psychosis involving a disturbance in awareness that results from changes in cerebral metabolism, as Romano and Engel demonstrated in their classic studies of adults.[28,78,79] Kanner[48] and Green[41] have provided clinical descriptions in children, and Goodman and Sours[37] and Prugh[73] have had the impression that children are more apt to respond to respiratory infections and fever with delirium states than are adults.

The clinical pictures may be gross and easily identifiable; they are characterized by wildly agitated or confused behavior and vivid hallucinations.[42] The hallucinations are usually visual (and they are more concrete than they are in childhood psychosis) although auditory hallucinations also occur. The child may have visual illusions of "witches" or "ghosts" in his room based on his misperception of shadows, or he may perceive gleaming instruments as the weapons of "killers"—the doctors and the nurses. Delusions may also develop, with the child resisting medications as "poison," tearing off dressings in fear of "being tied up," or believing that his parents are dead or that they have abandoned him because he was "bad." He may also have tactile illusions and somatic delusions.

A subclinical form, however, may be manifested by subtle disturbances in awareness and orientation or mildly stuporous states, withdrawn, difficult, or bizarre behavior, or irrational fears. In my experience,[75] cases of this type occur much more commonly than is believed, and they often go unrecognized. These cases include children who have high fever from any cause, those who have viral illnesses, such as measles or chickenpox, which usually have mild associated meningoencephalitis, diabetic children who have insulin reactions, and children who are taking antiepileptic medication or heavy doses of one or more tranquilizers.[63] In a recently published study of delirium in childhood and adolescents carried out by Prugh and his colleagues,[74] some ambulatory children who had chronic renal insufficiency who were being evaluated for kidney transplantation were found to show this subclinical form. They showed waxing and waning of their levels of attention, memory, and orientation, and at times bizarre behavior, leading to a mistaken impression of a functional psychosis. Subclinical cases may be difficult to recognize, and the clinician must keep the possibility in mind to avoid overlooking the delirium or to prevent a misdiagnosis of psychotic behavior on a nonsomatic basis. Both gross and subclinical forms of delirium are characteristically worse at night, with an increase in the child's misperceptions and fears of the dark. (Postoperative delirious states and those arising from sensory deprivation are described later.)

If a delirious process is suspected, the flexible type of mental status examination described in Chapter 7 may be used. In the study just referred to, Prugh and his colleagues attempted to identify a small number of standardized items in such an examination, adapted to different levels of development, which would reliably discriminate between a group of children and adolescents who had delirium and a control group. From the study it can be said that a number of the traditional items such as object identification, astereognosis, graphesthesia, and other "soft" neurologic signs, as well as subtraction of serial sevens (whose worth Milstein[66] has already questioned) did not discriminate between the 2 groups. But disturbances in memory and orientation and obviously confused copying of certain geometric figures,* as well as EEG slowing and disorganization, did discriminate significantly.

I have found an abbreviated informal clinical interview adapted to the child's developmental level to be most valuable in evaluating such cognitive functions as memory, orientation, and general reality testing. Hospitalized children tend to resist formal questioning and adolescents tend to be scornful of the classic proverbs and tongue-twisters used in a traditional mental-status examination. Once the physician has established a relationship with the child by asking the child how he feels, who is in his family, and similar questions, information will emerge spontaneously. In such an open-ended approach, the child often shows waxing and waning of attention and awareness, disorientation, lapses in memory, slurring of speech, or confusion in

---

*These include Bender-Gestalt item #4 (form and angulation) and Bender-Gestalt item #7 (overlapping parallelograms). Errors in examiner-transposition orientation also discriminated.

thought. The use of a few simple structured tasks, such as drawing geometric figures, that take into account the child's physical difficulties and developmental level help to confirm the physician's initial clinical impressions.

An EEG that reveals disorganization and large slow waves is of positive diagnostic help.[74] The EEG tracing ordinarily improves when the disturbance in cerebral metabolism has been corrected, although some abnormalities may persist for weeks or months. Perceptual-motor difficulties may persist for some time also, and they may lead to learning difficulties when the child returns to school even though the brain lesion has completely healed.

Much valuable though less formally diagnostic verbal information may be elicited by asking the child about his wishes, dreams, and future occupations. Cognitive and perceptual dysfunctions may be revealed. The content of the child's fantasies and feelings, as well as of his hallucinations and illusions, is strongly influenced by his past experience and present stress. Also important is the child's psychologic reactions to the experience of delirium. Regression is common, as are denial of illness, fear of loss of control of feelings, and guilt over what might have been said during a period of amnesia (generally retrograde amnesia, with preservation of some memory fragments, which may be distorted). Depression may occur, sometimes lasting far beyond the subsidence of the delirious process, at times causing reverberations within the family.[74]

Case Example. A 3-year-old boy was hospitalized for second-degree burns he sustained when gasoline that was in an open container was ignited (by matches that the boy's 7-year-old brother had been playing with). The boy's parents did not visit him for 2 days after his admission to the hospital. The boy became withdrawn, and he resisted attempts by the nursing staff to help him. A consultation with a child psychiatrist was arranged for the boy. The psychiatrist found much of the boy's speech unintelligible. Once the boy said clearly, "I'll be good," and another time he misperceived the psychiatrist as a "bad man who wants to kill me." He also had other signs of delirium.

The psychiatrist called the boy's parents and made an appointment to see them. During the psychiatrist's discussion with the parents, it became clear that they had not visited the boy because they were afraid that the hospital staff would look on them as bad or neglectful parents. The psychiatrist helped relieve the parents' feelings of guilt. Later he learned that the boy and his parents had been battling about toilet training. (The parents had sent the boy to bed when he soiled himself.) The fact that the parents had not visited the boy in the hospital, as well as the fact that he had been confined to bed in the hospital (as he was at home when he was "bad"), had made the boy fear that he was being punished and deserted. The psychiatrist helped the parents clarify the situation. Soon after that, the boy's delirium, which had been improving, subsided altogether. (The boy's 7-year-old brother, who had not been burned in the accident, also needed help with his feelings of guilt.)

Preexisting or underlying psychoneurotic, personality, or even psychotic disorders may become more apparent after such insults to the central nervous system, and reactive disorders or later developmental deviations in cognitive or other areas may result. Conversion disorders and dissociative states may be admixed with the symptoms of delirium during the convalescent phase. The differential diagnosis includes pseudo-delirious dissociative disorders, acute confusional states caused by psychologic stress or exhaustion, psychomotor equivalents, and psychoses of nonsomatic origin. The particular type of reactive disorder or underlying personality disturbance can be specified.

Head Injuries. Head injury in children can be followed by a variety of psychosocial disorders,[44] including acute functional psychosis.[87] A "catastrophic reaction" has been described in adults by Goldstein,[36] and occasional cases, with behavioral as well as neurologic responses, may be seen in older adolescents. The postconcussive syndrome,[25,71] involving persistent headaches, and certain emotional reactions has been mentioned. The prognosis for response to head injuries has been said to depend on the child's premorbid personality, his family's response to the injury, and other predisposing factors.[29,30,94] A recent long-term study by Black and his colleagues[7] of the effects of head injury in children found less evidence of headache. They described significant changes in the child's behavior; 3% of the children studied had difficulties in controlling their feelings of anger and their impulses. They were mostly children who had no history of previous emotional disturbance. This finding suggests not only that guilt and other factors of the family's response to the injury may be involved but also that chronic brain injury may persist in some cases and interact with interpersonal factors.

Chronic Brain Syndromes

Chronic brain syndromes result from "relatively permanent, more or less irreversible, diffuse impairment of cerebral tissue function."[42] Such impairment may occur as the result of (1) congenital cranial anomalies, (2) the cerebral palsies and other disorders that arise from prenatal or perinatal damage to the brain, (3) syphilis of the central nervous system, (4) other infections, including various encephalitides, (5) intoxication of various types, including poisoning from heavy metals, (6) brain trauma, (7) a protracted convulsive disorder, (8) a circulatory disorder, such as a subarachnoid hemorrhage or "stroke" (rare in childhood), (9) a severe disturbance of metabolism or nutrition, (10) an intracranial neoplasm, or (11) heredodegenerative factors, such as Schilder's encephalitis and Heller's disease. Some disturbances in memory, judgment, orientation, comprehension, concentration, affect, and learning capacity may remain permanently, at times acompanied by remarkable compensations in individual children during the course of development. Children who lack a corpus callosum have been reported to show no sign of cerebral dysfunction, and at least a few children who have definitive brain damage show no difficulties in learning.

Contrary to earlier impressions, no personality disorder seems to be specific to all chronic brain syndromes. Rather, the children so afflicted seem to be a heterogeneous group.[42,73,82] There seem to be different personality patterns, ranging from overly anxious through obsessive-compulsive to overly independent, frequent developmental lags in personality organization, and other developmental deviations. These psychologic factors appear in varying admixtures with the effects on behavior of the underlying brain damage. For example, some of the psychologic features may represent a reaction to the child's perceptions of his own limitations. Specific problems may include apparent deficiencies in cerebral controls or inhibiting mechanisms in certain children;[3,89] these may result in uncontrolled or aggressive behavior in ambiguous or anxiety-provoking situations. Such children usually feel very guilty about such outbursts and consequently have a greater need than other children for structure, predictability, and external controls. At times, these children may act out unconsciously to test adults or to invite controls.

Case Example. A 9-year-old boy, who was very tall and heavy for his age, had sustained diffuse damage to his cerebral cortex at birth because of complications during labor. The brain damage was evidenced by his low Apgar score, by his diminished sucking reflex, and by his other neurologic abnormalities. During the boy's late infancy and preschool-age period, the boy was overactive (but not truly hyperactive), and he had a shortened attention span, outbursts of aggressive behavior, and trouble socializing. His developmental milestones were not significantly delayed. During this period, the boy's parents found him difficult to manage, and they had trouble setting consistent limits on his aggressive behavior.

When the boy was 6 years old, he began his formal schooling. His EEG was still definitely abnormal, he had difficulties in coordination, as well as other soft neurologic signs. Psycho-

logic tests indicated that he had significant visuomotor impairment. His overall intelligence
seemed to be at least in the average range, and
there was some suggestion that he had a higher
potential. He now seemed rather anxious rather
than aggressive, and he was easily managed in
class and at home.

The boy was given special tutoring, and by
the time he was in fourth grade, he was performing at nearly average level, having only
some mild difficulties with reading and mathematics. However, he had developed major obsessive-compulsive symptoms and inhibited social behavior, and for that reason he was referred
for a psychiatric consultation. The psychiatrist
thought that the boy's symptoms were related
to an unconscious fear he had that he would
lose control of his aggressive impulses and that
he would hurt other children his age (because
he was so big and heavy). The boy underwent
psychotherapy for a year—successfully so.

Some children may be afraid of losing
control of their aggressive impulses—and
of being punished for doing so—to the
point that they withdraw into a world of
inner fantasy that seems to them to be safer
and more satisfying. A few children show
withdrawn and autistic behavior to a psychotic degree, with hallucinatory fears
about external reality.

As has been pointed out by a number of
clinicians, some children who have diffuse
brain damage show "clowning" behavior;
that is, they respond to ridicule of their
difficulties in coordination or learning by
pretending they are only play-acting, thus
settling for a less painful notoriety.[27] They
may show perseveration and confabulation
to cover up their deficits in concentration
and memory. Some try awkwardly to elicit
affection from others, often unsuccess-
fully. Other children may regress, even to
infantile levels, because they fear growing
up in a competitive world. Some may use
denial or projection to deal with their problems, while others may withdraw entirely
from competition and so fail to use the skills
they do have.[69] Most suffer from low self-
esteem and distortions in body image.

The majority have problems in perceptual functioning, such as difficulty in distinguishing figure-ground relationships,[33]

problems in coordinating eye, brain, and
hand that produce spelling and writing disabilities,[24] problems in "stimulus competition" and intersensory integration of
stimuli,[6] and limitations in abstract reasoning, as in mathematics. Most of these children have concomitant emotional problems, such as anxiety over performance,
feelings of failure or inadequacy, negative
self-images, and resistance to learning.
Their waxing and waning in attention,
short attention spans, limited frustration
tolerance, hyperactive, or aggressive behavior may result in problems in social adjustment in the school setting.

Many children who have chronic brain
syndromes are not significantly retarded in
intellectual development although some
very small premature infants may sustain
sufficient brain damage to function at a retarded level.[21,58] Some children may function at a mentally retarded level, with psychologic and social factors playing a role in
lowering their capacity to achieve their full
potential. If true mental retardation is present, that fact should be specified. A diagnosis of "chronic brain syndrome" is not
enough because these children have personalities, and they usually have some disturbance in personality development. A diagnosis should be made wherever possible
of the predominant personality picture associated with the brain syndrome, as in
developmental deviations of social or other
nature, or reactive, psychoneurotic, personality, or psychotic disorders[40]; individual symptoms can be listed.

The parents of brain-damaged children
react much like the parents of a child who
has any type of chronic illness or handicap.[31] Their initial reactions to the diagnosis often include denial of its implications or even of the condition itself; the
parents often have difficulty in accepting
what they cannot easily understand or what
they fear cannot be helped. Guilt and self-
blame for not protecting the child may lead
to depression. Or the blame may be projected onto the spouse, and serious marital

conflicts, even divorce, may result. The parents may feel hopeless and at the same time they may feel anger at the doctor, or the school system, or the world. Sometimes they go on protracted "shopping" tours for other opinions. But after they mourn for the "child that was to be," many parents can accept the disorder and plan for the future realistically although some may continue denial or may become over-anxious or overprotective, and a few may reject or ostracize the child.

As Rose[80] has indicated, infants who have sustained definite hypoxia or other perinatal trauma may elicit doubt, frustration, fear, depression, overprotection, withdrawal, or other reactions from the parents that may adversely affect the infant's personality development. Also, the limitations of the Apgar test in regard to its long-term prediction capability are not well enough known, and an unduly pessimistic prognosis based on that test may result in the "vulnerable child syndrome" or other parent-child problems. Not all children who have sustained definite perinatal damage show adverse effects,[49,60] and many show remarkable compensation.[39,95]

A particular syndrome can occur in preschool-age and young school-age children who are presumed to have sustained diffuse damage to the cerebral cortex during the prenatal or perinatal period. The syndrome is often characterized by hyperactivity, distractibility, impulsivity, and other features. Diffuse abnormalities are ordinarily present in the electroencephalogram and on the electromyogram. Difficulties in perceptual-motor functioning, spatial orientation, and cerebral integration or organizational capacities, with waxing and waning in effectiveness, are characteristic. They lead to problems in using symbols, as, for example, in reading and writing and in abstract concept formation. Performance I.Q.s are usually lower than verbal I.Q.'s, with much scatter in subtests, in contrast to the higher Performance I.Q.s and lower Verbal I.Q.s that often arise from anxiety or other psychologic problems. Specific neurologic lesions are rarely demonstrable (although soft neurological signs[3] are frequent), and there is rarely a definitive history of cerebral insult. The lesions do not seem to be part of the continuum of "reproductive casualty."[72a]

Due caution must be used in arriving at a diagnosis in such children. As indicated earlier, children who have significant psychologic disturbances may also have difficulties in regard to impulse control, distractibility, and hyperactivity. Some of these children exhibit delayed perceptual-motor development and dysrhythmic EEG patterns, with one or more soft neurologic signs (which may persist[88] or which may change from time to time) in the absence of a history of specific signs of brain damage. Thus careful differentiation must be made from reactive disorders or developmental lags or deviations in perceptual-motor functions or in cerebral integration. Signs of such *cerebral dysfunction* may not arise from somatic sources alone; therefore, diagnoses of "organicity" or minimal brain damage," based principally on behavioral manifestations seem to be very much open to question.[61] Unfortunately, minimal brain dysfunction (MBD)[16,96] tends to be a wastebasket category and is probably a myth, as Schmitt[86] and others[61] have indicated. The almost synonymous use of the terms hyperactive child[98] and hyperkinetic syndrome[55] has compounded the difficulty; several studies have shown that a significant number of definitively brain-damaged children who have some of these problems are not hyperactive or are hypoactive[39] and that hyperactive children often have no signs of brain damage. A factor analysis study by Werry[97] found that neurologic, medical-historical, behavioral, cognitive, and EEG dysfunctions were basically unrelated ones, each tending to be made up of measures from a different professional group. The finding of 1 or 2 "soft" neurologic signs (e.g., difficulties in graphesthesia, speech, coordination, position sense, balance, double simultaneous stimulation) in a number of the normal controls in several studies[45,50,102] renders such signs of dubious diagnostic value.[14,99] It is true, however, that children who have hard neurologic lesions tend to show more soft signs than do healthy children.[50] There is a pressing need for research to establish uniform methods of testing in this area to establish developmental norms in motor, sensory, perceptual, cognitive, and other dimensions.

Children who have developmental aphasia have problems chiefly in expressing themselves. Their receptive skills are relatively intact, they are usually fairly competent in other areas of development, and they usually develop some communicative speech by about 4 years of age, as Cohen[17] has pointed out. They often have abnormal EEGs, and they sometimes have convulsive disorders. Such children may be mistakenly diagnosed as having early infantile autism or as being mentally retarded. They often have emotional problems that may intensify their basic disorder. Children who have so-called congenital aphasia have been described as having impairment of both their expressive and receptive skills.[4]

Formal psychologic testing of the perceptual-motor type, although most useful in eliciting such problems,[33,83,93] by itself has not been successful in differentiating "brain damaged" children, emotionally disturbed children, and retarded children.[38,103] (The limitations in the diagnostic use of the EEG were discussed in Chapter 8.) Reasoning such as this led the International Study Group on Child Neurology to propose recently that the term minimal brain dysfunction be discarded in favor of more meaningful classification of disturbances of cerebral function, such as motor disorders, disorders of communication, and perceptual disorders. I agree with Zimet and Fishman[105] that since the syndrome of MBD as described originally by Strauss and Lehtenen[92] refers to behavior and not to

brain damage as such, the difficulties children who have MBD experience need to be described in psychoeducational rather than neurologic terms. The search for etiologic factors should go on, but in a systematic and rigorous fashion. New techniques of remedial education and other measures, such as speech therapy and the use of stimulant drugs when indicated, have been developed which can help these children, regardless of etiology.

It has been estimated that children who have so-called MBD comprise 5% to 20% of the school population. I believe with Abrams[1] and others (admittedly without proof as yet) that the majority of these children actually have developmental lags in the perceptual-motor, cognitive, sensory, motor and other aspects of their development, which may have become intensified as the result of problems in interaction with the environment. These lags occur more frequently in children from poverty and ghetto backgrounds; poorer prenatal care and a higher incidence of prematurity may be involved, but environmental factors (e.g., a higher incidence of family disorganization and less verbal environments) undoubtedly play a role as well. In addition, as McDermott and Harrison[64] have emphasized, white, middle-, and upper-class clinicians are inclined to diagnose brain damage and mental retardation more often and more easily in children who come from lower-class or minority backgrounds than in children who come from their own socioeconomic and ethnic background.

For all the reasons just discussed or implied, as well as because of my own clinical experience and that of others, I have come to require, for a definitive diagnosis of diffuse cerebral brain damage, that all the following criteria be met.

1. The child must have *a definite history of an insult* to the central nervous system (not just a one-day fever or a "bump on the head" but no loss of consciousness or other signs).
2. The child must have three or more

soft neurologic signs that are present over a period of time.

3. The child must show significant and persistent EEG abnormalities (not simply "borderline dysrhythmia consistent with _____") that are evaluated with due regard for developmental norms[65] (see Table in Chapter 5).

4. The child must show *definite perceptual-motor abnormalities* on psychological testing on several tests (not simply "suggestive" difficulties on one or two of the Bender Gestalt figures).

Children who have *cerebral palsy*, originally described by Freud,[32] exhibit motor disabilities that are predominantly extrapyramidal and exhibit spastic or choreiform and athetoid movements as well as frequent sensory and perceptual defects and visual and hearing deficits. All of these problems dispose the child to learning difficulties and to problems in achievement on intelligence tests. He often has speech problems, and associated emotional and social problems, and he may have seizures.[23] The close association between the extrapyramidal system and emotional reactivity, combined with the child's inability to discharge his tension through physical activity and play, may produce a temporary or long-lasting intensification of his motor disability, especially athetoid movements, as a result of anxiety or emotional conflict. Certain parents may feel guilty and handle the child overprotectively, while others may feel ashamed, resentful, or hopeless. Too little stimulation or a pessimistic appraisal of the child's future by his parents, physicians, and teachers may lead to inadequate education, in addition to the inherent learning problems. Early diagnosis is important,[46] because it may lead to early intervention that helps the child greatly.

Children who have cerebral palsy are often emotionally immature, introverted ("shut-in"), overly dependent, fearful of falling,[56] sudden noises, or strange situations, irritable, egocentric, and socially retiring or isolated.[70] They are painfully aware that they are different from others, and they often have a negative self-image. Emotional conflicts are usually most intense during adolescence, although children who have athetosis or ataxia often remain surprisingly cheerful and outgoing (often they deny their limitations to some extent). While some parents may give up on their child, others go to great lengths to help the child. Some parents may push the child toward normality, having unrealistic expectations for him, and they may embrace too readily "gimmicks" or cure-alls. The Doman-Delacato approach, for example, which involves a great deal of effort and money, has been recently shown by a controlled study to be of no greater value than other methods, and it may produce emotional problems from the pressures it puts on the child. The Academy of Pediatrics, in collaboration with a number of other organizations recently stated that there is no empirical evidence that the theory or the practice of "neurologic organization" has validity.[2]

As implied earlier, it is clear today that a specific post-encephalitic syndrome does not exist, as Bond once believed.[8] Children who have suffered from encephalitides of different causes show varying responses, from the chronic brain damage picture just described,[59] to an occasional picture that mimics a functional psychosis,[100] to no effects whatsoever. Prugh, Nellhaus, and Bryant (unpublished material) have seen several children who had elective mutism but no significant residual brain damage following encephalitis of uncertain origin. In one child, the elective mutism seemed to be part of a functional psychotic picture that responded to long-term residential treatment. A psychosis associated with recurrent herpes simplex has been described in which the child showed fairly normal behavior between episodes although with some mild intellectual deterioration. Brain

damage following subarachnoid hemorrhage has been described, but marked anxiety and depressive states have also occurred in the absence of brain damage.[91]
Responses to rare "pediatric strokes" are
also varied, as are the responses of children
who have recovered from tuberculous
meningitis. These children may have intellectual deterioration,[68] as may children
who have had lead poisoning.[13,67]

Most *brain tumors* in children are fairly
easily diagnosed on the basis of vomiting,
diplopia, vertigo, and unsteadiness of gait
although the initial disturbances in the
child's behavior may be confusing. Tumors
of the fourth ventricle are difficult to diagnose. Rheinhart and Succop[76] have reported 2 cases in which vomiting and anorexia that seemed to be related to
psychologic problems were the presenting
symptoms for a number of months. Psychiatric management should be offered in
such cases, but the clinician should be alert
to the facts that both psychologic problems
and pontine tumors can coexist and that
an intracranial tumor can cause behavioral
disturbances, such as regression, withdrawal, or aggressive behavior. Riser and
his colleagues[77] have described adolescents
who showed mood swings and impulsive
behavior during the early course of
craniopharyngiomas. As Langford and
Klingman[54] long ago indicated, the type of
behavior disturbance is related more to the
child's premorbid personality, his attempts
to deal with any deficits, and the reactions
of his parents than to the location of the
tumor.

I have been involved with 2 such cases,
in which early school-age children exhibited regressive, demanding, and, in one
instance, aggressive behavior for some
months, while at the same time complaining of a feeling of intense pressure inside
their head (prior to eyeground changes or
other physical findings), associated with
vomiting and anorexia that seemed to have
no psychosocial basis. Since young children localize pain poorly, such complaints

should raise the clinician's index of suspicion. As indicated in Chapter 8, if the
physician or psychiatric consultant cannot
elicit positive data to explain a behavioral
disturbance, he should search further for
physical factors even while giving appropriate attention to the manifest psychosocial problems.

Children who have definitive localized
brain injury or ablation or who have chronic
brain syndromes with "hard" neurologic
signs are at high risk for learning disabilities. There is little if any direct relationship,
however, between the degree of damage
or site of damage and the child's academic
performance.[53] Some children who have
damage to the cerebral cortex are able to
recognize words but have difficulty in understanding sentences. Some children are
able over a period of time to compensate
for their difficulty and to learn adequately,
and some children have no detectable
learning difficulties.

Treatment and Prognosis

The prognosis for children who have
acute brain syndromes depends of course on
how much structural damage remains, at
what developmental level the cerebral insult took place, and other factors. With
modern antibiotics, the various types of
meningitis, except the tuberculous type,
may leave little residual damage. The viral
encephalitides cannot be controlled as well,
but children who have been in coma even
for several months have been known to
recover almost completely, gradually "relearning" functions that range from walking to reading. In all acute brain syndromes, particularly *head trauma* from
accidents, the child's response is also influenced by his parents' reactions to his
condition, (including guilt), the nature of
the parent-child relationship before the accident, and other factors. A minor concus-
sion may touch off the parents' overprotective tendencies; or the child's

psychologic problems, including conversion "headache," pain, or school phobia, may persist during the child's convalescence even though his physical recovery is complete.

A cardinal problem from a psychosocial point of view is the management of *delirium* while the underlying cause of the delirium is being sought and treated. The central problem is to help the child deal with his visual illusions, which are based on his misperceptions of stimuli in his environment, and to help him deal with his hallucinations or delusions. As a general principle, the delirious child should be isolated as little as possible from human contact. If possible, a special nurse, a family relative, or a foster grandmother should be in the room with the child at all times (especially at night), in order to serve as the child's external or "auxiliary" ego by continually monitoring the child's mental experiences and interpreting the external world for him. By patiently explaining the child's misperceptions to him, by explaining what happened during his lapses of awareness, by preparing him for new experiences, and by providing physical contact in a supportive way, such a person can help the child control his fears, guilt, and other feelings that arise from his confused inner experiences. Such an approach will be much more effective than restraints of any kind, which even healthy children misinterpret as punishment.

Keeping the room well lighted at all times supports the child's contact with reality. The window shades should be kept raised at all times, and a light should be kept on at night. The light should ordinarily be brighter than that shed by a small bed lamp or a dim room light. A bright light will cut down on confusing shadows and other vague or ambiguous stimuli.

If a sedative is needed to help with agitated or uncontrolled behavior or for sleep, chloral hydrate is probably the best choice. Larger doses may be required to overcome the effect of anxiety on the sedation threshold. Paraldehyde given orally or rectally is the ideal sedative in adolescents although they may find the odor offensive. Barbiturates tend to cause confusion and paradoxic stimulation, and they should be avoided. (Tranquilizing drugs in modest doses can help an excessively anxious patient; they should be used as little as possible, in order to avoid contributing to confusion.[74])

Even more important is the maintenance of the child's tie with his parents, the only truly familiar figures in the delirious child's confused world. The mother should visit the child daily or even stay with him overnight—even the school-age child. The parents may need considerable support and help in understanding and dealing with the child's behavior. If a parent is ill or far away and so cannot visit the child regularly, substitute mothering is all the more important. A familiar blanket or toy from home or postcards from the family that can be read to the child are of some help. Dealing with the parents' anxieties and guilt is important, especially if an accident or poisoning is involved. If the child recovers completely from what had caused the delirium, the child's parents and his teacher should be told that the child's perceptual-motor deficits may last for some weeks and that a gradual return to full academic performance is indicated.

The prognosis for children who have chronic brain syndromes is not discussed in detail in this book. The prognosis is undoubtedly better than many clinicians believe, and many children have been the victims of discouragement or insufficient help. Even children who have arrested hydrocephalus (e.g., that resulting from meningomyelocele, in which brain compression occurs slowly), may have adequate intellectual functioning. Although some correlation between the thickness of the child's cortex (the cerebral mantle) and his I.Q. has been shown in infants who have treated hydrocephalus,[104] I have seen children who were of average intelligence even though their cerebral mantles were "paper thin" (less than 1 cm thick, as shown by pneumoencephalography). More recently, Macnab[62] has reported on several children whose cerebral mantles were only 0.5 cm thick who had I.Q.s of 85 to 100. Other follow-up studies have shown that if they survive, even children who have untreated hydrocephalus from various causes have about a 50% chance of developing normal intelligence and that there is no correlation among head size, cortical thickness, and duration of progressive disease. As mentioned, infants and children are able to compensate for diffuse damage to the cerebral cortex, especially if attention is paid to the psychosocial needs of the child and his parents.

The prognosis of children who have *cerebral palsy* is undoubtedly better than the available studies indicate. As Klapper and Birch[51] have indicated, opportunities for follow-up studies have been limited both by the methodologic and other difficulties inherent in longitudinal studies and by the fact that only recently have community services for cerebral palsied children become widely available. In 1959, Crothers and Paine[20] found that less than 25% of the people in their sample group were suitable for nonsheltered employment as adults. Several studies have shown that about one-third of children who have cerebral palsy have functioning levels of at least average intelligence, and a few of these are of superior intelligence. Most of the other two-thirds are in the mildly retarded or low-normal range, and about 10% have I.Q.s below 50.

Klapper and Birch's[52] follow-up study of children who had cerebral palsy (reported in 1967) indicated that, in general, children who had I.Q.s under 50 and those who have I.Q.s over 90 tended to show similar scores as young adults. The majority of those in the intermediate group (one-third of the total group), however, showed increases in test scores of 15 points or more over their childhood scores and the group

as a whole tended to show increases in I.Q. level from childhood to young adulthood. Klapper and Birch also found that although the educational achievement of the people they studied tended to reflect both their intellectual level and their social background, in some young people who had completed college there seemed to be little correlation between either of these factors and the attainment of economic independence.

About 50% of the group were totally unemployed; less than 20% were employed on a competitive level, and only 3 out of 80 persons had achieved complete economic independence. Although the group as a whole had done very well physically, many showed a marked degree of social isolation. Their levels of self-care correlated most highly with their degree of employability, school achievement, economic status, and degree of social integration. In general, those who had spastic hemiplegia did better in all these areas than did those who had ataxia or mixed cerebral palsy. The overall conclusion of the study was that cerebral palsied adults who are potentially employable and capable of social activity are typically unemployed and socially isolated.

As Paine[72] has indicated, the majority of "floppy infants" have later athetotic or spastic manifestations. Some of these infants suffer from malnutrition, and a few have mental retardation, rare myopathies, or heredodegenerative disorders. The infants who had "benign congenital hypotonia" tended to improve. One group had associated hyperextensible joints and often a family history of such problems. Their prognosis for normal motor functioning in adult life was good.

The management[35] of the child who has cerebral palsy (and the management of his family) is generally like that described for children who have other chronic illnesses or handicaps. (Chronic illness and handicaps are more fully discussed in Chapter 25.) Parents need help in accepting the diagnosis. If they see several consulting professionals, one person—the primary care physician or a member of an interdisciplinary team—should integrate the results of the various evaluations and communicate the overall picture to the parents.

From the foregoing discussion it can be seen that support for personality development and gradual encouragement of self-care, with realistic goals for social and functional independence, are as important as treatment of the physical disability and the provision of appropriate educational opportunities. Continuing and consistent counseling of the child's parents, while dealing with denial, guilt, or other feelings, should include a balanced home program that gives the parents a way to help their child that does not overburden them. Group discussions[101] and involvement by parents in community organizations for the cerebral palsied[19] may be very helpful.

Besides physical therapy (when needed), speech therapy, occupational therapy, drug therapy for seizure control, muscle relaxation, or other purposes, special educational measures, and, later, vocational training (in sheltered workshops if necessary), a supportive psychotherapeutic approach can be employed by the physician and health professionals with good results. In the opinion of Berenberg,[5] such a combination of approaches (which should be coordinated by the physician), now available in many communities, can make many more people independent and self-supporting.

Even in cases in which the infant has virtually no muscle control except that involved in swallowing, Bryant[12] and others have accomplished remarkable results using resourceful and playful methods of teaching the child tongue control, then babbling, then head control, and then other motor and speech skills. These methods can be taught to parents. If such a hopeful but not unrealistic approach is taken, the child, as he progresses in his motor and speech development, may show unsus-

pected intellectual potential. Many such children would not progress, or might die, in institutional settings. The child's parents should be told such an approach may not work, but many parents will want to try it anyhow, before they consider institutionalization. If the child's progress levels off or if the parents seem too burdened, it will usually be easier for them to place their child if they feel that they tried to help the child first.

A recent controlled study[85] in the United States has shown that physical therapy is correlated with definite improvements in motor, social, and management skills in infants under 18 months of age. It has been suggested that with very young infants, other kinds of stimulation besides motor stimulation (e.g., social and emotional stimulation) are required.

Besides treatment directed toward the basic cause of brain dysfunction and the other rehabilitative techniques available, the management of brain damaged children includes *remedial education*. Remedial education may involve placing these children in small "ungraded" classes with children who have developmental lags in their perceptual-motor functions or who have other learning problems. The children's progress should be reviewed regularly, so that children can move to normal classes as soon as possible. The need of many brain-damaged children for order and predictability, based on structure and limits, in the classroom has already been mentioned. *Individual tutoring*[34] may enable the child to remain in his "age-appropriate" classroom. (The tutoring should usually be done by a professional; most parents have problems tutoring their own child.) Special remedial teaching techniques that involve the use of auditory, tactile, and kinesthetic stimuli, may be of value.[9,18,57] Deutsch[24] and others have shown how important such psychologic factors as set, attention, and motivation can be to the learning success of such children. (The question of "mainstreaming" of these and other children who have special educational needs is discussed in Chapter 28.)

Some children may require special handling through high school, with arrangements for on-the-job training in a school-work program. Although the child's perceptual-motor and other problems may persist into his adolescence and young adulthood, as Silver[89] has shown and although the child who has problems in impulse control may later become overcontrolled or inhibited, a concentration on the child's strengths and patient handling of him can enable many of these children to make an adequate adjustment. With modern approaches, the myths about "brain damage" being a disorder that has a poor prognosis are being disproved and the stigma surrounding the diagnosis is being removed. A *supportive relationship* for the child and his parents with the physician or health associate, who works in close collaboration with the child's school and the other resources in his community, is a vital ingredient in the successful management of the child's problems.

Contrary to the view previously held, children who have brain damage and serious emotional problems (e.g., marked anxiety over performance, a very negative self-image, serious problems in impulse control, intense resistance to learning or a feeling of hopelessness, or other reactive, psychoneurotic, personality, or psychotic disorders that involve family problems related or not related to the child's brain damage) may respond to psychotherapy for themselves and their parents. Such therapy may at first be largely supportive in nature, directed toward helping the child establish a more positive self-image, develop impulse controls, and deal with his parents' denial, guilt, or other conflicts, but later it may take a true insight-promoting approach.[11,15] Psychotherapy may be needed before tutoring or educational approaches will work. A child who has problems in impulse controls and who has outbursts of uncontrolled behavior may,

during the course of therapy, begin to rely heavily on the use of compulsive behavior to maintain order and control. If he does, other problems then occur that need help.

An educational approach, including some tutoring, may be integrated with the psychotherapy in a psychoeducational approach, as in a day treatment program. For children who are very severely disturbed, inpatient or residential treatment may be indicated.

Recently, behavior therapy[43] has been tried with some brain damaged children. Positive social reinforcement by teachers and parents has been said to bring about an improvement in attention that leads to a better attitude in the child about learning. But some parents who have marked conflicts about the serious difficulties in their child's relationship with them may be unable to use behavior therapy, and psychotherapy may be necessary. As Ross[81] has indicated, behavior therapy carried out by mental health professionals may be useful if the target symptoms are defined.

Anticonvulsant drugs used as necessary may be of some value.[22] Hyperactivity, impulsivity, and distractibility may respond to the judicious use of stimulant drugs; if much free-floating anxiety or disorganized behavior is present tranquilizing drugs may be of help. The use of the anticonvulsant ethosuximide (Zarontin), which has been said to help increase the functional I.Q. level through its effect on verbal functions in children who have learning problems and "cortical brain dysfunction" remains to be further evaluated.

As indicated earlier, developmental screening may be of value in the primary prevention of learning problems, through identification and referral for further study and remedial help of high-risk children with perceptual-motor and related problems, some of which may be the result of developmental deviations and some of which may derive from previously unrecognized mild brain damage. The Brazelton Neonatal Scale[10] has been used successfully to delineate the newborn's capacities and temperamental characteristics. The scale is sensitive also to neurologic abnormalities. Recently it has been used to differentiate infants born to heroin-addicted mothers taking methadone from infants in a normal group, with significant implications for behavioral management.[90] Early identification of parent-infant interactions and intervention to help parents handle their feelings in the newborn period have been of value.[80] (The topic is discussed more extensively in Chapter 28.)

Bibliography

1. Abrams, L.A.: Delayed and irregular maturation versus minimal brain injury: recommendations for a change in current nomenclature. Clin. Pediatr., 7:344, 1968.
2. American Academy of Pediatrics, Executive Board. Statement: Doman-Delacato. Treatment of Neurologically Handicapped Children. (Prepared with the Assistance of the Committee on the Handicapped Child.) Evanston, Ill., American Academy of Pediatrics, 1972.
3. Bender, L.: *Psychopathology of Children with Organic Brain Disorders.* Springfield, Ill., Thomas, 1956.
4. Benton, A.L.: Language disorders in children. Can. Psychol., 7:298, 1966.
5. Berenberg, W.: The physician's responsibility in the education of the cerebral palsied child. Pediatrics, 43:483, 1969.
6. Birch, H.G., and Bortner, M.: Stimulus competition and concept utilization in brain damaged children. Dev. Med. and Child Neurol., 9:402, 1967.
7. Black, P., et al.: The post-traumatic syndrome in children. In: *The Late Effects of Head Injury* (A. Walker, W. Caveness, and M. Critchley, Eds.). Springfield, Ill., Thomas, 1969.
8. Bond, E.D., and Smith, L.H.: Postencephalitic behavior disorders: A ten year review of the Franklin School. Am. J. Psychiatry, 92:17, 1935.
9. Bortner, M.: *Evaluation and Education of Children with Brain Damage.* Springfield, Ill., Thomas, 1968.
10. Brazelton, T.B.: *Neonatal Behavioral Assessment Scale.* Philadelphia, Lippincott, 1973.
11. Brier, N.M., and Demb, H.B.: Psychotherapy with the developmentally disabled adolescent. (Paper presented at the annual meeting of the American Orthopsychiatric Association.) Washington, D.C., October, 1977.
12. Bryant, K.: Unpublished material.
13. Byers, R.K., and Lord, E.E.: Late effects of lead poisoning on mental development. Am. J. Dis. Child., 66:471, 1943.
14. Camp, J.A., et al.: Clinical usefulness of the NIMH physical and neurological examination for soft signs. Am. J. Psychiatry, 135:362, 1978.
15. Christ, A.E.: Psychotherapy of the child with true brain damage. Am. J. Orthopsychiatry, 48:505, 1978.
16. Clements, S.: Minimal Brain Dysfunction in Children. Department of Health, Education, and Welfare, NIND Monograph No. 3. Washington, Government Printing Office, 1966.
17. Cohen, D.J., Caparulo, B., and Shaywitz, B.: Primary childhood aphasia and autism. J. Am. Acad. Child. Psychiatry, 15:604, 1976.
18. Cruickshank, W.M.: *A Teaching Method for Brain-injured and Hyperactive Children; A Demonstration-Pilot Study.* New York, Syracuse University Press, 1961.
19. Cruickshank, W., and Raus, G.M.: *Cerebral Palsy: Its Individual and Community Problems.* Syracuse, N.Y., Syracuse University Press, 1955.
20. Crothers, B., and Paine, R.: *The Natural History of Cerebral Palsy.* Cambridge, Mass., Harvard University Press, 1959.
21. Dann, M., et al.: A long-term study of small premature infants. Pediatrics, 33:394, 1964.
22. Denhoff, E., Ed.: *Drugs in Cerebral Palsy.* London, Medical Education and Information Unit of the Spastics Society, 1964.
23. Denhoff, E., and Robinault, I.: *Cerebral Palsy and Related Disorders: A Development Approach to Dysfunction.* New York, McGraw-Hill, 1960.
24. Deutsch, C.P., and Schumer, F.: *Brain-Damaged Children: A Modality-Oriented Exploration of Performance.* New York, Brunner/Mazel, 1970.
25. Dillon, H., and Leopold, R.L.: Children and the post-concussion syndrome. JAMA, 175:86, 1961.
26. Drage, J.S., et al.: The 5 minute Apgar score and 4 year psychological performance. Dev. Med. Child. Neurol., 8:14, 1966.
27. Eisenberg, L.: The psychiatric implications of brain damage in children. Psychiatr. Q., 31:72, 1957.
28. Engel, G.L., and Romano, J.: Delirium: A syndrome of cerebral insufficiency. J. Chronic Dis., 9:260, 1959.
29. Fabian, A.A.: Prognosis in head injuries in children. J. Nerv. Ment. Dis., 123:428, 1956.
30. Fabian, A.A., and Bender, L.: Head injury in children: Predisposing factors. Am. J. Orthopsychiatry, 17:68, 1947.
31. Freedman, A.M., et al.: Family adjustment to the brain-damaged child. In: *A Modern Introduction to the Family* (N. Bell and E. Vogel, Eds.). Glencoe, Ill., Free Press, 1960.
32. Freud, S.: Infantile cerebral paralysis. In: *Handbuch.* (H. Hufnagel, Ed.). Vienna, 1897.
33. Frostig, M.: Visual perception in the brain-injured child. Am. J. Orthopsychiatry, 33:665, 1963.
34. Gallagher, J.J.: *The Tutoring of Brain-injured Mentally Retarded Children: An Experimental Study.* Springfield, Ill., Thomas, 1960.
35. Garrard, S., and Richmond, J.: The psychological aspects of the management of children with

defects or damage to the central nervous system. Pediatr. Clin. North Am., November, 1957, p. 1033.

36. Goldstein, K.: *The Organism*. New York, American Book Company, 1939.

37. Goodman, J.D., and Sours, J.A.: *The Child Mental Status Examination*. New York, Basic Books, 1967.

38. Graham, F.K., and Berman, P.W.: Current status of behavior tests of brain damage in infants and preschool children. Am. J. Orthopsychiatry, 31:713, 1961.

39. Graham, F.K., et al.: Development three years after perinatal anoxia and other potentially damaging newborn experiences. Psychol. Mongr., 76:3, 1962.

40. Graham, P., and Rutter, M.: Organic dysfunction and child psychiatric disorders. Br. Med. J., 3:695, 1968.

41. Green, M.: Delirium. In: *Ambulatory Pediatrics* (M. Green and R.J. Haggerty, Eds.). Philadelphia, Saunders, 1968.

42. Group for the Advancement of Psychiatry: *Psychopathological Disorders of Childhood: Theoretical Considerations and a Proposed Classification*. Report No. 62. New York: Group for Advancement of Psychiatry, 1966.

43. Hall, R.V., and Broden, M.: Behavior changes in brain-injured children through social reinforcement. Exp. Child Psychol., 5:463, 1967.

44. Harrington, J.A., and Letemendia, F.J.J.: Persistent psychiatric disorders after head injuries in children. J. Ment. Sci., 104:1205, 1938.

45. Hertsig, M.E., Bortner, M., and Birch, H.G.: Neurologic findings in childen educationally designated as "brain-damaged." Am. J. Orthopsychiatry, 39:437, 1969.

46. Illingworth, R.S.: Diagnosis of cerebral palsy in the first year of life. Dev. Med. Child Neurol., 8:178, 1966.

47. Ingram, T.T.: Soft signs. Dev. Med. Child Neurol., 15:527, 1973.

48. Kanner, L.: *Child Psychiatry*, 3rd Ed. Springfield, Ill., Thomas, 1957.

49. Keith, H.M., Norval, M.A., and Hunt, A.B.: Neurologic lesions in relation to the sequelae of birth injury. Neurology, 3:139, 1953.

50. Kennard, M.: Value of equivocal signs in neurologic diagnoses. Neurology, 10:753, 1960.

51. Klapper, Z.S., and Birch, H.G.: The relation of childhood characteristics to outcome in young adults with cerebral palsy. Dev. Med. Child. Neurol., 4:645, 1966.

52. Klapper, Z.S., and Birch, H.G.: A fourteen year follow-up study of cerebral palsy: Intellectual change and stability. Am. J. Orthopsychiatry, 37:540, 1967.

53. Klebanoff, L.G., Singer, J.M., and Welensky, H.: Psychological consequences of brain lesions and ablations. Psychol. Bull., 51:1, 1954.

54. Langford, W.S., and Klingman, W.O.: Behavior disorders associated with intracranial tumors in childhood. Am. J. Dis. Child., 63:433, 1942.

55. Laufer, M.W., and Denhoff, E.: Hyperkinetic behavior syndrome in children. J. Pediatr., 50:463, 1957.

56. Little, S.: Note on an investigation of the emotional complications of cerebral palsy. Nerv. Child, 8:181, 1949.

57. Loring, J.: *Teaching the Cerebral Palsied Child; Proceedings of a Study Group at Grey College, Durham, April 1965*. London, Spastics Society/William Heinemann, 1965.

58. Lubchenko, L., et al.: Sequelae of premature birth. Am. J. Dis. Child., 106:101, 1963.

59. Lurie, L.A., and Levy, S.: Personality changes and behavior disorders of children following pertussis. JAMA, 120:890, 1942.

60. Mabry, C.C.: Prolonged neonatal anoxia without apparent adverse sequelae. J. Pediatr., 55:211, 1959.

61. MacKeith, R.C., and Bax, M.C.O.: Minimal brain damage—A concept discarded. In: *Minimal Cerebral Dysfunction* (Little Club Clinic in Developmental Medicine) London, National Spastics Society Medical Education Unit, 1963.

62. Macnab, G.H.: Hydrocephalus in infancy. In: *Surgical Progress*, Vol. 2 (E.R. Carling, and J.P. Ross, Eds.) London, Butterworths, 1961.

63. Maruta, T.: Prescription-induced organic brain syndrome. Am. J. Psychiatry, 135:376, 1978.

64. McDermott, J.F., et al.: Social class and mental illness in children: The diagnosis of organicity and mental retardation. J. Am. Acad. Psychiatry, 6:309, 1967.

65. Metcalf, D.R., and Jordan, K.: EEG ontogenesis in normal children. In: *Drugs, Development and Cerebral Function* (W.L. Smith, Ed.). Springfield, Ill., Thomas, 1971.

66. Milstein, V., Small, J.G., and Small, I.F.: The subtraction of serial sevens test in psychiatric patients. Arch. Gen. Psychiatry, 26:439, 1972.

67. Moncrief, A.A., et al.: Lead poisoning in children. Arch. Dis. Child., 39:1, 1964.

68. Nickerson, G., and MacDermot, P.N.: Psychometric evaluation and factors affecting the performance of children who have recovered from tuberculous meningitis. Pediatrics, 27:68, 1961.

69. Nordan, R.: The psychological reactions of children with neurological problems. Child. Psychiatry Hum. Dev., 6:214, 1976.

70. Oswin, M.: *Behavior Problems Amongst Children with Cerebral Palsy*. Bristol, England, Wright, 1967.

71. Otto, U.: The postconcussion syndrome in childhood. Acta Paedopsychiatr., 27:6, 1953.

72. Paine, R.S.: *Neurological Examination of Children*. London, Spastics Society Medical Education and Information Unit, 1966.

72a. Pasamanick, B., and Knobloch, H.: Brain damage and reproductive casualty. Am. J. Orthopsychiatry, 30:298, 1960.

73. Prugh, D.G.: Toward an understanding of psychosomatic concepts in relation to illness in children. In: *Modern Perspectives in Child Development* (A.J. Solnit and S.A. Provence, Eds.). New York, International Universities Press, 1963.

74. Prugh, D.G., Wagonfeld, S., Metcalf. D., and Jordan, K.: A clinical study of delirium in children and adolescents. Psychosom. Med., 42:177, 1980.

75. Prugh, D.G., and Kisley, A.J.: Psychosocial as-

pects of pediatrics and psychiatric disorders. In: *Current Pediatric Diagnosis and Treatment*, 5th Ed. (C.H. Kempe, H.N. Silver, and D. O'Brien, Eds.) Los Altos, Calif., Lange Publishers, 1978.

76. Reinhart, J., and Succop, R.: Psychiatric picture in pontine tumors. J. Am. Acad. Psychiatry, 2:244, 1963.

77. Riser, T., et al.: Early psychiatric forms of craniopharyngiomas. Ann. Med. Psychol., *103*:241, 1945.

78. Romano, J., and Engel, G.L.: Delirium. I. Electroencephalographic data. Arch. Neurol. Psychiatry, *51*:356, 1944.

79. Romano, J., and Engel, G.L.: Physiologic and psychologic considerations of delirium. Med. Clin. North Am., *28*:629, 1944.

80. Rose, J.A.: The prevention of mothering breakdown associated with physical abnormalities of the infant. In: *Prevention of Mental Disorders in Children* (G. Caplan, Ed.). New York, Basic Books, 1961.

81. Ross, A.O.: Behavior therapy. In: *Psychopathological Disorders of Childhood* (H. Quay and J. Werry, Eds.). New York, Wiley, 1972.

82. Rutter, M., Graham, P., and Yule, W.: *A Neuropsychiatric Study in Childhood*. Philadelphia, Lippincott, 1970.

83. Santostefano, S.: Psychologic testing in evaluating and understanding organic brain damage and the effects of drugs in children. J. Pediatr., 62:766, 1963.

84. Schachter, F.F., and Apgar, V.: Perinatal asphyxia and psychologic signs of brain damage in childhood. Pediatrics, 24:1016, 1959.

85. Scherzer, A.L., Mike, V., and Ilson, J.: Physical therapy as a determinant of change in the cerebral palsied infant. Pediatrics, *58*:47, 1976.

86. Schmitt, B.D.: The minimal brain dysfunction myth. Am. J. Dis. Child., *129*:1313, 1975.

87. Selley, I.: Acute psychosis after head injury in children. Acta Psychiatry, 33:208, 1958.

88. Shapiro, T., et al.: Consistency of "nonfocal" neurological signs. J. Am. Acad. Child. Psychiatry, 17:70, 1978.

89. Silver, A.A.: Behavioral syndrome associated with brain damage in children. Pediatr. Clin. North Am., 6:687, 1958.

90. Soule, A.B., et al.: Clinical uses of the Brazelton scale. Pediatrics, 54:583, 1974.

91. Storey, P.B.: The precipitation of subarachnoid hemorrhage. J. Psychosom. Res., *13*:175, 1969.

92. Strauss, A.A., and Lehtinen, L.E.: *Psychopathology and Education of the Brain-Injured Child*. New York, Grune & Stratton, 1947.

93. Taylor, E.M.: *Psychological Appraisal of Children with Cerebral Defects*. Cambridge, Mass., Harvard University Press, 1959.

94. Teuber, H.L., and Rudel, R.G.: Behavior after cerebral lesions in children and adults. Dev. Med. Child. Neurol., 4:3, 1962.

95. Thomas, A., and Chess, S.: A longitudinal study of three brain damaged children: Infancy to adolescence. Arch. Gen. Psychiatry, 32:457, 1975.

96. Wender, P.: *Minimal Brain Dysfunction in Children*. New York, Wiley-Interscience, 1971.

97. Werry, J.: Studies on the hyperactive child. IV. An empirical analysis of the brain dysfunction syndrome. Arch. Gen. Psychiatry, *19*:9, 1968.

98. Werry, J., et al.: Studies on the hyperactive child. VII. Neurological status compared with neurotic and normal children. Am. J. Orthopsychiatry, *42*:441, 1971.

99. Werry, J.S., and Aman, M.G.: The reliability and diagnostic validity of the physical and neurological examination for soft signs. (PANESS) J. Autism Child. Schizophren., 6:253, 1976.

100. Wilson, L.G.: Viral encephalopathy mimicking functional psychosis. Am. J. Psychiatry, *133*:165, 1976.

101. Winder, A.E.: A program of group counselling for the parents of cerebral palsied children. Cerebral Palsy Rev., *19*: No. 23, p. 37, May-June, 1958.

102. Winkler, A., Dixon, J.F., and Parker, J.B., Jr.: Brain function in problem children and controls: Psychoneurotic, neurological, and electroencephalographic comparisons. Am. J. Psychiatry, *127*:94, 1970.

103. Yates, A.J.: The validity of some psychological tests of brain damage. Psychol. Bull., *51*:359, 1954.

104. Young, H.F., et al.: The relationship of intelligence and cerebral mantle in treated infantile hydrocephalus. Pediatrics, *53*:38, 1973.

105. Zimet, C., and Fishman, D.: Psychological deficit in schizophrenia and brain damage. Ann. Rev. Psychol., 21:113, 1970.

General References

Birch, H., Ed.: *Brain Damage in Children: Biological and Social Aspects.* Baltimore, Williams & Wilkins, 1964.

Cruickshank, W.M.: *The Brain-injured Child in Home, School, and Community.* Syracuse, N.Y., Syracuse University Press, 1967.

Eisenberg, L.: Behavioral Manifestations of Cerebral Damage in Childhood. Brain Damage in Childhood. (H.G. Birch, Ed.) Baltimore, Williams & Wilkins, 1964.

Ford, F.R.: *Diseases of the Nervous System in Infancy, Childhood, and Adolescence,* 5th Ed. Springfield, Ill., Thomas, 1966.

Friedlander, B.Z., Sterritt, G.M., and Kirk, G.: *Exceptional Infant,* Vols 1, 2, 3. New York, Brunner/Mazel, 1975.

Gomez, M.R.: Minimal cerebral dysfunction (maximal neurologic confusion). Clin. Pediatr., 6:589, 1967.

Graham, F., et al.: Behavioral differences between normal and traumatized newborns. Psychol. Monogr., 70:17, 1956.

Ingraham, F.D., and Matson, D.D.: *Neurosurgery of Infancy and Childhood.* Springfield, Ill., Thomas, 1954.

Livingston, S., and Pauli, L.L.: Neurological evaluation in child psychiatry. In: *Comprehensive Textbook of Psychiatry* (A. Freedman, H. Kaplan, and B. Saddock, Eds.). Baltimore, Williams & Wilkins, 1975.

Low, N.L., Correll, J.W., and Hamill, J.F.: Tumors of the cerebral hemispheres in children. Arch. Neurol., *13*:547, 1965.

Matson, D.D.: *Neurosurgery of Infancy and Childhood,* 2nd Ed. Springfield, Ill., Thomas, 1969.

Menkes, J.: *A Textbook of Pediatric Neurology.* Philadelphia, Lea & Febiger, 1974.

Nellhaus, G.: Neurologic and muscular disorders. In: *Current Pediatric Diagnosis and Treatment* (C.H. Kempe, H.K. Silver, and D. O'Brien, Eds.). Los Altos, Calif., Lange, 1978.

Pasamanick, B., and Knobloch, H.: Brain damage and reproductive casualty. Am. J. Orthopsychiatry, *30*:298, 1960.

Prechtl, H., and Beintema, O.: *The Neurological Examination of the Full Term New Born Infant.* London, Heineman, 1964.

Schilder, P.: *Contributions to Developmental Neuropsychiatry.* (L. Bender, Ed.). New York, International Universities Press, 1964.

Schulman, J.L., Kaspar, J.C., and Throne, F.M.: *Brain Damage and Behavior:* A Clinical-Experimental Study. Springfield, Ill., Thomas, 1965.

Stone, F.H.: Psychodynamics of brain-damaged children: A preliminary report. Child Psychol. and Psychiatry, *1*:203, 1960.

Teuber, H.L.: The premorbid personality and reaction to brain damage. Am. J. Orthopsychiatry, *30*:322, 1960.

23

Mental Retardation

Somewhere on the other side of despair.
(T.S. Eliot)

Energy set free by the magic agencies
of hope. . . .
(J.J. Putnam)

The diagnostic features of mental retardation are:

1. The child's intellectual functioning is significantly subaverage throughout the developmental period, as evaluated by repeated psychologic testing.
2. The child's lower intellectual functioning is associated with a concurrent impairment of his adaptive behavior.
3. In mild-to-moderate cases, the child's slower intellectual development is often associated with disturbances in his personality development or functioning of various types, from mild emotional problems to more serious psychopathologic disorders.

Since mental retardation has been well discussed in several excellent and recent monographs (see General References for this chapter), only the psychosocial aspects of mental retardation are emphasized in the discussion that follows.[43]

Until quite recently, the term mental retardation tended to evoke, in the mind of the physician, as well as of the child's parents and the general public, either an image of a severely retarded person who had a known clinical picture and often certain physical stigmata or an image of a person who had a markedly disfiguring kind of developmental defect.[23] In addition, until about the early 1960s, state institutions (which were often isolated from the community) were the chief and sometimes the only resources for the care and management of the mentally retarded, a circumstance that reinforced those images of mental retardation.[49] Other commonly held ideas about the mentally retarded are that mentally retarded adolescent girls are easily taken advantage of sexually and often become pregnant out of wedlock, that mentally retarded people have more children than the general population, and that the children of mentally retarded people are themselves usually retarded.

Actually, mildly retarded children (i.e., those whose I.Q.s are 50 to 70) comprise about 85%[36] of all retarded children. Mildly retarded children rarely have manifest physical abnormalities and by most criteria are indistinguishable from other children.[103] In addition, studies[72] have shown that retarded adolescent girls do not become pregnant more frequently than do girls in comparable socioeconomic groups. And mentally retarded people as a group do not have more children than do people who come from comparable socioeconomic backgrounds, and their children are usually not retarded.[60] (Some severely mentally retarded people cannot reproduce.) Although some states still have laws about compulsory eugenic sterilization, sterilization of the mentally retarded has been done only infrequently in recent years, largely because of the growing rejection of the view that mental retardation is hereditary. Today many legal authorities[77] feel there is no sound basis for sterilization, a procedure that is often regretted later by patients who have undergone it.[86] Many outstanding clinicians (e.g., Tarjan) have abandoned the practice.

These and other myths about the retarded have recently been laid firmly to rest. The current tendency to use the term mental retardation, rather than mental deficiency (high grade, low grade, etc.) indicates a more dynamic, humane, and expectant attitude, and such terms as idiot and moron are no longer used by knowledgeable professionals because they have opprobrious connotations. However, further education of the general public and even certain segments of the medical profession about these matters is needed.

About 3% of the population have functioning I.Q.s of 70 or below, the usual clinical point of designation today of a person as mentally retarded. Figure 23–1 shows how intelligence is distributed among the general population. (The categories of "borderline" and "dull normal" today are regarded as "normal variations" of intelligence and should no longer be used; see p. 401.)

In regard to the figure of 3% just mentioned, Tarjan has emphasized that a valid diagnosis of mental retardation requires that along with the impairment in intelligence, a similarly significant impairment in general adaption be present, and both must become manifest before the person is 17 years old.[105] Since the correlation between levels of intelligence and adaptation is high only during the school-age period, Tarjan has estimated that at any one point only 1% of the population would fit a clinical diagnosis of overt mental retardation.[103] Even so, the limitations of the I.Q. (discussed in Chapter 8) apply, and only an I.Q. range, not an exact I.Q., can be established for a given child, even when the child is repeatedly tested.

Mental retardation is not a disease, a defect, or a diagnosis. It is a symptom complex, that now is known to involve about 200 causative factors. As Phillips[72] has emphasized, the diagnostic term retardation tends to label the child in such a way that others tend to forget that he is a developing, learning person who comes from a particular background and who has his strengths and skills as well as his limitations. No one's intelligence is fixed or immutable,[91,97] and, on a particular day, depending on a variety of factors, the retarded child (like everyone else) may perform more or less well at school or in other settings.[124] In view of this fact and of the fact that there is a range of error of a few points in intelligence tests, it follows that a child who

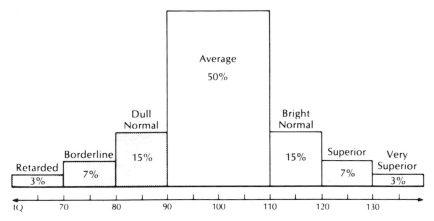

Figure 23–1. Classification of intelligence in the general population. (From G. Solomons: Counseling parents of the retarded: The interpretation interview. In: *Psychiatric Approaches to Mental Retardation* (F.J. Menascolino, Ed.). New York, Basic Books, 1970.)

scores near the top of one range may be actually capable of functioning as well as the child who scores in the lower portion of the next higher range and that a person may meet the criteria for mental retardation at one time or at one age and not at another time or at another age. Finally, it should be remembered that children who have mental retardation also have personalities.

Of the people who fit the criteria for a valid diagnosis of mental retardation, about 25% have so-called clinical types of mental retardation and concomitant somatic manifestations whose causal mechanisms are not clear in some cases. Nearly 75% have no demonstrable biologic or medical disorder, and psychologic and social factors seem mainly to be involved. Even among people who have the "clinical" type of mental retardation, most but not all of whom are moderately or severely retarded, psychologic and sociocultural factors are involved to some extent.

Figure 23–2 illustrates schematically the relative importance of the causative factors.

To summarize, nearly all people whose I.Q.s are below 50 have demonstrable brain disease or damage and their mental retardation is largely of "biologic" origin. These people belong to all social and economic segments of the population. In contrast, social or psychologic factors account for most cases of mental retardation in people whose I.Q.s are above 50. Their mental retardation has a largely psychosocial and sociocultural origin. These people come mainly from socially and economically deprived segments of the population.

Biologic Factors

The "biologic" factors that produce impairments of central nervous system functioning include somatic factors which affect the developing fetus (e.g., infection or dietary deficiencies[6]), metabolic disorders, or toxic influences that affect the mother, complications during the birth process (e.g., asphyxia neonatorum), and infections or trauma that occur immediately after birth. Severe, long-continued malnutrition during infancy can be a causative factor in intellectual impairment, in an environment that is unfavorable to intellectual development.[14,45] But an episode of severe malnutrition under favorable environmental conditions may not cause later intellectual impairment.[79] Besides such perinatal influences[70] there is a second set of factors, which involves pathologic conditions of the reproductive cells of the parents: heredi-

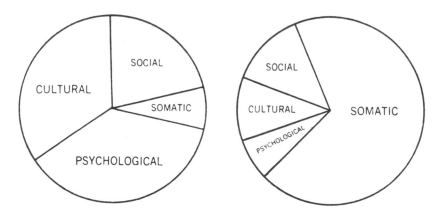

Figure 23–2.   The relative importance of etiologic factors in *A*, mild retardation and *B*, moderate and severe retardation. (From Group for the Advancement of Psychiatry: Basic Considerations in Mental Retardation: A Preliminary Report. New York, Group for the Advancement of Psychiatry, 1959, Report No. 43.)

tary disorders (e.g., enzymopathies), chromosomal aberrations (e.g., Down's syndrome), or the results of exposure to harmful external agents (e.g., ionizing radiation). Finally, a third group of factors includes conditions which damage the central nervous system during the course of development (e.g., trauma, infection, intoxications, marked malnutrition, new growths, and demyelinating or hypermyelinating disorders.

Such somatic factors are fully discussed in other works and are not elaborated on here. But it should be said that those factors cannot always be identified in the individual case of encephalopathy or chronic brain syndrome associated with mental retardation. Classification on the basis of pathogenesis is also difficult because the causes of some clinically well-defined syndromes that involve mental retardation have not yet been fully investigated. In phenylketonuria,[111] the precise manner in which intellectual impairment comes about is unclear, as is true in other enzymatic and biochemical abnormalities. Although some cases of mental retardation involve factors that are genetic in origin (e.g., inborn errors of metabolism, chromosomal abnormalities, and heredodegenerative disorders[13]) the old concept of "familial mental retar-

dation," which is based on examples like the Jukes and the Kallikak families and which assumes that a single hereditary or somatic factor is involved, is no longer valid today, as Kugel[56] has emphasized. Some people believe that the effects of poverty, lack of appropriate stimulation, and inadequate education of parents are probably more important in such cases than are any truly hereditary factors.

Different children respond in different degrees to the same central nervous system infection, and people who have inborn errors of phenylalanine metabolism but do not have significant mental retardation have been identified in families of retarded children who have phenylketonuria.[21] The "defect" concept is simply not adequate. Multiple factors, including a combination of biologic and psychosocial handicaps[118] (e.g., feelings of hopelessness on the part of the child's parents), undoubtedly contribute to the degree of manifest intellectual retardation, as well as to the degree of impairment in adaptation. Although most children who have such disorders fall into the severely retarded category, some may show only mild retardation, as do many children who have Down's syndrome. (A few people who have Down's syndrome and who have normal intelligence have been reported.[37])

Psychosocial Factors

The psychosocial factors that produce functional mental retardation in children whose intellectual potential is adequate include psychoneurotic disorders (often with learning inhibitions), severe reactive disorders (at times with negativism or depression), and personality disorders[24] (often with oppositional or aggressive behavior[16]). In these disorders of adaptive behavior, the individual functions may be variably normal or retarded. Psychotic disorders, which are often associated with bizarre or stereotyped behavior,[52] represent a special case. It is sometimes difficult to determine without a trial of therapy (which may not be totally decisive) whether the picture is primarily that of a psychotic disorder, with mental retardation being one of the several manifestations of the severe psychopathology or is primarily that of mental retardation (sometimes with associated brain damage), with a superimposed psychotic disorder.[63] Some clinicians use the term pseudo-retardation to refer to all patients in whom mental retardation seems to result from a psychopathologic disorder, including some patients who have severe emotional deprivation.[31,35] Although most of these patients are in the mildly retarded category, a few may function at a moderately retarded level.

Sociocultural Factors

By far the largest group in this second category, estimated by some to make up two-thirds or more of the group, are children who function at a retarded level because of what has been termed "sociocultural deprivation." (It has also been referred to as cultural, familial, or environmental deprivation and deprivation of a psycho-social nature.) The diagnosis is generally made at the time the child begins school. Retarded children tend to have higher verbal scores than performance scores in the preschool-age period and lower verbal scores than performance scores in the school-age period. When the child reaches maturity, the overt manifestations of retardation tend to disappear. These children are normal in appearance, and ordinarily have no concomitant physical disabilities. It has been conservatively estimated by Tarjan[106] that children who have economically, socially, and educationally deprived backgrounds, both urban and rural, have a risk of sociocultural retardation that is 15 times higher than that of children who have middle-class suburban backgrounds. Such children are more often unplanned and unwanted, and they tend to be raised in homes in which the father is absent and the mother is physically overworked and emotionally harassed. Many of these children come from ghetto families in which the parents feel hopeless and do not offer their children motivation toward academic learning. These children do not have the organized tactile and kinesthetic stimulation during infancy that middle-class children have. For example, they are often left unattended on the floor or in a crib. Their exposure to noises, odors, and colors is often chaotic and uneven, and their parents are said to use fewer words and often to speak in brief and "negative" sentences.[11]

The concept of "verbal deprivation" has recently been criticized. It has been pointed out that children from Spanish-speaking families in the barrio may hear a full and fluent version of their own tongue. It has also been pointed out that black children from the ghetto may receive a good deal of verbal stimulation but that they learn a special ghetto language, one that is different from the language of the majority. In either case, however, the child is penalized in the school if his teacher comes from a different background and so interprets his different way of speaking (or his anxious, mistrustful silence) as a sign of limited intelligence.[3]

It has also been pointed out that children who have sociocultural retardation come from socioeconomic groups in which malnutrition during pregnancy is common, prenatal care is limited or nonexistent, prematurity is high, nutrition and health care are inadequate during infancy and early development, and young children are often exposed to noxious stimuli (e.g., infections, trauma, poisons, and noise). Undoubtedly some of these "somatic noxae" help cause the sociocultural retardation. Some clinicians prefer to use a biomedical model that emphasizes these factors heavily. Other clinicians offer genetic explanations, which are based on the theory of "assortive mating" of the mentally retarded or on the theory of racial inferiority. (I and others strongly disagree with this point of view, as discussed in Chapter 5).

Although, as Tarjan and his colleagues,[106] Eisenberg,[24] Yarrow,[122] Prugh,[78] and others, have pointed out, much remains to be learned about the effects of deprivation (in regard to timing, quality, quantity, specificity, and other variables), and although some rather global conclusions have already been drawn, there are specific data concerning the effects of deprivation. (Some data regarding the positive effects of early enrichment on children who come from impoverished backgrounds[124] are mentioned in Chapter 28.) The beneficial effects of environmental stimulation in the preschool-age period on a group of orphanage children who were mildly retarded (reported on by Skeels[94]) have been shown in a follow-up study to have held up over a 20-year period. Stevens and Heber[100] have recently reported on a group of children of mentally retarded parents. The children had been in a special preschool program, and later they were able to function normally in school. The "culture-bound" qualities of intelligence tests have been mentioned, as has the "promotion" from retarded to normal of many

Spanish-surnamed children when they were given an I.Q. test in Spanish.

Finally, Scrofani, Suziedelis, and Shore[92] recently did an experimental test of Jensen's hypothesis that children who have poor socioeconomic backgrounds and who repeatedly score 15 to 20 points below middle-class children on conventional I.Q. tests have genetically determined limitations in their conceptual ability. Using special exercises, these investigators trained groups of children in concept formation. The children were matched for sex and race (white and black), and they came from all socioeconomic backgrounds. A significant number of the children who came from poor socioeconomic backgrounds achieved performance levels that were equal to those of middle-class children. No race or sex differences were noted; the child's developmental level seemed to be more important than his age. These findings are in opposition to Jensen's theory, and they support the belief of Cronbach and others that the conceptual ability of many lower-class children is equal to that of middle-class children if the lower-class children are given special training.

The criteria for classifying the degree of mental retardation that are used by such organizations as the American Association for Mental Deficiency,[42] the American Psychiatric Association,[9] and the World Health Organization (WHO) are somewhat discrepant and thus confusing for the clinician. The International Classification of Diseases[105] defines mental retardation on the basis of a set of standard deviations from a mean of 100. Thus mild mental retardation refers to an I.Q. range of 50 to 70; moderate retardation to an I.Q. range of 35 to 50; severe retardation to an I.Q. range of 20 to 35; and profound retardation (a designation that is rarely used in the United States) to an I.Q. that is below 20. Figure 23–3 shows the relative percentages of retarded people who fall into the mild, moderate, and severely retarded categories.

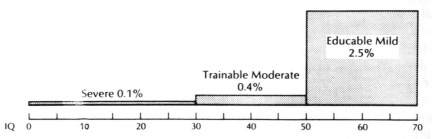

Figure 23–3. Classification of mental retardation. (From G. Solomons: Counseling parents of the retarded. In: *Psychiatric Approaches to Mental Retardation* (F.J. Menascolino, Ed.). New York, Basic Books, 1970.)

The use of the terms educable for the mildly retarded and trainable for the moderately retarded is common in the United States today. Those terms are used rather loosely sometimes, but they have some value. As Tarjan[103] and others[75] have pointed out, with adequate educational opportunity almost all children whose I.Q.s are above 50 (i.e., 85% of retarded people) can learn to read and write, can achieve at a useful level in other subjects (e.g., arithmetic), can become socially responsible citizens, and, if they do not have other gross handicaps, can become economically self-supporting. Some have, by adulthood, developed beyond expectation.[89] Several studies in the United States and Great Britain have shown that when these children become adults they tend to merge with the general population and that their children are not retarded. Very few have associated physical signs.

Some children whose I.Q.s are from 35 to 40 can acquire some rudimentary reading skills and are capable of working in "open" employment. There is a report[82] of an 11-year-old girl who had an I.Q. of 41 who was able to read and write fluently and who worked at a seventh-grade level. Most of these children, however, are able to work only in "sheltered" employment. Some of them have associated physical handicaps. Almost no children whose I.Q.s are below 35 are able to work outside an institution or to live independently. Most are able to perform only the most simple tasks, even with close supervision, and many have associated serious physical handicaps.

Although I.Q. scores have some educational value, their limitations are such that the Fifth World Health Organization (WHO) Seminar in Psychiatric Diagnosis, Classification, and Statistics (held in 1969) recommended (1) that I.Q. scores not be used as the sole measure of the degree of retardation, (2) that I.Q. scores be omitted from the category headings, and (3) that the categories be carefully defined in regard to the degree of social and adaptive handicap. Although assessment of social competence was mentioned earlier as a component of a valid diagnosis of mental retardation, such assessment has so far not been feasible on a rigorous basis. For example, the Vineland Social Maturity Scale, a standardized test, has been found to be a poor predictor of a child's scholastic performance and to be influenced by a child's deviant behavior. The clinician must still rely on making a thoughtful assessment of all the information he can gather about the child's intellectual functioning, the demands being made of him, his family and social situation, the motivational factors, and his adjustment in school, at work, and in social settings.

The WHO seminar also recommended that the categories borderline mental retardation (I.Q.s of 70 to 80) and dull normal (I.Q.s of 80 to 90) (see Fig. 23–1) be replaced by the category of normal variations in intelligence.

The *differential diagnosis* in mental retardation includes: (1) psychotic or other psychosocial disorders, (2) the effects of severe emotional deprivation, (3) sensory deficits (e.g., blindness,[25] and high-frequency hearing deficits), (4) developmental lags in cognitive, perceptual-motor, or language functions, in which some aspects of development are usually within the normal range, (5) chronic brain syndromes, (6) neuromuscular disorders in infancy, and (7) the psychosocial effects of chronic physical illness or debilitation, repeated or prolonged hospitalization, depression, and lack of environmental stimulation. The fact that intelligence tests of infants and young childhood have limited value as predictors of a child's later scholastic performance has been mentioned, as has the fact that group I.Q. tests also are of limited value. The need for prolonged observation and follow-up and for repeated testing has also been emphasized. Useful as it is as a screening procedure, the Denver Developmental Screening Test is not an intelligence test. If it raises a question about mental retardation in a child, the child should be referred to a competent clinical child psychologist. Besides a developmental history and physical studies, a psychosocial evaluation of the child in his family setting is needed to determine the child's adaptive capacity as well as the possible psychologic and social factors involved.

Recently some investigators have pointed out that having a white person test a black child may affect adversely the child's motivation and performance. Conversely, some black testers and white children have had similar difficulties. But as Engel[27] has indicated, social class background and value orientation probably have more bearing on the accuracy of the test results than do racial or ethnic factors.

Psychopathologic Problems and Mental Retardation

Until recently, the developmental characteristics and behavior of retarded chil-

dren were generally felt to derive solely from their intellectual limitations. But a number of studies have supported the observation of Potter, Jenkins, and other pioneers that retarded children are subject to anxiety and emotional conflicts—perhaps more so than children of average intelligence. The poor self-images, feelings of inadequacy, tendencies toward passive, inflexible, or negativistic behavior, "shutting out" of questions, constant "smokescreening" of questions, or "clowning" behavior observed in retarded children have been described as attempts the children make to cover up their limitations.

Some investigators (e.g., Webster[112]) have felt that the retardation has a relatively specific effect on the child's personality development, perhaps in respect to maturity or other kinds of readiness for experience. Others, (e.g., Chess[8] and Phillips,[75]) have felt that maladaptive behavior in a retarded child is more a function of his interpersonal relationships and the way in which he is reared and taught than of the retardation itself and that the emotional responses of the retarded child are essentially the same as those of the normal child. My experience inclines me toward the latter view in regard to most mildly retarded children. But there is probably some truth in the former view, and much more research must be done on the relationship between emotional disturbance and mental retardation.

Although estimates vary, it now seems clear that the incidence of disturbance in adaptation and in personality development is higher in retarded children than in those who are not retarded.[112] However, emotional disturbances in retarded children, when they occur, bear many similarities to those in other children although retarded children may be especially vulnerable to the development of withdrawn and autistic behavior (not necessarily of psychotic proportions) when faced with significant anxiety or emotional conflict.[65] Certainly, retarded children may show any of the clinical disorders of adaptation found in children of normal intelligence, including reactive, psychoneurotic, personality, and psychotic disorders.[32,75] Children with these disorders should receive a comprehensive evaluation, including a psychosocial evaluation as well as an intellectual evaluation, and appropriate physical studies.[102] These disorders have been shown by Woodward,[120,121] Chess,[8] Phillips,[75] and others to be responsive to treatment, regardless of the mental retardation involved. Although opinions differ, if mental retardation is seen as the basic disorder, it is probably best to give it as the primary diagnosis, but a personality diagnosis of any associated disorder should be added. If definitive brain damage is present, it may contribute to these disorders, as described in the preceding section.

Early placement of the child in an institutional setting in which he will be unable to establish close relationships with others may also adversely affect the child's personality functioning and intellectual potential. Menolascino[64] has shown that emotional disturbances of a variety of types occurred three times more often in a group of children with Down's syndrome who were in institutions than in a group of children with Down's syndrome who were outpatients. Other studies[4,62,90] have suggested that children with Down's syndrome* who were reared at home function generally at a moderately or at times mildly retarded level, while those reared in an institutional setting function within the severely retarded range. (As mentioned, a few children who have Down's syndrome have been said to have I.Q.s within the normal range.) In addition to the inadequate interpersonal relationships in large institutions, for a number of reasons[44] the child's contacts with his family and his

*Although in general I am opposed to the use of eponyms, I agree with those who dislike the term mongolism because it suggests that the disorder has a racial origin, and I support the effort to use instead the term Down's syndrome.

family's interest in him often diminish when the child is institutionalized.

As Zigler's[123] work has demonstrated, institutionalizing a mentally retarded chil can help cause not only problems in motivation that adversely affect his learning but also some of the behavioral patterns (e.g., head banging, rocking, rumination, and temper tantrums) long thought to be the result of the retardation.

Although, as one study has suggested,[110] mentally retarded children may be more "outer directed" in problem solving than are normal children, the "overaffectionateness" often described in children who have Down's syndrome is probably a device those children use to cope with the social and emotional deprivation that they often experience in large institutions. Mentally retarded children in institutions have been shown to have a heightened motivation to interact with supportive adults, but this characteristic seems to be coupled with wariness and mistrust at times. At best it seems to be a superficial and somewhat indiscriminate attempt at relatedness, without commitment to deep relationships, which is often seen in institutionalized children who are not mentally retarded. Actually, as Prugh and Harlow[78] and others have demonstrated, "masked emotional deprivation" may occur in intact though disturbed families, and various kinds of behavioral response may result, including those just described. Retarded children reared at home may also be exposed to such social and emotional deprivation more often than are normal children, because of the hopeless or negative attitudes of some parents.

The response of the child's parents and the other members of his family to the diagnosis of mental retardation is an important factor in the disturbances of personality development and even in the limitation of the child's functioning intellectual potential. (The responses may be similar to the responses to the diagnosis of any serious defect in a child.) The impact on the family of the birth of a child who has Down's syndrome or other obvious stigmata can be catastrophic, as Wolf and Lourie[115] and others[28] have pointed out. The reactions may include feelings of shock, denial, anger, guilt, worry about costs, and blame; and marital conflict and even separations or divorce are not uncommon outcomes. In a study by Gralicker and his colleagues,[39] about 50% of parents whose children had been given a diagnosis of mental retardation in a clinic setting had initially reacted with feelings of rejection of the child, associated with feelings of shame or guilt. Many of the other parents were intensely concerned about the reactions of their children, relatives, and friends to the diagnosis. Some parents, after first denying the problem, then mourning,[26,95] and then feeling guilt and other emotions, can accept the diagnosis fully (similar "phasic responses" by parents to the occurrence of illness or injury or the diagnosis of fatal illness in their children are described in Chapter 24). Other parents continue to show denial and disbelief and then embark on "shopping tours" to other agencies or cling to fantasies that the child will "grow out of it." Later overprotection of the retarded child and overpreoccupation or overinvolvement with his care[17] can result in the parents' neglect of his siblings or ambivalence toward them,[29,88] and the siblings may show varying types and degrees of behavioral responses.[34,40,41]

Another study by Koch and his colleagues[53] has indicated that parents are often intensely dissatisfied with the way pediatricians and general practitioners deal with their mentally retarded child. For example, some parents have felt that the physician did not spend enough time discussing the diagnosis and its implications or that the physician presented the diagnosis too abruptly. Parents have also said they felt that the physician's examination of their child was not thorough enough, that the physician was disinterested in their problem, that he made no suggestions about

handling the child, or that he held out no hope for the child, sometimes even recommending institutionalizing the child immediately. Koch's study was done over 15 years ago. Because more is now known about mental retardation, physicians, especially pediatricians, may be more interested in retarded children and less inclined to recommend early institutionalization, as one study of physicians' attitudes[109] has suggested. But complaints like these just listed are still heard from a number of parents.

When a newborn shows problems that suggest brain damage, his parents may fear mental retardation and other difficulties. Rose[84] has pointed out how the mother-infant interaction may be affected by a lack of responses or by strange responses from the infant toward the mother. The mother of such an infant may feel inadequate as a mother, remain cautious and detached, or show oversolicitous or other inappropriate behavior. The father also may be at least indirectly involved. Long-term adverse effects on the parent-child relationship and the child's later personality development and adaptation (including the "vulnerable child syndrome") may occur even if mental retardation or definitive brain damage do not occur. Other adverse effects may arise from false-positive tests for phenylketonuria, as Rothenberg[85] has indicated.

Management, Prognosis, and Prevention

As implied earlier, most mentally retarded children do not require institutionalizing, and they may be harmed emotionally and physically[69] by such a step. In the early 1960s, it was estimated that only about 4% of all mentally retarded persons were in residential settings and that at least 96% remained in the community. At that time, more than 50% of the mentally retarded who were in public institutions were only mildly retarded. This group included children who were put in institutions because of emotional disturbances or family problems and young adults who were so disturbed that they could not remain in the community. Most of the children who were in institutions had not had adequate psychiatric evaluation, and little consideration was given to alternatives to institutional care. Similarly, little attempt had been made to treat the young adults in the community during their childhood. Of the moderately and severely retarded children, about two-thirds were being cared for at home although there was little in the way of school or day care facilities at that time. Martin[60] has estimated recently that only about 1% of the mentally retarded require institutional care.

In the late 1960s, educational programs for the mildly and moderately retarded were begun in the public schools,[33,51,101] and the number of mentally retarded people in public institutions began to decrease. This "normalization shift"—from institutional to community and home care[20,47,57]—has paralleled but lagged behind the changes taking place in the care of the mentally ill. As Tarjan[104] has indicated, the trend toward decreasing the number of institutionalized patients continues, calling for both early discharge and alternatives to admission. The placement of institutionalized retarded persons in the community is going forward actively and successfully although many of these people have lost contact with their families[87] and although "transitional" jobs often must be found for these people before they are able to work and live independently in the community.[99] Both placing these people in the community and finding alternatives to admission initially depend on having certain community resources (e.g., health, educational, vocational, social, recreational, mental health, legal, welfare, and other supportive and protective programs) that have only recently begun to be available.[71,76,104,108] For severely retarded people who require continuing residential care, the trend is toward the breaking down of large institutions into smaller units that make possible more interpersonal contacts, special enrichment programs, and the development of self-care, and other improvements.[22,48,57]

Despite the trend toward community care of the vast majority of retarded persons, there are still ethical problems regarding the severely or profoundly retarded, especially those who have associated physical handicaps of a marked degree. With the recent change in attitudes toward abortion, the birth of some of those who have genetic defects has been prevented. But ever-improving techniques of perinatal care have inevitably resulted in the birth and survival of smaller premature infants, who are more likely to be retarded or damaged.[114] As mentioned, sterilization of mentally retarded persons in general has been opposed—on both clinical and legal grounds. Abuses in regard to the sterilization of the mentally retarded have been brought to the attention of the Department of Health and Human Resources. As Clifford[10] has emphasized, prevention of prematurity by better and more easily available prenatal care is the sine qua non for reducing the incidence of mental retardation and some neurologic disorders. (The ethical problems of active and passive euthanasia[83] are discussed in Chapter 26.)

I am opposed to active euthanasia for mentally retarded people (or for anyone). The mentally retarded cannot give informed consent, and consent given by their parents has ethical and moral, not to mention psychologic, ramifications. I believe that a democratic and humanistic society must give humane and humanitarian care to even its most profoundly damaged members. It should be remembered that in the Nazi regime, denying the right to live began with the mentally retarded.

The Physician's Feelings

In diagnosing and managing mental retardation in infants and children, the obstetrician, the pediatrician, or the family physician should remember that he as well as the parents may have feelings of guilt, helplessness, or hopelessness. The physician, feeling that he must do something, may be tempted to give his opinion and advice immediately, (e.g., about institutionalizing the child[38]). He may identify with the parents and conclude too readily that to keep the child in the home would be too heavy a burden for the family,[107] or he may overidentify with his retarded patients and try to protect them from stress.[1]

The physician should examine himself in regard to these feelings so that he can deal with them—and the situation—in a reasonably objective and realistic way. The younger pediatrician and health associate have more experience with less severely retarded children, perhaps in training programs in mental retardation that have become more common in pediatric settings. But the older physician may recall only a visit or two to an institution for the retarded that left him only with memories of severely damaged children and that may affect his reactions to all retarded children.

Some physicians may be interested mainly in treating infants who have phenylketonuria or other inborn errors of metabolism, that now can be helped by dietary or other methods. Since so much interest has been stirred up in metabolic disorders, it is easy for the physician to forget that these disorders are rare compared to the gamut of mental retardation. The physician should keep in mind that even a low-phenylalanine diet for an infant who has phenylketonuria (the diet is only part of the treatment) can be complicated by a lack of appetite, vomiting, and other feeding problems, as well as by retarded growth or weight gain, and other symptoms of malnutrition, not to mention the lack of uniformly effective prevention of the mental retardation itself. Thus the psychosocial components of the problem, including the feelings of the parents, must be considered even in what seems to be a primarily metabolic disorder.

Richardson and Normanly[80] have reported on a group of children who were referred for evaluation of possible mental retardation because they had learning disabilities or delayed development (the children comprised 9% in a pediatric outpatient clinic). About 40% of those children were found to be not retarded. Language, perceptual, and emotional disturbances, many of them related to developmental lags, were the most frequent causes of the pseudo-retardation in these children. Although in a study by Korsch and Cobb,[54] pediatricians' estimates of the intelligence of normally developing children were shown to come fairly close to the evaluation of an experienced psychologist, the pediatricians tended to underestimate the potential of children who had major physical illnesses (and to overestimate the intelligence of children who functioned at a subnormal level). As indicated earlier,[102] the evaluation of a child's mental development should not be based on the pediatrician's estimate alone or on the use of a screening test, such as the Denver Developmental Screening Test, but on a comprehensive study. If it is suspected that a child is retarded, the child should be referred to a competent clinical child psychologist or to a clinic where a multidisciplinary evaluation can be made. In any case, repeated follow-up visits over a period of time are necessary, because the child's performance on tests may change, especially the younger child's.

Telling the Parents

If the retarded infant has no physical stigmata, the retardation is usually only gradually suspected, often not until after the child is 1 year old. Parents who themselves bring up the question as to whether the child is developing normally have obviously been considering the possibility of retardation for some time, and they are less likely to use strenuous denial when the diagnosis is finally made. In some cases, the physician must ask the parents what their impression is of their infant's development, because the parents may have been afraid to bring up the question (the question refers to the parents' impressions as to whether their child is developing normally—not whether he is mentally retarded). The question may come up naturally during the use of the Denver Developmental Screening Test or some other screening device.

As Solomons[96] has emphasized, in the absence of definite neurological signs it is best not to make a specific diagnosis during the child's first year or two, even when he is behind in all developmental aspects. As was Crothers's practice long ago,[15] the parents should be told that the infant is "developing more slowly than others his own age" without any "serious" causes. The physician can also mention that many children are "late bloomers" or "catch up" later, that test results are not always accurate at this age, and that it would be wise to have another evaluation in 6 months or a year. The parents should not be reassured hollowly that the child will "grow out of it," and the physician should always spend time listening to and responding to the parents' concerns. They may have feelings of guilt or blame, or they may have unrealistic fears about their child. For example, they might be afraid that their child may turn into a juvenile delinquent or a "sex maniac."

As Solomons has indicated, in attempting to make a prognosis, the physician must remember that any child, no matter how retarded, will improve to some degree over a period of time. As Solomons has pointed out, the rate of improvement is determined primarily by the degree of retardation (although other factors may be involved), and the prognosis should reflect the physician's degree of optimism about the infant. Thus, if the infant's retardation is not more than 50% at about 1 year (i.e., if the infant can do about 50% of what a one-year-old child is expected to do), the physician is justified in encouraging the parents to be optimistic. If the infant's retardation seems to be more severe, the parents can be told the infant's developmental age in months (e.g., that an infant who is 12 months old is functioning "about like a child who is 4 months old." In such cases, the physician should be noncommittal, but he may hold out some hope that the infant will improve by the next evaluation.

After a follow-up of 2 years or more, the physician may feel justified in making a firm diagnosis of mental retardation (although a few children show developmental spurts at 3 years of age or even later). If the parents have not already brought up the subject of mental retardation, the physician should discuss the diagnosis with them, referring to the level at which the child is functioning. If the child is mildly mentally retarded, his parents can be told that the child will learn more slowly than other children and will need some help but that he can learn in school and that he can grow up to be "a happy and self-supporting person." The same prognosis can be given for an older child who is mildly mentally retarded but whose course the physician has not followed if the child's current test scores correlate with the scores of tests done previously by a competent psychologist. The physician can tell the parents their child's I.Q. range, but more meaningful to the parents is the child's mental age or the level at which he is functioning. If the child's earlier scores were higher, the physician should assume that the child has a higher potential than he now shows, and the physician should look for and deal with factors which have interfered with the child's potential (e.g., inappropriate hopelessness in the parents about the child's future, a poor self-image, an emotional disturbance, or a family conflict).

If such a child has had a chronic or an intermittent illness, has been hospitalized repeatedly, has a history of serious family problems, or has been in several foster homes, I automatically assume that the child potentially has an I.Q. that is 10 to 15 points higher than the test results indicate. I think also that the school-age child can reach his potential if he is helped, perhaps by psychotherapy. Children are resilient and they respond to an optimistic approach. In most such cases, my optimism has been justified.

If the child is moderately retarded, his parents can be told that he "will be able to learn" but that he will need a good deal of special help and that it is best to wait to see what his skills are. This advice is honest and it also gives parents some hope. Parents often ask how they should tell their other children about their retarded child's problem. Siblings should be told the truth, that their brother or sister is "slower" but that he has feelings just like theirs and that the parents love him very much. It is sometimes painful for parents to be honest with other relatives or people outside the family, but honesty is the best policy. Public acceptance of retarded people is gradually increasing.

If an infant is born with physical stigmata, such as those of clear-cut Down's syndrome,* or a serious neurologic defect, the parents should be told as soon as possible, preferably together. If possible, a diagnosis should be given, with a brief explanation but without confusing details. The parents usually react initially with shock, which is sometimes followed quickly by denial, feelings of guilt, or feelings of anger or blame toward the physician, as they try to deal with the shattering of their 9-month-long hope for a healthy child. Even though the experience is painful for everyone, the physician should allow enough time in the first conference to answer all the parents' immediate questions and, in subsequent conferences, to permit the parents to begin the vital process of

*"Diagnosis of borderline" cases with mosaicism requires chromosomal analysis and careful follow-up.

mourning for the "child that was to be." If the parents do not raise the question of guilt themselves, they should be helped to understand that the defect could not have been helped and that it was "nobody's fault."

Prognosis; Recommendation for Care

No matter what the child's defect is, the physician should not give a sweeping prognosis and he should not immediately recommend institutionalization or other residential care.[116] Although the prognosis may be guarded, any step toward institutional care should be taken gradually and the parents themselves should make the final decision. Even when their child is seriously damaged, parents often can take this step only after they feel that they have tried to care for the child at home, and that they "have done everything possible." Although today many workers believe that the physician should rarely recommend institutionalization, in the case of a severely damaged child, the possibility of institutional care for the child can be mentioned to the parents during follow-up visits for their consideration.

The tendency today is toward home care[20] for the child's first three years of life if at all possible, because home care permits healthier emotional development. As Meier[61] has emphasized, institutional care should be a last resort, even for a severely retarded child in a deprived home setting. Many children who have Down's syndrome can be reared in the home[37] and are trainable (some are educable or better); most will require sheltered workshop programs as adults. Such factors as considerable nursing care[117] for children who have associated defects of a markedly handicapping degree, lack of community day care facilities, family disintegration, the needs of siblings, or the complete inability of the parents to accept the child should be relevant considerations only after serious attempts have been made to deal with them. Follow-up care and much support for the parents are needed (even if they decide to institutionalize the child) to help them deal with later feelings of guilt or resentment.

Continuing supportive care of retarded children can be offered by the physician in private practice, with appropriate consultation with speech and hearing, dental, educational, mental health, and other professionals.[2,36,81] Such care also may be offered in a multidisciplinary setting of the type recently established in a number of universities if a team coordinator integrates the findings for the parents and one team member establishes and maintains a supportive relationship with the family. Continued close follow-up care is necessary, with visits at least every 6 to 12 months, to discuss ongoing problems, to offer support, and to help confused or troubled families take prompt advantage of the community facilities and thus avoid the "diagnostic-therapeutic gap" described by Meyer and his colleagues.[68] Home visits can be made by public health nurses or other personnel to offer training[19] in regard to feeding, toileting, or home management, and homemaker services have been most valuable. Pamphlets for parents, such as those developed by the National Association for Retarded Children, can be helpful, but they are not substitutes for parent counseling on a continuing basis by the same physician or health associate. The relationship between the physician and the family should be one in which questions can be asked and disturbed feelings can be brought out and dealt with constructively.[116]

Parents can receive much help from local chapters of the National Association for Retarded Children and the Association for Children with Learning Disabilities. These associations offer group support, information about resources or new developments, and parent education, and they are vehicles for community action and change. In some settings, such groups have re-cruited citizen advocates, volunteers who on a one-to-one basis assume responsibility for helping the family of a retarded child. These volunteers can help the parents take advantage of the educational, recreational, vocational, and other community resources while offering the child their interest and a support.

Today adequate home medical care of children who have associated physical defects is much more feasible than it was, and so the longevity of children with Down's syndrome (for example) is much better.

Freeman's critical review[30] has indicated that what is now known about the effects of drugs points up the similarities between mentally retarded persons and people of normal intelligence rather than their differences. The drugs used in the management of mentally retarded children add nothing to those children's behavioral repertoire; they merely stimulate or inhibit functions that are already present. Thus training and rehabilitative efforts are necessary in order to take full advantage of any benefits offered by psychopharmacologic drugs. General agreement exists that drug therapy should not be the only kind of treatment, nor should it be used as a substitute for comprehensive treatment approaches to the problems of retarded (or disturbed) children.

The major tranquilizers (e.g., chlorpromazine and thioridazine) have been reported to be useful in the relief of such symptoms as anxiety or agitated behavior, which may inhibit learning, but the drugs themselves may inhibit learning slightly. In nonpsychotic hyperactive children, both those who have definitive brain damage and those who do not, the stimulants may help reduce distractibility, improve attention, and enhance goal-directed behavior, and they seem not to inhibit behavior that is conducive to learning. The minor tranquilizers and sedatives have much more limited use for retarded children; and antidepressants are of questionable value (see Chapter 13 for a fuller discussion of psychopharmacologic treatment).

Although a number of attempts have been made over the last 25 years to bring about biochemical alterations in the learning or memory processes (e.g., with the use of drugs, vitamins, and proteins), the results are conflicting at best, as Freeman has indicated,[30] and no support for such "intelligence-enhancing" approaches can be offered at the present time.

Preschool-age children may benefit from attending nursery schools that have special programs.[119] Specially trained teachers who use an individualized approach can help retarded children develop greater independence and self-esteem, reduce their perceptual-motor deficits, improve their language skills, and solve other problems. These teachers can also help the parents help their children.

School-age children who are mildly retarded or educable can learn at their own pace in small, ungraded classes for slow learners or in special classes for the retarded, with individual tutoring if necessary. Yearly evaluation of the child's progress is needed to permit a child to move toward higher levels of achievement or to move to a regular class. Some school systems now provide educational programs for moderately retarded children. Other children can profit from programs for trainable children in day care centers, cerebral palsy centers, and private schools. Some mildly retarded adolescents may require school–work programs; many of the more severely retarded can benefit from working in sheltered workshops. Unfortunately, many communities still do not offer most of these educational opportunities, and many states have not provided their mentally retarded children with special education. Not enough teachers who have special training are available for the programs that do exist.

Until recently, child guidance clinics and mental health clinics tended to offer psychotherapy only to children whose I.Q.s were below average but who were felt to be pseudo-retarded as a result of a primary emotional disturbance.[5] Psychotherapy for these children sometimes resulted in a dramatic rise in their performance I.Q.s—20 to 40 points or more. (Such a case example is offered in Chapter 18.) Today mental health facilities are beginning to offer psychotherapy to children who are both retarded and emotionally disturbed. These children also may be able to achieve their potential. Treatment approaches must be individualized.[7,74,98] They may range from helping the child's parents accept his retardation[1,96] through relationship therapy for a moderately retarded child (which provides the child with structure, limits, and an opportunity to ventilate his feelings), with therapy for his parents as well, to an insight-promoting therapy for the child and his parents to help them uncover and deal with their unconscious and self-defeating neurotic conflicts.[12,50,98] Group therapy for parents has been helpful.[59,93] The use of behavior modification techniques by siblings has helped the siblings help the retarded children. Especially useful are the techniques that involve positive reinforcement.[113] The various individual and group psychotherapeutic approaches that can be used to help mentally retarded children and adolescents are well summarized in a book edited by Menolascino.[67] In that book, Woodward emphasized the importance of early intervention, basing her conclusions on her experience with therapeutic nursery school programs for preschool-age children who had retarded functioning. The functioning of a high percentage of the children in her programs, most of whom had no demonstrable brain damage, improved considerably, supporting the impression that psychosocial factors can play a major part in such developmental lags.

Some severely disturbed and retarded children may benefit from residential treatment, which is usually costly and available only in private settings.[67] In the past, state hospital treatment units for disturbed children often excluded children who had psychotic disorders and mental retardation, and institutions for the mentally retarded usually did not have facilities to treat them. Providing teachers and other personnel with special training in mental retardation to state hospital units and schools for the handicapped has been an answer in some settings, while institutions for the retarded are using child psychiatrists or other mental health professionals as consultants or staff members and are enlarging their pediatric staffs.

As Dybwad[22] has emphasized, small cottage-type group-living units or group foster homes should ultimately replace large institutions for those mildly-to-moderately retarded children who must live away from home, (chiefly because of family breakdown or other social problems) and for the more severely retarded. Half-way houses are being used for some of the retarded, until they can return to the community. All children should of course live as close as possible to their own families. Medical group foster homes that have adequate nursing care and opportunities for medical consultation may be useful in providing temporary placements for severely retarded children who have associated handicaps of a marked degree, for children whose families are in crisis, or for children whose families need time to work out a permanent arrangement.

Besides health, educational, recreational, mental health, and other considerations, the planning of community-based services for mentally retarded children and adolescents should take into account the need for more and better job opportunities.[104] That need is ignored by many states, and the result is that many retarded persons who have the potential to do so cannot become active, self-supporting members of the community.

Finally, as Philips[72] has emphasized, many of the private and governmental efforts to improve services for mentally retarded children tend to isolate these children rather than bring them into the mainstream of community care. Part of this problem stems from the past neglect of the retarded by most pediatric and child psychiatry facilities, a situation that is gradually being rectified.[18,66] In addition, although federal legislation has helped set up needed services, it has also helped support the separate development of mental retardation and mental health centers. (Recently there has been some integration of these centers.) Local, regional, and state planning should aim at coordination of services for all children, and should avoid competition among services. (The enactment by Congress of Public Law 94–142 required public schools to educate all handicapped children, but provided no funds.) The mentally retarded need services that other children also need, as well as some specialized services. As Philips,[72] Lourie and Lourie,[58] Hobbs,[46] and others have pointed out, in the future, programs should offer comprehensive services to all children, without overemphasizing diagnostic categories.

Prevention

Preventive measures include early and effective prenatal care. It should include good nutrition,[6] the management of infections or metabolic disorders, the avoidance of exposure to radiation or unnecessary drugs, and the prevention of rubella. Improved perinatal and postnatal care should also be available for everyone, especially for pregnant women in disadvantaged neighborhoods.[10,73,103] As Meier[61] has urged, in view of the large number of children who have sociocultural retardation, the pediatrician should advocate better nutrition, preschool enrichment programs in more— and more fully staffed—day care centers, more individualized education in school systems, better medical care in general for children who come from minority and poverty backgrounds.

Genetic counseling is becoming more widely available to married couples who have a retarded child in whose problem genetic factors may have played a role and to couples in whose families there is a history of mental retardation. Fortunately, many such conditions are rare and are inherited recessively. (For a fuller discussion of the psychosocial aspects of genetic counseling, see Chapter 25.)

Bibliography

1. Beck, H.L.: Casework with parents of mentally retarded children. Am. J. Orthopsychiatry, 32:870, 1962.
2. Bolian, G.C.: The child psychiatrist and the mental retardation "team." Arch. Gen. Psychiatry, 18:360, 1968.
3. Carlson, H.B., and Henderson, N.: The intelligence of American children of Mexican parentage. J. Abnorm. Soc. Psychol., 45:455, 1950.
4. Centerwall, S.A., and Centerwall, W.R.: A study of children with Mongolism reared in the home compared with those reared away from home. Pediatrics, 25:678, 1960.
5. Chandler, C.A., Norman, V.D., and Bahn, A.K.: The mentally deficient in outpatient psychiatric clinics. Am. J. Ment. Defic., 67:218, 1962.
6. Chase, H.P., et al.: Intrauterine undernutrition and brain development. Pediatrics, 47:491, 1971.
7. Chess, C.: Psychiatric treatment of the mentally retarded child with behavior problems. Am. J. Orthopsychiatry, 32:863, 1962.
8. Chess, S., and Hassibi, M.: Behavior deviations in mentally retarded children. J. Am. Acad. Child Psychiatry, 9:282, 1970.
9. Classification of Mental Retardation. Am. J. Psychiatry, 128 (Suppl.): No. 11, 1606, 1972.
10. Clifford, S.H.: Prevention of prematurity sine qua non for reduction in mental retardation and other neurologic disorders. N. Engl. J. Med., 271:243, 1964.
11. Coleman, R.W., and Provence, S.: Environmental retardation. Pediatrics, 19:285, 1957.
12. Cowen, E.L.: Psychotherapy and play techniques with the exceptional child and youth. In: Psychology of Exceptional Children and Youth (W.M. Cruikshank, Ed.). Englewood Cliffs, N.J., Prentice-Hall, 1955.
13. Crandall, B.F.: Genetic disorders and mental retardation. J. Am. Acad. Child Psychiatry, 16:88, 1977.
14. Cravioto, J., De Licardie, E., and Birch, H.: Nutrition, growth, and neurointegrative development: An experimental and ecologic study. Pediatrics, (Suppl.) 38:319, 1966.
15. Crothers, B.: Personal communication.
16. Crowcroft, A.: Psychogenic retardation. In: Modern Perspectives in International Child Psychiatry (J.G. Howells, Ed.). Edinburgh, Oliver and Boyd, 1979.
17. Cummings, S.T., Baylery, H.C., and Rie, H.E.: Effects of the child's deficiency on the mother: A study of mothers of mentally retarded, chronically ill and neurotic children. Am. J. Orthopsychiatry, 36:595, 1966.
18. Cytryn, L.: The training of pediatricians and psychiatrists in mental retardation. In: Psychiatric Approaches to Mental Retardation (F.J. Menolascino, Ed.). New York, Basic Books, 1970.
19. Dittman, L.L.: Home training for retarded children. Children, May-June, p. 32, 1957.
20. Dittman, L.L.: The Mentally Retarded Child at Home. Department of Health, Education, and Welfare, Children's Bureau Publication No. 374, Washington, Government Printing Office, 1959.
21. Dobson, J.C., et al.: Intellectual performance of 36 phenylketonuric patients and their nonaffected siblings. Pediatrics, 58:53, 1976.
22. Dybwad, G.: Changing patterns of residential care for the mentally retarded—A challenge to architecture. New York, Columbia University Press, 1967.
23. Edgerton, R.B.: The Cloak of Competence: Stigma in the Lives of the Mentally Retarded. Berkeley, Calif.: University of California Press, 1967.
24. Eisenberg, L.: Emotional determinants of mental deficiency. Arch. Neurol. Psychiatry, 80:114, 1958.
25. Elonen, A.S., and Zwarensteyn, S.B.: Appraisal of developmental lag in certain blind children. J. Pediatr., 65:599, 1964.
26. Emde, R.N.: Adaptation after the birth of a Down's syndrome infant: A study of 6 cases, illustrating differences in development and the counter-movement between grieving and maternal attachment. J. Am. Acad. Child Psychiatry, 16:299, 1977.
27. Engel, M.: Psychopathology in Childhood: Social, Diagnostic, and Therapeutic Aspects. New York, Harcourt, Brace, Jovanovitch, 1972.
28. Farber, B.: Effects of a severely retarded child on family integration. Mongr. Soc. Res. Child Dev., 24(2), 1959.
29. Farber, B., and Ryckman, D.: Family organization and parent-child communication: Parents and siblings of a retarded child. Monogr. Soc. Res. Child Dev., 28:7, 1963.
30. Freeman, R.D.: Psychopharmacology and the retarded child. In: Psychiatric Approaches to Mental Retardation (F.J. Manolascino, Ed.). New York, Basic Books, 1970.
31. Freedman, D.A.: The role of early mother-child relations in the etiology of some cases of mental retardation. In: Advances in Mental Sciences. I. Congenital Mental Retardation (F.G. Austin, Ed.). University of Texas Press, 1969.
32. Gardner, W.J.: Occurrence of severe depressive reactions in the mentally retarded. Am. J. Psychiatry, 124:386, 1967.
33. Garton, M.D.: Teaching the Educable Mentally Re-

tarded—*Practical Methods.* Springfield, Ill., Thomas, 1964.

34. Gath, A.: Sibling reactions to mental handicap: A comparison of the brothers and sisters of Mongoloid children. J. Am. Acad. Child Psychiatry, 15:187, 1974.

35. Gelinier-Ortigues, M., and Aubry, J.: Maternal deprivation, psychogenic deafness, and pseudoretardation. In: *Emotional Problems of Early Childhood* (G. Caplan, Ed.). New York, Basic Books, 1956.

36. Garrard, S.: Intellectual retardation. In: *Ambulatory Pediatrics* (M. Green and R.J. Haggerty, Eds.). Philadelphia, Saunders, 1968.

37. Golden, D.A., and Davis, J.G.: Counselling parents after the birth of an infant with Down's syndrome. Children Today, 3:7, 1974.

38. Goodman, L.: Continuing treatment of parents with congenitally defective infants. Soc. Casework, 9:92, 1964.

39. Graliker, B.V., Parmalee, A.H., Sr., and Koch, R.: Attitude study of parents of mentally retarded children. II. Initial reactions and concerns of parents to a diagnosis of mental retardation. Pediatrics, 24:2, 1959.

40. Gralicker, B., et al.: Teenage response to a mentally retarded sibling. Am. J. Ment. Defic., 66:838, 1962.

41. Grossman, H.J.: *Brothers and Sisters of Retarded Children.* New York, Syracuse University Press, 1972.

42. Grossman, H.J., Ed.: Manual on Terminology and Classification in Mental Retardation: 1973 Revision. American Association on Mental Deficiency. Special Publication No. 2, New York, 1975.

43. Group for the Advancement of Psychiatry: *Basic Considerations in Mental Retardation: A Preliminary Report.* New York, Group for the Advancement of Psychiatry, 1959, Report No. 43.

44. Hammond, J., Sternlicht, M., and Deutsch, M.R.: Parental interest in institutionalized children. Hosp. and Commun. Psychiatry, 20:338, 1969.

45. Hertzig, M.E., et al.: Intellectual levels of school children severely malnourished during the first two years of life. In: *Annual Progress in Child Psychiatry and Child Development.* (S. Chess and A. Thomas, Eds.). New York, Brunner/Mazel, 1973.

46. Hobbs, N.: *The Futures of Children.* San Francisco, Jossey-Bass, 1975.

47. Holt, K.S.: The home care of severely retarded children. Pediatrics, 22:74, 1958.

48. Joint Commission on Accreditation of Hospitals: Standards for Residential Programs for Mentally Retarded. New York, 1971.

49. Kanner, L.: *A History of the Care and Study of the Mentally Retarded.* Springfield, Ill., Thomas, 1964.

50. Kessler, J.W.: Psychotherapy with mentally retarded children. Psychoanal. Study Child, 31:493, 1976.

51. Kirk, S.: *The Education of Exceptional Children.* Chicago, University of Chicago Press, 1950.

52. Klein, J.J.: Child schizophrenia states simulating retardation and auditory impairment. Nerv. Child., 10:135, 1954.

53. Koch, R., et al.: Attitude study of parents with mentally retarded children. I. Evaluation of parental satisfaction with the medical care of a retarded child. Pediatrics, 23:582, 1959.

54. Korsch, B., Cobb, K., and Ashe, B.: Pediatricians' appraisals of patients' intelligence. Pediatrics, 27:990, 1961.

55. Kugel, R.B.: *Changes in the Concept of Training and Care for the Mentally Retarded Child Within the Family Group.* Department of Health, Education, and Welfare, Washington, Government Printing Office, 1961.

56. Kugel, R.B.: Familial mental retardation: Some possible neurophysiological and psychosocial interrelationships. In: *Modern Perspectives in Child Development* (A. Solnit and S. Provence, Eds.). New York, International Universities Press, 1963.

57. Kugel, R.B., and Wolfensberger, W., Eds.: Changing patterns in residential services for the mentally retarded. A President's Committee on Mental Retardation Monograph. Department of Health, Education, and Welfare, Washington, Government Printing Office, 1961.

58. Lourie, N., and Lourie, A.: Non-Categorical Funding. Unpublished material.

59. Mandelbaum, A.: The group process in helping parents of retarded children. Children, 14:227, 1967.

60. Martin, H.P.: Developmental problems of childhood. In: *Current Pediatric Diagnosis and Therapy.* (C.H. Kempe, H.N. Silver, and D.O'Brien, Eds.). Los Altos, Calif., Lange, 1978.

61. Meier, J.H.: *Developmental and Learning Disabilities.* New York, University Park Press, 1975.

62. Melyn, M.A., and White, D.T.: Mental and developmental milestones of noninstitutionalized Down's syndrome children. Pediatrics, 52:542, 1973.

63. Menolascino, F.J.: Emotional disturbance and mental retardation. Am. J. Ment. Defic., 70:248, 1965.

64. Menolascino, F.J.: Psychiatric aspects of Mongolism. Am. J. Ment. Defic., 5:653, 1965.

65. Menolascino, F.J.: Psychoses of childhood: Experiences of a mental retardation pilot project. Am. J. Ment. Defic., 70:83, 1965.

66. Menolascino, F.J.: Mental retardation and comprehensive training in psychiatry. Am. J. Psychiatry, 124:459, 1967.

67. Menolascino, F.J., Ed.: *Psychiatric Approaches to Mental Retardation.* New York, Basic Books, 1970.

68. Meyer, R.J., Stafford, R.L., and Jacobsen, M.D.: Patterns of family follow-up: A study of children with mental retardation and associated developmental disorders. Community Ment. Health J., 6:393, 1970.

69. Mossier, H.D., Grossman, H.J., and Dingman, H.F.: Physical growth in mental defectives: A study in an institutionalized population. Pediatrics, 36 (Suppl.):132, 1965.

70. Pasamanick, B., and Lilienfield, A.M.: Association of maternal and fetal factors with development of mental deficiency. I. Abnormalities of prenatal and paranatal periods. JAMA, 159:155, 1955.

71. Philips, I.: Children, mental retardation, and planning. Am. J. Orthopsychiatry, 35:899, 1965.
72. Philips, I.: Mental hygiene and mental retardation: Implications for planning. Ment. Hyg., 49:525, 1965.
73. Philips, I., Ed.: *Prevention and Treatment of Mental Retardation*. New York, Basic Books, 1966.
74. Philips, I., et al.: The application of psychiatric services for the retarded child and his family. J. Am. Acad. Child Psychiatry, 1:297, 1962.
75. Philips, I., and Williams, N.: Psychopathology and mental retardation: A study of 100 mentally retarded children. I. Psychopathology. Am. J. Psychiatry, 132:1265, 1975.
76. Potter, H.W.: The needs of mentally retarded children for child psychiatry services. J. Am. Acad. Child Psychiatry, 3:352, 1964.
77. President's Panel on Mental Retardation: Report of the Task Force on Law. Department of Health, Education, and Welfare, Washington, Government Printing Office, 1963.
78. Prugh, D.G., and Harlow, R.G.: "Masked deprivation" in infants and young children. In: *Deprivation of Maternal Care. A Reassessment of its Effects*. Public Health Paper No. 14. Geneva, World Health Organization, 1962.
79. Richardson, S.A.: The relation of severe malnutrition in infancy to the intelligence of school children with differing life disorders. Pediatr. Res., 10:57, 1976.
80. Richardson, S.O., and Normanly, J.: Incidence of pseudoretardation in a clinic population. Am. J. Dis. Child., 109:432, 1965.
81. Richardson, J.B., Tarjan, G., and Mendelsohn, R.S., Eds.: *Mental Retardation: A Handbook for the Primary Physician*. Chicago: American Medical Association, 1974.
82. Riese, H.: Academic work with an eleven year old girl with an I.Q. of 41. Am. J. Ment. Defic., 60:545, 1956.
83. Robertson, J.A., and Fost, N.C.: Passive euthanasia of defective newborns: legal considerations. J. Pediatr., 88:883, 1976.
84. Rose, J.: The prevention of mothering breakdown associated with physical abnormalities of the infant. In: *Prevention of Mental Disorders in Children*. G. Caplan, (Ed.). New York, Basic Books, 1961.
85. Rothenberg, M.B., and Sills, E.M.: Iatrogenesis: The PKU anxiety syndrome. J. Am Acad. Child Psychiatry, 7:689, 1968.
86. Sabagh, G., and Edgerton, R.: Review of sterilized mentally retarded. Eugenics Q., 9:213, 1962.
87. Saenger, G.: *The Adjustment of Severely Retarded Adults in the Community*. Albany, N.Y., New York State Interdepartmental Health Resources Board, 1957.
88. San Martino, M., and Newman, M.B.: Siblings of retarded children: A population at risk. Child Psychiatry Hum. Dev., 4:168, 1974.
89. Satter, G., and McGee, E.: Retarded adults who have developed beyond expectation. Train School Bull, 51:43, 1954.
90. Schipper, M.T.: The child with Mongolism in the home. Pediatrics, 24:132, 1959.
91. Schwartz, E.M., and Elonen, A.S.: I.Q. and the myth of stability: A 16 year longitudinal study of intelligence test performance. J. Clin. Psychol. 31:687, 1975.
92. Scrofani, K., Suziedelis, D., and Shore, M.: Experimental test of Jensen's hypothesis. Unpublished material.
93. Siegel, B., Sheridan, K., and Sheridan, E.P.: Group psychotherapy: Its effects on mothers who rate social performance of retarded. Am. J. Psychiatry, 127:1215, 1971.
94. Skeels, H.M.: Adult status of children with contrasting early life experiences. Monogr. Soc. Res. Child Dev., 31:77, 1966.
95. Solnit, A.J., and Starts, M.H.: Mourning and the birth of a defective child. Psychoanal. Study Child, 16:523, 1961.
96. Solomons, G.: Counselling parents of the retarded: The interpretation interview. In: *Psychiatric Approaches to Mental Retardation*. (F.J. Menolascino, Ed.). New York, Basic Books, 1970.
97. Sontag, L.W., Baker, C.T., and Nelson, V.L.: Mental growth and personality development: A longitudinal study. Monogr. Soc. Res. Child Dev., 23:10, 1958.
98. Sternlicht, M.: Psychotherapeutic techniques useful for the mentally retarded: A review and critique. Psychiatr. Q., 39:84, 1965.
99. Sternlicht, M., Hammond, J., and Siegel, L.: Mental retardates prepare for community living. Hosp. Community Psychiatry, 2:15, 1972.
100. Stevens, H.A., and Heber, R.: *Mental Retardation: A Review of Research*. Chicago, University of Chicago Press, 1964.
101. Stevens, M.: *Observing Children Who Are Severely Subnormal: An Approach to Their Education*. London, Armond, 1968.
102. Syzmanski, L.S.: Psychiatric diagnostic evaluation of mentally retarded individuals. J. Am. Acad. Child Psychiatry, 16:67, 1977.
103. Tarjan, G.: Mental retardation. JAMA, 182:617, 1962.
104. Tarjan, G.: Mental retardation and the organization of services. Psychiatr. Ann., 6:27, 1976.
105. Tarjan, G., and Eisenberg, L.: Some thoughts on the classification of mental retardation in the United States of America. Am. J. Psychiatry, 128 (Suppl.): 14, 1972.
106. Tarjan, G., et al.: Natural history of mental retardation: Some aspects of epidemiology. Am. J. Ment. Defic., 77:369, 1973.
107. Thayman, A.M., and Barclay, A.: Physician's attitudes toward institutionalization of mentally retarded children. Mo. Med., 62:209, 1965.
108. Tizard, J.: *Community Services for the Mentally Handicapped*. London, Oxford University Press, 1964.
109. Todres, I.D., et al.: Pediatrician's attitudes affecting decision-making in defective newborns. Pediatrics, 60:197, 1977.
110. Turnure, J., and Zigler, E.: Outer-directedness in the problem solving of normal and retarded children. J. Abnorm. Soc. Psychol., 69:427, 1964.
111. Umbarger, B., Berry, H.K., and Sutherland, B.S.:

Advances in the management of patients with phenylketonuria. JAMA, *193*:784, 1965.

112. Webster, T.G.: Unique aspects of emotional development in mentally retarded children. In: *Psychiatric Approaches to Mental Retardation.* (F.J. Menolascino Ed.). New York, Basic Books, 1970.

113. Weinrott, M.R.: A training program in behavior modification for siblings of the retarded. Am. J. Orthopsychiatry, *44*:362, 1974.

114. Werner, E.E., and Smith, R.S.: *Kauai's Children Come of Age.* Honolulu, University Press of Hawaii, 1977.

115. Wolf, S., and Lourie, R.S.: Impact of the mentally defective child on the family unit. Clin. Proc. Child. Hosp., *9*:25, 1953.

116. Wolfensberger, W.: Counselling the parents of the retarded. In: *Mental Retardation.* (A. Baumeister, Ed.). Chicago, Aldine, 1967.

117. Wolff, I.S.: Nursing Role in Counselling Parents of Mentally Retarded Children. Department of Health, Education, and Welfare (Maternal and Child Health Services), Washington, D.C., Government Printing Office, 1964.

118. Wood, A.C., et al.: Psychosocial factors in phenylketonuria. Am. J. Orthopsychiatry, *37*:671, 1967.

119. Woodward, K.F., and Siegel, M.G.: Psychiatric study of mentally retarded children of preschool age: Preliminary report. Pediatrics, *19*:119, 1957.

120. Woodward, K.F., and Siegel, M.G.: Psychiatric study of mentally retarded children of school age. Pediatrics, *19*:119, 1957.

121. Woodward, K.F., Siegel, M.G., and Enstis, M.J.: Psychiatric study of mentally retarded children of preschool age: Report on first and second years of a three-year project. Am. J. Orthopsychiatry, *28*:376, 1958.

122. Yarrow, L.: Separation from parents in early childhood. In: *Review of Child Development Research.* Vol. I. M.L. Hoffman and L.W. Hoffman (Eds.). New York, Russel Sage Foundation, 1966.

123. Zigler, E.: Motivational determinants in the performance of retarded children. Am. J. Orthopsychiatry, *36*:848, 1966.

124. Zigler, E., and Butterfield, E.C.: Motivational aspects of changes in I.Q. test performance of culturally deprived nursery school children. Child Dev., *39*:1, 1968.

General References

American Academy of Pediatrics: The Pediatrician and the Child with Mental Retardation. Committee on Children with Handicaps. Evanston, Ill., American Academy of Pediatrics, 1971.

Anastasi, A.: Psychological testing of children. In: *Comprehensive Textbook of Psychiatry.* (A. Freedman, and H. Kaplan, Eds.). Baltimore, Williams & Wilkins, 1967.

Baumeister, A.A., Ed.: *Mental Retardation: Appraisal, Education, and Rehabilitation.* Chicago, Ill., Aldine, 1967.

Bayley, N.: Value and limitations of infant testing. Children, *5*:129, 1958.

Benda, C.E.: *The Child with Mongolism.* New York, Grune & Stratton, 1960.

Clarke, A.D.B., and Clarke, A.M.: *Mental Deficiency: The Changing Outlook.* New York, Free Press, 1975.

Cruikshank, W., Ed.: *Psychology of Exceptional Children and Youth.* Englewood Cliffs, New Jersey, Prentice-Hall, 1963.

de la Cruz, F., and La Veck, G.D.: *Human Sexuality and the Mentally Retarded.* New York, Brunner/Mazel, 1973.

Dybwad, G.: *Challenges in Mental Retardation.* New York, Columbia University Press, 1964.

Escalona, S.: The use of infant tests for predictive purposes. Bull. Menninger Clin., *14*:117, 1950.

Federal Research Activity in Mental Retardation: A Review with Recommendations for the Future. Report of the Ad hoc consultants on mental retardation to the Directors of the National Institute of Child Health and Human Development and the National Institute of Mental Health, Alcohol, Drug Abuse, and Mental Health Administration, Department of Health, Education, and Welfare, Washington, 1977.

Friedlander, B.Z., Sterritt, G.M., and Kirk, G.E. (Eds.): *Exceptional Infant*, Vol. 3 (Assessment and Intervention). New York, Brunner/Mazel, 1975.

Group for the Advancement of Psychiatry: Basic Considerations in Mental Retardation: A Preliminary Report. New York, Group for the Advancement of Psychiatry, 1959, Report No. 43.

Group for the Advancement of Psychiatry: Mental Retardation: A Family Crisis—The Therapeutic Role of the Physician. New York, Group for the Advancement of Psychiatry, 1963, Report No. 56.

Group for the Advancement of Psychiatry: Mild Mental Retardation: A Growing Challenge to the Physician. New York, Group for the Advancement of Psychiatry, 1967, Report No. 66.

Hellmuth, J., Ed.: *The Exceptional Infant*, Vols. 1 and 2 (*The Normal Infant; Studies in Abnormalities*). New York, Brunner/Mazel, 1971.

Hutt, M.L., and Gibby, R.G.: *The Mentally Retarded Child: Development, Education, and Treatment.* 3rd Ed. Boston, Allyn & Bacon, 1976.

Knobloch, H., et al.: President's Panel on Mental Retardation. A Call for Action by the Pediatric Profession. Am. J. Dis. Child., *108*:315, 1964.

Koch, R., and Dobson, J.C.: *The Mentally Retarded Child and His Family: A Multidisciplinary Handbook.* New York, Brunner/Mazel, 1971.

Koch, R., and Fishler, K.: *Down's Syndrome: Family Management. Feelings and Their Medical Significance. 8*:37. Columbus, Ohio: Ross Laboratories, 1966.

Luria, A.R.: *The Mentally Retarded Child.* New York, Macmillan, 1963.

Masland, R., Sarason, S.B., and Gladwin, T.: *Mental Subnormality: Biological, Psychological, and Cultural Factors.* New York, Basic Books, 1958.

Menolascino, F.J.: Parents of the mentally retarded: An operational approach to diagnosis and management. J. Am. Acad. Child Psychiatry, *7*:589, 1968.

Menolascino, F.J.: *Challenges in Mental Retardation:*

Progressive Ideology and Services. New York, Human Sciences Press, 1977.

Mental Retardation Source Book. Office of Mental Retardation Coordination, Department of Health, Education, and Welfare, Washington, 1972.

National Association for Retarded Children. 386 Park Avenue South, New York, N.Y., 10016

Newman, R. Ed.: Institutionalization of the Mentally Retarded: A Summary and Analysis of State Laws Governing Admission to Residential Facilities and Legal Rights and Protection of Institutionalized Patients. New York, National Association for Retarded Children, 1967.

President's Panel on Mental Retardation: A National Plan to Combat Mental Retardation. Washington, Government Printing Office, 1962.

President's Panel on Mental Retardation: Report of the Task Force on Prevention, Clinical Services, and Residential Care. Department of Health, Education, and Welfare. Washington, Government Printing Office, 1962.

President's Panel on Mental Retardation: Action Against Mental Deficiency. Washington, Government Printing Office, 1964.

Robinson, H.B., and Robinson, N.M.: *The Mentally Retarded Child: A Psychological Approach.* New York, McGraw-Hill, 1965.

Szurek, S.A., and Berlin, I.N.: *Psychosomatic Disorders and Mental Retardation in Children.* Langley Porter Child Psychiatry Series, Vol. 3. Palo Alto, Calif., Science and Behavior Books, 1968.

Tjossem, T.D., Ed.: *Intervention Strategies for High Risk Infants and Young Children.* Baltimore, University Park Press, 1976.

Wright, S.W., and Tarjan, G.: Mental retardation: A review for pediatricians. Am. J. Dis. Child., 105:511, 1963.

24

Acute Illness and Injury: Psychosocial Aspects of Management

*Thus medicine is the science of agencies helpful
and harmful—the helpful being alike those
which conserve existing health and those which
restore it when deranged, while the harmful are
the opposite of these.*
(Galen, De sectis)

Illness Patterns

It was mentioned in Chapter 1 that the practicing pediatrician sees only a small percentage of children who have serious physical illnesses. It was mentioned also that the general physician (the internist and the family practitioner) still cares for more than 50% of the children in the United States. In 1963, the Children's Bureau published a report[14] that was based on information obtained by the National Health Survey. The report pointed out that the incidence of acute and chronic illness in children in the United States is much greater than had been realized and that many children who have chronic conditions and who come from low-income or rural families receive little or no medical care. This observation was more recently supported by the findings of the Head Start studies, which have indicated that 25% or more of children in poverty areas have an illness or a disability which has not received medical care. Other studies have indicated that malnutrition occurs more often in children who live in ghettos and rural areas than in children who live elsewhere.

Acute Conditions

According to the National Health Survey, acute conditions occur at a rate of 291.1 per 100 children, an average of 3 episodes a year for every child under 15 years old. More than 50% of these acute conditions are respiratory conditions. They occur more often in children than in adults, and they occur most often in children under 5 years old. Acute conditions occur more often in children living in urban areas, and they occur about as often in girls as in boys. Eleven percent of all acute conditions are injuries, and more than 50% of the injuries and accidents that occur happen in or around the home. Adolescents have more injuries away from home although only a relatively small percentage of adolescents are involved in motor accidents. (Accidents of all kinds are the leading cause of death in children.)

Chronic Conditions

The incidence of chronic conditions is surprisingly high. About 180 children and adolescents per 1000 children (nearly 1 out of 5 children) have one or more chronic illnesses or handicaps. Allergies and respiratory conditions are the most common (accounting for about 45% of all chronic conditions), orthopedic impairments are the next most common, and hearing difficulties, speech problems, heart disease, blindness, epilepsy, cerebral palsy, and other conditions make up the rest. The rate of prevalence of chronic conditions increases with age. One out of 10 children who have chronic conditions (more than 1 million children) is limited in normal activities by a chronic condition, and in one study[26] one-third of the chronic conditions were permanent. Various American and British studies indicate that nearly 10% of all children have chronic illnesses that are primarily physical, and many of these children have significant psychosocial and educational problems (more commonly boys than girls). Whether or not a child with a chronic condition receives medical care seems to be related to his family's income and place of residence. In the studies, a significant number of urban poor children (including many from minority families) and rural children received little or no medical care.

Dental Problems

Dental caries is the most common physical defect found in school-age children and adolescents. The survey indicated that 50% of people under 15 years of age in the United States have never been to a dentist. Children from lower-income urban families, nonwhite children generally, and children from rural areas are far more likely than other children to have never been to a dentist or to have received inadequate dental care. Girls seem to receive more dental care and preventive orthodontic services than boys do, probably for cosmetic reasons.

Total Incidence of Disorders in Childhood and Adolescence

Besides the estimate that 10% to nearly 20% of young people have chronic physical conditions, one must consider the estimates that 8% to 12% of children and adolescents have emotional and mental disturbances serious enough to require mental health services, that 3% are mentally retarded, and that 10% to 25% have learning problems. Using the lowest estimates and allowing for differences in the definition of the childhood age range and much overlapping in the statistics, one must still conclude that at least 25% to 35%[22] of young people have some long-term physical or psychosocial disorder. When the shocking lack of dental care is also considered, the functional well-being of children and adolescents in the United States is not impressive, to say the least.

The incidence of disorders is, of course, different in different age groups. In a recent survey of 19 pediatric clinics that care for adolescents, emotional disorders accounted for 25% to 50% of the diagnoses; of the rest, obesity, acne, allergy, seizures, and orthopedic disorders were the 5 most frequent disorders and many of the cases had emotional components, of course.

Reactions of Children and Families to Illness and Injury

In Chapter 4, the general patterns of response of the child and his family to stressful stimuli were sketched. In this chapter, the responses of the child and his family to acute or chronic illness, injury or handicap, and the attendant treatment are discussed in more detail, and specific suggestions are made for management and prevention from a psychosocial point of view.

The child's immediate response to illness or injury may vary somewhat according to the organ, the organ system (or systems) affected, and the consequences at the psychologic or social level. (For example, the local and systemic effects of acute rheumatic fever usually have a more severe temporary impact on the psychosocial functioning of the child and usually produce greater anxiety in the parents than does a simple greenstick fracture.) Children in general show certain broad patterns of response; and some differences in response are related to the child's individual differences and to his developmental level.

Whether a child's illness has a significantly adverse effect on his adaptation or on his family's equilibrium depends on (1) the child's developmental level, (2) the child's previous adaptive capacity, (3) the nature of the parent-child relationship before the illness, (4) the nature of the child's family's equilibrium, (5) the nature of the child's illness or injury (including the organ system affected and any residual defect or handicap), the type of treatment or home care, and (6) the meaning of the illness to the child and his family (to be evaluated in terms of the events that occurred immediately before the illness and their actual or fantasied connection with the illness, the previous experience of the child and his family with illness, the effect the illness has on the child's social, academic, and athletic or other physical capacities, and the effect it has on the child's siblings and other family members.

Direct Effects

The direct effects of illness include malaise, discomfort, or pain, which produce listlessness, prostration, disturbances in sleep and appetite, and irritability. Restlessness is more common in children, and hyperactivity often occurs when the illness is milder, particularly in preschool-age children although lethargy and withdrawal also occur. Anorexia and refusal of food may be marked in younger children. Well-meaning but overanxious parents may urge food on such a child, who responds to their urgings in a negativistic way. Such an interaction often leads to feeding problems that persist long after the illness subsides. Difficulties in falling asleep, nightmares, and night terrors are common. Sleeping problems also may continue as young children and their parents struggle for control.

Besides such direct effects, which may closely resemble or overlap with disturbances in behavior from primarily psychologic or interpersonal sources, other responses (reactive effects) may occur.

Regression

Emotional or behavioral regression is a universal pattern of response to illness. It is seen most strikingly in older infants and preschool-age children, but it occurs also in school-age children and adolescents (and, for that matter, in adults to a lesser degree). In infants and young children, regression may take the form of a return to thumb sucking, a return to the bottle, demanding, clinging, negativistic, or aggressive behavior, a return of earlier fears, and the temporary giving up of recently learned abilities, such as speech, walking, and bowel or bladder control. In an older child, regression is shown by the reappearance of more immature social patterns, including greater dependence on the parents, particularly the mother, demanding or aggressive behavior, limitations in the child's capacity to share with his siblings or others, and trouble in concentrating and learning. Such regression seems to stem partly from the direct effects of the illness on the child's ego and partly from the temporary falling back on earlier, more familiar modes of satisfaction or the giving up of more highly developed functions in an adaptive retreat and regrouping of forces.

Depression

Depression is another pattern of response to illness. It often is different in infants, children, and adolescents from depression in adults. Depression may arise partly from the direct effects of the illness, as in infectious mononucleosis or infectious hepatitis, and partly from the discouragement or restriction of activity the illness has brought. In young children who have been hospitalized, depression may arise from the child's separation from his parents. Eating and sleeping disturbances occur often in young children as depressive equivalents, as do changes from hypoactive behavior to hyperactive behavior. Wide mood swings often occur in older children and adolescents. Other emotional responses (often ones related to regressive trends) include the reemergence of primitive fears and of feelings of inadequacy or helplessness and hopelessness. Stereotyped behavior of a compulsive or ritualized nature may occur, as may transient hypochondriacal concerns.

Misinterpretation

The child commonly misinterprets the meaning of his illness or injury. The misinterpretation is related to the child's limited capacity for understanding and testing reality and the tendency (particularly of the young child) toward magical or animistic thinking. Young preschool-age children ordinarily view separation from the parents or pain or discomfort arising from illness or accident as a punishment for their real or imaginary transgressions. Older preschool-age and early school-age children show fears of bodily mutilation related to treatment procedures. Such fears are more intense when sensitive areas of the body, such as the head or the genitals, are in-

volved (fears of harm to the genitals in late preschool-age or early school-age children are related to sexual differentiation and psychosexual development). Older children and adolescents may have unrealistic fears of sudden death or severe disability. Those fears are related to guilt they feel about their aggressive impulses or other conflicts.

Physiologic Concomitants of Anxiety

Psychologic conflicts about the meaning of illness that are enhanced by regressive trends may result in the appearance of the physiologic concomitants of anxiety. Tachycardia, palpitations, hyperventilation, diarrhea, or other signs and symptoms of anxiety may be exhibited. Such psychophysiologic changes, which are ordinarily reversible, may compound the effects of the predominantly physical illness, as in the deleterious effects on diminished cardiac function in congestive failure[4] or the perpetuation of diarrhea originally arising from a bacterial infection or parasitic infestation.[27] At times, these physiologic concomitants may lead to diagnostic confusion with such conditions as hyperthyroidism or rheumatic fever.

Conversion Disorders

Conversion disorders are often seen in school-age children or adolescents. As indicated earlier, conversion disorders affect the voluntarily innervated striated musculature and the somatosensory apparatus, with their unconsciously symbolic expression of emotional conflict (conversion disorders are discussed more fully in Chapter 18), and they are to be differentiated from psychophysiologic disorders, which affect the involuntarily innervated systems and visceral end-organs and which do not have symbolic significance.

Conversion disorders are manifested in a variety of personality pictures, ranging from the relatively normal personality to the classic hysterical personality in older children and adolescents. Transient, mild-to-moderate conversion symptoms often occur during convalescence from a predominantly physical illness.[2] Such an illness may temporarily block a child's intense developmental need to achieve scholastically, athletically, or socially. The illness may precipitate a conflict between his regressive wish to continue to be cared for by the mother and his guilt about that wish as he feels pressure from within and without to return to the world of competition. Often the symptoms of the physical illness are unconsciously incorporated into the conversion symptoms, as in the continuance of pain, vomiting, headache, and dysphonia or, in a more general sense, weakness and easy fatigability. At times, other symptoms (e.g., certain types of syncope and disturbances in gait) may appear. Conversion reactions may also be admixed with physical disorders.[12] Many of these conversion reactions disappear in a few days or weeks, but they may persist chronically in a child who has a limited adaptive capacity or in a child whose family encounters special difficulty with the convalescent phase of the illness.

Dissociative Reactions

Dissociative reactions, such as amnesia, pseudo-delirious states, somnambulism, or fugue states, may also occur. These reactions may compound (or be compounded by) an actual delirium which is often of a subclinical nature. In children, delirium may arise in response to drug administration or from various insults to the central nervous system. Or even in the absence of a direct insult to the central nervous system, delirium may accompany a systemic disease that involves a marked fever or a disturbance in cerebral metabolism. Catatonic behavior unrelated to psychosis may be seen temporarily in normal or mildly disturbed children if the physical, psychologic, or social circumstances are sufficiently stressful.

Perceptual-Motor Lags

Other effects on behavior may be manifested in the convalescent phase. Meyer and Crothers[24] have described children who have shown lags in perceptual-motor functioning following poliomyelitis. Similar lags may occur following systemic illness, such as pneumonia or high fevers from any cause. The lags may persist for several weeks or months in the absence of any apparent damage to the central nervous system. Such children, who may have experienced a temporary disturbance in cerebral metabolism, often one compounded by regressive tendencies, may have learning difficulties after they return to school. If these difficulties are not recognized, they may become chronic and result in resistance to learning or some other behavioral disturbance. Early recognition of them allows the parents and the teachers to help the child to return gradually to full academic performance.

Differentiation of Reactions

Some difficulty may be encountered in separating the child's reactions to the illness or injury (which represent the effects of the stressful stimuli at the physiologic level) from his reactions to hospitalization, surgery, or other diagnostic or treatment measures (which represent stressful stimuli at the psychologic or social level of organization). For this reason, their management is discussed in detail in the section on hospitalization and surgery. (The handling of the convalescent phase of an acute illness or injury is discussed later.)

The reactions under discussion here may occur with any illness. They are largely nonspecific responses related to the way in which the child's environment—parental, familial, medical, social, or physical—helps him cope with the physical consequences and the symbolic meaning of illness or injury. Some reactions may be classified as healthy responses that are related to a situational crisis or that involve a developmental crisis touched off by the experience of illness. Other reactions may be reactive disorders although continuing developmental deviations, structured psychoneurotic disorders, chronic personality disorders, or even psychotic disorders may be touched off or exacerbated by such stresses in children who are biologically or experientially predisposed to them. (Illness and injury involving the central nervous system were discussed in Chapter 22.)

Major Acute Illness or Injury

Within broad limits, the nature of the child's illness and how it is treated significantly affect his response to it, particularly in catastrophic or overwhelming illnesses or injuries in which there may be a chronic illness or a handicap. In such situations, there is a generic human organismic response; it is related to the adaptive mechanisms that come into play during the phases of impact, recoil, and restitution. Such phasic responses may be seen most clearly in children of school age and older. Older preschool-age children tend to show similar but less clear-cut patterns, and the responses of younger preschool-age children are related more to separation from the parents. These same phasic responses were originally described in 1954 (by Prugh and Tagiuri[28]) in relation to respiratory poliomyelitis in children and adolescents, but they occur also in severe burns, accidents, and numerous other conditions.

Responses of Children and Adolescents

Impact. In older children and adolescents, the impact phase involves initially realistic fears of death (see Table 24–1). A child may have a specific fear related to the nature of his illness or injury. For example, a child who has a respiratory disorder may be afraid that he will suffocate. Such fears are basically a fear of "annihilation of the self." If present initially, as is often the case,

delirium may compound, distort, or intensify such fears.

Marked regression occurs. It is fostered in part by the child's physical dependence, and it is associated with his strong need for succor and nurturing. Various symptomatic regressive manifestations occur, such as wishes for special foods and a preoccupation with bodily needs. The child usually shows a massive or sweeping denial of the long-term implications of his illness. Primitive fantasies emerge (e.g., dreams of becoming a champion athlete or a world-famous ballet dancer). Such fantasies seem to help the child maintain the denial (which is adaptive at this point) and to cope with his enforced helplessness.

Even in conditions that do not directly involve the cerebral cortex, marked withdrawal, at times associated with mutism or catatonic behavior, may occasionally occur. The withdrawal may represent a stage of "psychic shock" that involves a temporary, nonspecific disorder of psychotic proportions that usually has a good prognosis. This state may occur in older infants as well as in children and adolescents. It may be mistakenly diagnosed as being due exclusively to brain damage. Brain damage may be involved to some extent in some so-called catastrophic reactions, but its residual effects may be minimal once the psychologic features respond to treatment.

The impact phase usually lasts some days or several weeks, but it may last much longer. The family's reactions and how the child is managed may help determine the child's capacity to "negotiate" this phase and the following phases in a reasonable length of time.

Recoil. The recoil phase involves a lessening of regression and denial, and the child begins to realize the seriousness of his situation. As such recognition proceeds, the child grieves ("mourns for the loss of the self"). Recoil is a constructive step—toward adaptation and coping with reality; the patient begins to turn his energies away from himself and toward his environment. The adaptive quality of his step may be masked by the attempts to achieve some control of the environment in the face of his continued helplessness. These attempts may take the form of demanding or "bossy" behavior toward the staff concerning details of his care, and they may be compounded by the child's projection of his fears of being disliked and by "testing-out" behavior, particularly on the part of the adolescent.

Another factor in such demanding and sometimes overtly hostile behavior seems to be the child's need to ward off serious depression during the mourning period. Such depression may sometimes break through for a moment and then become briefly manifested clinically. Or the child may have eating, sleeping, or elimination problems or other problems that may be depressive equivalents. Sometimes depression continues. It is related to the child's persistent feelings of hopelessness or loss of self-esteem, often heightened in school-age children by the almost universally present feelings of guilt or by regressive feelings that the illness was a punishment.

The recoil phase is generally the most trying one for the medical and nursing staffs, and often for the child's family as well. It may last for some weeks or several months, and feelings of grief may later recur in muted form.

Restitution. The restitution phase is one of gradual adaptation. It involves increasing acceptance of the situation and its possible outcomes and of any changes that have occurred in the patient or in his body image. The patient adjusts also to the fact that he will be different from his peers. Individual patterns of coping emerge that are related to and sometimes complicated by the patient's premorbid personality characteristics, (e.g., apprehensiveness, overdependence, or an unrealistic push toward independence). The patient's reactions to the acute illness or injury merge into the stage of the handling of chronic

illness or handicap. Patients who have sweeping physical limitations apparently must retain some measure of denial in order to maintain hope.

Management. The management of the patient should be geared to his progress through these phases. Acceptance and strong emotional support are vital in the impact phase, and, whatever the ultimate outlook for the patient, no attempt should be made to attack his denial or to challenge his fantasies. In cases of "psychic shock," attempts to break through the withdrawal and mutism are not indicated because they may intensify the reaction. Most children respond in several days when a supportive relationship is offered by a foster grandmother or someone else. A few children require long-term psychotherapy or even residential treatment, but the prognosis is generally favorable.

In the recoil phase, acceptance of the patient despite his physical and emotional limitations becomes even more important. Understanding the ramifications of the mourning process can help the staff members understand the patient's demanding and often seemingly hostile behavior and avoid responding personally to that behavior (although they must set some limits on the child's demands). The patient should be encouraged to participate in his management and self-care. (This participation may be limited at first to appropriate choices in management routines and minimum participation in self-help.) Such participation may be time consuming, but it can help patients overcome their feelings of helplessness. Emotional support of the patient must be continued, and the patient must be permitted or encouraged to talk about his feelings, particularly those connected with mourning.

Only after he has negotiated the first two phases successfully can the patient undergo rehabilitation successfully. The staff members must have an attitude of firm encouragement. A laissez-faire approach may reinforce the patient's feelings of worthlessness by making him feel he is not worth bothering about. On the other hand, there is little justification for forcing a patient to take steps toward rehabilitation; such an approach can produce severe depression or anxiety about failure. Psychiatric consultation may be needed if the patient becomes seriously depressed or has a significant conflict about his physical limitatons or his enforced dependence.

A somewhat similar set of phasic responses have been described in regard to adults who have serious burns (by Hamburg[13]), in adults who have spinal cord injuries (by Wittkower[35]), and in adults who had been told they had terminal cancer or some other terminal condition (by Shands[32] and Kübler-Ross[19]). Similar reactions of children and adults to civilian and military disasters have been observed by Silber and his colleagues,[34] and by Cobb and Lindeman.[5] In adults, who have more firmly established ego structures, the regressive manifestations may help them ward off feelings of helplessness and hopelessness. In some respects, such phasic responses are also characteristic of the "work of mourning" the death of a loved person, as described by Freud,[9] Lindemann,[20] and others.

Responses of Parents

Parents have parallel phasic responses to catastrophes in their children (see Table 24–1). As Richmond[29] has indicated, parents first enter the phase of *denial and disbelief*, which may last for days or weeks and which may involve "shopping" for other opinions. After the first shock, which is often followed by anger and self-pity, most parents feel "this can't be real" or "this can't be happening to us" or "this can't be happening to our child." A few parents show continuing or massive denial for weeks or months that often is related to unconscious feelings of guilt. This phase is followed by the phase of *fear and frustration*, during which parents must deal with their grief and undertake the work of "mourning for the loss of the child that was to be" as they prepare to cope with the long-term and often uncertain implications of their child's condition. Muted feelings of grief may recur for many months. Unrealistic guilt or self-blame about having "let the child down" by failing to protect him is commonly experienced by parents in this phase, and some parents are even unable to encourage the child to help himself. The blame may be projected onto the spouse, and a marital crisis or even divorce may result. Or the parents may blame others, including the hospital staff, for their child's lack of response to treatment. One or both parents may become severely depressed. The parents' previous experience with loss and bereavement may affect strongly their fears and other responses. After some weeks or several months, the parents generally reach the phase of *rational inquiry and planning*, in which they are increasingly able to accept the situation and the child's limitations, to handle their worries about the future, to live with some ambiguity, and to help the child take the appropriate steps toward rehabilitation and become as independent as possible.

Ideally, the physician discusses the child's illness and management with both parents together, both initially and in the later contacts. It is vitally important that the physician give the parents strong emotional support during the first phase. Attempts to help either parent or child to face the reality of the situation before they are ready tend to increase their denial. Indeed, parents and children may need some denial to maintain hope. Opportunities to discuss their grief and their feelings of guilt again and again (and to be "absolved" by the physician) must be available during the second phase. Such an approach helps the parents later to make realistic plans for the future. Both parents often do not go through these phases at the same pace, and they may react differently during each

Table 24–1. *Phasic Responses of Children, Adolescents, and Parents to Catastrophic Illness or Injury.*

Phase	Responses of Affected Children and Adolescents	Responses of Parents
Impact	Fears of death or of "annihilation of the self" (can be compounded by delirium) Marked regression in behavior associated with enforced dependence, needs for nurturance, etc. Denial assisted by primitive fantasy	Initial shock, with fears of child's death, anger at fate, etc. Denial and disbelief
Recoil	Lessening of regression and denial; misinterpretation of illness as punishment Appearance of "mourning for the loss of the self" Attempts to overcome helplessness by controlling the environment	Lessening of denial and disbelief Fear and frustration associated with guilt and need to deal with blame Appearance of "mourning for the loss of the child that was to be"
Restitution	Increasing acceptance of changes in the self and the uncertainty of the future Emergence of individual coping patterns, related to premorbid personality characteristics Utilization of rehabilitative measures in movement toward control of the future, but with measure of denial necessary for maintenance of hope	Increasing acceptance of the reality of the situation and the child's limitations Rational inquiry and planning now possible, with ability to live with some ambiguity Capacity to help child achieve appropriate rehabilitative steps but with measure of denial necessary for maintenance of hope

From D. Prugh. In: *Behavioral Advances in Pediatrics: A Research Annual* (B.W. Camp, Ed.). Greenwich, Conn., Jai Press, 1980.

phase. If one or both parents show continuing or massive denial or severe depression, psychiatric consultation may be necessary. (The management of denial and other aspects of the adjustment of parents to chronic illness in their child is discussed later.)

Case Example. A 9-year-old boy and his father were visiting a friend on his farm. The two were mulching cornstalks. The mulcher had stopped, and the boy reached inside it to loosen a stalk. As he did so, the mulcher suddenly started, and the boy's right arm was amputated just above the elbow. The boy was rushed to a medical center, where he was sedated and his arm was placed in traction. When his parents first saw the stump, they both exclaimed, "No, it can't be true." When the boy awakened, somewhat confused, he was told the story by his parents, and he sobbed, "I'm sorry—I should have been more careful." His parents reassured him and said he should not blame himself. No further discussion about the accident took place among the boy, his parents, or the hospital staff during the next several days. The boy became rather sad, less communicative, lost his appetite, and had nocturnal enuresis on 3 occasions.

During the second week, the boy stayed alone in his room, often crying softly. The nursing staff discovered from his parents that he had been an outstanding Little League pitcher, although when the boy was asked about sports, he said he liked soccer best. At the weekly psychosocial rounds, these facts were discussed, and the child psychiatry–pediatric liaison consultant was asked to see the boy.

In the first brief interview, the boy indicated his wish to win in competitive activities and his sadness that he would not be able to pitch. He also said that he and his father often did "scary" things together, such as climbing high rocks, but that he was afraid to admit to his father that he was frightened. The consultant continued to see the boy for 20 minutes or so each day. The boy began to talk, draw, and use puppet play, focusing on on themes about accidents and loss. He became less withdrawn, his appetite improved, he ceased to cry, he engaged in ward activities, and he worked with the rehabilitation team in getting ready to learn how to use his "iron hand."

During this time, the parents told the consultant about their initial disbelief on seeing the boy's stump. They said they now recognized the facts but were having difficulty with their feelings about their "different" son and had cried together about this. They said that they had blamed each other and the boy for the ac-

426   Specific Clinical Considerations

cident but had come to feel that "accidents do happen." The parents talked with some of the boy's baseball buddies who also played soccer. His friends wanted to make him a present of a soccer ball, which delighted both the parents and the boy. The consultant gradually withdrew from the case, leaving plans for follow-up and prosthetic adjustment to the orthopedic and nursing staffs.

Psychosocial Sequelae

In the "vulnerable child syndrome," a disturbance in the family's psychosocial development may be traced to the fact that when their child was much younger the parents had been told that he would probably not live (this syndrome was described originally in 1964 by Green and Solnit).[11] A recent systematic study by Sigal and his colleagues[33] that used siblings as controls has indicated that parents of a child who had severe croup in early childhood tended to have more difficulty in setting firm limits for the child after he recovered than they had setting limits for the child's siblings. They later perceived the child as having more problems controlling his behavior, as being more dependent, and as showing more testing of limits than the sibling closest in age. Concern about the child's survival and "parental preoccupation" with the child seemed greatest in parents of children who had had tracheotomies. Similar effects may occur when infants recover from severe blood-type incompatibilities and other perinatal complications. However, as Gibson[10] has shown, there is no exact correlation between birth defects and later disturbances in personality functioning. Because of their conflicts, a few parents may isolate or stigmatize the child within the family or may openly neglect or reject him.

Except under very unusual circumstances, the pediatrician must be cautious about giving a straight-out prognosis about the expected death of an infant. If such a prognosis has been given earlier by someone else, pending the results of treatment the pediatrician may wisely qualify his re-

marks on the outlook for the child while acknowledging the seriousness of the child's condition. If the child survives, the pediatrician should undertake preventive measures in order to avoid the "vulnerable child syndrome," overpermissive handling by the parents, or other negative effects of the experience. He should first assure the parents that the child's life is no longer in danger. He can then tell them that when a child has been so ill, parents tend later to handle the child "in a special way." He can give the parents some indication of the importance of "weaning" the child to his previous level of functioning, reassuring them that he will help them in later talks about the child's convalescence and development. Supportive measures and pediatric counseling should be continued for a number of months in at least monthly contacts, especially during the convalescent phase, and the parents should be given opportunities to work through their feelings, especially any feelings of guilt and anxiety.

Minor Acute Illnesses

In preschool-age children, acute minor illness (e.g., respiratory infections, otitis media, cervical adenitis, bronchitis, or contagious diseases) involve varying amounts of pain and discomfort. In some children, irritability, crying, fatigability, hyperactivity, or somnolence may be premonitory behavioral signs of an impending illness. Most preschool-age children can communicate their pain or marked discomfort to their parents although they may localize the pain poorly. With high fever, many children experience febrile delirium, with brief hallucinatory episodes and an occasional seizure, which may frighten the parents. During the acute phase of the illness, most children become less active (at times somnolent), and their appetite decreases. A few children, however, become overactive and restless and have trouble falling asleep or have frightening dreams.

Most studies of patients' reactions to acute illness have been carried out in the hospital, where it may be difficult to distinguish the reactions to the illness itself from the emotional reactions to hospitalization itself and to the treatment. In a recent study by Mattsson and Weisberg[23] of a group of children 2 to 4 years old who had minor acute infectious illnesses that were treated at home, reactions of the type just described were noted. In addition, all the children became somewhat more irritable in their relations with others, particularly with their mothers. All showed some transient regression. Two-year-olds commonly refused to cooperate in dressing and bathroom routines; those preschool-age children who sucked their thumbs or used comforters at night showed a marked increase in these habits in the daytime. In contrast to hospital studies, loss of bladder or bowel control was rare among children who had achieved toilet training. Some children under 4 years old showed the return of their earlier fears of animals, monsters, and the dark. Most regressive manifestations disappeared as the children improved.

Although all the children in the study, regardless of age, sex, and type of illness, showed some temporary setbacks in beginning independence and self-care, there were significant qualitative differences in the changes in the mother-child relationship. Those changes were categorized as Reaction No. 1 and Reaction No. 2. Reaction No. 1 was seen in most 2-year-olds. It was characterized by clinging dependence on the mother, with much whining and wishing to be constantly carried or held. The children exhibited an inability to occupy themselves and extreme irritability and intolerance to frustration. Reaction No. 2 was encountered only in children over 3 years of age. It was characterized by diminished interest in physical or verbal contact with the mother and other family members, often associated with rejection of the mother's attention, and withdrawal into a self-contained, relatively undemanding, quietly restful state. Children who showed Reaction No. 2 looked at picture books, colored, or watched television; occasionally they made simple demands (e.g., for a drink or a blanket) and they whined for only a short time if their wishes were not immediately gratified.

Almost all children over 4 years of age showed Reaction No. 2. Most of these children had shown Reaction No. 1 when they were ill at 2 or 3 years of age. No child changed from Reaction No. 2 to Reaction No. 1. Although there appeared to be no correlations with sex, ordinal position, type and severity of illness, deaths in the family or other factors, there was a significant correlation between age and type of reaction; Reaction 1 decreased and Reaction 2 increased as the children grew older. Many mothers of the 4- and 5-year-olds commented on the more self-confident attitudes their children had when they were ill at home. Thus, the reactions of preschool-age children to acute minor illness at home seemed to progress with age toward more self-contained and independent behavior.

A number of the parents of the 2- and 3-year-olds expressed frustration that they were unable to comfort their children or to protect their bodies and alleviate pain as they were accustomed to do at times of minor hurts or tensions. This suggested that a minor illness in a preschool-age child might help promote his growth toward independence and, in the face of his mother's helplessness, his beginning capacity to master responsibility for the care of his body. Of course, children who have developmental lags, overly dependent children, and significantly disturbed children may not show such an orderly progression toward independence in regard to their response to minor illness. Differences in temperament may also account for differences in response patterns.

Management of Acute Minor Illnesses

Carey and Sibinga[3] have pointed out that the physician's management of acute minor illness may affect the child's development as well as the emotional adjustment of the parent and the child. Carey and Sbinga emphasize the importance of avoiding diagnosing or treating "pseudo-disease" or "nondisease." (He may fall into such a trap either because he is anxious or uncertain about the diagnosis or because he is being pressured by the parents.) The pediatrician should nurture him without either overemphasizing or neglecting the child's illness.

Carey and Sibinga have indicated that overdomination of the parents by the physician, neglect of the parents, and incorrect handling of the parents can lead to significant problems. The physician should keep in mind the needs of the parents as well as of the child. He should give the parents adequate information about diagnosis and treatment, encourage them to ask questions, help them deal with any misconceptions or feelings of guilt, and help them cope with the realities of their child's illness. His approach should aim at promoting the parents' self-confidence in their capacity to handle illness in their child.

Common colds (most of which are caused by a group of rhinoviruses[25]) can be a special problem. Many parents do not know that the average child has 4 to 8 colds a year. According to a 10-year family study by Dingle,[8] colds occur more often among preschool-age children and they decline to 3 or 4 a year among adolescents. Some children and some families have very few or very many colds.

Although allergy and seasonal and environmental factors (e.g., forced hot-air heating) may help cause some colds, most children who have more than the average number of colds have no underlying abnormalities, and neither chilling nor excessive fatigue seems to affect one's susceptibility to colds significantly. But psychosocial factors[6] have been shown to be a factor in colds. In one study, some volunteers developed colds after the instillation of a placebo,[18] while the incidence of colds dropped 50% in a group[7] who had been given placebo vaccines. Dingle's study and a more recent controlled study have indicated clearly that frequent colds are not an indication for tonsillectomy and adenoidectomy.

Mortimer[25] believes that no therapeutic measures of proven effectiveness are available to help the child with frequent colds and that the most effective approach involves a sympathetic presentation of the facts to the parents, together with guidance about the management of individual episodes. This approach is often neglected although 15 minutes of explanation will save many hours later and can help allay the parents' feelings of guilt and anxiety. Mortimer includes in his brief discussion with the parents of the causes of colds, (1) the fact that viruses do not respond to antibiotics, (2) some information about the epidemiology of colds, including the information that there is no evidence that chilling and "low resistance" are predisposing factors, and (3) the facts that each cold must be treated individually and symptomatically and that there are no effective preventive measures (including tonsillectomy and adenoidectomy). Mortimer assures the parents that the child is not basically unhealthy, that a certain number of colds are a part of growing up, and that frequent colds are not a sign that the parents neglect their child's health.

Mortimer advises looking for sources of tension or family discord which might contribute to the frequency and severity of colds. He also believes that the physician should determine whether the parents are too concerned about sniffles, or keep the child home from school too easily. Dispelling unhealthy attitudes in the parents can prevent the child from becoming overdependent or developing school phobia.

Convalescence

Mention was made earlier of the phasic responses of the human organism to catastrophic illness or injury and of the need of the patient and his family to deal with any residual defect or handicap. Restitution, the final phase in that sequence, corresponds to the stage of convalescence from less serious illness. As Senn indicated in his classic paper[31] on convalescence, it is difficult to say exactly when convalescence begins or when it ends, just as it is hard to differentiate the signs and symptoms of an illness, a temporary breakdown in adaptation, and the indications of the reparative process. Senn says, "In a consideration of illness and of returning good health it is important that the child be considered as a living, changing person, whose mind and body jointly share in the progress of recovery and in the process of growth. An interplay of the forces of physiology and pathology, influenced by endogenous psychological factors and by various exogenous phenomena, produce the emotional reactions, and since all these powers are dynamic the resultant feeling tones are moving and changing."

Senn has also emphasized that while some children respond to illness with resistance, others respond with feelings of pleasure. Senn says, "It is quite likely that in all of us pleasure is mixed with pain, and that illness may foster emotions of relief and joy after initial feelings of pain and displeasure, and that convalescence may offer surcease from a life of struggle and turmoil. This is expressed in modern psychiatry as 'the secondary gain' of illness." Senn pointed out over 30 years ago some of the pitfalls of acute illness (these include many of those mentioned in the previous section on the management of acute major and minor illnesses), and he indicated that the physician must try consciously to avoid producing fear in the child, to avoid deception, and to take the time to listen to doubts and fears, thus exerting a reassur-

ing influence which can shorten the period of convalescence and prevent psychologic complications. Senn also described the strong emotional tie which can arise between the sick child and the nurse and which must be gradually deflected onto the child's parents.

Certain illnesses by their very nature seem to make convalescence difficult. For reasons which are not clear, infectious hepatitis and infectious mononucleosis often have depressive effects; and Sydenham's chorea can easily be intensified and prolonged by psychosocial factors. In addition, two controlled studies have demonstrated that loss of morale can lengthen convalescence from influenza[16] and brucellosis[15]. Another controlled study[21] has indicated that the speed of healing following an operation for a detached retina can be affected by how well the patient accepts his condition. Lags in perceptual-motor functioning that follow a high fever or an insult to the central nervous system have already been referred to as frequently unrecognized causes of learning problems during the convalescent phase.

The child's developmental stage may affect his convalescence. Problems in appetite, feeding, and sleeping are common in infants and very young children, especially in the hospital. These problems often disappear when the child goes home. "Addiction" to tracheostomy has been described in infants,[17] and behavior modification techniques[36] have been used to restore nasal breathing in such cases. In the study of reactions to minor respiratory illness done by Mattsson and Weisberg,[23] heightened irritability and short-lived anger were seen in all preschool-age children during the convalescent period, and they lasted 1 to 5 days. In the 3-year-old children who showed the self-contained, undemanding response during the acute phase, a temporary appearance of separation anxiety was common during convalescence. It was combined with the child's expectations of his mother's affection, bossiness, and easy frustration.

In the school-age period, the social and educational implications of the illness are usually predominant. For example, a child who recovers from acute rheumatic fever without adverse physical sequelae, may have a conflict about the need to return to the competitive world of school and his wish to remain safe at home, dependent on his mother. In such a situation, abdominal pain may persist on a conversion basis ("memory pain"); or weakness or some other symptoms may occur. In most such cases, a supportive psychotherapeutic approach usually helps the process of convalescence.

Examples of school phobia and of psychologic invalidism following acute illness were mentioned earlier in the book. In such conditions (e.g., anxiety and depression that can follow mild upper respiratory infections in older school-age children[30]) predisposing conflicts about the handling of dependence and aggression are ordinarily present, with the illness serving as a precipitating factor. In many of these cases, formal psychotherapy is necessary.

In adolescence, with its heightened concern over the integrity and functioning of the body, preoccupation with the physical sensations that are associated with minor illness may lead to problems during convalescence. The adolescent may hear his pulse beat while he lies in bed, or he may hear his heart beat during a fever, and so become concerned about heart disease, for example. The adolescent who has mild discomfort while urinating (associated with a higher specific gravity of the urine) may be afraid that he has a venereal disease or of abnormal or inadequate genitals. Ordinarily such fears pass quickly, but if they are associated with a move to a new school, a family crisis, or feelings of tension, uncertainty, or discouragement, they may persist and increase to an almost hypochondriacal degree. Fears of this nature are not uncommon in college students, even when

they do not have an acute minor illness, and the "medical students' syndrome" that appears during the study of pathology is well known.

Careful physical examination and judicious reassurance, combined with encouragement to talk about their life situation, are usually enough to help most young people with such problems. Again, the patient's premorbid personality is of significance during the convalescent period. People who have anxious, obsessive-compulsive, or overly dependent personality disorders may, if the circumstances are sufficiently stressful or the conflicts intense enough, develop lasting concerns about their health that amount to psychologic invalidism. Cases of "cardiac nondisease" have been known to develop in such convalescent patients.

Some adolescents may also resent the temporary loss of freedom that arises from respiratory infections or other acute minor illnesses. Struggles for control between the parents and an adolescent pushing for independence can arise if the parents continue to overemphasize bedrest.

Besides being contributory and perpetuating forces, psychologic and social factors may act as predisposing and precipitating forces in acute illness or injury. (These factors were discussed in Chapter 4.)

Bibliography

1. Association for Child Care in Hospitals. Unpublished material.
2. Brazelton, T.B.: The pediatrician and hysteria in childhood. Nerv. Child., *10*:306, 1953.
3. Carey, W.B., and Sibinga, M.S.: Avoiding pediatric pathogenesis in the management of acute minor illness. Pediatrics, *49*:553, 1972.
4. Chambers, W.N., and Reiser, M.F.: Emotional stress in the precipitation of congestive heart failure. Psychosom. Med., *15*:38, 1953.
5. Cobb, S., and Lindemann, E.: Neuropsychiatric observations. Ann. Surg., *117*:814, 1943.
6. Despert, J.L.: Emotional factors in some young children's colds. Med. Clin. North Am., *28*:603, 1944.
7. Diehl, H.S., Baker, A.B., and Cowan, D.W.: Cold

vaccines. Evaluation based on a controlled study. JAMA, *111*:1168, 1938.

8. Dingle, J.H.: The common cold and common cold-like illnesses. Med. Times, *94*:186, 1966.

9. Freud, S.: Mourning and melancholia. In: *Collected Papers. 14*:152. London, Hogarth Press, 1925.

10. Gibson, R.M.: Trauma in early infancy and later personality development. Psychosom. Med., *27*:229, 1965.

11. Green, M., and Solnit, A.: Reactions to the threatened loss of a child: A vulnerable child syndrome. Pediatrics, *34*:58, 1964.

12. Halper, I.J.: An occult conversion reaction superimposed on a facial nerve lesion. Psychosomatics, *7*:311, 1966.

13. Hamburg, D., Hamburg, B., and DeGoza, S.: Adaptive problems and mechanisms in the severely burned patient. Psychiatry, *16*:1, 1953.

14. *Illness Among Children.* Department of Health, Education, and Welfare. Washington, Government Printing Office, 1967.

15. Imboden, J.B., et al.: Brucellosis. III. Psychological aspects of delayed convalescence. Arch. Intern. Med., *103*:406, 1939.

16. Imboden, J.B., Canter, A., and Cluff, L.E.: Convalescence from influenza. Arch. Intern. Med., *103*:393, 1961.

17. Jackson, B.: Management of the tracheostomy in cases of tetanus neonatorum treated with intermittent positive pressure respiration. J. Laryngol., *77*:541, 1963.

18. Jackson, G.G., Dowling, H.F., and Muldoon, H.R.: Acute respiratory diseases of viral etiology. VII. Present concepts of the common cold. Am. J. Public Health, *52*:940, 1962.

19. Kübler-Ross, E.: *On Death and Dying.* New York, Macmillan, 1969.

20. Lindemann, E.: Symptomatology and management of acute grief. Am. J. Psychiatry, *101*:141, 1944.

21. Mason, R.C., et al.: Physical healing related to patients' attitudes. *J. Religion Health*, *8*:123, 1969.

22. Mattsson, A.: Long-term physical illness in childhood: A challenge to psychosocial adaptation. Pediatrics, *50*:801, 1972.

23. Mattsson, A., and Weisberg, I.: Behavioral reactions to minor illness in preschool children. Pediatrics, *46*:604, 1970.

24. Meyer, E., and Crothers, B.: The psychologic and psychiatric implications of poliomyelitis. J. Pediatr., *28*:324, 1946.

25. Mortimer, E.A.: Frequent colds. In *Ambulatory Pediatrics.* Edited by M. Green and R.J. Haggerty. Philadelphia, W.B. Saunders, 1968.

26. Pless, B.J.: Epidemiology of chronic disease. In *Ambulatory Pediatrics.* Edited by M. Green and R.J. Haggerty. Philadelphia, W.B. Saunders, 1968.

27. Prugh, D.G.: Natural history of children with chronic diarrhea. In: *Psychosomatic Aspects of Gastrointestinal Illness in Childhood.* Report of the Forty-Fourth Ross Conference on Pediatric Research (S. Buckingham, Ed.). Columbus, Ohio, Ross Laboratories, 1963.

28. Prugh, D.G., and Tagiuri, C.K.: Emotional aspects of the respirator care of patients with poliomyelitis. Psychosom. Med., *16*:104, 1954.

29. Richmond, J.B.: The pediatric patient in illness. In: *The Psychology of Medical Practice* (M.H. Hollender, Ed.). Philadelphia, Saunders, 1958.

30. Richter, H.G.: Emotional disturbances of constant pattern following non-specific respiratory infections. J. Pediatr., *23*:315, 1943.

31. Senn, M.J.E.: Emotional aspects of convalescence. Child, *10*:24, 1945.

32. Shands, H.: An outline of the process of recovery from severe trauma. Arch. Neurol. Psychiatry, *73*:403, 1955.

33. Sigal, J.J., et al.: Later psychosocial sequelae of early childhood illness (severe croup). Am. J. Psychiatry, *130*:786, 1973.

34. Silber, E., Bloch, D., and Perry, S.: Some factors in the emotional reaction of children to disaster. Am. J. Psychiatry, *113*:416, 1956.

35. Wittkower, E.E.: Rehabilitation of the limbless: A joint surgical and psychological study. Occup. Med., *28*:93, 1947.

36. Wright, L., et al.: Behavioral techniques for reinstating nasal breathing in infants with tracheostomy. Pediatr. Res., *3*:275, 1969.

General References

Apley, J., and MacKeith, R.: *The Child and His Symptoms.* Philadelphia, Davis, 1968.

Constanza, M., Lipsitch, J., and Charney, E.: The vulnerable child revisited: A follow-up study of children three to six years after acute illness in infancy. Clin. Pediatr., *7*:680, 1968.

Engel, G.L.: *Psychological Development in Health and Disease.* Philadelphia, Saunders, 1962.

Gallagher, J.R.: *Medical Care of the Adolescent.* New York, Appleton-Century-Crofts, 1966.

Glidewell, J., Mensh, J., and Gliden, M.: Behavior symptoms in children and degree of sickness. Am. J. Psychiatry, *114*:47, 1957.

Hollender, M.H., Ed.: *The Psychology of Medical Practice.* Philadelphia, Saunders, 1958.

Josselyn, J.M., Simon, A.J., and Fells, E.: Anxiety in children convalescing from rheumatic fever. Am. J. Orthopsychiatry, *25*:109, 1955.

Kanner, L.: The invalid reaction in children. J. Pediatr., *11*:341, 1937.

Korsch, B.M.: Psychologic principles in pediatric practice: The pediatrician and the sick child. Adv. Pediatr., *10*:11, 1958.

Langford, W.S.: Physical illness and convalescence: Their meaning to the child. J. Pediatr., *33*:242, 1948.

Lipowski, Z.J.: *Psychosocial Aspects of Physical Illness: Advances in Psychosomatic Medicine.* Basel, S. Karger, 1972, Vol. 8.

Little, S.: Psychology of physical illness in adolescents. Pediatr. Clin. North Am., *7*:85, 1960.

Maginnis, E.: Diagnosis and treatment: Organization for convalescence. Pediatrics, *41*:1131, 1968.

Peabody, F.W.: The care of the patient. JAMA, *88*:877, 1927.

Prugh, D.G.: Toward an understanding of psychosomatic concepts in relation to illness in children. In: *Modern Perspectives in Child Development*. (A. Solnit and S. Provence, Eds.). New York, International Universities Press, 1963.

Schiffer, C.E., and Hunt, E.R.: *Illness Among Children*. Department of Health, Education, and Welfare, Washington, Government Printing Office, 1963.

Sigal, J.J.: Enduring disturbances in behavior following acute illness in early childhood: Consistencies in four independent follow-up studies. In: *The Child in His Family: Children at Psychiatric Risk*. (E.J. Anthony and C. Koupernik, Eds.). New York, Wiley, 1974.

Werkman, S.L., Greenberg, L., and Lourie, R.S.: Symposium: coping with serious illness. Clin. Proc. Child Hosp. Washington, D.C., 22:118, 1966.

25

Chronic Illness and Handicap in Children*

. . . neither is it proper to cure the body
without the psyche.
(Plato)

A chronic illness is a disorder that is protracted (and sometimes exacerbated). It is associated with some impairment of functioning at the physical and often the psychologic or social levels. Some chronic illnesses are of course permanent, but they may be compatible with a fairly normal life span. Some chronic illnesses follow a progressive course, and have a fatal outcome. A chronic handicap may be congenital or acquired, and some congenital handicaps and some acquired handicaps may be reversed or repaired and thus may not be permanent. A chronic handicap, whether congenital or acquired, involves some impairment of functioning, and some chronic handicaps may be associated with a shortened life span. The onset of a chronic ill-

ness and a chronic handicap may be related to an acute or catastrophic illness or injury, or it may have been gradual and insidious.

Many of the considerations mentioned for acute illness and injury apply also to chronic illness and handicap, the major health problem of children today. The handling of the acute phase or the catastrophic response may in part determine what problems remain if a chronic phase develops. Although a chronic illness or handicap often has serious adverse effects on the child's personality development and on his family's functioning, many children so affected make a surprisingly good adaptation to or compensation for their disabilities. The child's previous adaptive capacity and the parent-child-family balance, or interpersonal equilibrium, seem to be more important than the type of disease or handicap. The child's stage of development, the severity of the illness or handicap, the prognosis, the treatment, and other factors are, of course, also significant.

*This chapter has been adapted from an article originally published as "Why Did It Happen to Us? A Psychiatrist Explores Chronic Childhood Disability," *The American Family* Unit II, Report 4, Smith Kline & French Laboratories, Philadelphia, 1978. With permission.

Special challenges to development exist for children who are blind or deaf (and those whose defects are congenital respond somewhat differently from those whose defects are acquired). Problems in sexual development occur in children who have pseudo-hermaphroditism or exstrophy of the bladder. Difficulties in adaptation arise for children whose movements are restrained in orthopedic casts or who require special prosthetic devices. The debilitation and discomfort produced by certain diseases affect the child's social or academic functioning and his parents' responses.

Different children and parents may respond differently to such conditions, however. The earlier concept that specific personality malformations result from particular chronic illnesses or handicaps has today been largely abandoned. Adler's[1] concept of "organ inferiority," which involves compensatory behavior, has some validity in certain cases. (Adler's concept involved the idea that each human being has a weakness, either congenital or acquired, in some bodily organ, and that efforts to overcome the feelings aroused by such a deficiency often involved behavioral attempts at overcompensation.) Compensatory behavior is only one form of response, however, and that behavior may also be seen in people who do not have physical defects. The personality disorders of children who have a variety of chronic illnesses or handicaps resemble closely those of children who have no physical disorders. The blind child's fear of loss of control over his environment, the fear of the child who has cerebral palsy that he will lose his balance and fall, and the deaf child's suspicion that he is being talked about are common, but those fears do not seem to be specific to blindness, cerebral palsy, or deafness.

Even a small and virtually unnoticeable defect may, for unconsciously determined reasons, have overwhelming significance in certain families. Although a visible cosmetic defect may be most troubling in some families, a hidden metabolic defect may, regardless of its severity, be more mysterious and threatening in other families.

Reactions of Children and Adolescents

The concept of coping behavior was mentioned earlier. As Mattsson[116] has emphasized, coping behavior involves all the adaptive mechanisms the child uses to master stressful stimuli at the physical, psychologic, and social levels of organization of his personality. Thus coping behavior includes cognitive behavior, emotional expression, psychologic defenses, and motor activity. If coping behavior is successful, adaptation is achieved, and the child functions effectively whatever the nature or degree of his disability.

The direct effects of chronic illness or handicap include malaise, discomfort, and pain caused by the disorder itself or by the attendant treatment, feelings of fatigue and irritability, as well as the effects of any physical limitations.

In young children, other responses center on resentment or complaints about interruption of play to take medicines or other treatments, dietary deprivations, and physical limitations which prevent the children from keeping up with others. As in acute illness, young preschool-age children who must be hospitalized are most concerned with being separated from their parents. Late preschool-age and early school-age children are more concerned with the conditions surrounding the illness or treatment procedures, and they tend to misinterpret pain or other symptoms as punishment. Children who have heart disease may think that their disability is the result of their having been too active, and those who have diabetes may think that their disability is the result of their having eaten too many sweets. Children who have a disorder that has a genetic component may blame a parent or relative who has a similar disorder for having "given" it to them. Fear of bodily mutilation in hospital settings is characteristic of children in this age group.

School-age children may become frustrated, anxious or frightened if they have been given too little information or conflicting information about their condition. That is especially true if their parents cannot discuss the facts with them because of their own feelings. Children may worry that they will die from their disorder although death does not become a "reality" for a child until he reaches later school age. Loss of control over their bodies, their behavior, or their environment is especially troubling to school-age children, especially in the hospital.

Late school-age children and adolescents may worry especially about the restrictions their disorder imposes on their social life, and they may be sensitive to "teasing" or other evidence that they are not accepted by their peers.[193] They may keep to themselves feelings of inadequacy, inferiority, bitterness, discouragement, helplessness, and depression, as well as recurring thoughts about "never growing up" and about being inadequate sexually.[19] Adolescents especially may be troubled by or ashamed of their illness or handicap, because of the limitations, embarrassing symptoms, painful treatment, or social stigma associated with it. They are often deeply concerned about how the disorder will affect their educational and vocational plans and their chances for marriage and parenthood, and they are confused about their identity and future independence. Adolescents do fear death, and certain adolescents handle fears of death by trying to disprove them, to the point of taking dangerous risks or acting in antisocial ways.

Emotional immaturity, overdependence, social inhibitions and other neurotic symptoms, pseudo-independence, learning difficulties, rebellious behavior at home and at school, and resistance to therapy may occur in some older school-age children and adolescents. Conversion symptoms may be interwoven with the basically physical symptoms of a chronic disorder,[84] increasing the disability, sometimes to a serious degree. Conversion mechanisms or other psychologic responses, such as depression, may lead to invalidism in children who are only slightly handicapped.[91] The acute phase of a chronic disorder may evoke a reactive disorder; the chronic phase may result in developmental deviations in motor, social, or other dimensions. In some cases, a structured psychoneurotic or personality disorder may be associated with a chronic illness or handicap, or, more rarely, decompensation may ensue and a psychotic disorder may occur.

A chronic disorder with associated impairment in functioning often limits the child's experience, particularly in regard to social activities and (in adolescents) interaction with the opposite sex. The child has fewer opportunities for positive feedback from others, and so he may fail to develop self-esteem. And his motivation for learning or for achievement in other ways may be affected adversely. School phobia is not uncommon in such a child, and it is often compounded by overly dependent tendencies. Since there may be a discrepancy between the child's aspirations and his capacities, it is often difficult for him to plan long-term goals and to act in a goal-directed way.

Effects on Personality Development and Functioning

Although specific personality malformations do not result from specific chronic illnesses or handicaps, certain patterns of personality development and functioning are apparent in people who have chronic illnesses or handicaps. In the past, emphasis was often put upon maladaptation on the part of child and family to such disorders. Studies indicate that there is a higher incidence of maladaptation among adults who have chronic illnesses or handicaps than in the general population, (Barker[10]) and the National Health Survey figures cited earlier seem to indicate that the same is true of children and adolescents. However, recent studies (summarized by Mattsson,[116]) indicate that a surprisingly large group of chidren are able to cope successfully and to achieve adequate adaptation, even to severely limiting or handicapping disorders. The patients studied, some of whom were followed into adulthood, seem to have functioned effectively in school, with their peers, and at home, and to have had a good understanding of their disorder and a realistic acceptance of their limitations. They showed an age-appropriate and realistic dependence on their parents and other family members, and generally they came to assume responsibility for their own care and for participating in the medical management of their disorder. They seem to have developed a sense of self-preservation, and to have had little need for secondary gains from their disorder. They seem to have achieved adequate, although sometimes modified, patterns of social interaction.

In coping with a chronic disorder, the patients studied seem to have found various compensatory activities—intellectual or physical pursuits—which offered them important satisfactions. They seem to have been able to express sad or angry feelings when they were frustrated and feelings of confidence or guarded optimism when those feelings were appropriate. Many of them used denial adaptively in order to maintain hope and to deal with the uncertainty of their future. Some dealt with their concerns in an altruistic way, wishing to become doctors or nurses and thus help others with problems similar to theirs. Younger children identified with other patients, and they not uncommonly wished for a miraculous cure for "anybody who has this problem" or "who is sick." The opportunity to associate with and to learn about others who have successfully adapted to similar problems was often important in the development of confidence and positive feelings about themselves.

The parents of the children who coped successfully were generally able to understand and to accept their child's limitations, to permit him appropriate dependence, and to help them make good use of their capacities and strengths.

Children and adolescents who have failed to make an adequate adaptation to their chronic disorders seem to fall along a continuum.[147] At one end is a group of children who are overly dependent on their parents, particularly their mothers. Children in this group show overanxiety and fearfulness, passive or withdrawn behavior, and inactivity or lack of outside interests; often they have strong unconscious secondary gains from their illness or handicap. Some children develop chronic personality disorders of the overly dependent or overly inhibited types. Although the parents of children in this group are often described as overanxious and overprotective and sometimes as overindulgent, there is no exact correlation between the parents' response to the child's disorder and the specific type of personality distortion in the child. Some children in this group have been rejected by their parents.[195] Rejection is a much less common response than overprotection.

Case Example. An 11-year-old boy was suffering from a mild form of an obscure variant of Charcot-Marie-Tooth disease. Although the muscles around his shoulder and pelvic girdles were somewhat weak, he had been able to function without help until his alcoholic father left the home (when the boy was 6). He then became very dependent on his mother, who had a mild form of the same disorder but who was able to support herself as a teacher. At times the boy would ask the mother to carry him around, a request that gradually she became too weak to fulfill, and he could not get to school unless she drove him. The mother talked with the clinic social worker. After some talks it became clear that the mother was preoccupied with the boy's needs because of her feelings of loneliness and guilt. As she became aware of these feelings, she became more able to set limits on the boy's behavior and to develop a life of her own. At the same time, the boy, in periodic talks with a child health associate, said that he wanted to have more contacts with his peers. He developed those contacts as he became more independent and better able to use his limited physical capacities.

At the other end of the continuum is a group of children who are overly independent. These children tend to deny their limitations, pushing themselves unrealistically or acting as if they were not sick, sometimes carrying such denial to unhealthy extremes. They often risk danger, as if to cover up their fear of being harmed or feelings of inadequacy. Such counterphobic behavior can result in repeated pathologic fractures in a child who has renal rickets or in frequent episodes of bleeding from injury in a child who has hemophilia. The disorders of a number of children in this group were either acquired or became manifest during their autonomy stage of development, and the negativism normal in that stage may have been involved in the development of the pattern of denial and rebellion against prohibitions. The parents of these children, particularly the mother, are often described as oversolicitous and guilt ridden. Again there is no exact correlation between the parents' response to their child's disorder and the child's personality malformation. The parents of some of these children have had difficulty in accepting their child's disability, often denying its extent while pushing the child beyond his capacities or occasionally rejecting, scapegoating, or isolating the child within the family unit.

Case Example. A 10-year-old-boy who had renal rickets was hospitalized several times over a year's time because he had pathologic fractures, which occurred while he was playing sandlot football. When counseling the boy and his mother did not help, a child psychiatry–pediatric liaison consultant was called in. In talking with the mother, the consultant learned that the boy's father, who had been said to have "kidney trouble," had died suddenly a year before of a myocardial infarction. It became clear that the mother feared that the boy would also die suddenly, a fear which the boy later said he had too. The mother had been trying to limit the boy's activity, while the boy had been trying to deny his fear by playing football, a sport his father had enjoyed. When it was pointed out to the boy and his mother that the boy had a different illness from his father, and it could not lead to a similar outcome for the boy, the mother's struggle for control and the boy's denial diminished markedly. The boy subsequently was able to find an outlet playing milder sports, and he had no more fractures.

Freud described a pattern of maladaptation in adults who have congenital deformities or handicaps, and Mattsson further described that pattern in regard to older children and adolescents. People who show such a pattern become shy and lonely, feel resentful toward people who do not have defects, and feel that society owes them a living. They often come from families who have isolated them or made them scapegoats because of their defects, and they have accepted their families' view of them as defective outsiders. In my experience, this pattern of maladaptation is uncommon in children and adolescents.

Effects on Body Image

Most children who have chronic illnesses or handicaps have problems establishing or maintaining their body image, the mind's picture of the body. But such problems may also be seen in children who have psychosocial difficulties but no physical limitations or disfigurement. Gellert[63] has shown that many healthy school-age children and even young adolescents have poorly crystalized and inaccurate images of their bodies, particularly in regard to the location and functioning of their internal organs. Thus children who have chronic or acute disorders may easily become confused and anxious about the effects of medical or surgical procedures on vital organs or on the genitals from inguinal operations.

As the foregoing discussion implies, the term body image focuses on the feelings as well as the attitudes a person has toward his body. The image of his body which a person acquires is influenced by his experience and development and by the attitudes of others toward him, and it is closely linked to his self-concept. Relatively few systematic studies have been done of the body image problems of chronically ill or handicapped children. In a controlled study,[174] children who had amputations tended in their drawings to represent realistically their bodies and the bodies of others. In another study children who had orthopedic handicaps[28] usually indicated the "area of insult" in their drawings, but the person who interpreted the drawings could not determine the type and degree of handicap without knowing the child's personal history. Children who have congenital heart disease have produced significantly smaller and more constricted human figure drawings than did children in a control group.[71] (But a group of emotionally disturbed children and a group of intellectually retarded children also produced smaller drawings.) Two studies[89,168] of the impact of obvious physical handicaps on self-concept in male and female adolescents have had conflicting results.

The foregoing studies seem to offer no consistent patterns in regard to body image and self-concept in handicapped children. But a recent study[49] offers some clarification. In that study, three groups of children were asked to make figures of people from plastic material. One group comprised children living at home who had handicaps resulting from spina bifida; another group comprised normal, nonhandicapped children also living at home. There was no significant difference in the measurements of the figures made by those two groups. The third group comprised children who had handicaps resulting from spina bifida living in an institution. The figures these children made had consistently smaller measurements and many of the figures lacked one or more limbs. (These findings are consistent with the perceptions by these children of themselves as "deformed" and insignificant persons.)

The foregoing would seem to support the conclusion that psychosocial factors are important in the development of the body image. This conclusion is consistent with the observation of Richmond[59] and his colleagues that how the child's family handles and accepts the child's chronic illness or handicap is the most important determinant of his adaptation and social adjustment. People who have hidden metabolic disorders (e.g., diabetes), thus may develop a distorted or negative body image and self-concept as a result of adverse psychosocial experiences. In a study[51] of adult medical inpatients who had respiratory, neurologic, musculoskeletal, skin, and other disorders, 20% of the patients were dissatisfied not only with those parts of their bodies that were affected by illness but also with a number of other bodily parts and functions. This extension of the patients' negative feelings toward their body as a whole correlated with their degree of emotional disturbance. It is my experience that the same phenomenon often occurs in children and adolescents.

Of course other factors also affect body image. The person's stage of development is important; for example, cosmetic defects on the face or on other visible parts of the body cause special problems for adolescents particularly, as McGregor[113] has shown. An adolescent who has a chronic disability may have a special problem developing intimate heterosexual relationships, and children who cope fairly successfully may have problems in adaptation during adolescence. Depression, marked denial, or other responses to a damaged body image may interfere with the child's acceptance of rehabilitative procedures during the late preschool-age period, when the body image of a male or female is being formed. The child's social or interpersonal situation may also be a significant factor.

Some adolescents may have trouble with identity if their limitations or defects are significantly different from those of other adolescents being treated for the same basic disorder. Some adolescents may feel too different from the others, while others may feel guilty if they are less seriously disabled or disfigured than others in the group. Recent studies[164] indicate that healthy people also differ in body image patterns (with some sex differences[50]) and suggest that the way people experience certain symptoms is influenced by their body image patterns.[29]

Even the treatment may influence the body image. Children and adolescents (adults too) who have been in respirators for long periods of time tend to incorporate the respirators into their body images,[150] and they often have trouble accepting their actual bodies when they are not in their respirators. Unfortunately, there has been too little concern among members of the medical profession, including many psychiatrists, about body image problems in illness, as Stone has lamented. The clinician should be aware of what a changed body means to a patient, giving due recognition to the importance of "somatopsychic" factors. Encouraging a child to talk about the meaning of his illness or injury, including changes in his body image, should be a part of the supportive psychologic components of total therapy in the acute as well as the chronic phase of his disorder. Children and adolescents who have chronic illnesses or handicaps must mourn at each stage of their development, the "self that was to be."

Other Considerations

Psychosocial factors have been observed to play contributory, perpetuating, and sometimes precipitating roles in certain chronic disorders. These disorders include the collagen diseases (particularly lupus[122]), infectious diseases (e.g., tuberculosis,[27,83]

chronic respiratory infections or sinus infections,[86] brucellosis,[81] infectious mononucleosis,[72] herpes simplex[18]), certain degenerative diseases (e.g., multiple sclerosis[127,143] and Parkinsonism,[21]), pernicious anemia,[105] and fungus infections.[80] Experienced clinicians have observed that marked depression and feelings of hopelessness adversely affect the course of fatal chronic diseases,[147] such as carcinoma and leukemia. Although many of these disorders contribute to depression through their debilitating effects, mononucleosis and infectious hepatitis seem to cause a specific depressive effect in a way that is poorly understood.

Supportive psychological measures should be a part of the total treatment approach for children and adolescents who have the disorders just mentioned; psychiatric consultation or more specific measures (such as hypnosis for verruca vulgaris) is often helpful.

As discussed in Chapter 4, illnesses such as leukemia and lymphoma in adolescents and adults have been observed to have their onset in association with actual or symbolic losses of key figures, suggesting that psychosocial factors may be involved in their precipitation, along with environmental and other factors of etiologic significance.

Reactions of Parents and Families

The phasic responses of parents to their child's catastrophic illness or injury (which often results in residual chronic illness or handicap) were discussed in Chapter 24. Even if the chronic illness or handicap began gradually, parents tend to have the same phasic responses: initial fear that the child might die associated with shock, resentment, or anger, and denial and disbelief of the diagnosis and its long-term implications. Complaints of incomplete information and "shopping around" for other opinions may accompany this phase. As the parents move into the phase of fear and frustration, in which they begin to accept the reality of the chronic disorder and to mourn, feelings of guilt over having failed to prevent the disorder or of having transmitted or somehow caused it are experienced. The parents may project their feelings of blame onto the medical or nursing staff, or one parent may project those feelings onto the other parent. One or both parents may become seriously depressed. When the parents can verbalize and cope with their feelings, they can move into the phase of rational inquiry and planning, in which they can begin to accept the reality of the serious disorder.

But even parents who have negotiated successfully the first phases may have significant problems when faced with the stresses of the illness, including financial burdens, physical strain or fatigue, discouragement, emotional depletion, and the necessary rearrangement of family patterns of living. Also, at each stage of the child's development, his parents need to mourn again the child that was to be.

One of the central difficulties for the parents of a child who has a chronic disorder is how to handle the child's dependence-independence needs. Some younger children tend to cling to dependency, and their parents may have difficulty helping them to "move out" physically, socially, and academically. Some parents may try to push their child toward unrealistic independence, and the child may become either clinging or defiant. Most parents also have trouble in talking with their child about his disorder, and some parents may even hide the facts of his disorder from him. The parents also may have trouble talking with each other about the child's disorder. The father may give the child's care over to the mother and stay away from the situation. (The impact on the parents of the birth of a retarded or otherwise defective child is discussed elsewhere.)

Parents may differ between themselves in how they perceive their child's limitations or capacities. This difference may lead to the situation in which one parent pushes

the child and the other protects the child, and serious marital problems may result, especially if the parents had had marital problems before the child's disorder began. Divorce occurs several times more often in families of children who have chronic disorders than in families in the general population, and sometimes neither parent wants custody of the child. Some parents search ceaselessly for new and miraculous treatments; they may also resent the child's failure to be grateful for their self-sacrifices, developing ambivalent feelings toward the child as a result.

All of the foregoing are potential problems, and in the past much attention was given to parents who have significant difficulty in accepting their child's disabilities and in caring for him and guiding him. But a surprisingly large group of parents adapt successfully to the problems involved in rearing a chronically ill or handicapped child. After the initial phasic responses, these parents come to understand and accept the child's limitations; they permit the child the degree of dependence he needs while helping him move toward independence and self-care. They encourage regular school attendance and help the child to develop compensatory physical and intellectual activities. These parents see that only the most necessary restrictions are placed on the child and that the child has adequate social and recreational opportunities.

The parents just described usually rear children who also cope successfully. Nevertheless, with the continuing strain of the child's situation, these parents tend to use some denial in dealing with the uncertainty of the future and in maintaining hope. They may also use denial and isolation of their feelings of helplessness and anxiety during an exacerbation of the child's illness or other medical crisis, and, as Mattsson has indicated,[116] they may experience later a "rebound phenomenon" characterized by feelings of depression or irritability. These parents may also rationalize; for example, they may have a conviction that the child's disability has helped the whole family (it may have but such a conviction may also help the parents ward off feelings of sadness or resentment). Many parents also use intellectual methods of coping; for example, they may read material or attend lectures dealing with the medical or psychologic aspects of their child's disorder. Many parents identify with other parents whose children have similar disabilities, and a number can offer help to other parents who are beginning to face a similar experience. All these responses can help the parties involved.

Maladaptive patterns of parents also fall along a continuum. The largest group of parents who show maladaptive patterns tend to be overanxious, overprotective, and overindulgent and to have trouble setting limits on their child's demands. These parents have usually been unable to deal successfully with their feelings of guilt about having failed to "protect" their child from becoming sick or disabled, about having transmitted the disorder to the child, or about not having wanted the child originally. The child's illness or injury may have reactivated a conflict the parent had about the death of another relative, or the child may have experienced a serious illness at birth or in infancy from which he was not expected to recover. Some children reared by these parents fall into the overly dependent group; other children rebel against the parents' overconcern and associated overcontrol and become overly independent, as described earlier. The child's temperamental differences, his developmental stage when the disorder appeared, and other factors may help to determine his response.

Case Example. A nine year-old boy was seen by a pediatrician. The boy had had acute rheumatic fever at age 7. Although the parents had been told that the boy had recovered completely, their anxiety over possible residual heart disease, which had occurred in both their families, was so intense that they had not been able to allow the boy to engage in any strenuous exercise or even in after-school activities. The

boy resented the parents' overprotection, but he could not verbalize his feelings, and he became demanding and obstinate, and had frequent temper tantrums. The tantrums terrified the parents, who feared they would be bad for his heart. As a result, they also overindulged the boy. He seemed to rule the family, and his younger sister, a quiet obedient girl, seemed to be pushed into the background.

The parents were given supportive psychotherapeutic help by the pediatrician. They talked about their guilt about their family histories and they admitted to themselves that they were angry about the boy and his behavior. They were then able to set limits on the boy's behavior. The boy seemed relieved. He said he had not been sure his parents loved him because they never said no to him. The parents were able to permit the boy more freedom and his domination of the family ceased.

At the other end of the continuum is a much smaller group of parents who cannot accept a disability. They experience the same feelings of guilt and resentment about their children's disorders as do the parents just described; but they react differently from them because of their personality patterns, previous experiences, marital conflicts, or other factors. Parents in this group may deny the extent of the child's disorder and may push him beyond his capacities. A few parents in this group may need to deny the child's illness because they fear that he may die suddenly (and they may transmit that fear to the child.) Other parents in this group may project the blame for the child's difficulties with his disorder onto the medical staff, and they may postpone seeking help, be reluctant to accept recommendations for treatment, or unconsciously "forget" them. Some of these parents may unconsciously perceive the child's defect as reflecting their own or as being "retribution" for their own transgressions. They may unconsciously wish the child had not survived, to stand as a reflection of their own limitations.

In some families, disease that may carry a social stigma (e.g., epilepsy) may be felt so keenly by the parents that they unconsciously isolate or scapegoat the child within the family. The parents' lack of knowledge about the cause of the disorder may contribute to such behavior, as may their cultural beliefs (e.g., about the "evil eye"). But the roots of the behavior are usually deeper, and they often reflect a conflict the parents had about the particular child that existed before the onset of his condition. Some families isolate themselves socially; others battle society about the child's disorder and its implications. A few parents blame the child for inconveniencing them, or they openly reject or neglect the child. Children reared by such parents may become either depressed and hopeless or angry and rebellious. In either case, the child's feelings may interfere with his self-care or his response to treatment.

Case Example. A girl, a first child, was born with a cleft palate. Her parents had it repaired surgically, but they felt that the girl's defect was a kind of punishment, because her conception had forced their marriage. As a result, they reared her in a large closet with a small window and kept her largely out of sight of visitors and even her twin siblings. When her existence was inadvertently revealed at age $3^{1}/_{2}$, she exhibited asocial behavior, failure to thrive, and limited speech. Placement in a foster home and play therapy produced considerable improvement, but the girl's prognosis for normal development was still guarded when the girl was five years old.

Reactions of Siblings

In certain families with a chronically ill child, one parent (usually the mother) may, out of unconscious needs, devote so much time to the care of that child that his siblings may feel left out or neglected. Occasionally the parent will "devote her life" to the care of the ill child, because of a marital conflict or her "need to be needed," with the result that the siblings, and even the husband, are neglected. Situations of this kind may lead to jealous and demanding behavior, open complaints, aggressive or destructive behavior, psychophysiologic disorders, learning difficulties, and other responses on the part of the siblings.

Younger siblings may even pretend to have the same illness, and older children and adolescents may unconsciously develop conversion symptoms which are similar to those of the ill child. Young preschool-age siblings may be expected to understand the handicapped child's problems before they are capable of doing so, perhaps at an age when they are too young even to notice the defect. Children and adolescents may become "too good," out of guilt that they are well, or they may develop self-sacrificing attitudes and behavior. Resentment and other negative responses are more common and more intense in families that tend to avoid open discussion of feelings of any kind. The physician should make sure initially that the siblings understand the illness or handicap of the patient, talking to them if necessary, and from time to time he should ask about their adjustment.

Reactions of Other Persons

The reactions of relatives, neighbors, teachers, and members of the child's peer group to the child's disorder may affect family functioning, the parents' attitudes, and the child's adjustment. Some common reactions are pity, oversolicitous behavior, curiosity, teasing, fear, disgust, or open rejection. Some of these responses may be based on social stigmas, such as that still associated with epilepsy or mental illness despite widespread public education programs. Many of the reactions can be ameliorated by information about the disorder although it is often hard to reach the persons involved to give them the information. A talk by the physician, nurse, or health associate, in which a noncritical approach is taken, with a relative who has such a reaction may help. The attitudes and manner of the teacher can help the child's classmates understand the problems his condition poses. If the teacher feels uncertain, anxious, or helpless about what may happen in class (e.g., with a child who is subject to seizures) her fears may be communicated to the child's classmates and to the child himself. Close communication and exchange of information between health-care personnel and educators is of obvious benefit to all concerned, but such an approach is often overlooked.

Congenital vs. Acquired Disorders

Whether a disorder is congenital or acquired may affect how the parents and the child respond to it. The effects of a congenital abnormality (e.g., a malformation of the heart) may become manifest only gradually, allowing the parents time to adjust to its significance. Some congenital disorders, however (e.g., an amputation or the abnormalities produced in utero by rubella, syphilis, or toxoplasmosis), pose an immediate problem, requiring the parents to deal immediately with guilt and other feelings and to go through the mourning process. Particularly in older children, an acquired disorder may result in an "acute dislocation of the self-image," with significant emotional conflict involved in the reestablishment of a self-image that is consistent with the change in bodily functioning. But it is often less difficult to determine the potential limits imposed by an acquired disorder than by a congenital one, and the management of an acquired disorder may be easier because of the existing parent-child relationship and the child's progress in personality development.

In a follow-up study by Gibson,[65] the personalities of children who had congenital obstructions of the alimentary tract that required early surgery were systematically compared with the personalities of normal children. Comparisons were also made of the emotional stability and attitudes of the mothers of the children in the two groups. The findings suggested that there is no unilateral relationship between trauma in early

infancy and later signs of emotional disturbance, at least those that occur in later childhood. Children born with atresia of the esophagus showed no significant differences in their later adjustment from the control group, whereas boys who had congenital pyloric stenosis and girls who had congenital imperforate anus showed significant signs of emotional disturbance. There seemed to be no correlation between the severity of disruption of the normal pattern of gastrointestinal activity or the amount of separation from the mother in early infancy and the signs of emotional disturbance on the part of the children or deviant attitudes on the part of the mothers. The reaction to and interpretation of the congenital disorder and its effects on the parents and on the parents' personalities seemed to be the determining factors in the response of the child. The long-term study by Engel and Reichsman[46] of the development of an infant born with a tracheoesophageal fistula seems to support this conclusion.

In another study (by Werner and his colleagues[194]) during pregnancy and a two-year follow-up period, biologic stress in utero had a far greater impact on children whose parents were poor and relatively uneducated than on children whose parents were well educated and had adequate incomes. Perinatal complications and deprived environment seemed to have had a cumulative effect on the physical, intellectual, and social development of preschool-age children.

Initial Management

Management begins with the onset of the disorder, whether the onset is acute or gradual. If the onset is acute, how the child and his family are helped to pass through the phases of impact and recoil and to begin the process of restitution affects their long-term adaptation. Similar though muted phasic responses occur when a chronic condition that began gradually is finally diagnosed. (The management of psychophysiologic disorders, which may produce states of chronic illness or handicap, has been discussed, as has the handling of the parents' initial response to the birth of an infant who has a congenital abnormality.)

Discussion of the Diagnosis with the Parents

When the parents first bring their ill child to the physician, the physician may suspect that the child's condition is a chronic, even fatal one. However, it is vital that the physician keep his diagnostic intuitions to himself—and at all costs he must avoid giving the parents a differential diagnosis. The physician may be wrong about the diagnosis. And even if he is correct, he only gives the parents information that they are not ready to face. If he is wrong, anxious parents may later remember only the threatened condition, even though it has been ruled out, and they may worry for years that the condition will one day manifest itself. If the child is obviously seriously ill, the physician should acknowledge that fact but not make an immediate prognosis. An off-the-cuff prognosis (e.g., "He probably won't pull through, but I'll do the best I can") covers the physician in a legal sense, but if the child does pull through, the parents may remember the prognosis and may make the patient a "vulnerable child" by overprotecting him. It is better to make a broad estimate of the chances of recovery, leaving the parents some hope to the last. If there is no hope for the child, the physician can say, "We'll do our best, but the final result is in the hands of God (or Providence)."

When the physician is sure that the child has a serious or fatal chronic condition, he should meet with both parents together. He does so to let them share—and help each other with —the impact of the diagnosis and to make sure that both have the same basic information. The discussion should be carried on in a quiet private area that is removed from intrusive or curious onlookers. The physician should allow himself enough time to explain the condition. He should explain it in broad outline, without too much detail. Using nontechnical language, he can describe the studies which led to his diagnosis. He should use the bare minimum of medical terms, explaining even them carefully. He should tell the truth in a straightforward but kindly and sympathetic manner. He should temper truth with judgment, however, and not give all the details of the expected course of the illness at once. Delay or hedging will only increase the parents' fears. Medical terms in general use (e.g., cystic fibrosis) may have to be used, but they should be explained in everyday language. For example, "Cystic fibrosis is an abnormality a baby is born with, in which the mucous glands don't work right; the mucus is too thick and plugs up the glands, which affects the way the lungs and other organs work." Unfamiliar terms (e.g., agammaglobulinemia and nephrotic syndrome) only confuse parents.

After explaining the diagnosis briefly, the physician may frankly but gently indicate that the condition is a chronic or serious one but that certain things can be done to help. At this point, he should pause to let the details of the prognosis and treatment be elicited through the parents' questions about the seriousness of the disorder, the outlook for the child, and related matters. One should not assume from parents' silence that they understand fully. Feelings of shock or confusion that arise from apprehension, guilt, or other feelings may keep them from asking questions. (As indicated earlier, time should be allowed for a parent to cry in a sympathetic atmosphere.)

As indicated earlier, a 50-minute hour is not usually needed for the initial explanation of the child's disorder. About 30 minutes will suffice for many parents, provided they have regular opportunities to talk with the physician afterward. Some parents will need more time initially, but the extra time will be well spent. As a general principle, the full interpretation of a chronic condition occurs over a number of meetings, and it depends on a trusting alliance of the physician, patient, and parents.

If the parents do not talk about guilt or self-blame in the initial meeting, the physician can give them an opening by asking what they think caused the illness. All parents have some theories about the cause, no matter how limited their knowledge. Often parents will respond with misconceptions, such as, "I let him eat too much," "I didn't make him rest enough," or "Maybe he inherited it from my father. He had the same illness." Replies such as these help the physician allay guilt by correcting misconceptions. Some ideas or theories about illness are personal, while others may be influenced by sociocultural beliefs (e.g., in the "evil eye"). If the parents do not respond, the physician may at that point or later attempt to "incise and drain guilt" by the technique of generalization, as discussed in Chapter 12.

A review of Chapter 10 will augment this discussion of the physician-parent interview and subsequent interactions.

The Approach to the Child

One cannot assume that the parents alone will be able to help the child or adolescent deal effectively with his feelings about his condition. The physician should interview the child alone to give him a chance to ask questions and to air any misconceptions, which may be damaging to his self-image. The child might think, for example, that his illness is a punishment or that he will not grow up to be an adult. Or he may have some of the other confusions about body-image mentioned earlier. Only by understanding the patient's thoughts, feelings, and fears can the phy-

sician or health associate offer specific rather than blanket reassurances and make sure the child understands his condition as fully as possible. As was pointed out earlier, some of these feelings may be elicited during the physical examination by judicious questions about how the child feels about his illness, about how his body functions, and about what he thinks made him sick. If the child resists treatment, he can be helped only by open discussion of his feelings about the treatment, his condition, his outlook for the future, and his parents' reactions. With adolescents, the problem should perhaps be discussed also in a family interview in order to promote open and supportive communication about how it should be handled.

Physicians or other health professionals are often reluctant to discuss a child's illness with him, because they fear the child may become depressed if he is forced to think about the implications of the illness. But as was indicated earlier, most older children and adolescents are preoccupied with various thoughts about their illness, and an opportunity to discuss them can only be beneficial. Usually they eagerly seize on the chance to ventilate their frustrations, fears, discouragement, and resentment. And after the discussion, the child often seems relieved to know the truth. Also, the physician can sometimes learn from the child facts about his illness or his family situation which did not come to light in the history taken from the parents.

The physician who asks the child about what is the most difficult thing about his illness, often gets valuable clues that can lead to significantly supportive measures. If the child says the other children tease him at school, the physician not only can give him emotional support but also can contact the teacher, to give information about the illness and to help the teacher tell the patient's classmates about it. If a child who has hemophilia says that his disorder was caused by his "running around too much," the physician can reassure him that the illness was not his fault and he can help the child's parents deal with their feelings of guilt and help them discuss the truth of the matter with the child. The use of figure drawings can help to uncover the child's body image or feelings about himself, his illness, or his family's responses.

The physician who says to a child, "Tell me 3 things you wish for," or, "Would you like to get married and have children?" or, "Tell me about a good (or a bad) dream," can ordinarily quickly get a good idea of the child's feelings about himself, his family, and his illness. If the child has a physical illness, often his first wish is to get well. If he wishes for something not directly connected with his disorder, this may mean that he fears getting well, having to be independent, or growing up or that he has some other conflict related to the unconscious secondary gain or other psychosocial aspects of the disorder.

Preschool-age children will ordinarily wish for things for themselves, but they may wish for something for their parents. Older children and young adolescents ordinarily include other family members in their wishes, but if they are emotionally deprived, they may wish only for themselves. A child or an adolescent with a physical disorder who wishes things only for others is exhibiting an excess of altruism. His behavior may arise from guilt about his illness or the expense of the treatment, but it may also indicate hopelessness about himself, an unconscious need to suffer, or an identification with an overly self-sacrificing parent.

A child or young adolescent who cannot think of any wishes at all is ordinarily very depressed. He may feel hopeless about getting well, may feel that nothing good can happen to him, or may have given up completely and have a wish to die. Depression is especially likely if the lack of wishes is coupled with a lack of interest in his future or with a feeling that he will not be able to hold a job, get married, or have children.

The failure of a child to report or even to imagine a good dream or the recounting of a series of dreams about sad events or death often indicates that he feels hopeless or depressed. In such cases, one can say to the child that perhaps he gets discouraged at times or does not think anything good will happen to him. If he breaks down and cries, he can ventilate his feelings of hopelessness or despair. Once he gets these feelings off his chest, he may be more hopeful.

Some children who are not depressed show a disinterest in work, marriage, or having children, because their parents' marital, financial, or vocational problems have "turned them off" toward such things. Asking a child whom he would take with him if he had to be on a desert island can be most revealing, particularly if he selects an animal and not a person. Some children who are chronically ill may wish to be small animals that can be taken care of. Others may disguise this wish and turn it into an altruistic channel by wishing for a small animal to take care of and protect. Children who have unhappy experiences with family members or others about their disorder may wish to be a wild animal, which does not have to depend on anyone. Other children may have a favorite animal "who likes me," indicating that they trust animals more than they do people.

Many children when asked what caused their disorder indicate feelings of guilt by their reply (e.g., "I ran too hard" or "I ate too much"). Some children and adolescents deny having thought about the cause. Usually, however, some gratuitous remark, such as, "I don't want to think about it," gives a clue to their feelings of guilt, despair, or hopelessness.

Psychologic Evaluation

A clinical child psychologist can be most helpful in setting up a management program for a child or adolescent who has a chronic illness or handicap. Periodic evaluation may be necessary if the child is having problems performing or adjusting in school or if the parents are discouraged or hopeless. An intelligent child who has a disfiguring handicap (e.g., a cleft palate) may be thought by his parents and his teacher to be mentally retarded. The preschool-age child who is chronically ill tends to test lower than his actual ability, especially if he has been hospitalized repeatedly. The prognosis for adequate academic performance by children who have such congenital anomalies as meningomyelocele has been shown recently by Gardner and her colleagues[162] to be relatively good, in contrast to the rather hopeless attitudes of most physicians. The same is true of many children who have cerebral palsy, as Crothers and Paine[37] have indicated. One British study suggests that most athetoid disorders in children can be prevented if treatment is offered by 18 months of age.

A psychologic evaluation that is made when the child is in the hospital should be repeated later. In my experience, the performance I.Q. of a child who has a chronic illness or handicap tends to be 10 to 15 points higher when he is outside the hospital than when he is hospitalized. Clinical child psychologists know this, but until recently, many training programs in clinical child psychology did not require their students to have much experience in a pediatric hospital. Other considerations regarding psychologic testing have been discussed in Chapter 8.

Long-term Management

As mentioned earlier the physician should see the parents of a child who has a serious chronic disorder together whenever possible. Of course, it is sometimes necessary to talk to one parent alone (e.g., if a parent requests it or if the physician wishes to talk to one parent about the other parent's feelings of guilt, depression, or fatigue). Other factors are also important, but continuity in the relationship between the parents and the physician or other health professional is the key to successful long-term management. In discussions, the strengths of the child should be emphasized wherever possible as his problems are faced openly and honestly.

Conferences with both parents can help provide support and counseling about some of the stresses mentioned earlier. For example, a family who considers moving soon after the diagnosis of a serious chronic condition, often does so as a result of feelings of guilt or denial. A move under these circumstances is almost always unwise. In the conference, the physician can help the parents think such a move through carefully and perhaps avoid taking an impulsive step they may regret.

Parents who show continuing massive denial of the diagnosis or prognosis often have strong unconscious feelings of guilt. They may not be able to accept the situation because the child has been overvalued (e.g., as an only child or as one awaited for many years) or for some other reason. A frontal attack on the denial usually intensifies it, but "incision and drainage" is occasionally helpful. A psychiatric or other type of mental health consultation may be useful if the parents are willing. Offering the parents a chance to obtain a second opinion from another physician may prevent "shopping." Supportive psychotherapeutic measures can be tried. Patient tolerance by the physician of the denial, with the gradual development of a trusting relationship, may be the only possible approach, and even this may occasionally fail. But if the door is left open, the parents may return.

Anticipatory guidance regarding problems the child or adolescent who has a chronic disorder will face can do much to prevent difficulties. The parents and the child should be carefully prepared for the necessary medical or surgical procedures or for new steps to be taken or new phases to be entered during the management. As Mattsson[116] has pointed out, preparation of the parents and the child can help to mobilize their psychologic defenses and intellectual functioning and thus help them cope with the stress that is anticipated.

In the course of the disorder, the physician can assess the parents' progress in handling their feelings about the child's disorder and in arriving at realistic measures of childrearing. Through pediatric counseling, he can help the parents become aware of any tendencies toward overprotective, overindulgent, overrestrictive, or neglectful behavior toward their child. The most effective way is to make a tactful observation (i.e., through a gentle confrontation) of it to the parents. The observation may be preceded by a generalization and followed by a question. The physician might say, for example, "Most parents with a sick child have trouble letting him try things on his own, like taking medications by himself. I've noticed that that's a problem for you sometimes. Have you thought about it?" Or he might say, "All parents with a sick child get tired and frustrated at times, and they may wish they could just walk away from the problem. I've noticed you get irritated sometimes. Is it hard to concentrate on what Johnny wants then?"

Overindulgent or overpermissive parents may need to be "given permission" to set limits on their child's behavior or demands. They can be helped to deal with their feelings of guilt by being told that limits will help, not harm, their child. The physician can offer these suggestions in the context of a discussion of the child's need to live as normal and as happy a life as possible, adding that all children need and want some limits and are not really happy if all their wishes are fulfilled.

If the father is distant or uninvolved in the child's rearing, the physician can talk to him alone about the importance of his relationship to his child. The physician can help the father find activities he can genuinely share with his child in order to help the child develop compensatory interests and skills. This is sometimes easier if the child in question is a boy, but the father can be helped to see that a daughter needs signs from him that he values her as a person and as a woman-to-be. By tactful questioning, the physician should also try to find out whether the child's siblings are being given appropriate attention and affection by the parents. If they are not, he can point out their needs to the parents in a sympathetic and noncritical fashion, and he can make suggestions as to how their needs can be met. Psychiatric consultation can be helpful for parents who show the maladaptive patterns mentioned earlier.

Work with the Child

Continuity in the relationship between the young patient and the physician is of great importance in the long-term management of the disorder. When the physician is out of town, any problems that arise should be handled by a professional whom the child and his parents know. If the child is in the hospital when the physician is about to go out of town, the physician should introduce the physician who will be covering for him to the child and parents. Continuity in the relationship between the physician and the patient enables the physician to offer more effective support and counseling about developing compensatory interests, handling the child's dependence-independence needs, and working toward significant long-range goals. Supportive psychotherapy may be needed for both the child and his parents.

A child who has a chronic condition which limits his activity often has intense feelings of anger or aggression which cannot be discharged through activity. It is important to let the child verbalize these feelings if he can and to permit him to discharge them through play. For example, a child immobilized in a body cast can be encouraged to make up stories or to draw pictures which will express his feelings. Or a child confined to bed at home can use "play dough" (made of flour and salt), which he can squeeze hard and thus act out regressive impulses to soil or mess (a plastic sheet can be used to cover the bed).

A variety of task-oriented activities can be of value in the hospital. These activities may be offered under the professional umbrellas of occupational therapy, recreational therapy, or activity therapy. The methods of these disciplines are somewhat different, but their goals are similar: (1) to help the child achieve pleasure and success, sometimes for the first time since he became ill or handicapped, (2) to encourage the child to participate in group activities, and (3) to prepare the child to return to task-oriented endeavors in school or in vocational programs. The activities are best integrated into a play program that gives the child opportunities for appropriate expression of feelings, as the work of Staub,[149] Planck,[144] and Azarnoff[9] indicates. Flexible educational programs are also important in hospital settings. Such programs can help the child retain his orientation toward learning. Rie and Boverman[154] have developed a program which involves tutoring and ventilation of feelings for the school-age child. Such approaches are discussed more fully in Chapter 27.

During the course of the chronic condition the child and his parents can be helped to take small day-to-day steps,[38] thus encouraging hope while not arousing unrealistic expectations. If the child is in the hospital, his parents' attention can be directed to the child's progress in physical therapy or an increase in activity to the point of being discharged. If the child is at home, encouragement can be offered toward gradual resumption of individual activities within realistic limits. Gradual redirection of the child's interests may help him come to excel in new activities and thus to compensate for being denied other activities. Giving the child a chance to ask questions freely and encouraging him to take an active role in taking his own medicine and regulating his diet (for example) can encourage a sense of confidence and mastery. All along, the child and his parents can be helped to ventilate any feelings of frustration, resentment, discouragement, confusion, fear, and guilt. Psychiatric consultation may be needed for children and parents who are having difficulty in coping, and intensive psychotherapy may be indicated, along with medical measures, for those who show signs of maladaptive patterns.

Green, a pediatrician well versed in psychiatry, has admirably summarized the basic ingredients of the management of children who have chronic illnesses or handicaps[70]:

1. Competence
2. Continuity and time
3. Availability
4. Family focus
5. Seeing the child as a child
6. Preparation for what is going to happen
7. Open communication
8. Collaboration
9. Promotion of a positive identity
10. Support and encouragement

Battle[12] has emphasized the role of the pediatrician as an ombudsman and coordinator in the health care of the handicapped child involving an interdisciplinary team approach, and Ames[6] has proposed that there be a department of rehabilitation in children's hospitals. Handicapped adults are now beginning to exert their rights, and affirmative action programs backed by the Department of Health, Education, and Welfare have begun to arrange for the installation of ramps and specially equipped bathrooms and for other features that would promote the hiring of handicapped persons. EPSDT, the screening program established under Medicaid, has been a failure in most states; screening has not led to diagnosis and treatment because the facilities are limited, uneven, and fragmented.

Alternatives to Hospitalization

Although orthopedic and other hospital schools or long-term residential rehabilitation units were popular in the past and still help many children, the trend today is toward alternatives to hospitalization. Convalescent hospitals have largely disappeared. Medical group foster homes that offer nursing service and pediatric consultations can offer important benefits to the child who cannot return to his home. (However, these homes are still rare.) Spagnuolo and his colleagues[176] have developed a successful program at the Irvington House Day Hospital in New York City for children who have rheumatic fever. These workers believe that children who have brittle diabetes, cystic fibrosis, or rheumatoid arthritis and children who are convalescing from heart surgery can also benefit from such a day hospital program, which offers continuity of medical care and school, which reduces the stress on the family while the child is living at home. Not incidentally, the cost is much less than that of full-time hospitalization.

At the Winnipeg Children's Hospital, a program of home care has been worked out for children who have cystic fibrosis. Their parents are taught to do physical therapy by medical and nursing personnel who visit the home. Such programs have also been tried for children who have cerebral palsy (e.g., by Bryant at the University of Colorado), and they have been used for children who have chronic disorders. Homemaker services and the help of foster grandparents have also been offered to families who have a chronically ill or seriously handicapped child at home. The use of medical foster homes has been mentioned. Summer camps for children who have diabetes or other chronic illnesses have been most successful.

The use of home teachers may enable the homebound child to keep up with his or her schooling, especially with the help of radio and television programs and school-to-home telephones. But to foster his social development, the child should attend school if at all possible, even on a part-time basis. He might attend a special class or, ideally, a regular class. If a home teacher's services are used, the child's situation should be reviewed at least every 3 months in order to avoid psychologic invalidism or school phobia in a child whose physical condition has improved. The trend today is toward putting handicapped children in regular classrooms ("mainstreaming") rather than in special classes. The concept is basically valid, but teachers tend to feel they do not have the training they need to teach these children.

Vocational training that is compatible with an adolescent's intellectual and physical capacities (no matter how limited those capacities are) can be arranged with the help of community resources. It may be of remarkable help in the habilitation or rehabilitation of even markedly handicapped young persons by developing in them a sense of mastery and accomplishment. As indicated earlier, more such training, along with more job opportunities, is needed. If the child has such a serious handicap that he cannot leave home (such handicaps are rare), a social club can be built around the child in his home or telephone games (e.g., of chess), can be arranged. Such approaches have been taken by family agencies and children's agencies, and they have helped prevent the child from feeling inferior, lonely, depressed, or resentful.

Group discussions, often with a social worker or other mental health professional acting as a co-leader with the pediatrician, have been of value in offering emotional support and understanding for parents of children who have similar chronic illnesses,[96,111,130] as well as for older children and adolescents who have hemophilia, muscular dystrophy,[13] diabetes, or other chronic disorders. Parents' organizations may give the parents valuable emotional support and the feeling that they are helping others. These organizations may also arrange for counseling. Rehabilitation centers may be most useful to older children and adolescents, and many such centers now offer psychiatric consultation, along with other services. Early intervention programs that offer stimulation to infants and young children and help for parents are most important.

Although reading is no substitute for a relationship with the physician, the nurse, or the health associate, parents can get valuable information about the approach to their child's problems from reading *Caring for Your Disabled Child,*[177] which deals sensitively with the feelings of parents and children and offers sensible advice about a great many things, including play activities in the home and agencies in the community that can offer help.

Comprehensive Care

The term comprehensive care has been variously defined. To some, it means care that takes into consideration the psychosocial aspects as well as the physical aspects of the problems of the child and his family (and also the psychologic reactions of the physician to those problems). To others, it refers to care given by an interdisciplinary team approach coordinated by a pediatrician (ombudsman). Of course, the two definitions are compatible with each other. In private practice, the pediatrician may draw on the consultative and collaborative help of professionals in other fields. In either case, the care given is family centered rather than child centered.

Although quantitative studies[106,142] of the effects of comprehensive care of handicapped children offered by a primary physician working with an interdisciplinary team have not demonstrated that there is a relationship between the amount of professional care given and improvement in patient and family functioning, no qualitative measures of patient and family satisfaction (or of physician satisfaction) were included. My experience and that of

others[4,66] indicate that patient and family satisfaction is much greater when continuity of contact with a primary and coordinating physician is maintained. In its *Standards of Child Health Care*, the American Academy of Pediatrics recommends that a primary physician be assigned at the outset of the child's hospitalization to act as a liaison with the parents, the medical and nursing staffs, and the consultants. In my opinion, the principles of continuity, communication, collaboration, consultation, and coordination should be maintained on an outpatient as well as an inpatient basis.

Problems Associated with Bed Rest

Some of the deleterious effects of chronic illness or handicap stem from the misuse of bed rest. The adverse metabolic effects of restricted activity in bed are unfortunately not well enough known.[126] Loss of nitrogen and calcium in particular occurs within a few days.[25,77] Easy fatigability and increasing generalized weakness are other results. Kidney stones have occurred in patients who are in respirators for long periods of time,[150] and osteoporosis has occurred in infants who have been hospitalized. Bed rest is often difficult to enforce in children and adolescents. Many resist it, and preschool-age and early school-age children may resist it to the point of becoming hyperactive. That behavior may actually increase the work of the heart or the cardiorespiratory system as the result of the activity itself or of the associated emotional tension. In fact, one study[82] indicates that simply lying down increases cardiac output, stroke volume, and the work of the heart. A recent quantitative study[11] showed no significant difference in activity between a group of school-age children who were confined to bed and a group permitted full activity.

Bed rest has been used as nonspecific treatment for almost any disorder in children, from the common cold to tuberculosis. In the past, children who had rheumatic fever and acute nephritis, especially, were confined to bed for many weeks or a number of months. However, controlled studies by Akerren and Lindgren[3] in Sweden and by McCrory and his colleagues[124] in the United States have demonstrated that bed rest has no long-term value in the treatment of nephritis. Lendrum and her colleagues[103] found that a program of "rapid rehabilitation" for a large group of children with rheumatic fever, involving a short period of bed rest (until temperature, pulse rate, leukocyte count, and sedimentation rate approached normal limits), followed by gradually increasing activity, did not produce a significant increase in residual cardiac damage, even in the follow-up period of several years. The results of the study were compared to the results of a study of a group of children generally subjected to prolonged bed rest, but the control group was not an adequate one. Nevertheless, Lendrum's findings support those of other clinicians[73] who have allowed children who have active rheumatic fever full activity in a hospital ward as soon as they were considered well enough (from 2 days to 2 or 3 weeks), apparently without any harmful results. In Lendrum's studies, the children permitted early ambulation made better adjustments to their illness and hospitalization and had less anxiety and fewer instances of psychologic invalidism.

In regard to respiratory infections, in one controlled study[64a] there was no difference in outcome between a group of children confined to bed for at least 3 days and a group of children allowed as much activity as they wished, whether or not they had a fever. Illingworth and his colleagues[87] have treated children who had tuberculous meningitis and miliary tuberculosis by allowing early ambulation after institution of treatment measures, apparently without any deleterious effects. There is even clinical evidence that bed rest may be harmful to children who have rheumatoid arthritis and that children who have muscular dys-

trophy may respond to bed rest with rapid and serious deterioration.

Complete bed rest thus seems to have no significant therapeutic value in the management of most serious illnesses. Furthermore it can be psychologically harmful as well as highly unphysiologic. Illingworth[88] believes that the only true indications for bed rest are infectious hepatitis, in which activity predisposes the patient to relapses, and the preparalytic stage of poliomyelitis, in which physical exertion in the 48 hours after the onset of meningismus increases the risk of paralysis. When bed rest is necessary, it should be discontinued as soon as possible. (Early ambulation and partial bed rest in hospital settings is discussed later.) A flexible approach to rest, one based on how the child feels, can be used at home. As Nadas[137] and Harrison[82] have pointed out, most children who have even severe forms of chronic heart disease do well on activity levels below the point at which symptoms occur (e.g., dyspnea or fatigue), and many children spontaneously limit themselves.

Illingworth's 3 questions[88] are relevant to the treatment of any medical or surgical condition: (1) What good will the treatment do? (2) What harm can the treatment do? (3) What harm can occur as a result of not giving the treatment?

The Psychosocial Aspects of Pain

Pain is now considered a complex phenomenon, a far cry from the earlier simplistic differentiation between "organic," or somatic, and "functional," or psychologic, types of pain. Recent reviews of studies of pain in adults have been made by Strain[179] and by Shanfield and Killingsworth,[169] although there has been little discussion of pain in children. Beecher's studies[15] of pain in soldiers injured in war revealed wide variations in pain awareness and tolerance that had little relationship to the severity of injury. The pain threshold in children and adolescents can be affected by such factors as biologic factors, the child's level of development, his previous experience with pain, the meaning the particular pain and the illness associated with it has for him, the part of the body involved, the child's emotional state, level of attention, and personality style, the circumstances under which he experiences the pain, and the reactions of his parents and other family members. The experience of predominantly physical pain includes the physical reaction to the noxious stimulus, the central registration of the reaction in the brain, and whatever psychologic elaboration may occur within the mental apparatus. Pain of psychologic origin involves no peripheral stimulus, but the two types of pain frequently overlap and co-exist. Finally, pain may be shared with or communicated to another person—in the case of a child's pain, to his parents.

In infancy, pain seems to arise from more global experiences and to be more poorly tolerated than at later stages, and pain is still poorly localized by young children. (Rare congenital indifference to pain[35] and its consequences were discussed in an earlier chapter.) Preschool-age children have "magical" views of the mother's capacity to soothe pain. In addition, in one study[34] young adults who as young children had been less protected and had been forced to be "independent" showed lower pain thresholds and poorer tolerance of pain than did those who had been permitted to be appropriately dependent. In the preschool-age child, pain and illness may be misinterpreted as punishment. As conscience develops in the early school-age child, pain may be associated with feelings of guilt, which may be influenced by interpersonal forces in the family and by sociocultural factors. Children's responses to pain are also influenced by the pain responses of other family members, especially the parents. Thus pain comes to have a personal signature (as Engel[45] has termed it), which is related to the young person's

experiences and the way he responds to discomfort and suffering.

As a result of the factors mentioned earlier, following the painful stimulus and its central registration, the psychologic responses within the mental apparatus may vary widely. Temporary behavioral regression is almost ubiquitous, especially in young children. Anxiety and fear are common, and they may intensify the perception of pain. People who are markedly or chronically anxious have a significantly lowered pain threshold. Feelings of guilt, helplessness, depression,[23] or other feelings may also intensify pain perception. Intense and persistent feelings of guilt may lead certain people to invite further pain, in order to satisfy their unconscious need for punishment or suffering.

Some older children and adolescents may have a high tolerance for pain because they have strong needs to deny any weakness or dependency, because they fear that the pain may have some catastrophic significance, or because of culturally determined or other reasons.

Specific types of painful stimuli (e.g., trauma from burns or accidents), the pain of malignancy, surgical pain, and specific pain syndromes (e.g., headache and abdominal pain), as well as congenital absence of pain, are discussed elsewhere in the book.

Diagnostic Considerations. A small group of older adolescents seem to be like the "pain-prone" adult patient Engel[44] described. The pain-prone patient suffers chronically, from a variety of painful disabilities, some that have recognizable lesions and some that do not. Often he has a history of having undergone various medical procedures or operations or having had painful injuries. (Atypical facial pain, a serious problem in adults,[43,104] is rarely seen in children and only occasionally in adolescents.) Often the patient elaborates pain symbolically, fearing some vaguely defined damage to the self or expressing an unconscious need to suffer.

Chronic pain becomes a way of life for such a person, who often has a history of defeat but who, out of feelings of guilt or unconscious and unresolved conflicts, cannot tolerate success.[45] Usually, such a patient comes from a disturbed or broken family, and he has a parent who also has chronic pain.

Pain comes to be a maladaptive way of dealing with conflicts. Some people who cannot accept healthy types of pleasure get an unconsciously masochistic enjoyment from suffering. The pain and the chronic illness also are a form of communication of the person's feelings of helplessness, frustration, loneliness, despair, and failure and of his wish for affection and support from other people, especially the physician, the nurse, and the other health associates.

Although such affection and support may be forthcoming, it cannot satisfy the patient's conflicting needs, the psychologic component of which he needs to deny. Thus most treatments do not relieve the patient's pain and suffering, and the patient tends to arouse feelings of frustration, anger, and occasionally rejection in the physician. Desperate attempts to admonish the patient to change his life-style are doomed to failure, and they may be interpreted by the patient as disinterest or hostility. In some cases, the hope of financial compensation in accident or other types of litigation helps to prolong the chronic illness pattern, while in other cases, the patient's need to control others, including the medical personnel, is deeply involved.

Pain of psychologic origin includes conversion pain, pain associated with reactive disorders, chronic anxiety, depression, hypochondriacal tendencies, and psychotic disorders in children and (as Shanfield and Killingsworth have indicated) in adults. As Strain has pointed out, although most physicians and patients tend to think that the presence of pain confirms the existence of physical disease, in one study of adults[39] carried out in a general medical setting, about 75% of the patients who complained of pain had no demonstrable physical disease. As suggested earlier, even when pain from basically somatic sources is present, pain of psychologic origin is often admixed in varying degrees.

As mentioned earlier in regard to other symptoms of psychologic origin, a diagnosis of pain of psychologic origin should never be made by a simple "ruling out" (or exclusion), because that type of pain is often fused with pain from obscure somatic sources. The use of placebos to distinguish types of pain is fraught with danger, such is the power of the placebo.[14] In his experimental studies of pain caused by radiant heat, Beecher was unable to distinguish any differences between the effect of morphine and the effect of a placebo. Thus placebos can diminish or do away with mild-to-moderate pain from either psychologic or physical origin or both. (In the management of very severe or protracted pain, analgesics are superior to placebos.) Finally, if older patients or parents find out that a placebo is being used, the doctor-patient-parent relationship may be seriously disrupted.[170]

Conversion pain, which represents an unhealthy and partial solution to an unconscious, unresolved conflict, may have its origin in the mechanisms discussed in an earlier chapter, including the revival of a memory trace of a previous bodily experience of generally painful nature, identification with a key figure who has suffered from a similar symptom, punishment for unacceptable wishes or impulses, or any combination of these. Conversion pain may be admixed with pain of psychologic or physical origin.

Pain associated with reactive disorders in young children is apt to be vague, shifting, and often transient although frequently recurring. It seems to be saying in physical terms, "I am hurting." Even children who have no psychologic disorder may have transient pains or aches, at times associated with fatigue, overstimulation, or mildly depressed feelings ("growing pains"?), and children undergoing developmental or situational crises may experience these pains and aches more frequently. Children who have chronic anxiety, usually children with psychoneurotic or personality disorders of the anxiety type or chronically tense children, may also show vague and shifting pain although it may be expressed in painful contractions of various muscle groups.

As indicated earlier, depression in children often takes different forms from depression in adults. Transient and mild depressive feelings of course occasionally occur in healthy children and adolescents, sometimes in association with transient aches and pains. Although overt depression, with sadness, slowing down of activity, and other signs, occurs more often in children than some have believed, as Poznanski[145] has noted, hyperactivity, changes in eating and sleeping patterns and other depressive equivalents still occur often in children and adolescents. Pain associated with depression is, in my experience, less common in children than in adults, even in psychoneurotic depressive disorders. Depression of psychotic proportions, often involving pain as a part of a somatic delusion (e.g., a delusion that one has a brain tumor) rarely if ever occurs in children and is quite rare in adolescents. Pain of psychologic origin that occurs in association with depression in school-age children and adolescents is often of a conversion nature and has a symbolic significance. Often it is related to the loss of a key person for whom the child or adolescent has not mourned in a healthy manner.

Hypochondriasis in the adult form occurs rarely in children. When it does, it may represent a prepsychotic phase of a schizophreniform disorder, when the child is gradually withdrawing and his perception of his world and himself is painfully breaking up. Hypochondriacal preoccupations with bodily functions may at times be seen in depressed adolescents.

Children who have psychotic disorders in the early childhood period ordinarily do not build delusional systems with which pain might be associated, and school-age children with the schizophreniform type of psychotic disorder rarely have hallucinations or delusions until they are 9 or 10 years of age. Systematized delusions associated with pain are uncommon, although self-mutilation based on isolated delusions may occur. Adolescents may show adult-like schizophrenic pictures, occasionally accompanied by delusions of a somatic nature (e.g., a belief that part of the body is painfully rotting away) or, more rarely, hallucinated pain sensations.

Management of Chronic Pain. At the heart of the approach to the child who has any type of pain is the relationship of the physician, the nurse, and the other health associates with the child and his parents. People who specialize in working with patients with chronic pain tend to agree that the principal reason for failure in treatment is that positive and trusting relationships do not develop, often because the medical personnel spend too little time with the patient and his family. With the rare adolescent pain-prone patient, the physician and those who work with him must be prepared to be available on a flexible basis and to study and deal with the life-style of the patient and the problems in the family—not just the pain. Treatment must be directed at helping the patient to substitute a life-style of positive adaptation for one of pain and chronic illness. Although management on an ambulatory basis is preferable, hospitalization may be necessary initially to make possible a comprehensive evaluation of the patient and his family and to begin treatment in a setting outside the home, where the perception of pain is often unconsciously reinforced by family members. Psychiatric consultation is frequently indicated, even though no formal psychotherapy may be required, and management should ordinarily be coordinated by the pediatrician.

If hospitalization is employed, the ward

management conference (described in Chapter 27) is especially important, because the collaborative roles of physician, nurse, health associate, and other specialists must be clearly defined, with much attention given to consistency in communication and coordination of overall management. (Such an approach can of course be adapted to an ambulatory setting.) Honest and realistic goals must be chosen and thoroughly discussed with the patient and his parents. A positive, hopeful, and nonjudgmental attitude, without unrealistic promises or expectations is vital. Gradually a trusting relationship can be developed with the patient and his family. The relationship involves much time spent in listening. Within that framework, a supportive psychotherapeutic approach will often suffice, with small, gradual steps toward mobilizing the patient taken daily. Intensive psychotherapy may be needed later, especially if the family's interactions seem to be unconsciously reinforcing the patient's chronic illness.

The pain itself is the first object of attention. If pain from physical sources is at least part of the picture, analgesics should be used, perhaps in combination with a tranquilizer if pain of psychologic origin is admixed. (The management of pain in dying patients is discussed in Chapter 26.) Tranquilizers alone are not a substitute for analgesics if the pain has a somatic component, and antidepressants are of little use in children and of limited use in adolescents. If analgesics are used, they should be given on a regular, fixed-dosage schedule rather than on an as-needed basis, which often reinforces the pain experience. If the pain seems to have a psychologic origin, some initial sympathetic discussion of its nature and impact is necessary, with a gradual shift to consideration of the patient's family and other problems. The pain must be accepted as "real" (not "in your head"), and it must not be challenged or interpreted early in the relationship. Analgesics are rarely helpful although a mild

one may have a placebo effect. (The use of placebos is unwise, as discussed.) Mild tranquilizers may help temporarily. With predominantly physical pain, a shift to related topics is usually possible once the pain has been somewhat relieved.

Biofeedback techniques (for adults) and behavioral therapy and hypnotic techniques (for adults and adolescents) have also been effective in relieving pain. Surgical treatment or nerve blockade for intractable pain seems to be not indicated or necessary in younger children. Approaches that may prevent lingering or chronic pain (e.g., preparation for operation and anesthesia), have been shown to be effective in controlled studies. They are discussed elsewhere in the book.

Case Example. A 15-year-old girl, an only child, had influenza at age 10. She recovered, but she continued to complain of pain in her muscles, back, and joints, although there were no objective physical findings. Little by little, her life became one of constant pain, with a gradual restriction of social contacts that was intensified by the use of a home teacher for several years. Her parents felt unable to deal with the girl other than as a pain-wracked invalid; they centered their lives on her, and a variety of treatments prescribed by a succession of doctors were of no avail. Pediatric hospitalization produced no pertinent medical findings, and the family would not agree to psychiatric consultations. One of the nurses developed a supportive relationship with the patient, accepting her complaints of pain and showing an interest in her as a person. Gradually, the girl confided in the nurse her fears that her parents' marriage would break up, telling of marital battles that had surfaced around the time she had influenza. A pediatrician and a psychologist, in a discussion of school planning, helped the parents to discuss their conflicts. They accepted marital counseling, and, over a period of several months, the girl gradually recovered.

Psychosocial and Psychophysiologic Factors in Responses to Treatment

Although most children who have chronic disorders respond well to the use of newly developed drugs and surgical procedures, a small group of children may show paradoxical responses: psychologic decompensations, marked conversion disorders, or other symptomatic responses.[147] If the child's invalidism has become central to the family equilibrium, the "precipitation into health" of the child by the treatment may upset that tenuous balance, making it difficult for the child to return quickly to a healthy role within the family and outside. Some parents of chronically ill children who have adjusted to a life of "care-giving" may actually decompensate psychologically when their child suddenly becomes "well." A gradual rehabilitative approach is necessary for such children, and psychiatric consultation is indicated. Intensive psychotherapy is often needed for the child and his parents.

In adolescents, as in adults, psychotic episodes occasionally occur in response to the administration of adrenocorticotropic hormone or cortisone during treatment for rheumatic fever, lupus, and other disorders.[157] Besides the direct effect of the drug on the brain (which is poorly understood), problems in the realignment of intrapsychic and interpersonal balance may also be involved.[147] Psychiatric consultation should form at least a part of the evaluation of such psychotic episodes. The clinical picture in adults has been said to often be one of euphoria. In adolescents, the psychotic episode appears more often to be a frankly depressive one although a schizophrenia-like picture may be seen. Most such episodes subside when the dosage is lowered or the drug is stopped. Since a few episodes may continue subclinically, good follow-up care is important. Psychiatric treatment should be given as indicated.

Resistance to therapy may be based on the patient's need to deny the seriousness of the illness because of its social implications, or it may reflect difficulties in communication within the family, marital battles about the patient's illness, or other problems. In more serious situations, resistance to therapy may signify that the patient has "given up," out of depression or hopelessness or a self-destructive, even suicidal, tendency that is related to serious family problems. Younger children may resist the use of prostheses because they have an intense need to deny the loss of a limb. (To the 4-to-6-year-old child, the thought of bodily mutilation is terrifying.) Older children and adolescents may resist the use of prostheses because of their difficulty in accepting an altered body, because of their rebellion against a troubled family, or because they have self-defeating unconscious needs. Encouraging the patient to talk about his feelings may help. If he cannot discuss his problems, a gentle confrontation may be useful. Supportive psychotherapy may help the patient and his parents. Psychiatric consultation is often indicated, and intensive psychotherapy may be necessary.

Another psychosocial factor in resistance to treatment of chronic disorders is the psychologic response of the physician. Acutely ill children usually recover fairly promptly and thus are an important source of satisfaction to the physician. Conversely, chronically ill children who do not respond to treatment or who respond minimally are a source of frustration to the physician. Responsibility for children who have serious and often life-threatening illness is demanding for the physician, nurse, or other professional, and it may be depressing, especially if the patient and his parents are depressed. Understandably, the physician sometimes feels irritated when a patient does not improve or when a patient or his parents are angry and demanding rather than grateful.

In such a situation, the physician must examine his feelings. If he understands his responses, he may be able to empathize more fully with the fears and frustrations of the parents and the child. He may be able to discuss his frustration with the parents in a nonjudgmental way, saying that it seems that he has not been able to meet their expectations. Such an admission may help him gain control of his feelings, and the parents' response may be surprising. Some parents may respond by saying that they realize how difficult it is for the physician, and the air may be cleared. Occasionally it may be wise to suggest in a nonjudgmental way that the parents have a consultation with another physician or that they might be happier with another physician. But before any such action is taken, it might be wise to discuss the case with a child psychiatrist or some other type of child mental health professional.

Genetic Counseling

Only the psychosocial aspects of genetic counseling are discussed here. (The reader who wishes sophisticated discussions of genetic probabilities is referred elsewhere.)

The genetic counselor does not make decisions for the people he counsels. He gives them as many facts and probabilities as he can, and on the basis of that information they must make their own decisions. But that information can change as knowledge about genetics grows. For example, a few years ago, it was felt that diabetic persons should not marry other diabetics, and that if two diabetics did marry, they should not have children. It now appears that the increased risk to children if both parents have diabetes is about three times that if only one parent is affected. Certain workers have felt that the impaired fertility of "double-diabetic" marriages may easily outweigh this "slight" numerical burden. Others feel that the congenital anomalies in children born to diabetic and prediabetic mothers are underreported and that some of the inborn defects of the heart, lung, and kidney may not become evident until later in life.

In other situations, the genetic data are more clear-cut. In autosomal recessive disorders (e.g., cystic fibrosis), the probabilities are that 25% of the children of a couple who have had one child with such a disorder will be affected (a risk of 25%). How-

ever, some workers have pointed out that the situation can be looked at another way: 75% of the children will probably be normal. (This is not assurance, only a probability.)

As the foregoing examples indicate genetic counseling has its sensitive areas. Some couples who have had a child with a defect want absolute assurance that the next child will not have a defect. Of course, such an assurance cannot be given and these couples should be advised to adopt if they wish more children. Some couples look at the optimistic side of the probabilities. Townes[185] feels that a somewhat optimistic approach toward genetic counseling is warranted, because the prognosis is frequently much better than the parents had imagined.

The genetic counselor must give the parents enough time to ask questions and to air their misconceptions. He must recognize and deal with feelings of guilt (e.g., those of a father of a child who had Down's syndrome and who was afraid that his earlier habit of masturbating had caused his child's defect.) The finding that such a disorder as classic hemophilia came from the mother's side of the family can bring about much guilt, leading to blame, marital conflict, and even divorce.

The genetic counselor also must be aware that some parents who want assurance that their next child will be normal may not wish to adopt because the adopted child would not be "part of ourselves." Thus the counselor must not let his feeling that the parents should adopt children come across so strongly that the parents feel he is critical of them.[181] He may also have to deal with his own frustration with a couple who are at serious risk and who insist on having children—or with a couple who cannot seem to reach a decision. In addition, he must be sensitive to differences in point of view between husband and wife and he should refer them for marital counseling when appropriate.[182]

The genetic counselor does not simply

give the parents facts. Taking into consideration their ages, religious beliefs, emotional resources, responsibilities, and other factors, he helps them examine their problems. Thus genetic counseling often takes a good deal of time, and it should involve a supportive psychotherapeutic approach. What seems factual is also a human interaction.

Special Problems

Although many of the reactions of the child and his family are nonspecific ones, some reactions have specific features related to the organ system involved, the symptoms, the child's developmental stage, the etiology, and other factors. Disorders that may evoke specific reactions are discussed in the pages that follow.

Birth Defects

Cleft Palate. Children who are born with a cleft palate or a cleft lip or both, experience development differently from normal children, as Tisza and her colleagues[184] have pointed out. The majority of such children had no opportunity as babies to suck because they had to be fed by special methods. Before surgical repair of their defects, these children often regurgitate food through their noses and have frequent episodes of choking. In the first 2 or 3 years of life often they must undergo several operations and the separation from the parents, pain in the oral region, and temporary restriction of movement of the arms and hands that the operations entail. Their speech development is usually delayed, and, when the child is able to say words, they are hard to understand. When the child enters school, he looks and sounds "different,"[160] and he may become isolated from his peers. Some children often show considerable drive for mastery, associated with postural tension, muscular rigidity, and manipulation of their arms and hands.

Their intelligence is normal, but they have some developmental lags in perceptual-motor functions that are related to their perceptions of their body images and their problems in verbalizing concepts.

Besides their feelings of grief and guilt, the parents[183] of a child who has a cleft palate feel frustrated about feeding the child, fear that the child may be mentally retarded because his speech development is delayed and because he drools, and feel shame about the child's appearance, particularly if he also has a cleft lip. Some parents continue to deny the defect and focus on the child's intelligence or other strengths, and a few parents reject their children. Thus special perspectives in management are indicated.[110]

Meningomyelocele. A significant number of children born with meningomyelocele still die from infection although survival rates have increased with improvements in therapy. The ventriculo-jugular shunt operation has diminished the incidence of serious hydrocephalus, and partial spinal ostectomy has been of help to some patients although it involves some months of immobilization in body spica casts. Some of these children are destined for a wheelchair existence. In the past, children who had meningomyelocele were regarded as having a poor prognosis in regard to their intellectual development. The birth of such a child puts severe stress on family integrity, and many of these children have been put in institutions or foster homes, with little chance of adoption. Recent studies by Gardner[162] and others[79,191] indicate that most of these children who live have the capacity for normal intellectual, educational and social functioning but that emotional deprivation and too little stimulation by the parents and the hospital staff seem to interfere with adequate development in a number of cases.

Exstrophy of the Bladder. The problems in ego development of children born with exstrophy of the bladder have been studied by Fineman[48] and by Feinberg and his colleagues.[47] Before the treatment approach involving uterosigmoidostomy and cystectomy was developed, children who had this defect were continually plagued with the problem of wetness and odor from urine. Since surgeons prefer to do these operations after bowel training (because the procedures modify the bowel contents), the child has to deal with the problem of being a "dirty, smelly thing" until he is 4 or 5 years old. In boys, the penis is short and stubby even after it has been reconstructed surgically. As adolescence approaches, fears of sexual inadequacy are common in both boys and girls, although if the condition is properly treated surgically, persons of both sexes can have adequate sexual experiences and are not sterile. Parents find it difficult to talk with their child about the defect, as do some medical personnel. Hypospadias and its surgical repair evoke special anxieties about sexual adequacy in the parents, the child, and the medical and nursing staff members.

Limb Deficiency. Limb deficiency (congenital amputation or malformation of the limb structure, as in phocomyelia resulting from the use of thalidomide) poses special problems for the child and his parents. Treatment should be instituted during early infancy.[74] The child's training in the use of prostheses should take into consideration the child's developmental stages; for example, more refined techniques should be offered when the child reaches higher stages of his mental and physical development. Children in the late preschool-age period and early adolescence may resist the use of prostheses. In both these periods, the child is sensitive about his physical appearance and has conflicts about independence. Apprehension or overcontrol on the part of the parents are often underlying factors. Children who have phocomyelia, especially those with arm deficiency, have been found to invest strongly their almost useless limbs,[158] and they sometimes resent or resist the use of prostheses. Mothers find it more difficult to caress their children when they are wearing their prostheses. In general, the parents' acceptance of the child helps the child to integrate the prosthesis into his body image.[17]

Congenital Heart Disease. Children who have congenital heart disease have been described variously. Earlier studies suggested that many are "nervous" but not seriously disturbed. In a more recent study (by Landtman and Valanne[102] in Sweden) 50% of children who had congenital heart disease showed signs of severe maladjustment. Children who have congenital heart disease are often overdependent and clinging and show little initiative. Many have been restricted in physical activity to an unnecessary degree. Glaser and her colleagues[67] have indicated that a number of mothers of children born with congenital heart defects recalled that before the diagnosis was made they had vague fears about their child's poor color, odd heart sounds, inactivity, or recurrent infections during the weeks or months after birth.

Glaser's study and other studies[8,108] describe the majority of mothers as being overprotective and overindulgent in their handling of these children and at the same time overrestrictive of their children's activity. Because of the widespread fear and lack of understanding of heart disease, many parents (and some children) fear a sudden heart attack or death. The child's behavior disturbances and the frequent family conflicts do not seem to be directly related to the severity of the cardiac lesion. There seems to be no relationship between the child's level of intellectual functioning and his level of arterial blood oxygen saturation[31] although children who have cyanotic heart disease[173] tend to have lower I.Q. scores than do children in general. After surgery, a rise in the I.Q. score of as much as 20 to 30 points is often observed.[109] The rise is not related to the degree of improvement (or lack of it) in the child's tolerance for exercise. It seems to be related to the child's improvement in initiative, concentration, activity, and mood, deriving principally from a decrease in the parents' anxiety and restrictiveness.

Congenital Rubella. Babies who have congenital rubella have problems similar to those of other multihandicapped children. Although children who have congenital rubella have often been given extremely pessimistic prognoses, a recent long-term follow-up study by Menser and his colleagues[128] indicates that the most such children adjust well in early adult life. Infants who have multiple handicaps that include cataracts[58] are more likely than those who have only auditory defects to be significantly delayed in their psychomotor and neuromuscular development; a significant number show autistic behavior, as well as other more subtle behavioral abnormalities (described by Chess and her colleagues[32]). Besides the reduction these infants have in sensory input because of defective end organs, their environmental stimulation is often diminished because they often assume bizarre postures, which, coupled with the possibility of contagion, render their handling by the mother extremely difficult in the early months.

Congenital Insensitivity to Pain. Children who have congenital insensitivity to pain often have burns and other injuries. Sometimes the injuries are so serious that their fingers or other parts of their bodies must be amputated.[35] The parents of these children are apt to be overprotective and overrestrictive, and the children are apt to be dependent and anxious (although in one child, rebellion seemed to lead to increased injury). In another child, the auditory, visual, and kinesthetic stimuli seemed to be sufficient to permit the child to develop a warm attachment to his mother, to show separation anxiety, and to respond to positive or negative social stimuli at age-appropriate points in his development.[52]

Parents' Response. The parents' response to the birth of a child who has a defect is an important part of the management. Telling the parents about the defect is the responsibility of the pediatrician.

While telling the parents, the pediatrician might hold the baby and look at it with the parents, as Battle[12] has suggested. This approach demonstrates the physician's acceptance of the child as well as his concern for it. In a recent study, the longer the delay in telling the mother that her newborn had a cleft lip, the more vividly she recalled being told.

In regard to the broader aspects of management, Gellis[64] has written, "The technical advances which have emerged in the treatment of birth defects have made the care of the child highly specialized. Care becomes even more complicated when defects are multiple. As a result, there has been little attempt at comprehensive care for the birth-defect child, the neurosurgeon assuming primary responsibility for the hydrocephalic, the orthopedist for phocomyelia, the urologist for exstrophy of the bladder, the psychiatrist for the mentally retarded." Gellis has suggested that the pediatrician serve as the ombudsman for the handicapped child and his family, whether serving as coordinator of a team of specialists in a medical center or by working with others in private practice. The pediatrician should be responsible for periodically reviewing all aspects of the child's functioning with the specialists involved and with the child's family, the school authorities, and the community agencies.

The rest of the chapter is concerned with special problems associated with other chronic disorders (most of these are acquired, though some are congenital). The discussion follows the outline of organ systems used in Chapter 3.

Cardiovascular Disorders

As Kennell[94] has emphasized, *rheumatic fever* is still poorly understood by many parents, particularly those who have a limited education, and it poses a special challenge in adaptation. Even after the child has fully recovered, many parents fear that he will die suddenly; the coronary attack (which occurs rarely in children) is still the stereotype of "heart trouble," and symbolic references to the heart ("My heart stopped when I heard. . . ") are common in everyday conversation.

Josselyn,[90] Shirley,[171] and others long ago indicated that children who have rheumatic fever can become anxious as a result of restriction of their physical activities, separation from home during periods of long-term hospitalization, and the fear of death. Although the prognosis for rheumatic fever has improved greatly and methods of management have changed since penicillin has been used to prevent recurrences, Glaser and her colleagues[112] have shown that school-age children who have established cases of rheumatic fever associate their illness with pain, punishment, physical restrictions, heart disease, social handicap, crippling, and death to a significantly greater degree than do children matched for age, sex, and socioeconomic status who are suffering from mild, self-limiting, and short-term illnesses.

Although long-term hospitalization was formerly the approach of choice in rheumatic fever, short-term hospitalization with early ambulation[73,103] and referral for day treatment[176] or even home treatment in certain cases[196] is now preferred and there has been no apparent change in the long-term outlook. The child's parents are often overprotective,[68] and the child may respond either with overdependence and anxiety or with denial and rebellious behavior, both of which can adversely affect his cardiac functioning. Rheumatic fever is more common in poverty-stricken, urban environments, and some clinicians[85] have the impression that emotional stress can be a precipitating factor. A number of factors, including a change in the child's immunity to streptococci and some hereditary predisposition, are probably involved.

(Other chronic disorders involving the cardiovascular system are discussed elsewhere in the book.) They include congenital heart disease and essential hyperten-

sion, migraine, and other disorders dealt with in Chapter 21.

Respiratory Disorders

Cystic Fibrosis. Cystic fibrosis (mucoviscidosis) is now ordinarily diagnosed earlier and has a better prognosis than was formerly the case. Newer methods have helped, and it is now known that some patients have little respiratory involvement. The problems for the child and his parents in dealing with an ultimately fatal illness, sometimes after the child has been ill for years, are discussed elsewhere, as are the problems involved in genetic counseling of parents of these (and other) children. In the course of cystic fibrosis, the child is often quite irritable, probably as a result of debilitation, fatigue, and difficulty in breathing, perhaps compounded by fears of suffocation or by other feelings.[7] The child's sleep problems are sometimes related to his fear that he will die while asleep. Stunting of growth can occur with any chronic condition, but it may be especially marked in children who have cystic fibrosis of early onset.

Cramps, flatulence, and malodorous bowel movements, as well as coughing, may occur if treatment is not well accepted. Preoccupation with thoughts of death, depression, or rebellious feelings may interfere with the adolescent's acceptance of therapy.[60] The adolescent may also worry about lack of acceptance by his peers and by limitations in his social life. In a study by Tropauer and his colleagues,[186] nearly 75% of a group of patients showed some indications of emotional disturbance in drawings they made of human figures. (This finding is disputed by Gayton and his colleagues.[61]) Denial is used by most patients to maintain hope. Children who are openly uncooperative about therapy generally come from families in which there are marital problems and problems in communication.

The parents of a child who has cystic

fibrosis must do nebulization and postural drainage. Postural drainage can be difficult and exhausting and can leave the parents emotionally depleted.[123] Mothers especially may become depressed and discouraged. A number of parents are overprotective and overly restrict the child's behavior, and a few may be openly rejecting. The hereditary component of the disorder poses problems for parents in regard to handling their feelings of guilt. Denial of the severity of the child's illness is a not infrequent mechanism. Some denial is needed to maintain hope, however, and many parents can come to help their children make an adequate adjustment. Because the patient needs time-consuming home treatments, his siblings are often demanding and complaining and they may even pretend to have the illness. The siblings may also have learning problems and engage in acting-out behavior. (But again, more systematic studies by Gayton and his colleagues[61] indicate that there is less emotional disturbance and greater strength in parents and siblings than the more impressionistic investigations indicate.)

Tuberculosis. Tuberculosis in children occurs less frequently today than formerly although the illness is still not completely under control. Morbidity and mortality have fallen dramatically since 1900, but the incidence of new reported cases has increased recently, and tuberculosis is still more common among black children than among white children. Sleep disturbances, nighmares, depression, and resistance to enforced rest are often encountered, as is the adolescent's preoccupation with the possibility of death. Parents and children share the stigma of tuberculosis, which has been stereotyped as being associated with unsanitary conditions and "weakness," and they may feel that the disease is unclean and shameful.

In the past, as Dubos[40] has indicated, children who had tuberculosis resented the isolation and long periods of bed rest its treatment entailed. Some rebelled against the rules, while others dreamed of engaging in almost constant activity. The limitations of the child's opportunities to learn and other factors, including depression, often resulted in his scoring lower on I.Q. tests, and sometimes the child was mistakenly said to be mentally retarded. There is no specific personality picture associated with tuberculosis, as was formerly believed. The association of emotional crises with the onset and exacerbations of the illness has been reported by Holmes[85a] and others; the changes in immunochemical mechanisms which take place in response to stress are not yet understood. (A graphic picture of the treatment of tuberculosis patients in sanitariums is offered by Thomas Mann in *The Magic Mountain.*)

The parents of the child who has tuberculosis may have great difficulty in accepting the diagnosis, partly because of the stigma associated with the disease but more intensely because of the possibility that they have given the disease to the child. The refusal of a parent who has tuberculosis to be hospitalized for treatment has led to the death of several children in the family from tuberculous meningitis. With modern treatment, death occurs infrequently, but parents still may fail to report a tuberculin test that had positive results, and routine follow-up measures are important. Enforced bed rest is no longer felt to be necessary in the treatment of tuberculosis, and early ambulation can help prevent emotional and other problems.

Other chronic respiratory disorders are discussed elsewhere in the book. They include bronchial asthma, allergic rhinitis, chronic sinusitis, and cystic fibrosis.

Gastrointestinal Disorders

Chronic disorders that involve primarily the gastrointestinal system are discussed elsewhere in the book. They include peptic ulcer, ulcerative colitis, mucous colitis (the "irritable bowel syndrome"), regional enteritis, anorexia nervosa, obesity, periodontal disease, megacolon, celiac disease, failure to thrive, and cleft palate.

Genitourinary Disorders

Today children who have chronic kidney disease tend to be considered early for kidney transplantation. (Some of the problems involved in kidney transplantation in childhood will be discussed in the section dealing with reactions to surgery.) It is my opinion that the medical management of children who have chronic kidney disease is not being taught as well as it could be to medical students and residents in pediatrics and family practice, because of the popularity of the kidney transplantation operation. If a child or adolescent is not considered to be a candidate for kidney transplantation, the tendency is to feel that even with dialysis, he will not live long. However, in the days before dialysis and kidney transplantation, many children who had chronic kidney disease were helped to survive and to live in reasonable comfort for a number of years. The study of medical management should not be neglected today.

It was commonly observed that children who had chronic kidney disease often developed signs of increased intracranial pressure related to cerebral edema. (Magnesium sulfate given intravenously can be quite effective in dealing with the increased pressure.) However, it was not commonly observed that long before the signs of increased intracranial pressure appeared, children who had chronic kidney disease sometimes were confused and mildly disoriented. Prugh and his colleagues[148] recently observed carefully some patients who were confused and disoriented. The observations were part of a clinical study of delirium in childhood and adolescence, a type of study that had not before been done systematically in regard to patients in these age groups. The observations showed clearly that the metabolic disturbances that occur in chronic kidney disease often pro-

duce a state of delirium that is frequently not recognized as such. The patient's tendency to misperceive external stimuli, his disorientation, and his confused thought processes, along with other signs of delirium discussed earlier, are often subtle, and gross agitation or semi-stuporous states are not common. Waxing and waning of the delirious, fearful, or aggressive behavior and other signs of the subclinical delirium are apt to be interpreted by the parents and the medical and nursing staffs as simply odd behavior. If the behavior is sufficiently deviant, it may be misinterpreted as being a manifestation of an intermittent psychotic disorder of psychologic origin.

A diagnosis of subclinical delirium will usually be confirmed by the results of a mental status examination. If it is, parents and staff will be able to view the patient's behavior much more objectively. A psychologic approach to the management of the delirious state, combined with medical procedures, may help the patient return to normal.

Other chronic disorders of the genitourinary system are discussed elsewhere in the book. They include menstrual disturbances, habitual abortion, certain types of polyuria, vesical paralysis, and congenital anomalies, such as exstrophy of the bladder.

Hemic and Lymphatic Disorders

Hemophilia. Hemophilia and other chronic bleeding disorders present special challenges to the child's development. The diagnosis is ordinarily made around the latter part of the first year or the early part of the second year, as the infant begins to creep or walk and to explore his environment. Thus the parents must monitor and at times judiciously restrict the infant's behavior as he enters the stage of the establishment of a sense of autonomy. In classic hemophilia,[151] the mother knows that she has transmitted the frightening and life-threatening disorder to her child. It is terribly difficult for her (and for the father also) not to be overrestrictive and overcontrolling toward the child during this early phase, which is characterized by oppositional behavior as he works toward autonomy.

The young child who has hemophilia has a constant fear of bleeding[119] and the associated pain, together with the fear of separation and the treatment that frequent hospitalization entails. Older children and adolescents often deal with their fears of fatal bleeding through denial and isolation of feelings.[24] Besides the bleeding caused by cuts and other injuries, Mattsson[120] and others[24,151] have described episodes of "spontaneous" bleeding that occur in relation to emotional stress. There may be an autonomic response to stress in such episodes, involving increased fragility of the capillary wall. Also, fibrinolytic activity and blood coagulability have been known to be affected by anxiety. The actual mechanisms are not fully understood.

It appears from the literature[2,69,92] that in a number of families, the mother has continued to overprotect and overrestrict the child, a pattern that developed after the diagnosis was made in infancy. Often the mother had experienced the death of a relative from hemophilia. In such families, the father has often blamed the mother and has paid little attention to the child, and divorce sometimes occurs. Some boys respond to their mothers' handling of them by becoming passive and overly dependent, manifesting depression at times or showing anxiety or phobic patterns. Others, perhaps for temperamental reasons, rebel. They may act out their feelings or manipulate the parents and use denial heavily, repeatedly putting themselves into risky situations. They thus cover up their fears with the use of counterphobic mechanisms, sustaining injuries often and having frequent episodes of bleeding. A few parents show marked denial of their worries, manifesting an attitude of unconcern and offering little or no supervision of the child. A few parents may openly reject the child.

With the help of their pediatrician, most of the mothers Mattsson studied[118] had been able to master their guilt and anxiety and to mourn. They were able to accept the fact that their child would have some episodes of bleeding, and they kept their supervision of him within reasonable limits. Such mothers kept denial of the dangers of the illness also within reasonable limits, and they isolated much of their anxiety, using an increasingly intellectual approach. They discussed the nature of the disorder with the patient and his siblings at an early age, and they could communicate their feelings to other family members and to the pediatrician. The fathers, after their initial feelings of sadness and sometimes of blame of the mothers, were able to help care for their children and to provide a model for masculine identification. These parents were able to cooperate with medical care, and they tended to identify and associate with other parents of hemophiliac children, both informally and in organized meetings. The successful adaptation to the task of raising a child with hemophilia did not seem to be related to the severity of the disorder, the child's age at diagnosis, whether another child in the family had hemophilia, or whether the parents knew about the genetic risk before they married.

Children in families that had adapted successfully had begun to cope cognitively with the illness by the time they reached the early school-age period. They showed an understanding of the relationship between injuries and bleeding and they had begun to set limits on their own activity and to get involved in their medical management. By adolescence, these children had developed appropriate compensatory motor activities and intellectual pursuits, but they were able, usually with the help of their fathers, to participate in a surprising range of play activities and sports. They were able, with their parents' support, to express sadness, anxiety, anger, confidence, and hope appropriately. They also used appropriately such defense mechanisms as denial, isolation and intellectualization of feelings, and identification with other patients and with medical personnel. They were able to maintain hope and to develop positive images of themselves—as productive and socially competent people who had hemophilia. In this series, small groups exhibited both the passive-dependent and risk-taking responses described earlier.

Although recent advances in the management of hemophilia have made it possible for patients to live longer and fuller lives, many physicians are still reluctant to be involved in their continuing treatment because of the sometimes stormy course, and the frequent physical and emotional complications. In a recent article, Bowden and Rothenberg[22] described in great detail a comprehensive approach to the management of a mildly mentally retarded and disturbed hemophiliac adolescent boy who had a tongue-biting tic. They pointed out that problems can rise from (1) the child's psychosocial status, (2) the individual psychodynamics of the physicians, and (3) the group dynamics of the medical team.

Supportive psychotherapeutic measures of the type described by Bowden and Rothenberg can be useful in many situations. In some cases, intensive psychotherapy for the child and his parents, along with medical measures, is needed to deal with the child's risk-taking or self-destructive behavior. Mattsson[117] has used group therapy for parents.

LaBaw[100] has used light hypnosis ("suggestive therapy") for older children and adolescents. He reported a striking drop-off in accidents, bleeding episodes, and hospitalizations. LaBaw teaches the children in a group to induce a light trance-like state in themselves using a code word; the children apparently are able to achieve greater calm and relaxation with self-hypnosis.[101] The support of the group and the group leader is an important part of the approach, even though these regular weekly sessions are not structured formally as group therapy.

Methods of home care for patients with hemophilia have been developed recently. In a controlled study of hospitalization as opposed to home care given by a nurse practitioner, Strawczynski and his colleagues[180] showed that most episodes of bleeding do not need to be treated by hospitalization. When home care was given, more episodes of bleeding were reported and they were reported earlier. Children and parents preferred home care to hospitalization, and the home care approach was an excellent model for teaching.

With the use of anticipatory guidance and pediatric counseling, the physician can offer much in the way of prevention in the early years which can minimize difficulties later.

Sickle Cell Anemia. Sickle cell anemia is found predominantly but not exclusively among members of the black race. The longevity of children who have sickle cell anemia is better than was originally believed. The literature contains little about the emotional development of the child who has this disorder. As Duckett[41] has indicated, the child is faced with many problems, including repeated episodes of pain or other sickle cell "crises," which may require frequent hospitalizations, clinic visits, and school absences. Competition in strenuous sports must be curtailed and there is danger of infection. Some children seem to be crisis prone, having recurrent episodes at brief intervals (sometimes associated with emotional stress and other factors), while other children may be symptom free for months. The parents are subject to stresses similar to the stresses of parents who have children with other types of chronic disorders. Some parents are overprotective of their child, and others are more flexible.

I have had experience with several cases of sickle cell anemia in which a conversion component seemed to be involved in the pain, intensifying mild pain or continuing long after the crisis had subsided. In one case, psychotherapy for child and parent brought about relief of the conversion component.

Indiscriminate screening for the sickling trait may have its problems, and the possibility of widespread genetic screening raises ethical, psychologic, and medicolegal questions. Equal access, individual rights to privacy, freedom of choice in childbearing, and avoidance of stigmatization are only a few of the issues which must be dealt with in community screening programs.

Other chronic disorders of the hemic and lymphatic system (e.g., leukemia and lymphoma) are discussed in Chapter 27.

Musculoskeletal Disorders

Children who have orthopedic handicaps often have special problems in regard to their body image and their self-concept. The way in which the parents react to their child's deformity can affect how well the child integrates the defect into his developing body image and self-concept. As Shechter[167] has pointed out, most children regard the handicap or the illness leading to it as punishment for some misdemeanor on their part, with the injured part of the body being an external representation of the punishment. Many of the problems related to depression, hopelessness, apathy, and learning difficulties (described earlier) arise in part from the long periods of time the child spends in the hospital, often without adequate recreational and educational programs. Patients who have muscular dystrophy,[175,189] dystonia musculorum deformans[97] (which may present with conversion symptoms,[146]), and dystrophia myotonia[192] may need psychotherapy. Conditioning has been helpful in the management of dystonia.[33]

Long periods of immobilization in body or other casts, as in osteogenesis imperfecta,[121,153] interfere with the child's need to move to discharge tension, to release aggression, and to master his environment.[16] Also, the child feels helpless and vulnerable when he is unable to move and is forced to remain passive and dependent, with the result that his anxiety and aggression are increased. This observation is especially valid in regard to the late preschool-age child, who is unable to comprehend fully the reason for his immobilization. He may develop temper tantrums and demanding behavior, or he may withdraw into a depressed or apathetic state and have a delay in speech articulation.[172] Older children and adolescents can better understand the need for immobilization, but often they have some of the same feelings. The child who can verbalize his feelings is apt to cope better with the immobilization. Opportunities to talk, to play games competitively, or to read or hear stories which have some aggressive fantasy content (e.g., "Jack, the Giant Killer") can help children release some of their aggression and achieve a feeling of mastery or control.

An example of the problems orthopedic handicaps pose for adolescents is offered by the recent study (by Myers and her colleagues[135]) of adolescent girls who had structural scoliosis and who were treated with the Milwaukee brace. More than 50% of the girls expressed overt distress over the recommendation that they wear the brace. They went through a period of withdrawal and depression, which was followed by a conscious decision to wear the brace and do the exercises that were prescribed. Most of the girls eventually wore the brace; only 2 out of 25 continued to refuse to wear it. Some mothers described their daughter's first night in the brace as frightening for the daughter; some of the girls were afraid they would choke or fall out of bed. All the girls found it hard to face their friends for the first time wearing the brace, which called attention to a defect that was not noticeable before.

About 50% of the girls had a a good relationship with their mothers, and all the girls were able to be responsible for doing the prescribed exercises. The other 50% of the girls, who had been overly dependent on their mothers, relied heavily on their mothers to help them with the exercises and other aspects of their daily life. For a small number of girls in this second group, their relationship with their mothers had been characterized by overdependence and mutual resentment. This interaction was made worse by the demands of the exercise program, and the exercises were done haphazardly and intermittently. Psychologic tests suggested that most girls perceived the experience as a threat to their bodily integrity but that they had minimal disturbance of their body images.

It was the impression of Myers and her colleagues that the girls who displayed overt distress (an "initial storm") and then made a conscious decision to accept the brace and the exercise program showed a better overall adaptation than those who were not able to express their distress. Other factors that helped the girl cope included: (1) a good understanding on the part of the girl and her mother of scoliosis and the need for the brace, (2) the active decision by the girl and her parents to wear the brace, (3) the continuing support and encouragement of the girl's family, (4) the hope for a successful outcome, a definite termination time, and some signs of progress, and (5) continuity, coordination, interest, and support in regard to the girl's visits to the medical staff.

In the process of coping, all the mothers closely identified with their daughters. The daughter's attitude toward the brace reflected the mother's, and both people became "stronger" when their attitudes were positive ones. Mothers and daughters both used some denial and intellectualization (as well as other defense mechanisms), although only one family used denial to the point that it interfered seriously with the treatment. Parents often helped their daughters make creative adaptations to

their problem; for example, by helping them find comfortable writing positions and by shopping with them for clothes that made them feel more attractive.

Myers and her colleagues wondered whether the relatively good adaptation that most of these girls made was partly a result of the fact that their handicap appeared later in childhood, after their body images were fairly well formed. Two of the girls who had had handicaps since early childhood had especially serious problems in adapting to the brace. But as mentioned earlier, the question is hard to answer. Perhaps the response to a brace designed to help a handicap that appears early in childhood is different from the response to a disfiguring defect that appears later in childhood. Individual differences and other factors also are involved.

Myers and her colleagues emphasize that besides detecting the scoliosis early, the pediatrician can help the family by showing his continued interest and support and by preparing the family for referral. He can also offer anticipatory guidance by explaining in advance the disorder, how it can be managed, and the expected psychosocial problems.

Other chronic disorders of the musculoskeletal system that have been discussed elsewhere in the book include rheumatoid arthritis, tension headaches, and limb deficiency.

Skin Disorders

Chronic disorders affecting the skin have been discussed elsewhere in the book. They include neurodermatitis, psoriasis, pruritus, alopecia, eczema, urticaria, angioneurotic edema, verruca vulgaris,[187,188] herpes simplex, and acne (see Chapter 21).

Endocrine Disorders

Children who are unusually short for no apparent somatic reason often have associated delays in sexual maturation. Short children are often teased as "runts" at school and babied as "dwarfs" at home.[116] Some of these children may try to cope by using massive denial of their problems; they may become aggressive and assertive or they may try to act the clown. Others show dependent or withdrawn tendencies, at times associated with enuresis or learning inhibitions. A few are able to cope fairly well, finding acceptance by developing compensatory skills. (See Chapter 21.)

The Committee on Drugs of the American Academy of Pediatrics recently stated that psychologic management is the approach of choice for most short children. The committee also stated that if drug treatment is attempted, it should be carried out in conjunction with counseling.[5] In my opinion, the same is true for the use of drugs to treat delayed puberty.

Money[133] and Patton and Gardner[141] have discussed cogently the principles of counseling short children and their parents. Parents need to be helped to build up their child's confidence. They should spend time with him each day, helping him develop compensatory skills that can bring him recognition and success. The parents and the child are often reassured to learn that ultimately the child will show some growth and will be normal sexually. (Although a delayed growth spurt can be predicted, the extent of growth cannot. Often the parents themselves are short.) In some cases, the child's withdrawal, aggressiveness, or other disturbance in behavior or the parents' conflicts about him may be intense enough to warrant referral for intensive psychotherapy. Children who have dwarfism of hypopituitary origin often show emotional immaturity, distorted body images, difficulties in expressing aggression, depression, and problems in identity formation.[159] Some develop obsessive-compulsive defenses and rigid personality structures.[99] Their parents are often overprotective.

Children who are unusually tall may be unusually tall as adults. For girls, the tallness may be a social handicap and a cause of much anxiety. Krims[98] feels that if the probability is great that the child will be excessively tall as an adult, and if hormonal intervention is considered, thorough interviews are indicated before treatment in order to help the girl accept her body more comfortably. Children who show precocious puberty[78,132] may be unusually tall during the preschool-age and early school-age years although as adults they are shorter than the average. Their size, combined with their unusual strength during these years, may cause problems in their social interaction with other children, and their early sexual development may arouse apprehension and conflict in their parents.

Other chronic disorders that involve the endocrine system are discussed elsewhere in the book. They include thyrotoxicosis, diabetes, hyperinsulinism, and pseudocyesis.

Central Nervous System Disorders

Poliomyelitis. Children and adolescents who have had poliomyelitis, now a rare disorder, may have many of the reactions already discussed. Even if no paralysis results, many children show difficulties in cognitive functioning for several weeks to several months after recovery, as Crothers and Meyer[36] long ago demonstrated. These difficulties seem to be the result of the meningoencephalitis which occurs, often on a subclinical basis, during the acute stage. It is manifested by drowsiness, severe headaches, a slightly stiff neck, and signs of mild disorientation—symptoms that may occur with other viral disorders, including measles, mumps, and chickenpox. Convalescent problems most often involve perceptual-motor difficulties, as manifested by difficulty in copying forms, drawing, remembering design, and doing formboard tests. Irritability, fatigability, and problems in concentration are also frequent. Such problems may also be observed in the convalescent stage of contagious diseases mentioned, and of course in other disorders producing delirium discussed in Chapter 22. Such problems may lead to other problems when the child returns to school, particularly if pressure is put on him by parents or teachers to achieve at his previous level. Part-time attendance when he first returns to school, special tutoring, or other preventive methods are important.

When paralysis is present, the child may later experience difficulty in competing socially, either because of overdependence or overrestriction by his parents.[165] Or he may show unrealistic denial of the defect (often related to the parents' response to his disorder) and push himself too hard.[150] As in other handicaps, the family may scapegoat or psychologically extrude the child, usually without actually rejecting him.[114,156a] Conversion symptoms can be admixed with the paralysis caused by the polio.[197]

Sydenham's Chorea. Children who have Sydenham's chorea show an acute onset of choreiform movements, emotional lability, decreased attention span, and frustration, sometimes to the point of agitation, over their inability to control the movements. I am inclined to the view that Sydenham's chorea is an acute benign encephalopathy based on the child's hypersensitivity to streptococci, which may occur in the absence of the other hypersensitivity phenomena involved in the syndrome of rheumatic fever. About 50% of the patients who have Sydenham's chorea do not develop clinical rheumatic fever. The onset of the chorea has frequently been observed to be associated with various types of emotional crises.[115] These crises may affect immunity to streptococci in susceptible children in a manner not yet understood. Psychophysiologic effects on host resistance to disease are discussed more fully in Chapter 4. Some reports suggest that a high percentage of children who have Sydenham's chorea later develop psychotic disorders and, as adults, schizophrenia.

Freeman and his colleagues[56] did a long-term follow-up study of patients hospital-

ized during childhood for Sydenham's chorea. The results of psychiatric interviews and evaluations were compared with those from a control group composed of patients hospitalized during childhood for rheumatic fever, glomerulonephritis, and osteomyelitis. The average length of "post-illness" time was 25 to 30 years in both groups. A high incidence of psychologic disturbance in the patients who had Sydenham's chorea was found to exist at the time of follow-up examination and, from the history and the hospital record, was determined to have existed before the chorea began. This finding is in contrast to what happened in the control group, which showed an incidence of disturbance about equivalent to that found in the general population. Twenty-five percent of the chorea patients had suffered the loss of a parent before the chorea began, and about 65% had suffered significant emotional trauma as judged by stringent standards.

Although I question the absolute accuracy of such retrospective data and would raise some questions about the methods used to evaluate the follow-up data, the chorea patients on follow-up study clearly had an incidence of psychologic disturbance that was about 3 times that of the control group. However, it is also clear that although there was a surprisingly high incidence of chronic personality disorders in the group—and a lower incidence of psychoneurotic disorders—there were no schizophrenic or otherwise psychotic patients in the "postchorea" group, contrary to what some believed would occur. Keeler's[93] study bears this out.

In my experience, children who develop Sydenham's chorea today are not so disturbed as the group reported on by Freeman and his colleagues, nor did they have as much early emotional trauma. Nonetheless, I agree with their conclusion about the need to consider psychosocial factors in the evaluation of Sydenham's chorea.[190]

Nelhaus[138] considers Sydenham's chorea a self-limiting disorder which may last from a few weeks to approximately 2 years. He says that about 65% of the patients have relapses but the relapses do not seem to affect the ultimate outcome.

Children who have Sydenham's chorea used to be treated by sedation, bed rest, and diminution of stimuli in a darkened room, and they were kept in the hospital for a number of months. It was Senn's impression[166] that this treatment intensified the choreiform movements and produced further motor restlessness and (sometimes) depression. Senn believed that the problem was not one of sedation but of looking at the child and meeting his needs. He reported on several cases in which this supportive psychotherapeutic approach resulted in a dramatic subsidence of the choreiform and related symptoms.

I have followed Senn's supportive psychotherapeutic approach, and I have seen some children so treated lose their choreiform symptoms within a few days after their admission to the hospital—and before sedation was tried. Nelhaus and others recommend the use of tranquilizing drugs, particularly Thorazine. Drug therapy may be of real help, but it should not blind the physician to the need to evaluate and deal with the psychosocial aspects of the case. I have seen cases in which a relapse appeared to be related to the lack of resolution of the psychosocial problems of the child in the family. It is my impression that the disorder would in many cases subside in a few weeks to several months if such a comprehensive approach is adopted. In some cases, the choreiform movements actually subside but conversion symptoms continue; they resemble somewhat the original symptoms. Conversion symptoms of a motor nature may also be admixed with the choreiform movements in the course of the illness. Intensive psychotherapy may be needed if conversion symptoms continue.

Infectious Mononucleosis. Infectious mononucleosis is a viral disorder that affects adolescents and college students in particular. It is said to be common among medical students. It often appears during periods of especially fatiguing work or long-continued emotional stress, and so psychophysiologic factors may act as contributory or precipitating forces through a shift in immunochemical mechanisms that is not yet understood. Besides the characteristic pharyngitis and lymphadenitis, fatigability is common. The spleen is enlarged, but hepatitis is a rare complication.

Bed rest had ordinarily been prescribed until the fever has disappeared and the laboratory values have returned to normal. With such an approach, slight fever and marked fatigability have often continued for weeks and sometimes months, and relapses have not been uncommon. I think that bed rest has been overused. Immobilizing an active young person, who may have been somewhat depressed as well as exhausted when the illness began, may help cause further listlessness and depression and may intensify or perpetuate the feelings of exhaustion and a continuing mild fever of psychophysiologic origin. Some college physicians have the impression that infectious mononucleosis is ordinarily a self-limited condition, lasting at most a few weeks, and many college physicians now tell patients to gear their activity to their levels of personal comfort. They caution the patients against contact sports only as long as the spleen is enlarged. If hepatitis occurs, bed rest is indicated.[72]

Other chronic disorders that involve the central nervous system have been discussed elsewhere. They include idiopathic epilepsy, narcolepsy, chronic brain syndromes, and meningomyelocele.

Familial Dysautonomia. Familial dysautonomia (Riley-Day syndrome) is a disorder that has complex symptoms referable to the central nervous system. Disturbed functioning of the autonomic nervous system, with episodes of vomiting and hypertension, and sensory defects, involving pain and problems in proprioception, taste, and temperature, are characteristic. Emotional lability, limited frustration tolerance, and temper outbursts are common.[155] Such children generally do poorly in school, and many are thought to be mentally retarded. Hereditary factors are involved; familial dysautonomia often occurs in Jewish children.

As Freedman and his colleagues[57] demonstrated, the picture seems to be at least partly the result of the interplay between the affected child, his family, and his environment. The parents' feelings of frustration, helplessness, anger and guilt may reinforce the child's feelings of inadequacy and guilt, with the resultant conflicts intensifying the autonomic instability. Testing in the study of Freedman and his colleagues and in other studies[161] led to the conclusion that the children were not grossly retarded in their overall intellectual capacity but that motor problems interfered with their performance. Much supportive work must be done with the parents and the child. Placing the child in a residential treatment center has helped in several cases.

Adolescents who have spinal cord injuries[131] are intensely concerned with fears of total sexual dysfunction, sometimes more so than with fears of being unable to walk or to work. But if an interdisciplinary rehabilitative approach is taken, most patients are able to achieve some degree of sexual functioning.

Disorders of the Organs of Special Sense

Blindness. A person whose vision is less than 20/200 after correction is usually considered blind from the point of view of education. Partially sighted persons are those whose vision is 20/70 to 20/200 after correction. Marked defects in visual fields may be equally handicapping. Estimates of the number of blind children in the United States vary. About 0.3 children per 1000 are said to be blind. The incidence was a little higher (0.37 per 1000) during the early 1950s

as a result of the number of children who had retrolental fibroplasia. Approximately 2 children per 1000 are partially sighted (about 100,000). Most are blind at birth, and most of the rest become blind during their first year of life, as the result of infectious disease, trauma, neoplasms, or other causes. The rate is higher in boys than in girls.[139,140]

Special tests are needed to measure the intelligence of blind children. The tests available are oral, touch, or Braille in nature; some are of questionable validity. Apparently there is no difference in learning ability between blind children and seeing children who are equal in intelligence. However, the average I.Q. of blind children is slightly (about 10 points) below that of seeing children, partly because of the problems in rearing a blind child toward independence and in teaching him and partly because a greater number of blind children are also brain injured and/or deaf, particularly blind children who have retrolental fibroplasia.

Blind children develop some skills later than do normal children although they develop them in an orderly sequence. Speech usually develops later, and speech defects are common.[55] Developmental lags in motor and other capacities are also common.[42,53] Some children who have a number of lags or great unevenness in development are pseudo-retarded,[75] sometimes as a result of insufficient sensory or emotional stimulation. Blind children require more time in school to cover the same amount of work. Those who became blind before the late preschool-age period have difficulty in forming visual images of objects or of themselves. Some blind people are said to dream in color. Although blind people do necessarily cultivate their senses of touch, hearing, smell, and taste, they are not innately equipped with these capacities to a greater degree than are seeing people.[30]

"Blindisms" are almost universal. They include rubbing the eyes, shaking or rolling the body, poking at the eyes and ears, flapping the hands, or, if the child has partial vision, fanning the fingers in front of the eyes. Blindisms seem to be attempts at self-stimulation or to use primitive rhythmic movements for gratification.[26] But since they may be intensified by anxiety, they may be mistaken for signs of early infantile autism.[76] A few blind children do show a type of psychotic disorder in early childhood that resembles autism.[93a] It is sometimes admixed with brain damage or mental retardation, and it is often associated with emotional deprivation. These children can be treated effectively in a therapeutic nursery school, with concomitant play therapy for the child and therapy for the parents. The earlier the intervention, the better the results.[42,54]

Many otherwise normal blind children are overly sensitive and overly dependent. A few may be angry and demanding. Their adjustment depends on their parents' ability to accept the defect, to use speech and touch effectively to stimulate and teach them about the world, and to provide appropriate social contacts. (Fraiberg[54] has provided a particularly helpful program of assistance for parents in these areas.) Nursery school programs can be most valuable to parents and child. There are some special programs, but most blind children can attend programs with seeing children. Observation of the child in a nursery setting can help the physician evaluate the child's capacities.

Although nearly 50% of the blind children in the United States are educated in special schools, the trend is toward their attending Braille classes in the same day schools as normal children.[152] This mainstreaming approach seems to offer the child important emotional benefits, from home care to social contact with nonhandicapped persons. Over 50% of the blind people in the United States are self-supporting or better, and only 20% are completely dependent. With better emotional prepara-

tion and vocational training, many in the latter group could be independent. Some blind people will always need sheltered workshops, but blind children should not be reared in the largely custodial institutions still found in some communities. Special units may be needed for psychotic blind children. Most state hospitals will not accept such children although they could handle them if trained teachers were available.

Two blind parents often have difficulty in rearing their seeing children, but some are able to do so remarkably well.

Although specialists and special programs play important parts in the education of the blind child and in working with his parents, the physician or health associate can be of help to them in evaluating the child's capacities and, through pediatric counseling, in preventing pseudo-retardation and other problems.

Hearing Defects. The term hearing defect refers to (1) total deafness, (2) a hearing impairment that makes aural communication unfeasible, and (3) partial deafness, in which hearing is defective but functional, with or without a hearing aid. The human range of hearing is from about 20 to 20,000 cycles per second. Hearing losses are computed by the decibel loss in the speech range. A hearing loss in the range of 15 to 30 decibels is considered mild; 31 to 50, moderate; 51 to 80, severe; and 81 to 100, profound. A low-tone loss is the most common defect found in both sexes. High-tone deafness is more common in boys than in girls. Hearing deficits are now classified as sensorineural (if the auditory nerve or cochlear cells are damaged); conductive (resulting from blocked sound transmission from the external auditory canals to the inner ear); and mixed.

In the United States, the actual prevalence of deafness is 1.2 to 1.4 per 1000 children, and 2% to 3% of all school children have a significant degree of hearing loss.[136] In about 50% of these cases, the cause of the child's hearing loss is unknown. In most of the other cases, deafness occurred as a result of prenatal factors (e.g., rubella), perinatal factors (e.g., kernicterus in premature infants), or postnatal factors (e.g., infections). (Deafness from otitis media now occurs rarely.) The administration of streptomycin to a pregnant woman may cause deafness in her child.[178]

Audiometric techniques of measuring hearing acuity for sounds of varying pitch and loudness are, of course, more accurate than ordinary clinical methods (involving the use of whispered words, hand clapping, the sound of a watch, rattle, or bell, or watching for a turn of the head or a pupillary reflex in response to the use of a tuning fork). Children under 5 years of age, can only occasionally participate in audiometric testing to the extent necessary. But newer tests involving a conditioned psychogalvanic skin response, the use of standardized HEARometer amplifiers, and a technique based on EEG-evoked responses seem of value in testing the hearing of young children and even infants. But careful history taking and evaluation of the child's development may be of even more help in the early diagnosis of a hearing impairment. From the time he is 5 to 6 months old, the infant should move his eyes in the direction of sound. Quietness, failure to begin to laugh and vocalize, monotonal vocalization, or failure to imitate the mother's sounds may be important signs that a hearing problem exists.

The Moro reflex in response to the sound of a wooden clacker will establish gross hearing ability within a few hours after birth. Newborn infants respond most keenly to higher tones in the mother's voice. Children who have severe mental retardation or emotional disturbance, particularly early childhood psychosis, may fail to respond normally to sound. Psychotic children who have normal hearing may show abnormal evoked auditory potentials on the EEG, possibly because they shut out ("tune out") the stimulus.

A defect involving the loss of less than 66% of hearing capacity, properly treated, will not significantly interfere with a child's ability to learn in school.[136] However, deaf children score slightly lower on I.Q. tests than do hearing children, even on specially adapted tests. This phenomenon may be related to a child's difficulties in language development, lack of stimulation, or, in certain cases, to brain damage associated with the cause of the deafness. No significant differences in intellectual capacities exist between children who have congenital deafness and those who have acquired hearing defects. Speech development is slower, but it follows the same sequence as in hearing children. With the use of oral methods (lip reading and speech), most deaf children can be taught to speak.[134] Even in children taught to communicate by manual methods, there is no ultimate interference with mental development; although language is important in learning to think, a person's intellectual capacity is not dependent on speech. The age at which the hearing loss occurs is significant, however. Obviously, if a child was once able to hear and to recognize speech, his ability to develop language skills will be facilitated accordingly.

Deaf children learn more slowly than do hearing children. Lack of sensory experience or emotional deprivation may produce pseudo-retardation[62] in some deaf children. There is no specific psychology of the deaf although some deaf people may be overly suspicious that they are being talked about. Most personality problems of the deaf can be explained by a deficiency in experience and/or a lack of opportunity. Some deaf children are shy, anxious, or overdependent, while others exhibit oppositional and rebellious behavior. Some children may bluff or respond irrelevantly to remarks they cannot hear. Many parents find it difficult to teach a deaf child to speak. Most parents of a deaf child tend to be overattentive and overprotective. Hearing aids are useful when indicated, and, if properly fitted, may result in better hearing than a fenestration operation. Some children can use hearing aids by the time they are 2 or 3 years old, and most children can use them by school age; some infants can be fitted with hearing aids. A few children may resist using hearing aids or may use them to manipulate the parents (e.g., by turning the hearing aids off[129]). Some children in disturbed families who have mild hearing loss may exhibit pseudo-deafness.[62,95]

Speech and language training should be begun in the preschool-age years. Some school systems provide such training, and preschool programs that use speech and hearing specialists are available in speech and hearing centers and other settings. Behavior-oriented treatment methods have been said to be of help.[20] Home training has been helpful also; a correspondence course is available for parents of deaf children from the John Tracy Clinic in Los Angeles.

Special classes for the deaf are now included in the curriculums of a number of public schools, and many children who have a hearing loss can eventually move into regular classrooms. Some totally deaf children must be placed in residential schools. However, state hospitals and schools for the deaf often do not take mentally ill deaf children. Adding specialists in teaching deaf children to the staffs of state hospitals would solve that problem.[156]

If given adequate opportunities, most deaf children can learn to support themselves. Some deaf people have graduated from "hearing" colleges. Gallaudet College, in Washington, D.C., is maintained for deaf students by the federal government. Even multiply handicapped deaf adolescents and adults have been successfully rehabilitated at the Hot Springs Rehabilitation Center, in a program offering special psychologic evaluation, counseling, and vocational training. As with other handicaps, better vocational rehabilitation and job counseling are needed, and there are still too few job opportunities for people who have hearing impairments.

The pediatrician can help both the child with hearing loss and his family by being alert to the possibility of a hearing loss and by making early referral for a thorough otologic and audiologic evaluation. He can reassure the parents that most children who have a hearing loss can be taught to talk and understand speech—which is usually the parents' central anxiety—and, working with other specialists, he can be of supportive help through pediatric counseling throughout the child's development.

Other chronic disorders, which cannot be considered in relation to a single organ system, are discussed elsewhere in the book. These include mental illness, mental retardation, some inborn errors of metabolism, and sex chromosome abnormalities.

Bibliography

1. Adler, A.: *The Neurotic Constitution: Outlines of a Comparative Individualistic Psychology and Psychotherapy.* New York, Dodd Mead, 1926.
2. Agle, D.P.: Psychiatric studies of patients with hemophilia and related states. Arch. Intern. Med., *114*:76, 1964.
3. Akerren, Y., and Lindgren, M.: Investigation concerning early rising in acute hemorrhagic nephritis. Acta Med. Scand., *151*:419, 1955.
4. Allen, J.E., and Lelchuk, L.: A Comprehensive Care Program for Children with Handicaps. Am. J. Dis. Child., *111*:229, 1966.
5. American Academy of Pediatrics, Committee on Drugs: Counselling and synthetic steroids in short stature without organic disease. Pediatrics, *53*:285, 1974.
6. Ames, M.D.: Proposals for a department of rehabilitation for children. Pediatrics, *36*:277, 1964.
7. Andersen, D.H.: Cystic fibrosis and family stress. Children, *7*:9, 1960.
8. Apley, J., et al.: Impact of congenital heart disease on the family. Br. Med. J., *1*:29, 1964.
9. Azarnoff, P., and Flagel, S.: *A Pediatric Play Program.* Springfield, Ill., Thomas, 1974.
10. Barker, R.O., et al.: *Adjustment to Physical Handicap and Illness: A Survey of the Social Psychology of Physique and Disability.* New York, Social Science Research Council, Bulletin No. 55, 1953.
11. Bass, H.H., and Schulman, J.L.: Quantitative assessment of children's activity in and out of bed. Am. J. Dis. Child., *113*:242, 1967.
12. Battle, C.U.: The role of the pediatrician as om-

budsman in the health care of the young handicapped child. Pediatrics, 50:916, 1972.

13. Bayrakal, S.: A group experience with chronically disabled adolescents. Am. J. Psychiatry, 132:1291, 1975.

14. Beecher, H.H.: The powerful placebo. JAMA, 159:1602, 1955.

15. Beecher, H.K.: The measurement of pain in man: A re-inspection. Work of the Harvard group. In: Pain. (A. Soulairac, J. Cahn, and J. Charpentier, Eds.). New York, Academic Press, 1968.

16. Bergmann, T.: Observation of children's reactions to motor restraint. Nerv. Child, 4:318, 1945.

17. Blakeslee, B.: The Limb Deficient Child. Berkeley, Calif.: University of California Press, 1963.

18. Blank, H., and Brody, M.W.: Recurrent herpes simplex: A psychiatric and laboratory study. Psychosom. Med., 12:254, 1950.

19. Blos, P., Jr., and Finch, S.M.: Sexuality and the handicapped adolescent. In: The Child with Disabling Illness. (J.A. Downey and N.L. Low, Eds.). Philadelphia, Saunders, 1974.

20. Bolton, B.: A behavior-oriented treatment program for deaf clients in a comprehensive rehabilitation center. Am. J. Orthopsychiatry, 44:376, 1974.

21. Booth, G.: Psychodynamics in parkinsonism. Psychosom. Med., 10:1, 1948.

22. Bowden, D.M., and Rothenberg, M.B.: Comprehensive care of a mentally retarded adolescent hemophiliac with a tongue-biting tic. Pediatrics, 43:19, 1969.

23. Bradely, J.J.: Severe localized pain associated with the depressive syndrome. Br. J. Psychiatry, 109:741, 1963.

24. Browne, W.J., Mally, M.A., and Kane, R.P.: Psychosocial aspects of hemophilia: Study of 28 hemophiliac children and their families. Am. J. Orthopsychiatry, 30:730, 1960.

25. Browse, N.L.: The Physiology and Pathology of Bed Rest. Springfield, Ill., Thomas, 1965.

26. Burlingham, D.: Some problems of ego development in blind children. Psychoanal. Study Child, 20:194, 1965.

27. Calden, G., et al.: Psychosomatic factors in the rate of recovery from tuberculosis. Psychosom. Med., 22:345, 1960.

28. Cassell, W.A.: Body perception and symptom localization. Psychosom. Med., 27:71, 1965.

29. Cath, S.H., Glud, E., and Blane, H.T.: The role of the body-image in psychotherapy with the physically handicapped. Psychoanal. Rev., 14:34, 1970.

30. Code, N.J., and Taboroff, L.H.: The psychological problems of the congenitally blind child. Am. J. Orthopsychiatry, 25:627, 1956.

31. Chazan, M., et al.: The intellectual and emotional development of children with congenital heart disease. Guys Hosp. Rep., 100:331, 1951.

32. Chess, S., Korn, S.J., and Fernandez, P.B.: Psychiatric Disorders of Children with Congenital Rubella. New York, Brunner/Mazel, 1971.

33. Cleeland, C.S.: Conditioning and the dystonias. In: New Applications of Conditioning to Medical Practice. University of Wisconsin Press, 1972.

34. Collins, L.G.: Pain sensitivity and ratings of childhood experience. Percept. Mot. Skills, 21:349, 1964.

35. Critchley, M.: Congenital indifference to pain. Ann. Intern. Med., 45:737, 1956.

36. Crothers, B., and Meyer, E.: The psychologic and psychiatric implications of poliomyelitis. J. Pediatr., 28:324, 1946.

37. Crothers, B., and Paine, R.S.: The Natural History of Cerebral Palsy. Cambridge, Harvard University Press, 1959.

38. Day, H.: Setting small goals: An effective way of providing nursing care for children. Hosp. Community Psychiatry, 23:126, 1972.

39. Devine, R., and Mersky, H.: The description of pain in psychiatric and general medical patients. J. Psychosom. Res., 9:311, 1965.

40. Dubos, S.: Psychiatric study of children with pulmonary tuberculosis. Am. J. Orthopsychiatry, 20:520, 1950.

41. Duckett, C.L.: Caring for children with sickle cell anemia. Children, 18:227, 1971.

42. Elonen, A.S., and Cain, A.C.: Diagnostic evaluation and treatment of deviant blind children. Am. J. Orthopsychiatry, 34:625, 1964.

43. Engel, G.L.: Primary atypical facial neuralgia. Psychosom. Med., 13:375, 1951.

44. Engel, G.L.: Psychogenic pain and the pain-prone patient. Am. J. Med., 26:899, 1959.

45. Engel, G.L.: Guilt, pain, and success. Psychosom. Med., 24:37, 1962.

46. Engel, G.L., Reichsman, F., and Segal, H.L.: A study of an infant with a gastric fistula. I. Behavior and rate of total hydrochloric acid secretion. Psychosom. Med., 18:374, 1956.

47. Feinberg, T., et al.: Questions that worry children with exstrophy. Pediatrics, 53:242, 1974.

48. Fineman, A.D.: Ego development in boys with a congenital defect in the genitourinary system. J. Am. Acad. Child Psychiatry, 2:636, 1963.

49. Fisher, S.: Body image and psychopathology. Arch. Gen. Psychiatry, 10:519, 1964.

50. Fisher, S.: Sex differences in body perception. Psychol. Monogr., 78:1, 1964.

51. Fisher, S.: Organ awareness and organ activation. Psychosom. Med., 29:643, 1967.

52. Ford, F.R., and Wilkins, L.: Congenital universal indifference to pain. Bull. Johns Hopkins Hosp., 62:448, 1938.

53. Fraiberg, S.: Parallel and divergent patterns in blind and sighted infants. Psychoanal. Study Child, 23:764, 1968.

54. Fraiberg, S.: Intervention in infancy: A program for blind infants. J. Am. Acad. Child Psychiatry, 10:381, 1971.

55. Fraiberg, S., and Freedman, D.A.: Studies in the ego development of the congenitally blind child. Psychoanal. Study Child., 19:113, 1964.

56. Freeman, J.M., Aron, A.M., and Collard, J.E.: The emotional correlates of Sydenham's chorea. Pediatrics, 35:42, 1965.

57. Freedman, A.M., et al.: Psychological aspects of familial dysautonomia. Am. J. Orthopsychiatry, 27:96, 1957.

58. Freedman, D.A., et al.: A multi-handicapped ru-

bella baby: The first 18 months. J. Am. Acad. Child Psychiatry, 9:298, 1970.

59. Garrard, S.D., and Richmond, J.B.: Psychological aspects of the management of chronic diseases and handicapping conditions of childhood. In: *The Psychological Basis of Medical Practice.* (H.I. Lief, K.F. Lief, and A.R. Lief, Eds.). New York, Harper & Row, 1963.

60. Gayton, W.F., and Friedman, S.: Psychosocial aspects of cystic fibrosis. Am. J. Dis. Child., 126:856, 1973.

61. Gayton, W.F., et al.: Children with cystic fibrosis. I. Psychological test findings of patients, siblings, and parents. Pediatrics, 59:888, 1977.

62. Gelinier-Ortigues, M., and Aubry, J.: Maternal deprivation, psychogenic deafness, and pseudo-retardation. In: *Emotional Problems of Early Childhood.* (G. Caplan, Ed.). New York: Basic Books, 1955.

63. Gellert, E.: Children's conceptions of the content and functions of the human body. Genet. Psychol. Monogr., 65:293, 1962.

64. Gellis, S.S.: Prospects for patient care of birth defects. In: *Congenital Malformations.* (F.C. Fraser, and V.A. McKusick, Eds.). Amsterdam, Excerpta Medica, 1970.

64a. Gibson, J.P.: How much rest is necessary for children with fever? J. Pediatr., 49:256, 1956.

65. Gibson, R.M.: Trauma in early infancy and later personality development. Psychosom. Med., 27:229, 1965.

66. Glaser, H.H., et al.: Comprehensive medical care for handicapped children. Am. J. Dis. Child., 102:344, 1961.

67. Glaser, H.H., Harrison, G.S., and Lynn, D.B.: Emotional implications of congenital heart disease in children. Pediatrics, 33:367, 1964.

68. Glaser, H.H., Lynn, D.B., and Harrison, G.S.: Comprehensive medical care for handicapped children. I. Patterns of anxiety in mothers of children with rheumatic fever. Am. J. Dis. Child, 102:344, 1961.

69. Goldy, F.B., and Katz, A.H.: Social adaptation in hemophilia. Children, 10:189, 1963.

70. Green, M.: The management of children with chronic disease. Proc. Inst. Med. Chic., 31:51, 1976.

71. Green, M., and Levitt, E.E.: Constriction of body image in children with congenital heart disease. Pediatrics, 29:438, 1962.

72. Greenfield, N.S., et al.: Ego strength and length of recovery from infectious mononucleosis. J. Nerv. Ment. Dis., 128:125, 1959.

73. Grossman, G.J.: Early ambulation in the treatment of acute rheumatic fever. Am. J. Dis. Child., 115:557, 1968.

74. Gurney,, W.: Congenital Amputee. In: *Ambulatory Pediatrics.* (M. Green, and R.J. Haggerty, Eds.). Philadelphia, Saunders, 1968.

75. Hallenbeck, J.: Pseudo-retardation in retrolental fibroplasia. N. Outlook Blind, 48:301, 1954.

76. Hallenbeck, J.: Two essential factors in the development of young blind children. N. Outlook Blind, 48:308, 1954.

77. Hamilton, M.: Factors influencing excretion of calcium. Am. J. Dis. Child., 36:450, 1928.

78. Hampson, J.G., and Money, J.: Idiopathic sexual precocity in the female. Psychosom. Med., 17:16, 1955.

79. Hare, E.H.: Spina bifida cystica and family stress. Br. Med. J., 2:727, 1966.

80. Harris, H.J.: Fungus infection of feet. A case report illustrating a psychosomatic problem. Psychosom. Med., 6:336, 1944.

81. Harris, H.J.: *Brucellosis: Clinical and Subclinical.* New York, Hoeber, 1950.

82. Harrison, T.R.: Abuse of rest as a therapeutic measure for patients with cardiovascular disease. JAMA, 125:1075, 1944.

83. Hawkins, N.G., Davies, R., and Holmes, T.H.: Evidence of psychosocial factors in the development of pulmonary tuberculosis. Am. Rev. Tuberc. Pulmon. Dis., 75:5, 1957.

84. Herman, M.N., and Sandock, B.A.: Conversion symptoms in a case of multiple sclerosis. Milit. Med., 132:816, 1967.

85. Holder, R., Brazelton, T.B., and Talbot, B.: Emotional aspects of rheumatic fever in children. J. Pediatr., 43:339, 1953.

85a. Holmes, T.H., et al.: Psychosocial and psychophysiologic studies of tuberculosis. Psychosom. Med., 19:134, 1957.

86. Holmes, T.H., et al.: *The Nose: An Experimental Study of Reactions Within the Nose in Human Subjects During Varying Life Experiences.* Springfield, Ill., Thomas, 1949.

87. Illingworth, R.S.: Why put him to bed? Clin. Pediatr., 2:108, 1963.

88. Illingworth, R.S.: Indications for bed rest. In: *Ambulatory Pediatrics.* (N. Green, and R.J. Haggerty, Eds.). Philadelphia, Saunders, 1968.

89. Johnson, F.A.: Figure drawings in subjects recovering from poliomyelitis. Psychosom. Med., 34:19, 1972.

90. Josselyn, I.M.: Emotional implications of rheumatic heart disease in children. Am. J. Orthopsychiatry, 25:109, 1955.

91. Kanner, L.: The invalid reaction in children. J. Pediatr., 11:341, 1937.

92. Katz, A.H.: Social adaptation in chronic illness: A study of hemophilia. Am. J. Public Health, 53:1666, 1963.

93. Keeler, W.R., and Bender, L.: A follow-up study of children with behavior disorder and Sydenham's chorea. Am. J. Psychiatry, 109:421, 1952.

93a. Keeler, W.R.: Autistic patterns and defective communication in blind children with retrolental fibroplasia. In: *Psychopathology of Communication.* (P. Hoch, and J. Zubin, Eds.). New York, Grune & Stratton, 1958.

94. Kennell, J.H., et al.: What parents of rheumatic fever patients don't understand about the disease and its prophylactic management. Pediatrics, 43:160, 1969.

95. Knapp, P.H.: Emotional aspects of hearing loss. Psychosom. Med., 10:203, 1948.

96. Korsch, B., Fraad, L., and Barnett, H.L.: Pediatric discussions with parent groups. J. Pediatr., 44:703, 1954.

97. Kraft, J.A.: A psychiatric study of two patients with dystonia musculorum deformans. South. Med. J., *59*:284, 1966.

98. Krims, M.B.: Psychiatric observations on children with precocious physical development. J. Am. Acad. Child Psychiatry, *1*:397, 1962.

99. Krims, M.B.: Observations on children who suffer from dwarfism. Psychiatr. Q., *42*:430, 1968.

100. LaBaw, W.L.: Regular use of suggestibility by pediatric bleeders. Haematologia, *4*:419, 1970.

101. LaBaw, W.L.: Auto-hypnosis in hemophilia. Haematologia, *9*:103, 1975.

102. Landtman, B., and Valanne, E.: Psychosomatic studies of children with congenital heart disease. Acta Paediatr., (Suppl.) *48*:146, 1959.

103. Lendrum, B.L., Simon, A.J., and Mack, I.: Relation of duration of bed rest in acute rheumatic fever to heart disease present 2 to 14 years later. Pediatrics, *24*:389, 1959.

104. Lesse, S.: Atypical facial pain syndromes of psychogenic origin: Complications of their misdiagnosis. J. Nerv. Ment. Dis., *124*:346, 1956.

105. Lewin, K.K.: Role of depression in the production of illness in pernicious anemia. Psychosom. Med., *21*:23, 1959.

106. Lewis, C.: Symposium: Does comprehensive care make a difference: What is the evidence? Am. J. Dis. Child., *122*:469, 1971.

107. Lewis, M.: Mental health and illness in chronic non-life threatening disorders. Unpublished material.

108. Linde, L.M., et al.: Attitudinal factors in congenital heart disease. Pediatrics, *38*:92, 1966.

109. Linde, L.M., et al.: Mental development in congenital heart disease. J. Pediatr., *71*:198, 1967.

110. Lis, E., et al.: Cleft lip and cleft palate: Perspectives in management. Pediatr. Clin. North Am., *3*:995, 1956.

111. Luzzatti, L., and Dittman, B.: Group discussions with parents of ill children. Pediatrics, *13*:269, 1954.

112. Lynn, D.B., Glaser, H.H., and Harrison, G.S.: Comprehensive medical care for handicapped children. III. Concepts of illness in children with rheumatic fever. Am. J. Dis. Child., *103*:120, 1962.

113. MacGreagor, F.C., et al.: *Facial Deformities and Plastic Surgery: A Psycho-social Study.* Springfield, Ill., Thomas, 1955.

114. Maginnis, E.: When a child has polio. Children, *15*:166, 1951.

115. Markey, O.B.: Emotional factors in chorea. Ohio Med. J., *32*:36, 1936.

116. Mattsson, A.: Long-term physical illness in childhood: A challenge to psychosocial adaptation. Pediatrics, *50*:801, 1972.

117. Mattsson, A., and Agle, D.: Group therapy with parents of hemophiliacs: Therapeutic process and observations on parental adaptation to chronic illness in children. J. Am. Acad. Child Psychiatry, *11*:558, 1972.

118. Mattsson, A., and Gross, S.: Adaptational and defensive behavior in young hemophiliacs and their parents. Am. J. Psychiatry, *122*:1349, 1966.

119. Mattsson, A., and Gross, S.: Social and behavioral studies on hemophiliac children and their families. J. Pediatr., *68*:952, 1968.

120. Mattsson, A., Gross, S., and Hall, T.V.: Psychoendocrine study of adaptation in young hemophiliacs. Psychosom. Med., *33*:215, 1971.

121. Mattson, A., discussion of Reite, M., et al.: Osteogenesis imperfecta: Psychological function. Am. J. Psychiatr., *128*:1545, 1972.

122. McClary, H.R., et al.: Observations on the role of the mechanism of depression in some patients with disseminated lupus erythematosus. Psychosom. Med., *17*:311, 1955.

123. McCollum, A.T., and Gibson, L.E.: Family adaptation to the child with cystic fibrosis. J. Pediatr., *77*:571, 1970.

124. McCrory, W.W., Fleisher, D., and Sohn, W.B.: The course of acute nephritis in children allowed early resumption of normal activity. Am. J. Dis. Child., *96*:576, 1958.

125. McGregor, F.C.: *Transformation and Identity: The Face and Plastic Surgery.* New York, Quadrangle (New York Times Book Co.), 1974.

126. Mead, S.: Century of abuse of rest. JAMA, *182*:344, 1962.

127. Mei-Tal, V., Meyerowitz, S., and Engel, G.L.: The role of psychological processes in somatic disorder: Multiple sclerosis. I. The emotional setting of illness onset and exacerbation. Psychosom. Med., *32*:67, 1970.

128. Menser, M.A., Dods, L., and Harley, J.D.: A twenty-five year follow-up of congenital rubella. Lancet, *2*:1347, 1967.

129. Miller, A.A., et al.: Psychological factors in adaptation to hearing aids. Am. J. Orthopsychiatry, *29*:121, 1959.

130. Milliken, S.: Group discussions with parents of handicapped children from the health education standpoint. Am. J. Public Health, *43*:960, 1953.

131. Molnar, G.E., and Taft, L.: Pediatric rehabilitation. I. Cerebral palsy and spinal cord injuries. Curr. Probl. Pediatr., *7*:114, 1977.

132. Money, J., and Hampson, J.G.: Idiopathic sexual precocity in the male. Psychosom. Med., *17*:1, 1955.

133. Money, J., and Pollitt, E.: Studies in the psychology of dwarfism. II. Personality maturation and response to growth hormone treatment in hypopituitary dwarfs. J. Pediatr., *68*:381, 1966.

134. Morkovin, B.V.: *Through the Barriers of Deafness and Isolation: Oral Communication of the Hearing-Impaired Child in Life Situations.* New York, Macmillan, 1960.

135. Myers, B.A., Friedman, S.B., and Weiner, J.B.: Coping with a chronic disability: Psychosocial observations of girls with scoliosis treated with the Milwaukee brace. Am. J. Dis. Child., *120*:175, 1970.

136. Myklebust, H.R., Ed.: *The Psychology of Deafness.* New York, Grune & Stratton, 1960.

137. Nadas, A.S.: *Pediatric Cardiology.* Philadelpha, Saunders, 1957.

138. Nelhaus, G.: Neurologic and muscular disorders. In: *Current Pediatric Diagnosis and Treatment* (C.H. Kempe, H.K. Silver, and D. O'Brien, Eds.). Los Altos, Calif. Lange, 1978.

139. Norris, N., Spalding, P., and Brodi, F.: *Blindness in Children*. Chicago, University of Chicago Press, 1957.

140. Parmalee, A.H., and Liverman, L.: Blindness in infants and children. In: *Ambulatory Pediatrics* (M. Green and R.J. Haggerty, Eds.). Philadelphia, Saunders, 1968.

141. Patton, R.G., and Gardner, L.I.: *Growth Failure in Maternal Deprivation*. Springfield, Ill, Thomas, 1963.

142. Perrin, J.C.S., et al.: Evaluation of a ten year experience in a comprehensive care program for handicapped children. Pediatrics, 50:793, 1972.

143. Philippopoulos, G.S., Wittkower, E.D., and Cousineau, A.: The etiologic significance of emotional factors in onset and exacerbations of multiple sclerosis. Psychosom. Med., 20:458, 1958.

144. Planck, E.N.: *Working with Children in Hospitals*. 2nd Ed. Cleveland, Case Western Reserve University Press, 1975.

145. Poznanski, E.: Childhood depression: Clinical characteristics of overly depressed children. Arch. Gen. Psychiatry, 23:8, 1970.

146. Prugh, D.G.: Unpublished material.

147. Prugh, D.G.: Toward an understanding of psychosomatic concepts in relation to illness in children. In: *Modern Perspectives in Child Development* (A.J. Solnit, and S.A. Provence, Eds.). New York, International Universities Press, 1963.

148. Prugh, D.G., et al.: A clinical study of delirium in children and adolescents. Psychosom. Med., 42:177, 1980.

149. Prugh, D.G., Straub, E., et al.: A study of the emotional reactions of children and families to hospitalization and illness. Am. J. Orthopsychiatry, 23:70, 1953.

150. Prugh, D.G., and Tagiuri, C.K.: Emotional aspects of the respirator care of patients with poliomyelitis. Psychosom. Med., 16:104, 1954.

151. Ratnoff, O.D.: Classic hemophilia. In: *Bleeding Syndromes: Clinical Manual*. Springfield, Ill., Thomas, 1960.

152. Reed, H.: The school child and defective vision. Pediatr. Clin. North Am., 12:885, 1965.

153. Reite, M., et al.: Osteogenesis imperfecta: Psychological function. Am. J. Psychiatry, 128:1540, 1972.

154. Rie, H.E., and Boverman, H.: Tutoring and ventilation: A pilot study of reactions of hospitalized children. Clin. Pediatr., 3:581, 1964.

155. Riley, C.M.: Familial dysautonomia. Adv. Pediatr., 9:157, 1957.

156. Robinson, L.D.: Treatment and rehabilitation of the mentally ill deaf. J. Rehabil. Deaf, 4:44, 1971.

156a.Robinson, M., Finesinger, J.E., and Bierman, J.S.: Psychiatric considerations in the adjustment of patients with poliomyelitis. N. Engl. J. Med., 254:975, 1956.

157. Rome, H.P., Braceland, F.J.: The psychological response to ACTH, cortisone, hydro-cortisone, and related steroid substances. Am. J. Psychiatry, 108:641, 1952.

158. Roskies, E.: *Abnormality and Normality: The Mothering of Thalidomide Children*. Ithaca, N.Y., Cornell University Press, 1972.

159. Rotnem, D., et al.: Personality development in children with growth hormone deficiency. J. Am. Acad. Child. Psychiatry, 16:412, 1977.

160. Ruess, A.L.: A comparative study of cleft palate children and their siblings. J. Clin. Psychol., 21:354, 1965.

161. Sak, H.G., Smith, A.A., and Dancies, J.: Psychosometric evaluation of children with familial dysautonomia. Am. J. Psychiatry, 124:136, 1967.

162. Scherzer, A.L., and Gardner, G.G.: Studies of the school age child with meningomyelocele. I. Physical and intellectual development. Pediatrics, 47:424, 1971.

163. Schilder, P.: *Image and Appearance of the Human Body*. London, Kegan, Paul, Trench, and Trubner, 1935.

164. Schonfeld, W.A.: Body-image in adolescents: A psychiatric concept for the pediatrician. Pediatrics, 31:845, 1963.

165. Seidenfeld, M.A.: Psychological aspects of poliomyelitis. Pediatrics, 4:309, 1949.

166. Senn, M.J.E.: Emotional aspects of convalescence. Child, 10:24, 1945.

167. Schechter, M.D.: The orthopedically handicapped child: Emotional reactions. Arch. Gen. Psychiatry, 4:247, 1961.

168. Schwab, J.J., and Harmeling, J.D.: Body image and medical illness. Psychosom. Med., 30:51, 1968.

169. Shanfield, S.B., and Killingsworth, R.N.: The psychiatric aspects of pain. Psychiatr. Ann., 7:24, 1977.

170. Shapiro, H.K., and Struening, E.L.: The use of placebos: A study of ethics and physicians' attitudes. Psychiatry Med., 4:17, 1973.

171. Shirley, H.F.: Meeting the emotional and social needs of children with rheumatic heart disease. J. Child. Behav., 4:289, 1952.

172. Sibinga, M.S., and Friedman, C.J.: Restraint and speech. Pediatrics, 48:116, 1971.

173. Silbert, A., Wolff, P.H., and Mayer, B.: Cyanotic heart disease and psychological development. Pediatrics, 43:192, 1969.

174. Silverstein, A.B., and Robinson, H.A.: The representation of physique in children's figure drawings. J. Consult. Psychol., 25:146, 1961.

175. Solow, R.A.: Psychological aspects of muscular dystrophy. Except. Child., 32:99, 1965.

176. Spagnuolo, M., Gavrin, J., and Ryan, J.: A day hospital for children with rheumatic fever. Pediatrics, 45:276, 1970.

177. Spock, B., and Lerrigo, M.O.: *Caring for Your Disabled Child*. New York, Fawcett World Library, 1965.

178. Statloff, J.: Hearing defects in children. Pediatr. Clin. North Am., 43:679, 1957.

179. Strain, J.J.: The problem of pain. In: *Psychological Care of the Medically Ill: A Primer in Liaison Psychiatry* (J.J. Strain and S. Grossman, Eds.). New York, Appleton-Century-Crofts, 1975.

180. Strawczynski, H., et al.: Delivery of home care to hemophiliac children: Home care vs hospitalization. Pediatrics, 51:986, 1973.

181. Tips, R.L., and Lynch, H.T.: The impact of ge-

netic counselling upon the family milieu. JAMA, *184*:183, 1965.

182. Tips, R.L., et al.: *The "Whole Family" Concept in Clinical Genetics*. Birth Defects Reprint Series. New York, The National Foundation–March of Dimes, 1964.

183. Tisza, V.B., and Gumpertz, E.: The parents' reaction to the birth and early care of children with cleft palate. Pediatrics, *30*:86, 1962.

184. Tisza, V.B., et al.: Psychiatric observations of children with cleft palate. Am. J. Orthopsychiatry, *28*:416, 1958.

185. Townes, P.L.: Genetic counselling. In: *Ambulatory Pediatrics* (M. Green and R.J. Haggerty, Eds.). Philadelphia, Saunders, 1968.

186. Tropauer, A., Franz, M.N., and Dilgard, V.W.: Psychologic aspects of the care of children with cystic fibrosis. Am. J. Dis. Child., *119*:424, 1970.

187. Ulman, M.: On the psyche and warts. I. Suggestion and warts: A review and comment. Psychosom. Med., *21*:473, 1959.

188. Ulman, M., and Dudek, S.: On the psyche and warts. II. Hypnotic suggestion and warts. Psychosom. Med., *20*:68, 1960.

189. Vignos, P.J., Spencer, J.E., and Archibald, K.C.: Management of progressive muscular dystrophy of childhood. JAMA, *184*:89, 1963.

190. Walker, E.R.C.: Psychological and social aspects of Sydenham's chorea. In: *Modern Trends in Psychosomatic Medicine* (D. O'Neil, Ed.). London, Butterworth, 1955.

191. Walker, J.H., Thomas, M., and Russell, I.T.: Spina bifida and the parents. Dev. Med. Child. Neurol., *13*:462, 1971.

192. Wallerstein, R.S., and Rubin, S.: Some psychosomatic implications in dystrophia myotonica. J. Nerv. Ment. Dis., *120*:277, 1954.

193. Waston, E.J., and Johnson, A.M.: The emotional significance of acquired physical disfigurement. Am. J. Orthopsychiatry, *28*:85, 1958.

194. Werner, E.E., Bierman, J.M., and French, F.H.: *The Children of Kauai*. Honolulu, University of Hawaii Press, 1971.

195. Westlund, N., and Palumbo, A.Z.: Parental rejection of crippled children. Am. J. Orthopsychiatry, *16*:271, 1946.

196. Young, D., and Rodstein, M.: Home care of rheumatic fever patients. JAMA, *152*:987, 1953.

197. Young, R.H., and Herman, H.T.: Hysterical paralysis associated with poliomyelitis. JAMA, *147*:1132, 1951.

General References

Adams, J.F., and Lindemann, E.: Coping with long-term disability. In: *Coping and Adaptation* (G.V. Coeltho, D.A. Hamburg, and J.E. Adams, Eds.). New York, Basic Books, 1974.

Agle, D.P., et al.: Multidiscipline treatment of chronic pulmonary insufficiency. I. Psychologic aspects of rehabilitation. Psychosom. Med., *35*:41, 1973.

Anthony, E.J., and Koupernick, C., Eds.: *The Child in*

His Family: The Impact of Disease and Death. New York, Wiley, 1973.

Balint, M.: *The Doctor, the Patient, and His Illness*. 2nd Ed. London, Pitman, 1971.

Barsch, R.H.: *Parents of the Handicapped Child*. Springfield, Ill., Thomas, 1968.

Beers, N.: Helping the blind child in the hospital. Hospitals, *32*:32, 1958.

Brolley, M., and Hollender, M.H.: Psychological problems of patients with myasthenia gravis. J. Nerv. and Ment. Dis., *122*:178, 1955.

Caldwell, B., and Stedman, D. (Eds.): *Infant Education: A Guide for Helping Handicapped Children in the First Three Years*. New York, Walker, 1977.

Carter, V., and Chess, S.: Factors influencing the adaptations of organically handicapped children. Am. J. Orthopsychiatry, *25*:627, 1955.

Colman, M.D., Dougher, C.A., and Tanner, M.R.: Group therapy for physically handicapped toddlers with delayed speech and language development. J. Am. Acad. Child Psychiatry, *15*:395, 1976.

Combs, R.H.: Effects of labels on attitudes of educators toward handicapped children. Except. Child., *33*:399, 1967.

Crussi, F.G., Robertson, D.M., and Hiscox, J.L.: Pathological condition of the Lesch-Nyhan syndrome: Report of two cases. Am. J. Dis. Child., *118*:501, 1969.

Dowling, S.: Seven infants with oesophageal atresia: A developmental study. Psychoanal. Study Child, *32*:215, 1978.

Downey, J.A., and Low, N.L.: *The Child with Disabling Illness: Principles of Rehabilitation*. Philadelphia, Saunders, 1974.

Eissler, R.S., et al.: *Physical Illness and Handicap in Childhood: An Anthology of the Psychoanalytic Study of the Child*. New York, International University Press, 1974.

Findlay, I.I., et al.: Chronic disease in childhood: A study of family reactions. Br. J. Med. Educ., *3*:66, 1969.

Fisher, S., and Cleveland, S.: *Body Image and Personality*. New York, Van Nostrand, 1958.

Freedman, D.A.: Congenital and perinatal sensory deprivation: Some studies in early development. Am. J. Psychiatry, *127*:1539, 1971.

Freeman, R.D.: Emotional reactions of handicapped children. In: *Annual Progress in Child Psychiatry and Child Development* (S. Chess and A. Thomas, Eds.). New York, Brunner/Mazel, 1968.

Freud, A.: The role of bodily illness in the mental life of children. Psychoanal. Study Child, *7*:69, 1952.

Gardner, L.I.: *Endocrine and Genetic Diseases of Childhood*. Philadelphia, Saunders, 1969.

Gerver, J.M., and Day, R.: Intelligence quotients of children who have recovered from erythroblastosis foetalis. J. Pediatr., *36*:342, 1950.

Goldie, L.: The psychiatry of the handicapped family. Dev. Med. Child Neurol., *8*:456, 1966.

Green, M., and Solnit, A.J.: Reactions to threatened loss of a child: A vulnerable child syndrome. Pediatric management of the dying child. III. Pediatrics, *34*:58, 1964

Green, M.: Care of the child with a long-term life-threatening illness: Some principles of management. Pediatrics, *39*:441, 1967.

Green, M.: The management of long-term non-life-threatening illness. In: *Ambulatory Pediatrics* (M. Green, and R.J. Haggerty, Eds.). Philadelphia, Saunders, 1968.

Hayden, P.W., Shurtleff, D.B., and Broy, A.B.: Custody of the myelodysplastic child: Implications for selection for early treatment. Pediatrics, *53*:253, 1974.

Holdaway, D.: Educating the handicapped child and his parents. Clin. Pediatr., *11*:63, 1972.

Houpt, J.L., Gould, B.S., and Norris, F.H.,Jr.: Psychological characteristics with amyotrophic lateral sclerosis. Psychosom. Med., *39*:299, 1977.

Jennings, C.D., and Whittaker, C.K.: Pediatric strokes. Mo. Med., *64*:483, 1967.

Johnson, F.A.: Figure drawings in subjects recovering from poliomyelitis. Psychosom. Med., *34*:19, 1972.

Jordan, T.E.: Research on the handicapped child and the family. Merrill-Palmer Q., *8*:243, 1962.

Kessler, J.W.: Parenting the handicapped child. Pediatr. Ann., *6*:654, 1977.

Kimmel, J.: A comparison of children with congenital and acquired orthopedic handicaps on certain personality characteristics. Dissert. Abstr., *19*:3023, 1959.

Kivowitz, J., and Keirn, W.: A genetics counselling clinic in a mental health setting. Hosp. Community Psychiatry, *24*:156, 1973.

Korsch, B.: Psychological principles in pediatric practice: The pediatrician and the sick child. Adv. Pediatr., *10*:321, 1958.

Korsch, B., and Barnett, H.L.: The physician, the family, and the child with nephrosis. J. Pediatr., *58*:707, 1961.

Langford, W.S.: Physical illness and convalescence: Their meaning to the child. J. Pediatr., *33*:242, 1948.

Lasagna, L., et al.: A study of the placebo response. Am. J. Med., *16*:771, 1954.

Lesser, A.: *Emotional Problems Associated with Handicapping Conditions in Children*. Department of Health, Education, and Welfare, Washington, Government Printing Office, 1952.

Little, S.: Psychology of physical illness in adolescents. Pediatr. Clin. North Am., *7*:85, 1960.

Linder, R.: Mothers of disabled children—the value of weekly group meetings. Dev. Med. Child Neurol., *12*:202, 1970.

Lowenfield, B.: *Our Blind Children*. Springfield, Ill., Thomas, 1956.

Martmer, E.E.: *The Child with a Handicap: A Team Approach to His Care and Guidance*. Springfield, Ill., Thomas, 1959.

Mattsson, A., and Gross, S.: Social and behavioral studies on hemophilic children and their families. J. Pediatr., *68*:952, 1966.

McMichael, J.K.: *Handicap: A Study of Physically Handicapped Children and Their Families*. Pittsburgh, University of Pittsburgh Press, 1977.

Merskey, H., and Spear, F.G.: *Pain—Psychological and Psychiatric Aspects*. London, Bailliere Tindall, 1967.

Meyer, E.: Acute psychological disturbances in the course of hospitalization: patients with chronic illness. J. Chron. Ill., *3*:111, 1956.

Meyerson, L.: Somatopsychology of physical disability. In: *Psychology of Exceptional Children and Youth* (W.M. Cruickshank, Ed.). Englewood Cliffs, N.J., Prentice-Hall, 1955.

Minde, K.K., et al.: How they grow up: 41 physically handicapped children and their families. Am. J. Psychiatry, *128*:1554, 1972.

Money, J.: Questions and answers in counselling. Rehabil. Lit., *28*:134, 1967.

Money, J.: Psychologic counselling: Hermaphroditism, endocrine, and genetic diseases in childhood. In: *Endocrine and Genetic Disease of Childhood* (L. Gardner, Ed.). Philadelphia, Saunders, 1973.

Mould, P.C.: *Hemophilia: A Bibliography of Mental Health and Social Service References*. Michigan, National Hemophilia Foundation, 1977.

Myers, B.A., Friedman, S.B., and Weiner, J.B.: Coping with a chronic disability. Am. J. Dis. Child., *120*:175, 1970.

Parmalee, A., Jr.: The doctor and the handicapped child. Children, *9*:189, 1962.

Pless, I., and Douglas, J.W.B.: Chronic illness in childhood. I. Epidemiological and clinical characteristics. Pediatrics, *47*:405, 1971.

Pless, J.B., and Pinkerton, P.: *Chronic Childhood Disorders: Promoting Patterns of Adjustment*. Chicago, Year Book, 1975.

Pless, J.B., and Roghmann, K.J.: Chronic illness and its consequences: Observations based on three epidemiologic surveys. J. Pediatr., *79*:351, 1971.

Pless, J.B., Satterwhite, B., and Van Vechten, D.: Chronic illness in childhood: A regional survey of care. Pediatrics, *58*:37, 1976.

Prugh, D.G.: Psychological and psychophysiological aspects of oral activities in childhood. Pediatr. Clin. North Am., *3*:1047, 1956.

Prugh, D.G.: Psychophysiological Aspects of Inborn Errors of Metabolism. In: *The Psychological Basis of Medical Practice* (H. Lief, V. Lief, and K. Lief, Eds.). New York, Hoeber, 1963.

Prugh, D.G., and Eckhardt, L.O.: Children's reactions to illness, hospitalization, and surgery. In: *Comprehensive Textbook of Psychiatry* (A. Freedman, H. Kaplan, and B. Sadock, Eds.). 2nd Ed. Baltimore, Williams & Wilkins, 1975, Vols. 1, 2.

Richardson, S.: Some social psychological consequences of handicapping. Pediatrics, *32*:291, 1963.

Richmond, J.B.: Self-understanding for the parents of handicapped children. Public Health Rep., *69*:702, 1954.

Richmond, J.B.: The pediatric patient in illness. In: *Psychology of Medical Practice* (M.H. Hollender, Ed.). Philadelphia, Saunders, 1958.

Robinson, A.: Genetic and chromosomal disorders. In: *Current Pediatric Diagnosis and Treatment* (C.H. Kempe, H.K. Silver, and D. O'Brien, Eds.). Los Altos, Calif., Lange, 1972.

Romano, J.: On those who care for the sick. J. Chronic Dis., *1*:695, 1955.

Rothenberg, M.B.: Reactions of those who treat children with cancer. Pediatrics, *40*(Suppl.):498, 1967.

Rothschild, E., and Owens, R.P.: Adolescent girls who

lack functioning ovaries. J. Am. Acad. Child Psychiatry, *11*:88, 1972.

Ruess, A.L.: Behavioral aspects of the physically handicapped child. J. Am. Phys. Ther. Assoc., *42*:163, 1962.

Rutter, M., Tizard, J., and Whitlemore, K.: *Handicapped Children: A Total Population Prevalence Study of Educational, Physical, and Behavioral Disorders.* London, Longmans, 1968.

Sandberg, S.: Psychiatric disorders in children with birth anomalies. Acta Psychiatry Scand., *54*:1, 1976.

Schnaper, N., and Cowtey, R.: Overview: Psychiatric sequelae to multiple trauma. Am. J. Psychiatry, *133*:883, 1976.

Schonfeld, W.A.: Body-image in adolescents: A psychiatric concept for the pediatrician. Pediatrics, *31*:845, 1963.

Schwab, J.J., and Harmeling, J.D.: Body image and medical illness. Psychosom. Med., *30*:51, 1968.

Selected References on Handicapped Children: An Annotated Bibliography. 2nd Ed. Committee on Handicapped Children. Evanston, Ill., American Academy of Pediatrics, 1968.

Silverstein, A.B., and Robinson, H.A.: The representation of physique in children's figure drawings. J. Consult. Psychol., *25*:146, 1961.

Shapiro, M.: Intensive assessment of the single case. In: *The Psychological Assessment of Mental and Physical Handicaps.* (P. Mittler, Ed.). London, Methuen, 1970.

Shrand, H., and Lightwood, R.: Organized home care for sick children. Courrier, *14*:353, 1964.

Smith, D.W., et al.: The mental prognosis in hypothyroidism of infancy and childhood. Pediatrics, *19*:1011, 1957.

Stubblefield, R.L.: Psychiatric complications of chronic illness in children. In: *The Child with Disabling Illness* (J.A. Downey, and N.L. Low, Eds.). Philadelphia, Saunders, 1974.

Sultz, H.A., et al.: *Long-term Childhood Illness.* Pittsburgh, University of Pittsburgh Press, 1972.

Tisza, V.B.: Management of the parents of the chronically ill child in pediatrics. Am. J. Orthopsychiatry, *32*:55, 1962.

Travis, G.: Chronic Illness in Children: Its Impact on Child and Family. Stanford, Calif., Stanford University Press, 1976.

Valadian, J., Stuart, H.C., and Reed, R.B.: Studies of illnesses in children followed from birth to eighteen years. Monogr. Soc. Res. Child Dev., *26*:No. 3, 1961.

Wallace, H.M., et al.: The homebound child. JAMA, *158*:158, 1955.

Wenar, C.: The effects of a motor handicap on personality. I. The effects on level of aspiration. Child Dev., *24*:123, 1953.

Wenar, C.: The effects of a motor handicap on personality. II. The effects on integrative ability. Child Dev., *25*:287, 1954.

White, G.: The role of the medical social worker in the management and control of rheumatic fever and rheumatic heart disease. Am. J. Med., *2*:618, 1947.

Wills, D.: Problems of play and mastery in the blind child. Br. J. Med. Psychol., *41*:213, 1968.

Wolf, S.: Effects of suggestion and conditioning on the action of chemical agents in human subjects: The pharmacology of placebos. J. Clin. Invest., *29*:100, 1950.

Wolf, S., and Pinsky, R.H.: Effects of placebo administration and occurrence of toxic reactions. JAMA, *155*:341, 1954.

Wolff, H.G., and Wolf, S.: *Pain.* Springfield, Ill., Thomas, 1958.

Wolff, J.M., and Anderson, R.M.: *The Multiply Handicapped Child.* Springfield, Ill., Thomas, 1969.

Wolfish, M.G., and McLean, J.A.: Chronic illness in adolescents. Pediatr. Clin. North Am., *21*:1043, 1974.

Work, H.M.: The role of the psychiatrist. In: *The Child with a Handicap: A Team Approach to His Care and Guidance.* Springfield, Ill., Thomas, 1959.

Wright, B.: *Physical Disability: A Psychological Approach.* New York, Harper & Row, 1960.

26

Psychosocial Aspects of the Management of Fatal Illness

A good Doctor can foresee the fatal outcome of an incurable illness; when he cannot help, the experienced Doctor will take care not to aggravate the sick person's malady by tiring and injurious efforts.
(Hermann Boerhave)

One of the most difficult tasks facing the physician and other health professionals is that of helping a family deal with a fatal illness in their child. In such a case, the physician, the nurse, and the other medical professionals who understand what stresses the family faces and the coping responses the family members are likely to make can give the family valuable support. A knowledge of the family history, including the family's experience with illness and death and how the family has responded in the past to stressful situations, can help the physician. Such knowledge may not be readily gained, however, and attempts to elicit it during a crisis may be difficult or unwise. Thus awareness of the problems the child, his parents, and his siblings face is vital, and, as Friedman[9] has indicated, the concept of anticipatory guidance is a central one.

Coping Responses

Kaplan[21] sees a family's coming to grips with a fatal illness in one of its members as a "family coping process" that is related to the family's patterns of communication, mutual support, and cohesion in times of crisis. The ultimate outcome of the process seems to be based on "family coping responses" (adaptive or maladaptive), which become manifest in the weeks following the diagnosis. Kaplan considers the phasic responses of parents to catastrophic experience as part of the family coping process. However, he broadens concepts such as those of Richmond[38] and Kübler-Ross,[23] and discusses the need for all family members to deal with the initial feelings of shock and anger, using the coping mechanisms of denial and disbelief, and then to experience a "grief period" of shared family mourning that brings mutual consolation, support, and relief from guilt. The family mourning includes the fatally ill child. Such an adaptive family coping response leads to a final grief response after the child's death which may take some months, with the ultimate acceptance of the loss of the loved one.

Maladaptive family coping responses, which fail to support realistic communication, anticipatory or "partial" grief responses, and mutual consolation among family members, occur often. Some responses are similar to the responses to the diagnosis of catastrophic illness or injury (see Chapter 24). Although marked psychologic decompensation by a parent or family member is only rarely precipitated by such an illness in a child, in the study by Kaplan and his colleagues, more than 75% of families faced with fatal illness failed to cope successfully with its consequences. Divorce, illness, and school problems among the healthy siblings occur often, as Bozeman's[4] has indicated. In Binger's[3] study, more than 50% of the families required psychiatric treatment for at least one member. A controlled study in Britain by Rees and Lutkins[36] confirmed and extended other observations (regarding adults[34]) that the death of a family member significantly increases the mortality among parents, siblings, and other close relatives within the following year, as the result of suicide or increased susceptibility to illness.

Reactions of Parents

Adaptive Responses. Although maladaptive responses of parents are frequent, more recent observations suggest that under "optimal" circumstances, most parents are able to adjust, however painfully, to the death of a child. Factors that may affect the adjustment include the length of time the parents have to prepare for the child's death and the degree to which the death is anticipated (sudden, unexpected deaths

seem to be more difficult for the parents to cope with[10]). Recent observations also suggest that the degree of candor about the diagnosis, prognosis, and management of the child's illness and the parents' response are also factors in adjustment.

Studies differ somewhat in regard to the family's use of denial and disbelief after the initial feelings of shock and anger. In the study by Friedman and his colleagues[9] of parents of children who had leukemia, most parents, after their initial shock, seemed to accept intellectually the diagnosis and its implication although most parents said that it took some days for the diagnosis to "sink in." These parents seemed to be using intellectualization and isolation of feeling to a greater extent than did those described earlier by Natterson and Knudson[33] and by Bozeman and his colleagues.[4] Among those parents, denial and disbelief continued for some weeks at least. Perhaps the public's greater awareness of leukemia, an earlier suspicion about its presence, and differences in referral patterns and sample groups contributed to the differences. In Friedman's group, a few parents openly denied the seriousness of their child's illness and its prognosis; these parents seemed to have used similar defenses to cope with stress in the past.

In the groups studied by Natterson and Knudson and Friedman and his colleagues, after an initial expression of guilt, the parents gradually moved toward emotional acceptance of their child's outlook. The mothers in particular seemed to be able to deal with fear and frustration, as well as with guilt, by participating actively in the overall care of the children.[2] In Friedman's study, the grandparents (and friends and other relatives) showed more denial of the diagnosis and prognosis than did the parents. As a result, a paradoxical set of pressures arose. The parents felt uncomfortable about "defending" their child's diagnosis and prognosis. And although the parents were not allowed (by society) to give up hope and to express feelings of hopelessness, they were also expected to appear grief stricken and to avoid pleasurable experiences for themselves and their other children.[11]

Parents did at times obtain valuable emotional support and offers of help from friends and relatives, but they seemed to get the best support from parents of similarly afflicted children who were undergoing similar emotional experiences. Most parents looked for meaning in their child's illness, sometimes by considering recent theories regarding the cause of leukemia. A religious orientation was helpful to some, but some parents began to doubt (although not actually to renounce) their religious beliefs.

In both groups, hope was important to parents, and it was often associated with a mild degree of denial. Gradually, hope began to dissipate or to narrow itself to the hope for a remission rather than a cure. If their child was still alive by the fourth month, parents in both groups seemed to be actively involved in the process of mourning or anticipatory grief. The signs of the grief included complaints of somatic symptoms, weakness, apathy, and sighing, with occasional crying at night and preoccupation with thoughts of the ill child. At other times, parents showed an increase in motor activity combined with tendencies to talk at length about the ill child. As anticipatory mourning progressed, the parents often seemed to detach themselves somewhat from their child, to appear resigned to the outcome, and at times to wish "it were all over." (Most parents have such feelings, and verbalizing them may be helpful.) In these studies, as in the earlier study of Richmond and Waisman,[38] anticipatory mourning seemed to be of definite value in preparing the parents for the eventual loss. In both studies, parents who displayed such anticipatory reactions grieved again after the child's death but with a calmer acceptance of the death and with only transient feelings of guilt and self-blame. In Friedman's groups, the final

mourning became much less pronounced after 3 to 6 weeks.

Maladaptive Responses. Some maladaptive coping responses of parents are similar to those described earlier. Massive denial of the diagnosis, often based on guilt about past conflicts in the parent-child relationship, may occur, leading to "shopping" for other opinions, with at times disastrous financial effects on the whole family. The parents may be unable to accept or discuss the diagnosis, and that inability may be associated with intense hostility toward the physician or the hospital staff, who may not realize that the hostility is based on feelings of guilt or other feelings and is not directed toward them personally. Or the parents may accept the diagnosis but not the prognosis. They may be unable to believe that the illness is fatal, or they may deny even obviously worsening symptoms or the side-effects of treatment, such as the "moon face" that results from the use of steroids.

Some parents may desperately try to keep the child from knowing that he is seriously ill, permitting no one to give the child any information about his illness. Other parents cannot even talk to each other about the child's illness, each fearing that the other will break down or otherwise lose control if the topic is broached. "Discrepant parental coping" may also occur, with parents unable to agree on the diagnosis or prognosis or on what is to be communicated to whom. In such a situation, the other family members cannot cope and family relationships may be weakened. Still other failures in family coping may result from the inability of the grandparents or other influential family members to accept the diagnosis or prognosis. (The impact on siblings is discussed more fully later.)

Some parents may be unable to set limits on the sick child's demands, because they fear they will hurt the child. They may overindulge him, wishing to make the remainder of his life happy. A few parents may be able to accept the diagnosis but may show their inability to cope by "early abdication" of their responsibility for the child's care. Divorce, psychiatric illness in one or both parents, and other maladaptive responses have already been mentioned.

As Friedman has pointed out, the parents' coping behavior may be evaluated from two points of view. One view involves the determination of whether the parents' coping behavior permits them to carry out certain socially desirable goals, such as fulfilling family responsibilities while participating appropriately in the care of their ill child. The other view evaluates the parents' coping behavior in terms of its effectiveness in helping the parent to tolerate the stressful circumstances without disruptive anxiety, depression, or ego disintegration. Friedman and his colleagues[13] studied the hormonal and behavioral responses of parents of children who had neoplastic disease. These workers found that both pathologic and socially desirable coping responses were associated with stable excretion rates of 17-hydroxycorticosteroid if such responses protected the parent from seriously disruptive feelings. Coping behavior thus enables the parent to deal with stress and keeps the emotional distress within tolerable limits. The dynamic balance between both functions determines the adaptive outcome, which may shift during the course of the child's illness.

Reactions of Children and Adolescents

Children who have fatal illnesses may show positive coping responses; they may also show the maladaptive responses seen in children who have chronic, nonfatal illness, namely, denial, depression, withdrawal, overdependence, poor school performance, and other behavioral disturbances.

The responses of children to the idea of death follow a developmental sequence, as Nagy[32] long ago indicated in a study of healthy children. More recently, Natterson and Knudson[33] have confirmed and elaborated Nagy's findings in regard to a group of hospitalized children who ranged from 1 year to 12 years of age and who had leukemia, neuroblastoma, lymphosarcoma, and other fatal illnesses. Children in the early preschool-age period generally think of death as a temporary separation. When they talk of dying, they express mainly their fear of separation from their parents and a fear of loss of affection and of not being cared for. The older preschool-age child is concerned about pain and about burial and its consequences although still in the context that death causes a temporary interruption of familiar relationships. The early school-age child thinks of death as a person who may be strange and take him from the familiar. When he talks about dying, he expresses his fear of pain and bodily mutilation and of being alone and helpless in the presence of the unfamiliar. The concept of death as adults know it becomes fully developed in the later school-age period (around 9 to 10 years of age), in relation to the developing sense of the self and the beginning mastery of abstract concepts. Even then (as with adolescents and many adults), the fear of pain and of being alone is intermingled with the fear of the obliteration of the self.

In the past, a nearly universal concern of parents has been what the ill child knows or should know about his illness. In the past, most parents, even though gradually able to accept their child's illness, tended to shield the child from hearing the word leukemia or any other reference to the illness. Even the hospital staff members have at times participated in this unconscious "conspiracy of silence" because of their fears of upsetting the children; and without realizing it, they may even stay away from the child to avoid the topic (or to protect their own feelings). Actually, children know soon after their parents have been told the diagnosis that something is seriously wrong with them. Their entire environment changes, and they easily sense that the people they love and trust are keeping something frightening from them. Some children fear something even more terrible than the truth, and some children (over the age of 9) have verbalized to staff members their awareness[41] of the nature of their illness—often to the distress of their parents.

Some children who have leukemia or other fatal illnesses may openly reject their parents. Often they do so after they have been ill for some time, as if they blamed their parents for being unable to prevent the illness and the painful procedures associated with it. Like children who have other illnesses, younger children especially tend to equate their illnesses with punishment for real or fantasized transgressions. Some children and adolescents, reacting to the secrecy surrounding their illness, may feel left out and resentful, or they may show apprehension, depression, withdrawal, refusal to take their medications, or other behavioral disturbances. During periods of remission some adolescents may have trouble dealing with the questions or the sometimes thoughtless comments of their friends.

Psychologic disturbance may also arise from the physical effects of the illness itself and of the treatment. Fatigue, malaise, anemia, and cachexia (as well as pain) may result in apathy, withdrawal, or depression. Deranged functioning of the organ in which a metabolic change occurs can produce mental changes, and brain tumors may cause delirium in certain stages. Changes in physical appearance caused by the illness or drugs (e.g., loss of hair) may pose special problems for adolescents. As indicated in Chapter 4, serious depression or hopelessness may even intensify the basic disorder and thus hasten the progression of the illness.

Reactions of Siblings

Siblings also perceive quickly that something serious has occurred. They too may feel the parents are hiding something dreadful from them, especially if they have been given little information. The special treatment given the ill child may arouse resentment or jealousy, particularly in younger siblings, thus jeopardizing the family's coping responses. Siblings will ask questions about illness and death; and their stages of development, their relationships to the patient, and other factors will help determine their responses to the information they are given.

School-age children particularly may show little response immediately; they use denial and avoidance of feeling as coping mechanisms. These mechanisms may reach maladaptive proportions, as may depression, fear of their own deaths through misconceptions about the illness, and guilt about past arguments or other conflicts with the ill sibling. A drop in school performance, stealing, regressive behavior, and other disturbances in adaptation have also been encountered, and may point to the need for a psychiatric consultation. Feinberg[8] has described a form of brief preventive therapy for school-age siblings of a child who has leukemia. The therapy gives the children an opportunity to ventilate their feelings, to engage in "immunizing" discussions, and to begin anticipatory mourning.

The death of a child is a situational crisis, and the siblings may react to it with various immediate behavioral responses. These responses include loss of appetite, nightmares, enuresis, speech disturbances, and states of anxiety or confusion. In some cases the siblings may show no overt sadness or grief, or (just the reverse) they may talk incessantly about the death. If adequate family coping responses are forthcoming, most children can share in the mourning process and their behavioral responses are not enduring. If the parents cannot give the siblings enough information to permit them to talk about their feelings or to ask about the death, the siblings are likely to have lasting maladaptive responses. These responses may include guilt about their survival, suicidal thoughts, punishment-seeking or testing behavior, depression, withdrawal, poor school performance, acting-out behavior, fear of not growing up, fear of death, and fear of doctors and hospitals, as Cain and his colleagues[6] have indicated. These workers have also pointed out the similarity between these and other responses of siblings to other types of losses, including the death of relatives and friends, as well as the loss of siblings through divorce or placement in foster homes or institutions. Anniversary episodes of depression, conversion pain, paralysis, and convulsion-like states have been described as resulting from the sibling's identification with the dead child or his fantasied manner of death.

As Cain has pointed out, part of the impact of the death on the sibling may stem from the parents' reactions to the death. If the family's coping process is not effective, withdrawal, depression, or preoccupation with thoughts about the dead child on the part of one or both parents may leave little time for them to help the siblings. Fears on the part of the parents that a young sibling will also die, often combined with feelings of guilt, may lead them to become overprotective and even to the development of the vulnerable child syndrome.[16] Parents may misinterpret a sibling's lack of open mourning as unfeeling behavior, and a few parents may show hostility and little affection for the surviving child, leading him to feel guilty that he is alive when his sibling is dead. Idealization of the dead sibling by the parents may lead to feelings of guilt or bitterness or to other feelings in the survivors. Later, the parents may conceive a "replacement child,"[35] or occasionally the parents may "misidentify" a sibling with the dead child, making him an open substitute. In either case, serious problems for the replacement child's self-concept and identity result. Indirect reverberations on the family's adaptive equilibrium may also occur (a father who deeply needs a lost

only son may unconsciously masculinize a daughter, or a mother may displace her blocked need to mother a lost baby onto an adolescent son). It is obvious that both reactions will bring problems.[5]

Management

Telling the Parents About a Fatal Illness

Before explaining the illness to parents, the physician should be sure of the diagnosis. Mistaken diagnoses[43] have resulted in the development of the vulnerable child syndrome and have had other unpleasant consequences. As Friedman[9] indicates, the parents should be given enough information. Too little information can contribute to the parents' later confusion and doubts about the physician's competence. Since fatal illnesses in children are not common, the physician may not be thoroughly familiar with their management. But he should be ready to make use of referrals or consultations where indicated, permitting shared responsibility for the management, as Green[15] has emphasized.

Parents may suspect that their child has a fatal disorder before learning of it from the physician. But the physician should not list or even discuss differential diagnoses with the parents before he has arrived at the final diagnosis. As Friedman emphasizes, the physician should be available to the parents if they need to confront him with their fears, and he should be willing to answer their questions honestly and openly. Physicians may wish, consciously or unconsciously, to avoid such a confrontation until the diagnostic tests are completed. But a wait may only increase the parents' anxiety or provoke their anger, and it may interfere with the parent-doctor relationship. Also, airing their fears in an open fashion may help the parents to prepare themselves for the diagnosis they fear.

Explaining a child's fatal illness to his parents is a complicated and delicate task. However, as Green emphasizes, not to explain the illness is a disservice to the child and his family. Knowing the individual child and family and understanding the child's concept of death may give the physician some guidelines for the explanation. He should meet with the parents together if at all possible. The meeting place should allow for privacy, enough time should be set aside for the parents' questions and answers, and the parents' feelings should be respected. If there is a language barrier, an interpreter should be brought in.

Physicians vary in how they discuss a fatal diagnosis. Many physicians are frank in describing the illness as fatal. Others are realistic in describing the illness and its prognosis but are eager to support hope by talking about a possible research breakthrough or by focusing the family's hopes on long remissions, during which the child will be comfortable and can live at home. Some physicians have advocated telling the parents the prognosis some time after they have told them the diagnosis. But the studies of Friedman and his colleagues[9] and the results of the more recent system of management developed by Lascari and Stebbins[26] indicate that giving the parents frank and complete information about the diagnosis and prognosis at the outset is the best way to help the parents mourn, to support the family's coping, to achieve effective communication, and to help the child and his family in other ways. The physician discusses the possibility of remission with the family and he helps them keep up their hopes.[31] Friedman and his colleagues have written a pamphlet for parents[12] that is helpful, but written material is not a substitute for a good relationship between the physician and the parents.

In Lascari and Stebbins' approach, 75% of the parents studied were able to carry out their normal family responsibilities during their child's illness and 95% of the parents and all of the siblings had normal grief reactions, without special professional intervention, after their child died. These findings are in contrast to those of the earlier studies cited, in which 50% or more of the families studied required some form of psychiatric intervention.

The parents' earlier reactions to their child's illness may give the physician some clues as to how to begin the interview in which he tells the parents about the diagnosis and prognosis. If the parents had told him earlier that they feared their child had cancer or some other fatal illness, he may start by saying, "I'm sorry to say that Johnny has a very serious illness" and then pausing briefly. The pause may give the parents time to brace themselves and even to ask, "Is it leukemia?" or "Will it be fatal?" The answer initially need be no more than a sympathetic nod. If the parents do not say anything, the physician can say something like, "All the tests confirm that it's leukemia, and I guess you know that although we can do a lot for him, it will take him away eventually." If the parents are able to ask, their initial feelings of shock and anger may be lessened and they may be able to accept the diagnosis more easily.

The physician should give the parents a chance to express their shock and anger and to break down and cry if they are able to do so. He can offer the parents tissues and wait sympathetically, offering no more than a simple reflection of their feelings (e.g., "It is very hard"). In the discussion that ensues, if the parents ask whether the disease could have been prevented or if they express feelings of guilt or self-blame, the physician should reassure them. If he feels that this is not the time to "incise and drain" the parents' feelings, he should at least give them "absolution" by saying at an appropriate point, "It couldn't be helped" or "These things can't be prevented." The parents may respond to his comment by verbalizing their feelings of guilt. If they do not, they will ordinarily bring up these and other misconceptions in later interviews.

Since many children who have a fatal illness do not seem especially ill at the time the diagnosis is made and since with treatment they may go promptly into remission, the physician may use anticipatory counseling to help the parents with denial. As Friedman suggests, the physician might tell the parents that it is natural for them to have trouble believing the diagnosis when the child seems well. Such counseling can also help the parents deal with the unbelieving responses of relatives and friends mentioned earlier.

It is generally considered unwise to estimate how long the child will live. But the parents need detailed answers to their questions about possible overnight stays in the hospital, how to care for the siblings at home, and other aspects of the management of the illness.

Dealing with the Impact of Sudden Death

Mention was made earlier of the difficulty parents have in coping with unexpected death. Next to accidents, the most common cause of death in children as a whole, the sudden infant death syndrome (SIDS), has been identified as the principal cause of death in infants from 1 month to 1 year of age (the peak incidence occurs at 2 to 3 months of age). A number of theories about the causes have been discredited. Bergman and his colleagues[1] believe that SIDS may be a reflex or "threshold" phenomenon that ends in laryngospasm or apnea and that it is precipitated by a number of interrelated factors (e.g., respiratory inflammation from a mild viral disorder, the constitutional reactivity of the infant's autonomic nervous system, which is just maturing at 2 to 3 months of age, the season of the year, and the child's sleep-wake rhythms). SIDS is more common among families from lower socioeconomic backgrounds and among nonwhite families,

which suggests that poverty is related to a greater susceptibility to respiratory infection. It has been suggested, but not proved, that occasional cases of SIDS are related to the infant's emotional deprivation and to maternal postpartum depression.

As Friedman[10] has noted, the immediate reaction of the parents to the discovery of their dead or moribund infant is one of disbelief, acute grief, rage, guilt, and, ordinarily, projection of blame. Mothers, who often are the ones who find the baby, are especially prone to blame the father, a sibling, a babysitter, or a physician who has recently examined the child. They do so because they feel responsible or because they feel guilty about conflicting feelings they have had about the infant or because of fears about their maternal adequacy. Unexplained deaths invite inquiry into possible child abuse, which makes the parents feel angry and resentful as well as grief stricken.[42] Often parents have separated after such a death, and the siblings whether blamed or not, tend to feel guilty and fearful about the infant's death and the parents' rage and grief. Often parents become overprotective and overconcerned about the surviving siblings. It has been suggested that the death of an infant comes as a greater shock today than in the past, when the death of a child was more common.

As the National Institute of Child Health and Human Development[37] indicates, in counseling parents in regard to SIDS the pediatrician must find out what the parents think happened and elicit any feelings of guilt, fear, and blame, using "incision and drainage" if necessary. He should give them reassurance or "absolution" in dealing with their misconceptions. Since the emergency room nurse may be the first health professional the parents encounter after the infant's death, she has an important role in dealing with the parents' immediate reactions. Psychiatric consultation may be indicated for the parents. The social worker can help the family manage their grief, deal with the emotional problems of siblings, and handle any other resulting problems. Bergman and his colleagues[1] and Weinstein[42] believe that autopsies should be available for all such infants regardless of the family's ability to pay (that is not the case in some parts of the country). In Seattle, the parents are notified immediately of the autopsy results, which an informed health professional discusses with them. The families may need psychologic support for months or even longer. Intensive psychotherapy in a child mental health clinic or on a private basis may be needed for a sibling who is blamed for the death, and marital counseling or other forms of therapy may be needed for the parents.

In Seattle and some other communities, local committees of parents who belong to the National Foundation for SIDS make themselves constantly available to newly bereaved parents who wish to talk with parents who have had the same experience. In some communities, dissemination of information about SIDS has been part of a preventive approach, to alleviate guilt and blame. Formal SIDS information and counseling centers have been set up (e.g., at the Children's Hospital in Denver).

Telling the Child About His Illness

In line with the developmental concept of death discussed earlier, it is usually not necessary to tell the preschool-age or early school-age child his diagnosis; the younger child is more afraid of separation and pain than of death itself. Some physicians have felt that no child should be told that he has a fatal illness. (The inconsistency and, often, the impossibility of this approach has already been mentioned.) Other physicians have felt that only some patients, particularly teenagers, should be told of the diagnosis and that only the patients who seem to want to know should be told.

In the mid-1960s, Vernick and Karon[40] instituted a policy at the National Cancer Institute of telling children over 9 years old who had leukemia (sometimes even younger children) the diagnosis as soon as it had been verified. The manner in which the children were told varied with their ages and backgrounds. The policy was based on the assumption that the best way to meet the emotional needs of the seriously ill child was to provide an atmosphere in which the child could feel free to express his concerns and to receive honest answers to his questions. The staff knew that all the children were worried about their condition and that most had some knowledge of the seriousness of their illness. Some children knew exactly what was wrong. Thus the staff members were able to abandon the more traditional attempt to "protect" the child from worry by being secretive and to become actively involved in helping children and parents cope with their concerns.

The policy had good results. In a group of 51 patients, all were able to function relatively normally, and the withdrawal, depression, and other manifestations often observed were said to occur very infrequently and were always transient in nature. It should be noted that the approach involved other components of management (to be discussed later), which may be used effectively in a hospital ward of leukemia patients only but may be more difficult to use in the usual pediatric unit, where only a few patients may have a fatal illness. Nevertheless, the policy seems to me to have important implications for all patients and all families.

Most clinicians agree that when a child is told of his disease (whether or not a diagnostic term, such as leukemia, or a generic term, such as cancer, is used), he should be given an explanation of it in simple terms and some idea of its chronicity. For example, a child who has leukemia can be told that he has something wrong with his blood which makes him bleed easily and get tired. If he does not ask why he has the disease, he can be told that it was no one's fault and that it could not be helped. He should be offered some hope for the immediate future (e.g., that treatment will help him feel better if that is the case). With leukemia and some other disorders, the child can be told that he will be able to go home and resume his normal activities even though he may have to return to the hospital from time to time. Older children may get some help from the knowledge that research is being done to help children who are ill.

Although as Green[15] points out, most seriously ill children do not ask directly whether they are going to die, some children 4 years old or older may ask. Parents, physicians, and nurses may have different ideas about how to answer. When the question is raised, the physician should determine what exactly the child is asking. The physician might ask the child what he means by dying or why he thinks he might die. He may find out that the child is worried about whether he will be alone when he dies or whether the doctor will take care of pain. The physician should not tell the child that he will die without first discussing the matter with the parents and obtaining their permission. The parents may wish to answer the child's question themselves, or they may wish help from the physician or nurse or religious counselor. A few parents are terrified of the child's question and may not wish it answered at all. In that case, it is best to tell the parents that the child knows that something is seriously wrong and that he needs to know at least something about what is wrong. It may help to tell the parents about the young child's concept of death.

If the parents give permission, the child's question about dying may be answered by the statement that he may die but that everything possible will be done to help him get better and go home. The older school-age child or the adolescent who knows the diagnosis may also know the prognosis although he may not ask directly about death. It is best to answer questions of older children and adolescents simply and honestly; they are usually relieved to know the truth. If the patient expresses a fear of death openly, he can be assured that relief from pain will be available and that he will not be alone when he dies. He should not be told that his parents will be with him, because his condition may change suddenly without the opportunity for his parents to be there. If his fear of death is intense or persistent, a psychiatric consultation may be valuable.

Management of the Illness

The management of the illness itself is somewhat similar to the management of chronic illness or handicap. The principal difference is that the parents of a fatally ill child need help in moving through the phase of denial and disbelief into the phase of anticipatory mourning, in preparation for the phase dealing with the child's terminal illness and actual death. The use of anticipatory guidance during remission in leukemia has been discussed. While the child is in the hospital, the physician should see the child and parents for at least brief periods daily, to answer their questions, to deal with their feelings of guilt and self-blame, and related misconceptions and to help them in the coping and mourning processes. The physicians and the nurses should be ready to accept the parents' expressions of feelings and to support their anticipatory mourning wherever possible. They should also consider the siblings' needs, and they should encourage the parents to visit and talk with staff about their sadness, and other feelings, particularly if the patient had been a favored child or a child with special problems. Family conferences may help promote communication, support shared family grief, or deal with other problems. Psychiatric consultation may be valuable.

For the preschool-age child who is hospitalized, living-in by the mother or the father is especially helpful in the early stages of the illness. But parents should not be pushed to live in if they cannot bring themselves to do it. Unrestricted visiting is of course vital. Knudson and Natterson[22] and others[2] have demonstrated the worth of having parents participate in the care of fatally ill children. With that approach, discharges against medical advice have been rare and the turnover in the hospital staff has been low. Knudson and Natterson believe that the mother's participation in care reduces separation anxiety in the pre-school-age and early school-age child and helps the mother resolve her feelings of guilt and denial, accept the diagnosis, and engage in anticipatory grieving. In their study, the parents seemed to have less need to participate in the program after about 4 months, by which time much of the work of grieving was usually accomplished and the parents had come closer to accepting the fact that their child would die.

Various workers have noted the supportive value to parents of informal "leaderless" group discussions held in the hospital's lounge areas.[17] Vernick and Karon[40] held regular group sessions for parents who happened to be visiting the pediatric unit. The sessions were led by the chief pediatrician with the assistance of a medical social worker. The meetings were informal and unstructured, and they focused on how parents can best help the entire family cope with a serious or fatal illness. Vernick and Karon noted that the sessions usually began with the parents' expressing a desire for more medical information but they invariably ended with the parents' discussing such emotionally charged issues as what to tell the ill child about leukemia. Much group support was evident, and the parents benefited from the opportunity to see how others had handled similar problems. Other workers have tried the same approach and have had equal success. Various authorities have cautioned, however, that such groups should be restricted to discussions, ventilation of feelings, and helpful comments; direct interpretation of the parents' behavior should be avoided.

Group sessions are not a substitute for the parents' having frequent individual contacts with the physician and the nurse. Occasionally a parent becomes upset in a group discussion; he can be seen supportively in an individual interview. As indicated earlier, psychotherapy is sometimes needed for one or both parents or for the patient.[44] LaBaw[25] has taught children to use self-hypnosis to control pain.

Other community resources can also be used to help parents express their feelings rather than maintain an unrealistic silence. The parents' friends often have trouble talking to the parents about the ill child, and parents often fear criticism for having a good time outside the home. Parents' organizations can help supply information and group support. Members of the clergy and mental health consultants may be helpful.

The family should be permitted to mourn in the manner to which they are accustomed, even to mourn in the presence of the child, if ethnic patterns apply.

In the course of a fatal illness, the focus should be kept on day-to-day steps. Some hope for temporary improvement can be kept alive with the use of new drugs and treatments. The child should be encouraged to maintain as many normal activities as possible. Whether the child is at home or in the hospital, recreational and occupational therapy activities are important, and parents may need home visits to help plan them. Such extreme measures as reverse isolation for children who have leukemia may confuse and depress the child; I agree with those who think that ordinarily the suffering involved is not worth the possible slight prolongation of the child's life.

If a child is at home, parents often have great difficulty in setting limits on his behavior. They often overprotect or overindulge the child, particularly if they feel guilty or fear unrealistically that the child will die suddenly. The guilt and the unrealistic fear must be dealt with, and the parents should be helped to understand that the child will be happier with their usual methods of discipline. The parents may need psychotherapy to help them deal with severe discipline problems, marked denial, or other difficulties. Children and (especially) adolescents have "reentry" problems[20] after they leave the hospital. Some previously disturbed children develop symptoms of conversion pain or weakness, hyperventilation, or other symptoms of emotional disturbance. These symptoms may be admixed with the symptoms of the basic illness, and psychotherapy for the child and his parents may be indicated. Psychotherapy may also be needed for parents who, after months or years of struggle, have given up mourning and have become detached from their child and his care. Such parents may not visit the child if he is in the hospital, or they may neglect the child's home treatments or office visits if he is at home. Without help, these parents usually feel intense guilt when the child dies.

Management of the Terminal Phase

The terminal phase may be the most agonizing one of all, for the staff as well as for the parents, particularly if the child lingers for days, weeks, or even months in a stuporous or comatose state. Recently, there has been much discussion among the public as well as among professionals of euthanasia and of "death with dignity" (i.e., a death in which no heroic measures are taken to prolong life). Seminars on death, dying, grief, and related matters are offered at medical centers throughout the country. A number of books dealing with death or dying have been published.[23] Euthanasia and "good death" societies are being formed, and sample wills are being distributed that ask that no heroic measures be taken in the testee's terminal phase.

Death, long a difficult subject to talk about, is now being discussed openly, and attitudes toward death and dying are changing. This change is in contrast to the way physicians have been trained in the last 30 to 40 years. The physician has been taught to maintain the patient's life at all costs and to the last moment.[39] Also, the physician is reluctant to admit that he is helpless in the face of death. Of course, the physician has saved many lives using modern techniques (e.g., cardiac massage and stimulation and organ transplantations). But the physician must come to terms with the changes in attitudes toward death and reconcile them with his own attitudes.

Some parents want everything possible done to keep their seriously ill child alive; some parents ask their physicians not to use heroic measures to keep their child alive (and thus prolong his suffering); and a few parents ask the physician "not to do anything more" in the way of treatment. The physician is responsible for making decisions about treatment; he should not let the family bear the burden alone. Parents who say "No more treatment" or who ask "Can't we do something to prevent further suffering?" may later become intensely guilty about having done so.[7]

I consider active euthanasia unthinkable. It implies an unwarranted assumption of infallibility on the part of the physician (spontaneous remissions have occurred in the sickest patients). No ethical physician would respond to the irresponsible (and uninformed) calls for euthanasia for the mentally retarded, and no moral society would follow the path of Hitler. Passive euthanasia (negative euthanasia) is a different matter. I agree with those who think that last-minute heroic measures to save a comatose, terminally ill child should be avoided. The physician can avoid taking heroic measures and still say truthfully to the parents, "Everything possible is being done."

I believe also that it is ethical and humane to avoid giving the child who is suffering the "ultimate" antileukemia drug if it will increase or prolong his suffering. The parents should be told that such a drug exists but that in the physician's opinion it will only cause the child more suffering. I have never known or heard of parents who questioned the physician's advice in such a situation if he handled it properly.

Although I consider active euthanasia unacceptable, I agree with Howell[18] that no child should be allowed to die in agony. As Howell and Marks and Sachar[28] point out, one does not need to fear addiction in a terminally ill patient, and appropriate drugs and narcotics, such as morphine, should be used to help the child who has intense pain to achieve a state of sleep. Death during sleep is peaceful for the patient and much more bearable for the family. Also, as Howell points out, sleep, whether induced or natural, does not interfere with other continuing therapeutic measures or with the natural course of life. Hypnosis for terminally ill patients has been used successfully to control pain by both LaBaw[24] and Gardner.[14]

During the terminal phase, the child's parents should be permitted to visit him whenever they want and for as long as they want. It can be arranged in a ward management conference that both parents can live in if they wish to do so. In Colorado some parents from Spanish-surnamed families ask to take their child home to die. Such a request often upsets pediatric residents,[39] but I have encouraged compliance with it. These families have their own ways of mourning, and the child is happier if his family deals with death in their traditional way. Other families wish to bring members of the extended family, dressed in black, into the hospital to mourn openly, sometimes with a priest present. Again, the custom should be respected. It brings comfort to both the patient and his family. Recently, some middle-class Anglo families have asked to take their child home to die. If home visiting by a nurse or physician is undertaken, there are fewer problems than when the child dies in the hospital.[29]

Some parents wish to stay with their child until he has died. Others parents wish to remember their child as he was in life and they prefer to leave if he is comatose or peacefully asleep. Certainly someone should stay with the child until the actual moment of death; the child may have a lucid interval and may be frightened if he is alone. I believe that the parents should not be pushed to stay with their dying child if they do not wish to do so or if they feel conflicting responsibilities. But they should be helped to reflect on a decision to leave. If the decision is made hastily, they may regret it later. Sometimes one parent decides to stay, while the other decides to leave. I believe also that parents should not be kept from staying with the child for fear they will be upset. Even a child who is dying of cystic fibrosis can be helped with drugs to achieve reasonable sleep; his parents will not see him die in agony. They should be permitted to stay if they wish. If they are not permitted to stay, they may later blame themselves for having deserted the child or they may blame (justly, I think) the hospital staff for preventing them from sharing their child's last moments. The value of having a member of the clergy sit with the parents for at least part of the time is real. He is a "shared presence" as well as a "religious presence." A member of the hospital staff can also be such a shared presence from time to time.

If a child dies suddenly or unpredictably in the hospital or if he suddenly enters the terminal phase, it is best to call the parents, no matter what the time of day or night, and ask them *both* to come to the hospital immediately. As Dr. William Berenberg advised me during my pediatric training, when the parents arrive, the physician should simply say "I'm afraid I have bad news for you" and then wait for the parents' questions. The pause gives the parents a few moments to prepare themselves for the worst; they can assimilate the news better if they themselves ask, "Is he worse?" or "Is he dead?" thus facing the possibility themselves rather than having it come from another person. The physician should let the parents break down as much as they need to. He can sympathet-ically indicate he knows how much they are suffering—it is a terrible shock—and wait until they have controlled their shock and initial grief well enough to ask ques-tions. Their shock may include anger that arises out of helplessness; the physician must accept their reactions and not take them personally.

I believe that the methods just described for helping parents handle the terminal phase are much more effective in helping them accept also the recommendation of the doctor (a sympathetic ally) that an au-topsy be done than the traditional argu-ments for having an autopsy done (namely that the parents would want to help other children and would want to know the pre-cise cause of death).

Parents frequently need an ongoing sup-portive relationship after their child has died, and an opportunity to form one should be routinely available to them. An appointment should be made to see them in 3 to 4 weeks to answer (sometimes for the second or third time) any questions they have. One can also see how the parents are progressing in their work of mourning and can schedule another appointment for sev-eral weeks later if one is indicated. Such an opportunity to "work through" their feelings may help the parents avoid con-ceiving another child to take the place of the lost one. Parents who ask about having another child should be advised to wait for some months before making a decision. They should be helped to understand that the grieving process goes on for a number of months and that the role a "replacement child" must play is a difficult and confusing one for him.[5,27,35]

Bibliography

1. Bergman, A.B., Miller, J.D., and Beckwith, J.B.: Sudden death syndrome: The pediatrician's role. Clin. Pediatr., 5:711, 1966.
2. Bierman, H.R.: Parent participation program in pediatric oncology: A preliminary report. J. Chronic Dis., 3:632, 1956.
3. Binger, C.M., et al.: Childhood leukemia: Emo-tional impact on patient and family. N. Engl. J. Med., 280:414, 1969.
4. Bozeman, M.F., et al.: Psychological impact of cancer and its treatment. I. The adaptation of mothers to the threatened loss of their children through leukemia. Cancer, 8:1, 1955.
5. Cain, A.C., and Cain, B.S.: On replacing a child. J. Am. Acad. Child Psychiatry, 3:443, 1964.
6. Cain, A.C., Fast, I., and Erickson, M.E.: Chil-dren's disturbed reactions to the death of a sib-ling. Am. J. Orthopsychiatry, 34:141, 1971.
7. Duff, R.S., and Campbell, A.: On deciding the care of severely handicapped or dying persons. Pediatrics, 57:487, 1976.
8. Feinberg, D.: Preventive therapy with siblings of a dying child. J. Am. Acad. Child Psychiatry, 9:644, 1978.
9. Friedman, S.B.: Care of the family of the child with cancer. Pediatrics, (Suppl.) 40:498, 1967.
10. Friedman, S.B.: Psychological aspects of sudden unexpected death in infants and children. Pe-diatr. Clin. North Am., 21:103, 1974.
11. Friedman, S.B., et al.: Behavioral observations on parents anticipating the death of a child. Pedi-atrics, 32:610, 1963.
12. Friedman, S.B., Karon, M., and Goldsmith, G.: *Childhood Leukemia. A Pamphlet for Parents.* De-partment of Health, Education, and Welfare, Washington, Government Printing Office, 1963.
13. Friedman, S.B., Mason, J.W.,. and Hamburg, D.A.: Urinary 17-hydroxycorticosteroid levels in parents of children with neoplastic disease: A study of chronic psychological stress. Psychosom. Med., 25:364, 1963.
14. Gardner, G.G.: Childhood, death, and human dignity: Hypnotherapy for David. Int. J. Clin. Exp. Hypn., 24:122, 1976.
15. Green, M.: Care of the dying child. In: *Care of the Child with Cancer* (A.B. Bergman, and C.J.A. Schulte, III, Eds.). Pediatrics (Suppl.), 40: 1967.
16. Green, M., and Solnit, A.J.: Reactions to the threatened loss of a child: A vulnerable child syn-drome. Pediatrics, 34:58, 1964.
17. Hoffman, I., and Futterman, E.H.: Coping with waiting: Psychiatric intervention and study in the waiting room of a pediatric oncology clinic. Compr. Psychiatry, 12:67, 1971.
18. Howell, D.A.: A child dies. J. Pediatr. Surg., 1:2, 1966.
19. Jacobs, S., and Ostfeld, A.: An epidemiologic re-view of the mortality of bereavement. Psycho-som. Med., 39:344, 1977.
20. Kagen-Goodheart, L.: Reentry: Living with child-hood cancer. Am. J. Orthopsychiatry, 47:651, 1977.
21. Kaplan, D.M., et al.: Family mediation of stress. In: *Coping with Physical Illness* (R.H. Moss, Ed.). New York, Plenum, 1977.
22. Knudson, A.G., and Natterson, J.M.: Participa-tion of parents in the hospital care of fatally ill children. Pediatrics, 26/2:482, 1960.
23. Kübler-Ross, E.: *On Death and Dying.* New York, Macmillan, 1969.

24. LaBaw, W.L.: Terminal hypnosis in lieu of terminal hospitalization: An effective alternative in fortunate cases. Gerontol. Clin., *11*:312, 1969.
25. LaBaw, W., et al.: The use of self-hypnosis by children with cancer. Am. J. Clin. Hypn., *17*:233, 1975.
26. Lascari, A.D., and Stebbins, J.A.: The reactions of families to childhood leukemia. Clin. Pediatr., 12:210, 1973.
27. Legg, C., and Sherick, I.: The replacement child: A developmental tragedy. Child Psychiatry Hum. Dev., 7:113, 1976.
28. Marks, R.M., and Sachar, E.J.: Undertreatment of medical in-patients with narcotic analgesics. Ann. Intern. Med., *78*:173, 1973.
29. Martinson, J.M., et al.: Home care for children dying of cancer. Pediatrics, 62:106, 1978.
30. Melamed, B.G., et al.: The influence of time and type of preparation on children's adjustment to hospitalization. J. Pediatr. Psychol., *1*:31, 1976.
31. Menninger, K.: Hope. Am. J. Psychiatry, *116*:481, 1959.
32. Nagy, M.: The child's theories concerning death. J. Genet. Psychol., 73:3, 1948.
33. Natterson, J.M., and Knudson, A.G., Jr.: Observations concerning fear of death in fatally ill children and their mothers. Psychosom. Med., 27:456, 1960.
34. Parkes, C.M.: The first year of bereavement: A longitudinal study of the reaction of London widows to the death of their husbands. Psychiatry, 33:444, 1970.
35. Poznanski, E.O.: The "replacement child": A saga of unresolved grief. J. Pediatr., *81*:1190, 1972.
36. Rees, W.D., and Lutkins, S.G.: Mortality of bereavement. Br. Med. J., 4:13, 1967.
37. Research Planning Workshops on the Sudden Infant Death Syndrome. I. Behavioral Considerations. National Institute of Child Health and Human Development, 1972.
38. Richmond, J.B., and Waisman, H.A.: Psychologic aspects of management of children with malignant diseases. Am. J. Dis. Child., *89*:42, 1955.
39. Schowalter, J.E.: Death and the pediatric house officer. J. Pediatr., 76:706, 1970.
40. Vernick, J., and Karon, M.: Who's afraid of death on a leukemia ward? Am. J. Dis. Child., *109*:393, 1965.
41. Waechter, E.H.: Children's awareness of fatal illness. Am. J. Nurs., 70:1168, 1971.
42. Weinstein, S.E.: Sudden infant death syndrome: Impact on families and a direction for change. Am. J. Psychiatry, *135*:831, 1978.
43. Winkelmayer, R., Judd, A.B., and Stearns, R.P.: Two mistaken diagnoses of fatal illness in brothers. Pediatrics, *40*:390, 1967.
44. Zuehlke, T.E., and Watkins, J.T.: The use of psychotherapy with dying patients: An exploratory study. J. Clin. Psychol., *31*:729, 1975.

General References

Airing, C.D.: Intimations of mortality. An appreciation of death and dying. Ann. Intern. Med., *69*:137, 1968.

Anthony, S.: *Discovery of Death in Childhood and After.* New York, Basic Books, 1972.
Bergman, A.B., and Schulte, C.J.A., Eds.: Care of the child with cancer. Pediatrics, (Suppl.) 40:487, 1967.
Chodoff, P., Friedman, S.B., and Hamburg, D.A.: Stress, defenses, and coping behavior: Observations in parents of children with malignant disease. Am. J. Psychiatry, *120*:743, 1964.
Cobb, B.: Psychological impact of long illness and death of a child on the family circle. J. Pediatr., 49:746, 1956.
Easson, W.M.: *The Dying Child: The Management of the Child or Adolescent Who is Dying.* Springfield, Ill., Thomas, 1970.
Erickson, M.H.: Hypnosis in painful terminal illness. Am. J. Clin. Hypn., 1:117, 1959.
Friedman, S.: Care of the family of the child with cancer. In: *Ambulatory Pediatrics* (M. Green and R.J. Haggerty, Eds.). Philadelphia, Saunders, 1968.
Friedman, S.B.: Management of fatal illness in children. In: *Ambulatory Pediatrics* (M. Green and R.J. Haggerty, Eds.). Philadelphia, Saunders, 1968.
Friedman, S.B., et al.: Behavioral observations on parents anticipating the death of a child. Pediatrics, 32:610, 1963.
Furman, R.A.: Death and the young child: Some preliminary considerations. Psychoanal. Study Child, *19*:321, 1964.
Futterman, E.H., and Hoffman, J.: Crisis and adaptation in the families of fatally ill children. In: *The Child in His Family: The Impact of Disease and Death* (E.J. Anthony and C. Koupernick, Eds.). New York, Wiley, 1973.
Goldfarb, C., Driesen, J., and D. Cole: Psychophysiologic aspects of malignancy. Am. J. Psychiatry, *123*:1545, 1967.
Greene, W.A., Jr.: Role of a vicarious object in the adaptation to object loss: I. Use of a vicarious object as a means of adjustment to separation from a significant person. Psychosom. Med., *20*:344, 1959.
Greene, W.A., Jr.: Role of a vicarious object in the adaptation to object loss. II. Vicissitudes in the role of the vicarious object. Psychosom. Med., *21*:438, 1959.
Group for the Advancement of Psychiatry. Death and Dying: Attitudes of Patient and Doctor. Symposium No. 11. New York, New York Mental Health Materials Center, 1965.
Hamovitch, M.B.: *The Parent and the Fatally Ill Child.* Duarte, Calif., City of Hope Medical Center, 1964.
Hollingsworth, C.E., and Pasnau, R.O., Eds.: *The Family in Mourning. A Seminar in Psychiatry Monograph* (M. Greenblatt, Series Ed.). New York, Grune & Stratton, 1977.
Krupp, G.R., and Kligfield, B.: The bereavement reaction: A cross cultural evaluation. J. Religion Health, *1*:222, 1962.
Kübler-Ross, E.: *Death: The Final Stage of Growth.* Englewood Cliffs, N.J., Prentice-Hall, 1975.
Mitchell, W.M.: Etiological factors producing neuropsychiatric syndromes in patients with malignant disease. Int. J. Neuropsychiatry, *3*:464, 1967.

Norton, J.: Treatment of a dying patient. Psychoanal. Study Child, *18*:544, 1963.

Orbach, C.E., et al.: Psychological Impact of Cancer and Its Treatment. III. The Adaptation of Mothers to the Threatened Loss of Their Children Through Leukemia. Cancer, *8*:20, 1955.

Parkes, C.M., Benjamin, B., and Fitzgerald, R.G.: Broken Heart: Statistical study of increased mortality among widowers. Br. Med. J., *1*:740, 1969.

Pritchard, E., et al., Eds.: *Social Work with the Dying Patient*. New York, Columbia University Press, 1977.

Renneker, R., and Cutter, M.: Psychological problems of adjustment to cancer of the breast. JAMA, *148*:833, 1952.

Rochlin, G.: Loss and Restitution. Psychoanal. Study Child, *8*:231, 1953.

Rothenberg, M.B.: Reactions of those who treat children with cancer. Pediatrics, (Suppl.) *40*:498, 1967.

Samaniego, L., et al.: Exploring the physically ill child's self-perceptions and the mother's perceptions of her child's needs. Clin. Pediatr., *16*:154, 1977.

Shands, H.C., et al.: Psychological mechanisms in patients with cancer. Cancer, *4*:1159, 1951.

Solnit, A.J.: The dying child. Dev. Med. Child. Neurol., *7*:693, 1963.

Solnit, A.J., and Green, M.: Psychological considerations in the management of deaths on pediatric hospital services. I. The doctor and the child's family. Pediatrics, *24*:106, 1959.

Solnit, A.J., and Green, M.: The pediatric management of the dying child. II. The child's reaction to the fear of dying. In: *Modern Perspectives in Child Development* (A.J. Solnit and S.A. Provence, Eds.). New York, International Universities Press, 1963.

Toch, R.: Management of the child with a fatal disease. Clin. Pediatr., *3*:418, 1964.

Weissman, A.D.: *On Dying and Denying: A Psychiatric Study of Terminality*. New York, Behavioral Publications, 1972.

27

Reactions of Children and Families to Hospitalization and Medical and Surgical Procedures

If you take a sick child from its Parent or Nurse,
you break its Heart immediately.
(George Armstrong—in the eighteenth century)

A careful examination of the 1971 edition of *Care of Children in Hospitals*[8] published by the American Academy of Pediatrics shows that sweeping changes have taken place in the philosophy of the care of children in hospitals and in the types of treatment facilities and programs for children. Topic areas include visiting patterns, parent participation and overnight stay, preparation for disturbing procedures, recreational programs, adolescent facilities, day treatment, and planning for ambulatory services.

But despite the changes, it seems to me that in the last 20 years there has been very little overall change in the way most children are handled when they are hospitalized. Individual pediatric units, some in academic settings, some in community programs, do an outstanding job of meeting the emotional needs of children and families during hospitalization. However, in the United States today, the majority of hospitalized children are not even handled in separate pediatric units. Even when separate facilities are available, many give only lip service to the concepts endorsed by the American Academy of Pediatrics. I base that statement on what I saw when I visited many of the major pediatric units in the United States.

Prugh and Jordan have discussed[228] a number of explanations for this unfortunate situation:

1. Changes in the reason for hospitalization have followed upon important advances in medicine; as a result, hospitalization for chronic illnesses or handicaps, diseases of genetic origin, complications of accidents, and emotional disorders has largely replaced hospitalization for acute physical illnesses.

2. Medicaid has made hospitalization possible for poor and minority group youngsters. These children are often admitted for the treatment of acute infections, diseases, and nutritional deficiencies, conditions now rarely seen in children from middle- and upper-class families.

3. The technologic revolution in medicine has produced many new complex and sophisticated laboratory tests which have important constructive implications. Because of convenience, and/or the problems connected with medical insurance, children are often unnecessarily hospitalized for these tests, which could otherwise be done on an outpatient or a day care basis. Such tests are also often ordered to rule out what seems to be a physical disorder in children who are in fact emotionally disturbed. All too often these children are hospitalized for extensive (and expensive) laboratory tests to rule out a physical disorder, such as a kidney problem or a brain tumor.

4. As the statistics imply and as outstanding pediatricians (e.g., Kempe[141]) attest, thousands of children are still admitted to hospitals each year for unnecessary tonsillectomies.

Also, the number of children admitted to hospitals has undoubtedly increased with the decline of the family physician (who is just now being resurrected) and the trends toward specialization and increased family mobility, all of which have had an adverse impact on continuity in medical care. Thus a sick child is often taken to a doctor who knows little or nothing about his past history or present circumstances, and if the parents are upset about the child's illness, they may not be able to recall pertinent details. If the doctor has any significant doubt about the nature of the illness or its seriousness, he may hospitalize the child—"to be on the safe side."

Of course it is not indifference to the welfare of children that has resulted in the present state of affairs. Many of the practices now regarded as more liberal could be found in children's hospitals to some degree 50 or 60 years ago. They were discontinued with the rise of "scientific pediatrics" in the 1930s and 1940s, largely because of the fear of cross infection and the belief of nurses and physicians that the presence of parents tended to disrupt ward routines.

It should be noted that pediatricians, pediatric nurses, and other professionals involved in hospital programs are usually kind and compassionate people who love children and who make great sacrifices to obtain the long and arduous training needed to treat their illnesses and injuries. The fear that the visits of parents and siblings increase the risk of cross infection has been laid to rest (most cross infections[230] with "staph" come from "staff"—dedicated people who come to work when they should stay at home because they have colds or sore throats); and various controlled studies have proved what every mother knows—that children have emotional needs which must be met, preferably by their parents. Therefore, only inertia and the difficulty of changing the "system" prevent the inauguration of more "liberal" practices in most hospitals. As Cooke[51] has pointed out, emotional trauma is a greater danger to children in hospitals than the possibility of infection or of accidents (although accidents are a serious hazard).

The preparation and care of children before, during, and after hospitalization—a problem of monumental proportions—are important parts of pediatric practice. Approximately 25% of patients hospitalized each year in the United States are 15 years of age or younger. Statistically, this means that every child in the United States has a chance of being hospitalized once before he reaches the age of 15 years. In actual fact, these figures do not distinguish between one-time admissions and multiple admissions of one child. Nevertheless, it is a fair estimate that 33% or more of all young people will have been hospitalized at least once before they reach adulthood. Since 50% of the U.S. population is now under 25 years of age, the projected increase in hospital admissions in coming years is staggering. Even if the experience of hospitalization were only occasionally harmful, a large number of children would be affected. In fact, in my opinion, hospitalization very often has a negative impact on a child and his family. Children do not need any more problems added to the problems they already face. At least 25% of all children in the United States must cope with poverty and racism, with the instability of contemporary family life (divorce occurs in 25% to 35% of families), with frequent moves (1 family in 5 moves each year, and young families move more often), and with a way of life that permits them little contact with extended family members.

There is much talk about preventive approaches to mental health problems of children. Yet in one area in which it is known how to forestall problems— deleterious reactions to hospitalization—very little is being done. Many hospitals continue to limit parents' visits to short periods several times a week. These are general hospitals without separate pediatric units, or, if they have such units, there is often no pediatrician to administer them. According to a 1960 survey,[257] only about 28 out of 5000 general hospitals had facilities for mothers to stay overnight with their infants and preschool-age children. Today most children's hospitals permit parents to live in, but some arrangements are makeshift.

Many other hospital policies and programs also show a lack of concern for (or at least a lack of understanding of) the special needs of children at different ages. Toddlers who can move about are not provided with play pens. Many times children 4 to 5 years old or even older are put in cribs for fear they will fall out of adult beds onto a hard floor. If an older child becomes disturbed at being confined "like a baby" and tries to climb out of the crib, a net is likely to be placed over him. Or at other times, the child may be tied down while he is receiving an intravenous infusion.

Recreational areas for free play are rarely provided for preschool-age and early school-age children, and many hospitals lack educational facilities for school-age children and adolescents. Children confined to bed are not given play materials to help work off tensions or just to enjoy themselves. Most hospitals are still bed-oriented and use enforced bed rest too freely. In confining children to bed, often in an impersonal and embarrassing hospital gown, hospital personnel fail to consider the fact that most children are not acutely ill. More important, such treatment tends to promote a "regressive sick role"— which children both resist and are tempted by—and which can complicate convalescence.

Even when visits from parents are permitted, they are often regarded as "getting in the way" of rigid hospital routines. Rigid diets are still prescribed too frequently. Children instinctively (and wisely) resist rigid diets, which have been proved to be unnecessary for most children and adolescents suffering from diabetes, obesity, and other disorders. Restraints and sedatives are still used to excess, supposedly to keep the child quiet, but in practice they serve only to confuse and agitate him more. Isolation of children to prevent cross infection continues to be used although it is often ineffective, and it is frequently prolonged unnecessarily, despite the child's lonely, frightened feelings.

The problem is not simply that most hospital programs deprive children of the attention and support of their parents, as well as the facilities and opportunities to play and learn in an age-appropriate manner. Also involved is the fact that most hospital personnel do not expect children to be particularly upset by these deprivations. Furthermore, they usually expect ill children to readily accept living in an unfamiliar hospital environment, where frightening or painful procedures are performed on them. Children are not "little people." They do not automatically adjust to the reality of illness and hospitalization under particularly stressful circumstances. Even adults find this difficult, as a study of adult reactions to care in a coronary unit indicates.[110]

The unhappy fact is that many hospitals have become tightly knit, hierarchical, regimented institutions run by administrators (some of them doctors) who often exhibit little concern for people in general, let alone children. Many hospital regulations stem from blind adherence to tradition rather than from a rational concern for the needs of children. "Adultomorphic" policies are commonly applied to children, and many hospital personnel give the impression that they would like to do a "parentectomy" so that they could handle the child without interference.

Like many others, I have worked throughout my career to change the treatment of children in hospitals. I feel that my work has given these children little benefit. Of course, some hospitals in the United States have developed good methods of handling children. But the treatment of children in many hospitals causes unnecessary problems for both the children and their parents. James Robertson, an English investigator, has done much work to show that the parents of infants and young children should be able to live with their children while the children are in the hospital. Like Robertson, I feel that parents must demand changes in the treatment of their children in hospitals. Parents in England[237] and in the United States[46a] are beginning to make such demands. It seems that only parents' demands can cause changes in the treatment of children in hospitals and bring about real respect for the rights of children.[89,281]

Like other members of the medical profession, Dr. Irving Berlin, past president of the American Academy of Children's Psychiatry, has agreed publicly[22] with the statements that I and my colleague Jordan have made. Azarnoff, who was recently the president of the Association for Child Care in Hospitals, has agreed privately with those statements.[9] However, Azarnoff also pointed out the important changes that have occurred recently in methods of treating children in hospitals.[11] I am not satisfied with those changes for children. Some physicians, nurses, and administrators may feel these statements are not fair to the excellent programs they have developed. However, they must feel as anguished as I do about poor programs.

Reactions of Infants, Children, and Adolescents

Hospitalization, because it involves separation from home and often unpleasant treatment procedures, may cause a variety of reactions in children.[45,99,159,223,230,297] The type of reaction depends on the child's level of psychosocial development, his previous adaptive capacity, the parent-child relationship, the meaning of the illness and hospitalization to the child and his family, the events that immediately preceded the hospitalization, the nature of the illness and its treatment, and the reverberations within the family when the child returns home. The older the child, the more he will be able to understand the real meaning of his experience and to interpret properly its significance.

All children, even very young infants, show at least some temporary response to the experience of hospitalization—from a rise in blood pressure[47] to emotional and behavioral responses—insofar as these can be differentiated from a specific response to the illness or operation. Such reactions take different forms at different age levels, but severe reactions are more intense and prolonged in younger children. Thus developmental issues are of major significance in evaluating the effects of hospitalization.

As Schaffer and Calender[246] have proved, even infants under 5 months of age show a kind of global reaction to hospitalization, even though they have not yet developed a close attachment to the mother. For example, changes in the infant's patterns of feeding, sleeping, and elimination seem to be responses to a disruption in the continuity and nature of care; that is, responses to the fact that the handling and stimulation provided by the nursing staff differ from the handling and stimulation provided by the mother. Such responses ordinarily last from a few days to several weeks after an infant's return home, and they may arouse anxiety or guilt in the mother, who feels that she is a stranger to her own infant. Her response may lead her to try to prove she is an adequate mother, perhaps by urging feedings on the infant. Thus a negative feedback system may develop between mother and infant, involving feeding problems, sleeping problems, or other difficulties, which may deepen or expand unless there is some therapeutic intervention. Anticipatory guidance of the parents before the infant goes home can prevent many of these problems.

Infants in the second half of their first year, a time when children begin to develop a close attachment to the mother and an awareness of "self" as separate from the mother, may exhibit true anxiety in reaction to hospitalization. As Benjamin[19] has pointed out, such anxiety surfaces in the form of "stranger" anxiety when the child is 5 to 7 months old, and it is followed by "separation" anxiety when the child is about 7 to 9 months old. In the second half of his first year, the infant is engaged in developing a "sense of trust," as Erikson terms it (see the schematic developmental chart in Chapter 5), and the experience of the separation from the mother can arouse not only anxiety but also a "sense of mistrust." In addition to anxiety, depression

may occur (as Spitz and Wolf[273] have pointed out), regression in behavior may develop, or there may be psychophysiologic reverberations, such as headaches, diarrhea and vomiting.

Children from 1 through 3 years of age are engaged in establishing a "sense of autonomy," as Erikson puts it. They are beginning to establish feelings of independence and mastery. The separation involved in hospitalization is a serious threat to the adaptive balance of children in this age group. The separation may be more significant than the illness or the medical or surgical procedures they must undergo. The young child may, of course, misperceive the procedures themselves as "attacks" by strangers, and aggressive "fighting off" is often seen. The young child's sense of autonomy can be undermined by the separation anxiety or by the primitive fears aroused by the procedures. As Anna Freud[91] has pointed out, the child may experience a kind of "objective anxiety" based on a fear of loss of the mother and reinforced by his limited capacity to understand reality, his inability to judge the passage of time, and his tendency to misinterpret the disappearance of the mother as punishment for "being bad." Regressive behavior is also common. Increased thumb or finger sucking, feeding difficulties, a need to return to the bottle, and loss of bladder or bowel control frequently occur in 2- to 3-year-old children hospitalized for a short time.

The sequence of *protest, despair,* and *detachment* (described by Robertson[238]) is the characteristic response of the young child to anxiety over separation. When that sequence occurs—and the child tends to ignore the mother for a time—particularly when he returns home from the hospital, it can be most upsetting for the parents. The child's regressive or demanding behavior may result in struggles or other continuing problems between the child and his parents; sadness, outbursts of anxiety, nightmares, and fears of doctors and needles are common. If the parents are prepared by anticipatory guidance to give the child a period of time to "warm up" and to offer him regressive satisfactions before "weaning" him back to his previous level of performance and adaptation, these post-hospitalization problems may be avoided.

In the older preschool-age child (from 4 to 6 years of age), separation anxiety is still present to some degree although regression is still manifest and aggressive behavior may occur, particularly in boys. In Erikson's view, the child in this phase is engaged in establishing a "sense of initiative" related to sexual differentiation and social autonomy. The child's fear of punishment, which is related to his developing capacity for fantasy, together with his still limited ability to test reality, lead to the beginning of "mutilation anxiety," based on fear of bodily harm of a more subjective nature. Those fears of harm are related especially to developmentally important body parts (e.g., the genitals) and sensitive areas (e.g., the head and eyes). Thus the child often misinterprets the meaning of various procedures, particularly painful ones, and preparation for such procedures becomes more vital and effective for the child in this age group, even though his ability to understand is limited.

Separation anxiety is much more muted in the school-age child than in the younger child, except in relation to regressive tendencies in the early phase (from ages 6 to 8). Nadas and his colleagues,[205] in a study of the psychologic impact of cardiac catheterization, confirmed the regression in various respects in this age group described in earlier studies.[230] Mutilation anxiety is still high, and although the child's capacity to comprehend reality is greater than that of the preschool-age child, the early school-age child in particular still exhibits fears, fantasies, and misconceptions of a more subjective nature. Children in the early school-age phase are preoccupied with establishing a sense of industry and accomplishment, as Erikson puts it. Fear of gen-

ital inadequacy, muscular weakness, loss of body mastery, and loss of control of impulses are accordingly intense, as the studies of Jessner and her colleagues[134] indicate, particularly in connection with the experience of undergoing anesthesia. Anxiety may be compounded by the school-age child's fear of potential harm to his body in situations in which he is not in control. He may fear what was done to him under anesthesia without his knowledge or what he might have said during the procedure while he was unconscious.

As conscience formation, a process that began in the preschool-age phase, is consolidated, with the associated repression of unacceptable thoughts or feelings, the school-age child tends to unconsciously invest various diagnostic or treatment procedures with punitive significance related to his guilt about his past transgressions; thus, as Anna Freud[91] has suggested, a type of "super-ego anxiety" arises. Such anxiety may also compound the difficulties that arise during convalescence as the child experiences guilt about the regressive satisfaction of his dependent wishes and, at the same time, the conflicting need to return to the competitive world of school and of his peer group.

The adolescent is engaged in establishing a "sense of identity," in trying to complete the unfinished "tasks" of earlier developmental stages, and in reaching ahead toward achieving independence, choosing a career, and learning to function in a heterosexual role. Thus, hospitalization may make him anxious that he will lose his still shaky identity among a new group of peers and adults. The forced dependency of illness may be unconsciously perceived as threatening. Abnormalities in his bodily functioning and the way they are dealt with by the hospital staff may arouse anxieties about his newly changed body and about his adequacy as a potential adult in relation to the opposite sex. Accepting the authority of the hospital staff and the need to "yield" to hospital rules and treatment procedures may be difficult for him as well, depending on his relationship with his parents and how well he is able to control his aggressive impulses.[249]

Reactions of Family Members

The *parents' reactions* are similar in some respects to those that parents have during acute illness. Denial and disbelief are usually less marked when the illness is less serious. Many parents fear criticism from the hospital staff regarding their role in the illness or their effectiveness as parents. Some parents may show strong rivalry with the nurses or physicians, interpreting professional competence in handling the child as a reflection on their abilities as parents. A feeling of being left out or unwanted is also common among parents. A few parents may project their feelings of guilt onto the hospital staff and blame them for minor difficulties. Difficulty in accepting recommended treatment occasionally leads to their removing the child from the hospital against the advice of their physician.

Other children in the family may react to the hospitalization of a sibling with guilt or undue anxiety, depending on their stage of development, their relationship to the ill child, and the circumstances that led to the illness or accident. Grandparents and other family members may respond appropriately to the hospitalization, dealing with the illness and posthospitalization behavior of the child as a family crisis. In less well-balanced families a preschool-age child who shows regressive, demanding behavior or returns to soiling or bedwetting on his return home may pose an adaptive challenge which the parents cannot meet. The parents' guilt may lead them to become overly indulgent, overly permissive, or (at times) overly demanding or restrictive toward the child. Jealousy in a slightly older sibling may touch off rebellious or regressive behavior. Struggles for control

between the child and his parents or disagreements between the parents about the sick child's temporarily changed behavior may become chronic or pervasive.

Long-Term Hospitalization

With proper treatment, long-term hospitalization or institutionalization is rarely necessary for chronically ill or handicapped children. The studies of Bakwin,[13] Spitz,[272] Bowlby,[35] and Provence[221] in particular have indicated the likelihood of serious emotional deprivation for such children. Especially in large institutions, children show chronic depression and detachment, which often lead to shallow social relationships, distorted time concepts, limited capacities for learning, a lowered resistance to disease, and rebellious or antisocial behavior. Mortalities in orphanges, now largely abandoned, used to reach 50%. In such settings, children who have especially appealing qualities can "win the hearts" of the often too-small staff and have their emotional needs met, but most children cannot and they suffer significant personality distortions. Frequent hospitalizations can have much the same effects, especially on young children. When it is clear that hospitalization will be prolonged, early supportive interventions can have real preventive value.[223,235]

Although some reactions of the type just described are virtually universal, most children are able to adapt successfully to the experience of a brief hospitalization, showing self-limited reactions that ordinarily subside after several weeks to several months. A recent long-term follow-up study by Douglas[64] indicates that for children between the age of 6 months and 4 years, a single admission to a hospital for more than a one-week stay, as well as repeated hospital admissions, is associated with an increased risk of behavior disturbance and poor reading in adolescence. Hospitalization is not necessarily a traumatic experience for the child, but it should be used as sparingly as possible. During the course of his development, a child may pass through especially vulnerable ("sensitive") phases. One such phase comes in the second half of the first year of life, as mentioned earlier. Children under 4 years of age have special vulnerabilities, as do previously disturbed children of any age, children experiencing a family crisis at the time of hospitalization, and children who are undergoing developmental crises. The incidence of continuing emotionally traumatic reactions (variously estimated at 5% to 15%[64,230,279,296]) is great enough to indicate the need for (1) careful thought before recommending hospitalization, (2) the use of psychologic preventive measures if hospitalization is clearly indicated, and (3) choosing alternatives to hospitalization whenever possible.

Post-Hospitalization Behavior

As indicated earlier, most young children show some regression for a few days or weeks after returning home from the hospital. The regressive behavior may persist if it is reinforced by parental anxiety or guilt feelings. Anticipatory guidance and support for the parents and a weaning of the child from regressive behavior can be valuable in preventing the regressive behavior from becoming deep seated and/or unnecessarily prolonged. Certain children may not be able to easily relinquish the greater dependency they developed in the acute phase of their illness, and they may fear a return to a competitive environment. (See Chapter 24 for a fuller discussion of convalescence and possible learning problems.) The parents' patience may be taxed considerably during this period, and they may need help in understanding that the child may be reacting to the previous separation experience. Flexibility may be needed in regard to bed rest and other treatment routines. Rest in an area where

contact with other people is possible may be more therapeutic than rest in the bedroom, where a lack of interaction may prolong or intensify the regressive behavior. The child should return to an integrated family life and to school as quickly as possible. He should also be given responsibilities gradually as he returns to normal.

Preparation for Hospitalization and Medical Procedures

The child should be told simply and truthfully—and in terms appropriate to his developmental level—why he is going to the hospital. He should be given a general idea of what being in a hospital is like, an indication that hospitalization is for his welfare, some awareness of what will be done to make him comfortable, and, most important, reassurance that his parents will remain in contact with him. The preparation of the parents for their child's hospitalization has been shown to be of positive value to them[100] and their children.[303] When the physician decides that hospitalization is necessary, he should tell the parents what to tell the child, and he should help them deal with their own apprehension, guilt feelings, or conflicts.

Preschool-age children should be prepared for elective hospitalization no more than a few days in advance.[195,226] This approach avoids allowing too much time for anxiety to build up, but it permits enough time for questions. For older children and adolescents, a longer advance preparation is appropriate. In some instances, a group session with physician, parents, and child may help support anxious parents and give the child a feeling of being involved in the planning. Even in emergency admissions, some preparation of the parents and child is usually possible and should not be overlooked.

A tour of the hospital is useful for older preschool-age and school-age children. This approach has been taken by Azarnoff and her colleagues.[12] The children are shown the hospital on a pre-admission visit and are encouraged to "play out" their feelings in advance. Booklets about "going to the hospital" that the parents can read to the older preschool-age and younger school-age child can be of value if the parents give the child a chance to ask questions. (Two such booklets are now available in Spanish.) Films for children and the staff are available. Lists of such books and films are included at the end of the section on General References in this chapter. Such helps are not really helps if they give the impression that being in the hospital is like "going to a party" where there are all sorts of entertainment. Visits to the home have also been found to be helpful in preparing the child for the hospital stay.[95]

Preparation of the child for potentially frightening or painful medical or minor surgical procedures should begin shortly after the child is admitted to the hospital. A thorough explanation of such procedures is not necessary for most children, but older school-age children and adolescents may be given more details if they express an interest. Simple but practical discussions of (for example) when and how meals are served, the doctors' and nurses' uniforms, and the use of the bedpan can be of value to older preschool-age children. "Playing out" hospital situations with a toy doctor's or nurse's kit may help the child master his anxiety. Controlled studies, employing puppet therapy for children undergoing cardiac catheterization (Cassell[41]), by Minde and Mahler,[201] and by others for children undergoing surgical procedures have demonstrated the effectiveness of early preparation in diminishing anxiety, and, possibly, reducing the length of the hospital stay.[201,230]

Painful procedures, such as venipunctures, subcutaneous or intramuscular injections, and lumbar punctures, are frightening to young children and may present difficulties for the physician. Very young children cannot be expected to cooperate.

Older children may be able to cooperate if the procedure is first explained to them. Or they may be led to take an interest in the physician's instruments, which will permit them to have a sense of mastery and control in the face of the anticipated pain. It should be emphasized that if a procedure will be painful, the physician should tell the child that some pain will occur, without minimizing or exaggerating it. The physician should tell the child when and where it will hurt and should encourage him to cry if he wants to. When necessary, restraint should be firmly but kindly applied, with the explanation that it will help the child hold still so that "it won't hurt so much." The idea to be conveyed is that the patient, the doctor, and the nurse are working as a team to get the job done with as little pain as possible.

Positive Use of Hospitalization

The positive use of hospitalization for infants and young children who have certain psychologic or psychophysiologic disorders has been discussed by Solnit.[265] These disorders may involve severe feeding problems, diarrhea, vomiting, marked toilet training difficulties, failure to thrive, rumination, and other problems. Guerin[109] has discussed hospitalization of poor children from chaotic families as a positive experience, one that offers structure and support as well as medical benefits. Hospitalization has been used as a form of crisis intervention by Galdston.[93] With the use of a mother substitute (a nurse, a nurse's aide, or a foster grandmother[174]), symptomatic improvement can result in several weeks. Therapeutic work with the parents by a social worker, pediatrician, or psychiatrist can often help to maintain gains after the child has been discharged from the hospital. In addition to improved physical health as a result of hospitalization, some older children benefit from the experience of relating to other children and adults outside the home, especially if the family has been disturbed or isolated. Not infrequently, previously unrecognized psychologic problems in a child with a predominantly physical illness may come to light as a result of a comprehensive evaluation done in a hospital setting, where the behavior of the child and the interaction with his parents can be observed at greater length and in more detail.

As Rose and Sonis[240] have pointed out, older children caught in a family crisis or engaged in a struggle for control with parents can frequently profit from the more neutral emotional climate of the hospital, and the family can, in the meantime, begin to work out its interactional problems. In such cases, if the family or some other financial resource can bear the cost, it may be prudent to keep the child in the hospital a few days or weeks longer in order to consolidate his initial gains. The use of pediatric hospitalization in an adolescent "suicidal crisis" is discussed in Chapter 28.

Planning Hospital Programs

Maintaining the tie between the child and his family is the central consideration and the most vital mental health need of the child while he is in the hospital. To maintain that tie, a "therapeutic alliance" must be formed between the parents and the hospital staff.

The staff must consider the needs of the parents as well as of the child and must strive to avoid feelings of rivalry with the parents and of possessiveness toward the child, which are so easy to fall into. If the parents are given the necessary emotional support, they can help not only their own child but other children as well. (However, parents must not be used as time savers for the hospital staff.)

The needs of the hospital staff must be kept in mind also, particularly their need for some uninterrupted time alone with the child to carry out certain diagnostic and treatment procedures. There are some procedures for which the presence of parents can be used constructively, such as the taking of blood and the induction of anesthesia. It is generally unwise for parents to be in or near the treatment room when major procedures are being carried out. Many parents are quite upset by the normal consequences of certain procedures—for example, by the child's vomiting when coming out of anesthesia—and they need a great deal of support and an individualized approach to the amount of participation they can offer in the child's care. The first contact with the admission staff, whether professional or clerical, is significant, and a warm and welcoming manner is important. Interpreters for Spanish-speaking families should be available if necessary.

Visiting Arrangements

Sir James Spence[271] developed the first mother-child unit in England more than 45 years ago. Today there is no reason why flexible visiting on a daily basis should not be permitted in pediatric units. In a controlled study completed long ago, Prugh and his colleagues[230] showed daily visiting to be effective in minimizing traumatic responses in school-age children. The danger of cross infection from hospital visitors has been shown to be minimal.[230,305] Unrestricted visiting (parents should not be considered visitors) is permitted in some units, and provision should be made for "living-in" by the mother (and at times the father) of children under 5 years of age. (The Platt Report[104] has recommended that such facilities be provided in all new hospitals constructed in England.)

Two controlled studies[38,80] have shown living-in to be the only truly effective preventive measure for hospitalized infants and preschool-age children. And animal studies[119] suggest that such practices are important for the child and for his parents. However, for a number of reasons, some parents cannot or do not wish to take full advantage of living-in or unrestricted visiting opportunities, and thus individualized planning about visiting should be part of the total therapeutic program. Flexible programs cannot be legislated into existence. They should be well planned and inaugurated gradually, not created by fiat. The hospital staff has to feel comfortable about unrestricted visiting and overnight stays and convinced of the importance of the therapeutic alliance, with due consideration to the needs of the patient, the parent, and the staff. If this is not the case, the programs will not work.

If unrestricted visiting is permitted, siblings also should have this privilege. A hospitalized child is often adversely affected by the absence of a sibling, sometimes only because he does not know what is happening to a brother or sister at home. A child may have feelings of guilt about an argument he had with his sibling just before he left for the hospital, and he may misinterpret the argument as a cause of his illness. Twins, especially, should see each other. If a child has had an accident in which a sibling was involved, he should be able to meet with the sibling and with the help of a staff member, talk out his feelings. If a baby brother or sister is born during the course of a long hospital stay, the mother should be able to bring the baby to visit the child. Siblings may be worried about the patient and seeing him may be important for their mental health, as well as for the good of the patient.

Arbitrarily limiting sibling visitors to children over 12 or 15 years of age is not justifiable. Several units have developed plans for visits by siblings 3, 4, or 5 years of age. If the child is ambulatory (at least 50% of the children in hospitals are), visits with family members in the outpatient area or in some other part of the hospital set aside for this purpose will help minimize the small risk of cross infection. This is not to deny that younger children should be checked for a history of recent exposure to contagious disease or that other precautions should be taken before they visit. Every hospital should have a visiting room and baby-sitting facilities. There are many imaginative ways in which such arrangements can be worked out once it is acknowledged that the solution of the problem using a truly family-centered approach[123] is important for the mental health of both the child and his family.

Flexible visiting arrangements are important in other ways. One or both parents may be able to come only in the evening, and they should be encouraged to visit then—not just permitted to do so. Significant benefits may be derived from visits by college or high-school students or other volunteers. Parents should be encouraged to be present at the child's bedtime, and they can be helpful in certain aspects of the child's care.

During hospitalization, a child's "life space" should be as wide as possible, and his ties with life outside the hospital should be maintained. Recreational, educational, and other relevant considerations must be kept in mind in planning hospital programs.

The Role of the Nurse

Over the years, changes in nursing education have emphasized the positive contributions the nurse can make to the emotional well-being of the hospitalized child, helping to meet his total needs, not just offer him physical care.[28,304,308] A more recent trend is toward "case assignment" rather than "task assignment," so that a nurse has a continuing relationship with the children under his or her care.

Nursing assistants and foster grandmothers now do many of the tasks formerly assigned to nurses. This is a positive development that permits the nurse to enjoy the professional aspects of meeting the patient's medical and human needs. Nurses learn much more about growth and development today than formerly, and they should be responsible for in-service training programs for other members of the hospital staff, from foster grandmothers to maids and janitors, since all these people have an impact on a child in the hospital setting. Besides having technical knowledge, the nurse must be able to communicate effectively and must develop empathy in dealing with sick and dying children and their parents. The head nurse, who is responsible for the smooth operation of the hospital ward, must be mature and capable. In some hospitals, when a child is admitted, his parents are asked to fill out a checklist that covers such items as the child's nickname, religion, eating, sleeping, and elimination habits, favorite toys, school grades, special interests or hobbies, favorite books, and the names and ages of his siblings. An example of such a checklist is listed under Appendix G in "Care of Children in Hospitals," published by The American Academy of Pediatrics.[8]

Nurses have also helped develop booklets for parents, and have helped make admission procedures more flexible, recognizing how important it is for the mother, with the support of one particular nurse, to accompany the child to the ward and help "settle him in" with a toy from home. In some hospitals, the child is permitted to wear his own clothes, and the nurses wear street clothes or colored smocks rather than the emotionally sterile white uniforms.

Nurses have encouraged early ambulation for the child (in carts if necessary). Being able to move around helps the child gain a feeling of mastery and stimulates his appetite. Nurses have also played a part in developing family-style eating arrangements, which provide a social experience, improve appetite, and hasten convalescence. Erickson[77] has developed a standardized doll play kit that includes toy transfusion sets and other equipment that can help nurses help children "play out" their feelings about hospital procedures and personnel, as well as about separation and other emotional experiences. Recently, nurse clinical specialists have made important contributions to clinical work and teaching of nurses in particular areas in pediatrics.

Recreational Programs

Recreation for the hospitalized child involves more than simply finding things for him to do which will keep him quiet and occupied, as important as that may be for the child who requires rest as a part of his total therapy. It is more important, however, that recreational activities provide the child with an outlet for his emotional tensions and an opportunity to master and work through the feelings aroused by his illness and hospital experience.[32,285] Play is a child's busy-ness,[213] and it is serious and purposeful as well as joyful.

A well-meaning but inexperienced volunteer "play-lady" is woefully equipped to organize an important program of this type, but in recent years, a variety of professional persons have developed skills and understanding which equip them to work in the recreational area in hospital settings. A nursery school teacher may be able to make a vital contribution to programs for preschool-age children, perhaps working together with an occupational therapist who has special experience in dealing with older children and adolescents. Nurses who have special training in child development have functioned effectively in this area, as have social group workers who have a special knowledge of group interaction and its therapeutic use. In the past two decades, the new discipline of recreation therapy has evolved, in which professionals are trained to work with hospitalized children.

An ideal program would be one based on developmental grouping.[206] Such a program, like the ones developed by Plank[216,217] and Azarnoff,[12] could include a nursery school teacher[39] for toddlers and preschoolers, an occupational therapist[230] for older children, and a social group worker[53,148] for adolescents and for special groups activity projects with school-age children. A recreational therapist working in close collaboration with the teacher would be the coordinator of the program. Such a program would necessitate that the nurses understand the respective contributions of the other professionals and that each nurse have an active and planned part in some phase of the program. Volunteers who can agree to a regular and moderately extensive commitment to such a program can be of real value, but only if they work under appropriate professional supervision.

Educational Programs

The teacher has a diagnostic and therapeutic role that goes beyond the part she plays in the hospitalized child's academic learning.[178] It is easier to see the benefits of a program designed to forestall disruption of the educational process in a long-term hospital setting, in which the child's life-space needs, including his need for academic advancement, are more clear-cut and are obviously pressing. However, the same needs are often present in the case of short-term hospitalization.

Although the number of children who openly ask for the help of a teacher in order to keep up with their school work during short-term hospitalization is not large, many children wish for such help, not only because they are worried about falling behind but also because the presence of a teacher provides them with a tie to their world outside the hospital. Thus it is appropriate and necessary to provide a teacher, and some professional or semi-professional teacher's assistants, in a short-term hospital unit even though the average length of stay is only 7 or 8 days.

An arbitrary rule that requires a child to have an anticipated hospital stay of a certain number of weeks or months before he is offered a teacher's services is out of touch with educational and psychologic realities. The same is true of archaic laws in some states that restrict the reimbursement for educational services provided by public schools to children hospitalized for physical illnesses. Such laws deny a vital experience to children admitted to the hospital for psychologic problems and, many times, force the physician to compromise his integrity by manufacturing a physical diagnosis. Laws of this kind ignore as well the relationship between physical and psychologic disorders discussed earlier.

The approach to education in a short-term hospital setting must be very different from that in a long-term unit. It should be standard procedure to ascertain the grade level of each child admitted, as well as pertinent details about the child, such as his academic performance, social relationships, acceptance of authority, and family background as perceived by the school. This information, which can usually be obtained from the child's classroom teacher, will help the teacher in approaching and working with the child and may lead to some diagnostic considerations that would otherwise be missed. The teacher should approach each child of school age even if the background information is available. In discussing the child's school and other experiences, the teacher may collect other data of diagnostic significance, and, more important, can learn of the child's educational concerns and offer a relationship with a familiar figure.

In working with a child who is hospitalized on a short-term basis, the teacher must be extremely flexible and creative. Even if the child is to be in the hospital for several weeks, the goal should not be a rigid one. That is, it should not be insisted that the child keep pace with his classmates. The emotional regression shown by physically sick children, particularly in response to the anxiety they have about hospital procedures, makes it impossible, at least initially, for them to learn as effectively as they would at home or in a regular classroom. In addition, the perceptual-motor difficulties that may be a feature of various illnesses, including systemic disorders unrelated to the central nervous system, may temporarily render learning difficult. This difficulty may be enhanced by regressive trends, which can themselves produce perceptual-motor problems.

In some instances, the child may spontaneously reach out to the teacher (rather than the nurse or other members of the medical staff) as the one person on the ward to whom he can relate. Such an attempt to establish a relationship should always be responded to, ideally by a person assigned to continue the relationship on a supportive basis. In such an instance, the teacher may function more as a recreational therapist at first, shifting to a more academic role later. In every case, the child should know from the first that the teacher is a teacher, and no attempt should be made to hide this fact in a misguided effort to prevent the child from becoming anxious or guilty about his inability to study or learn. The teacher can reassure the child by telling him that because of his illness, he is not quite ready for much instruction and that they will spend some time getting to know each other and will begin to do some school work together later, when he feels better.

The extent to which the teacher works with the child individually or draws him into a classroom group will, of course, depend on a number of variables, including the nature of his illness, his degree of physical mobility, and his ability to socialize (which may be affected detrimentally by his illness). Other factors, including the physical set-up, the number of patients, and the number of teaching assistants, must also be considered. If the child is ambulatory when he is admitted to the hospital, he can and should go directly into some type of group situation. This will provide a continuity of experience on the ward which will tie him to his past and his fu-

ture. If he is forced to remain in bed, the teacher may work with him individually. If he can be partially mobilized (in a wheelchair or a cart), the teacher can plan for him to join a group on a modified basis.

Classroom groups established in hospitals should ordinarily be smaller (not more than 6 to 8 children per teacher) and much more flexible in regard to planning and performance than in the regular school. Much mixing of age groups must take place, and the teacher must have special training and experience in adapting orthodox teaching techniques to these circumstances and the physical and psychologic limitations of the group members. The importance of coordinating conferences with other staff members and the need to apprise the teacher of the degree of activity and mental alertness she can expect from each child cannot be overemphasized. (This information should be given to all nonmedical professional personnel who have not been trained in a medical setting.) Schools of education are beginning to see the value of having teacher trainees work with physically ill or handicapped children as well as with emotionally disturbed children. The pediatrician in charge of the ward can often be of great help in arranging for an affiliation with a university department of education or a teachers college, thus offering such experience to students.

Hospitalization— A Learning Experience?

Much has been said[258,295] about hospitalization as a constructive learning experience for children. In my opinion, some of this thinking stems from an overly sentimental appraisal of the hospital setting. Of course, any new experience can be a learning experience for a child, but studies of children's reactions to hospitalization indicate that very few, if any, children find the hospital experience completely constructive. Some exceptions may be found among children who have special problems or who come from very poor homes. There is little doubt that most children would be better off emotionally if, as Sir James Spence has attempted to do, treatment could be carried out in the home. Recent studies of the hazards of adverse drug reactions in the hospital add other sober reflections.[33,194] Hospitalization can sometimes be avoided—and should be whenever possible—by judicious examination of the indications[208] and contraindications (including psychologic) and by greater use of home visits by medical and nursing personnel. Nevertheless, many children have serious illnesses that require the diagnostic and treatment facilities of a hospital.

When hospitalization is necessary for a child, the hospital staff should make the experience as positive and educational a one as possible while recognizing that a hospital cannot be a home.[223] With proper planning, the negative aspects of hospitalization can be minimized, and the total experience can be largely constructive for some children and partially constructive for others.

Coordination of Planning

It is estimated that at least 26 different people a day come in contact with a child in the hospital. The most basic challenge in the hospitalization of children is to coordinate the activities of these people. A weekly or a semi-weekly conference can provide the 5 Cs of ward management: coordination, communication, continuity of contact, collaboration, and consultation. These conferences should be chaired by a clinical director who is a senior pediatrician dedicated to patient care and who sees "patient-care research" (e.g., study of the effectiveness of certain kinds of inpatient and outpatient treatment methods) as a respectable, worthwhile activity. He also communicates with the pediatricians or

family physicians who may be involved in a case. A nonmedical person could perform these functions, but lacking the medical knowledge or the authority of the physician, he may encounter difficulties because of the hospital's status system. In some situations, an interdisciplinary "psychosocial" conference can be held without the pediatrician. He should be present, however, in order to add the full team quality of a true "ward management" approach, as is usually the case in an intensive care unit, burn unit, etc.

A ward management conference should include a review of the child's medical progress and his and his family's adjustment to the hospitalization. Observations of the child's behavior and of the parent-child interactions should be provided by the ward personnel, drawing on the janitor, maid, or ward volunteers if they have something to contribute. If the child's parents are not visiting him, perhaps out of guilt or fear of criticism, a visit to the home may be arranged. If the parents cannot visit, it can be arranged that they call the child or write him letters. If parents cannot be involved in preparing a child for a diagnostic or surgical procedure because of geographic or other problems, one nurse (or a person with whom the child has developed a good relationship) may be assigned to prepare the child and accompany him to the treatment or operating room and to be with him when he returns to his own room. This person should also be prepared to deal with the child's feelings about the parents' absence, and later with the parents' feelings as well. If the father has not visited a child who seems to need him, a visit can be arranged. Arrangements can be made for the child to have familiar toys and clothes from home. These objects serve as important "transitional objects"[313] in the process of separation-individuation.

In the case of children from special ethnic backgrounds, food prepared by the mother can be brought in.[225] If the child's condition permits, temperature, pulse, and respiration checks can be held to once daily. If a 2-year-old child resists a rectal thermometer, axillary temperature readings can be substituted. Rather than extruding demanding or hostile parents, as so often happens, the social worker or some other professional person can plan to work with these parents, helping them deal with their feelings of guilt.[251] Arrangements for volunteer help can be coordinated in ward management conferences. If mothers who are "living in" become ill, arrangements can be made for members of the hospital staff outside of the pediatric unit to handle this problem effectively. The principle of bringing the consultant to the child, rather than having the patient go from one consultative service to another, can be implemented in such a conference. Or with some preparation and support it can be planned for a mother to be with the child during some procedures.

If a child has a favorite live animal, it may be brought into the hospital. Bradford[37] in Rochester has shown that hamsters and other small animals can be kept in the hospital without danger to patients, and volunteer groups have brought larger animals to the hospital for children to play with. Other hospital routines can be changed if sufficient thought is given. If a physician or nurse with whom the child has an important continuing relationship goes on vacation, a substitute can be introduced. If a child is transferred to another ward, a familiar staff person can go with him and arrange tapering-off transitional visits.

The Hospital Management of Extremely Disturbed Children

Modern children's hospitals may need a small ward for children who have serious emotional problems and physical illness.[280] This psychiatric unit can be used flexibly, as are those at the Boston and Denver children's hospitals. Of course, it is of great importance that the nursing staff assigned to this unit be trained to deal with disturbed children and have access to appropriate consultants. With the use of a ward management conference and child psychiatrists and other mental health consultants, most children can be helped to deal with emotional problems in the usual pediatric ward setting. This includes some aggressive children, some who show acute anxiety or bizarre behavior, and some adolescents who have attempted suicide.[185,312] However, a separate ward is necessary for children who are too disturbed to be handled properly by the pediatric staff. These include children who become acutely delirious, those who have developed a psychosis while undergoing steroid therapy, extremely aggressive children, children who have severe psychophysiologic disorders, such as anorexia nervosa and ulcerative colitis, and children who may easily regress to borderline psychotic states which may involve extremely violent behavior. A relatively short stay in a psychiatric unit may enable many of these children to return to the pediatric ward.

In a children's hospital, the special psychiatric unit may be operated by the child psychiatry staff. In a general hospital, it may be an inpatient component of the child psychiatry division in the psychiatry department. In the latter, children from the pediatric ward who require temporary psychiatric care may be handled as "boarders" or may participate in the program as day patients. A few may require formal transfer to the child psychiatry inpatient service for longer-term care or other disposition. Preferably, the child psychiatry unit should be contiguous to the pediatric unit. Not only does this arrangement offer coordinated patient care, it also brings the child psychiatry staff into close contact with the pediatric staff and in touch with developments in clinical functions. "Curbstone consultation," teaching around crisis intervention, and participation by child psychiatrists in pediatric ward rounds[184] can be more readily arranged. Pediatric–psychiatric consultation liaison units with a suite of offices in pediatric settings, as at the University of Colorado Medical Center, or as described by Chess and Lyman,[46] offer constructive opportunities.[6,167,227]

Planning Hospital Construction

Drawing on some of the foregoing considerations, certain important points can be made about hospital planning.[8,257] Most of them apply principally to short-term hospital units although some may also apply to long-term hospital or institutional settings. Architects who are engaged in drawing up plans for pediatric facilities should work closely with medical and nursing personnel to achieve the goals discussed in the following pages. Flexibility, expansibility, convertability, and the concepts of "child-centered space" and family participation are some of the fundamental principles.

Inpatient Facilities

In regard to inpatient facilities, the following principles should be kept in mind:
1. There should be space for parents and children to visit comfortably and pleasantly. Small cubicles save space but cramp visiting. For ambulatory children, visiting can take place in large playrooms. There is some advantage in this type of arrangement, for the parents' own children and for other children whose parents are not present and who can benefit from the visit. Some privacy for family groups is essential, however. Thus multiple-bed units should have large enough cubicles to permit both parents to sit comfortably on chairs (not on the bed) and should have curtains that draw easily. Carpeting on hospital floors is more homelike and less expensive to maintain than is vinyl flooring.

2. Provision should be made for overnight stays or living-in by the mothers of infants and preschool-age children. The Platt report in England[104] stipulated that for every 20 patient beds there should be at least 4 beds for mothers. Some hospitals simply place a cot for the mother in a conventional single room, sometimes adding a dresser and an easy chair. The unit developed by Kempe at the University of Colorado provides a Pullman-type, pull-down bed for each of two parents in a double room for infants and preschool-age children. If distance permits, the mother can go home for visits with siblings. If it does not, the father may bring the other children to visit. At times, the mother and the patient may go home for weekends.

The English program decribed by MacCarthy[179] includes such features as a lounge and a central kitchenette, where mothers can prepare their own and some of their children's meals. Such facilities should not be too far from the ward since opportunities for frequent supportive contacts with mothers by the nursing staff are important. The Tufts–New England Medical Center has a "family participation unit," with "homelike" facilities where mothers can stay at no charge. The Care-by-Parent Unit at the University of Kentucky[128] is a ward where "minimally ill," largely ambulatory children can be cared for by their parents. No nurses are assigned, and therapeutic and diagnostic procedures are scheduled in advance, thus achieving a considerable reduction in costs. A full-time pediatrician directs the unit, and the parents can be taught how to handle some medical and other problems. Each room is equipped like a motel room, with a private bath, and a well-equipped utility room for the parents is available. Both parent and child are served meals in the room.

3. Age grouping of children and adolescents should be handled flexibly, both

because children need to interact with children of different ages and because it is impossible to predict day-to-day shifts in the ages of new patients. Nevertheless, the following broad considerations are applicable:

a. Newborn and premature units have their merits but they should include planned facilities for parent "rooming-in," as developed in the United States by Jackson[124] and others. Rooming-in can be accomplished by providing individual rooms or space in a special unit where babies can be near their mothers.

b. Rocking chairs should be provided for mothers of infants up to 1 year of age (these chairs can be used by nurses also). They lend a homelike touch and can provide comforting experiences for both infants and mothers.

c. Units for toddlers from 1 to about $1^1/_2$ years of age should have playpens or other protective arrangements for children who are not acutely ill. Beds that can be raised and lowered will protect against injuries and eliminate the need for nets or other protective devices that many children find upsetting.

d. Preschool-age children need special play areas adapted to their needs. Beds that can be raised and lowered can also be helpful for this age group; they eliminate the need for nets if the child is frightened or delirious.

e. School-age children have their own special needs for educational and recreational activities, as discussed earlier.

f. As the Platt report suggested, adolescents should have separate facilities, either in a special unit or in one part of the ward, including a room for group activities.[248]

In planning room units, the 2-to-4-bed unit seems to provide the necessary opportunity for social interaction without overstimulation. Individual cubicles afford privacy when needed. A few single rooms should be provided for seriously ill children in order to facilitate the special medical and nursing care they need and to minimize the impact on other children as well. The child's need for "ownership" should be respected, and drawers should be provided where he can keep his special belongings inviolate. It is no longer necessary that beds be grouped around the nurse's station; there should be enough nurses to move around among the patients' rooms.

Other Considerations. The following principles are also important in planning inpatient facilities:

1. There should be sound-proof treatment areas separate from living areas or play space. Special consideration should be given to traffic flow so that children on their way to treatment or operating rooms need not pass other patients or visitors.

2. Age-appropriate recreational space that is not used for treatment purposes is of great importance. Separate areas for preschool-age, school-age, and adolescent patients should be available in order to allow for appropriate programming and congregation by age group. Space should be provided for wheel toys for ambulatory preschoolers, group games for school-age children, and activity and lounge rooms for adolescents. Outdoor play space and equipment should be available as well. With proper coordination, some physical therapy or occupational therapy can be carried on in these settings; however, separate areas off the ward are required for specialized treatment. Age group separation should not be carried to the point where adolescents are not permitted to help in the care of younger children or to work in laboratories if they wish or to the point where other flexible arrangements could not be made.

3. There should be family-style eating ar-

rangements, possibly in play or recreational areas, for ambulatory children or children who can be mobilized in carts or wheelchairs.

4. Classroom facilities for school-age and adolescent age groups are essential. Some informal teaching can be done at the bedside or in the recreational areas. However, regardless of the amount of formal learning involved, even children hospitalized for short periods can benefit from moving from the bed to the classroom and from contact with the teacher, who is a representative of the world outside the hospital. Schoolrooms should have doors wide enough to admit the beds of chronically ill or handicapped children.

5. Space near the ward is needed for interviewing parents and older ambulatory children; it may include offices for social workers or psychologists. Rooms should be available for private interviews with ward physicians or consulting psychiatrists, for psychologic testing, and special examinations by neurologists and other consultants. A comfortable waiting space (and toilet facilities) should be provided for parents. Informal discussions may be carried on in these areas,[153] or more formal discussions may be carried on in a conference room.[98]

6. Meeting rooms are needed for ward management and other conferences. The main part of the discussion of ward rounds can take place in these rooms, thereby keeping bedside discussion of patients to the minimum necessary for examination and interviewing. Conference rooms should be sufficiently removed from living and play areas so that discussions cannot be overheard by children or parents, yet near enough to permit easy access to the patient who is to be presented or interviewed.

7. Office space and lounge areas for hospital staff should be close enough to the ward to permit quick responses to emergency calls but far enough away to permit the staff to relax without fear of being overheard by children or parents.

8. Day hospital facilities should be provided for local children who require long and complicated treatment programs. These facilities may be integrated with existing ward programs or may be separate for children with special types of handicaps. They may be tied in with outpatient programs as well.

9. The decor of pediatric facilities should be warm and should include appropriate pictures. The colors should be bright but not overstimulating. Light-brown, beige, creams, and light-yellow tend to degenerate quickly into "institutional buff," while dark colors can be depressing. Children can decorate their rooms and the hall walls with their own pictures; this is a constructive activity for which adequate provision should be made. Furniture should be as homelike as possible. Professional decorators who understand children should be consulted,[27] not volunteer artists.

Outpatient Facilities

Many of the principles discussed apply also to outpatient planning. Outpatient clinics should be supervised by an experienced clinical director and should be located in a central area. Specialty clinics should be nearby so that visiting and treatment may be coordinated. One person should be assigned the responsibility for continuity of care; that is, coordinating the use of outpatient and inpatient facilities and arranging for home care and appropriate community services. Some factors that warrant special considerations are as follows:

1. Adequate, attractive waiting space should be provided for parents and children. Seating is best broken up into small social units rather than arranged in long rows. Moveable chairs permit family units to segregate or interact as

desired. If the appointment system is effective, less space will be required, families will be happier, and the behavioral aspects of diagnosis will be more accurate than when the patient is observed after a long wait that has left him fatigued and resentful.

The waiting area should be close enough to the clinical offices so that the pediatrician, the nurse, and the clerical personnel can observe how the child behaves toward his parents, other adults, and other children. Toilet facilities should be immediately adjacent.

2. Both indoor and outdoor play space and facilities should be located near the waiting area. In addition to reading materials, shelves of toys should be provided in a sheltered corner of the waiting room. During the waiting period, skilled nursery school teachers or recreational therapists can help young children by engaging them and their parents in discussion of their concerns and fears while observing the behavior and the physical capacities of the patients.[10,116] Many years ago, Elizabeth Staub, a pioneer in the field, established an observation nursery in a well-child unit,[276] and Green[105] has suggested that such a unit be incorporated into hospital ambulatory services. Clinical nurse specialists in child development and other professionals can help in developing a parent education program.

3. For adolescents, there should be a separate entrance, waiting space, and examining area whose decor is suited to adolescents.

4. The examining rooms should be sufficiently soundproof to insure privacy. They should be large enough to permit a small child some room to play while the parents give the history, and there should be enough chairs to accommodate both parents and any other family members present. Some play materials should be kept in a cupboard in each examining room, and a small table and

chair should be provided so that the development of older infants and young children can be evaluated.

5. Treatment rooms should be soundproof and sufficiently removed from the waiting areas and the examining and conference rooms that procedures can be carried out without disturbing other patients or parents. Simple immunizations, blood counts, and other uncomplicated procedures can be done in the examining rooms, ordinarily with the parents present. However, there should be a waiting area somewhat near the treatment room so that parents may wait not too far from the child when more complicated procedures are necessary.

6. Conference rooms should be sufficiently removed from waiting or examining areas so that patients will not overhear discussions taking place.

7. Adequate office facilities should be provided for medical, nursing (clinical and public health), and social work staff, for individual psychologic testing, and for interviewing by psychiatrists and other kinds of consultants.

8. Ideally, motel-type facilities should be adjacent to the clinic. As Green[106] pointed out, such facilities can be used for the child also if actual hospitalization is not necessary (as in the case of an ambulatory child undergoing diagnostic study of a congenital abnormality). Siblings or other family members could stay in such facilities. These facilities also can be tied in with a day hospital program and with baby-sitting provisions.

Green[106] developed the Baxter Parent-Care Pavilion at the Riley Hospital in Indianapolis. There family-centered health care is offered that combines the medical care of the child with the health needs of the parents and other siblings. Green points out that the parent-care unit should not be isolated, even if it is a separate building. Rather it should be integrated with other ambulatory medical, developmental, and rehabilitative services. Although economy may be a welcome by-product of this innovative approach, it is not its primary justification. In fact, with the necessary supporting services, there may be little difference in the per diem cost.

The Children's Inn at the Children's Medical Center in Boston is a modern motel, separated from the hospital. In this facility, parents of hospitalized patients are offered accommodations at low cost. When the child is able to leave the hospital, he may remain at the inn with his parents during convalescence. The inn is managed for the medical center by the Marriott corporation, an example of innovative cooperation between private enterprise and voluntary hospitals.

9. Emergency room facilities should include rooms where children may stay overnight for observation or brief treatment. These should be combined with facilities where the mother can remain overnight if the patient is an infant or a very young child.

Alternatives to hospitalization should be taken whenever possible. Day care can be planned for children who have chronic illnesses or diagnostic problems which do not require hospitalization. Greater use can be made of home care[168] if a "family team"[20] is available for this purpose. A controlled study by Shrand[266] in England indicates that such an approach to the treatment of young children reduces the amount of anxiety, regression, and depression.

The Surgical Experience

The possibility that children will show deleterious emotional responses to surgical experiences was noted by Langford[158] in 1937 and by Pearson[212] in 1941. Such responses in adult patients were described by Lindemann[169] in 1941, by Deutsch,[62] in 1942, and by Menninger[196] in 1946. Levy's[164]

classic paper, published in 1945, and the studies on children's reactions to tonsillectomy by Jessner and her colleagues[135] and by Faust and his colleagues in the early 1950s[81a] crystalized professional interest in this important question. In the 1950s, articles dealing with the recognition and management of traumatic emotional reactions in children appeared in pediatric[44] and otologic[136] journals, and in the Ross Conference report on the nonoperative aspects of pediatric surgery.[222,283] A chapter on this subject by Loomis,[173] a child psychiatrist, was included in a major textbook on pediatric surgery, and a book, *The Surgeon and the Child*, by Potts,[219] a leader in pediatric surgery, was published. In 1958, the *American Journal of Surgery*[85] carried an article by a child psychiatrist dealing with consultative contributions in liaison with a children's surgical service, and several other articles have been published more recently in psychiatric periodicals.[96,121,170] By the 1960s this topic was beginning to be discussed in journals for general practitioners,[127] surgeons,[102] and research nurses.[180]

Although articles dealing with the reactions of children and families to illness and hospitalization have appeared in surgical journals, including the *Journal of Pediatric Surgery*, in my experience, many general surgeons, who do much children's surgery, and even some pediatric surgeons, are not familiar with the literature. Perhaps because of the nature of their work, surgeons may find it more difficult to spend as much time with their patients as do physicians in other specialty fields. Yet a number of leading pediatric surgeons do show extraordinary understanding and concern for the emotional well-being of children and parents. In my opinion, with the recent extension of psychiatric consultation–liaison programs to surgical services, other surgeons can and should learn much more about this vital aspect of the art of surgery, which, in addition to preventing emotional problems that can affect recovery, may even have some bearing on morbidity and mortality.

General Reactions of Children to Surgery

The reactions of children to surgery are often very similar to their reactions to hospitalization and medical procedures. However, since surgery is a definite event for which the child is usually admitted to a hospital, a separate discussion is warranted. Perhaps it is best to discuss the surgical experience in three phases: preoperative, operative, and postoperative (as Hackett and Weisman[111] have done in discussing the surgical experience of adults). (Toker[287] and Reinhart and Barnes[234a] have prepared the most complete reviews of the literature concerning surgery in children. This literature deals especially with open-heart surgery.)[1,7]

In the preoperative phase, a variety of reactions have been described in children and adults. Anxiety of varying degrees, panic reactions, denial, depression, psychophysiologic symptoms, and regressive/aggressive and overly dependent or passive behavior have been observed. Kimball[147] has reduced the 6 groups of adult reactions described by Kennedy and Bakst[144] to 4 groups:

1. The adjusted group, made up of patients whose level of functioning in the past, in the period immediately preceding hospitalization, and at the time of surgery was judged to be realistic and coping. Such patients were usually able to express some anxiety and even fear of dying; their defenses appeared intact, however, and they expressed confidence about the outcome of surgery and their future life.
2. The symbiotic group, made up of patients who had adapted to their illness and who were living in a "symbiotic" relationship with it, with unconscious secondary gains related to long-time dependence on parents, spouses, or other key figures.
3. The anxious group, made up of patients who had generally coped adequately. They had used much denial, but at the time of the operation this defense seemed shaky. They could not verbalize their anxiety, but they showed hyperalertness, hyperactivity, suspicion, and often sleeplessness.
4. The depressed group, made up of patients who had often had difficulty coping. Although they used some denial, they had difficulty in verbalizing anxiety and they were clinically depressed, had little orientation toward the future, and often openly expressed fears that they would not survive.

Reinhart and his colleagues divided their patients, aged 5 to 14 years, into 3 groups: (1) a severely anxious group, made up of children who showed frequent overactive motor or verbal behavior or, occasionally, marked constricted behavior, (2) a mildly anxious group, made up of children who showed a capacity to socialize and to verbalize some anxiety but not fear of dying, and (3) a coping group, made up of children who could verbalize or play out mild anxiety and fear reasonably comfortably. The majority of the children who were not accepting of surgery were in the severely anxious group.

In Kimball's and Kennedy and Bakst's groupings, correlations could be established between preoperative reactions and outcomes in the operative phase. Mortality was highest in the depressed group and was next highest in the anxious group. Reinhart and his colleagues observed individual children who were extremely fearful, agitated, and at times openly depressed. These children expected to die during cardiac surgery, and actually did die during induction of anesthesia or during the operation itself.

In a prospective study of 72 adults scheduled to undergo open-heart surgery, Kilpatrick and his colleagues[146] administered a battery of tests, including intellectual and personality tests and neuropsychologic tests with instruments. The patients were also rated as to the degree of cardiac impairment. Statistical evaluation of these data enabled these investigators to identify in advance all the fatalities and nearly 90% of the survivors.

During the postoperative period, vomiting, delirium (often transient and often seen only at night), depression, fear of doctors, other psychologic reactions complicating convalescence (e.g., conversion symptoms and negativistic, overly dependent, or disruptive behavior), and even psychotic disorders have been described in adolescents and adults. Children seem to have a lower incidence of postoperative delirium[71] and psychoses. Postoperative delirium is poorly understood, but, like psychosis, it seems to be related more to preoperative personality[36] and family problems than to drugs or electrolyte disturbances although these can be involved (at times in an interactive fashion with anterospective psychosocial variables). In one study of adults,[290] depression in the postoperative period involved a high risk of operative death which could not be accounted for solely on the basis of a worsened cardiac status. In another prospective study, Throughman and his colleagues,[284] using personality rating scales, were able to predict significantly both successful and unsuccessful postoperative outcomes in surgery for patients who had intractable peptic ulcer.

Reactions to Anesthesia. Relatively few systematic studies have been done on the reactions of children to loss of consciousness during anesthesia.[126] The available data indicate that young preschool-age children react adversely to the strangeness of the induction area and the operating room. The absence of the mother is the factor causing the greatest stress.[294] Many children resist being held down. Jessner[133] has indicated that older preschool-age and school-age children may fear that they will

do or say "something bad" when they are not in control and that they may also be concerned about what may be done to their bodies while they are helpless. Some children are afraid that they will awaken before the operation is over; others may interpret the onset of unconsciousness as impending death.

Bothe and Galdston[34] noted difficult inductions (i.e., those involving loud crying, shouting, or physical resistance) in 14% of children 4 to 14 years of age, and excited or delirious emergence in 13% of children from 3 to 9 years of age. In a similar study, Smessaert[267] reported an excited or delirious emergence in 8% of children from 10 to 17 years of age. The incidence of difficult inductions and excited emergences is undoubtedly influenced by the type and amount of premedication,[239] the anesthetic used, the child's developmental level, and a number of other factors, such as the meaning of the operation to the child, his previous adaptive capacity, the parent-child relationship, the child's previous experience with anesthesia, the psychologic preparation, and even the personality of the anesthesiologist.

Since oral barbiturates may have a stimulant effect on young preschool-age children unless given in large doses, Smith[268] and others recommend the use of basal anesthetics (e.g., thiopental) for children of all ages in order to relax the child before he is taken to the operating room.

Long ago, Jackson,[125] a pediatric anesthesiologist, adopted the practice of visiting the child in his room on the day before the operation, accompanying him to the operating room, explaining the mask and other instruments, and providing personal support during induction in order to reduce possibility of emotional trauma. In a controlled study, Jackson showed that these methods were effective in cutting down the amount of anesthesia necessary and in ameliorating postoperative reactions, such as vomiting. (More recently, special nursing support[69] has also been shown to be effective in diminishing post-operative vomiting.) A controlled study by Schulman and his colleagues[252] demonstrated that the mother's presence during the induction of anesthesia significantly reduced fear, aggression, and other mood responses in children from 2 to 5 years of age, and the mothers themselves were not significantly disturbed. The greatest difference between the responses of the two groups—those with their mothers and those separated from their mothers—came at the time of greatest stress, when the mask was held above the child's face. Swenson[283] has indicated that allowing the young child to sit up in a nurse's arms during induction rather than making him lie down and feel helpless, and using play methods in administering the anesthesia results in much less crying and fighting. The induction is smoother, and there is less bronchial secretion and possibly less respiratory irregularity.

Considerations of this kind apply not only to psychosocial responses but also to the question of the *margin of safety*. Although, as Janis[130] has suggested, some anticipatory anxiety, with appropriate preparation, may be beneficial in facing surgical procedures, marked anxiety may significantly raise the sedation or anesthesia threshold,[256] while at the same time reducing the margin of safety in patients who have serious heart disease or other debilitating conditions. Price and his colleagues[220] showed that in adults urinary corticoid levels were elevated in preoperative states, and they believed that especially high levels were associated with poor psychologic defenses. Reinhart and his colleagues[234a] showed that 17-hydroxycorticosteroid levels were elevated preoperatively in children, and they were able to demonstrate elevated levels later—when the sutures were removed and even on return visits. McFarlane and Biggs[188] have reported that preoperative anxiety and fear in adults seemed related to "spontaneous" fibrinolysis which occurred in 14% of a group of

patients; they suggest that this phenomenon is part of the "alarm" reaction (discussed elsewhere in the book). Many more studies of this important topic are needed, particularly in regard to children and, as Reinhart and his colleagues emphasized, in regard to the family also.[72]

Some problems regarding the responses of children and families to the experience of anesthesia remain unresolved. The majority of studies to date have described the types of morbidity observed in a significant number of children. However, the inferences are inconclusive. For example, one study indicated that routine operative experiences had little effect on children.[59] In another study, the responses of adults undergoing mitral surgery[198] were found to be little different from responses to other types of surgery although the investigators speculated that the study itself could have had a prophylactic effect. For a variety of reasons, systematic long-term follow-up investigations have been difficult to carry out. The percentage of patients who have continuing responses of an emotionally traumatic nature is hard to estimate although anecdotal reports and retrospective studies suggest that the incidence of this type of reaction to anesthesia is at least as high as, if not higher than, reactions to hospitalization. Even mortality studies, both retrospective and predictive, involve relatively small groups of patients. Nevertheless, in my opinion, the various clinical and neuroendocrine investigations I have cited lead to several valid conclusions: (1) anesthesia has a stressful effect on children at physical, psychologic, and social levels, (2) the child's response differs in accordance with his developmental patterns, and (3) there is some overlapping in stress deriving from the preceding illness and hospitalization.

Such distinguished pediatric surgeons as Gross and Swenson are reluctant to subject a markedly depressed or anxious patient to an elective surgical procedure, particularly a physically taxing procedure, such as a colectomy or open-heart surgery, without preparatory psychotherapy or other specially supportive measures. Outstanding cardiologists, such as Nadas,[205] have felt that preparative and supportive measures during cardiac catheterization help to minimize the effects of anxiety on cardiac functioning and management. Bothe and Galdston[34] (and I) feel that psychiatric consultation is indicated if a child cannot talk about impending anesthesia and surgery, and Haller[113] has urged consideration of the emotional reactions of children who are to undergo surgical treatment for physical trauma. Swenson[283] and other pediatric surgeons believe that in-hospital play programs and other methods of preparation are vital for children scheduled for surgery. Correction of minor surgical problems on a day-case basis,[161] with appropriate preparation of the child and his parents, and the development of day surgical units (as in the Denver Children's Hospital) are steps toward avoiding the potential trauma and risks of hospitalization, with a not-incidental cost saving.

Preparation for Surgery

In preparing a child and his parents for surgery, one should know in advance certain things about both the child and his parents. If the child, his parents, or other close relatives have previously undergone surgery (or hospitalization), it is important to determine the nature of the child's (and the parents' or relatives') reaction to the experience. The nature of the family's normal adaptive equilibrium should be known generally, as should the nature of the parent-child relationship and the child's adaptive capacity. This last may be one of the most important factors in determining the child's response. Thus in preparing a child for major surgery the surgeon should take a history and make an evaluation of the whole child—not just an organ system— if he is to avoid morbidity and possibly death. If a clinical study reveals that the family

equilibrium is disturbed or chaotic or if the study suggests that the parent-child relationship is unhealthy, preoperative psychiatric consultation is indicated. If the child is markedly agitated, fearful, openly depressed, or expects to die, if he is manifestly severely anxious despite the use of denial, or if he cannot talk at all about the procedure or shows no response, psychiatric consultation is urgently needed. In emergency situations, the psychiatric consultant may recommend special preparatory psychologic measures; if the operation is elective, he may recommend that it be postponed and that the child undergo preparatory or intensive psychotherapy of suitable duration.

The approach to preparation of the child (and his family) for elective surgery by the surgeon,[52] anesthesiologist,[125] pediatrician,[193,195] nurse,[303] or child psychiatrist[49,287] has been discussed in a number of publications. Particular approaches used in preparing children include the use of puppet shows,[88] explanations of hospital equipment,[217] and the use of motion pictures.[293] It has been recommended[135] that school-age children be admitted to the hospital a day before the operation in order to permit them to adjust to the ward staff and setting. In a controlled study by Brain and Maclay[38] disturbances in behavior in preschool-age children who had been hospitalized for tonsillectomy were significantly reduced if the mothers were permitted to remain in the hospital with the children. Vaughn,[292] a child psychiatrist in England, demonstrated in a controlled study that a preoperative interview helps to reduce deleterious responses in school-age children undergoing eye surgery. In controlled clinical nursing experiments, Mahaffy[180] and Skipper and her colleagues[264] concentrated preparatory and supportive intervention on the mothers rather than on the children. The mothers who received such special information and emotional support in caring for their children had significantly less distress and felt more satisfied and helpful than did the control mothers. Their children showed less emotional distress, better adaptation and recovery (in terms of behavioral ratings, blood pressure and pulse at stress points, length of time to first voiding, emesis in the recovery room and amount of fluid intake), as well as fewer behavioral problems on returning home than did control children.

In a major recent study,[303] Visintainer and Wolfer, a nurse and a psychologist, provided a partial replication and extension of the two studies just cited. These investigators provided information and emotional support for both the parents and children during periods of stress. The results of their study supported the findings of Mahaffy and Skipper that children and parents show less emotional distress and better adjustment if supportive intervention is offered.

Visintainer and Wolfer went further in an effort to ascertain whether it was the information giving and play rehearsal or the emotionally supportive and trusting relationship between the nurse and the child that provided the stress-reducing effects observed in the experimental intervention. To answer this key question, they divided children (aged 3 to 14) who were to undergo minor elective surgery and their parents into 4 groups:

1. A stress-point preparation group, in which a single nurse gave information and emotional support to the children and their parents (using play techniques for younger children), at 6 critical times: on admission, before blood tests, late in the afternoon, before preoperative medication, before transport to the operating room, and on return from the recovery room.
2. A single-session preparation group, in which information, support, and play rehearsal if indicated were offered to the child and his parents only shortly after admission.
3. A consistent supportive care group, in which a nurse gave warm support and reassurance to the child and his

parents at the 6 critical times listed in No. 1, answering questions but providing no other information or play opportunities.
4. A control group, in which the routine preoperative procedures only (e.g., blood tests and preoperative medications) were offered by any nurse without special support or preparation except on specific request or unless problems arose. In this group, the anesthesiologist did not routinely see the parents or child preoperatively, and the parents were not permitted to accompany the child to the operating room. Contact with the surgeon occurred late in the afternoon after surgery.

The children's responses were measured by a nurse observer, using (1) pretested and reliable "manifest upset" scales and cooperation scales, (2) blind measures of medications the children needed in the recovery-room, and the ease of the children's fluid intake. In addition, standardized and reliable questionnaires designed to evaluate the child's posthospital behavior and adjustment were sent to the parents. The parents' experiences during their children's hospitalization were assessed with the use of an information questionnaire, an anxiety questionnaire, and a satisfaction questionnaire. Comparisons of ratings by age groups indicated that younger children showed more negative responses in the hospital and after discharge than did older children although there were significant differences relating to birth order, sex, or the socioeconomic status of the family.

Overall, the results of the study supported the thesis that systematic preparation and support increase children's cooperation, decrease their disturbed behavior and problems in posthospital adjustment, and result in less anxious, better informed, and more satisfied parents. The response to the combination of information and consistent supportive care offered in the stress-point preparation group was significantly superior to the responses observed in the other three groups. These findings therefore suggest that even for younger children, a need for information and a desire to maintain control over the environment are important factors underlying reactions to stressful stimuli. They also support the thesis that parents need preparation and understanding to help them respond positively to their children's behavior and needs.

In this study, single-session preparation was less effective overall than stress-point preparation. This finding is difficult to square with Vaughn's findings (mentioned earlier). But Vaughn's interviews may have been different, and his subject population did not include younger children. In general the findings of Visintainer and Wolfer are in agreement with results of earlier studies of hospitalized children and their families, and they ratify the thesis that systematic preparation and support afford substantial benefit to both child and parent.

As stated earlier, in preparing the child for elective surgical procedures the physician should include a careful assessment of the previous adaptive capacity of both the child and his parents.[226] The child's capacity to master anxiety depends on his adaptive capacity, his developmental level, and his available defenses. The adaptive capacity of each parent, the character of the parent-child relationship, and the previous and current family adaptive equilibrium are also important. The type of surgical approach, the particular parts of the body involved, the related fears and fantasies of the child and his parents, and the meaning the surgical procedure has for them in relation to immediately antecedent and distant past events also influence the child's response. Of course, preparation for surgery also includes preparation for hospitalization unless day surgery can be done.

For the preschool-age and early school-age child, explanations should be simple,

concrete, and brief, and presented no more than a week or so in advance. This will permit time for questions and the mobilization of defenses, but not so much time that excessive anxiety builds up. Procedures should be described in terms appropriate to the child's developmental level, and the child should also be told of the sensory experiences he will undergo. The child can be asked what he thinks will happen. That will provide an opportunity to correct any misconceptions, using the child's own words. For a tonsillectomy, for example, the young child can understand that his tonsils are "little lumps" in his throat that make his throat sore, that he does not need them, and that taking them out will make his throat get better. His throat will hurt for a little while after the operation.[102] The child should be permitted and encouraged to ask as many questions as he wants, both before and after surgery. Many older children can understand better if a simple drawing is used. If the child does not ask questions, he should be asked if he has any; usually fears and concerns will then be uncovered. Preschool-age and early school-age children should be told, even if they do not ask, that "nothing else" will be done or "taken out" during surgery. It is important that the child feel the operation is necessary. Surprise and confusion should be avoided as much as possible, and the child should have time to build his defenses.[215]

Real equipment and toy equipment can be used to demonstrate procedures in advance. Puppet shows and puppet "therapy" also help to prepare the child for coming procedures. Special equipment, such as masks for anesthesia, intravenous equipment, and traction apparatus, can be demonstrated in the shows. This type of preparation can be offered individually or on a group basis. The person putting on a puppet show should know how much each patient knows about why he is in the hospital and what part of his body is sick, what his family has told him, and what questions he has. If other units, such as physical therapy, occupational, or intensive care units, are to be used during the treatment program, it should be arranged for the child and his parents to visit these areas and to ask any questions they may have. School-age children can be helped to adjust to the ward and staff by being admitted a full day in advance of an elective operation. But early admission does not ordinarily help preschool-age children, because they have a more limited understanding and greater separation anxiety.[135]

As for painful medical procedures (including catheterization, lumbar punctures, venipunctures, etc.), the child should be told that he will have some pain, without minimizing or exaggerating it. Ideally the person carrying out the procedure should tell the child when and where he will feel pain, and should encourage him to express his feelings about it (e.g., "It's all right to cry"). Very young children cannot be expected to cooperate voluntarily, and firm but kindly restraint is often necessary. One should try to assure the young child that the doctor and nurse are working together to get the procedure done with as little pain as possible. An appropriate explanation often helps older children achieve a sense of mastery and control when undergoing a procedure in which pain can be expected.

Preparation for surgery should include a special explanation of possible presurgical and postsurgical experiences. Preoperative medication, induction of anesthesia, and recovery states should be thoroughly explained. Preschool-age children feel much more secure if a familiar person—a nurse or, ideally, his mother—accompanies him to the anesthesia room and is present during the induction and recovery periods. Some children need reassurance that they will not awaken before the surgical procedure is completed. Others may mistake the onset of unconsciousness for impending death, and need to be told in advance that the induced sleep is only temporary and will be followed by awakening and re-

covery. Here again, the child's questions are the best guide to his specific fears. Postoperative pain, confusion, and the necessary restrictions of activity should also be discussed and explained. The difference between the anesthetic mask and the oxygen mask which may be used during the recovery should also be pointed out.

It is difficult for younger (and some older) children to understand special postoperative procedures, such as tracheostomy, deep suctioning, or the use of a pacemaker.[63] If these procedures will be performed, the child should be forewarned and told that he will be helped to understand any special problems. Such an approach avoids too much preoperative anxiety, and reassures the child that the staff will be ready to help him whenever necessary.

At all levels of preparation, the physician can rely on the child's need to share and confide his feelings about things to come. A positive relationship between the parents and the doctor and nurse will make it possible for the younger child to extend to them the confidence he has in his parents and to talk openly without a conflict of loyalty. Older children may use the same process, but may form an independent alliance with the staff more easily. When an atmosphere of trust and understanding exists, the staff, parents, and child can work together in a therapeutic alliance to prepare the child for what may be a painful and frightening experience. The pediatrician should make sure that appropriate preparation takes place, no matter whether he, the surgeon, or a nurse carries it out.

Case Example. A 5-year-old boy watched a boy puppet receive a shot and have a mask placed over its face. The puppeteer explained that the mask would not hurt the puppet but that something that smelled sweet would put the puppet to sleep. It was said that after the operation, a tonsillectomy, the puppet would wake up and be all right although his throat would hurt somewhat and he would feel funny for a little while. The boy played for some time with the mask, placing it on the puppet's face and finally on his own. The play seemed to help him feel less anxious and uncertain. The next day the preoperative medication and anesthesia induction went well although the boy's mother could not be present. When the boy woke up in the recovery room, however, he screamed in alarm when the nurse was about to place an oxygen mask on his face. When the use of the oxygen mask was explained to the boy, he gradually calmed down and accepted the procedure. It was later learned the boy feared something had gone wrong with the operation and that the mask would put him back to sleep.*

The indications for psychiatric preparation for surgery were discussed earlier. Children may also require mental health consultation and treatment for problems that arise postoperatively. A child psychiatrist, child clinical psychologist, or social worker can frequently help the physician and other staff members understand and manage the problems of the child and his family that interfere with the child's recovery or convalescence. In my experience, brief daily visits with the child and his family are more effective than longer but less frequent visits. Daily communication should be maintained between members of the hospital staff and the mental health worker with regular group ward management meetings chaired by a senior surgical staff member. Group meetings with children and with parents can also be helpful in airing fears and fantasies, in discussing ward policies, and in other ways.

Case Example. A 9-year-old boy was referred to the hospital's child psychiatry consultant because he had intense chronic anxiety, marked apprehension about new experiences, and a number of fears, including the fear of dying. The boy was to be operated on for a patent ductus arteriosus, and the pediatric surgeon was worried about the boy's reaction to the impending surgery. The boy was seen in weekly sessions for 3 months; he underwent psychotherapy that focused on his fear of surgery and death. A technique suggested by Levy[164] for anxious preschool-age children was used. It was

arranged that the boy receive thiopental as a basal anesthetic in his room with his mother present. The child psychiatrist assured the boy that he would accompany him to the operation, would remain with him throughout the operation, would come back with him to his room, and would be there with the mother when the boy awakened. While the boy was in the anesthesia room, another patient, who had a congenital cardiac abnormality, died suddenly on the operating table, presumably of a vasovagal crisis, and the surgeon felt emotionally unable to operate on the boy. When the boy awoke, he was told that he had not been operated on because another patient had died, but that the patient had a different kind of heart abnormality with special complications. The psychiatrist was concerned about the boy's possibly adverse reaction to the postponed surgical experience, but the previous preoperative procedures were repeated, and the boy underwent the surgery without any immediate ill effects. Postoperatively, he expressed fear that his heart would not work right, and he complained of weakness and chest pain. Supportive psychotherapy was instituted after his discharge, primarily because of conflict between the parents about his activity level. Later, he and his parents underwent more intensive long-term psychotherapy for his longstanding personality problems.

Special problems may arise in connection with any type of surgical intervention, but particularly following operations in which a body part is removed or lost (as in an amputation) or in which a body part is added or substituted (as in a renal transplantation). These and other special problems are discussed in the rest of the chapter.

Reactions of Children to Amputation

Although many studies of adult reactions to amputation have been reported over the years,[211,233] studies that cover the responses of children to loss of a visible body part are more limited and are of recent origin.[43,117,137,218,260,277,309]

According to reports in the literature the child's developmental level at the time of injury is especially important. Children as young as 3 years of age, who have a fairly well-formed self-concept but a still-shaky body image, must integrate the change

*This material was adapted from a chapter by Eckhardt, L.O., and Prugh, D.G.: Preparing children psychologically for painful medical and surgical procedures. In E. Gellert, Ed.: *The Psychosocial Aspects of Pediatric Care.* New York: Grune & Stratton, 1978.

brought about by amputation into their mental picture of themselves and should experience some mourning for the lost part of themselves. This crisis is, of course, more challenging to school-age children and adolescents, who have a more fully established although still evolving body image and who are engaged in finding their place in their peer group.[43] The phasic responses to catastrophic injury or illness are, of course, involved; initial denial and regression is more prominent in younger children. The school-age child must struggle with feelings of inferiority and inadequacy,[137,260] while the adolescent must grapple with feelings of dependence, doubts about his sexual attractiveness, and fears about how his handicap will affect his vocational and other life aspirations.[277,309] Guilt about an accident affects all ages, and the parents' phasic responses profoundly affect the child's attitude toward himself.[117]

The phantom limb phenomena[149] and postmastectomy "breast phantoms"[131] that occur in adults are uncommon in children and adolescents, although they may occur.[261]

Strenuous denial at any age, depressive equivalents (e.g., hyperactivity, apathy, and aggression), and open depression in adolescents may interfere with their acceptance of prosthetic devices or rehabilitative measures. The child and his parents must be allowed time for denial to give way to mourning and for restitution and compensation to begin before the use of a prosthesis is urged. Considerations such as these have led me and others to the conclusion that most, perhaps all, children who are about to undergo a planned amputation should have psychiatric consultation and a month or two at least of preparation. Plank[218] and Healy[117] have described such an approach using prosthesis dolls (they are helpful but not necessary). Other children, such as those who have experienced a traumatic amputation, may also require consultation and psychotherapy.

Case Example. A girl suffered a traumatic loss of her left arm in an automobile accident at age 3 years, 8 months. She was said to have fallen through the rusted floor boards of her mother's station wagon while the car was moving. The mother said that she did not know that the girl had fallen through the floor until she looked in her rear view mirror and saw the girl lying in the road. The girl lost her entire left arm up to the shoulder. She was taken to the emergency room for the amputation, and she subsequently spent several weeks in the hospital.

The mother contacted the psychiatric clinic 6 weeks after the accident. The mother seemed to be expressing a blandness and lack of concern about the problems that were likely to develop in the child as a result of the experience. But the mother seemed to be quite eager to visit the clinic herself, and the focus at the time of the evaluation shifted to her own very intense needs for help in this situation and also for her chronic depression, which had exacerbated around the time of the accident.

Although the problem was alleged to be the girl's difficulty in accepting the loss of her arm and her refusal to accept a prosthesis (a prosthesis had been fitted during the evaluation), the mother stated that the girl had no trouble with adjustment. She felt the girl seemed to accept the loss although physicians in the amputee clinic at Children's Hospital and her own pediatrician, as well as other individuals involved, stressed that the girl was showing serious denial and that her mother was having trouble helping her accept what had taken place.

The mother tended to deny that her daughter had any significant problems connected with the accident or that the girl had earlier shown evidence that suggested that she was somewhat hyperactive and accident prone. (The girl had again and again gotten into situations in which she got hurt, she had had 2 or 3 incidents of accidental poisoning, and she had had several serious falls.)

In the evaluation, the girl seemed to be an extremely hyperactive but sensitive child who was having significant difficulties in integrating the accident in terms of her own experience and in being able to use her mother to get some support through this difficult time. She had had unclear speech for the last year, and she had been placed in a preschool language development program. She seemed to be a rather pleasant and likeable youngster and she seemed to have the capacity to relate.

The girl was seen weekly in play therapy, beginning 3 months after the accident. Initially, therapy focused on helping her accept the fact that her arm was irreparably lost. Throughout the therapy, her play focused on being in the hospital, building hospitals, and babies' getting sick, and hurt and damaged. When children pointed at her artificial arm and asked what it was, she finally began to talk about it. She became able to talk about her feelings and to be more open about her anger and sadness about losing a part of herself. Her therapy centered on her bringing out her anger at people for not being taken care of and on becoming able to talk about her own hospital experience and how frightening it was. She was finally able to deal with her anger and her rage at her mother for allowing her to get hurt. The mother was initially seen periodically by the child's therapist, but later she asked for a therapist of her own to help her with her dependency and other problems. She talked about her feelings of guilt about the accident, and then she seemed to be able to talk with her daughter and to help her deal with her problems. At the present time, the girl uses her prosthesis appropriately. She is in the first grade. She has some mild educational problems but no social problems. In conjunction with her treatment, there were numerous contacts and conferences with the surgeon, pediatrician, amputee clinic, speech and language clinic, nursery school, and nursery school teachers.

Reactions of Children to Organ Transplantation

In recent years, surgical transplantation of various organs has become possible. Although cardiac transplantations are still undertaken, most surgeons think that the problems involved in the operation are insurmountable, and surgeons are awaiting the development of an artificial heart. Although there have been reports of the successful resolution of the significant emotional reverberations in child and family following hepatic,[214] lung,[300] bone marrow,[94] pineal, and other kinds of transplantations, problems arising as a result of renal transplantation have received the most attention. As Starzl and his colleagues[274] have pointed out, renal disease in children usually involves only a single organ system; therefore it is children who should benefit most as renal transplantation and hemodialysis techniques are

improved. A number of studies concerning the adjustment of children undergoing dialysis and transplantation and of the reactions of their families have been reported on recently. Although these studies differ somewhat as to reactions encountered and conclusions drawn, all report special significant emotional challenges to the child and his parents.

Renal Transplantation. Renal transplantation cannot be discussed apart from hemodialysis.[151] Some children and adolescents suffering from end-stage renal disease have conditions that rule out transplantation, and some reject transplanted kidneys (sometimes more than once),[83] and must return to hemodialysis on a temporary or permanent basis.

Children and adolescents who undergo *hemodialysis*—and their parents as well—exhibit many of the reactions characteristic of a chronic disease. Younger children often show regression, denial, and withdrawal,[2,140,151] as well as fear of pain and immobilization. Older children may show denial and withdrawal, but less regression, and, in addition, exhibit anxiety about changes in their bodies, delayed growth, and conflicting feelings of frustration and anger at being dependent on "the machine."[2] A few show oppositional or resistive behavior, as did a 9-year-old girl who repeatedly picked at or pulled out the shunt.[243] Sampson[244] described a group of children whose coping mechanisms were characterized by a readiness to interact with others, a greater tolerance of pain, and less conflict over enforced dependence (perhaps a type of "adaptive" regression[298]). Adolescents have even more intense conflicts related to dependence, fear of sexual inadequacy,[165] and missing much school. Occasionally when a transplantation is not possible, some adolescents,[192] like adults, have "given up" and covertly decided to die.[250] Some have attempted suicide.[5,103] Azotemia has produced subclinical delirium, with concomitant bizarre behavior mistaken for functional psychosis,[229] or even frank toxic psychosis,[278] in older children and adolescents.[229] Psychotherapy,[60] modified group therapy,[122] and hypnosis[254] have been helpful in certain instances.

The parents of a child undergoing chronic dialysis find it hard not to be overprotective, particularly if the child has a long history of renal disease; and a special interdependence often develops between the mother and child. As a consequence, some fathers have felt displaced (as have siblings)—occasionally to the point of divorce. Some closely knit families become even more cohesive.[244] Most observers have found that previously disturbed children and families, children who have a long history of serious medical problems, and children in whom renal failure occurs suddenly have the most difficulty adapting to the experience of chronic dialysis. In reviewing the histories of patients who require dialysis, Evans[78] has found withdrawal, depression, and school failure to be the most prevalent problems.

It is the hope of most parents of children with end-stage renal disease that *kidney transplantation* will be possible. But even if this comes to pass, families must grapple with the fact that few children have functioning first grafts after 5 or 6 years,[61,84,275] and second grafts are generally shorter-lived. Nevertheless, most children who have a functioning graft survive for 5 to 10 years after the development of end-stage renal disease—a remarkable decline in mortality. The difference in morbidity between patients on chronic hemodialysis and those who have transplants is less impressive.[156] Although the quality of life of successful renal transplantation patients is generally regarded as superior to that of patients on chronic renal dialysis, complications of surgery, rejection episodes, the side-effects of immunosuppressive drugs, and the number of days of hospitalization suggest that the benefits of transplantation may be less than originally hoped for. The survival time for patients receiving kidneys from related donors is longer than that for patients receiving cadaver kidneys,[14,108] but donorship itself gives rise to certain problems.

Korsch[154] has used the term "critical periods" in discussing the problems of children and their families which can arise in the periods of hemodialysis and transplantation. When the decision to transplant is made, the child and his parents may already be in the process of mourning a long terminal illness and may have difficulty shifting gears. The child who is to receive a transplant has a shorter period of dialysis, but time almost stands still[244] during the uncertain wait, and anxiety builds up as the date for the transplantation approaches.[166] Most children and parents are almost convinced that all problems will be solved by the operation: the "new kidney" will make a "new person." However, they are usually ambivalent about the operation, primarily because of the known effects of drugs on growth and appearance, the fear of death,[17] and apprehension about the effects of the procedure on sexual development. The bilateral nephrectomy preceding the transplantation poses the usual problems related to the loss of body parts, and uncertainty about integrating a new part[16] poses an additional problem. After the transplantation, some depression is often experienced, because "rebirth" has not occurred. The fear of rejection begins, never to be lost, and it is intensified by crises although denial mechanisms may be used. Decrease in the level of activity, fear of rejection by the peer group, and identity and body image problems often contribute to the child's difficulties when he returns to school. These problems may be intensified by the parents' fears and protectiveness. Severe anxiety and regression in children or adolescents, as well as depression[234] and other serious responses,[151] may necessitate psychotherapy in the post-transplantation period.[66] Psychotic episodes have been reported in adults, sometimes related to steroid medication. Such episodes seem less common in adolescents and rarely occur in children. Group discussions have been helpful for parents in this phase.

The foregoing suggests that the periods before and after the transplantation procedure are generally quite stressful for most children and their families. In fact, the impact on the family is often intense. Kahn and his colleagues[145] and Sampson[244] have commented on the impact on siblings, who often feel pushed aside and resentful toward the patient and their parents, with the consequent appearance of hostile or withdrawn behavior. Kemph and his colleagues[143] and Bernstein[23] have identified shifts in family dynamics which have occurred as a result of the stresses of surgery.

Family responses have frequently been complicated by the donor-patient relationships. Although most parents, especially mothers, have been regarded as willing donors, many parents have second thoughts and sometimes feel that they have been pushed to the decision.[82] A number of parents exhibit ambivalence about the loss of a kidney.[23,48] Lack of communication within the family has been reported.[262] Some parents have threatened to "take back the kidney" in an effort to control adolescent behavior. At times, a quasi-symbiotic relationship develops between the patient and the donor; the results are increased dependence on the part of the patient and a feeling of displacement on the part of the other spouse.[143] Crammond[55] found that the relationship between the donor and the recipient was hostile and dependent if the prior relationship had been disturbed or ambivalent. These and other interactions may necessitate psychotherapy for both the donors and the recipients of the transplants.[142] Children have developed conflicting fantasies related to their having a parent's kidney inside them,[244] and brothers who have received a kidney from their sisters have developed some confusion about their sexual identity.[55] Guilt and worry about the donor's welfare are common. Some medical centers will not permit children or adolescents to donate a kidney. Also, there are medicolegal problems involved.[245] In one study,[24] however, it was found that a year after the operation, adolescent donors were more likely than adults to have experienced a boost in self-esteem and a feeling of reward rather than regret.

In regard to cadaver transplants it is obvious that an ambivalent relationship does not occur between the donor and the recipient. However, adolescents and adults may have some conflicts; they include guilt about the death of the donor, ambivalent feelings about having a "dead" organ in their bodies, and a feeling of "twinship" with another patient who has received a kidney from the same cadaver.[3] Some observers hold that the cadaver donor should remain anonymous although anonymity may be hard to achieve in the face of persistent questions. Castelnuovo-Tedesco,[42] Ford and Castelnuovo-Tedesco,[86] and Muslin[204] have emphasized that the integration of a new body part—an "emotional transplant"—and the incorporation of a part of another person into the body image may present some serious difficulties for predisposed patients, even to the point of psychosis.[42] Many of the early postoperative problems arising from family-related[183] or cadaver transplants[3] can be ameliorated in the late postoperative period, but some will continue, and may result in serious family problems and even divorce. Psychotherapy for both donor and recipients may be necessary.[142] Group discussions may be helpful for parents; they may include patients and staff. When patients have rejected kidneys, individual or group psychotherapy may be necessary.[269]

In the few available long-term studies of the problems encountered by children and families in adapting to kidney transplantation,[23,145,155,286] the major problems of a psychosocial nature were related primarily to fear of rejection, fear of death, damaged self-esteem, depression, and the visual consequences of immunosuppressive therapy (persistent short stature, weight gain, and cushingoid facies). In the only controlled large-scale follow-up study (carried out by Korsch and her colleagues[155]), only 13% of the recipients who had a currently functioning graftwere not engaged in any meaningful activity. The remaining 87% had returned to their individual and family pre-illness condition in about one year. The results of personality tests given the transplant recipients in this study were similar to those of a control group of chronically ill children, but the transplant recipients were significantly more restricted in social adaptation and social activities than were a group of well children of the same ages.

In Korsch's study, in the 43 cases followed for more than 5 years there were 8 cases of noncompliance.[152] They involved interruption of immunosuppressive therapy leading to irreversible reduction in allograft function or allograft failure. Most of the cases of noncompliance involved adolescent girls who had deep-seated social and emotional problems, a finding which was consistent with the observations of Uehling and his colleagues.[291] The reasons for noncompliance included (alone and in combinations) conflicts about the cosmetic side-effects of corticosteroid treatment, significant adolescent rebellion, depression, and a wish to deny the entire experience. In addition, individual case reports[73,288,299] have indicated that there is some association between kidney transplant rejection and grief over the loss of a key figure around the time of the operation, hate for the donor, or other negative factors. Although no incontrovertible proof exists and the need for further research is clear, it is possible, as Solomon[270] has speculated, that immune mechanisms in such cases may be affected psychophysiologically by the "giving-up–given-up" syndrome described by Engel and Schmale.[76]

Staff and Patient Interactions in Hemodialysis and Renal Transplantation. As the foregoing suggests, staff-patient interaction in dialysis and transplantation programs is shaped by the needs of the individual child and his family. In their devoted attempts to deal with these constant concerns, fears, and demands, which are sometimes intensified by projected guilt or other feelings, it is only realistic to expect that the staff will sometimes feel frustrated, resentful, or angry, even to the point of wishing a difficult patient or family would leave.[139] When the medical and surgical challenges are intense, it is hard for the staff to provide suitable stimulation even if there is an intensive care unit. Certain patients seem to derive an unconscious secondary gain[58] from a hospital dialysis or transplantation program, and they have difficulty moving on to the rehabilitation program, which will lead to convalescence and more healthy independence. Obviously, the pediatric nephrology team, which already involves professionals from different disciplines, must be expanded to a truly multidisciplinary team[50,118] that includes adult psychiatrists,[54,182] child psychiatrists,[244,286] other kinds of mental health professionals,[24] and psychologically trained and sophisticated pediatricians (such as Korsch[155]). The programs devised by the mental health specialists may include direct consultation, brief psychotherapy[289] or other direct help for the patient or his family, and/or collaborative work with the staff.

Clinical, Moral, Ethical, and Economic Considerations in Hemodialysis and Renal Transplantation. Some years ago, Riley,[236] Reinhart,[234] and Prugh,[224] on the basis of the limited data then available, began to question whether renal transplantations were really worth the emotional price children (especially adolescents) and their families had to pay. In addition, there were moral and ethical problems that still have not been fully solved.[236] These problems are related to getting a truly informed consent from parents, older children, and relatives, a valid definition of cadaver death, and choosing candidates for transplantation, without being influenced by economic and other factors that should not ethically apply.[82,166,253,317]

Although more recent data indicate that the picture has improved considerably, I still feel that transplantation should not be regarded as a panacea and pushed too aggressively, as many residents still believe. There is room for improvement in transplantation results, both in regard to morbidity and mortality. More sophisticated hemodialysis and peritoneal dialysis techniques and the advent of home dialysis (although that is not without problems) now make a true choice of therapeutic modalities possible. Earlier detection of kidney disease and good medical management may stave off end-stage renal disease in a considerable number of cases.[70] If a patient is doing well on dialysis and the patient and his family have not expressed a wish for a renal transplantation, I agree with Krumlovsky[156] that suggesting a transplantation only because one is available may have serious repercussions. The following case example is pertinent.

Case Example. An 11-year-old girl faced terminal renal failure due to progressive chronic glomerulonephritis. She rejected an initial cadaver transplant and tolerated a second one for several months. A third transplantation was quite successful for nearly 5 years before the transplant failed because of the toxic effects of phenobarbitol taken in a suicide attempt. During those 5 years, the girl was able to live at home with her family in rural Colorado. Her family, poor Spanish-Americans with limited education, had had many psychosocial difficulties, in addition to those related to the girl's illness. The girl's adjustment was affected by a mild mental retardation, and an only moderately controlled seizure disorder, which was unrelated to her renal disease. Following her suicide attempt, she lived in foster homes in Denver, but she was depressed and hostile toward her foster mothers. Careful selection of a firm but supportive foster mother and the use of brief psychotherapy, during the course of which she came to recognize that she was displacing onto the foster mothers her anger toward and sadness about her own mother, resulted in remarkable stabilization. One year after the suicide attempt, the girl was considered to be doing well. She had few physical problems

with dialysis, was developing well in special education classes in a public high school, and appeared to be no longer depressed.

When offered the opportunity to have another cadaver transplant, however, the girl and her family quickly agreed. The transplantation was done, but the transplant was rejected. She received 3 more transplants within 2 months. The girl died of infection and debilitation from the transplantation procedures and medications.

As with donors,[74] attempts have been made to predict which patients are the best candidates for successful transplantation.[3] But the results to date are inconclusive. In view of the present state of the art, it is essential that a comprehensive health care team, including suitable mental health professionals, be involved from the start in the evaluation of patients with end-stage renal disease and in planning their treatment program. All available methods of treatment should be considered. (Failure to have considered all methods of treatment may account for some of the differences in the available long-term outcome studies.[145,151]) With this type of approach, the resources, strengths, and coping mechanisms as well as the problems and vulnerabilities of children and families can be identified before therapeutic intervention is required.[155]

Burns

Burns are among the most common types of accidents in children under 2 or 3 years of age.[242] Accidents often occur in relation to a family crisis, and prompt intervention in such crises, in addition to basic safety measures, may help prevent them.[132] A study in England[319] and one in the United States[301] showed that most burned children over 3 years of age experience fear of loss of their parents' love and guilt feelings about the accident. Those feelings often last for years. These and other studies[92,172] also indicate that serious depression often occurs. Depression, accompanied by anorexia and other emotional responses, may be a factor in poor wound healing and poor responses to grafting procedures.[114] In older children and adolescents, the depression may be associated with fears of disfigurement and dying. Regression and withdrawal are also seen. In one study,[203] early psychiatric intervention markedly reduced later social withdrawal in children and adolescents.

Parents of burned children tend to feel exceedingly guilty and often blame themselves or each other for inadequate supervision of the child. As a matter of fact, the lack of supervision that may occur in disturbed families and families in crisis often results in burn accidents. In a small percentage of cases, burns are caused by actual neglect or abuse.

The parents of a burned child are often frustrated because they cannot hold their child and thus demonstrate their affection. They may also fail to visit the child because of fear of criticism or because of guilt about their feelings of revulsion at the child's changed appearance.[318]

As with other accidents, a careful but sympathetic history should be taken and the parents and children should be helped to express their feelings. If a sibling was involved in the accident, he should be permitted to visit and also helped with his inevitable guilt feelings, no matter how irrational. The heavy costs of treatment may burden the parents and at times result in ambivalence toward the child.

The development of special facilities and specially trained teams of professionals represents a significant advance in the treatment of burns. In addition to pediatric surgeons, clinical nurse specialists, physical and occupational therapists, psychologists, and social workers, burn teams should include a child psychiatrist.[26] He may offer direct consultation and formal psychotherapy for the child and/or his parents, or he may work collaboratively with other members of the team. In ward management conferences, a child psychiatrist or some other mental health professional can provide support to the staff in encouraging them to discuss the feelings of discouragement and frustration, as well as the distressing problems which often arise in dealing with severely burned children and their parents.[232,255] Discussion of the preparation of the burned child and his parents and related matters can also take place in these conferences.

Some child psychiatrists (e.g., Bernstein[25]) have used hypnosis to minimize the excruciating pain[209] of debridement, dressing changes, or the passage of a bougie. LaBaw[157] has used trance therapy for this purpose and also for regressive encopresis and enuresis, which can be serious complications. Following a burn accident, the child's return to school may require special consideration. For adolescents, vocational planning should be a part of the comprehensive approach to burn care.

Case Example. A 3-year-old boy was burned over the lower part of his body and legs by a fire that broke out when the boy's 7-year-old brother was playing with matches near an open gasoline can. The can had been left unguarded by the father, who was somewhat distracted over the loss of his job several days before. The boy was treated with silver nitrate, then still in use because of the excellent eschar it produced. The parents did not visit the boy for nearly a week after his admission to the hospital; the boy was exceedingly anxious and agitated, and he fought against staying in bed, especially in the evening. The child psychiatrist on the burn team saw the boy in consultation. He noted the boy's confusion and incoherent speech and concluded that the boy was delirious, with the delirium compounded by excessive separation. In addition, the boy's electrolyte metabolism appeared to be deranged as the result of loss of fluid into the eschar. Intravenous fluid therapy was only partially helpful, as was having a nurse sit with the boy in the evening with the lights on. The psychiatrist called the parents. When they came to visit the boy, the psychiatrist learned that they had been staying away for fear of being judged as bad parents. He learned also that the mother had been struggling with the boy about toilet training and that her method of punishing him for being "dirty" was to put him to bed. The psychiatrist dealt with the parents' guilt, helping the mother stop blaming the father and understand his concern about losing his job. He also helped them reassure the boy that he was not bad because his buttocks were black and he was made to stay in bed. The boy's behavior immediately became more manageable. In a follow-up interview with the parents and the 7-year-old brother, the psychiatrist was able to deal successfully with the problems of blame and guilt.

Although not arranged for in the case just described, a foster grandmother can be virtually a life saver for a seriously depressed hospitalized child whose parents are having trouble handling their feelings.[175] Even though a foster grandmother may not be able to hold the child, she can show him pictures, read to him, sing to him, and offer other types of stimulation. At times simply a touch with a finger or a light pat on a nonpainful area may be of significant symbolic import. Even with current methods of treatment, delirium may be present in the early stages of burn therapy, and a foster grandmother may play a part in the treatment. Careful explanation and preparation and abundant opportunities for questions are especially important for all children and their parents. Used in conjunction with the remarkable recent advances in treatment by burn teams, the psychosocial aspects of management described can minimize lasting emotional problems for most children with serious burns, and support rehabilitation.[101]

Other kinds of surgery that deserve special discussion are genitourinary surgery, plastic surgery, certain orthopedic procedures, and a miscellany of surgical procedures that generally involve organ removal, including colectomy,[65] mastectomy,[129,306] and other types of cancer surgery.[171,282] These topics are discussed in the following paragraphs.

Reactions of Children to Genitourinary Surgery

Although Wolff's[316] large-scale studies in England have indicated that operations on the genitalia are particularly disturbing to young children and although Blotcky and Grossman[31] have indicated that there is a significant association between childhood genitourinary surgery and emotional disturbance, the evidence is not conclusive. According to Witmer[314] children who have cryptorchidism seem to be far more susceptible to emotional disturbances (anxiety, restlessness, and immaturity) than are the general population. If these disturbances are unchecked at an early stage, their long-range effects are depression, passivity, poor self-concept, and confusion about body image and sexual identity. In their study, Cytryn and his colleagues[56] found that body-damage anxiety was often intensified by concern, anxiety, and guilt on the part of the parents. Like Blos,[30] these investigators found a family constellation composed of a dominant mother and a passive, withdrawn, or absent father to especially predispose a child to the development of emotional difficulties. Falstein and his colleagues[81] reported a high incidence of frightening fantasies centering on damage to the genitals in children about to undergo surgical correction of a hernia in the genital region, which frequently occurs with cryptorchidism.

According to Gross's study,[107] in dealing with bilateral cryptorchidism in the past, the general practice was to wait for spontaneous testicular descent until a boy was 11 or 12 years of age. If it did not occur, a medication with human gonadotropic hormone was instituted for a short period, or orchiopexy was done, with a good chance that the patient would have some degree of fertility. However, recent evidence[120,160] indicates that when an undescended testis is not brought down into the scrotum by the time a boy is 5 or 6 years of age, the cytology of the organ will definitely suffer. Bilateral cryptorchidism now seems to be less common than the unilateral condition. Moreover, there is a greater risk of neoplasm in an undescended or ectopic testis.[57] In addition, Lattimer (a surgeon) and her colleagues[160] cite the psychoanalytic studies of Bell and her colleagues[18] regarding the importance of testicular and scrotal, as well as penile, stimulation for psychosexual development. Thus they believe that, if at all possible, on histologic, cellular, kinetic, and psychologic grounds, both testes should be in the scrotum by the child's fifth birthday. Some experts prefer to delay correction until the boy is 9 or 10 years of age, while others advocate correction at 2 or 3 years of age. Most experts prefer the late preschool-age period.

In the past, many child psychoanalysts (I among them) believed that all elective surgery should be avoided in boys 4 to 6 years old, the period encompassing the oedipal stage, when boys are vulnerable to castration anxiety (or, more broadly, mutilation anxiety). It now appears that this period is the best one for orchiopexy, both psychologically as well as physically, and the studies of Cytryn and his colleagues,[56] which indicate that emotional problems increase with postponement, seem to support the conclusion. Obviously, appropriate preparation, including information and support for the child and his parents, and other preventive measures are especially important, since the psychosocial vulnerabilities cited earlier exist.

Perhaps the foregoing considerations also apply to surgical repair of a number of other abnormalities of the genitourinary tract in children, such as exstrophy of the bladder, epispadias, and genital trauma,[302] and concern for the consequences of developmental pathophysiology must take precedence over the psychologic concerns. Nevertheless, the latter should be taken into account, and appropriate preventive and supportive measures should be undertaken. Simple uncomplicated herniorrhaphies might be postponed until the most vulnerable period has passed. (Kidney transplantations, a special case, have already been discussed.) Hysterectomy, which occasionally is needed in adolescents, poses special problems for the development of sexual identity; and depression and other responses may result.[197,315]

Vasectomy, rare in even late adolescent males, seems less deviant than formerly but may still have psychosocial and psychosexual repercussions.[310,320]

Circumcision, one of the oldest operations on record, is also the most common operation performed in hospitals in the United States. Recently questions have been raised about its necessity.[177] Emdee and Harmon[75] have shown that there is significant pain associated with the operation, and that infants often respond to this pain by becoming quiet. Daniel and his colleagues[57] have come to believe that circumcision should be reserved for the treatment of phimosis, in which the preputial narrowing restricts urinary flow. In the opinion of these investigators, circumcision of newborns should be done only if the parents desire it, and phimosis, penile carcinoma, or cervical malignancy in the female whose sexual partner is uncircumcised are not significant risk factors. Daniel and his colleagues, along with others, have identified some disorders, such as penile abnormalities and blood dyscrasias, as contraindicating circumcision. They believe, as I do, that circumcision of older boys incidental to another operation requiring general anesthesia is likely to be emotionally traumatic, and that full explanation and preparation are vital if circumcision is indicated in a school-age or adolescent boy. In a program instituted at the University of Colorado Medical Center, parents of newborn boys were queried about their attitudes toward routine circumcision. Most parents had made up their minds and the majority chose circumcision. Attitudes change slowly.

Tonsillectomy and Adenoidectomy

Next to circumcision, tonsillectomy with adenoidectomy is the most common operation performed on children. In the 1920s, when Kaiser[138] began his pioneering studies of the end results of this operation in Rochester, New York, many physicians advocated routine removal of tonsils and adenoids for all children. Kaiser's large-scale studies showed that these operations result in some improvement in children suffering from repeated tonsillitis, cervical adenitis, and nasal blockage resulting in mouth breathing but little or no change in children with a history of repeated colds, laryngitis, bronchitis, and otitis. Studies by McCorkle and his colleagues[187] and McKee[190] in Britain indicated no decrease in respiratory infections following the operation, although McKee did find significantly fewer cases of sore throat and otitis media in young children. A second study by McKee[191] revealed that adenoidectomy alone resulted in the same reduction in the incidence of otitis media as the combined operation but no significant reduction in the incidence of throat infections.

Although there were some methodologic problems in the studies just described and in other studies, Haggerty[112] was able to conclude in 1968 that although 30% to 40% of all children in Rochester underwent tonsillectomies and adenoidectomies (sometimes in family groups), probably no more than 2% to 3% required the operation. Haggerty summarized the estimates of complications of these operations; out of 1.5 million children undergoing tonsillectomies and adenoidectomies each year in the United States, 300 die, primarily as a result of blood loss, 30,000 or more develop transient bacteremia; some develop pneumonia or lung abscesses, and many have psychologic trauma.[135,164] What to tell a young child about tonsillectomy was spelled out on page 525, and the puppet approach to preparations for anesthesia for T & A is included in a case example on page 526.

In an attempt to develop guidelines for the clinician, Haggerty suggested that the surgical approach be limited to (1) children under 5 or 6 years of age who have persistent nasal and/or pharyngeal obstruction and clear evidence of enlarged adenoids or tonsils, (2) children under 8 years of age

who have repeated and proved episodes of bacterial tonsillitis over the course of the past year, (3) children with otitis media and threatened deafness, who should undergo only adenoidectomy. Haggerty felt that with rare exceptions, no children under 2 years of age should be operated on for these conditions and that the combined operation should rarely be done before a child is 4 years of age. Even in older children who have the indications just discussed, Haggerty recommended waiting for a year in most cases. He saw no reason for surgical treatment of children who have repeated respiratory infections nor of children who have rheumatic fever or nephritis, who can be treated medically with antibiotics. He also recommended that the primary physician, rather than the surgeon, should usually make the decision and that all children scheduled for surgery receive a competent medical work-up and careful preparation and that provision for overnight stay for parents and other preventive psychologic measures be emphasized.

Haggerty's measured appraisal of the relatively small place of tonsillectomy and adenoidectomy in the treatment of children has been widely noted, particularly by some third-party insurers. The consequence has been a noticeable decline in the popularity of such operations in this country during the past decade. In Vermont, for example, tonsillectomies and adenoidectomies decreased by 46% over a period of 5 years with the use of feedback and review.[307] But the number of such operations is still unacceptably high, and Paradise[210] has called for further investigation, including blind prospective studies.

Facial Surgery

The psychologic and social importance of facial surgery was well recognized by surgeons by at least the end of the sixteenth century. Cosmetic considerations are, of course, very important to parents and even more so to adolescents. Such operations usually go smoothly, and the results are very beneficial to the child and his parents. However, as McGregor[189] has shown, paradoxical reactions may occur even in response to apparently small changes, such as a change in the contour of the nose, especially in an older child or adolescent who is having difficulty in creating a solid body image or whose parents have pushed so hard for the procedure that the patient feels they do not accept him "as he is" or like him for himself.

In adolescents and young adults, apparently simple requests for alterations in facial contours (particularly of the nose in males) may mask deep uncertainties about sexual identification.[199] Occasionally a psychotic episode may ensue, as if unconscious fears had been realized and inadequacies exposed by the surgeon's agreement to what was in reality a "test" request.[176] In the opinion of some surgeons, psychiatric consultation should be routine in such situations in order to avoid the possibility of an unexpected untoward response.

Orthopedic Restraints

Orthopedic procedures sometimes involve the restraint of movement, as with the use of body casts and traction.[202] Frustration,[21] aggressive feelings,[40] stereotyped movements, tics, and dammed-up hyperactivity[163] have been described. Some very young children subjected to chronic restraint have shown problems in speech development.[259] Opportunities for release and mastery of feelings in fantasy, through talking, reading, movies, and doll play activities, in addition to a significant supportive relationship with a nurse, recreational therapist, teacher, or some other person, can be of important preventive and therapeutic value to such patients.[216]

Appendectomy

Appendicitis is a common diagnosis, but in fact an appreciable number of the appendices removed are normal. The majority of the misdiagnosed cases of appendicitis occur in female patients between the ages of 10 and 29.[200] Some symptoms may be related to a ruptured ovarian follicle. Most such patients have recurrent abdominal pain associated with various emotional problems, hysterical personalities with conversion pain, and events related chronologically to birth experiences[79] or to other stressful experiences.[29] Although any causal relation to appendicitis is unproven, a pattern of recurrent abdominal pain calls for at least psychiatric consultation prior to surgery. In some patients, an unconscious need to suffer because of guilt or other conflicts may lead to a pattern of "polysurgical addiction," as Menninger[196] has termed it, a condition in which the urge for frequent operations can be diminished only by intensive psychotherapy.

Intensive Care Units: Psychosocial Considerations

In recent years, the use of intensive care units has become widespread in pediatric programs, particularly in teaching centers. Units have been set up for premature infants, for newborns who have hyaline membrane disease and other high-risk problems, for patients undergoing hemodialysis, kidney transplantations, and open-heart surgery, for children and adolescents who have catastrophic illnesses or injuries as a result of infection, accident, and attempted suicide, and for patients who have severe respiratory difficulties. There are real advantages in establishing special units for patients who have the same illness. This type of arrangement permits a concentration of staff people who have special training and skills, the development of special emergency and other treatment procedures, and the specialized use of monitoring systems and other newly developed methods. However, the fact that such units result in special problems is not widely recognized.

One such problem arises from the very existence of a highly trained group of specialists who must work as an efficient team to meet the special challenges and crises in the lives of their patients. The members of such teams must work together and lean heavily on one another in mutual cooperation and trust. In so doing, they inevitably face real and human problems of getting along with one another. However, sometimes without realizing it, they often establish an in-group relationship which can be supportive and satisfying but which results in the relegation of nonteam members to an out-group (although not necessarily inferior) status.

Certain "bridges to the outside world" are more easily maintained than others. On a pediatric intensive care unit, the consultative services of others who must help deal with emergency situations are desperately needed, and relationships with surgeons specializing in cardiac, kidney or neurosurgical problems, neurologists, and metabolic specialists are relatively easily maintained. Relationships with those who do not provide such urgent physical help (e.g., psychiatrists and pediatricians with other interests) are less easily maintained. In fact some professionals are often regarded with disinterest, if not mistrust. Ironically, parents are often treated as members of an out-group. It is true that parents are in a special position (have a special bridge) since theoretically they can visit their child at any time because he is on the danger list. In many intensive care units, however, special visiting privileges do not accord the parents special status, and the parents may feel shut out by the busy in-group even though the child being cared for so efficiently is their own.

Perhaps the clearest insights into the problems of intense in-group specialization

are contained in a paper entitled "Problems of Neonatal Intensive Care Units," which was presented at the 59th Ross Conference on Pediatric Research. The participants in the conference were distinguished; they included most of the outstanding pediatricians engaged in research in the United States. The report deals with the latest and most sophisticated methods of physical care—from methods of monitoring through prolonged nasotracheal intubation to catheterization of the umbilical vessels. However, there are no references at all in the report to the parents of the patients although death rates are discussed. The patients' siblings are mentioned, but only as controls. Of course, this does not mean that these outstanding pediatricians do not deal with parents. They do, and many of them do so with compassion and support. But the omission is a measure of a rather exclusive in-group intellectual excitement about methods of saving babies' lives.

Unfortunately, physicians, medical students, and other professionals who read publications reflecting such attitudes come away with the feeling that methodology is all that counts and that meeting the needs of parents to see their infants and to help care for them if possible is not urgent. In my opinion, meeting such needs is a real challenge to be taken up by those who are entrusted with delivering health care to the public. Some efforts designed to meet this challenge are already underway.

Recently, a few neonatal intensive care units have begun to admit parents for overnight stay and to permit them to touch, as well as to see, their infants. A few leaders in the field, (e.g., Lubchenko at the University of Colorado Medical Center) are convinced that it is important for parents, especially the mothers, to participate in feeding their infants, and they provide rocking chairs for the mothers to use while doing so. Klaus, Kennell,[147a] and others believe it is vital that all infants, especially premature infants, receive positive social as well as tactile, rhythmic, and other types of stimulation from adults, especially the mother since providing such care also supports her bonding or attachment to her infant. Studies of newborns carried out by several investigators generally support these recommendations. For example, Lubchenko[177] and several others suggest removing one side of an Isolette in order that such stimulation may be provided by staff members as well as by parents.

Some intensive care programs for older children and adolescents have begun to recognize the need for a "therapeutic alliance" of staff and parents and to observe some of the principles mentioned earlier in this chapter. Cotton, who is a clinical director of a respiratory intensive care unit, has set up regular ward management conferences in order to foster collaborative planning, to permit discussion of the feelings of the staff about the stresses to which they are inevitably subjected, and to provide an opportunity for the staff to bring up new ideas about ward procedures, including the handling of relationships with parents. Rosini and his colleagues[241] have reported on the use of group meetings in a pediatric intensive care unit. Drotar[67] has described the evolution of the ward management conference from its roots in the requests of nurses in an intensive care nursery for ad hoc consultations with a mental health specialist. The conference approach is based on the principles developed by a rehabilitation team more than 30 years ago and was described long ago in papers by Fox and her colleagues,[87] by Prugh and Tagiuri[231] and by others. The rehabilitation team approach was developed in the 1940s by Howard Rusk and his colleagues at a rehabilitation center in New York City.

It is easy to have compassion for the staffs of modern intensive care units, which are so much more complex technologically than those that existed years ago.[186] The stresses on the nurses are especially intense.[115] They must work with seriously ill, sometimes terminal, patients, applying modern treatment techniques with great efficiency. It is impossible not to fear making mistakes in applying emergency procedures, and it is difficult to attend to the needs of anxious, sometimes desperate, sometimes angry parents while meeting the child's urgent needs. Nor can physicians, who must decide on the methods to be employed, avoid such feelings. Under such conditions of pressure, it is only normal that the people involved will sometimes feel discouraged, depressed, and even helpless. (And guilt is often attached to these "secret" feelings.) Specialists from outside, even those who have a special bridge, may arouse feelings of rivalry in the ward staff at times, because they may be seen as competing in the care of the child and, in fact, sometimes disagree with the ward staff about the treatment approach being taken. Their sudden appearance and disappearance, after dispensing what may seem arbitrary judgments, may lead to feelings of resentment as well. Even differing opinions as to what to tell the parents and the child about the illness may lead to skirmishes, particularly if the outside expert recommended that they should be told very little, and, at the same time, both the child and his parents are beseiging the staff with questions. In addition, the staff, who are often called upon to treat a patient whose prognosis is apparently hopeless,[68] are often confronted with moral and ethical dilemmas.

In situations such as these, it is easy to see what contributions regular ward management conferences can make. During such conferences, which should be chaired by a senior pediatrician acting as clinical director, planning can be coordinated and thus carried out more effectively. If any staff members must absent themselves from the conferences because of an emergency, the clinical director can contact them later and fill them in on the discussion and any decisions made. Consistent plans can be made as to what to tell parents or patients and for the assignment of a particular nurse or other professional to work individually with a parent or patient who has a special problem.[150] Feelings of frustration, helplessness, discouragement, or depression can be shared openly without feelings of guilt, with the group's providing important support. Consultants without bridges, such as psychiatrists and psychologists, can meet with the ward medical, nursing, and social work staffs, to plan the management of special problems. Arrangements can be made to rotate the nurses after some months on the unit, in order to permit them to enjoy the rest and recreation essential to their demanding work. Experiments with rotating shifts, part-time collateral experiences in clinic areas, regard for maintenance of support systems outside the hospital, and informal "debriefing" sessions before going off duty are among the other efforts to avoid "burnout" of nursing staff.[115]

Plans can be made to install dividers or otherwise to rearrange large units in order to reduce the amount of confusing stimuli, which can be overwhelming to patients, parents, and staff. Conversely, both experimental research and clinical experience indicate that people require a steady stream of external stimuli of varying types if they are to maintain a healthy awareness of and contact with reality. Some stimuli are present even in intensive care units but many come from machines, and they may be insufficient, monotonous, or confusing. More important, in intensive care units there are often far too few consistent contacts with concerned people, and on an open ward, inconsistent contacts with staff and machines may result in a feeling of invasion of privacy that is especially threatening to some patients and their parents. Thus, even in the midst of activity, an anxious patient can at the same time feel isolated, dehumanized, and invaded and, as a consequence, can develop a special type of sensory deprivation.[1] In predisposed adults[181] and occasionally in older adolescents,[162] the deprivation can lead to psychotic episodes (sometimes compounded by the effects of

steroid medication). These episodes are usually transient, but they can be seriously disruptive to treatment regimens. Such episodes can often be prevented by appropriate preparation and consistent postoperative care.[162]

In the ward management conference, plans can be made for continuity in relationships (or for a tapering off) when a patient improves and is moved to an ordinary ward. This is a most important consideration, since some children may become worse physically or in their behavior when they must break off an important relationship with a staff member. In some units arrangements are made for the intensive care unit staff to continue in the care of a transferred child. At a minimum, arrangements should be made for a familiar staff person to accompany the child to the new ward and introduce him to the new staff or to visit the new ward with him before the transfer. Thereafter, an intensive care staff member can be assigned to visit the transferred child every day, tapering off as the child develops relationships with the new staff. Later, if the child remains in the hospital for some time, he can return to the intensive care unit for brief visits. These principles also apply to the staff's relationships with parents and other family members.

When a patient is transferred, the effect of the transfer on the remaining patients must be considered. A particularly likeable child or adolescent may be keenly missed; or a particular adolescent or young adult may have developed an older-sibling or parent-substitute relationship with a younger patient. Prugh and Tagiuri[231] described one such situation, in which the majority of patients in a polio unit had to return to their respirators for at least several days following the discharge of a young man who had been the most supportive figure in the unit and two patients had bouts of asthma, a disorder they had not had since early childhood. Having the young man return for visits and making him the editor of the unit's newspaper helped both him and the remaining patients. Similar principles apply to the transfer of staff members to another unit or to their leaving the hospital to work elsewhere.

If a child dies, other children on the ward should be told about the death. They inevitably sense that something serious has happened even if the death occurred during the night. "Epidemics" of depression or conversion symptoms based on identification with the missing child have often occurred. In addition to the opportunity to express their grief, the other children may need to be reassured that their condition is different, if at all possible, from that of the child who died.

Reverse Isolation

A few years ago, some observers advocated the use of reverse isolation for children suffering from leukemia or taking immunosuppressive medications. Githens[97] has since come to feel that the negative emotional effects of reverse isolation outweigh its value, and the procedure is not popular today. More recently, reverse isolation has been used for children receiving bone marrow transplants for leukemia and aplastic anemia. In the United States and in Germany reverse isolation from birth on has been employed in the cases of several infants suffering from combined immune deficiency.

The psychosocial problems of 4- to 15-year-old children (and of their families) undergoing bone marrow transplants have been described by Gardner and her colleagues.[94] In their studies, these investigators encountered problems similar to those related to kidney transplantations, such as fear of rejection of the transplant and death, increased dependence on the part of the patients, guilt on the part of the parents, and guilt on the part of the sibling donor if the procedure was unsuccessful

and the patient died. In addition, the patients exhibited anxiety and depression related to the 6 weeks or so of isolation. These patients showed intermittent withdrawal and uncooperativeness, anger toward both the staff and parents, and depression that lasted for several months after discharge. No child in the group studied suffered profound deterioration, and there were no episodes of psychotic or suicidal behavior. Special psychologic evaluation of patients prior to the isolation (and of donors after the procedure) led to individualized methods of psychologic support for both groups. Staff members at the Denver Children's Hospital, where isolation lasts for 2 to 4 months, have developed a facility for reverse isolation. It consists of a special room within a room. Visitors in the outer room can leave their faces uncovered, and patients can talk through an intercom and can have some control over lights and drapes in the inner room. Sterilization protocols are less irksome for patients, parents, and staff, and the patients' sense of social isolation seems to be reduced.

In Germany, fraternal twins who had congenital combined immune deficiency states were reared in strict reverse isolation until they were 28 and 32 months old.[263] These infants were studied by Simons and his colleagues, who found that at 2$\frac{1}{2}$ years of age, both children had significant learning disorders. They also had evidence of what the observers concluded was a lasting intellectual impairment attributable to their extended stay in the isolator.

The single infant known to have been reared in isolation in the United States has been the subject of two reports, one of the child at 48 months of age[311] and one of the child at 52 months of age.[90] At 8 to 9 months of age the infant showed some disregard of his environment, a delay in language development, and a persistent involvement in rhythmical self-stimulating behavior. These manifestations led to a reevaluation of the quality of his care. As a result, a campaign of intensified stimulation was undertaken. It included a systematic program of prespeech stimulation, the placing of a television set near his isolator, and the assignment of a specific person to care for him when he was in the hospital. Systematic efforts were made to play with him through the isolator's glove openings, both in the hospital and when he was at home (about 50% of the time). Within a few weeks the child responded with an increase in babbling and better word comprehension. His speech development still lagged, but his emotional expression became more varied and appropriate and his social behavior more outgoing. By the time the child was 24 months old, his speech therapist estimated his ability to communicate to be at least on a par with his age level.

From that point on, the child's development progressed more rapidly, and he showed a clearer attachment to his mother and, later, to other persons. At age $2^1/_2$, he showed some resistance to bowel control and to weaning, but he had achieved full continence by the time he was 33 months old, and he accepted weaning at about the same time. At 35 months, he began to talk occasionally about getting out of his isolator but had not made any attempts to do so. At 3 years of age, he showed some spontaneous masturbatory behavior. At 53 months, his mental developments seemed normal. Freedman and his colleagues[90] point out, however, that this child has inevitably experienced some forms of sensory deprivation, never having felt another person's skin, or smelled another person's breath or body, or experienced the process of molding his body to that of a caretaker. As these investigators point out—and as Shiller's[247] work with chimpanzees affirms—the sensory deprivation and the idiocratic experiences to which this child has been subjected could color his later psychologic development. Nevertheless, these investigators conclude that reverse isolation is not incompatible with normal emotional and intellectual development if the child is offered a special program of stimulation.

Bibliography

1. Abram, H.S.: Adaptation to open heart surgery: A psychiatric study of response to the threat of death. Am. J. Psychiatry, *122*:659, 1956.
2. Abram, H.S.: Survival by Machine: The psychological stress of chronic hemodialysis. Psychiatr. Med., *1*:37, 1970.
3. Abram, H.S.: The psychiatrist, the treatment of chronic renal failure, and the prolongation of life. III. Am. J. Psychiatry, *128*:1534, 1972.
4. Abram, H.S.: Psychiatric reflections on adaptation to repetitive dialysis. Kidney Int., *6*:67, 1974.
5. Abram, H.S., Moore, G.L., and Westervelt, F.B., Jr.: Suicidal behavior in chronic dialysis patients. Am. J. Psychiatry, *127*:1199, 1971.
6. Adams, P.L.: Techniques for pediatric consultation. In: *Consultative Psychiatry* (J. Schwab, Ed.). New York, Appleton-Century-Crofts, 1968.
7. Aisenberg, R.B., et al.: Psychological impact of cardiac catheterization. Pediatrics, *51*:1051, 1973.
8. American Academy of Pediatrics: *Care of Children in Hospitals*. Evanston, Ill., American Academy of Pediatrics, 1971.
9. Azarnoff, P.: Personal communication.
10. Azarnoff, P.: A play program in a pediatric clinic. Children, *17*:6, 1970.
11. Azarnoff, P.: The care of children in hospitals: An overview. J. Pediatr. Psychol., *1*:5, 1976.
12. Azarnoff, P., and Flegal, S.: *A Pediatric Play Program*. Springfield, Ill., Thomas, 1975.
13. Bakwin, H.: Loneliness in infants. Am. J. Dis. Child., *63*:30, 1942.
14. Barnes, B.A., et al.: The 10th report of the transplant registry. JAMA, *221*:1495, 1972.
15. Barnes, C.M., et al.: Measurement in management of anxiety in children for open heart surgery. Pediatrics, *49*:250, 1972.
16. Basch, S.H.: Intrapsychic integration of a new organ: A clinical study of kidney transplantation. Psychoanal. Q., *42*:364, 1973.
17. Beard, B.H.: Fear of death and fear of life: The dilemma in chronic renal failure, hemodialysis, and renal homotransplantation. Arch. Gen. Psychiatry, *21*:373, 1969.
18. Bell, A.I., Strocbel, C.F., and Prior, D.D.: Interdisciplinary study: Scrotal sac and testes: Psychophysiological and psychological observations. Psychoanal. Q., *40*:415, 1971.
19. Benjamin, J.D.: Some developmental observations relating to the theory of anxiety. J. Am. Psychoanal. Assoc., *9*:652, 1961.
20. Bergman, A.G., Shrand, H., and Oppe, T.E.: A pediatric home care program in London—ten years' experience. Pediatrics, *36*:314, 1965.
21. Bergmann, T.: Observations of children's reactions to motor restraint. Nerv. Child, *4*:318, 1945.
22. Berlin, I.N., Ed.: Editorial comment on physical illness and injury: The hospital as a source of

544   Specific Clinical Considerations

emotional disturbance in children. In: *Advocacy For Child Mental Health* (N. Berlin, Ed.). New York, Brunner/Mazel, 1975.

23. Bernstein, D.M.: After transplantation—the child's emotional reactions. Am. J. Psychiatry, *127*:1189, 1971.
24. Bernstein, D.M., and Simmons, R.G.: The adolescent kidney donor: The right to give. Am. J. Psychiatry, *131*:1338, 1974.
25. Bernstein, N.R.: Observations on the use of hypnosis with burned children on a pediatric ward. Int. J. Clin. Exp. Hypn., *13*:1, 1965.
26. Bernstein, N.R., Sanger, S., and Fras, J.: The functions of the child psychiatrist in the management of severely burned children. J. Am. Acad. Child. Psychiatry, *8*:620, 1969.
27. Birren, F.: *Color Psychology and Color Therapy*. New York, McGraw-Hill, 1950.
28. Blake, F.G.: *The Child, His Parents, and the Nurse*. Philadelphia, Lippincott, 1954.
29. Blanton, S., and Kirk, R.: A psychiatric study of sixty-one appendectomy cases. Ann. Surg., *126*:305, 1947.
30. Blos, P.: Comments on the psychological consequences of cryptorchidism: A clinical study. Psychoanal. Study Child, *15*:395, 1960.
31. Blotcky, M.J., and Grossman, I.: Psychological implications of childhood genitourinary surgery. J. Am. Acad. Child Psychiatry, *31*:488, 1978.
32. Blumgart, E., and Korsch, B.M.: Pediatric recreation. Pediatrics, *34*:133, 1964.
33. Boston Collaborative Drug Surveillance Program: Drug surveillance—problems and challenges. Pediatr. Clin. North Am., *19*:117, 1972.
34. Bothe, A., and Galdston, R.: The child's loss of consciousness: A psychiatric view of pediatric anesthesia. Pediatrics, *50*:252, 1972.
35. Bowlby, J., et al.: The effects of mother child separation: A follow-up study. Br. J. Med. Psychol., *29*:211, 1956.
36. Boyd, I., Yeager, M., and McMillan, M.: Personality styles in the postoperative course. Psychosom. Med., *35*:23, 1973.
37. Bradford, W.: Personal communication.
38. Brain, D.J., and Mclay, I.: Controlled study of mothers and children in hospitals. Br. Med. J., *1*:278, 1968.
39. Brooks, M.: Constructive play experience for the hospitalized child. J. Nurs. Educ., *12*:7, 1957.
40. Burlingham, D.: Notes on problems of motor restraint during illness. In: *Drives, Affects, Behavior* (R.M. Lowenstein, Ed.). New York, International Universities Press, 1953.
41. Cassel, S., and Paul, M.H.: The role of puppet therapy on the emotional responses of children hospitalized for cardiac catheterization. J. Pediatr., *71*:233, 1965.
42. Castelnuovo-Tedesco, P.: Organ transplant, body image, psychosis. Psychoanal. Q., *42*:349, 1973.
43. Centers, L., and Centers, R.: Peer group attitudes toward the amputee child. J. Soc. Psychol., *61*:127, 1963.
44. Cermak, E.G., and Brutt, M.M.: Behavior changes indicating emotional trauma in tonsillectomized children. Pediatrics, *12*:23, 1953.

45. Chapman, A.H., Loeb, D.G., and Biggons, M.J.: Psychiatric aspects of hospitalizing children. Arch. Pediatr., *73*:77, 1956.
46. Chess, S., and Lyman, M.S.: A psychiatric unit in a general hospital pediatric clinic. Am. J. Orthopsychiatry, *39*:77, 1969.
46a. Children in Hospitals, 31 Wilshire Park, Needham, Mass., 02192. A group of parents and professionals.
47. Clayton, G.: Variations in blood pressure in hospitalized children. J. Pediatr., *40*:462, 1952.
48. Cleveland, S.E.: Personality characteristics, body image, and social attitudes of organ transplant donors versus nondonors. Psychosom. Med., *37*:313, 1975.
49. Cline, F.W., and Rothenberg, M.B.: Preparation of a child for major surgery: A case report. J. Am. Acad. Child Psychiatry, *13*:78, 1974.
50. Collins, J.L.: Multidisciplinary collaboration for a renal dialysis–kidney transplantation unit. J. Natl. Med. Assoc., *66*:277, 1974.
51. Cooke, R.E.: Effects of hospitalization upon the child. In: *The Hospitalized Child and His Family* (J.A. Haller, Jr., Ed.). Baltimore, Johns Hopkins University Press, 1967.
52. Cooper, H.: Psychological aspects of congenital heart disease. S. Afr. Med. J., *33*:349, 1959.
53. Coyle, G.L., and Fisher, R.: Helping hospitalized children through social group work. Child, *16*:114, 1952.
54. Crammond, W.A., Knight, P.R., and Lawrence, J.R.: The psychiatric contribution to a renal unit undertaking chronic haemodialysis and renal homotransplantation. Br. J. Psychiatry, *113*:1201, 1967.
55. Crammond, W.A., et al.: Psychological aspects of management of chronic renal failure. Br. Med. J., *1*:539, 1968.
56. Cytryn, L., Cytryn, E., and Rieger, R.E.: Psychological implications of cryptorchidism. J. Am. Acad. Child Psychiatry, *6*:131, 1967.
57. Daniel, W.A., Jr., et al.: Diseases of the reproductive system. In: *Principles of Pediatrics: Health Care of the Young*. (R.A. Hoekelman, S. Blatman, P.A. Brunell, S.B. Friedman, and H.M. Seidel, Eds.). New York, McGraw-Hill, 1978.
58. Dansak, D.A.: Secondary gain in long-term hemodialysis patients. Am. J. Psychiatry, *129*:352, 1972.
59. Davenport, H.T., and Werry, J.S.: The effect of general anesthesia, surgery and hospitalization upon the behavior of children. Am. J. Orthopsychiatry, *40*:806, 1970.
60. De-Nour, A.K.: Psychotherapy with patients on chronic hemodialysis. Br. J. Psychiatry, *116*:207, 1970.
61. Deshazo, C.V., Simmons, R.L., and Bernstein, D.M.: Results of renal transplantation in 100 children. Surgery, *76*:461, 1974.
62. Deutsch, H.: Some psychoanalytic observations in surgery. Psychosom. Med., *4*:105, 1942.
63. Dlin, B.M., Fischer, H.K., and Huddell, B.: Psychologic adaptation to pacemaker and open heart surgery. Arch. Gen. Psychiatry, *19*:599, 1968.
64. Douglas, J.W.B.: Early hospital admissions and

later disturbances of behavior and learning. Dev. Med. Child Neurol., *17*:456, 1975.

65. Druss, R.G., O'Conner, J.F., and Stern, L.O.: Psychologic response to colectomy. II. Adjustment to a permanent colostomy. Arch. Gen. Psychiatry, *20*:419, 1909.

66. Drotar, D.: The treatment of a severe anxiety reaction in an adolescent boy following renal transplantation. J. Am. Acad. Child Psychiatry, *14*:451, 1975.

67. Drotar, D.: Consultation in the intensive care nursery. Int. J. Psychiatry Med., *7*:69, 1976.

68. Duff, R.S., and Campbell, A.G.M.: Moral and ethical dilemmas in the special care nursery. N. Engl. J. Med., *289*:890, 1973.

69. Dumas, R., and Leonard, R.: The effect of nursing on the incidence of postoperative vomiting. Nurs. Res., *12*:12, 1963.

70. Edelman, C.M. Jr., and Barnett, H.L.: Chronic renal disease. In *Ambulatory Pediatrics*. (M. Green and R.J. Haggerty, Eds.). Philadelphia, Saunders, 1968.

71. Egerton, N., and Kay, J.H.: Psychological disturbances associated with open heart surgery. Br. J. Psychiatry, *110*:433, 1964.

72. Eickenhoff, J.E., Kneale, D.H., and Dripps, R.D.: Incidence and etiology of postanesthetic excitement. Anesthesiology, *22*:667, 1961.

73. Eisendrath, R.: The role of grief and fear in the death of kidney transplant patients. Am. J. Psychiatry, *126*:281, 1967.

74. Eisendrath, R.M., Guttman, R.D., and Murray, J.E.: Psychologic considerations in the selection of kidney transplant donors. Surg. Gynecol. Obstet., *129*:243, 1969.

75. Emde, R.N., et al.: Stress and neonatal sleep. Psychosom. Med., *33*:491, 1971.

76. Engel, G., and Schmale, A.: Psychoanalytic theory of somatic disorder. J. Psychoanal. Assoc., *15*:344, 1967.

77. Erickson, F.: Play interviews for four-year-old hospitalized children. Monogr. Soc. Res. Child Dev., *23*:3, 1958.

78. Evans, R.W.: Children of dialysis patients and selection of dialysis setting. Am. J. Psychiatry, *135*:343, 1978.

79. Eylon, Y.: Birth events, appendicitis, and appendectomy. Br. J. Med. Psychol., *40*:317, 1967.

80. Fagin, C.M.: *The Effects of Maternal Attendance During Hospitalization on the Post-Hospital Behavior of Young Children: A Comparative Study.* Philadelphia, Davis, 1966.

81. Falstein, E.I., Judas, I., and Mendelsolin, R.: Fantasies in children prior to herniorraphy. Am. J. Orthopsychiatry, *27*:800, 1957.

81a.Faust, O.A., et al.: *Reducing Emotional Trauma in Hospitalized Children.* Albany, N.Y., Albany Research Project, Albany Medical School, 1952.

82. Fellner, C.H.: Selection of living kidney donors and the problem of informed consort. Semin. Psychiatry, *3*:1, 1971.

83. Fine, R.N., et al.: Second renal transplants in children. Surgery, *73*:1, 1973.

84. Fine, R.N., et al.: Long-term results of renal transplantation in children. Pediatrics, *61*:641, 1978.

85. Fineman, A.D.: Child psychiatry on a children's surgical service. Am. J. Surg., *95*:64, 1958.

86. Ford, C.V., and Castelnuovo-Tedesco, P.: Hemodialysis and renal transplantation—psychopathological reactions and their management. In: *Psychosomatic Medicine: Its Clinical Applications* (E.D. Wittkower and H. Warnes, Eds.). New York, Harper & Row, 1977.

87. Fox, R., Rizzo, N.D., and Gifford, S.: Psychological observations of patients undergoing mitral surgery: A study of stress. Psychosom. Med., *16*:186, 1954.

88. Frain, B.: Personal communication.

89. Fraser, B.: The pediatric bill of rights. South Texas Law J., *16*:245, 1975.

90. Freedman, D.A., et al.: Further observations on the effect of reverse isolation from birth on cognitive and affective development. J. Am. Acad. Child Psychiatry, *15*:593, 1976.

91. Frend, A.: The role of bodily illness in the life of the child. Psychoanal. Study Child, *7*:74, 1952.

92. Galdston, R.: The burning and the healing of children. In: *Annual Progress in Child Psychiatry and Child Development* (S. Chess and A. Thomas, Eds.). New York, Brunner/Mazel, 1974.

93. Galdston, R., and Hughes, M.C.: Pediatric hospitalization as crisis intervention. Am. J. Psychiatry, *129*:721, 1972.

94. Gardner, G.G., August, C.S., and Githens, J.: Psychological issues in bone marrow transplantation. Pediatrics, *60*:625, 1971.

95. Geis, W.: Home visits help prepare preschoolers and their parents for hospitalization. AMA Regional Clinical Conference, Chicago, American Medical Association, 1967.

96. Geist, R.A.: Consultation on a pediatric surgery ward: Creating an empathic climate. Am. J. Orthopsychiatry, *47*:445, 1977.

97. Githens, J.: Personal communication.

98. Glaser, H.H.: Group discussions with mothers of hospitalized children. Pediatrics, *26*:132, 1960.

99. Gofman, H., Buckman, W., and Schade, G.: The child's emotional response to hospitalization. Am. J. Dis. Child., *93*:157, 1957.

100. Gofman, H., Buckman, W., and Schade, G.: Parents' emotional response to child's hospitalization. Am. J. Dis. Child., *93*:629, 1957.

101. Goldberg, R., Bernstein, N., and Crosby, R.: Vocational development of adolescents with burn injury. Rehabil. Counselling Bull., *18*:140, 1975.

102. Goldman, H., and Bohcali, A.: Psychological preparation of children for tonsillectomy. Laryngoscope, *76*:1698, 1966.

103. Goldstein, A.M., and Reznikoff, M.: Suicide in chronic hemodialysis from an external locus of control framework. Am. J. Psychiatry, *127*:1204, 1971.

104. Great Britain Platt Committee: The welfare of children in hospital. London, Her Majesty's Stationery Office, 1959.

105. Green, M.: Integration of ambulatory services in a children's hospital: A unifying design. Am. J. Dis. Child., *110*:178, 1965.

106. Green, M.: A new arrangement for hospital services: The parent-care pavilion. Pediatrics, 43:486, 1969.

107. Gross, R.E., and Jewett, T.C., Jr.: Surgical experiences from 1,222 operations for undescended testes. JAMA, 160:634, 1956.

108. Grushkin, C.M., Korsch, B.M., and Fine, R.N.: The outlook for adolescents with chronic renal failure. Pediatr. Clin. North Am., 20:953, 1973.

109. Guerin, F.S.: Hospitalization as a positive experience for poverty children. Clin. Pediatr., 16:509, 1977.

110. Hackett, T.P., Cassem, N.H., and Wishnie, H.A.: The coronary care unit: An appraisal of its psychologic hazards. N. Engl. J. Med., 279:1365, 1968.

111. Hackett, T.P., and Weisman, A.D.: Psychiatric management of operative syndromes. I. The therapeutic consultation and the effect of non-interpretative intervention. Psychosom. Med., 22:267, 1960.

112. Haggerty, R.J.: Diagnosis and treatment: Tonsils and adenoids—A problem revisited. Pediatrics, 41:815, 1968.

113. Haller, J.A.: Newer concepts in emergency care of children with major injuries. Pediatrics, 52:485, 1973.

114. Hamburg, D., Hamburg, B., and De Goza, S.: Adaptive problems and mechanisms in the severely burned patient. Psychiatry, 16:1, 1953.

115. Hay, D., and Oken, D.: The psychological stresses of intensive care unit nursing. Psychosom. Med., 34:109, 1972.

116. Hefferman, M., and Azarnoff, P.: Factors in reducing children's anxiety about clinic visits. HSMHA Health Report, 86:1131, 1971.

117. Healy, M.H., and Hansen, H.: Psychiatric management of the limb amputation in a preschool child: The illusion of "like me—not me." J. Am. Acad. Child Psychiatry, 16:684, 1977.

118. Hemodialysis and renal transplantation in children: The role of the pediatric nephrology team. Pediatrics, 53:864, 1974.

119. Hinde, R.A., and Davies, L.: Removing infant rhesus from mother for 13 days compared with removing mother from infant. J. Child Psychol. Psychiatry, 13:227, 1972.

120. Hinman, F., Jr.: The implications of testicular cytology in the treatment of cryptorchidism. Am. J. Surg., 90:381, 1955.

121. Hockaday, W.J.: Experiences of a psychiatrist as a member of a surgical faculty. Am. J. Psychiatry, 117:706, 1961.

122. Hollon, T.H.: Modified group therapy in the treatment of patients on chronic hemodialysis. Am. J. Psychother., 26:501, 1972.

123. Hymovich, D.P.: Nursing of Children: A Family-Centered Guide for Study. Philadelphia, Saunders, 1974.

124. Jackson, E.B., et al.: A hospital rooming-in unit for four newborn infants and their mothers: Descriptive account of background, development and procedures with a few preliminary observations. Pediatrics, 1:28, 1948.

125. Jackson, K.: Psychologic preparation as a method

126. Jackson, K., et al.: Behavior changes indicating emotional trauma in tonsillectomized children. Pediatrics, 23:964, 1953.

127. James, F.E.: The behavior reactions of normal children to common operations. Practitioner, 185:339, 1960.

128. James, V.L., and Wheeler, W.E.: The care-by-parent unit. Pediatrics, 43:488, 1969.

129. Jamison, K.R., Wellisch, D.K., and Pasnan, R.O.: Psychosocial aspects of mastectomy. I. The woman's perspective. Am. J. Psychiatry, 135:432, 1978.

130. Janis, I.L.: Psychological Stress: Psychoanalytic and Behavioral Studies of Surgical Patients. New York, Wiley, 1958.

131. Jarvis, J.H.: Post-mastectomy breast phantoms. J. Nerv. Ment. Dis., 144:266, 1967.

132. Jensen, G.: Preventative implications of a study of 100 children treated for serious burns. Pediatrics, 24:623, 1959.

133. Jessner, L.: Personal communication.

134. Jessner, L.: Some observations on children hospitalized during latency. In: Dynamic Psychopathology in Childhood (L. Jessner and E. Pavenstedt, Eds.). New York, Grune & Stratton, 1959.

135. Jessner, L., Blom, G.E., and Waldfogel, S.: Emotional implications of tonsillectomy and adenoidectomy in children. Psychoanal. Study Child, 7:126, 1952.

136. Jongkees, L.B.W.: The psychic effect of hospital and surgical interventions on children. Ann. Otol. Rhinol. Laryngol., 63:145, 1954.

137. Jorring, K.: Amputation in children. Acta Orthop. Scand., 42:178, 1971.

138. Kaiser, A.D.: Children's Tonsils In or Out: A Critical Study of the End Results of Tonsillectomy. Philadelphia, Lippincott, 1932.

139. De-Nour, A.K., and Czaczkes, J.W.: Emotional problems and reactions of the medical team in a chronic haemodialysis unit. Lancet, 2:987, 1968.

140. De-Nour, A.K., Shaltiel, J., and Czaczkes, J.W.: Emotional reactions of patients on chronic hemodialysis. Psychosom. Med., 30:521, 1968.

141. Kempe, H.: Personal communication.

142. Kemph, J.P.: Psychotherapy with donors and recipients of kidney transplants. Semin. Psychiatry, 3:145, 1971.

143. Kemph, J., Berman, E., and Coppolillo, H.P.: Kidney transplants and shifts in family dynamics. Am. J. Psychiatry, 125:39, 1969.

144. Kennedy, J., and Bakst, H.: The influence of emotions on the outcome of surgery: A predictive study. Bull. N.Y. Acad. Med., 42:811, 1966.

145. Khan, A.U., Herndon, C.H., and Ahmadian, S.Y.: Social and emotional adaptations of children with transplanted kidneys and chronic hemodialysis. Am. J. Psychiatry, 127:1194, 1971.

146. Kilpatrick, D.G., et al.: The use of psychological test data to predict open-heart surgery outcome: A prospective study. Psychosom. Med., 37:62, 1975.

147. Kimball, C.P.: Psychological response to the ex-

perience of open heart surgery. I. Am. J. Psychiatry, *126*:3, 1969.

147a.Klaus, M.H., and Kennell, J.H.: *Parent-Child Bonding.* St. Louis, C.V. Mosby, 1976.

148. Konopka, G.: *Group Work in the Institution.* New York, Whiteside & Morrow, 1954.

149. Kolb, F.: *The Painful Phantom.* Springfield, Ill., Thomas, 1954.

150. Koop, C.E.: The seriously ill or dying child: Supporting the patient and the family. Pediat. Clin. North Am., *16*:555, 1969.

151. Korsch, B.M., et al.: Experiences with children and their families during extended hemodialysis and kidney transplantation. Pediat. Clin. North Am., *18*:625, 1971.

152. Korsch, B.M., Fine, R.N., and Negrete, V.F.: Noncompliance in children with renal transplants. Pediatrics, *61*:872, 1978.

153. Korsch, B.M., Fraad, L., and Barnett, H.: Pediatric discussions with parent groups. J. Pediatr., *44*:703, 1954.

154. Korsch, B.M., Francis, V., and Fine, R.: Critical periods for children and their families in a hemodialysis and kidney transplant program. Pediatr. Res., *3*:346, 1969.

155. Korsch, B.M., et al.: Kidney transplantation in children: Psychosocial follow-up study. J. Pediatr., *88*:399, 1973.

156. Krumlovsky, F.A., et al.: Morbidity of chronic hemodialysis and transplantation. Trans. Am. Soc. Artif. Intern. Organs, *21*(Suppl. 10): 102, 1975.

157. LaBaw, W.L.: Adjunctive trance therapy with severely burned children. Int. J. Child Psychiatry, *2*:163, 1973.

158. Langford, W.S.: Anxiety states in children. Am. J. Orthopsychiatry, *7*:210, 1937.

159. Langford, W.S.: Physical illness and convalescence: Their meaning to the child. J. Pediatr., *33*:242, 1948.

160. Lattimer, J.K., et al.: The optimum time to operate for cryptorchidism. Pediatrics, *53*:96, 1974.

161. Lawrie, R.: Operating on children as day cases. Lancet, *2*:1289, 1964.

162. Lazarus, H.R., and Hagens, J.H.: Prevention of psychosis following open-heart surgery. Am. J. Psychiatry, *124*:1190, 1968.

163. Levy, D.M.: On the problem of movement restraint: Tics, stereotyped movements, hyperactivity. Am. J. Orthopsychiatry, *14*:644, 1944.

164. Levy, D.M.: Psychic trauma of operations in children and a note on combat neurosis. Am. J. Dis. Child., *69*:7, 1945.

165. Levy, N.B.: Sexual adjustment to maintenance hemodialysis and renal transplantation: National survey by questionnaire: Preliminary report. Trans. Am. Soc. Artif. Intern. Organs, *19*:138, 1973.

166. Lewis, M.: Kidney donation by a 7-year-old identical twin child. J. Am. Acad. Child Psychiatry, *13*:221, 1974.

167. Lewis, M.: Child psychiatric consultation in pediatrics. Pediatrics, *62*:359, 1978.

168. Lightwood, R., et al.: Home care for sick children. Lancet, *1*:313, 1957.

169. Lindemann, E.: Observations in psychiatric sequelae to surgical operations in women. Am. J. Psychiatry, *98*:132, 1941.

170. Lipowski, Z.J.: Psychiatric liaison with neurosurgery. Am. J. Psychiatry, *129*:136, 1972.

171. Locke, B.: Psychology of the laryngectomee. Milit. Med., *131*:593, 1966.

172. Long, R.T., and Cope, O.: Emotional problems of burned children. N. Engl. J. Med., *264*:1121, 1961.

173. Loomis, E.: The child's emotions and surgery. In: *Pre- and Post-Operative Care in the Pediatric Surgical Patient* (W.B. Kiesewetter, Ed.). Chicago, Year Book, 1956.

174. Loomis, W.G.: The use of a foster grandmother in the psychotherapy of a preschool child on a pediatric ward. Clin. Pediatr., *6*:384, 1967.

175. Loomis, W.G.: The management of children's emotional reactions to severe burns. Clin. Pediatr., *9*:362, 1970.

176. Lorand, S.: The body image and the psychiatric evaluation of patients for plastic sugery. J. Hillside Hosp., *10*:224, 1961.

177. Lubchenko, L.: Personal communication.

178. Lucas, W.P.: Education for hospitalized children. Med. Women J., *56*:22, 1949.

179. MacCarthy, D., Lindsay, M., and Morris, L.: Children in hospital with mothers. Lancet, *1*:603, 1962.

180. Mahaffey, P.R.: The effects of hospitalization on children admitted for tonsillectomy and adenoidectomy. Nurs. Res., *14*:12, 1965.

181. Margolis, G.J.: Postoperative psychosis on the intensive care unit. Compr. Psychiatry, *8*:227, 1967.

182. Marshall, J.R.: Effective use of a psychiatric consultant on a dialysis unit. Postgrad. Med. J., *55*:121, 1974.

183. Marshall, J.R., and Fellner, C.H.: Kidney donors revisited. Am. J. Psychiatry, *134*:575, 1977.

184. Mattsson, A.: Child psychiatric ward rounds on pediatrics. J. Am. Acad. Child Psychiatry, *15*:357, 1976.

185. Mattsson, A., and Naylor, K.A.: Psychiatric emergencies on the pediatric ward: Clinical characteristics and suggestions for management. In: *Emergencies in Child Psychiatry* (G.C. Morrison, Ed.). Springfield, Ill., Thomas, 1975.

186. May, J.G.: A psychiatric study of a pediatric intensive care unit. Clin. Pediatr., *11*:76, 1972.

187. McCorkle, L.P., et al.: Study of illness in a group of Cleveland families. III. Relation of tonsillectomy to incidence of common respiratory diseases in children. N. Engl. J. Med., *252*:1066, 1955.

188. McFarlane, R.G., and Biggs, R.: Observations on fibrinolysis: Spontaneous activity associated with surgical operations and trauma. Lancet, *2*:862, 1946.

189. McGregor, F., et al.: *Facial Deformities and Plastic Surgery: A Psychosocial Study.* Springfield, Ill., Thomas, 1953.

190. McKee, W.J.E.: Controlled study of the effects of tonsillectomy and adenoidectomy in children. Br. J. Prev. Soc. Med., *17*:49, 1963.

191. McKee, W.J.E.: The part played by adenoidectomy in the combined operation of tonsillectomy with adenoidectomy. Br. J. Prev. Soc. Med., 17:13, 1963.

192. McKegney, P.F., and Lange, P.: The decision to no longer live on chronic hemodialysis. Am. J. Psychiatry, 128:267, 1971.

193. McKeith, R.: Children in hospital: Preparation for operation. Lancet, 2:843, 1953.

194. McKenzie, M.W., et al.: A pharmacist-based study of the epidemiology of adverse drug reactions in pediatric medicine patients. Am. J. Hosp. Pharm., 30:898, 1973.

195. Mellish, R.W.P.: Preparation of a child for hospitalization and surgery. Pediatr. Clin. North Am., 16:543, 1969.

196. Menninger, K.: Polysurgery and polysurgical addiction. Psychoanal. Q., 3:173, 1946.

197. Menzer-Benaron, D., et al.: Patterns of emotional recovery from hysterectomy. Psychosom. Med., 19:5, 1957.

198. Meyer, B.C., Blacker, R.S., and Brown, I.: A clinical study of psychiatric and psychological aspects of mitral surgery. Psychosom. Med., 23:194, 1961.

199. Meyer, E., and Edgerton, M.T.: Psychology of patients seeking plastic surgery. Bull. Johns Hopkins Hosp., 100:235, 1957.

200. Meyer, E., Unger, H.T., and Slaughter, R.: Investigation of a psychosocial hypothesis in appendectomies. Psychosom. Med., 26:671, 1964.

201. Minde, K., and Maler, L.: Psychiatric counselling on a pediatric medical ward: A controlled evaluation. J. Pediatr., 72:452, 1968.

202. Mittelman, B.: Psychodynamics of motility. Int. J. Psychoanal., 39:196, 1958.

203. Molinaro, J.R.: The social fate of children disfigured by burns. Am. J. Psychiatry, 135:979, 1978.

204. Muslin, H.L.: On acquiring a kidney. Am. J. Psychiatry, 127:1185, 1971.

205. Nadas, A.S.: Personal communication.

206. Neubauer, P.B., and Flapan, D.: Developmental groupings in latency children. J. Am. Acad. Child Psychiatry, 15:646, 1976.

207. The Non-operative Aspects of Pediatric Surgery. Report of the Twenty-Seventh Ross Conference on Pediatric Research. Columbus, Ohio, Ross Laboratories, 1958.

208. North, A.F., Jr.: When should a child be in the hospital? Pediatrics, 57:540, 1976.

209. Nover, R.A.: Pain and the burned child. J. Am. Acad. Child Psychiatry, 12:499, 1973.

210. Paradise, J.L.: Why T and A remains moot. Pediatrics, 49:648, 1972.

211. Parkes, C.M.: Components of the reaction to loss of a limb, spouse or home. J. Psychosom. Res., 16:343, 1972.

212. Pearson, G.H.J.: Effect of operative procedures on the emotional life of the child. Am. J. Dis. Child., 62:716, 1941.

213. Peller, L.E.: Libidinal phases, ego development and play. Psychoanal. Study Child, 9:178, 1954.

214. Penn, I., et al.: Psychiatric experience with patients receiving renal and hepatic transplants. Semin. Psychiatry, 3:1, 1971.

215. Plank, E.N.: Preparing children for surgery. Ohio Med. J., 59:809, 1963.

216. Plank, E.N.: Working with Children in Hospitals. 2nd Ed. Cleveland, Case Western Reserve University Press, 1975.

217. Plank, E.N., Coughey, P.A., and Lipson, M.F.: A general hospital child care program to counteract hospitalization. Am. J. Orthopsychiatry, 29:94, 1959.

218. Plank, E., and Horwood, C.: Leg amputation in a four-year-old: Reactions of the child, her family and the staff. Psychoanal. Study Child, 16:405, 1961.

219. Potts, W.J.: The Surgeon and the Child. Philadelphia, Saunders, 1959.

220. Price, D., Thaler, M., and Mason, J.: Preoperative emotional states and adrenal cortical activity. Arch. Neurol. Psychiatry, 77:646, 1957.

221. Provence, S., and Ritvo, S.: Effects of deprivation on institutionalized infants. Psychoanal. Study Child, 16:189, 1959.

222. Prugh, D.G.: Emotional reactions to surgery. In: The Non-Operative Aspects of Surgery. Report of the Twenty-Seventh Ross Conference on Pediatric Research. Columbus, Ohio, Ross Laboratories, 1958.

223. Prugh, D.G.: Emotional aspects of the hospitalization of children. In: Red Is the Color of Hurting: Planning for Children in the Hospital (M.F. Shore, Ed.). Department of Health, Education, and Welfare. Washington, Government Printing Office, 1965.

224. Prugh, D.G.: The immediate and prolonged psychological implications of transplants in children. In: The Effects of Hospitalization on Children (E.K. Oremland and J.P. Oremland, Eds.). Springfield, Ill, Thomas, 1973.

225. Prugh, D.G.: First Elizabeth M. Staub Memorial Lecture. One of the pieces: respect for the cultural heritage of the hospitalized child. J. Assoc. Child Care Hosp., 4:1, 1975.

226. Prugh, D.G., and Eckhardt, L.O.: Preparing children psychologically for painful medical and surgical procedures. In: Psychosocial Aspects of Pediatric Care (E. Gellert, Ed.). New York, Grune & Stratton, 1978.

227. Prugh, D.G., and Eckhardt, L.O.: Child psychiatry and pediatrics. In: Basic Handbook of Child Psychiatry (J.D. Nospitz, et al., Eds.). New York, Basic Books, 1979.

228. Prugh, D.G., and Jordan, K.: Physical illness or injury: The hospital as a source of emotional disturbance in children. In: Advocacy for Child Mental Health (I. Berlin, Ed.). New York, Brunner/Mazel, 1975.

229. Prugh, D.G., Wagonfeld, S., Jordan, K., and Metcalf, D.: A clinical study of delirium in children and adolescents. Psychosom. Med., 42:177, 1980.

230. Prugh, D.G., et al.: A study of emotional reactions of children and families to illness and hospitalization. Am. J. Orthopsychiatry, 23:78, 1953.

231. Prugh, D.G., and Tagiuri, C.K.: Emotional aspects of the respirator care of patients with poliomyelitis. Psychosom. Med., 16:104, 1954.

232. Quinby, S., and Bernstein, N.: Identity problems and the adaptation of nurses to severely burned children. Am. J. Psychiatry, 128:58, 1971.

233. Randall, G.G., Ewalt, J.R., and Blair, H.: Psychiatric reaction to amputation. J. Am. Med. Assoc., 128:645, 1945.

234. Reinhart, J.B.: The doctor's dilemma: Whether or not to recommend continuous renal dialysis or renal homotransplantation for the child with end-stage renal disease. J. Pediatr., 77:505, 1970.

234a.Reinhart, J.B., and Barnes, C.: Measurement and management of anxiety of children undergoing open heart surgery. Pediatrics, 49:250, 1972.

235. Rie, H., Boverman, H., Grossman, B., and Ozoa, N.: Immediate and long-term effects of intervention early in prolonged hospitalization. Pediatrics, 41:755, 1968.

236. Riley, C.M.: Thoughts about kidney transplantation in children. J. Pediatr., 65:797, 1964.

237. Robertson, J.: *Hospitals and Children: A Parent's Eye View.* New York, International Universities Press, 1963.

238. Robertson, J.: *Young Children in Hospitals.* New York, Basic Books, 1968.

239. Root, B.: Problems in evaluating effects of premedication in children. Anesth. Analg., 41:180, 1962.

240. Rose, J.A., and Sonis, M.: The use of separation as a diagnostic measure in the parent-child emotional crisis. Am. J. Psychiatry, 116:409, 1959.

241. Rosini, L.A., et al.: Group meetings in a pediatric intensive care unit. Pediatrics, 53:371, 1974.

242. Rowntree, G.: Accidents among children under two years of age in Great Britain. J. Hyg., 48:323, 1950.

243. Salisburg, R.E.: Behavioral responses of a nine-year-old child on chronic dialysis. Am. Acad. Child Psychiatry, 7:282, 1968.

244. Sampson, T.F.: The child in renal failure: Emotional impact of treatment on the child and his family. Unpublished material.

245. Santiago, D., et al.: Medico-legal management of the juvenile kidney donor. Transplant. Proc., 6:441, 1974.

246. Schaffer, H.R., and Callender, W.M.: Psychologic effects of hospitalization in infancy. Pediatrics, 24:528, 1959.

247. Schiller, P.H.: Innate motor action as a basis of learning. In: *Instinctive Behavior* (C.H. Schiller, Ed.). New York, International Universities Press, 1957.

248. Schowalter, J.E., and Ford, R.D.: Utilization of patient meetings on an adolescent ward. Psychiatry Med., 1:197, 1970.

249. Schowalter, J., and Ford, R.: The hospitalized adolescent. Children, 18:4, 1971.

250. Schowalter, J.E., Perhott, J.B., and Mann, M.M.: The adolescent's decision to die. Pediatrics, 51:97, 1973.

251. Schulman, J.L.: The management of the irate parent. J. Pediatr., 77:338, 1970.

252. Schulman, J.L., et al.: A study of the effect of the mother's presence during anesthesia induction. Pediatrics, 39:111, 1967.

253. Schreiner, G.E., and Maher, J.F.: Hemodialysis for chronic renal failure. III. Medical, moral, and ethical, and socioeconomic problems. Ann. Int. Med., 62:531, 1965.

254. Scott, D.L.: Psychiatric problems of hemodialysis: Treatment by hypnosis. Br. J. Psychiatry, 122:91, 1973.

255. Seligman, R., Carroll, S., and MacMillan, B.C.: Emotional responses of burned children in a pediatric intensive care unit. Psychiatry Med., 3:591, 1972.

256. Shagass, C., and Naiman, J.: The sedation threshold. Psychosom. Med., 17:480, 1955.

257. Shore, M.F., Ed.: Red is the color of hurting: Planning for children in the hospital. Department of Health, Education, and Welfare, Washington, Government Printing Office, 1967.

258. Shore, M.F., Geiser, R.L., and Wolman, H.M.: Constructive uses of a hospital experience. Children, 12:3, 1965.

259. Sibinga, M.S., and Friedman, C.J.: Restraint and speech. Pediatrics, 48:116, 1971.

260. Siller, J.: Psychological concomitants of amputation in children. Child Dev., 31:109, 1960.

261. Simmel, M.L.: Phantom experience following amputation in childhood. Neurol. Neurosurg. Psychiatry, 25:69, 1962.

262. Simmons, R.G., and Klein, S.D.: Family noncommunication: The search for kidney donors. Am. J. Psychiatry, 129:687, 1972.

263. Simons, C., et al.: The impact of reverse isolation on early child development. Psychother. Psychosom., 22:300, 1973.

264. Skipper, J.K., Leonard, R.C., and Rhymes, J.: Child hospitalization and social interaction: An experimental study of mothers' feelings of stress, adaptation and satisfaction. Med. Care, 6:496, 1968.

265. Solnit, A.J.: Hospitalization: An aid to psychological and physical health in childhood. Am. J. Orthopsychiatry, 99:155, 1960.

266. Shrand, H.: Behavior changes in sick children nursed at home. Pediatrics, 35:604, 1965.

267. Smessaert, A., Scher, C.A., and Artusio, J.F.: Observations in the immediate postanesthesia period. II. Mode of recovery. Br. J. Anaesthesiol., 32:181, 1960.

268. Smith, R.M.: *Anesthesia for Infants and Children.* 3rd Ed. St. Louis, Mosby, 1968.

269. Smyrl, R.: Personal communication.

270. Solomon, G.F.: Emotional stress, the central nervous system and immunity. Ann. N.Y. Acad. Sci., 164:335, 1969.

271. Spence, J.C.: The care of children in hospitals. The Charles West Lecture. London, Royal College of Physicians, November, 1946.

272. Spitz, R.: Hospitalism: An inquiry into the genesis of psychiatric conditions in early childhood. Psychoanal. Study Child, 6:255, 1951.

273. Spitz, R., and Wolf, K.: Anaclitic depression. Psychoanal. Study Child, 2:313, 1946.

274. Starzl, T.E., et al.: The role of organ transplantation in pediatrics. Pediatr. Clin. North Am., 13:381, 1966.

275. Starzl, T.E., et al.: A decade follow-up in early

cases of renal homotransplantation. Ann. Surg., *180*:606, 1974.

276. Staub, E.: Personal communication.

277. Steensma, J.: Problems of the adolescent amputee. J. Rehabil., *25*:19, 1959.

278. Stenback, A., and Haapanen, E.: Azotemia and psychosis. Acta Psychiatr. Scand. (Suppl.) *43*, 66, 1967.

279. Stocking, M., et al.: Psychopathology in the pediatric hospital: Implications for the pediatrician. Psychiatry Med., *1*:329, 1970.

280. Stocking, M., et al.: Psychopathology in the pediatric hospital: Implications for community mental health. Am. J. Public Health, *62*:551, 1972.

281. Suran, B.M., and Lavigne, J.V.: Rights of children in pediatric settings: A survey of attitudes. Pediatrics, *60*:715, 1977.

282. Sutherland, A.M., and Orback, C.E.: Psychological impact of cancer and cancer surgery. II. Depressive reactions associated with surgery for cancer. Cancer, *6*:958, 1952.

283. Swenson, O.: Play programs for surgical patients. In: *The Nonoperative Aspects of Pediatric Surgery*. Report of the Twenty-Seventh Ross Pediatric Research Conference. Columbus, Ohio, Ross Laboratories, 1957.

284. Thoroughman, J.C., et al.: Psychological factors predictive of surgical success in patients with intractable peptic ulcer. Psychosom. Med., *26*:618, 1964.

285. Tisza, V.B., and Angoff, K.: A play program and its function in a pediatric hospital. Pediatrics, *19*:293, 1957.

286. Tisza, V.B., Dorsett, P., and Morse, J.: Psychological implications of renal transplantation. J. Am. Acad. Child Psychiatry, *15*:709, 1976.

287. Toker, E.: Psychiatric aspects of cardiac surgery in a child. J. Am. Acad. Child Psychiatry, *10*:156, 1971.

288. Tourkow, L.: Psychic consequences of loss and replacement of body parts. J. Am. Psychoanal. Assoc., *22*:170, 1974.

289. Tuckman, A.J.: Brief psychotherapy and hemodialysis. Arch. Gen. Psychiatry, *23*:65, 1970.

290. Tufo, H.M., and Ostfeld, A.M.: A prospective study of open-heart surgery (Abstr.). Psychosom. Med., *30*:552, 1968.

291. Uehling, D.T., et al.: Cessation of immunosuppression after renal transplantation. Surgery, *79*:278, 1976.

292. Vaughn, G.F.: Children in hospitals. Lancet, *272*:1117, 1957.

293. Vernon, D.T.A., and Bailey, W.C.: The use of motion pictures in the psychological preparation of children for induction of anesthesia. Anesthesiology, *40*:68, 1974.

294. Vernon, D.T.A., Folley, J.M., and Schulman, J.L.: Effect of mother-child separation and birth order on young children's responses to two potentially stressful experiences. J. Pers. Soc. Psychol., *5*:162, 1967.

295. Vernon, D.T.A., and Schulman, J.: Hospitalization as a source of psychological benefit to children. Pediatrics, *34*:694, 1964.

296. Vernon, D.T.A., Schulman, J.L., and Foley, J.M.: Changes in children's behavior after hospitalization. Am. J. Dis. Child., *3*:581, 1966.

297. Vernon, D.T.A., et al.: *The Psychological Responses of Children to Hospitalization and Illness*. Springfield, Ill., Thomas, 1965.

298. Viederman, M.: Adaptive and maladaptive regression in hemodialysis. Psychiatry, *37*:68, 1974.

299. Viederman, M.: Psychogenic factors in kidney transplant rejection: A case study. Am. J. Psychiatry, *132*:957, 1975.

300. Viersieck, J., Barbier, F., and Derom, F.: A case of lung transplant: Clinical note. Semin. Psychiatry, *3*:1, 1971.

301. Vigliano, H.S., et al.: Psychiatric sequelae of old burns in children and their parents. Am. J. Orthopsychiatry, *34*:753, 1964.

302. Vincent, H.B., Jr., and Rothenberg, M.B.: Comprehensive care of an 8-year-old boy following traumatic operation of the glans penis. Pediatrics, *44*:271, 1969.

303. Visintainer, M.A., and Wolfer, J.A.: Psychological preparation for surgical pediatric patients: The effect on children's and parents' stress responses and adjustment. Pediatrics, *56*:187, 1975.

304. Wallace, M., and Feinauer, V.: Understanding a sick child's behavior. Am. J. Nurs., *48*:517, 1948.

305. Watkins, A.G., and Lewis-Faning, E.: Incidence of cross-infection in children's wards. Br. Med. J., *2*:616, 1949.

306. Wellisch, D.K., Jamison, K.R., and Pasnau, R.O.: Psychosocial aspects of mastectomy. II. The man's perspective. Am. J. Psychiatry, *135*:543, 1978.

307. Wennberg, J.E., et al.: Changes in tonsillectomy rates associated with feedback and review. Pediatrics, *59*:821, 1977.

308. Wessel, M.A.: The pediatric nurse and human relations. Am. J. Nurs., *47*:213, 1947.

309. Wesseling, E.: The adolescent facing amputation. Am. J. Nurs., *65*:90, 1965.

310. West, W.M., and Janke, L.D.: A methodological critique of research on psychological effects of vasectomy. Psychosom. Med., *36*:438, 1974.

311. Williamson, A.P., et al., Eds.: A special report: Four year study of a boy with combined immune deficiency maintained in strict reverse isolation from birth. Pediatr. Res., *2*:63, 1977.

312. Wilson, J.A.: Joint pediatric and psychiatric care of the hospitalized child. Am. J. Orthopsychiatry, *28*:539, 1958.

313. Winnicott, D.W.: Transitional objects and transitional phenomena. Int. J. Psychoanal., *4*:29, 1953.

314. Witmer, H.L.: *The National Picture of Children's Emotional Disturbance*. New York, Child Development Center, 1962.

315. Wolf, S.R.: Emotional reactions to hysterectomy. Postgrad. Med., *47*:165, 1970.

316. Wolff, S.: *Children Under Stress*. London, Allen Lane, 1969.

317. Wolstenholme, G.E.W., and O'Connor, M.: *Ethics in Medical Progress: With Special Reference to Transplantation. Ciba Symposium*. London, Churchill, 1966.

318. Woodward, J.M.: Parental visiting of burned children. Br. Med. J., *1/2*:1656, 1962.
319. Woodward, J., and Jackson, D.: Emotional reactions in burned children and their mothers. Br. J. Plast. Surg., *13*:316, 1961.
320. Ziegler, F.J., Rodgers, W.A., and Prentias, R.J.: Psychological response to vasectomy. Arch. Gen. Psychiatry, *21*:46, 1969.

General References

Ack, M.: Considerations regarding the organization of a children's hospital. J. Assoc. Child Care Hosp., *4*:27, 1963.

Association for the Care of Children in Hospitals. *Hospitalized Child Bibliography*) P.O. Box H, Union, W. Va. 24983.

Azarnoff, P.: The care of children in hospitals: An overview. J. Pediatr. Psychol., *1*:5, 1976.

Bakwin, H.: The hospital care of infants and children. J. Pediatr., *39*:383, 1951.

Bell, J.E.: *The Family in the Hospital: Lessons from Developing Countries.* Department of Health, Education, and Welfare, Washington, Government Printing Office, 1969.

Bergmann, T.: *Children in the Hospital.* New York, International Universities Press, 1965.

Bernstein, N.R.: *Emotional Care of the Facially Burned and Disfigured.* Boston, Little, Brown, 1976.

Bishop, R.: Toys prescribed. The Modern Hospital, *2*:63, 1949.

Blake, F., and Wright, F.H.: *Essentials of Pediatric Nursing.* Philadelphia, Lippincott, 1963.

Blau, A., et al.: The collaboration of nursing and child psychiatry in a general hospital. Am. J. Orthopsychiatry, *29*:77, 1959.

Blom, G.: The reactions of hospitalized children to illness. Pediatrics, *22*:590, 1958.

Bowlby, J.: The nature of the child's tie to his mother. Int. J. Psychoanal., *39*:350, 1958.

Bowlby, J.: Separation anxiety. Int. J. Psychoanal., *41*:89, 1960.

Cassell, S.E.: *The Psychologic Responses of Children to Hospitalization and Illness.* Springfield, Ill., Thomas, 1965.

Castelnuovo-Tedesco, P.: *Psychiatric Aspects of Organ Transplantation.* New York, Grune & Stratton, 1971.

Dembo, T., Leviton, G.J., and Wright, B.A.: Adjustment to misfortune—A problem of social-psychological rehabilitation. Artif. Limbs, *3*:4, 1956.

Dimock, H.G.: *The Child in Hospital: A Study of his Emotional and Social Well Being.* Philadelphia, Davis, 1960.

Donnelly, M., et al.: *Hospitalized Child Bibliography.* Union, W. Va. Association for the Care of Children in Hospitals, 1976.

Edelston, H.: Separation anxiety in young children: A study of hospital cases. Genet. Psychol. Monogr., *28*:3, 1943.

English, O.S.: Psychosomatic medicine and dietetics. J. Am. Diet. Assoc., *27*:721, 1951.

Erikson, E.H.: Sex differences in the play configurations of pre-adolescents. Am. J. Orthopsychiatry, *21*:667, 1951.

Faust, O.A., et al.: Reducing emotional traumas in hospitalized children. Albany, N.Y., Albany Research Project, Albany Medical School, 1952.

Fox, H.M., Rizzo, N.D., and Gifford, S.: Psychological observations of patients undergoing mitral surgery: A study of stress. Psychosom. Med., *16*:186, 1954.

Fuller, T.E.: *Ethical Issues in Medicine: The Role of the Physician in Today's Society.* Boston, Little, Brown, 1968.

Geist, H.: *A Child Goes to the Hospital: The Psychological Aspects of a Child Going to the Hospital.* Springfield, Ill., Thomas, 1965.

Gofman, H., Buckman, W., and Schade, G.H.: The child's emotional response to hospitalization. Am. J. Dis. Child., *93*:157, 1957.

Gofman, H., Buckman, W., and Schade, G.H.: Parents' emotional response to child's hospitalization. Am. J. Dis. Child., *93*:629, 1957.

Greene, M.E., and Segar, W.E.: A new design for patient care and pediatric education in a children's hospital. Pediatrics, *32*:825, 1961.

Hall, J.H., and Swenson, D.D.: *Psychological and Social Aspects of Human Tissue Transplantation: An Annotated Bibliography.* Department of Health, Education, and Welfare, Washington, 1968.

Haller, J.A., Jr., Ed.: *The Hospitalized Child and His Family.* Baltimore, Johns Hopkins University Press, 1967.

Hardgrove, C.B., and Dawson, R.B.: Parents and children in the hospital: The family's role in pediatrics. Boston, Little, Brown, 1972.

Hartley, R.E., and Goldenson, R.M.: *The Complete Book of Children's Play.* New York, Crowell, 1963.

Heinecke, C.M.: Some effects of separating two-year-old children from their mothers: A comparative study. Human Relations, *9*:105, 1956.

Hofmann, A.D., et al.: *The Hospitalized Adolescent: A Guide to Managing the Ill and Injured Youth.* New York, Free Press, 1970.

Illingworth, R.S.: Children in hospital. Lancet, *2*:165, 1958.

Jackson, E.B.: Treatment of the young child in the hospital. Am. J. Orthopsychiatry, *12*:56, 1942.

Jackson, K., et al.: Problem of emotional trauma in hospital treatment. Pediatrics, *12*:23, 1953.

Jessner, L.: Some observations on children hospitalized during latency. In: *Dynamic Psychopathology* (L. Jessner and E. Pavenstedt, Eds.). New York, Grune & Stratton, 1959.

Kaplan, S.M.: Psychological aspects of cardiac disease: A study of patients experiencing mitral commissurotomy. Psychosom. Med., *18*:221, 1956.

Kemph, J.P.: Renal failure, artificial kidney and kidney transplant. Am. J. Psychiatry, *122*:1270, 1966.

Kimmel, M.R.: The use of play techniques in a medical setting. Soc. Case Work., *33*:30, 1952.

Langford, W.A.: The child in the pediatric hospital: adaptation to illness and hospitalization. Am. J. Orthopsychiatry, *31*:667, 1961.

Lewis, M.: The management of parents of acutely ill children in the hospital. Am J. Orthopsychiatry, *32*:60, 1962.

Mason, E.A.: The hospitalized child—His emotional needs. N. Engl. J. Med., 272:406, 1965.

Moncrief, J.A.: Burns. N. Engl. J. Med., 288:444, 1973.

Oremland, E.K., and Oremland, J.D., Eds.: *The Effects of Hospitalization on Children: Models for Their Care.* Springfield, Ill., Thomas, 1973.

Petrillo, M., and Sanger, S.: *Emotional Care of Hospitalized Children: An Environmental Approach.* Philadelphia, Lippincott, 1972.

Potts, W.J.: *The Surgeon and the Child.* Philadelphia, Saunders, 1959.

Powers, G.F.: Humanizing hospital experience. Am. J. Dis. Child., 76:365, 1948.

Provence, S.A., and Lipton, R.C.: *Infants in Institutions.* New York, International Universities Press, 1963.

Prugh, D.G.: Emotional aspects of the hospitalization of children. Child Family, 12:1, 1973.

Prugh, D.G., and Eckhardt, L.O.: Children's reactions to illness, hospitalization, and surgery. In: *Comprehensive Textbook of Psychiatry.* 2nd Ed. (A. Freedman and H. Kaplan, Eds.). Baltimore, Williams and Wilkins, 1975.

Rigg, C.A., and Fisher, R.C.: Some comments on current hospital medical services for adolescents. Am. J. Dis. Child., 120:193, 1970.

Robertson, J.: *Young Children in Hospital.* 2nd Ed. London, Tavistock, 1970.

Robins, A., and Sibley, L.B.: *Creative Art Therapy.* New York, Brunner/Mazel, 1976.

Roudinesco-Aubry, J., David, M., and Nicholas, J.: Responses of young children to separation from their mothers. Cour. Centre Int. Enfance, 2:66, 1952.

Saunders, L.: *Cultural Differences and Medical Care: The Case of the Spanish-Speaking People of the Southwest.* New York, Russell Sage Foundation, 1954.

Siegal, L.J.: Preparation of children for hospitalization: A selected review of the literature. J. Pediatr. Psychol., 1:26, 1976.

Skipper, J.K., Leonard, R.C., and Rhymes, J.: Child hospitalization and social interaction: An experimental study of mothers' feelings of stress, adaptation and satisfaction. Med. Care, 6:496, 1968.

Smith, R.M.: Children, hospitals and parents. Anesthesiology, 25:461, 1964.

Spence, J.C.: Care of children in hospital. Br. Med. J., 1:125, 1951.

Stacey, M., et al.: *Hospitals, Children and Their Families.* London, Routledge & Kegan Paul, 1970.

Titchener, J.L., and Levine, M.: *Surgery as a Human Experience: The Psychodynamics of Surgical Practice.* New York, Oxford University Press, 1960.

Vernon, D.T.A., et al.: Changes in children's behavior after hospitalization. Amer. J. Dis. Child., 111:581, 1966.

Wilson, J.: Joint pediatric and psychiatric care of the hospitalized child. Am. J. Orthopsychiatry, 28:539, 1958.

Wessel, M.A.: The pediatric intern. J. Pediatr., 29:651, 1946.

Books for Children

Altshuler, A.: *Books that Help Children Deal with a Hospital Experience.* Department of Health, Education, and Welfare, Washington, Government Printing Office, 1975.

Azarnoff, P.: *It's Your Body—Es Tu Cuerpo.* California, University of California, Los Angeles Hospital, 1973.

Chase, F.: *A Visit to the Hospital.* New York, Grosset & Dunlap, 1958.

En El Hospital: El Hospital Neuva York–El Centro Médico de Cornell, El Departmente de Pediatria. New York, The Society of the New York Hospital, 1970.

Margaret's Heart Operation. Philadelphia, Children's Hospital, 1969.

Misterrogers Talks About Going to the Doctor. New York, Platt & Munk, 1974.

Olshaker, B.: *Tommy's Tonsillectomy.* Washington, D.C., Marko Books, 1962.

Rey, M., and Rey, H.A.: *Curious George Goes to the Hospital.* Boston, Houghton Mifflin, 1966.

Sever, J.A.: *Johnny Goes to the Hospital.* Boston, Houghton Mifflin, 1953.

T.L.C. in the Life Support Unit. Minneapolis, Minnesota Children's Health Center, 1975.

Your Child in the Hospital. Denver: University of Colorado Medical Center, E. 9th Ave., Denver, Colo. 80220.

Films for Children

A Hospital Visit with Clipper. 15 minutes, 16 mm, color. Media Center, Children's Hospital, National Medical Center, Washington, D.C. 20009.

We Won't Leave You. 17 minutes, color. Edward A. Mason, M.D., Films. 58 Fenwood Road, Boston, Mass. 02115.

Films for Staff

Children in the Hospital. 44 minutes, black & white. Edward A. Mason, M.D., Films. 58 Fenwood Road, Boston, Mass. 02115.

Linda: Encounters in the Hospital. University of California, Los Angeles. UCLA Instructional Media Library, 405 Hilgard Avenue, 1 Royce Hall No. 8, Los Angeles, California 90024.

To Prepare a Child. 32 minutes, 16 mm, color. Media Center, Children's Hospital, National Medical Center, Washington, D.C. 20009.

Robertson, J.: A Two Year Old Goes to Hospital. 45 minutes, 16 mm, black & white. New York, New York University Film Library. (Also an abridged version, 30 minutes.)

Robertson, J.: Going to Hospital with Mother. 40 minutes, 16 mm, black & white. New York, New York University Film Library.

Robertson, J.: Guide to the Film "Going to Hospital with Mother." London, Tavistock Publications, 1958.

28
Family and Developmental Problems

*Freud's discovery of the importance of the
experiences of early infancy for the subsequent
development of the personality has profoundly
influenced our conception of human nature, and
has had lasting effects on ethics.*
(W. Russell, Lord Brain)

*Let us speak less of the duties of children and
more of their rights.*
(Jean Jacques Rousseau)

Pregnancy and
the Postpartum Period

Pregnancy, the event which transforms a married couple into a family, is not simply a biologic event. Pregnancy is also a psychosocial experience and an adaptive process for the mother and, less directly, for the father. Bibring[47] has pointed out that pregnancy is a developmental or maturational task for the mother. And in the view of Benedek[34] and Erikson,[145] parenthood is a developmental task for both parents.

Marital conflicts, lack of support from the husband, and stressful events, such as the death of a parent during pregnancy, may influence the course of pregnancy[360] and labor and the nature of delivery,[302] and they can have a lasting effect on the woman's adjustment as a mother and on her perception of her infant and her interaction with him. The woman's feelings about her own experiences of being mothered are related to her ability to feel confident about being a wife and mother. In a controlled study, prenatal counseling, especially anticipatory guidance, enabled the group of people who were counseled to cope better with labor, delivery, and the early post-

553

natal period than the group of people who were not counseled. Current "natural" practices (e.g., natural childbirth, the Lamaze method, rooming-in, allowing the father to be in the delivery room, and encouraging both mother and father to hold the baby immediately after delivery) can make the experience of pregnancy and delivery more satisfying for the mother and can involve the father more fully. Current practices also allow the siblings of the newborn infant to visit him in the hospital in a special visiting room. Such practices can also cut down on drug responses in the newborn[65] and thus both prevent interference with feeding and support the mother's bonding to the baby (which, I believe, begins during pregnancy, when the fetus begins to move).

Miscarriage

When a miscarriage occurs, besides being disappointed, the woman may fear that she is incomplete, and she may feel guilty about any minor deviations she made from her doctor's instructions during the pregnancy or because of other even less rational reasons. The husband may have similar feelings, and he may project his guilt onto his wife, with resulting marital conflict. A preschool-age child in the family may think that the miscarriage was his mother's fault or his own, and he may be affected by the mother's withdrawal from him as she mourns her loss. Even if the child is not told about the miscarriage, he will sense the disturbance in the family.[70] Children going through such a crisis may react in the ways described in Chapter 11. Counseling can help the parents air their feelings and discuss the problem openly with the child, rather than hide it. The child can be helped to talk also or to play out his feelings, and any misinterpretations he may have made may thus be corrected.

Habitual Abortion

Studies by Mann[287] of young women who have habitual abortions suggest that those women have greater dependency needs than do other women and that they experience difficulty about their femininity and about motherhood. The mothers of these women were generally dominant and possessive, and their fathers were generally passive. Psychologic factors seem to be involved in habitual abortion; psychoanalysis has helped several such women to deliver normal infants. Mann and his colleagues[288] used supportive psychotherapy in a number of cases; successful pregnancy was achieved in about 80% of the cases. A fuller discussion is offered in Chapter 21.

High-Risk Parent-Infant Relationships

Various approaches have been devised to anticipate problems in the parent-infant relationship and to predict "high-risk" situations. No absolute predictions can be made. I have designed an approach to elicit potential problems in a brief interview. The approach involves asking the patient 5 questions (see Appendix B). The questions have been standardized but not yet validated. Others are working in the same direction. Fletcher has gathered data (unpublished) using a somewhat similar questionnaire approach. Her approach seems to be promising in identifying high-risk situations. Kaplan and Mason[228,294] and Kennell and his colleagues[149] have developed a method of counting the visits or contacts of the parents (especially the mother), to an infant who must remain in the hospital longer than usual after birth. The method has useful results, and it permits early preventive steps to be taken in the home.

A number of potential high-risk situations can be identified from clinical impressions. They include a recent death or the death of a key family figure during the pregnancy, teenage pregnancy, out-of-wedlock pregnancy, marital conflicts, desertion by the husband during pregnancy, and extreme poverty. Evidence is available from the studies of Klaus and Kennell[248] and Leiderman and his colleagues[254a] that separation of a mother from a newborn who must remain in the hospital can interfere with the ongoing process of attachment or bonding of the mother and the newborn. In the view of these workers, various clinical problems (from difficulties in feeding and sleeping to failure to thrive and child abuse) may have their origin in this separation of the mother and her infant. They believe, as do Lubchenko, Prugh, and others (including those whose views are reflected by a recent statement[405] by the American Medical Association), that permitting mothers (and fathers) to see and touch their infants even in high-risk nurseries, giving them emotional support, and encouraging them to participate in the care of their infants can help prevent disturbances of attachment and, if the infant dies, can help the parents mourn.[242] Research to examine these impressions more systematically is underway. Cross-infection does not seem to be a problem.[456]

Postpartum Psychosis

In recent years, evidence gathered in England and in the United States indicates that postpartum mental illness is usually related in part to a woman's problems in assuming the mothering role with a particular infant,[199,367] but that the more familiar postpartum "blues" may have more physiologic components.[463] The practice of admitting to the psychiatric hospital both the mother who has a postpartum psychotic disorder and her infant was developed in England,[283] and it has been followed in some centers in the United States. As Luepker[281] has pointed out, there seems

to be a direct correlation between the success of the practice and how central the mother-child relationship is to the mother's illness.

The mother who is so treated seems to look to the nurses as mothering models, and her baby's presence seems to be a helpful link between the mother and her family and friends. The timing of the mother's admission to the hospital seems to be important. Mothers have some conflicts between their wishes to be cared for themselves and their obligation to care for their babies. The staff may also have some conflict about the approach at first.[6] When appropriately handled, the experience seems to contribute to the mother's recovery by helping her to reorient herself to reality and to gain confidence in her ability to mother. Some workers attribute an earlier discharge from the psychiatric hospital to this approach. (Men can also have a postpartum reaction, and postpartum psychosis has been reported in seriously disturbed fathers.)[425]

Prematurity

In the view of Caplan[81] and Kaplan and Mason,[228] prematurity is a family crisis, and the crisis may be resolved or it may produce parenting disorders. Blau and his colleagues[54] studied a group of women who delivered prematurely for no accountable medical reason. Compared with mothers of full-term infants, the mothers of the premature infants had significantly more negative attitudes toward their pregnancies, greater emotional immaturity, and a poorer resolution of oedipal problems. A high incidence of emotional problems has been said to occur in children born prematurely, and low birth weight is more often associated with a higher rate of handicap than is any other common perinatal complication.[110,126,280]

Caplan and his colleagues[82] found that a group of children born prematurely had significant deficits in cognitive organization and were more likely to show personality disturbances than were children in a control group. A clear preponderance of children who had emotional problems and families who had overprotective, oversolicitous, and growth-inhibiting home environments was found in the premature group, in contrast to a preponderance of well-adjusted children and "growth stimulating" families in the control group. Some prematurely born children adapt more successfully as they grow older, and some parents can handle these children constructively.

De Hirsch, Jansky, and Langford[116] compared a group of prematurely born children with a group of maturely born children of average intelligence. The prematurely born children showed a poorer performance on a battery of kindergarten tests; their later progress was uneven, and they continued to lag in academic achievement well into the eighth year of life. This finding fits with those of other studies (by Harper, Fischer, and their colleagues[202]) which showed a high frequency of reading disabilities in prematurely born children, who seemed to show developmental lags in perceptual-motor and other types of cognitive development without actual brain damage. Thus even though they catch up physically during their first two years or so, children born prematurely seem to be at high risk for the development of emotional and learning problems.

As Kennell and his colleagues[149] have pointed out, reports of of infants who show failure to thrive in the absence of physical disorder and of children who have been abused show a disproportionally high incidence of prematurity; 25% to 41% of infants who fail to thrive are premature, and 23% to 31% of abused infants are premature or have been separated from their mothers because of serious illness. These workers believe that difficulties in maternal attachment related to the infant's longer stay in the hospital are involved. As mentioned earlier, Kaplan and Mason,[228] Mason,[294] and Kennell and his colleagues have developed a method of predicting high-risk families by counting the number of visits mothers made to their infants who were in the hospital's premature unit. A drop in the number of visits or in the regularity of visiting toward the end of an infant's stay indicated that the parents were having difficulty dealing with their anxiety and guilt about the prematurity.[228] Fanaroff and his colleagues[149] counted the total number of visits and telephone calls made by the mother during her premature infant's stay in the hospital. Disorders of mothering, including battering and failure to thrive, later occurred in 9 cases out of 38 in which the combined number of phone calls and visits was less than 5 in a two-week period. In the Kaplan and Mason study, preventive intervention through home visits made by a mental health professional within a week after the infant's discharge helped resolve parent-infant problems during the first year. At the University of Colorado Medical Center, homes in which the parent-infant interactions are considered high risk, either on the basis of interviews of the parents or because the infant remained longer than usual in the hospital, are visited by a public health nurse or a child health associate. Kempe and his colleagues (personal communication) and Dawson and his colleagues (personal communication) are using home visits more routinely, as happens in Britain, New Zealand, and other countries.

The practice referred to earlier of encouraging mothers to visit their premature infants in the hospital and to help care for them, no matter how small or how much at risk the infants are, supports maternal attachment. If the infant dies, the practice makes it easier for the mother to mourn for her infant because she has seen, touched and cared for him. Experiments have been undertaken with sending home babies who weigh at least $3\frac{1}{2}$ pounds, rather than waiting for the babies to reach the traditional

5-pound figure. The practice seems to be both safe for the baby and helpful to parents who have been screened properly.

Problems in the Family

Separation and Divorce

Divorce has increased rapidly in the United States in recent years; the prevalence now approaches one in three marriages. More than two-thirds of divorces occur in the first 14 years of marriage, and the median duration of marriage is about 7 years.[120] Counseling services are more readily available to parents who are concerned about the effects their divorce will have on their children. Separation and divorce present problems for children that are both similar to and different from problems presented by the loss of a parent from death.[300] As Wallerstein and Kelly[438] have pointed out, in both death and divorce, the external loss may not be fully assimilated emotionally by the child as a result of his unresolved ambivalent feelings toward the lost parent. But in divorce, the departed parent is still "available" to the child, and the child may have both longing for and conflicted feelings about the parent. Rutter[372] believes that the child can have more difficulty with divorce than with the death of the parent. The child of divorced parents must mourn[60] the loss of the departed parent, his former relationship with that parent, and the family as he knew it, and he must accept a more circumscribed relationship with the departed parent (still usually the father). Such painful adjustments take some months at least, and the child requires considerable help from his parents or other persons. If help is not forthcoming, adverse consequences may follow, and depression or antisocial behavior may occur later.[120]

During their mourning, children may become involved in arguments about custody. Those arguments usually arouse conflicting loyalties in the child however they are resolved. Parents sometimes unconsciously use children as extensions of their anger and wishes for vengeance, fighting battles over custody that may actually have little to do with the children. At times, parents experience social and emotional isolation following the disruption of the family, and they depend heavily on their children for solace. Some parents try to "catch up" on their sexual lives after a separation or divorce, and they seem to be oblivious to the fact that their activities can be both stimulating and anxiety provoking to young children and teenagers. The efforts some parents expend to enlist a child's loyalty and turn him against the other parent can be confusing and conflict provoking to the child. Some children show anger toward the custodial parent, and some adolescents withdraw in their attempts to deal with their feelings of divided loyalty and love. Most children feel devalued, and many wish to reunite the parents. Parents may feel hurt by their children's resentment or seeming disinterest.

The meaning of divorce to the child is related to his level of emotional development and capacity for understanding, as Wallerstein and Kelly pointed out in a series of articles about the effects of divorce on preschool-age children,[436] early school-age children,[239] late school-age children,[437] and adolescents.[435] Regression, clinging, fears of abandonment, and other responses are seen in preschool-age children. School problems, aggressive behavior, or depression may be seen in older children, and adolescents often exhibit anger toward one parent, and they frequently take sides. The preschool-age child's "magical" thinking often makes him feel he caused the divorce; school-age children and adolescents, although they can understand better, still have feelings of guilt. Early and late preschool-age boys, because of their stages of psychosocial and psychosexual development, are most vulnerable to the "man of the house" syndrome.[323,424] At times, children caught in conflicting loyalties and marital battles may show reactive disorders or even psychoneurotic or other disorders, and they may need intensive psychotherapy[167] as well as counseling.

The general practice of most divorce courts has been to award the custody of young children to the mother and to let adolescents choose which parent they wish to live with, a decision that may require professional help. Such custodial arrangements are beginning to be less common, although 1 out of 6 children under 18 years of age live in a one-parent family and the mother is the principal parent in over 95% of the cases.

Goldstein, Anna Freud, and Solnit[182] in an excellent discussion of the interests of the child, who may be caught in the struggle between the parents, think that in some cases it is better for the child to be placed with the psychologic parent (the parent most appropriate to his needs), and that his relationship with the other (often disturbed) parent be terminated. They go so far as to say that "the noncustodial parent should have no legally enforceable right to visit the child." But children whose parent suddenly disappears forever may be confused, may blame themselves for the parent's disappearance, and may have difficulty mourning their loss constructively. If the absent parent lives in the same city, it may be difficult for the child not to see him.

I believe that it is usually wiser for the child to see the noncustodial parent, because he must somehow come to terms with the image of the parent. I agree with Benedek and Benedek[35] that the child has a right to postdivorce visitation. If he does not see the parent, his picture of the parent may be seriously distorted. If the parent lives in the vicinity, it is wise for the young child to visit a day or so a week and for the older child or the adolescent to visit several days a month. If the parent has moved to another city, holiday visits and summer visits can be arranged. Regularity and predictability are important; dividing the year between two parents tends to divide loyalties. Joint custody is a recent development that, at the least, calls for mature and objective parents. At the worst, it can be very destructive. Parents should be counseled not to yield to the temptation to try to turn the child against the other parent; counseling in family or marital agencies or divorce counseling centers or psychotherapy given by mental health professionals may be wise for parents whose bitterness makes it difficult for them to follow such advice.[438]

Sometimes the mother does not wish to have custody of the children, and the father may need special help—perhaps of a female relative or a homemaker—in meeting his children's needs.

The pediatrician should not act as a marriage counselor unless he has the necessary training. But he can identify marital conflicts early, and by making the appropriate referrals perhaps he can help prevent divorce. (Lawyers still have little training in child development and family interactions. Divorce is becoming easier to arrange, and only a few lawyers or judges recommend marital counseling before the final decision is made.) Also, he can listen to the children of the divorcing couple sympathetically and objectively. In accordance with their developmental levels, he can help them express their feelings of anger, fear, guilt, or depression, and he can help them understand that they have not caused the separation or divorce. He can help the parents work out explanations geared to their children's levels of comprehension, as well as support their understanding of their children's conflicts and their worries about their parents and themselves.[362] He can detect and manage, sometimes directly, sometimes by referral, the emotional problems of children, before, during, or after the divorce,[44] and he can help parents understand their children's need to see the noncustodial parent. The importance of contacts with the father has been underscored in several studies of both boys[211] and girls.[203,205] The pediatrician should know of the existence of such organizations as Parents Without Partners, and Grandparents Anonymous, of homemaker services,[90] and of other helpful community programs. The physician's role is a difficult one, but it is most important.

Death in the Family

How the death of a parent affects a child depends on (1) the child's age and developmental level, (2) the quality of the relationship the child had with the parent, (3) the circumstances under which the parent died, (4) the emotional support the child receives from the surviving parent and other family members, and (5) the way the family deals with their feelings of loss and the process of mourning. The death of a parent need not be pathogenic in itself if the child is permitted to mourn the loss, an active process which takes some months and which may be revived briefly at later stages of the child's development. (Insufficient or unsuccessful mourning has usually been involved in the disorders in which there is a history of parent loss, such as schizophrenia and delinquency.[212] If the family has a religious framework within which it can mourn, the child's mourning may proceed effectively.

Many middle-class Anglo families do not have meaningful religious ties, and they find mourning difficult. It is even more difficult for them to permit their children to mourn openly. A few families even treat mourning as a "family secret," sometimes with harm to a particular child and with increased family alienation.[146]

The recent revival of freedom to talk about death is reflected in the existence of "good death" societies and wills which specify that heroic efforts not be made to keep consenting adults alive when their condition is hopeless.

Although, as Furman[164] has pointed out,

there are great individual differences in how children mourn, there are certain commonalities in how they mourn. The child's work of mourning differs considerably from that of an adult. The child's more limited reality testing ability allows him more opportunity for misinterpreting the meaning of events, particularly if his parent was killed in an accident in which the child was also involved.[32,449]

As indicated earlier, a child does not comprehend death as permanent until he is 9 or 10 years of age even though he may feel grief and loss before that point. A child can mourn a loss on his or her own developmental level after he has internalized the mental representation of the parent.[59] The child usually achieves this capability in the second half of his first year although his internalizations are not constant until the second half of his second year. The response of the infant at that age is principally to the disappearance and loss of the parent. By his third or fourth year, the child tends to misinterpret the death of a parent as a desertion possibly caused by the child's having done "something bad." By his fourth to sixth year, the child is capable of feeling guilt, and he tends to misinterpret the death of a parent of the same sex in terms of the oedipal phase, and he may feel that the death is a result of his past rivalrous or angry feelings toward the parent. School-age children are freer of such irrational feelings of guilt, but they may feel responsible in some fashion, as indeed adolescents and adults often do.

Although the initial reaction of most children to the death of a parent can be a healthy response, involving a situational crisis, with adequate mourning (see Chapter 15), children who have limited adaptive capacities or prior emotional disturbances may show reactive disorders, the crystalization of a psychoneurotic disorder, or (occasionally) the precipitation of a psychotic disorder. Some parents seem to know intuitively how to help their child handle the loss of the other parent.[29] If the surviving parent cannot do so naturally, he or she can be helped with counseling to explain to the child in simple terms the cause of the parent's death (how the child is told is more important than what he is told), to help the child realize that he was not responsible for the death, to permit him to cry openly, and to encourage him to talk about the dead parent and thus to carry on the work of mourning.[163] "Incision and drainage" of guilt in individual interviews may be necessary. Psychiatric consultation may be helpful. Some parents may need psychotherapy themselves to help them with the work of mourning, and to help them help their children to mourn.

In the case of a parent who commits suicide,[72,270] the child may be helped to understand that the parent was "sick" and that the suicide was "no one's fault." The death of a sibling should be handled somewhat like the death of a parent; a child's past feelings of sibling rivalry may lead him to misinterpret his sibling's death as a punishment and he may feel guilty.[73,452]

In general, school-age and older children should be permitted to attend the funeral of a parent and to participate in the family's mourning.

Mentally Ill Parents

Mental illness in a parent may have various effects on the child's development and behavior. Some workers have suggested that specific syndromes result from serious depression in the mother or from manic depression in the parents. The multifactorial theory of etiology (see Chapter 2) would argue against such specific effects, and in fact the literature supports the theory. The effects of heredity are definite though limited, and the child's response is largely to the parent's disturbance although the child's identification with the disturbed parent as a way of maintaining contact with the parent may play a partial role (as in folie à deux[14]). In a Scandinavian study, Mednick and Schulsinger[306] dem-

onstrated that the children of schizophrenic parents who break down have more obstetrical complications than do normal children and that they exhibit deviations in the functioning of the autonomic nervous system.

Children who have seriously depressed mothers may suffer from a lack of attention to their needs if other adults are not able to help them. In certain children, the lack of attention may produce environmental retardation, with the children able to make little use of the developmental skills they possess. However, some depressed patients cling to their children for support, and encourage their children to cling to them. Children of parents who have manic-depressive psychotic disorders may show depression, sensitivity to loss, and mood swings. Children who have schizophrenic mothers have been described as showing language distortions and lags in language development.[445]

In an ongoing extensive study, Anthony[16] has indicated that a relatively small percentage of the children who have psychotic parents may themselves have psychotic disorders. A much larger percentage of such children have exhibited a variety of emotional and behavioral disturbances, some of them apparently reactive disorders although in psychologically predisposed children more structured disorders may be precipitated by disturbed and chaotic behavior in their parents. Many of the children felt guilty because they feared that they had somehow contributed to their parent's illness.

The striking fact shown by Anthony's[16] study and by other studies[324] is that a significant number of children in these families did not show definitely disordered behavior. Not all these families were alike, and the premorbid adjustment of the family, the gradual or sudden shifts within it, and other factors were all important.[17] The children who were least affected were mainly those families in which only one parent had a psychotic disorder. The determining factor seemed to be whether the sick parent's disorder was inclusive of the child, as it is in a symbiotic relationship or in a delusional system involving the child. If the parent's disorder did not include the child, the child was usually able to develop a relationship with the healthier parent or (occasionally) with another family member that was satisfying enough to permit him to develop and function adequately. The child often could "tag" signs that the affected parent was decompensating (e.g., clothing strewn over the house), and he was able to turn to a healthier family member for emotional support.

The absence of a mentally ill parent who has been hospitalized for treatment poses a special problem for the child, as Rice and her colleagues have pointed out.[139,355] The absence represents a family crisis, and the level of the child's development, his previous adaptive capacity, and the nature of the substitute parenting are among the factors which determine the degree to which the child is affected. If the parent was reasonably well adjusted before the hospitalization, the child may mourn the loss; if the parent had had a long period of chaotic behavior, the hospitalization might be somewhat of a relief for the child.[17] The community mental health movement and the development of tranquilizing drugs have resulted in the emptying out of once crowded state hospitals. Unfortunately, state legislatures have often cut hospital budgets and have thus cut the amount of money available for follow-up care of discharged patients and for community services for their families.

Although former mental patients have often resumed productive lives, many have found reentry into their families difficult. Their impact on the behavior and development of their children has not been measured. Without adequate follow-up care, many former patients do not take advantage of the help of community mental health centers and other facilities, and it is my impression that their children often

suffer as a result. If the former patient is a mother, homemaker service provided by family and children's agencies may be helpful in keeping the family together and functioning. Custody contests[285] often center on the competence of a parent, usually the mother.

The physician should be aware of the effect a mentally ill parent can have on his children. Often a mentally ill parent brings a child to the pediatrician, focusing on the child's behavior as the problem. Although the pediatrician may recognize depressed, agitated, confused, paranoid, or other disturbed behavior in the parent, it may not be easy to persuade the parent to seek help. Psychiatric consultation can be helpful in this regard and in determining whether the child requires treatment also.

Adoption

Early placement for adoption (within the first 1 or 2 months or before 6 months) has become a standard practice since the work of Goldfarb,[181] Spitz,[400] and Bowlby.[58] Early adoption is better for the child, who has not yet developed an attachment to a parent figure, and for the adoptive parents. Nearly two million children under 18 years of age (2% of all children) are adopted children, and nearly 50% are adopted by relatives.

The placement of a baby for adoption is a complicated matter, particularly when there is mental illness in the baby's family. Modern genetics supports the view that mental illness is not strongly influenced by heredity although parents should be told of the chances of such a possibility in a susceptible child. The unpredictability of tests of intelligence in infancy has been mentioned, and the presence of mild retardation in an older infant who has experienced some deprivation is not necessarily a contraindication to adoption. Even babies who have certain physical and mental handicaps have been adopted in recent years. The most recent statement by the American Academy of Pediatrics[10] is helpful, particularly regarding the collaborative approach of the physician, the social worker, and the lawyer. The pediatrician often acts as a consultant for adoptive agencies in cases of adoption, and he can guide them in the use of community health facilities, visiting nurse services, and institutional facilities. Children awaiting adoption may be eligible for health services under Medicaid, the Elementary and Secondary School Education Act, and other new programs.

A careful and long-drawn-out appraisal of adoptive parents (on the basis of race, ethnic background, and social class) was the rule in the past. The present scarcity of potentially adoptive babies (originally because of the "gray market" but more recently because of the decreased stigma regarding out-of-wedlock pregnancies and the increasing tendency of even teenage unwed mothers to keep their babies) has affected the appraisal practices. Today, screening procedures have become more flexible, and even single-parent adoptions are considered. The need to evaluate the motivations of the potentially adoptive parents for adopting is obvious. Those candidates who have rigid ideas about the sex or characteristics of the infant may be neurotic or otherwise unhealthy. Probably the most basic criteria are (1) why the couple wishes to adopt, (2) the capacity of the couple to form easy and loving relationships with others, and (3) the nature of the couple's marriage relationship (the ability of the couple to meet their own needs and the needs of each other). Discussion of this last criterion is often avoided because it is a sensitive one, but the parents' ease (or lack of ease) in discussing the topic may be revealing.

If these criteria are used in a flexible way most adoptions can work out well for the child and the parents. But continued support for the parents after the adoption is vitally important in preventing problems;

adjustment is significantly better in agency-handled adoptions than it is in independent placements.[91] Inadequate staffing and poor financial support of public (and often private) agencies often prevent effective follow-up care from being given. Contrary to popular impressions, conception of a baby following an adoption by apparently sterile parents does not happen on a large scale although it does occur.[200]

Adoptive parents may have certain problems.[385] They include worry about their sterility and about the adopted child's ultimate development because they lack detailed knowledge about his biologic heredity—the "bad seed" fear. Since most children who have been adopted by relatives have been conceived out of wedlock, adoptive parents often fear that the adoptive child, like his parents, may have trouble during adolescence controlling his sexual impulses. Also, adoptive parents may try too hard to deal with the child's normal developmental problems because they fear criticism about their parenting ability.

As several studies[356,377,451] have indicated, adopted children generally have difficulties similar to those of other children in the same age groups but often in a more intensified form. They really have two sets of parents (one usually fantasied), which may compound the "family romance" in the late preschool-age period and which permits adoptive children to "split the parental images" when problems arise, seeing one set of parents as good and one set as bad. They may test out adoptive parents in various ways to make sure they are wanted and loved. Children adopted after infancy tend to have more problems adjusting to their adoptive families.[198]

In their desire to spare the child hurt, adoptive parents may have serious difficulties telling him that he was adopted. It is now generally agreed that it is best to tell the child about the adoption at an early age. In any event, the child usually finds out about the adoption by adolescence, and he may show significant emotional disturbance if he is told by "outsiders" or if he is told during his adolescent search for identity.[305] The parents' responses to the child's questions about where babies come from can lead to revelation of the adoption on a recurrent and gradual basis, beginning in the preschool period. Some parents find reading books to the child about adoption helpful. (*The Chosen One* by V. Wasson is one such book.)

Studies in the United States of the incidence of significant emotional disorders in adopted children as compared to the general population have shown conflicting results. A recent Scandinavian study suggests that the incidence of mental illness and criminal behavior is not higher among adopted children. Special problems face the black or other minority child in regard to adoption. Only 1 out of 20 black infants is adopted, compared to 7 out of 10 white infants. Efforts to break low-income cycles can increase the number of adoptions by minority families. Transracial adoptions of minority children by majority families pose some problems, but the numbers of such adoptions are increasing.[92]

Adoptive children are a high-risk group, and they need special supportive and counseling measures. (The majority of adopted children adjust well, but the risk of problems is real.) As Richmond[356] and Wessell[451] have indicated, the physician or health associate can help parents express and come to grips with feelings common to adoptive parents, and he can help them deal with related misconceptions. Mental health consultation by mental health professionals or in family and children's agencies may be necessary for some families who are having special difficulty (particularly about telling the child he is adopted), which may lead to or reflect problems in the marriage. Psychotherapy may be needed for the child.[130] Group discussions in a mental health setting for adoptive parents have been found to be helpful. The parents' relationship with the adoptive child may be especially important during adolescence, when he seeks to determine who he is, where he came from, and what he can become. Recently many adoptees have begun to search for their biologic parents. When they have found their parents, most adoptees have not been upset even when the encounters with their parents have not been pleasant. Most adoptees who have found their biologic parents have felt more satisfied with their adoptive families.[10]

Foster Home Placement

Thirty percent to 40% of children in the United States at some time in their lives must live at least temporarily in a broken family.[94] Although a significant decline in the number of orphans has occurred in the United States (the number is less than $\frac{1}{16}$ of the number in 1920), in 1977 approximately 330,000 children were living in other than their own homes.[150] Nearly one-third of these children were in institutions for dependent children, and the remainder were in foster homes. Of these children, about 1 in 4 is placed in foster care because of death, illness, or economic hardship in the family; the rest are placed in foster care for social reasons that involve family breakdown, or parental abandonment or abuse or for disturbed behavior on the part of the child. The classic study of Maas and Engler[295] focused attention on the difficulties interfering with the effectiveness of foster care. The majority of foster children are separated from their parents in the preschool-age period. Once placed in foster care, most children have remained in foster care from 2 to 5 years. (Siblings are often placed together.[40]) Only about 25% ever return to their own homes,[133] and 8% of foster children are adopted. Thus about 67% of these children remain in foster care until they are adults. Even more strikingly, about 25% of such children are moved at least four times during their stay in foster care, (the average number of moves is between

2 and 3), and a significant number of children have 10 to 15 or more moves.

Well over 50% of foster children show more psychopathology than do children who live in their own homes.[134] Aggressive behavior is common, and intellectual blunting, inarticulateness, poor judgment, poor time sense, apathy, disorganized habits, poor self-image, and mistrust are often seen.[444] Preplacement factors (e.g., abandonment) are of course involved in such psychopathology. Postplacement factors are also significant, and symptomatic behavior correlates positively with the number of different moves, not with the length of time in foster care. To some extent, the number of moves is related to the child's behavioral response to placement, (he may test the foster parents) and, if a child has had a series of moves, his behavior becomes increasingly mistrustful and disturbed.[272] Other factors may also be operative. They include lack of diagnostic services,[137] inadequate temporary shelter care, poor preparation for placement, lack of understanding by foster parents, and changes within the foster family. Well-motivated and capable foster parents are hard to find, particularly for children from minority groups.

Strenuous measures should be taken to keep families in crisis together. Those measures include the use of homemaker services[90] and financial aid offered by family and children's agencies and welfare or social service departments. If a child must be placed in foster care, the foster parents should be carefully selected and both the child and the foster parents should be carefully prepared for the move. The child should be encouraged to identify with his own parents and to keep in contact with them if possible. Follow-up help should be given to the foster parents and the child, and efforts should be made to help the child return to his home (or, if necessary, to help his parents relinquish him for adoption). Such measures help prevent emotional deprivation in the child,[174] which stems mainly from discontinuity in the parent-child relationship. Placement of a child in a foster home to help him with disturbed behavior often fails if the foster parents have not had special training and are not given considerable support. Children over 10 or 11 years old and adolescents rarely do well in an ordinary foster home.

Since the staffs of many public placement agencies are too small and are underpaid, group foster homes[426] and cottage or "family" type institutions staffed by trained foster parents[455] may be better than most individual foster homes, as the Child Welfare League has suggested. Social grouping can be of help to dependent children who are in institutions; the children can be grouped into smaller "family" units. There is an urgent need for "medical" foster homes (those that provide adequate nursing care and medical supervision) for seriously ill or handicapped children who must be removed from their homes. Medical foster homes are preferable to large institutions, such as the convalescent hospital, which is dying out. Children who cannot return home and who cannot be adopted need well-planned and permanent foster care. Certainly some sort of vigorous action must be taken, because these children will grow up to be inadequate parents if they receive inadequate family care. Many of these children urgently need intensive psychotherapy[114,229] on an ambulatory or a residential basis. The pediatrician can help both as a professional—by detecting problems in children and arranging for their treatment—and as an informed citizen—by recognizing and helping to meet the needs of displaced children from the United States and from abroad.[83,89]

Child Abuse

In cases of the "battered child syndrome," described by Kempe and his colleagues in 1962,[241] the relationship between the abusing parent and the child has usually been distorted as a result of the impact of the parent's experiences as a child. Parents who abuse their children are often young, immature people who have received inadequate parenting themselves (and who often were battered or otherwise abused as children). They have problems about their unsatisfied dependency needs, and often they cannot give emotionally to their children. They have unrealistic expectations of their children and their discipline is often inconsistent. Such parents usually are deeply resentful of their own parents, and they submit their children to traumatic experiences similar to those they endured during their own childhood.

As Steele[406] has indicated, abusing parents may unconsciously use role reversal, a mechanism in which the parents turn unrealistically to the child for the satisfaction of their dependency needs. Such parents often have problems in impulse control, and they may lash out at their child (as if to strike back at the world) and thus scapegoat the child, particularly parents who have been left alone by their spouses and who feel deserted and helpless.

The conceptual model shown in Figure 28–1 is that of an ideal support system for the mother of a newborn. It involves the newborn's father, the new mother's mother, and gratification for the mother from her infant's responses to her care. Breakdowns in the system may come from a lack of support from the father, the mother's mother, or other female relatives or friends, or from the mother's inability to receive positive signals from the infant, because of the infant's temperament or the mother's role reversal or both.

Kempe and his colleagues estimate that approximately 80% of abusing parents fit the description given earlier, and that about 20% of abusing parents are seriously mentally ill or psychotic.[207] The baby who is battered may have been born at a particularly stressful time into a rather chaotic family or he may have been unwanted.

Kennell's observation that one-fourth to one-third of abused children or children who show failure to thrive have been kept at the hospital for prematurity or other problems following delivery (a condition that interfered with the mother's attachment) is supported by the results of a recent prospective study of premature infants in a newborn intensive care unit.[217]

The term child abuse when used broadly includes not only battering but also the use of inappropriate methods of disciplining the child, such as burning him. Sexual abuse and serious neglect also frequently occur, sometimes in association with physical abuse. Child abuse occurs at all levels of society although its incidence is slightly higher among poor people (because of the greater number of crises associated with poverty). Job loss, bitter arguments and other events often touch off the abuse. Women who abuse children outnumber men. In a recent study at the Denver General Hospital, child abuse was shown to be less common in black and Chicano families than in Anglo families.

Kempe's group has estimated that nearly one million cases of child abuse, sexual molestation, and serious neglect occur each year in the United States although only about 300,000 cases are reported. In addition to failure to thrive, mental retardation may be associated with the abuse. If they survive, children who are abused grow up with feelings of loneliness and little personal worth. Withdrawn behavior, mistrust, fear of separation, and demanding and aggressive behaviors are common; some children are depressed, passive, and pseudo-adult in their behavior. Primitive defenses (e.g., denial and projection), impaired self-concepts, impaired impulse controls, and self-destructive behavior have also been described in these children.[186] In some cases, as Coppolillo[107] has indicated, the child's temperament may be a factor in the parent's first instance of battering. After they have been battered, some children may strike out or rebel, and they may un-

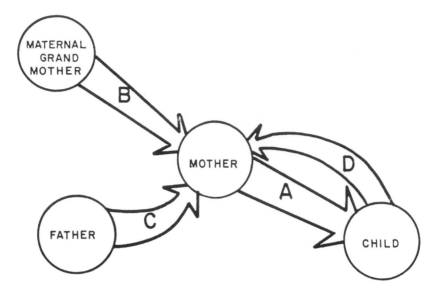

Fig. 28–1. A model of the ideal support system for the mother of a newborn. Homeostasis is established and maintained by the relationships between the mother, the father, the mother's mother, and the newborn. (From H.P. Coppolillo: A conceptual model for study of some abusing parents. In: *The Child in His Family: Vulnerable Children* (E.J. Anthony, C. Koupernik, and C. Chiland, Eds.). New York, Wiley, 1978.)

consciously invite further battering because of guilt or other feelings.[313] This is particularly true of adolescents, who make up nearly 30% of the group who are abused. Follow-up studies[291] of abused children have shown speech problems, emotional disturbance, growth failure, and poor school achievement in many and physical handicaps and delinquent behavior in some.

In cases in which a child was killed by battering, the child and his siblings had often been seriously mistreated before the death. In most such situations, a parent (usually the mother) or the mother's male friend commits the act in an impulsive rage. The child in question is usually a preschool-age child who was born out of wedlock. The assailants usually have backgrounds of assaultiveness and social deviance. When a child has died as a result of abuse, the responses of his siblings are like those of children who suffer the death of siblings or parents from illness, except that they are confused and anxious about the violence involved.

Parents who batter or otherwise harm or abuse their children require special handling. If it is suspected that a child being treated in an emergency room[216] has been battered, the child should be hospitalized immediately so that a full evaluation of the child and his family can be made with the help of a psychiatrist, a psychologist, and a social worker.[369] All 50 states have mandatory child-abuse reporting laws although these laws are not yet sufficiently invoked by physicians, particularly in "borderline" cases. The battered child may have to be removed from his home, a step that can be arranged by court order. A nonjudgmental, nonpunitive approach should be taken by the physician who makes the diagnosis, even though he must report the diagnosis. Such an approach may help the parents recognize or discuss their handling of the child as a problem, and it often leads to psychiatric counseling and referral to appropriate mental health facilities and other community[381] agencies. The physician may give the parents an opening by indicating that many parents have trouble controlling their tempers with young children. The use of such an approach, which is based on criteria for evaluating further abuse, has enabled programs such as that of Fontana[159] to keep two-thirds of children who have been abused safely in the home during the treatment program.

Once the problem of child abuse has been brought out into the open, a variety of approaches may be taken. Besides psychotherapy for the parents, Kempe and his colleagues and others have used successfully a 24-hour crisis center where parents who realize they are close to losing control of themselves may leave an infant or young child. A therapeutic play school for abused children is in session in the center for 6 hours a day. Family aides or lay therapists are available in the center to help put together a disorganized family or offer a telephone lifeline. These workers can also give "mothering therapy" in home visits to a mother who needs help. The therapists also encourage parents to participate in meetings of Parents' Anonymous. A live-in approach for families has been used experimentally, and a residential program for children that gives parents unlimited visiting rights is being developed. Helfer and Schmitt[208] have listed the basic components of an interdisciplinary community-based child abuse program: acute care and diagnostic evaluation, long-term treatment, and education, training, and research.

Kempe believes that with such a multifaceted approach, more than 80% of parents can be helped, sometimes over a period of years, to avoid future abuse and that most of the children will eventually be able to return to their homes. Close collaboration of the courts, welfare and other placement agencies, practicing physicians, and other community resources is a necessity in difficult cases. One central agency, ideally the juvenile court, should bear the ultimate responsibility for implementing

the plan arrived at, including the custody arrangements.[209] In Colorado, a lawyer is appointed as an advocate (guardian ad litum) for a child whose family is brought to court for battering or other kinds of child abuse. At the National Center for the Prevention and Treatment of Child Abuse and Neglect in Denver, established by Kempe, the staff includes a full-time lawyer, as well as pediatricians, public health nurses, psychiatrists, psychologists, social workers, and nursery school teachers. Psychotherapy is not employed for every abused child. Other approaches, involving consistent pediatric care, physical therapy, speech therapy, day care, attendance at a therapeutic nursery school, or special educational help in school are sometimes considered more appropriate. In my opinion, however, psychotherapy should be considered for every child. Play therapy for preschool-age and school-age children, interview therapy for adolescents, and, in some cases, group therapy for children or adolescents may be indicated. Therapy for the child should be coordinated with therapy for the child's parents, as described by Green.[185]

Similar results may be achieved with parents who are so preoccupied with their own problems or so disturbed that they neglect their children. Consultation by a mental health professional or in a public or private welfare or family agency is usually necessary. Such methods are preferable to legal ones since anything short of serious neglect is often difficult to prove in court. The same is true of "emotional abuse," a concept that is itself open to interpretation. A unified revision of legal statutes regarding children that takes into account the needs and rights of the child as well as those of the parents is badly needed in the United States although some encouraging steps have been taken recently. Pediatricians and child psychiatrists should use their influence as professionals and as informed citizens to help achieve the revision. Predicting battering or other forms of abuse is not yet possible although Kempe and his colleagues[184,292] are working on a broad-gauge predictive approach. High-risk situations may be suspected in cases in which the parents were battered as children, in which a newborn must remain in the hospital, as mentioned earlier, and in other cases. The use of the Five Questions interview approach (see Appendix B) may help identify high-risk parent-infant relationships that involve a number of problems, including battering.

Failure to Thrive

The effects of psychosocial (not just maternal) deprivation on the young child have been studied.[74] Some effects stem from the child's early separation from his parents and inadequate parent-substitute relationships,[345,465] and some stem from masked emotional deprivation[344,348] in intact families. Much of this deprivation is preventable,[26] as has been stressed, and much of it can be reversed.[5,401] Failure to thrive is only one result of psychosocial deprivation;[141,156,255] psychosocial deprivation may also overlap with child abuse.[249] In a recent study of mothers of children who suffered from failure to thrive,[245] some mothers were shown to be apathetic, dependent, passive, and isolated, and they seemed to be distant and at times hostile to their children. Other mothers were shown to be more vigorous and self-confident but to have weak family ties, controlling relationships with men, and a tendency to ignore or overstimulate their babies. Obviously, parents of infants who fail to thrive are not a homogeneous group.

Since failure to thrive is a psychophysiologic disorder, its management is discussed in Chapter 21.

Sexual Abuse

Parental seductiveness of an unconscious nature has been mentioned in relation to younger children; it may involve some conscious sexual stimulation of the child from infancy onward, and it may also occur during adolescence, with much fondling, kissing, or wrestling between the parent and the young person of the opposite sex. In some instances, the parent may be treating the adolescent as a younger child, without being aware of the seductive significance of such behavior, but in other instances, the parent may be aware of the sexual excitement. Parental seductiveness may also arise (1) in families in which one parent is absent, (2) as substitute gratification in an unsatisfying marital relationship, or (3) as a "localized neurotic interaction," often one involving a parent who had a similar relationship in his or her own childhood. The adolescent may enjoy the interaction, but usually feels anxious and guilty about it. Disturbed behavior may result, or the adolescent's relationships with the opposite sex may be distorted. At times, the adolescent may use the interaction to manipulate one or both parents. Disturbed adolescents may unconsciously invite seductive behavior by a parent.

Although the incidence of actual seduction in families or *incest* is difficult to estimate, there have been a number of discussions of the topic[1,321,366,375] since the studies of Kaufman and his colleagues[235] in 1954. Incest seems to be more common than formerly believed. Data compiled by Kinsey's colleagues[170] indicate that brother-sister incest is the most common type of incest although it is less often reported clinically than is father-daughter or stepfather-stepdaughter incest.[153] Mother-son and mother-daughter incest are rare,[432] and father-son incest is exceedingly rare although a recent study suggests it may be underreported.[122] Girls incestuously involved with their fathers or stepfathers are often the first daughters in the family and they are in preadolescence or early adolescence.[240]

Often there is a long-standing active or passive collusion in incest, especially in father-daughter incest, in which there is usually a *silent agreement* to the incest on the part of the mother, who often is dependent and frigid, has a history of desertion in her childhood, and sees the incest as the only way she can keep her husband in the family. The fear of family disintegration is shared by all family members. The father may be using the incest as a hostile act toward the mother. If the daughter makes complaints (she rarely does), her complaints are often ignored by her mother and even the physician, as Kempe[240] has indicated. The physician tends to think of the daughter as seductive or indulging in fantasy. In some cases, the family seems healthy although in other cases the incest appears to be only one of many family problems, as Nakashima and Zakus[321] have pointed out.

Girls who have incestuous relationships with their fathers seem less emotionally disturbed if the relationships occur when they are children, although these girls usually show depression and guilt. Adolescent girls who have an incestuous relationship with their fathers feel dirty, contaminated, anxious, and guilty. They may have psychophysiologic disorders, disturbances of appetite, conversion disorders, indulge in promiscuous behavior (occasionally), be depressed, attempt suicide, and attempt to run away from home (to escape the situation). Children born of incest have a higher mortality as infants, more congenital malformations, and lower I.Q.s.[321] Genetic risks seem to be involved but the complications of teenage pregnancy combined with poor prenatal care and a minimally nurturing environment may contribute to the disadvantages of these children.

A preschool-age child who has been raped shows regression, fears, night terrors, and other responses. In school-age girls, anxiety, depression, school problems, conversion disorders, and running away are among the most common responses to rape. Adolescents show much guilt, phobic responses, anxiety, depression, and mistrust of men. Although, as

Carol Nadelson[320] has indicated, adolescent and young women do have unconscious rape fantasies, actual *rape* is a life-threatening situation. Many rapes of children and adults have gone unreported because of embarrassment on the part of the victim and her family, but that picture is changing. Adult rapists of children are often disturbed persons who are inhibited about sex in their daily lives. They may be impotent, exhibitionistic, voyeuristic, and other kinds of pedophilic adults (as well as child murderers).[301,386] But many offenses against children are perpetrated by someone who is well known to the child, and force may play only a small role. Group rapes by adolescent males often are attempts to prove their masculinity. Adolescents may also seduce, molest, or rape younger children; such adolescents are usually quite disturbed, have distorted family relationships, and may be quite sadistic.

In dealing with parental seductiveness, discussing the overstimulating nature of the parent's behavior and the parent's need to treat the adolescent more maturely may help a parent who is unaware of the significance of his behavior. In more serious cases, psychiatric consultation is indicated, and psychotherapy for the adolescent and both parents is often necessary. In incest, treatment must be individualized, to the individual and the family's pathology. Courts, child welfare agencies, and mental health agencies or professionals most often are involved. Separation of the child and parent may be necessary, and sometimes the father is hospitalized. Individual, marital, or family therapy[282] may also be provided although some severely pathologic families are most difficult to treat.

If a child or adolescent has been raped or has undergone some other type of sexual assault, the family should discuss their feelings about the incident with the physician or health associate or with a mental health professional. Many families avoid such a discussion out of guilt, or negligence, or some other reason.[267] If such a discussion is held, the incident generally does not have a seriously adverse effect on the child's personality development. If the incident is not discussed, problems may arise immediately or later. More intensive psychotherapeutic measures may be indicated. Rape crisis centers have been set up in some medical centers. If the child must testify in court, it is best for a mental health professional to prepare the child and his family for the experience and to be in court with the child and his family. Efforts should be made to speed legal proceedings and to insure privacy in court procedures. Adults who molest children more than once should be given an indeterminate sentence and treatment. Mandated therapy on a long-term basis in a closed psychiatric treatment unit has been quite effective in California, and the rate of recidivism is very low.

Adequate sex education for the child is an important preventive measure, ideally offered by parents, but if necessary by physicians or school personnel.

Working Mothers: Day Care and Head Start Programs

Since so many mothers work and since at least one-sixth of children live in one-parent families, most of them headed by mothers, the question of the care of children outside the home has become more and more pressing. The studies of Poznanski and her colleagues[341] indicate that young children of working mothers, especially boys, tend to be somewhat more dependent but to achieve better grades in school than do the children of nonworking mothers. Day care centers have existed in the United States for many years. Although in the past, many mothers did not send their children to school until they were of nursery school age (about 3 years old) or elementary school-age, today more and more mothers are searching for good day care services for infants.

Head Start programs, which were begun in 1965 by Julius Richmond, were not meant to be day care programs. They concentrated on preschool-age children, and they were based on the premise that early intervention in the form of social, emotional, and cognitive enrichment and stimulation for children from economically disadvantaged families could help them better realize their intellectual potential. Although Head Start programs were originally summer programs, many became year-round preschool programs. At first, not enough trained nursery school teachers were available to supervise other personnel, and many Head Start programs were understaffed and varied greatly in content and goals. The early results of evaluation of these programs were accordingly uneven and contradictory. But the programs became better articulated and replication became better controlled, and it now seems clear that increased cognitive development consistently results from Head Start programs that have clearly developed models and that actively involve the parents.[49,237] Evaluations of the physical, psychologic, and social development of children in these programs have found that a number of children have problems. As has happened in other screening programs, follow-through with treatment has been uneven. Some Head Start programs have become associated with mental health clinics, and the results are promising.[102,183,365,384]

Day care programs involving infants and young children have been regarded ambivalently. These programs also have varied greatly, and some have been frankly custodial. But Caldwell and her colleagues[75] found that in well-run, well-staffed programs there was no more evidence of social or emotional deficits in infants who had entered these programs at 1 year, than in children in a matched control group who were reared at home.[76] Cognitive stimulation in day care centers has been studied. Caldwell and Richmond[75] showed that day care children from lower income families gained an average of 5.6 points in their developmental I.Q., while the developmental I.Q.s of a matched control group declined, with a significant spread. Heinecke and his colleagues[206] have provided an excellent description of the approach to organization of day care programs from the point of view of the support of the mental health of the child and family. Not only is well-organized day care not detrimental to children,[414] there is evidence that some children may benefit from day care, especially if their home environments are not optimal.[237]

Provence[343] has provided good guidelines for the care of infants in groups and some states have set reasonable standards for day care programs in homes and centers, but there are no federal standards. Cohen and Zigler,[98] (Zigler was formerly the head of the Office of Child Development) have discussed the 1972 revision of the standards proposed in 1968. The revision recognizes that most day care takes place in homes, rather than in centers. In addition to specifications for day care settings, staff competency, accountability, and methods of parent participation, the 1972 standards specify the ratio of child to staff according to the age of the child and the type of day care; for example, one caregiver is allowed to care for no more than 3 infants or toddlers. Pediatricians, in addition to their role as physicians in day care,[334] should work with other professionals to see that the federal standards are adopted.

Prejudice

The effects of prejudice begin to be felt keenly by children in the school-age period. Awareness of racial differences is present by 3 years of age. Awareness of ethnic and religious differences develops later (by the early school-age period); such awareness involves more complex perceptions and concepts. Associated value judgments come from the parents and from the attitudes of the family and the culture. They reach their peak in the late school-age and early adolescent periods, as identifications are consolidated, social stereotypes are encountered, and racial or ethnic self-preferences appear.[299] Although black children and children from other minority groups tended in the past in doll play to identify with the majority group, the tendency disappeared by adolescence and it has nearly vanished today.[403] Envy, frustration, and bitterness, as well as negative self-pictures and loss of self-esteem, become increasingly prominent in the victims of prejudice. Those feelings are accompanied by varying patterns of activity, aggression, and compensatory striving or by apathy, hopelessness, submission, and passive sabotage.[335] Adolescents from different ethnic groups have the same health concerns.[330]

Although children easily pick up social bias or stereotypes of minority groups, there is evidence that the most prejudiced children and adults are those who are insecure, jealous, hostile, suspicious, and distrustful of others. They frequently have been reared in rigid, autocratic families, and they tend to have "authoritarian" personalities.[93] The prejudiced person in North American society unconsciously pays penalties—restriction of his social contacts, the need to rationalize his inconsistent attitudes, anxiety over ambiguity, and guilt about his aggressive or hostile impulses.

Experiments have shown that prejudice can be combated successfully by positive contacts with people from other groups. But the current problems in attempted integration arise predominantly from de facto segregation in housing and education, limited job opportunities, and the current polarization of attitudes, which are circular and which tend to bind minority groups rather than to free them.

Poverty

The destructive effects of severe poverty on children and families have been referred to throughout this book.[48] Since many minority families are victims of unemployment, poor housing, poor nutrition, and poor health care, as well as prejudice, there is an obvious overlapping between the problems caused by poverty and those caused by racism.[376] Even within the poverty range, however, there are some families that are better off economically and that manage to hold themselves together more effectively than others.[331] However, even in the poorest group, some families become more disorganized than others.[332] The reason for the difference is not clear although it has been observed that severe urban poverty[314] seems to be more disorganizing than severe rural poverty.[275] The solutions to the problems of poverty are largely political although poverty seems to have psychosocial components.[43] Generally speaking, the poor are not lazy but hopeless, and a national health insurance scheme would be only one step in combating that hopelessness. As Coles[100] has pointed out, even children from affluent families have problems. One of them is coping with a surfeit of material goods.

Developmental Problems

The common developmental problems of infants, children, and adolescents were presented in schematic fashion in Table 5–1. The outstanding and difficult problems are discussed in the following paragraphs. (The reader who wishes more information should consult the reference material listed at the end of Chapter 5 or other sources.[18,101]) Some developmental problems, such as failure to thrive and reactions to hospitalization, are discussed in other chapters. (The feeding, weaning, sleeping, toileting, and other milder developmental problems such as those related to stranger[419] and separation anxiety,[420] are well discussed in other sources.)

Special Problems in Infancy

The following pages discuss some special developmental problems in infancy that are not discussed elsewhere in the book: colic, habit disturbances (e.g., head rolling, head banging, and body rocking, rumination, spasmus nutans, breath-holding spells, pica, and trichotillomania), and hyperactivity.

Colic. Most infants cry or fuss periodically in their first few weeks of life, most often in the evening. "Heavy" fussing sometimes builds up to a crescendo, and the infant often draws his legs up on his abdomen and seems to be relieved when he passes flatus. The condition ordinarily is manifested by 2 to 3 weeks of age, and it disappears by 10 to 12 weeks of age—it is the so-called three months' colic.[220] It seems likely (as Benjamin hypothesized,[36] with some support from the studies of Tennes and her colleagues[418]) that the infant's overready response to stimulation in this "sensitive" phase may be involved in the colic, as may irregular gastrointestinal peristalsis and other as yet unintegrated autonomic functions characteristic of the first 2 to 4 months.[142] Although the term colic has been widely used, the problem does not seem to be basically a gastrointestinal one. Rather, the basic problem seems to be a developmental vulnerability to stimulation, with air-swallowing, secondary gastrointestinal reverberations, and possibly peristaltic irregularity. Thus the term "paroxysmal fussing," which Wessel and his colleagues used,[450] seems more descriptive. Other contributory factors may be that in the evening the infant receives more stimulation from his father, that the mother is more anxious about the infant's sleeping, and that both parents are worried about criticism from relatives and neighbors about the infant's continual crying.[329,410]

Clinical observations suggest that prolonged and severe colic, which often persists until the latter part of the first year, occurs most commonly in infants who are overactive and tense from birth[84]—so-called hypertonic infants. As mentioned earlier, there may be some relation to the activity of the infant in utero and to the levels of anxiety in the mother during pregnancy. Maternal and family tension, as well as possible allergic tendencies, have also been implicated.[450] Such factors may be involved in many cases of pylorospasm, representing the interaction of innate and experiential forces.

Anticipatory guidance about avoiding overstimulation of an active infant may be helpful in minimizing developmental colic or paroxysmal fussing. Knowing that a certain amount of "unsatisfiable crying" will occur[64] can be reassuring to young, earnest parents, as can knowing that such fussiness ordinarily disappears by 3 months.[220] The use of a pacifier can be soothing to the infant; it does not promote more intense sucking or overdependency unless it is used too freely by an overanxious mother to prevent crying altogether as a substitute for tactile, rhythmic, and other important kinds of stimulation. Swaddling the infant in a receiving blanket may help a tense, fretful infant, as may rocking the infant in a baby carriage. If prolonged and severe colic supervenes, the infant's sucking time during feeding should be checked; the infant may need more than strictly nutrient sucking for emotional satisfaction. As Levine[260] has shown, a pacifier may help considerably if one was not used previously. Counseling is important. The parents should be given time to think out loud with the nonjudgmental help of the physician about the resolution of superficial family tensions centering on (for example) living arrangements, schedules, overstimulation of the infant by the father in the evening, arguments at night over handling the infant, and the criticisms of relatives, friends, and neighbors. Drugs are usually of no value.

Habit Disturbances. Other disturbances in behavior include repeated and prolonged bouts of marked *head rolling, head banging,* and *body rocking*. Such phenomena are referred to as habit disturbances, and they represent an intensification of the normal patterns of rhythmic satisfaction[278] involving unhealthy methods of substitute gratification in infants who have received too little extraoral stimulation. These disturbances may be also seen in infants who have been overstimulated, in which case they are ways of discharging tension, or in infants who have suffered emotional deprivation, in which case they are possibly attempts at self-stimulation.[250] Habit disturbances can be extremely disturbing to parents, whose desperate attempts to anchor the bed or tie the child down fail to affect the head rolling or rocking. Management is based on finding the source of the problem and in helping the parents achieve healthy stimulation of their infant. If the symptoms continue beyond the age of 3 years or if significant emotional deprivation seems to be involved, psychiatric consultation can be helpful. Drugs are usually of no value.

Another unhealthy substitute gratification for unmet basic needs is *rumination*, the mouthing of regurgitated food.[166,359] This habit disturbance occurs only after the infant is capable of voluntary behavior, at around 3 months of age. It occurs in infants who have had too little stimulation or who have had discontinuous or insufficient mothering because of maternal depression, preoccupation with marital conflict, or other conditions producing emotional deprivation. The infant may initiate the regurgitation by sticking his hand into his throat, or he may be able to bring up the food using the upper two-thirds of his esophagus (which receives some voluntary innervation), the pharyngeal muscles, the accessory muscles of respiration, and the diaphragm. The infant loses a considerable amount of food through drooling, and the resultant weight loss may be severe and even life threatening. Rumination may be associated with air swallowing (aerophagia), which sometimes leads to explosive vomiting.

Rumination ordinarily responds well to the positive use of hospitalization and "replacement therapy" for the emotional deprivation using a mother-substitute, especially a foster grandmother, and certain types of stimulation. Special work with the parents is needed to help them deal with their guilt about their child's problem as well as to help them deal with the basic problem in the parent-infant relationship. Play therapy is occasionally needed for a seriously disturbed infant or a preschool-age child.[407]

Spasmus nutans (nodding spasms, head tilting, infantile spasma) has its onset during the first year of life, after the infant is 3 or 4 months old. The disorder is characterized by sudden and frequent nodding or tilting of the head, together with nystagmus. It must be differentiated from hypsarrhythmia, which has a poor prognosis. Spasmus nutans generally subsides within a few months, and its prognosis is favorable. Lack of visual stimulation resulting from poorly lighted surroundings has been thought to be involved in the genesis of the disorder.[188] Maternal deprivation may be more fundamentally involved, however, and spasmus nutans can also appear in the context of overly anxious, immature, somewhat helpless attitudes on the part of the mother, with overstimulation of the child's face during feeding.[154] Management involves counseling or supportive psychotherapy, and psychiatric consultation is often helpful.

Breath-holding spells usually are of either the cyanotic or the pallid type.[274] They are usually touched off by situations involving angry or frustrated feelings.[172] The child's initial voluntary response of crying and holding his breath, a method of controlling the parents (by frightening them), may become involuntary, with syncope and even clonic-like seizures occurring in the pallid type. But the spells seem to have no relationship to epilepsy or brain damage, and the prognosis is good.

Explaining the phenomenon reassuringly to anxious parents and counseling them not to respond to the attacks will ordinarily suffice. Throwing water on the child frightens the child, and it is not recommended. Giving parents a formula to say to the child (e.g., "I'll just wait until you calm down") may help the parents to be firm. The infant's need to establish his autonomy and his need to have limits put on his behavior should be discussed with the parents. If the breath-holding spells are part of a serious struggle for control between the child and his parents, psychiatric consultation may be helpful and psychotherapy may be necessary.

Overactive, "overexploratory" infants may have repeated *accidents* or *poisonings* (beyond the occasional one that may occur during infancy), the stage during which most cases of accidental poisoning occur[370,393]). Studies indicate that repeated phenomena of this type usually occur in families in crisis[194] or in disturbed families[266,392] in which the parents are too preoccupied to take precautions or to offer the constant supervision a toddler needs. Education about accident prevention can be helpful in healthy families, but supportive help or more intensive psychotherapy for the parents may be necessary.

The symptom of *pica* is seen in almost all cases of lead poisoning in young children,[187] and children who are hospitalized for accidental poisoning also have a high incidence of pica. Pica is the persistent ingestion of inedible substances; for example, dirt or paint from woodwork, coated with lead paint.[62] Pica occurs in mentally retarded and brain-damaged children, and it occurs also in older infants or children of normal intelligence.[106] Beginning around the middle of their first year, normal infants explore their environment by mouthing, and they sometimes ingest inedible substances. Discontinuous or insufficient parenting, usually with maternal deprivation,[256] seems to shunt the child to oral satisfaction or "addiction" as an unhealthy substitute for basic emotional gratifications, as Millikan[312] and Lourie[277] have pointed out. Identification with a parent who shows (or showed) pica may also be involved. Marked and persistent pica in a child older than 18 months is suggestive of psychopathology. Coprophagia, beyond the first year or so, when it may be seen in normal infants, occurs occasionally in psychotic or profoundly mentally retarded children. The positive use of hospitalization and mother-substitute therapy, together with help for the parents, can be of value. Psychiatric consultation may be necessary, and intensive psychotherapy for the child and his parents may be indicated.

Somewhat similar mechanisms appear to be involved in *trichotillomania*, pulling of the hair of the head and occasionally of the eyebrows or eyelashes. The symptom ordinarily develops in the latter part of the child's second year, and it may continue for months and years, with exacerbations related to anxiety-producing events. It occurs more frequently in girls than in boys. Young children seem little concerned about the hair pulling, although children older than 7 are concerned about the teasing or rejection by their peers.[289] Nail biting, nose picking, masturbation, and social and academic problems, together with passive behavior, are often associated with pica. Often the mother is unavailable to the child because she is depressed, and the father is often detached from the family. The hair pulling seems to give substitute gratification, possibly derived from pleasurable experiences the child had during feeding or sucking in infancy when the infant may stroke his hair.[69] An unconscious need for and masochistic enjoyment of pain may also be involved. Occasionally older infants and young children eat the hair,[4,252] a habit that leads to the formation of a trichobezoar (hairball) that can gradually obstruct the stomach to the point of requiring surgical intervention, occasionally repeat-

edly.[113] Obviously, psychotherapeutic intervention for the child and his parents is indicated once the condition is diagnosed.

Hyperactivity. Hyperactivity has been discussed in several sections of this book. It has been emphasized that hyperactivity is regarded by me and others[136,257] as a symptom and that it may or may not be associated with distractibility and impulsivity.[428] It does not seem to be a syndrome, as some have implied.[78,253]

Hyperactivity may arise from multiple sources: constitutional or temperamental sources, resulting in "developmental hyperactivity,"[383] anxiety, depression, and certain cases of diffuse cerebral cortical brain damage. It has been emphasized that many children who have definitive brain damage do not exhibit hyperactivity but may show hypoactivity, withdrawal, or aggressive behavior not related to hyperactivity.[383] (My view, and that of others, that minimal brain dysfunction, in which hyperactivity is involved, is now recognized as a myth was mentioned earlier.)

It is true that about 50% of hyperactive children respond to the short-term use of stimulant medication, but there is no homogeneity even among the group who respond.[428] The dangers to growth of the long-term use of stimulants[99] were mentioned earlier, as was the view that drugs should be used only adjunctively in the context of a comprehensive program of management based on extensive evaluations of the child and his family.

Special Problems in the Preschool-Age Period

The following paragraphs discuss some of the special problems of the preschool-age period that are not discussed elsewhere in the book: sleep disturbances, speech disorders, and accidents. (The feeding, sleeping, toileting, and other milder developmental problems such as temper tantrums, excessive thumb and finger sucking, sibling rivalry, fears, and problems about sexual development encountered in this period are well discussed in other sources.)

Sleep Disturbances. *Nightmares.* Although most dreams that preschool-age children have involve either wishes or daytime activities, children of this age also often have nightmares. The nightmares involve intensely vivid experiences with frightening monsters or giants, often accompanied by a sense of helplessness. The child is fully awake following a nightmare; he can ordinarily recall at least fragments of the nightmare although he may be afraid to tell them for fear they will come true. Nightmares may be stimulated by disturbing or overexciting experiences, and ordinarily they contain a residue of the day's experience. As responses to single traumatic experiences, nightmares seem to be attempts to work over or desensitize the experiences during sleep. Their more basic origin in the preschool-age period lies in the child's need to repress unacceptable feelings of hostility, rivalry, or sexual attraction he feels toward a parent. Such feelings, together with self-punitive feelings, may break through in disguised form in the nightmare. The preschool-age child often comes into the parents' bedroom after a nightmare or asks to be taken into their bed. Repeated nightmares call for study.

Night Terrors. Night terrors (pavor nocturnus) have sources similar to those of nightmares.[398] They are less common than nightmares, however, occurring only occasionally in healthy children and after stressful or overfatiguing events. Repeated night terrors usually occur in a tense and anxious child who has overrestrictive or sometimes overindulgent parents or whose family situation is troubled. Night terrors represent a dissociated state of awareness. The child is not fully awake, he appears to be hallucinating, he cannot be awakened or comforted, sometimes for as long as half an hour, and ordinarily he has no memory of the experience, which is always a harrowing one for the parents. The parents

can usually be reassured about the transitory character of night terrors. They can be advised to hold the child comfortingly until he goes back to sleep or awakens fully, rather than throw water on him or use other extreme measures. Discussion of family tensions or conflicts may be necessary if the problem is marked and persistent. An occasional child and family require psychotherapy in a child guidance clinic or from a private mental health practitioner.

Deviations or Disturbances in Speech Development. A number of deviations or disturbances in speech development are discussed in the following paragraphs. They involve both physical and psychologic factors, but in most of the disorders, emotional factors are predominant.

Absence of Speech (Mutism). Mutism may occur in association with (1) severe mental retardation, (2) a congenital defect in or damage to the organs of articulation, (3) damage to those areas of the brain concerned with language or involved with the muscles of articulation, and (4) severe and persistent early infantile autism. Even in severe brain damage, however, there is usually an emotional component in mutism. Elective mutism may appear in children who have learned to speak.

Delayed Onset of Speech. The failure of a child 2 to 2½ years old to develop speech may be related to mental retardation, deafness, or blindness acquired during late infancy, to a developmental deviation in speech capacity that is associated with a family history of delayed development, or to a lack of adequate social, emotional, or sensory stimulation due to insufficient mothering. Other possible factors are marked negativism, in which a serious struggle with a parent over toilet training has been displaced onto speech, infantilism, with the child being handled like a baby and no demands made on him, and behavioral regression (due to physical illness or separation) at the time when speech is being developed. Aphasia of the expressive type may interfere with speaking but not with comprehension; it is rare and usually not clear-cut, with much overlapping with emotional influences. So-called tongue-tie (a tight frenulum) does not cause a delay or dysfunction in speech.

Disorders of Articulation. Disorders of articulation involve the omission, substitution, or distortion of speech sounds. They are the most common of all speech difficulties, occurring in about 5% to 10% of early school-age children and 2% of college freshmen. Disorders of articulation are occasionally related to brain damage or mental retardation, or they may arise from a full or partial (regional) hearing defect. But by far the majority of these disorders seem to represent immaturities in articulation, such as difficulties in handling consonants, the omission of final sounds, and lisping. In young children most of these disorders seem result from the persistence of infantile patterns in speech, and often they are associated with emotional immaturity. Some disorders of articulation derive from inborn developmental deviations in speech capacities.

Disorders of Phonation. Disorders of phonation involve marked deviations in loudness, pitch, quality, or flexibility of voice or intonation. Physical causes of these disorders include cleft palate, harelip, congenital deformities of the soft palate, enlarged adenoids, bulbar paralysis, encephalitis, and myopathies. Disorders of phonation are often associated with defects in articulation or other aspects of speech functioning; some of them may involve emotional components.

Many disorders of phonation have a predominantly psychologic basis. Voice changes in adolescents begin with physiologic changes, but they may occasionally persist on emotional grounds. Loud speech often occurs in emotionally anxious children or in tense, hyperactive children; strident speech may be associated with demanding behavior. A monotonous tone may be related to partial deafness, such as that produced by chronic otitis media,

which may also delay language development. Like loud or strident speech, however, a monotonous tone may also be a result of the child's imitation of or identification with a parent who has similar voice qualities. A high-pitched falsetto voice may occur in emotionally immature children, or it may be associated with early childhood psychosis. Aphonia of nonphysical origin usually is seen in late school-age children or adolescents; it is usually a conversion disorder related to repressed and unresolved emotional conflicts.

Disorders of Rhythm. Disorders of rhythm involve mainly stuttering (stammering), which occurs in 1% to 2% of the population in the United States and which occurs predominantly in males, often those whose families have a history of stuttering. Stuttering is characterized by disturbances or interruptions in the flow of speech; there may be blocking (inability to articulate certain sounds) or repetitions of sounds due to tonic and clonic spasms that affect respiration and phonation. Stuttering tends to begin when the child is between 2 and 5 years of age; a significant percentage of stutterers do not develop symptoms until they reach the early school years, and the incidence of stuttering decreases as puberty approaches. Stuttering becomes worse under conditions of emotional tension involving anxiety, feelings of pressure, or self-consciousness. The stutterer may make associated movements, including twisting his neck, protruding his tongue, or stamping his feet. Initially these movements are devices to prevent speech blocking although they may have some unconscious symbolic significance.

Stuttering seems to be a disorder of civilization; it is not known among primitive people. Although the mixed cerebral dominance theory of the origin of stuttering was popular,[53] most stutterers are in fact not ambidextrous or lefthanded. The changing of handedness does not seem to be significantly associated with stuttering. A certain group of stutterers do have a history of delayed speech development,[88] lags in the establishment of handedness, motor awkwardness, and cluttered (rapid, confused, and jumbled) speech during the initial phase of acquisition of language. Children in this group seem to be those who have developmental deviations in maturational patterns and who may also have visual-motor and auditory problems connected with reading or with other aspects of learning.

Aside from the constitutional predisposition, emotional factors in time come to assume the dominant role in stuttering. The developmental roots appear to lie in the normal hesitations and repetitions in the speech of the child in the "practicing stage" (from 2 to 4 years of age). Those phenomena largely disappear by the early school-age period. The current interactional theory of stuttering[224] emphasizes the part played by parental criticism of the child's speech and undue pressure on the child, during this critical phase of the development of speech fluency, to speak perfectly. This pressure is often the result of the parents' concern about their own speech in the past.

The mothers of stutterers appear often to dominate the child in a variety of ways, and their fathers are generally passive and retiring. In such a family constellation and under such developmental circumstances, the child who has a constitutional predisposition to stuttering may have difficulty establishing autonomy and initiative.[460] The child's initial anxiety about his speech can be compounded by an emotional conflict related to the prelogical thinking characteristic of the early school-age period.[46] The conflict may also further invade this vulnerable period of speech development, with words coming to stand symbolically and magically for hostile or sexual feelings the child has toward his parents.

As such conflicts become unconscious and internalized, the stuttering may later acquire the unhealthy adaptive character of an internalized symbolic psychologic symptom, aiding in the repression of unacceptable and conflicting thoughts or feelings by blocking the words that stand for them. Such a mechanism (which is a conversion mechanism) may operate especially heavily in children who do not stutter until the early school-age period. These children often begin to stutter in response to emotionally traumatic experiences. Regression as a result of a failure to accomplish the psychosocial tasks of the preschool phase may also be involved. Often the child is outwardly passive or inhibited or shows overly dependent personality patterns. The fear of stuttering (of losing control of speech under embarrassing social circumstances) is another factor in this latter group. Such a fear produces feelings of inferiority, which arise easily during the school-age period.

Disorders of Comprehension and Symbolization. Disorders of comprehension and symbolization are rare, and they are not easily evaluated. Receptive aphasia, aphasia of mixed receptive-expressive type, so-called central or global aphasia, or auditory verbal imperception (word deafness without a defect in hearing), may occur occasionally on a developmental basis, with disturbances in the comprehension of word differences or the symbolic meaning of words. It is difficult to find gross or subtle neurologic lesions to account for these phenomena. Emotional factors (e.g., shutting out or failing to hear the parent under conflictful circumstances and so-called psychogenic deafness) seem to be important in many cases.[41]

Idioglossia[23] (private speech), is an uncommon speech disorder. Siblings may invent a language which they use among themselves and which their parents cannot understand. Often the basis of the speech is a formula for changing the words. Occasionally an only child will invent a completely original language. Idioglossia sometimes occurs in twins, who are closely intertwined in their psychologic development. It may also occur in children with so-called auditory verbal imperception and in children whose speech development lags for some time after speech appears.

Anticipatory guidance may help prevent some developmental speech disorders. Knowing that there are individual variations in the rate and character of speech in the early stages of the acquisition of speech may help parents to be more relaxed and to avoid criticizing or pressuring their children in regard to the hesitations and repetitions that are normal in the speech of 2- to 4-year-olds. Mental retardation, significant brain damage, a defect in the articulatory organs, deafness, blindness, and early infantile autism as causes of absent speech, or delayed speech require certain therapeutic measures and the help of specialists. Children who have persistent elective mutism ordinarily have fairly severe personality disturbances, and they should be referred for psychiatric consultation. Counseling the parents in regard to individual developmental deviations, regression, negativism, infantilism, or lack of adequate social, emotional, or sensory stimulation as factors associated with delayed speech may be of value. Speech therapy given without pressure may help the child who has a developmental lag in speech mechanisms, and psychotherapy may be needed for marked negativism, infantilization, or too little stimulation.

Disorders of articulation often respond to speech therapy given in a relaxed manner. Counseling the parents may help them understand children with developmental disorders of articulation or persistent infantile speech patterns related to overindulgence, overprotectiveness, or overrestrictiveness. Psychotherapy may be required for children who have infantile speech patterns, because speech therapy, unless it is given in a psychotherapeutic context, does not ordinarily touch the family problems. Many disorders of phonation may respond readily to speech therapy, although a falsetto voice or aphonia usually

occurs in the context of psychosocial problems that call for psychotherapy.

Stuttering that appears in the early preschool-age period may be helped by counseling or by speech therapy, which is often given at this age principally through work with the parents. Wyatt[460,461] has had outstanding success with early and brief intervention in this age group, using psychodynamically oriented speech therapy involving parents and children. In older preschool-age and school-age children in whom the symptom has acquired conflictful emotional connotations, psychotherapy for child and parents should be undertaken early; speech therapy at this point is often difficult for the child to use effectively although lingering speech defects following psychotherapy may later be dealt with successfully by speech therapy. In adolescents, psychotherapy may not be helpful (and may even be harmful) if a markedly passive, overdependent personality is present. It is best to refer such patients to experienced speech therapists. Although tranquilizers are occasionally helpful in mild cases, they usually do not make a significant difference.

Aphasia of various types and auditory verbal imperception that is definitively present require sophisticated speech therapy. Psychotherapeutic measures may be needed later to deal with the frequent emotional components.

Accidents. As Meyer and his colleagues[308] have indicated, accidents in preschool-age children seem to occur at times of family crises, such as a move, the loss of a job, or a serious illness in the family. Sobol's[392] study of accidental poisonings shows that the factors involved in poisonings are (1) the child's developmental characteristics, (2) the mother's emotional resources, (3) the family's organization, (4) the availability of the poison, and (5) the quality of the parent-child relationships. In regard to children who are 18 to 30 months old, who are at the height of normal negativistic and imitative behavior and who have well developed climbing and manipulative skills but a poorly developed sense of danger, the family environment and interactions combined with the mother's state of emotional depletion are often factors in the child's ingestion of poison. In regard to children who are 2½ to 4 years old, the child's contribution to the poisoning ordinarily involves persistent heightened negativism and attempts to cope with feelings of envy or loss, such as those related to the birth of a sibling or the mother's pregnancy.

In regard to preventing accidents, the recommendations of the Academy of Pediatrics and other organizations regarding precautions to be taken in the home should be followed, and developmental and family dynamics must also be considered. Other preventive measures are the use of homemaker services when a parent is ill, the use of sitters to supervise the children during a move or some other preoccupying events, the referral of disorganized families and families with marital problems to mental health services, and the use of parent-child counseling or therapy.

Special Problems in the School-Age Period

The eating and sleeping problems of the school-age period are well discussed in other sources, as are persistent thumb sucking, nail biting, and other habit disturbances, teeth grinding (bruxism), lying, stealing, daydreaming, and other milder developmental problems. The psychophysiologic disorders which may appear in the school-age period (e.g., peptic ulcer, essential hypertension, epilepsy, narcolepsy, rheumatoid arthritis, and thyrotoxicosis) are discussed elsewhere in the book. Psychoneurotic disorders, personality disorders, psychoses, and mental retardation, which may become manifest in this phase, are also discussed in other chapters, as are such disorders as tics and disturbances in

sexual orientation and gender. The special problems discussed in the following paragraphs are headaches, sleep talking and sleep walking, accident proneness, school phobia, learning problems, enuresis, and encopresis.

Headaches. Headaches are not usually a complaint until the school-age period, because preschool-age children generally localize pain poorly. The most common type of chronic, recurrent headache in childhood is the "tension" headache (or muscle contraction headache). It is usually generalized, and it may be described as a "band around the head" or a feeling of pressure, at times accompanied by nausea and vomiting. Such a headache may be mild or severe, and it may last for days or weeks. If it is severe, it may, like headaches from other causes, be associated with spasm of the muscles of the neck and shoulders. The differential diagnoses should include migraine headaches, conversion headaches, post-traumatic headaches, headaches from eyestrain, and headaches from intracranial tumor and other physical causes. Tension mechanisms may be admixed with migraine headaches or headaches from physical causes. Positive psychologic data should be present, in addition to the absence of other causes.

Children who develop tension headaches are generally overconscientious and unusually sensitive and sometimes perfectionistic and compulsive. Their parents often have similar characteristics and have high expectations for their child. The headaches often occur in association with unacceptable and at times unconscious anger or hostility. Counseling or supportive psychotherapy for the child and his parents is often effective, with some ventilation of feelings for the child and help for the parents in tolerating feelings and alleviating undue pressure on the child. In a few instances, more intensive psychotherapy may be necessary. Analgesics may be required temporarily.

Headaches resulting from migraine are

discussed elsewhere in the book, as are headaches of post-traumatic origin. Conversion headaches are not common until the late school-age period or early adolescence. They do not usually involve throbbing sensations or a band-like pressure; they are more often described as localized and sharp, ("like a knife") or they may be described as feeling "like somebody took the top of my skull off and was looking in." The symbolic meaning often includes a memory trace of some bodily experience of the patient or of a member of his family, and the patient often identifies with a parent who had headaches from any cause. Milder conversion headaches may be seen frequently during convalescence, and conversion mechanisms may be admixed with headaches from other causes. Supportive psychotherapy may be of value, but if the child is more seriously disturbed, intensive psychotherapy for the child and his parents may be necessary. The need for the finding of positive psychologic data, beyond the "ruling out" approach, applies as discussed in regard to conversion disorders, as treated in Chapter 18.

Sleep Talking and Sleep Walking. Sleep talking is usually mumbled and relatively unintelligible; it is concerned with the day's activities or it occurs in association with a nightmare in light (Stage 1) sleep.[351] It occurs also in preschool-age children, often involving the calling of the mother's name in apparent fright or screaming during the course of a night terror, a dissociative state occurring in deep (Stage 3 or Stage 4) sleep. In school-age children, the condition is usually a dissociative disorder rather than simply a physiologic comitant of disordered sleep. Temporal lobe epilepsy must be ruled out.

Sleep walking, often referred to as somnambulism, another kind of dissociative state, occurs most often in school-age children.[395] Many relatively normal children have one or two episodes of sleep walking, usually following some crisis, such as an examination failure, illness in the family,

or intense fatigue. Sleep walking can also be associated with delirium from high fever arising suddenly during the night. Recurrent episodes may be encountered in anxious, guilty, or overly tense children, sometimes in association with night terrors or enuresis; a few children have more serious emotional disturbances. Although a familial tendency exists, sleepwalking in most instances is not associated with epilepsy. The child who sleep walks may go to the bathroom to urinate or to the parents' room, possibly out of anxiety or because of curiosity about the sexual act. A few children may endanger themselves during a sleep walking episode although their muscular coordination and unconscious awareness of objects is usually good.[421] A child may speak appropriately during a sleep walking episode, but ordinarily he has no memory for the event.

Occasional sleep talking or sleep walking may respond to a supportive, counseling approach dealing with disciplinary approaches or other family tensions. (Drugs alone are of limited value.) Parents may ask whether to awaken the sleep walker; if he is in danger (he occasionally is), it is better not to awaken him. Awakening him may disrupt his unconscious coordination. Calm and firm guidance of the child away from the danger is indicated. More severe or recurrent symptoms call for psychiatric consultation and may require intensive psychotherapy.

Accident Proneness. No one personality or family pattern prevails among school-age children who have repeated accidents (the "accident habit"). Some children are overactive, restless and impulsive, and they show an insistence on unrealistic independence which contains elements of oppositional behavior or defiance of parental authority.[161] Their parents are often dominating and overly strict, but they are overly casual about accidents. They often show less than the usual warmth toward their children without rejecting them openly. Accidents often occur to other members of the family, and they occur to the accident-prone child in family conflict situations that evoke reckless, impulsive, disorganized behavior.[218] In another group of accident-prone children, the family background seems to be much more disorganized, with a high incidence of marital conflict, broken homes, violent behavior, and serious personality disturbance in one or both parents and, at times, open rejection of the child.[68]

Accidents[290] such as scalds and burns often occur when the child feels helpless, inferior, deserted, or angry, and they may involve an unconscious wish for attention from parents in intact but strict families. Still other children seem to have strongly repressed and internalized their conflicts about aggressive impulses. Accidents may arise when the child feels guilty about having done something forbidden, and they may involve a turning inward of aggression in a self-punitive fashion. Whether or not such unconscious feelings are present, the child may look on an accident as punishment for unacceptable thoughts or wishes, and the parents also have intense feelings of guilt. Epidemics of accidents sometimes occur in institutions or summer camps after a favorite counselor or attendant has had an accident. Pediatric counseling or supportive therapy may help some parents to be less strict in handling their child, and to have more realistic expectations of their child. Psychiatric consultation is usually wise, and in a number of cases intensive psychotherapy is needed for the child and his parents.

School Phobia. School phobia is a morbid or an irrational dread or fear of some aspect of school life, such as a particular teacher or pupil or taking showers in gym. Somatic complaints (abdominal pain, nausea, vomiting, headaches, feelings of weakness, or low-grade fever) may be present. They usually appear on school days and often disappear if the child remains home (although the child is not malingering). These complaints have led Schmitt to call school phobia "the great im-

itator."[382] The basic fear is not of going to school but of leaving home.[131] Many normal children show mild fears and abdominal pain on first going to school, but their parents encourage them to overcome them, and they soon disappear.

School phobia generally occurs in an overdependent, shy, anxious child who has been handled during the preschool-age period in an overprotective or overcontrolling fashion by an anxious mother. His father is generally more passive and distant. A family move or an actual or symbolic loss may help precipitate the disorder. The mother often fears the child's growing away from her, and she communicates to him her anxiety[131] about his welfare or her mistrust of the school setting during the initial process of separation for full-time schooling. The child's fear of separation is displaced onto the school, which he perceives as a dangerous place, and he projects his resentment about his parent's overcontrol and his fear of retaliation for that resentment, (in the form of punishment, harm, or attack) onto the school. The mother and sometimes the father tend to take the child's fears too seriously, and an unhealthy and reverberating equilibrium is set up.[284] The longer the child remains at home, the more guilty, socially isolated, and afraid of failure he becomes. And the helpless parent, to whom he clings, becomes increasingly frustrated and impotently angry.

When school phobia occurs in first-grade or early school-age children, it ordinarily involves prolonged separation anxiety, a delayed developmental crisis over the move toward initiative,[457] or milder forms of phobic psychoneurotic disorders.[457] School phobia in junior- and senior-high-school students (and college students), is usually a manifestation of a more severe personality disorder or occasionally a disturbance of near psychotic proportions.[104] Job phobia in adolescents and adults is psychodynamically similar to school phobia.

The pediatrician may play an important role in the management of children who have school phobia. The condition is one of the few psychiatric emergencies, and certain first-aid measures are ordinarily indicated. The emergency situation represents the first phase of treatment, which may be carried out by the pediatrician if he understands the background of the difficulty and has the time he needs to work with the parents, the child, and the school authorities.

Early return of the child to school is the immediate goal.[132,434] The pediatrician should first make a thorough physical appraisal of the child. If the child has had abdominal pain or other gastrointestinal symptoms for some weeks or for several months, the pediatrician should have a barium x-ray series done to rule out peptic ulcer. Peptic ulcer, which is often of the acute type, is more common than was formerly believed, and occasionally it coexists with school phobia. If the findings are within normal limits, the pediatrician should reassure the overanxious parents that no physical abnormalities are present, and he should indicate that emotional tension can cause such symptoms. He should further indicate, in a noncritical, nonjudgmental way, that the child seems to be easily frightened by new experiences and starting school is certainly a milestone. Rather than immediately determining the parents' role in the problem, he should ask them what factors they feel might be involved.

With such an approach, many parents can begin to realize, without feeling very defensive or guilty, that they have kept their child too close to them. The pediatrician can suggest that they think out loud with him about ways to help the child become more independent. As a first step, he can indicate the importance of the child's early return to school, pointing out that continued delay will only make the steps of mastery harder for the child.

The pediatrician should have talked with the principal or (with the principal's permission) with the teacher, the school social worker, or the school psychologist in order to get the school's impression of the problem. Having discussed and cleared with the school authorities his plan for returning the child to school, the pediatrician should suggest to the mother that she take the child to school and, if necessary, to the classroom, even remaining there briefly. If the mother is too anxious to do this, the father may go also, or he may take the child himself. If neither parent feels able to carry out the plan, the pediatrician, working with the school authorities, can arrange for an adult relative, some other adult (e.g., the school nurse), or even an older child to take the child to school. If trouble arises, the pediatrician can talk by telephone with the parents and the child, or he can ask that the child be brought to the office, or he or a health associate can take the child to school. Once in the classroom, the younger school-age child usually settles in and does well. Some children may at first be able to attend school on a part-time basis only or to attend one class only. Some children may need to be excused from gym or even to be transferred to another teacher or another school. Such measures are usually not indicated in other disorders. Behavior therapy has been successful with less disturbed children who have school phobia.[128]

Once at school, some children may be unable to remain for long in the classroom, and they may ask to go home because they have abdominal pain or some other symptom. The doctor can have arranged with the school authorities to have the teacher send the child to the school nurse's office, where the child can lie down briefly. Then the nurse can reassure and encourage the child and return him to his classroom. If the child is permitted to call his parents, they may not be able to resist his appeals to come and take him home. No matter how worried the child's parents are, the physician should not give a medical certificate for home teaching for the child. Such a step may result in psychologic invalidism or a more pervasive kind of psychopathology.

In some cases, the ties between the parents and the child are so intense or the parents' fears of physical illness or harm to the child are so vivid that such emergency measures are not effective and early referral to a psychiatric clinic is warranted. With more intensive therapy for the child and his parents, the same results may be accomplished. In a few cases, the possibility that the truant officer will be called may galvanize helpless parents into action.[132]

Even if early return of the child to school is achieved (as it commonly is with younger school-age children), referral for psychotherapy should usually be undertaken to work out underlying conflicts and to prevent the return of symptoms. If the parents are reluctant to undertake psychotherapy following the resolution of the immediate symptoms, the pediatrician can take comfort from follow-up studies by Waldfogel and his colleagues,[433] which show that most such children are able to remain in school and to perform adequately although some psychologic problems may remain. With children who are in junior high school or high school, who are usually more severely disturbed, the first-aid approach should be tried. It may be successful,[457] but often it is not, and many adolescents who have school phobia require long-term intensive psychotherapy.[104] Some of these will respond only to psychiatric hospitalization or residential treatment. In a mildly disturbed adolescent, the positive use of brief pediatric hospitalization, involving psychiatric consultation and the help of a social worker, may mobilize the child and help his parents permit his gradual return to school. School phobia may arise in many children who have chronic physical illnesses, even mild ones. A case example of the pediatric approach to the management of an adolescent boy with mild asthma and an associated school phobia is presented in Chapter 25. The principles of management mentioned previously apply to these cases also.

Learning Problems. Since the invention of writing, the major advances in civilization have been based on man's ability to read. Today, however, 50% of the adult population of the world is illiterate. Despite the fact that in the United States basic education is available to everyone, 11% of the adult population cannot read beyond the third-grade level. From 15% to 30% or more of children in our school systems are said to suffer from some type of significant educational handicap.[178] At least 8% to 10% of these handicaps are said to involve perceptual-motor or related problems, and 8% to 12% of children are said to exhibit emotional problems that require treatment. There is some overlapping between these two groups of children and with children in other groups, such as those who have language disorders. Many children from Spanish-surnamed and other minority families suffer from a language barrier in the early learning years, which are crucially important ones.

In some underprivileged urban areas, nearly one-third of the children in sixth grade are at least two years behind in their reading levels. The figure is higher for boys than for girls,[39] and it is three times higher for blacks than for whites.[135] In ghettos and barrios, the percentage of school dropouts before completion of high school is 20% to 80%.[258] These figures are staggering when one considers that there are about 60 million children under 14 years of age (more than 30% of the population) and that by 1985 the percentage under 20 years of age should be 50%.

Reading is fundamental to all learning, and Eisenberg's classification[135] of the sources of reading retardation is helpful in discussing and coping with learning problems. Eisenberg divides these sources into sociopsychologic (psychosocial) and psychophysiologic sources. The following discussion is adapted from Eisenberg's approach.

Psychosocial Sources of Learning Problems. *Inadequate Opportunities for Formal Education.* This factor affects children of rural or migratory working families, who may be late in beginning school, who may attend school irregularly, and whose school year may be shortened to conform to the farming season. Children from disorganized urban families may have similar problems, because they move often from one school district to another. Even if children of poor urban or rural families attend school regularly, their schools are generally overcrowded and are staffed with less highly trained teachers. The teachers may be pessimistic about the educability of their poorly motivated and often difficult students, and so the students may be placed in low-ability classes.

Children from affluent families may suffer also, including children who have serious physical handicaps, children whose parents are in the military service and who move frequently, and children who have seriously disturbed parents who keep their children at home or who move nomadically around the country.

Inadequate Cognitive Stimulation in Preparation for Learning. When he starts school, the child from the ghetto has a more limited vocabulary than does the middle-class child. He is also less responsive to verbal instruction, and he often has difficulties in auditory attention and perception. He has learned the skills of survival in his neighborhood, but their aggressive qualities penalize him in the classroom, and he has had little contact with books, magazines, verbal or written games, or more general cultural pursuits that would prepare him for formal learning.

Other children, including those from middle-class families, may receive inadequate stimulation during infancy and the preschool-age periods as the result of emotional deprivation. Such lacks may stem from inadequate mothering, due to maternal depression or rejection, or from discontinuity in relatedness, due to the child's having been placed in a number of foster home.

Deficiencies in Motivation. Deficiencies in motivation may arise from the failure of parents to praise or reinforce the child for good academic performance or to chastise him for misbehavior in school. Some parents give the child the impression that success in school has little bearing on job success, or they may seem suspicious of or resistant to school authorities. Such parental attitudes, which lead to poor motivation on the part of the child, are common in disadvantaged families, and they overlap with too few opportunities for learning and too little early stimulation. For such families, particularly those from minority backgrounds, defeat, alienation, and too few job opportunities are problems for the parent are well as for the child. Teachers often share the child's feeling of hopelessness. They may accept his poor self-image and hold out little expectation that he can learn, sometimes placing him in a low-ability class that gives him no opportunity to break out of the vicious cycle. Parental attitudes that work against the child's motivation may be encountered also in certain middle-class families. The attitudes are related to the parents' early experiences. Certain working-class parents may have little motivation to see their children move toward the middle-class, and they put little emphasis on the children's finishing high school or on academic learning in general.

Psychopathologic Disorders. The adverse effect of psychopathologic disorders on the development of reading skills or other aspects of learning may arise from family conflict, broken homes, and disturbances in parent-child relationships. Children in the early grades who have been identified by screening procedures as being emotionally handicapped generally continue to show difficulties.[413] A longitudinal study has shown that without help such children tend to have emotional and behavioral problems as adolescents and young adults. They are usually problems in receiving (taking in) knowledge and in reproducing (giving out) knowledge.

The kinds of children who have problems in taking in knowledge include the shy, inhibited, and often socially isolated child who withdraws into fantasy or day-dreaming, the child who exhibits passive resistance and tunes out the teacher, the child who is truant because he resists adult authority, the hyperactive child who is easily distractible and who has trouble concentrating, the child who has such severe conflict and anxiety about competition, self-assertion, or even curiosity (derived from an overly strong inhibition of his aggressive or sexual impulses) that he develops emotional blocking, with limited or no comprehension during reading or other activities, the child who has low self-esteem (usually a boy) that is derived from his identification with a parent who is himself a failure, the child who is depressed or apathetic and has little energy for learning, the child who has difficulty in testing reality, and the psychotic child, who is unable to comprehend the reality of his experiences, academic or otherwise.

Difficulties in reproducing knowledge may arise in certain types of children who have negativistic or oppositional trends, the child who has examination anxiety or emotinal blocking, who forgets what he knows because he has an exaggerated fear that he will be punished if he fails, the aggressive or rebellious child, who defies adult authority to examine what he knows, the extremely shy child, who needs help in speaking up, and the child with elective mutism, who is unable to speak at all in class.

A syndrome of learning inhibition has been described. Although no specific type of personality is always involved in the syndrome, it usually occurs in an anxious, inhibited child (usually a boy) whose fear of the aggressive implications of competition is so intense that he is led unconsciously to "renounce and deny"[399] his competitive strivings by failing to read and to learn. Disturbances in heterosexual development are frequent, as are the associated inability to engage in boyish activities and the assumption of more passive, even feminine, attitudes and interests. Signs of anxiety may lead to restlessness, difficulty in concentration, and hyperactivity, but the usual picture is that of a "frozen" child, one who is afraid to commit himself and to acquire the learning skills which would lead to competitive engagement. The mother is often the dominant figure[210] (she is overprotective and controlling toward the child), while the father[190] is usually more distant and passive.

In such children, the psychologic mechanisms appear to involve constriction of activity and motility and an unconscious inhibition of the capacities for reading and learning. These are neurotic symptoms which resolve (unhealthily) the child's conflict, but which also cause him pain and suffering, with the added of social stigma that arises from failure to learn. The child may develop negativistic or oppositional tendencies in response to pressure at home or at school.

Predominantly Physical Problems. Children who have reduced vision rarely complain of it, and the defect may not be recognized. To interfere with learning, vision must be considerably reduced. Aniseikonia (inequality of images in both eyes) can prevent fusion of the two images, and it may be involved in a small number of learning disorders.

Children who have mild-to-moderate hearing defects often have learning problems, and they may attempt to bluff in class when they do not understand fully. Regional deafness (involving certain wave lengths in the speech range) may interfere with learning. Even children who have normal pure tone auditory thresholds may suffer from perceptual handicaps in discriminating speech sounds and from defective intersensory integration (e.g., in converting auditory signals to visual signals). Such deficits may result from pathology of the central nervous system, from faulty auditory experience, or from developmental lags. Remedial education can be of help in all those cases. Speech disorders may of course interfere with the child's capacity for concept formation and with his ability to communicate his knowledge or express his ideas.*

Developmental Deviations. Other causes of learning difficulty are mental retardation, brain injury (discussed elsewhere), and developmental lags in perceptual-motor and other cognitive functions or in cerebral integration. In the opinion of Snyder[391] and Prugh, developmental lags account for the majority of reading problems. Children who have developmental lags in cerebral integration are seen frequently in the early school grades although the exact incidence is not known. This type of cerebral dysfunction should be distinguished from definitive brain damage[243] although making the distinction is often not easy. Congenital word blindness,[125] primary reading retardation, developmental dyslexia,[108] and perceptual handicap are terms which have been used for the condition. Some children have been described as exhibiting a specific spelling or arithmetic disability.[389]

Such children often show a relative inability to comprehend letters, words, and numbers as symbols. This difficulty shows itself in visual perceptual problems, such as in reversal of words (e.g., was for saw), mirror writing, confusion of certain letters (e.g., b and d and p and g), omitted or added words, perseverations, and skipped, split, or repeated lines. In some, the perceptual problem is mainly auditory, leading to problems in spoken language.[439] Those problems have been termed developmental language disorders with interference in concept formation. There may be considerable overlapping. Such problems occur about four times as often in boys as in girls. Usually the children come from intact homes and have had adequate opportunity, stimulation, and motivation for education. They have normal intelligence, and no gross neurologic defects. Besides their reading problems, they usually have

*See Chapter 25 regarding learning problems in chronically ill or handicapped children.

trouble handling such abstract concepts as those related to time, size, numbers, and spatial organization; some also have motor clumsiness or distortions in writing that sometimes are related to tactile perceptual problems. Low performance scores on the Wechsler-Bellevue Intelligence Scale are common although the verbal scores are usually satisfactory. Secondary emotional problems arising from feelings of frustration, inferiority, a poor self-image, guilt, anxiety over competition, and depression often occur.[350]

Left-handedness (or, more especially, delayed or inconsistent laterality or incomplete establishment of cerebral dominance) and delayed right–left orientation, with disturbance in body image, occur more often in these children than among average children. But determination of laterality is not simple, and "brainedness" is not necessarily consistent with "handedness,"[148] nor is handedness necessarily consistent with "eyedness," or "footedness." Left-handedness (4–8%) occurs more often in males than in females and in twins than in nontwins (although it may not be concordant), and it may be culturally influenced. Once left-handedness is established, it is best left unchanged although change is not strongly involved in speech problems, as was once believed.[327] The apparent association between delayed establishment of laterality and reading other learning problems seems to be related to a common underlying developmental antecedent rather than having any causal significance.

The types of reading, spelling, writing, arithmetic, and other developmental lags in perceptual-motor function, with limitations in intersensory integration, that these children have are similar to those shown by normal children as they learn to read and write. As the child develops, however, those early immaturities in cognitive and integrative functions that were present at a "sensitive" stage in the learning process often seem to disappear (but they may persist into adolescence). The child may be left, however, with a residue of his early learning difficulty or even with a habit of reading or writing inappropriately. With the current pressure in most Western nations for early academic learning, the child is often far behind, and he has ordinarily acquired emotional difficulties of the types described which interfere with his using effectively his now adequate capacities for learning. As mentioned earlier, premature infants show a high incidence of such developmental lags until they are 8 to 9 years old; 4% of school children in the United States today were born prematurely.

In Russia and Scandinavia, children do not begin formal academic work until they are about 7 years old. Certain observers have the impression that this late start allows children who have developmental lags to catch up and that the children in these countries have fewer reading problems. Accurate data are not available. A recent study indicates that the incidence of reading problems in Japan is about 1%, as compared with 10% in the United States, Great Britain, and New Zealand. Much more remains to be learned from transcultural investigations, which might take into account the syntax and structures of languages and other variables.

The biologic source of developmental lags in cerebral maturation is not clear although in line with their tendency to mature more slowly generally, boys appear to be more susceptible than girls. Many clinicians are impressed with the regularity with which a history of reading difficulty is obtained from the parents and other collateral relatives of the child who has this type of learning disability. An extensive survey[415] has suggested the likely presence of genetic factors in some instances.

As Synder,[390,391] Prugh, and others have emphasized, children who have developmental lags in cognitive, perceptual-motor, and integrative functions do not suffer from permanent perceptual-motor handicaps. The tendency to label some of these manifestations as "soft" neurologic signs in-

dicative of minimal brain damage is to be decried, as indicated earlier. There are of course some children with diffuse damage to the cerebral cortex who have a definitive history of insult to the central nervous system, together with some true neurologic deficits, and who show learning problems with perceptual-motor components. (There are also some with such diffuse brain damage who learn to read without serious difficulty, compensating with remarkable effectiveness.) Prugh and others believe, however, that the majority of middle-class children who have learning problems fall into the group with developmental lags.

Birch and his colleagues[48] identified in Scotland a group of boys who were retarded readers and who showed lower verbal scores and average-to-above average performance scores on the Wechsler Intelligence Scale for Children, when compared to a group of normal readers in the classroom (rather than in a clinic referral population). Their studies suggest that in the early grades, reading seems to be related more to auditory-visual (perceptual) integrative capacities than to intelligence, with more general intellectual factors most important for the later elaboration of reading skills. Other workers have identified groups of children with reading disabilities who come from families in whom family pathology is significantly greater than in a control group of competent readers. Thus sampling problems, age levels, and epidemiologic as well as cross-cultural factors need to be taken into account in future studies.

Eisenberg[135] and others have shown that reading retardation in the United States is linked statistically to social class, and Birch and his colleagues[48] have demonstrated social-class differences in auditory perception. The problems of inadequate cognitive stimulation and problems in motivation interact with the higher incidence of prematurity, low birth weight, perinatal complications, and malnutrition to bring about, in a way not clearly understood, a significant lack of preparation for school achievement by children growing up in poverty, as Richmond has pointed out.

Underachievement, the failure of the child to achieve at the level expected by his I.Q., may arise from any of the sources just discussed. It may also occur in the child caught up in a family crisis, with the child struggling for control and showing oppositional, oversubmissive, or aggressive behavior that spreads into areas involving studying or learning. Underachievement may also arise in the child who is being pushed too hard toward extracurricular or social activities, as well as in the somewhat dependent child who requires considerable supervision and direction, which he may not obtain in some permissive school situations. Overconcern is not indicated in the early grades, however, because late bloomers often catch fire. Also, neurotic problems, such as mild-to-moderate obsessive-compulsive tendencies, may, in some children of average ability, actually serve later as an overly strong spur toward achievement (overachievement), in an attempt to compensate or obtain satisfactions through academic performance.

The handling of *gifted children* (those whose I.Q. is over 140, 0.5% of the population) presents special challenges. Such children become bored in a conventional classroom,[378] and they often require special stimulation.[115] They can be pushed too fast, however, and their social and emotional development may lag behind their intellectual development.[193]

Many of the principles of the management of school problems were outlined in the foregoing discussion. Early identification of children who have developmental lags in cerebral maturation, brain damage, or social and emotional problems that predispose them to learning difficulty is fundamental. Such identification may be made in Head Start or kindergarten programs by physicians, psychologists, teachers, nurses, or other personnel or by the pediatrician in his private office. An educational diagnosis should be made as soon as possible, and remediation should be offered for perceptual, motor, cognitive, or other defects.

A number of screening tests have been developed to identify at the preschool-age level children who will have difficulties in reading, spelling, and writing. (Care must be taken to avoid labeling such children, because they may improve spontaneously in time.) The tests include the Frostig test, which is based on the child's capacity to discriminate between figure-ground relationships and other techniques, and the Predictive Index of DeHirsch, Jansky, and Langford[117] (which is being validated), which evaluates children's developmental capacities in perceptual, motor, and language behavior. Sachs[409a] has also developed a set of predictive tests that are being validated, and Hitchman[213] has worked out screening tasks for teachers. The Reading Readiness Test, which is routinely administered to all New York City children in kindergarten or early in the first grade, has successfully predicted reading disabilities. Attempts have also been made to validate predictive tests of social adaptation in preschool-age children.[269]

Pediatricians have sometimes used adaptations of the Gesell Developmental Schedules, those developed by Provence, or the Catell or other infant tests. All these tests take much time to administer, and they have certain limitations. Screening tests, such as the Denver Developmental Test and the Thorpe tests, have already been discussed. Once early perceptual-motor or other problems are identified, the pediatrician must make sure that the child receives treatment or remedial education as soon as possible. For a variety of reasons, that has not always been the case.

Children who have developmental lags in perceptual-motor functioning or who have cerebral dysfunction can be helped in kindergarten to gain reading readiness in an unpressured way using auditory, tactile, or kinesthetic sensory techniques for learning. These children can be placed in an ungraded class in their first year of elementary school. If ungraded classes are not available, these children can be given individual or group tutoring of the types developed by Frostig, Dubanoff, and others. Most children who are given such help can catch up after one or more years and then move into normal classrooms if their progress is reviewed regularly.

Studies by Bower[57] and Glidewell and Swallow[178] demonstrated clearly that the identification of emotionally disturbed children in the classroom and the use of preventive and early treatment measures is feasible.[468] In a study in which the New York City Reading Readiness Test was used as a screening device, teachers of the first three grades and parents of the children in those grades met with a mental health consultant in separate weekly small discussion groups. The reading levels of these children showed a significant increase over those of a group of children not so handled. If emotional problems are not identified until the child is older, he may need intensive psychotherapy or placement in a class for emotionally disturbed children.[427] Tutoring may help some mildly disturbed children and may have therapeutic implications.[19,152]

The physician shares the responsibility with educators or other professional persons for helping children who exhibit various kinds of problems in learning of psychosocial origin. (In ghetto or barrio schools, the majority of children may have potential problems, for reasons mentioned earlier.) In his role as a physician, he can offer only limited help to children who have inadequate opportunity for formal education, inadequate cognitive stimulation in preparation for learning, or deficiencies in motivation, unless these conditions have arisen as a result of neurotic or other types of problems in the parents. But as a private citizen, the physician can play an important part in the development of community programs to remedy many of these problems and to provide opportunities for screening and early intervention for children from poverty backgrounds. Despite some controversy, integrated schooling offers minority children the best chance for learning, and it offers Anglo children the opportunity for social interaction with minorities. Biracial-bilingual programs have helped children of Spanish-speaking and other minority backgrounds learn to read.

With individual children who show behavioral or psychopathologic disturbances in learning, the pediatrician may be of greater help through his study of the child in the family. Children who show underachievement because of depression, shyness or withdrawal, passive resistance to learning, or truancy may, with their parents, respond to a supportive, counseling approach.[394] Behavior modification has also been used successfully.[368] Those who have well-established learning inhibitions, emotional blocking of a neurotic type, elective mutism, or chronic personality disorders should generally be referred for psychiatric evaluation and treatment. Mental health consultation with the teacher in the classroom by a mental health professional[42,80] may be of great value in the management of the child with behavior problems or the minority child.[7] Individual psychologic testing should be a part of the diagnostic work-up of any child who has a school problem, because group tests done in school by teachers have limitations, as was noted earlier.

With the passage of the Education for All Handicapped Children Act of 1975, schools offer an unparalleled opportunity for handicapped children and have some special problems. Actually, since no federal funding was included, the public schools cannot afford to pay for expensive programs for seriously handicapped children. Some parents are suing the schools for such aid. As Low[279] has pointed out, there is danger of the pediatrician's not being included in the planning. Also the concept of mainstreaming children who have any learning handicaps has become popular, with special educational consultants being brought in to the classroom instead of the child's being singled out for placement in a special class, as he was in the past. Although mainstreaming has much to recommend it, difficulties arise from the lack of special consultants, and the teacher who has a large class and too little help faces real problems in meeting the special needs of children who have emotional disturbances, mental retardation, brain damage, and developmental lags in learning. In my opinion and that of others[143,244] ungraded classes for slow learners and special classes for the emotionally disturbed and mentally retarded will be needed until the teacher-child ratio increases and teachers acquire more special training. Perhaps some children will always need such classes.

Enuresis. As Glicklich[177] has indicated, enuresis appeared with the dawn of civilization, and the continuing study of enuresis in modern times has produced a voluminous literature. A great number of diverse and conflicting theories about what causes enuresis have been offered, and much confusion has resulted. Bakwin[21] remarked that enuresis has been cured by a host of remedies that bear no relationship to its cause. The symptom of enuresis is not necessarily associated with any specific clinical picture. It may represent a normal pattern of urinary incontinence until the expected age of control through training (the age has changed over the years), a failure to achieve control, a regressive component of a reactive disorder in late preschool-age children, a developmental deviation in control mechanisms, a conversion symptom as part of a psychoneurotic disorder, or one of a constellation of symptoms in a chronic personality disorder or psychosis.

Continuing enuresis has been variously defined. In the large-scale anterospective study of enuresis by Harper and his colleagues in 1968,[326] over 30% of children representative of the metropolitan area in Baltimore were enuretic to some degree at ages 3 and 4. By age 6, nearly 90% of the entire group had achieved initial nighttime dryness. By age 12, only about 3% were enuretic. Occasional relapses occurred at all levels, but the general impression was that the enuresis usually disappeared by puberty. In military studies, about 1% of recruits were found to be enuretic.[319] These figures are slightly higher than those reported from other countries (e.g., Britain and Sweden), but methodologic factors probably account for the difference. Much higher estimates of enuresis[2] have been made for children in institutions and in foster homes; social and cultural factors also seem to play a role.[409]

In Harper's study, nearly 90% of all children had achieved initial daytime dryness by age 4, 95% at age 5, and 99% by age 7. Occasional relapses occurred.

Besides age, the child's developmental level and the intensity of the enuresis should be taken into account. If a 6-year-old child seems somewhat immature in other aspects of his development and wets a good deal of the time, a policy of "expectancy" should be followed. That is, the parents should be encouraged to handle the child supportively in the expectation that he will achieve essential dryness by the age of 7 or so. If a 6-year-old child wets every night, especially if he wets more than once a night, or if a child who has some dry nights has not achieved full control by about age 7, clinical investigation would seem to be called for. Similarly, clinical intervention is indicated for a 4-year-old child who wets often during the day and for a child of age 5 who wets occasionally during the day. But concern, anxiety, or shame on the part of the parents may make it hard for them to adapt such a relaxed attitude. Parents from families[409] in which little toilet training has taken place, parents from rural backgrounds,[268] and parents who themselves wet the bed may be much less concerned, however.

As indicated, *nocturnal enuresis* occurs much more often after age 4, and especially after age 6, than does diurnal enuresis. *Diurnal enuresis* is frequently associated with nocturnal enuresis, although in a small group of cases it also occurs independently. Like nocturnal enuresis,[56] diurnal enuresis is frequently associated with early and coercive toilet training, but unlike nocturnal enuresis, diurnal enuresis is associated with a high incidence of encopresis. The term diurnal enuresis refers to constant dribbling during the day, not to occasional accidents caused by anxiety or a momentary "forgetting" to empty a full bladder when preoccupied, as often occurs in late preschool-age children. Diurnal enuresis may become a problem when the child enters nursery school, or it may remain mild or unnoticed until the child enters formal school. Diurnal enuresis may be influenced by shyness about asking to go to the toilet, fear of strange toilets, negativistic tendencies, or chronic anxiety. It also may have its origin in a bout of cystitis, with the frequency and urgency continuing in relation to anxiety or other psychosocial factors. Occasional cases have been associated with petit mal attacks although even in these, as in epileptic attacks, psychosocial factors may play a role. In older school-age children, diurnal enuresis is most often encountered in chronically anxious children, some of whom have personality disorders of the anxious type, and in children who have oppositional personality disorders. Generally, diurnal enuresis is more difficult to treat with the usual methods, described below, than is nocturnal enuresis.

In considering nocturnal enuresis, it is helpful to distinguish between continuing enuresis (the child is never dry) and relapsing (regressive) types of enuresis, because the prognosis for response to treatment, particularly in the older school-age child, is generally better in the regressive types. Regressive enuresis, which occurs in response to hospitalization, the birth of a sibling, or other situations in the preschool-age period, was discussed earlier.

Both types of enuresis must be differentiated from voluntary enuresis, which may occur at night if the child's room is too cold, the child has fears of the dark, or the toilet is inaccessible. Voluntary wetting may occur in the daytime also in a few disturbed children, whose resentment toward their parents' domination of them is masked by a submissive exterior. Such voluntary enuresis is a "revenge" type of enuresis; it is a conscious, volitional act that is usually carried out in secret.

Children who have nocturnal enuresis have been variously reported to be more immature, tense, restless, anxious, irritable, excitable, timid or fearful, and dependent than other children and to have a higher incidence of nail biting, temper tantrums, aggressiveness, thumb sucking, stealing, and other behavioral disturbances.[196,326] Their parents have been variously reported to be overcontrolling, rejecting, overly punitive, seductive, and overly affectionate. Nocturnal enuresis has been said to be more frequent in boys than in girls although the opposite has also been reported. Some studies, like Bakwin's[21] and Harper's, show no sex difference. In a small percentage of cases, enuresis is associated with encopresis. Enuresis has variously been said to derive from constitutional, genetic, somatic (urologic and neurologic), and psychologic factors. Such findings are conflicting, and many of the studies involve individual case reports or small groups of cases and few controls.

Various systematic investigations have laid to rest some myths about enuresis. Children who have nocturnal enuresis seem to have a more urgent response to bladder distention during sleep than do those who do not have nocturnal enuresis,[21,195] but their bladder capacity is not significantly diminished,[412] as some have believed. Psychophysiologic studies of adults (see Chapter 21) have shown that some people have a tonic response (involving some bladder spasm) to stressful psychosocial stimuli, while others have a response that involves relaxation and dilatation of the bladder musculature. Although the results of cystometrographic studies are somewhat conflicting, it may be that in certain children a constitutional tendency toward an "irritable bladder" response pattern serves as a biologic factor that predisposes those children to a developmental lag in bladder control mechanisms, as Bakwin[21] has suggested. That pattern acts to make the children more prone to develop enuresis under emotional stress or if their toilet training is neglected. Muellner[318] has postulated the existence of a constitutional lag in the sensorimotor coordination of the several muscle groups involved in the act of micturition; presumably that lag could be corrected by Muellner's training program, which involves high fluid intake and forceful and complete voidings. Werry's study[448] did not support Muellner's postulate.

The sleep of enuretic children is not significantly deeper than the sleep of normal children, at least as measured by EEG studies.[61] Nocturnal enuresis is not related to epilepsy, except in those cases of urinary incontinence accompanying a nocturnal seizure. Most epileptic children are not enuretic. Although abnormal EEG tracings were reported in the past in enuretic children, they are not diagnostic, and many would not be considered abnormal by modern interpretative criteria.

As Bakwin[21] has indicated, there is no relationship between enuresis and mental retardation although some profoundly retarded children, often those who have associated physical defects, may have difficulty in achieving bladder control. Moderately retarded children can be trained at about the same age as normal children can.[21] There is no significant difference in I.Q. between enuretic and nonenuretic children.[2]

Several studies, notably Hallgren's[197] in Sweden, have consistently demonstrated that the frequency of enuresis among parents and siblings of enuretic children is significantly higher than that in the general population. As Breger[66] has emphasized, however, even those who believe that enuresis results from an inherited condition of bladder irritability have stated that only a potential is transmitted genetically, and symptoms develop only under certain environmental conditions. Such arguments do not stand up well in the face of the suggestions that a type of "psychic inheritance" rather than genetic transmission is involved, and Kanner[227] believes that no adequate proof exists that it is not family tradition that is passed on.

The involvement of somatic abnormalities in the etiology of enuresis has been a matter of controversy for many years. Minor urologic abnormalities have been described in some enuretic children and adolescents, particularly those whose conditions have been refractory to medical treatment. Bakwin[21] reported that only a very small proportion of cases involve somatic factors. He believed that the etiologic significance of such coexisting conditions as balanitis, phimosis, and adherent prepuce is doubtful and that cures following the correction of such problems are attributable to a psychic rather than a physical effect. Karlin[231] has stated that spina bifida occulta occurs in some non-enuretic children, and Hallgren[195] and others, including Prugh, believe that urologic abnormalities are very infrequently associated with enuresis, and at most may be contributing factors. The problem seems to be one of external sphincter control; abnormalities higher in the urinary tract seem not to play a significant role. Urinary incontinence, as distinguished from enuresis, may of course be a symptom of a neurologic condition that can interfere with bladder and sphincter innervation, such as cord tumor, exstrophy of the bladder, and transverse myelitis.

Faulty training in bladder control has been implicated as a cause of enuresis. Coercive toilet training that took place before the child was 6 months old and that involved punishing or shaming, is a frequent finding, with a struggle for control at times arising between the child and his parents. Failure to toilet train, because of the parents' preoccupation or neglect (sometimes associated with inadequate toilet facilities in poverty areas) is involved in some cases of continuing enuresis. Toilet training may not be achieved if a child is infantilized or handled too permissively. Those who view enuresis from the point of view of learning theory stress pathologic toilet training techniques heavily. Toilet training is not the only factor, however; some children who had too early or coercive toilet training do not have enuresis although they may have other problems— and in some cases there is no history of faulty toilet training.

I tend to agree with Breger[66] that a number of factors cause enuresis. Somatic factors seem to be rare, and when they are present, they are usually precipitating or contributory rather than primary. A constitutional factor involving a predisposition to the "irritable bladder" or a developmental lag in bladder control mechanisms seems likely in a number of cases although environmental factors are needed to activate a predisposition. Psychosocial factors appear to be significantly involved in the majority of cases, with cultural and socioeconomic factors playing a role in some, including lack of toilet training or a certain type of toilet training. When psychosocial factors are predominant, the symptom of enuresis can have a different dynamic basis in different children, and the meaning of the symptom can change as the child's development proceeds. I agree with Lourie[277] that the symptom may lose its original meaning and continue as an isolated, learned psychophysiologic response.

From a psychosocial point of view, children who have nocturnal enuresis fall into several groups, which may help to account for the conflicting findings in the literature regarding personality pictures and parent-child relationships. These groups are discussed in the following paragraphs.

Developmental Lag in Control Mechanisms. As the result of a developmental lag in control mechanisms,[21,25] which is related perhaps to irritable bladder responses (which can be intensified by anxiety or guilt), a continuing struggle for control can arise between the child and his parents. The children in question are not usually seriously disturbed although they may be timid, and anxious and show immature behavior. The symptom tends to become "encapsulated," with a failure to achieve conditioned nighttime control. The child consciously wants to achieve control, and he is ashamed of his bedwetting. Some of these children may not bedwet when they stay overnight at a friend's house or at a summer camp; perhaps they are responding to a less charged atmosphere.

Reactive Disorders. A second group is composed of children who have achieved nighttime control during the preschool-age period but who relapse or regress during the late preschool-age or early school-age period. Enuresis reappears usually in relation to some event or set of events that are stressful for the particular child, such as hospitalization or other kinds of separation from the parents, illness in the mother, the birth of a sibling, the transition to regular school, and peer group problems. Other regressive symptoms, such as tantrums, oppositional behavior, fears of separation, and nightmares, are often initially associated with the enuresis as part of a reactive disorder. Previous struggles over toilet training are common although often they were less intense than the current struggle. The parents tend to overreact to the enuresis, responding with punishment or scoldings. As with children in the first group, a struggle for control may arise. Similar mechanisms help to perpetuate the symptom on an encapsulated basis, and at times oppositional or negativistic behavior or other regressive manifestations also continue. Constitutional factors may help to determine the reappearance of enuresis, and a family history is not infrequently obtained. Previous pressure from the parents is usually also an additional predisposing factor, however, as are socioeconomic factors in some cases. Some children in this group may be difficult to distinguish from those in the first group, except on the basis of the history.

The children in these first two groups constitute the majority of the cases of enuresis seen by the practicing physician. Lourie[277] has estimated that in 80% of all cases the symptom is a superficial one and often responds readily to a variety of treatment approaches. Spontaneous remissions sometimes occur. A few children who have not had any toilet training also have enuresis as a superficial symptom, and they respond readily to treatment.

Psychoneurotic Disorders. Enuretic boys in this group are usually passive, somewhat inhibited, and often overly dependent or with phobic trends. They are often distractible at school and sometimes have difficulties in achieving and showing clown behavior.[173] They may identify with a more dominant mother or be fearful of a critical or punitive father. The enuresis seems to be of a conversion nature, involving a relaxation of the external sphincter in relation to unconscious sexual conflicts, often expressed in terrifying nightmares during which loss of control occurs.[336]

Enuretic girls in this group seem to be more active, sometimes overly independent, and competitive toward boys, with a tendency toward more masculine identification in an attempt to handle sexual fears. The enuresis seems to have more of an unconsciously hostile component toward the mother or toward men who could injure the girls.[173]

In my experience, children in this group, much like children in the second group, often show the onset of enuresis in a reactive disorder in relation to a separation or some other traumatic experiences in the late preschool-age period. The parents are more disturbed, however, and the child seems to be unconsciously selected by the parents to work out their own problems and the child seems thus to be locked into the later development of a psychoneurotic disorder. A history of coercive toilet training is often present, and a constitutional component may also be involved (other children who have similar neurotic pictures do not have enuresis). A family history of enuresis is occasionally present. Since the enuresis is a part of the neurotic process, not a superficial, encapsulated symptom, it is usually much more difficult to treat.

Tension Discharge Disorders. This group, which was first described by Michaels,[310] contains many more boys than girls. Some of them show impulse-ridden personality disorders, as well as problems in control in a number of areas, from sphincter control to impulse control, and many become delinquent. They often have dysrhythmic EEGs although the dysrhythmias seem to be related more to immaturity in central nervous system development, possibly representing a biologic predisposition toward motor discharge of tensions, than to other causes. A history of homes broken by separation, desertion, divorce, or death and of frequent moves to different foster homes, with serious emotional deprivation, is often present in this group, with neglect of toilet training or relapses in the face of stress. Some children in this group who have personality disorders involving previously repressed neurotic conflicts engage in fire setting and have dreams of firemen or firehoses putting out fires. Some show the triad of enuresis, fire setting, and stealing. If the fathers of these children are present, they often are overly punitive toward the boys, and their mothers ordinarily show little warmth. Enuretic delinquents have been said to be more submissive, to be lacking in dominance and leadership, to have less interest in sex, and to have a larger number of siblings than nonenuretic delinquents.[408]

Other Disorders. This general category includes some very seriously disturbed children, including some who have psychotic disorders. Some children who develop psychoses in the preschool-age period may have had too little contact with reality to respond appropriately to toilet training, while others may show relapses. In any case, the enuresis is only one of a constellation of symptoms of seriously disturbed behavior. In some very disturbed (almost chaotic) families, neither parent may be able to give toilet training to their children because of a serious disruption in the parents' personality functioning and all the children in those families may never have achieved bladder control. The same may occur in families who live in severe poverty and who are preoccupied with financial and housing problems and other overwhelming stresses. A few disturbed children, in whom resentment underlies passive-aggressive behavior, demonstrate the conscious, volitional type of "revenge" enuresis referred to earlier.

Diagnosis. Diagnostic studies should ordinarily go no further than a urinalysis to rule out cystitis (which might produce urinary urgency) or at most an intravenous pyelogram if abnormalities are seriously suspected. The use of retrograde cystoscopy in children whose urine specimens are normal should be avoided, because the procedure can be seriously anxiety-provoking to early school-age children, who have fears of bodily mutilation, especially in regard to their genitals. If the procedure is carried out without general anesthesia in neurotic adolescents, the experience may be paradoxically pleasurable, particularly for girls who have hysterical trends and masochistic needs. As indicated earlier, even if urinary tract abnormalities are found, they are rarely related to the enuresis; most children who have even serious kidney or urinary tract abnormalities do not have enuresis.

Treatment. The treatment of enuresis should be suited to the child's personality and his family picture. The pediatrician or health associate can use several methods to treat children who have continuing enuresis in which a developmental lag in bladder control mechanisms (often compounded by a struggle for control) seems to be involved and children who have relapsing enuresis, that appears as part of a reactive disorder. These two groups of children usually have superficial symptoms, and they represent the vast majority of children who have enuresis. The child is usually disturbed by the enuresis, and he may be ready to give it up if he is helped to do so by someone outside his family. Giving the child gold stars to put on a chart or using some other kind of reward or positive reinforcement for dry nights is often effective. "Picking up" the child and taking him to the bathroom before 11:00 P.M. or so may help the child if he awakens fully and if the parents can handle him in a relaxed manner. Restricting large amounts of fluids after 7:00 P.M. or so may also help. (But the results of the restriction are usually intermittent or temporary, and the approach should not be continued if it is not effective quickly. The restriction may be frustrating to the child, and he may feel he is being punished.)

Other methods of therapy include drug therapy, conditioning, and bladder training. Anticholinergic drugs (e.g., atropine, which has been said to inhibit or relax the detrusor muscle of the bladder), sympathomimetic drugs, (e.g., benzedrine, which is believed to have an antidepressant or stimulant effect on the central nervous systems), and other drugs (e.g., placebos) have been used with some success. In recent years, imipramine hydrochloride (Tofranil) has been said to create an increased level of awareness of a full bladder in sleeping children. As indicated earlier[121] in controlled studies it has been reported to be highly effective. Other studies have not shown such beneficial results; bedwetting ceased only after a number of months in some children, and relapses were frequent.

(The serious adverse side-effects and toxicity of imipramine, especially in young children, were discussed elsewhere.)

Conditioning instruments (e.g., the Enurtone apparatus) involve the use of a moisture-sensitive device that is placed under the mattress. When the child begins to wet the bed, the urine causes a bell or buzzer to sound and the noise awakens the child. The approach has had its successes. Werry[448] has shown that the "bed buzzer" is more effective than brief counseling or no treatment, but even so, he has noted that relapses are common, and he thinks that other methods should be tried first. Some children and some parents resist this approach. And mechanical failures can occur. Behavior modification therapy has also been reported to be successful.[225]

For many years, psychologic approaches have been used to treat enuresis. Play therapy[214] has met with some success, and intensive psychotherapy[45] and analytic methods[397] have been used successfully to treat more severely disturbed children in the psychoneurotic and other groups. Residential treatment or other may be needed for children who have psychotic pictures or marked personality disorders.

Bladder training therapy[318] is based on the theory that many children with enuresis have small bladder capacities and immature coordinational capacities in the elements of micturition. The child is directed to drink large amounts of water and then to hold in the urine for long periods of time. He is given some sort of positive reinforcement for improvement. But the holding-in process is somewhat uncomfortable, and conflicts between parent and child may arise accordingly.

In general, the methods used to treat enuresis have reflected the physician's theoretical orientation. As Bakwin[21] has remarked, perhaps the most important ingredient in the treatment approach is the physician's degree of conviction that his method will work. The concern of some psychoanalysts that simple relief of the symptom of enuresis without dealing with the underlying conflicts would result in the substitution of another symptom has not been borne out by most studies. Such studies have usually been carried out on less disturbed children, in the first two groups, however; for obvious reasons basic conflicts must be dealt with in more severely disturbed children. Even in these children, who are treated by intensive psychotherapeutic methods, the use of positive reinforcement or other methods of symptom relief is sometimes necessary to stop the bedwetting.

Over the years, I developed great respect for methods of symptom relief in the treatment of enuresis and certain other problems that trouble children and parents. Of course, the treatment techniques should not be ones that are psychologically harmful to the children, and any other problems the child has should not be overlooked. The gain in confidence and self-respect that children who have overcome bedwetting feel can be of great help to their development.

In all treatment approaches, the most basic ingredient is a good doctor-parent-patient relationship. In the context of such a relationship, the physician should explain to the parents that the child cannot help the enuresis. They should be assured that the problem is not "their fault," that the bedwetting is a developmental problem to which some children are more susceptible than others, and that bedwetting can be aggravated by nervous or emotional tension. The parents should be encouraged in a noncritical way to give up pressuring or punishing the child and to follow the physician's recommendations, whatever they may be. The physician can lift the burden of guilt from the parents and the child and can thus bring them much relief. He can point out some of the child's strengths to the parents, and he can help build up the child's confidence. The physician who has a good relationship with the child can help the child deal with feelings of guilt, shame, or resentment and can help him work with the method to overcome the enuresis. I find it helpful to start with positive reinforcement, using the gold-star chart or some other method of reward for early school-age children. I reserve other methods for use later if necessary or for use with older children. In some instances, bladder control has been gained during the evaluation period, even before a prescription has been given.

Psychiatric consultation or referral to a mental health facility is ordinarily indicated for the three groups of more disturbed children who have enuresis (those with psychoneurotic disorders, those with personality disorders, and those who are very seriously disturbed or psychotic). Together children in those groups make up about 20% of the cases. For children who have early and milder psychoneurotic or personality disorders, especially those who have a history of relapse or regression, the physician may be able to help the enuresis with the supportive approach described. Attention should be paid to the disorder of which the enuresis is a part, however, and referral for psychotherapy may still be indicated. Anticipatory guidance and pediatric counseling in regard to toilet training can be effective in preventing some cases of enuresis, as may supportive intervention in dealing with a developing struggle for control that centers on toilet training. Anticipatory guidance and counseling may also help parents to understand and deal with the regressive type of enuresis that appears in young children in relation to the birth of a sibling, hospitalization, or other potentially stressful situations.

Encopresis. Like enuresis, encopresis (repeated, involuntary fecal soiling) may be (1) a normal pattern of fecal incontinence until the expected age of control through training, (2) a failure to achieve control, (3) a regressive component of a reactive disorder in late preschool-age children, (4) a developmental deviation in control mechanisms, (5) a conversion symp-

tom as part of a psychoneurotic disorder, or (6) one of a constellation of symptoms in a chronic personality disorder or psychosis.

In deciding when the incontinence of stool has persisted long enough to be considered encopresis, it is helpful to look at the sources of the normative data available. In the large-scale anterospective study that Roberts and Schoelkopf[361] carried out in conjunction with Spock and Aldrich, 88% of young children whose bowel training began toward the end of the second year achieved bowel control by about $2^1/_2$ years. All the children attained control by 3 years, the girls slightly sooner than the boys. The results of this study, which were reported in the early 1950s, contrast with the results of an examination of the records of the subjects in a longitudinal study carried out by Stuart and his colleagues. Examining the available data on this group of children, who were bowel trained in the early 1930s and whose bowel training began before the end of their first year, Prugh, with the help of Jackson, found that the majority had achieved bowel control by 18 months and that all of them had attained control before $2^1/_2$ years.[346] There were more instances of temporary breakdown in control in the group trained earlier than in the group trained more than 15 years later, for whom the later and more relaxed methods of bowel training were used, methods that were advocated especially by Spock. In the Minnesota study and in several other studies, boys resisted bowel training more often than girls did. In most studies, daytime control was usually achieved several months earlier than nighttime control.

The historical perspective offered by these two studies indicates that children can achieve bowel control earlier than expected by present methods although the hazards of breakdown and struggle for control between child and parent are greater. Brazelton found that in his practice, 75% of the children of upper-middle-class, well-educated parents were more than 2 years old when they achieved bowel control, while 12% were more than 3 years old.[63] It should be noted that the earlier investigations of Havighurst and Davis[204] showed significant differences in bowel training, as well as in other child-rearing practices, in families from different socioeconomic and cultural backgrounds. Those differences seem to be diminishing today.

In considering encopresis, the distinction Anthony[15] made between continuous encopresis and discontinuous (relapsing or regressive) encopresis is useful. (The distinction some make between encopresis that occurs without constipation and encopresis that occurs only with constipation does not seem realistic to me on either conceptual or clinical grounds). In most studies of encopresis, boys outnumber girls by at least 3 to 1.[30] Encopresis often occurs at night, but it may occur in the daytime. Although it is generally involuntary, an occasional volitional revenge type of encopresis may occur.

In the light of the foregoing, Prugh and others have come to feel that, as in enuresis, several factors determine when a clinical investigation of encopresis should be undertaken. Since with current methods of training, virtually 9 out of 10 children achieve bowel control by the age of 3 years, the physician is certainly justified in taking a relaxed view of soiling up to that age. He should further recognize that normal children vary in the age at which they attain bowel control, and that some normal children do not achieve full control until $3^1/_2$ to 4 years of age. If a child is still soiling regularly by 4 years of age, clinical intervention would seem justified, as it may be in the case of some 3 year olds, whose soiling seems to be clearly related to a struggle between the child and his parents. Again, some parents can accept such a relaxed approach comfortably, while others may become very concerned if the child has not achieved control by two years of age or even earlier. Encopresis is ordinarily more upsetting to parents in North American so-

ciety, which emphasizes cleanliness and freedom from body odors, than is enuresis although a few parents may not show even appropriate concern.

As in enuresis, the decision to investigate encopresis clinically will be influenced by the physician's relationship with the parents, his knowledge of the child's development and family relationships, the degree of the parents' concern, and other factors.

Fecal incontinence can of course result from neurologic conditions which interfere with bowel and sphincter innervation, usually in association with urinary incontinence. Examples of such conditions are cord tumors, spina bifida with meningomyelocele, and transverse myelitis. Children who show congenital aganglionic megacolon (Hirschsprung's disease), with absence of parasympathetic ganglion cells (usually in the rectum or rectosigmoid segment of the colon), show fecal retention but they may or may not have encopresis.[157]

The actual incidence of psychosocial encopresis is not known. It is far from rare in childhood, however, and it may persist into adolescence. In the practice of Woodmansey[459] in Great Britain, of 384 children who were seen for psychiatric problems, 60 were soiling when they were seen or had soiled at some time after the age of 4 years.

As in enuresis, different groups of children exhibit encopresis, a fact that has led to much confusion in the literature.

Developmental Failure to Establish Bowel Control Mechanisms. As Fleisher[157] points out, temperamental differences in infants include fussiness, which may be misinterpreted by anxious parents as difficulty with bowel movements. Bowel movements are often irregular in the first several months of life, and an apprehensive parent (usually the mother), fearing constipation may mistake the grunting and straining of the infant during a bowel movement as a sign of constipation. Laxatives, suppositories, and enemas are often used from the second or third month, particularly in "bowel-oriented" families, in which a history of constipation or diarrhea may reflect a combination of autonomic patterns of inheritance and a psychic inheritance regarding the importance of bowel regularity and stool consistency. In some cases, the infant may inhibit defecation because of pain from an anal fissure or from the passage of hard or inspissated feces. Or the infant may fear defecation because he once had an explosive diarrheal illness. In any case, a struggle for control between the child and his parent over defecation may have begun before toilet training was begun.

As Spock[402] pointed out, many parents in U.S. society fear having conflicts with their children about toileting, and these fears are often heightened in bowel-oriented families. Toilet training is often given in a coercive manner, as determined by Husckha's[219] criteria; that is, it is given early (before 6 months) and in a rigid manner, with the child being shamed and punished and kept on the toilet for long periods. The child often develops what Pinkerton[338] terms bowel negativism, expressed originally as a persistent refusal to defecate or sometimes as defiant soiling. Obviously there is some overlapping between excessive anxiety and compulsive rigidity in the parents. The mother is most often the involved and dominating parent and she shows little warmth for the child; the father is usually more distant, but occasionally he becomes the central figure.

In most cases, the bowel negativism becomes more intense during the second and third year of life, when the child's need to establish a sense of autonomy, involving the so-called normal negativism, reaches its peak. A few cases have their onset during this period, when fear or inhibition of defecation arises from the sources mentioned earlier, with predisposing parental attitudes or personality traits leading to continued withholding of stools. The toddler's normal and temporary anxiety about

"losing" the stool—a part of his body—down the toilet can be compounded by his negativistic refusal to "give up" the body part to the mother. As the struggle deepens, the child may fear that he will be flushed down the toilet in retaliation for his rebellious behavior, or he may come to fear that one or both parents will be flushed down the toilet as a result of the child's guilt about his angry feelings toward them.

If the stool withholding continues into the preschool-age period, the original voluntary act becomes involuntary, and most children develop increasing constipation. Efforts to avoid painful bowel movements may be added to the withholding, and inhibition of the defecation reflex occurs. Anal fissure, perianal dermatitis, or rectal prolapse may be complications, producing fear of defecation and intensifying the withholding and the constipation. Voluntary withholding thus gradually becomes automatic, or habitual retention may occur. The parents usually become more concerned as actual constipation occurs. The constipation is manifested by infrequent bowel movements, and abdominal distention. When the stools are passed they are often large and firm (some are even large enough to plug the toilet). The parents may become more frustrated, and they may try to remove a bolus of feces with their hands or in some other way. The anorectal manipulation may produce much anxiety, resentment, or guilt in the child.[31]

As constipation increases, soiling, originally an occasional voluntary act related to the bowel negativism, may begin to occur as a displacement phenomenon from an overdistended rectum that still has some capacity for reflex emptying. The soiling may show itself as continual staining of underwear or clothing or as the dropping of small pellets of feces at various times and places.

In the case of a $5^1/_2$-year-old boy with constipation and soiling, the pediatrician noted that the mother, who was using frequent enemas and other desperate measures, seemed afraid of the boy's bowel "clogging up." When asked about this fear, the mother told him she blamed herself for the death of a previous infant from intus-susception. The pediatrician was able to give her focussed reassurance and abso-lution, and the mother was able to stop her approach, with the prompt subsidence of the boy's soiling.

In cases in which the colon and rectum have become more inactive, soiling may represent the involuntary passage of rela-tively liquid material, around a large im-pacted mass of feces. The phenomenon is variously referred to as overflow diarrhea, pseudo-diarrhea, and paradoxical diar-rhea.[111]

As chronic and severe constipation de-velops and the resultant soiling gets out of the child's control, his tendency to with-hold his stools persists. Although such children are usually ashamed of their symptom by the time they reach school age and although they have developed a poor self-image because they have been pun-ished, shamed, or teased, their opposi-tional and negativistic behavior patterns often persist. Guilt over such patterns, which include the stool withholding, may lead some children unconsciously either to invite punishment or shaming or to test people by showing their worst side (a self-defeating maneuver[15]). Other children seem to become more compulsive, inhib-ited, or anxious. Such problems are more intense in the child who soils outside the home or at school. The problem is more encapsulated and "private" if the child soils only at home; the struggle for control re-mains localized, and the prognosis for re-sponse to treatment is better. When the problem becomes public, the dynamics are usually more complicated and obscure, and such cases are harder to treat, especially if the problem continues into adolescence (as it occasionally does).

Usually only one child in the family ex-hibits soiling associated with marked con-stipation. But parents in such bowel-ori-ented families, who have overly anxious and often compulsive tendencies, often have difficulties in toilet training their other children, and these children may show milder constipation, diarrhea, abdominal pain, vomiting, or other gastrointestinal symptoms.

In a few families, several children exhibit constipation associated with soiling, some of them giving up the symptom earlier than others. At times, virtually no toilet training has been given, because the parents have been preoccupied with the effects of pov-erty or other stresses. In a few families, marked overpermissiveness on the par-ents' part, including poor bowel training, is involved. In some families, toilet training has been markedly coercive for all of the children, and other aspects of childrearing have been punitive. In such cases, strug-gles for control between the parents and several children may have become so in-tense and so pervasive, with oppositional behavior in a number of cases, that the par-ents have more or less given up. They may resign themselves to soiling and other problems, feeling they cannot control their children. But they often defend their chil-dren if the school authorities or other peo-ple complain of the soiling or the behavior of the children.

Other factors are involved in soiling, par-ticularly the soiling of one child in a family. Besides the parents' personalities and at-titudes about bowel functioning, there may be factors related to the marital or family situations or to events that surrounded the child's birth and early infancy that led the parents to be more concerned about him than others. Such events may also have affected the toilet training or, even more important, the parent-child interaction. Studies done by Prugh,[346] Pinkerton,[338] and others support the conclusion that the per-sonality of the parent and the quality of the parent-child relationship are more impor-tant than the techniques of toilet training alone in the development of disorders of bowel functioning.

Children who have so-called *psychogenic megacolon*, the syndrome first described by Garrard and Richmond,[168] often show the overflow type of soiling. (I prefer the term psychophysiologic megacolon, for the reasons given earlier.) A systematic study by Pinkerton[338] has demonstrated family dynamics similar to those just described. Using a control group of children who had constipation without somatic causes and who responded to routine treatment measures without relapse, Pinkerton found that the parents of the children who had non-aganglionic megacolon showed excessively rigid and/or excessively anxious personalities, showed fears and prejudices related to constipation and frequent overvaluation of the child, and had engaged in coercive toilet training in a significantly higher proportion than had the parents of the children in the control group. He observed bowel negativism and other evidences of disturbed behavior in virtually all the children who had megacolon, but he found such evidence to be significantly present in only about 25% of the children who had constipation.

I studied a group of children who had severe *constipation* without soiling,[346] and I found somewhat similar personality pictures and parent-child interactions, with a high incidence of coercive toilet training although the families seemed generally less disturbed than the families of children who showed soiling with or without psychophysiologic megacolon. In my opinion, children who develop this type of megacolon have some type of autonomic predisposition since there are no developmental or familial features to distinguish them from children who have marked constipation and soiling.

Reactive Disorders. In contrast to continuous encopresis, certain children seem to attain bowel control by $2\frac{1}{2}$ to 3 years of age, but they return regressively to soiling at $3\frac{1}{2}$ to 4 years of age in the face of stressful events, such as illness and hospitalization, the birth of a sibling with whom

the mother becomes preoccupied, the serious illness of a parent, the accentuation of marital conflicts, and other events. In the histories of such children there is often some evidence of mildly coercive bowel training or a brief struggle for control between the child and his parents during this period, but these children do not usually belong to bowel-oriented families. If the parents become upset by the regressive soiling, however, and use punishment, shaming, or other coercive approaches, a significant struggle for control may arise, and the soiling may continue for months or years. The soiling may represent an attempt to resist growing up or regressive wishes to remain a "baby." Some children use their bowel functions to control the parent, insisting that the mother (occasionally the father) supervise toileting behavior while resisting their supervision.

Psychoneurotic Disorders. A smaller group of children who have encopresis have psychoneurotic disorders, often of the mixed type. They are usually inhibited, dependent, and rather compulsive in regard to all areas other than soiling. The mother tends to be the dominating person in the family and usually she has some compulsive tendencies; the father is often passive and retiring. Often the mother has been depressed during the pregnancy because of the loss of a parent or some other close person, a marital problem, or some other stressful event. In this context, the mother tends to make the infant the center of her life, showing strong interest in the infant's bowel functioning as the result of experiences in her own childhood.

Toilet training takes place in an atmosphere of domination and control, and it is often early and coercive. The dominance of the parents seems to inhibit the child's more than mildly negativistic feelings and passive resistance, and the mother's interest in the child's bowel movements often take on unconsciously seductive implications. Soiling usually has its onset regressively in the late preschool-age or early school-age period, often in relation to traumatic events and occasionally in relation to a physical illness, especially diarrhea. The soiling upsets the parents, who may try desperate measures to stop it. The symptom soon seems to have a conversion character, with the anal sphincter's failing to contain the stool in situations of conflict, usually ones involving unconscious hostility toward the parent. As in other conversion symptoms, the child is unaware of the soiling at the moment it occurs, and he usually shows little anxiety or concern. Soiling rarely occurs at school. The child who hides the stool at home, perhaps wrapped in underwear, is expressing hostility toward the parent. The stool is usually soft and formed, the rectum is empty, and there is no paradoxical diarrhea.

Very Seriously Disturbed Children. Another group who have encopresis are much more seriously disturbed. They may manifest deep personality disorders of the overly inhibited, overly dependent, compulsive, isolated, or mixed type, at times with serious defects in reality testing. Certain children in this group have been known to show revenge encopresis. In some cases, a deeply disturbed parent, most often the mother, may be involved in a symbiotic or other deeply interlocking interaction with the particular child. In several families I have known, the parent was so deeply involved in the interaction, with intense unconscious needs centered on "cleaning out" and caring for the child, that when the child responded to treatment by cessation of soiling and greater independence, the parent had a temporary psychotic decompensation. Some of these children have been frankly psychotic since infancy, failing to comprehend bowel training and control and showing continuous encopresis. Others have developed encopresis as one of a group of bizarre symptoms involved in a schizophreniform disorder that appeared in the school-age period. Withholding of the stool and paradoxical diarrhea may or may not be present. A few

may have psychotic parents who have not been able to offer the child toilet training. The parents of most of these children are seriously disturbed, and they may at times interfere with treatment because of their fears or suspicions.

Diagnosis. The diagnostic differentiation between congenital aganglionic megacolon (for which the pull-through operation was developed by Swenson) and megacolon of psychophysiologic nature is well discussed by Richmond, Eddy, and Garrard.[358] In the experience of Woodmansey[459] and Prugh, the clinical distinction is not always an easy one to make. Children who have aganglionic megacolon with a later onset of symptoms may have encountered negative parental attitudes, coercive toilet training, or other environmental experiences that led them to soil. If these conditions are not changed, the children may continue to soil after operation, even in the absence of neurologic complications. In cases in which there is doubt, the final diagnosis must rest on rectal biopsy and histologic evidence of aganglionosis.

Treatment. Davidson[112] feels that most children who have severe constipation or related problems should not be hospitalized initially and subjected to repeated sigmoidoscopy, x-rays, and other laboratory studies. He recommends a combined treatment and evaluation program, on an ambulatory basis if possible.

The treatment should take into account the type of soiling, the personalities of the child and his parents, and the family's patterns of interaction, as Fleisher[157] has advised in his helpful classification of the disorders of defecation. The prognosis is generally best for children who develop regressive soiling in the preschool-age or early school-age period.

For a number of children who have continuous soiling of the developmental failure type, supportive psychotherapy for the child and his parents undertaken by the pediatrician combined with special measures of management can be effective. The first step after the history taking and the physical examination is to help the parents understand the nature of the disorder and the treatment. It should be emphasized to them that the symptom is not the child's nor their fault; they can be told that the soiling is a developmental problem to which some children are more susceptible than others and that the problem can be aggravated by nervous or emotional tension. The physician should encourage the parents not to pressure or punish and to follow the regimen he proposes. The burden of guilt is thus lifted from the child and his parents, and the responsibility for the treatment is transferred to the physician. The physician should see both parents together initially, to be sure they both understand the problem and its treatment.

It is not easy for the physician to reassure parents who are especially anxious about bowel functioning that the soiling can be treated. Their concern about bowel regularity, which has been reinforced by advertisements for laxatives and perhaps by advice from other physicians, compounds their distaste for the soiling. If the child has a fecal impaction and paradoxical diarrhea, his parents should be told of the likelihood of overflow or leakage and of the measures to be taken initially.

Some parents are already aware of the child's withholding of stools and even of the struggle for control. If they are not aware, they can be told about the phenomenon and that it can become a habit that may be intensified by pressure or punishment. It is important not to criticize parents about their past behavior and not to point out too soon their role in the struggle. Initially the focus should be kept on the child's symptom. It is wiser to sympathize with the desperation that led them to try any means and to deal with any misconceptions. Later the parents may spontaneously come to see that their behavior played a part. If the child's abdomen is visibly distended, his parents can be told that, contrary to popular belief, no per-

manently harmful effects will come from constipation or "stretching" of the bowel. (I know of a child who had no bowel movements at all for 8 months and who had no adverse effects). If an anal fissure or some other complication is present, it should be explained to the parents as stemming from the withholding and constipation. Some very anxious parents may not be able to accept reassurance, and some, out of guilt, may resist the explanation. Psychiatric consultation may be helpful in some cases at this point, but with some resistant parents, it is better to try the supportive approach first. If a referral is necessary, it may be more effective to suggest one later, when the parents have developed a more trusting relationship with the pediatrician.

It is important for the pediatrician to see the child separately at some point during the evaluation, in order to begin a supportive relationship. The child is usually embarrassed or ashamed and guilty about his soiling. If asked what the trouble is, many children will deny the symptom, even if they are asked directly about soiling. It is wise, however, to let the child know at this point that the physician is aware of his symptom; otherwise the child may fear he will be disliked when the symptom becomes known. If the child initially denies having any problems, the physician can say later, in a matter of fact way, that the parents told him about the child's trouble with his bowels or his "trouble going to the toilet." He should add that other children have the same problem, that it is nobody's fault, and that there are ways of helping him to get over the problem. In a case seen recently, an 8-year-old boy stopped soiling within several days after I reassured him that he was not "bad" and could be helped. Some opposition and mildly aggressive behavior appeared that required several months to work out.

If the child has a fecal impaction, hypertonic phosphate or oil retention enemas can be used after they have been explained to the child and his parents. The enemas can be given on an ambulatory basis, as Davidson[112] has recommended. If the parents are very worried or upset, it may be necessary to admit the child to a pediatric hospital unit in order to start the treatment program in a more neutral environment. Later, mineral oil can be prescribed; some children and parents are upset by the "leaking" mineral oil causes, and a mild laxative may be tried. The further use of enemas or strong purgatives is contraindicated. In the context of an ongoing individual relationship, the child can be helped to participate in the reestablishment of bowel routines and control. He can be encouraged, in an unpressured way, to try to have an evacuation each day; drawing on the action of the gastrocolic reflex after breakfast or a particular meal may help to reestablish bowel habits. (The doses of mineral oil used by Davidson[112] should result in several bowel movements a day.) The soiling needs to be discussed very little in this approach. Positive reinforcement (praise) for an evacuation or for diminished soiling is important. Asking the child how he has felt about past enemas, laxatives, and other treatment approaches may be helpful although probing for deep feelings about his parents is unwise. The child may be asked to draw a picture of how he felt, or other supportive techniques may be used. Sometimes much resentment and other negative feelings may be brought out, resulting in lessened tendencies toward stool withholding.

In this approach, the parents must be seen regularly, in order to help them avoid pressure, too much "checking up," or punitive measures. They should be encouraged to pay as little attention as possible to any soiling, and to praise the child when he reports an evacuation. Rewards for continued evacuations and diminished soiling can be helpful.[169] The parents should be encouraged to talk with the pediatrician and not the child about how they feel about the soiling, their past disagreements over its handling, and their misconceptions

about constipation. Such an approach can help them view and handle the child more objectively and work together more effectively.

The approach just described can be surprisingly effective in dealing with early school-age children in the developmental failure group (such as those with psychophysiologic megacolon). Levine and Bakow[259] have reported success with most of the children in their series, as have Richmond and his colleagues.[358] In regard to encopresis (and enuresis), I have come to have great respect for symptom relief. Children who overcome soiling feel more confident, have a better self-image, and sometimes perform better in school. But the child may have other problems besides the encopresis (e.g., negativistic behavior in other areas, or serious difficulties in peer relationships), and those problems should not be overlooked. Psychiatric consultation and even referral for more intensive psychotherapy may be indicated even though the soiling has ceased.

For some children who have developmental failure of control, particularly older school-age children who may have developed personality disorders, the supportive approach described will not be effective. However, in my opinion a trial of supportive psychotherapy is often warranted, with psychiatric consultation and referral later if necessary.[349] Davidson[112] recommends hospitalization for further studies to rule out neurogenic or anatomic obstruction if regular bowel movements are not achieved in 2 or 3 weeks. In my experience, a positive response without some recurrent constipation or occasional soiling often takes somewhat longer to occur.

Pediatric counseling can help parents understand the appearance of regressive soiling as part of a reactive disorder in a 4-year-old following the birth of a sibling, the illness of the mother, or other potentially stressful events. Encouragement of the parents to permit regressive behavior within limits and to offer emotional support to the child can usually help to avoid a struggle for control and can enable the parents to wean the child to his previous level of adjustment, usually with prompt cessation of soiling. If the reactive disorder has become chronic, supportive psychotherapy by the pediatrician or referral for more intensive therapy may be necessary. Anticipatory guidance regarding the probability that regressive behavior will occur during or after hospitalization can help parents understand and deal with soiling or other regressive manifestations as they occur.

A supportive approach to management can be effective in achieving control of soiling in late preschool-age or early school-age children who have beginning or mild psychoneurotic disorders that involve generally regressive soiling with conversion mechanisms or in early school-age children who have early or mild oppositional or other personality disorders. My feeling is that if the pediatrician is interested in undertaking it, a trial of supportive psychotherapy combined with medical management should be made when there is a history of a regressive onset of soiling. The child can be referred for intensive psychotherapy later if the soiling continues or other problems indicate the need for it. Children who have severe psychoneurotic disorders should have a psychiatric consultation as a part of the diagnostic workup if possible. In most cases, long-term intensive psychotherapy is needed for the child and his parents.

For children who have severe personality disorders or near-psychotic or psychotic pictures, the prognosis in regard to the soiling depends on the prognosis for the underlying disorders. The child or his parents may resist "cleaning out" procedures and the establishment (or reestablishment) of bowel routines because they fear harm or because they have other serious misperceptions. Intensive psychotherapy and, sometimes, placement of the child, resi-

dential treatment, or other measures are indicated.

Various kinds of psychotherapeutic approaches have been tried with more seriously disturbed children (often the reports do not specify the type of disorder). Using individual psychotherapy with children and group therapy for their parents, Pinkerton[338] was able to obtain remissions in 21 out of 30 cases, and most of the remissions were lasting ones. Others[77,254,346] have reported success with different types of individual psychotherapy, as well as with therapy for the parents. Psychotherapeutic sessions between parent and child have been combined with behavioral reward systems,[12] and combinations of individual psychotherapy, behavior modification, and family therapy have been used in situations involving deeply interlocking relationships.[238]

In a few cases, the parents of seriously disturbed children, because of their marked rigidity, disorganization, strong need to deny their involvement, feelings of hopelessness, or other reasons, cannot accept referral of the child for intensive psychotherapy. The positive use of pediatric hospitalization can be attempted; if the child has been excluded from school because of soiling, the parents occasionally accept psychiatric hospitalization of the child or residential treatment. If all other measures fail, the pediatrician can sometimes enter into a supportive relationship with an older school-age child or adolescent without working with the parents if the parents will permit him to do so. Discussion of such an approach with a child psychiatrist or some other type of mental health professional can be most helpful. In such cases, the pediatrician needs great patience and must avoid responding negatively to any "testing-out" behavior the child may show. Sometimes the pediatrician can help the older child or adolescent enter into a nonjudgmental relationship with him that can help the child develop a better self-image and greater motivation to overcome the problem of soiling.

Close collaboration between the pediatrician and child psychiatrist may be needed to coordinate the medical management with the psychotherapeutic approach, as well as to avoid misunderstandings that might lead overanxious or rigid parents to take the child out of therapy before he has responded to it. In psychotherapy, the symptom of soiling in seriously disturbed children must be tolerated for a longer period of time until the underlying conflicts in child and parents have been worked out. The pediatrician may be tempted to continue standard treatment measures, as Pinkerton has pointed out. If he yields to the temptation, the parents may misinterpret his behavior as showing a lack of confidence in the psychotherapeutic approach, and the child may be affected also.

Special Problems in the Adolescent Period

The developmental problems of adolescence, including those related to prepuberty and puberty, the achievement of identity, performance in school, and others, are well discussed in other books and in articles. The psychophysiologic disorders that may appear in adolescence (e.g., anorexia nervosa) are discussed elsewhere in this book, as are other psychopathologic disorders characteristic of adolescence (e.g., the acute confusional state and schizophrenia). The special problems of adolescence that are discussed in the following paragraphs are: suicide attempts, drug abuse, smoking, automobile accidents, dropping out of school, unwed motherhood, abortion, fire setting, running away from home, delinquency, and homicide.

Suicide Attempts. Threats of suicide are common in school-age children; they often occur as attempts to punish the parents ("You'll be sorry if I die"). These threats are in keeping with the inability to comprehend the reality of death until the age of 9 or 10 years. Actual suicide attempts are rare among school-age children. Those that do occur usually stem not from a serious wish on the part of the child to die, but rather from the child's need to punish himself or his parents. However, such attempts can be serious ones, and they may even accidentally be successful. Suicide attempts among children under 12 years of age seem to be increasing. Suicide attempts among children older than 14 years of age rise rapidly although the majority of such attempts are not successful.[404] Although suicide attempts among children are not reported accurately (physicians and parents often cover them up), suicide seems to be the third most frequent cause of death in older adolescents (ages 15 to 24) and the second most frequent cause of death in upper-middle-class college students.[215] In the past 20 years, suicide has more than doubled among people who are 15 to 19 years old and 20 to 24 years old. The increased incidence probably cannot be explained simply by the fact that suicide is diagnosed and reported more accurately.

Suicide rates among adolescents vary from country to country (Japan, Hungary, Czechoslovakia, and Finland have the highest suicide rates) and from region to region (the Rocky Mountain and the Pacific coast states have the highest suicide rates in the United States). Suicide seems to be more common in middle-class and urban areas. Suicide rates show some seasonal variations in temperate countries (they are highest in the spring) and some variations in relation to historical epochs and social crises. Suicide rates have increased most rapidly among young American Indians, many of whom feel hopeless and trapped.[123] Adolescent boys most commonly commit suicide by shooting, hanging, or poisoning themselves. Adolescent girls most commonly commit suicide by taking poison or an overdose of drugs (although recently it has become more common that they shoot themselves or destroy themselves with explosives). The suicide rate among boys particularly may even be higher if automobile accidents are considered, in some of which self-destructive or suicidal motives may be involved.

In the United States, the suicide rate formerly was highest among adolescent females. More recently, the rate of successful suicide among adolescent males is at least double that among adolescent females, although adolescent females make more suicide attempts. Among adolescents in general, the ratio of attempted suicide to "successful" suicide is about 120 : 1 (as opposed to 8 : 1 among adults). (The highest rate of successful suicides occurs in middle-aged melancholic men who are caught in a developmental crisis of middle life.) Occasionally a parent murders his children and then commits suicide. Double suicides and even epidemics of suicide among adolescents are also known to occur.

In addition to (1) the social, economic, or historical factors within the community or nation, (2) the popular attitude toward suicide, and (possibly) (3) childrearing approaches that stress shame, guilt, or achievement, in most specific suicide attempts individual, family, or situational factors are involved.[175,417,423] Those factors are significantly different in adolescents than they are in adults. A small proportion of adolescents who attempt suicide are psychotic, and these attempts may be bizarre attempts at self-mutilation rather than actual suicide attempts. Some adolescents who attempt suicide have chronic hysterical or other types of personality disorders, and their suicide attempts may clearly be attempts to manipulate their parents or peers. About 50% of adolescents who commit suicide come from broken homes and from families who have much psychopathology.[221,296]

A number of adolescents who commit suicide are somewhat immature, oversensitive, shy, anxious, and emotionally labile people who have low self-esteem; they are frequently in the midst of a serious identity crisis, and they are vulnerable to external events that are stressful for them. They may come from disorganized or disturbed families, but they themselves are not necessarily seriously disturbed. In the suicide attempts of these adolescents and those of reasonably healthy adolescents, situational factors are prominent. A sudden or a threatened loss of a key relationship or of self-esteem (e.g., in a broken love affair, a bitter fight with a parent, or school failure), an unwanted pregnancy, depression about chronic illness, hopelessness about poverty, dejection or guilt about a parent's illness, attempts to gain affection and esteem or to punish a parent or close friend of either sex, marked depression, feelings of unworthiness, or internalized anger at another (with guilt and depression), or even the acting out of an unconscious wish of a parent, of an identification with a parent who has committed suicide, or of a desire to join a dead relative may be involved in the suicide attempt (and usually more than one factor is involved). In a controlled study by Stanley and Barten,[404] loss of a parent by a child younger than 12 years old, and (more often) threats of loss implied in parents' talk of separation or divorce were the two major distinguishing features.

In adolescent suicide attempts, the adolescent's wish to die may be real, but it usually contains an element of a cry for help, indicating that the adolescent is hurting badly. Most adolescents who attempt suicide have shown open sadness,[340] withdrawal, decreased school performance, and "masked depression"[176] with loss of self-esteem, decreased activity, and sleep disturbances for at least one month before the attempt, while a number have shown disturbed behavior or neurotic depression[286] for nearly a year. The adolescent often tells the parent about his suicide attempt, and he may change his mind in the middle of the attempt (sometimes too late). If his bluff is called, he may feel backed into a corner by his suicide threat, and he may think that he has to carry out his threat in order to be true to himself. The available studies suggest that the adolescent who is alienated from his family, who does not live at home, and who has poor peer relationships and an unsatisfying social life is at high risk for suicide even after he has been hospitalized.

Many parents of adolescents who attempt to commit suicide feel ashamed and guilty, and their physician may unconsciously be led to conspire with the parents to forget the incident or to sweep it under the rug. Any suicide attempt—and even a suicide threat—should be taken seriously, no matter how superficial or manipulative it appears. If a suicide attempt produces no response from his parents or other adults, the adolescent may well try again, with tragic results. Even if a suicide attempt is not made, a suicide threat indicates that the adolescent is hurting, and a response should be made to his veiled cry for help.

One study has indicated that approximately 50% of adolescents who attempt suicide have consulted a physician about physical or emotional problems shortly before the suicide attempt.[441] The problems may contribute to the suicide attempt, but they also may be cries for help. For that reason, an adolescent who asks to talk with a physician, a teacher, or another adult should be given the chance to do so promptly, even if for only a few minutes (follow-up care can be planned). The chance to talk right away is more important than the amount of time spent talking. Even a brief talk may help prevent a suicide attempt or other kinds of impulsive behavior. The physician might tell the adolescent who seems seriously depressed that many people who feel low have thoughts of harming themselves. If the teenager does not respond spontaneously to this remark, the physician might ask if he also has had such thoughts. A number of adolescents will be relieved to be able to talk about their thoughts of suicide, to be able to discuss the problem, and to know that help is available. (Hollow reassurances or "pats on the back" from the physician or others are not helpful.)

Some communities have opened suicide prevention centers,[230] where telephone therapists are on duty around the clock. Such therapists are often able to help those who have threatened suicide but have not determined to die. Some people who call these therapists have made previous suicide attempts or have seen a psychiatrist; many others are acutely depressed and wish to talk to someone who cares whether they live or die.

If the adolescent has made a suicide attempt, the physician should ordinarily see the adolescent first (with his parents' permission) in order to attempt to build a trusting relationship with him. However, the adolescent may prefer to see the physician together with his parents. If the adolescent is obviously psychotic or seriously disturbed, he should be admitted to an adolescent psychiatric ward. In many cases, however, admission of the adolescent to the adolescent section of a pediatric ward can buy time during which the parents can be helped to communicate with the adolescent. The parents can usually be helped both to recognize the seriousness of their child's plea for help (however unrealistic the plea may seem to them) and to overcome the temptation to sweep the conflict under the rug. Kempe and Prugh have used such a technique, as have Lewis and Solnit.[265] Supportive counseling or environmental rearrangement may suffice, or more intensive psychotherapy can be begun at once if it is indicated. The management, with psychiatric consultation, of an adolescent boy who had made a suicidal attempt, and of his parents, by a pediatric resident is described earlier. Follow-up care should be planned carefully and in collaboration with community agencies when it is appropriate to do so.

Often an adolescent who has made a suicide attempt—especially an adolescent who has made a patently superficial and manipulative suicide attempt, such as by slashing his wrist superficially or by taking a small amount of a drug known to the public to be innocuous or a dose of barbiturates which can easily be dealt with by gastric lavage—is sent home from the emergency room. Such a practice is unwise. The adolescent's family often will not return for follow-up care, and the adolescent may make another, more serious, suicide attempt. If the adolescent seems seriously disturbed, emergency psychiatric hospitalization may be needed, and individual, tandem, or family therapy may be employed.[316] Survivors of adolescents who commit suicide need much help in dealing with their guilt, anger, and mourning.[71]

Drug Abuse. The use of drugs by adolescents is a controversial topic, as is drug addiction, or, more appropriately, drug dependence. Psychic dependence may be developed on any substance. Physical dependence occurs more strongly with certain drugs, and withdrawal symptoms are a factor. Drug tolerance (a diminished response to the same quantity of drug) is a frequent response to the continued use of many drugs. Drugs used include heroin, marijuana, the amphetamines (including methedrine, or speed), the barbiturates, the hydrocarbons (including glue, plastic cement, cigarette lighter fluid, and gasoline fumes), the hallucinogens or psychedelics (e.g., LSD, DMT, DET, STP, mescaline, peyote, and psilocybin), alcohol, and tobacco in various forms, and more recently angel dust (phencyclidine), about which little is known.

The biologic effects of LSD and related hallucinogens[105] resemble those of sympathomimetic drugs; the psychologic effects may last from several hours to more than a day. The physiologic effects usually last 4 to 8 hours. The effects are highly varied, and depend on the person taking the drug, his expectation of what will happen, his previous experience, the social setting, and other factors. Changes in perception (especially visual perception), synesthesias, changes in mood (including depression, euphoria, lability of mood), anxiety, sometimes amounting to panic, feelings of depersonalization, and changes in thinking (including flight of ideas, a feeling of having insight into universal and transcendental phenomena— the "psychedelic experience"), changes in time sense, and difficulty in logical thinking and concentration are among the reported effects.

Untoward psychologic effects involve "bad trips." These include the precipitation of psychotic episodes, usually in previously near-psychotic people,[155] prolonged depressive reactions, occasionally leading to suicide, intermittent return ("flashbacks") of hallucinatory experiences, and serious injury or death in an occasional person who feels he can perform such feats as controlling traffic or flying. Preliminary reports suggested that an increase of "breaks" in chromosomes, lasting at least 6 months, occurs in LSD users, and that children of mothers who have taken LSD early in pregnancy also exhibit such chromosomal breaks. The validity of these findings in vivo has recently been challenged, but many young people have taken them seriously. Caution in the use of LSD during pregnancy seems warranted.

The incidence of LSD use is difficult to determine since the drug is relatively easy to manufacture and readily available from illegal sources. The limited and possibly inaccurate studies that have been done indicate that 1 to 15% of college students tried the drug in the late 1960s. Many of these tried it only once—"for kicks." Some anxious and conflicted persons continued to use it, as did others who felt empty, alienated, or were "looking for answers." Although feelings of universal insight occur in some people who take LSD, these insights can rarely be described clearly to others. There is no evidence that LSD changes one's personality for the better or that users turn their insights to any personal or societal benefit. The use of LSD as an adjunct to psychotherapy for chronic alcoholism must be evaluated. The experimental use of LSD with autistic children was discussed in Chapter 13.

Marijuana (cannabis, hashish, pot) is more widely used than the psychedelic drugs. It is estimated that 20% of college students (perhaps many more) use marijuana. A national commission recently estimated that 26,000,000 adults and youths in the United States used marijuana. Marijuana seems to make the user more relaxed and to promote in him an introspective attitude, an elevation of mood and a lessening of inhibitions, particularly if he takes marijuana in a pleasant social setting.[55] The drug does not seem to be significantly involved in episodes of antisocial, destructive, or criminal behavior. It is not physically addictive, and, contrary to many fears, it does not seem to predispose the user to other types of drug dependence. Many young people give it up eventually although some adults continue its use. A recent study by the National Institute of Mental Health indicates that the effects of marijuana are no more harmful than those of alcohol although contaminants in poor-quality preparations may help to produce occasional psychotic episodes[416] or may evoke other deleterious responses.

Heroin seems to have addictive qualities.[470] Physical dependence on heroin or other addictive drugs, which is characterized by a great desire for the drug and an increasing tolerance of it, seems to be associated with certain psychologic needs for escape from reality, fear of withdrawal symptoms, or a conditioning process.[454] People who have addictive personalities of the dependent or other types often shift back and forth from alcohol to hard drugs. Antisocial acts (e.g., stealing) are often committed in order to pay for the drug. Death has occurred from overdosing and various infections, such as hepatitis, tetanus, malaria, and syphilis, have resulted from the use of unsterile needles. The use of heroin has long been fairly widespread among frustrated and alienated residents

of ghetto neighborhoods although exact figures are unavailable. Infants born to women addicted to heroin during pregnancy have been reported to have a high incidence of intrauterine growth retardation and neonatal abstinence syndrome.[96,469] The latter is characterized by signs of central and autonomic nervous system dysfunction, and the infants in question may be considered at risk for neurodevelopmental dysfunction. Wilson and his colleagues[458] followed a group of heroin-exposed children for 3 to 6 years and found that the infants weighed less, were shorter, made poorer adjustments, and had more perceptual-motor problems than did infants in control groups matched for age, race, sex, birth weight, and socioeconomic status. Thus heroin-exposed infants seemed to be vulnerable to growth, behavior, and learning problems. They are also often abandoned or placed outside the home during infancy because of the mother's addiction or may be placed later if the family unit breaks up.

The use of *the hydrocarbons* (glue, gasoline fumes, or cigarette lighter fluid) by children and adolescents seems to produce a state that resembles alcoholic intoxication. When they are inhaled, the hydrocarbons initially produce a "jag" characterized by exhilaration, euphoria, and excitement. Ataxia, slurred speech, diplopia, drowsiness, and stupor gradually appear later. Increasing tolerance may occur easily. Nausea, anorexia, weight loss, irritability, and somnolence, along with increased tolerance, may result from glue sniffing, but lasting serious physiologic effects on the brain[124] and other organs do not seem to occur. Gasoline sniffing, which has been reported in children as young as 18 months old, has occasionally caused accidental deaths. Although not physically addictive, the hydrocarbons offer easy habituation (psychic dependence). The hydrocarbons, particularly glue, are used principally by boys who have significant psychosocial problems that have led them to the habituation.[293] The same may be said of the young users of amphetamines, barbiturates, or alcohol. If amphetamines are taken intravenously, they may cause psychotic reactions or hepatitis.

Arrests of narcotic violators have increased severalfold in recent years although accurate statistics on so-called addiction in adolescents are difficult to obtain. Hard drugs have been used for years in ghetto neighborhoods. More recently, drug use has increased in young people from middle- and upper-income families, and parents and and other laymen who were once unconcerned about the problem are now creating a furor. Recent trends indicate that among high school and college youths the use of heroin, LSD, amphetamines, and hydrocarbons is decreasing, the use of barbiturates is increasing, and the abuse of alcohol is a serious problem.

Approaches to combatting the use of drugs by adolescents have generally been made in a frightened or frantic manner. Narcotics should of course not be available to teenagers, and peddling or pushing narcotics should be treated as a serious offense. LSD is relatively easy to manufacture, and marijuana is universally available, as are various hydrocarbons. Thus, in spite of realistic concerns about the use of the psychedelic drugs in particular, there is no simple and easy way to control these drugs legally or to detect them in the body.

The management of drug abuse should be medical, psychologic and social, rather than restrictive or punitive. Often multiple treatment modalities are necessary.[119,162,162a,171,446] Even alcoholism has been recognized recently by the courts as an illness that requires treatment, not primarily as an offense. Methadone programs for addiction in adolescents have had their problems, but they can be effective.[87] An understanding approach by the parents to general guidance and discipline, with some limits but with some flexibility, will prevent many from habitual use of drugs of any kind, or at least from more than an

experiment "for kicks." For those who have had "bad trips" or other untoward effects of drug use, or those in higher income families who use drugs chronically because of emotional disturbance or rebellion, psychiatric treatment is usually indicated, and individual and often family therapy and occasional hospitalization is often helpful. One study has developed the categories of (1) experimental drug users, who may be in a developmental crisis but do not continue more than social usage of alcohol or marijuana; (2) depressive drug users who feel isolated from family or society; (3) characterologic drug users, a small group, who are deeply disturbed.[342a]

The largest group of users among middle-class youth are those who are also rebelling against the established order, and many are unwilling to come to hospitals or clinics unless they are seriously ill. Therapeutic communities or programs in the community have offered help to those who are well motivated to stop taking drugs although many have relapsed. Some of the most successful results have been obtained in neighborhood clubs, where teenagers using drugs can come on their own for help in group discussions with sympathetic adults. Mixed group discussions with teenagers, and sometimes parents also, have been more effective in drug education than lectures by police or school principals. A recent study shows that drug education programs in junior high schools and senior high schools are not effective. For those who have had bad trips or other untoward effects of drug use, pediatric hospitalization with psychiatric consultation may be indicated on an inpatient or outpatient basis. Younger adolescents who have indulged in glue sniffing or in the abuse of other substances because of milder psychologic problems or sometimes because of conflicts about physical problems may often be successfully treated by the pediatrician, with the help of psychiatric consultation and therapy for the parents by a social worker or some other type of mental health professional. Other social and economic measures are needed to deal with the fundamental problems of poverty and discrimination which foster the use of drugs by adolescents in disadvantaged neighborhoods.

Quite recently, some legislators in Colorado have pointed out the harm to young people of the present legal and punitive approach to the use of marijuana. They have joined an increasingly large segment of the public who recognize that the effect of marijuana is like that of alcohol and that marijuana is widely used by adults as well as by youths, and they have proposed that marijuana be legalized, that it be standardized in regard to grade, and that it be sold in licensed liquor stores under the legal statutes pertaining to alcohol. It will be some time before the general public accepts these ideas, but their ultimate acceptance seems likely. Several states have already decriminalized the possession of small amounts of marijuana, and similar proposals have been made at the national level.

Alcohol Abuse. Analyses of surveys of the drinking practices of high-school students conducted between 1941 and 1975 (e.g., the analysis of Blane and Hewitt[52]) indicate that the prevalence of drinking rose steadily from World War II until the mid-sixties and thereafter remained fairly stable. Boys drank more often than girls, and the average age at first drink still remains relatively constant (about 13 years of age). A number of variables seem to influence adolescent drinking behavior, ranging from the drinking attitudes of peers, the parents' attitudes and behavior, environmental and social factors, and the adolescent's own personality with much interlocking among such variables. Alcoholism is a term which has been used loosely in various studies of adolescents.[85] Alcohol use seems to be higher in children of alcoholic parents,[85] in delinquent adolescents,[50] and perhaps in other subgroups. Ethnic factors also are involved, however, and several studies have shown that black students and students in certain other ethnic groups at all economic levels drink less alcohol than do white students,[85] although some students from poor families in some ethnic groups may use drugs more frequently.

In the early 1970s the minimum drinking age was lowered in a number of states,[304] and the data are conflicting as to how the change may have affected the recent drinking practices of adolescents. Thus the public belief that adolescents are using more alcohol today may not be correct. Much has been learned recently about the "fetal alcohol syndrome"[226] as a major cause of congenital cerebral and physical defects of infants born to alcoholic mothers, and teenagers are known to have more complications of pregnancy than have older women. Sander[373] has recently suggested that drinking during pregnancy may have significant adverse effects on newborn "state" regulation.

Many teenagers who have a drinking problem will respond to a supportive psychotherapeutic approach by the pediatrician although some with true alcoholism may need to be referred to mental health specialists. Alcoholism in adults can be treated more effectively today than it could formerly (although Alcoholics Anonymous still has a better success record than do most psychiatrists). But knowledge about preventing alcoholism, like that in accidents, smoking, and other self-destructive behaviors, is still limited.

Smoking. Smoking in adolescence represents a complex set of issues. Although teenagers and college students have repudiated many of the values of their parents' generation, they have accepted the cigarette-smoking habit. The hazards of smoking are now well known, and smoking seems to be a causative factor in carcinoma of the lung and cardiovascular disease, with emphysema and other pulmonary conditions at least more common in smokers.[51] Despite the ban on cigarette commercials on television, the great numbers of physicians (especially surgeons) who have stopped smoking, and the various antismoking campaigns, about 42% of the adult population still smoke, and children are more likely to smoke if their parents or older siblings smoke.

Most youngsters have their first experience with smoking between 11 and 14 years of age; the median age is about 12. (The youngest habitual smoker I have known was a 7-year-old boy, who started to inhale at $3^1/_2$ years of age, when his parents reinforced his "cute" behavior—smoking—by showing amusement at it.) By the time they enter their teens, about 14% of children are smokers; by the time they leave their teens, about 75% of adolescents have tried cigarettes, and the percentage of young smokers equals the percentage of adult smokers. Teenage smokers smoke fewer cigarettes than do adults; more boys smoke than do girls, and boys smoke more cigarettes than do girls. Teenage smoking varies little with social class; those who start early seem to be more tense and less well adjusted within the family and in relation to adult authority than do nonsmokers. Smoking is more common among students who have lower academic achievement although smoking is probably the result of the lower achievement, not its cause. Teenagers who smoke are more likely to associate with a peer group in which smoking is the norm and to have parents who smoke, unlike nonsmoking adolescents in the same schools.[20] Recently a relationship between heavy smoking in the pregnant mother and the health of the fetus has been pointed out.[11]

Many antismoking campaigns have not succeeded. Warnings of danger of death from serious disease has been met with denial in both adults and teenagers in most health education programs. In fact many teenagers take such warnings as dares. The example of adults who give up smoking and the promotion of the rights of the nonsmoker in public places should gradually have a positive effect. The Committee on Environmental Hazards of the American Academy of Pediatrics[11] has suggested playing up the antiestablishment feelings many young people have by pointing out the ridiculousness of most cigarette advertisements, which imply that smoking brings cars, wealth, and sexual attractiveness. A few peer leadership programs in schools have begun to show some effect.[297] The problem needs much more study, however.

Automobile Accidents. Automobile accidents are a growing problem among young people. Attempts to raise the age for getting a driver's license are of little help since the highest incidence of serious accidents is in males 19 to 25 years of age, in many of whom independence promotes recklessness. The influence of cultural values which stress speed as well as aggressive competition and risk taking may be compounded by the use of alcohol and drugs, and by unconscious self-destructive trends. Driver education has been shown to be effective in reducing accidents. Academic performance, particularly in high school boys, has been shown to be adversely affected by the possession of a car, and for that and other reasons parents would be wise not to offer this indulgence to their children, which is in line with the tendency of some adults to shower their children with material possessions. Possessions are not substitutes for love or for setting limits on behavior.

Dropping Out of School. The greatest problem in school adjustment during adolescence is dropping out of school. In 1962, about 36% of students in the United States did not finish high school; the percentage is higher today. Most of these students were from families in the lower socioeconomic group, many of whom all but officially dropped out before the legal age (in most states) of 16. In some ghetto neighborhoods the dropout rate has been as high as 80%, and the rate is nearly as high in some barrios. These students have usually not done well academically for years; they often have had moderate-to-severe reading problems, have not participated in extracurricular activities because of their alienation, and are not popular. Thus even though they know they are jeopardizing their economic future, many drop out because they cannot meet the demands of the student role. Boys are especially vulnerable to pressures to drop out since the student role is more central to their present and future self-image and since they are more autonomous than girls. To continue to be students when they are failing is to identify themselves as failures.

Although most high-school dropouts come from seriously impoverished families who have inadequate educational opportunities (often the result of racism), some come from working-class, often rural, families in which the parents do not value education strongly and are satisfied to have their children drop out of school and work to help support the family. Others come from middle-class families; they have not been successful in school and they strongly dislike it. Some have fought a continuing battle with their parents, who have overly high aspirations for their children; others have identity problems; often they develop a negative identity, one that opposes their parents' wishes. Some of these identity problems may be worked out later. Many adolescents who drop out, especially those who drop out for psychologic reasons, are not completely happy with the step. They may hang around the school, "dropping in" at times at a school club. Many of those who drop out for economic reasons and who apply for Job Corps status suffer from eye defects, subtle auditory impairments, dental neglect, poor oral hygiene, physical or mild neurologic problems, marked reading problems, and gross psychologic difficulties.

Various measures can help prevent dropping out. Some of these measures have been discussed earlier in relation to school problems. Work-study programs for adolescents beginning at age 15 can help motivate those from underprivileged backgrounds to complete high school. The emphasis on academic subjects, particularly science, in high school today has tended to make the large group of young people, who have not had adequate preparation at home and in the early school years, feel like second-class citizens. More status should be conferred on vocational schools, and more blue-collar jobs should be available for young people.

For those largely middle-class teenagers whose performance in high school drops off and who may become dropouts, counseling and support may be effective, or more formal psychotherapy may be necessary. Parents can be helped to ease the pressure on a possible late bloomer or an underachiever, and individual tutoring can be arranged. Special education in a community day school for adolescents who have learning problems can be of value. For those over 15 years old whose parents can afford it, a boarding school may promote independence and motivation. For those who have disorganized behavior patterns, a school that has a structured program and close supervision may be recommended. For those who have strongly oppositional attitudes toward studying and responsibility, a school that offers flexible and individual support may be best. If such a change of schools is considered, the adolescent should have a chance to participate in the decision.

The number of college dropouts has been increasing in recent years, perhaps to as many as 40% of the college population. Students drop out of college because of academic difficulty, sexual involvement, rebellion against parents or society, and psychologic disorders. Students who drop out because they have psychologic disorders constitute the largest number although they also show the highest rate of return.[151] Some show a depressive reaction ("work paralysis") that is related to their awareness that their ideal self—uniquely gifted intellectual achiever—does not match their real self— one of thousands struggling in a vigorously competitive environment. Others are confused about their identity as they move away from their parents' control for the first time. Sometimes after a year or two of work, they "find themselves" and return to college.[422] Still others become alienated and drop out of society. Others remain around the college, on the fringe of the group, and some return home and are caught up in unhealthy interaction with their families.[258]

Unwed Parenthood. The number of children born out of wedlock in the United States increased threefold from 1940 to 1968, when the figure reached 23.5 per 1000; recent estimates have ranged much higher, up to 16% of all births. Most of these children are born to adolescents. Until recently, the problem was assumed to be confined to nonwhite, lower-income, inner city people. Recent data indicate that teenage pregnancy is involving more and more middle-class white youngsters from suburban and rural backgrounds.[466] Marriage is no longer a prerequisite to parenthood for many youngsters, and adoption is no longer the rule.

Early reports by Battaglia[28] and others have indicated that pregnant adolescents show the highest rates of prematurity and other complications, including serious emotional problems relating to unplanned and unwanted infants.[303,431] More recent reports[440,466] show fewer significant differences in obstetrical complications or outcome for adolescents who have been given "comprehensive care," and they indicate some positive responses to psychosocial care.[298] Pregnant adolescents, especially younger ones, are still a group at special risk, but recent differences in access to good prenatal care, which are related to socioeconomic and ethnic factors, have become a more significant factor in influencing obstetrical outcome.[466] As indicated earlier, most unwed mothers are not mentally retarded.

Before the liberalization of abortion laws, psychiatric studies of unwed motherhood reported largely on middle-class young women.[127,189,273] The studies emphasized the following as factors in unwed motherhood: hostility toward and rebellion against overly restrictive parents, wishes for self-punishment, identification with a pregnant mother, relative, or friend, flight from a relationship with a seductive father, and a search for a meaningful relationship outside the family in order to achieve security or avoid depression. Other factors have also been described, including an attempt to pressure the "father" into marriage, an unconscious attempt to make up for previous emotional deprivation by "giving to a baby," an attempt to replace the actual or symbolic loss of a key figure (e.g., a parent, relative, or friend), a search for identity through a relationship with a person of the opposite sex, and the production of a baby as an unconsciously motivated gift to a mother who is uncaring or who wants a baby to care for.

In such situations, which involved largely neurotic disturbances in family relationships, most such girls were not promiscuous, and the pregnancy was usually a by-product of the girls' unmet and often overlapping emotional needs. The girls were pressed often to give up their babies for adoption or sometimes to marry the boy involved. Few of the marriages that resulted were successful. The stigma of unwed motherhood was real and intense, and the girls were ostracized from school.

In recent years, with the more open discussion of sexuality, the changes in sexual mores, the weakening of the double standard, the percentage of sexually active males and sexually active females has become more similar, and teenagers from all segments of society are becoming sexually more active and at an earlier age. (But it should be noted that it is hard to gather accurate statistics.[8]) Although an ambivalent mother-adolescent bond and an absent father are often factors in out-of-wedlock pregnancies, many teenage pregnancies now seem to be the product of more frequent sexual activity, ignorance about contraception, concern about spontaneity, and even a "risk-denial" syndrome, especially among younger teenagers. In most studies, teenagers are shown to be generally not promiscuous and to confine their sexual relations to a single partner in a "monogamous" relationship that extends over a long period of time.[8] Psychologic factors are not involved so often as they were formerly,[467] and the stigma of unwed motherhood has considerably lessened. More babies are kept, there is more successful coping,[165] and there are even more marriages following the pregnancy than was the case formerly. But broken homes, financial hardships, family problems, and the need for stability and love are still factors. A few severely narcissistic young women have conceived babies which they had planned from the start to rear themselves, a plan which usually involves difficulties later for the child. Anxiety about the impending labor is still frequent, and teenage girls still have some anxiety about the responsibility of becoming mothers.[322] They are still a high-risk group but much less so than formerly.

Unmarried young women 19 to 35 years old, particularly those who have several children, still show psychopathologic problems that involve intense hostile-dependent struggles with the mother and hatred toward the father, who is distant. A disinterest in motherhood is characteristic of these young women. Those who marry seem to do so principally to meet their dependency needs; they are lonely young women who have personality disorders of a hysterical, overly dependent, or mixed type.

Unwed fathers have been less well studied. Many of them do not have an adequate masculine model, and they often meet the needs of immature teenage girls immaturely. Neither the boys nor the girls have a clear identity nor even the beginning of a capacity for intimacy. In 1973 the Committee on Adoption and Dependent Care[9] supported the attempts of the courts to recognize the rights of the unwed father but only in cases in which the fathers have acknowledged paternity or that have been so adjudicated.

Management. In a statement published in the June, 1964, newsletter of the American Academy of Pediatrics (and approved by the American Academy of Pediatrics, the American College of Obstetricians and Gynecologists, the Child Welfare League of America, and the Children's Bureau), the need for the close collaboration of the physician, the social worker, and the lawyer in the care of the unwed mother was emphasized. It was pointed out that the physician is responsible for the physical and mental health of the mother. He must diagnose the pregnancy, determine the expected date of delivery, decide where the delivery should take place, give the mother information about the physiology of pregnancy, labor, and the puerperal period, and counsel the mother about breastfeeding or other methods of feeding. He must keep the information the mother discloses confidential, except as provided for by the laws of the state; he must make sure that the consent the mother gives for any disclosures, treatment, or procedures is valid. He should not become involved with the placement of the infant, nor should he act as an intermediary.

The statement pointed out that the social worker is responsible for helping the unwed mother with the social and emotional problems related to having a child out of wedlock. The social worker should work closely with the appropriate social agencies and other community resources, and she should use her social and diagnostic skills to determine what help the mother needs. Early referral for competent obstetrical care and support of the physician's recommendations for antenatal and postnatal care are important. The social worker counsels the mother about her plans for her future and that of the infant, makes sure that the interests of the child are safeguarded, provides psychologic help and support while supporting the legal obligations of the doctor, and offers counseling about the mother's need for legal advice.

The lawyer is responsible for counseling the mother about her legal rights in regard to the putative father and the legal consequences of keeping or giving up her child. If the mother decides to release the child for adoption, he must see that the legal requirements are met. He should avoid becoming involved with the placement of the child, acting as an intermediary, or representing the prospective adoptive parents.

The statement emphasized that the representatives of the three disciplines should recognize the right of the unwed mother to make decisions for herself and her child, except when such rights are terminated by the court. In order to avoid confusion, the collective counseling must be collaborative and harmonious, and any differences of opinion should be resolved in prior conferences. Each case must be handled individually in regard to particular questions, including whether the parents of the mother or the putative father should be told, whether the parents should marry, whether the mother should be allowed, urged, or forbidden to see, breastfeed, and otherwise care for her child, whether the mother should be told of any deformity or handicap the infant has, and if so, by whom, whether the mother should have psychiatric help, and at what point in the pregnancy or puerperium a decision should be made about the infant's future and related matters.

I heartily endorse the main thrust of the statement, but I would add to it the following comments. When a teenage mother consults a physician, he may have to seek legal advice immediately about the local laws since laws vary from state to state and even within states. Generally, a distinction is made between juveniles (those 15 years of age or younger) and minors (those 16 through 18 or 21 years of age). If the pregnant girl is a juvenile, the physician usually must tell her parents that she is pregnant.

(The decision as to whether to tell the putative father is more difficult.) Ideally, the physician is able to persuade the girl to tell her parents herself. In the case of a minor from another state who wishes to keep her pregnancy a secret from her parents, however, the situation is more complicated, partly as the result of inconsistency in attitudes, laws, and the implementation of laws.

The physician in private practice generally does not have a social worker working with him (but a social worker may be associated with doctors in group practice). He thus must be familiar with the appropriate social and legal agencies in the community or with private practitioners in social work and law. Whether or not the young woman becomes his patient, her initial visit to the physician is most important. His words and manner convey his attitudes; in her anxiety, the young woman may not even hear his confirmation of her pregnancy. Thus he must play the role of counselor, and he must spend some time listening to the young woman (and the putative father if he is available). If the parents are involved, he must help them deal with their feelings of shock, anger, or bitterness. It is important for the physician to help all parties avoid making hasty decisions. In this regard, the social worker and the lawyer or the appropriate agencies can be most helpful. If the girl (or others) is very disturbed, the physician may wish to seek a psychiatric consultation. A direct or an indirect consultation with a mental health professional or a religious counselor may be wise in the majority of cases; and various forms of psychotherapy for the girl, the boy, and/or their families may be necessary. Psychotherapy may involve a private practitioner, a mental health facility, a family or a children's agency, or some other community resource.

In her first contacts with the physician, the young woman may resist planning as she attempts to deny her pregnancy. A sympathetic approach, combined with sufficient time for the interview, often helps her to come to grips with her situation, whereas attempts to force her to face reality usually only increase her denial. When she admits to herself that she is pregnant and that she needs help, the young woman often becomes mildly depressed. Particularly if the putative father or her relatives are not available to her, she may feel that she cannot make a final decision about keeping or giving up her child until after the child has been born. In such a case, pressure should not be put on the young woman to make a decision. Contrary to popular views, the woman's decision seems to be more lasting if the mother sees her child, can help in its care, and, if she decides to relinquish her child, has time to begin her "work of mourning." If she does not see her infant, she may have fantasies that her baby has some defect. Also, she will find it difficult to mourn the loss of a baby she has never seen. She may try to find the child, or she may conceive another child to take its place or to make up to it for her abandonment. Rigid policies about the length of time she must or may care for her child are also unwise. If a woman who is planning to relinquish her baby gives birth to a baby who has a defect, she should be told of the defect; seeing her baby will help her to deal better with the problem since her fantasies may be worse than the reality.

Contacts between the mother and the physician or other professional during pregnancy may help the young woman to lead a more mature sexual life after the delivery and to improve her maternal skills. Although counseling about contraception should be offered routinely to teenage mothers, there is evidence that such counseling is not effective unless the mother has a continuing relationship with a helping person for some time after the delivery.[317] Young women who have repeated out-of-wedlock pregnancies obviously need intensive psychotherapy if they are to change their lives. Regular group meetings of these

women with an experienced and "giving" social worker who is able to help them deal with a variety of feelings, questions, and problems in a nonjudgmental atmosphere have been helpful. Group therapy meetings and individual counseling for the mothers of these girls have helped the mothers change their attitudes and behavior toward their daughters. Other group approaches have also had success with other groups of unwed mothers.[236]

Recently it has been recognized that continued schooling during and after pregnancy is important for teenage unwed mothers. Most of these mothers have been excluded from school in the past, and many of them, particularly those from lower socioeconomic backgrounds, do not return to school after their babies are born. Some community agencies have set up special educational programs for such girls. Some of the programs are combined with medical supervision. Schools are beginning to plan for their needs by setting up special classes and other approaches.[38]

Prevention of out-of-wedlock pregnancies should include anticipatory guidance, pediatric counseling, early identification and referral of disturbed families, and the development of more community health and mental health programs. Education for parenthood and sex education in schools is increasing,[13] partly in response to the increase in venereal disease.[158,271] But many teenage unwed mothers are not helped by an educational approach because they deny that they can get pregnant. For a number of teenage unwed mothers, the best preventive approaches involve the elimination of poverty, unemployment, racial discrimination, and segregated schools and housing.

Abortion. With the advent of more liberal abortion laws, the number of illegal abortions has dropped from its previously estimated number of one million to less than 100,000 per year in the United States. The danger of serious infection, even death, and the possibility of later sterility for the woman who has an illegal abortion are well known, as is the guilt the woman experiences whether or not the abortion is successful. The dangers for children who are unwanted—of rejection, abandonment, or physical abuse—are well known, as are the resentment and psychologic stresses for women who have children they do not want.[192] However, the legalization of abortion has not done away with many problems. For one thing, the majority of legal abortions have been performed on private as opposed to clinic patients. Thus the pattern of abortions shows a socioeconomic and to some extent an ethnic bias. The Supreme Court decision has helped to clarify the woman's legal right to have an abortion but anti-abortion groups are trying to limit this right, and again an ethnic bias is the result.

Since abortion became legal in the United States, there have been reports of women who have had psychotic episodes, made suicide attempts, and had severe guilt reactions following an abortion. These reports parallel those of several Swedish investigations. Some psychiatrists have become convinced that every abortion is an emotionally traumatic experience, and they are concerned that therapeutic abortion may be a two-edged sword, with the risk of guilt or other emotional trauma in some instances outweighing the risk of continuing the pregnancy.

The most recent studies of abortion in the United States and other countries (where abortion laws are generally more liberal) are more systematic than were the earlier impressionistic case reports. They seem to agree with the findings of a study of a legalized abortion program in New York State in which patients demographically reflected the community at large. The general conclusion of the study was that therapeutic abortion has few adverse objective psychologic sequelae in psychologically healthy women.[396] Even in a group of women who had a history of previous emotional disturbance, the incidence of unhealthy postabortion emotional reactions was no greater than that in a control group of women who did not have such a history.[147] In another study of women who had moderate-to-severe psychiatric problems, it seemed that the more serious the psychiatric diagnosis was, the less beneficial the abortion was.[328] In such cases it seems necessary to give the woman psychotherapy before the abortion is done. If an abortion is decided on, the psychotherapy should be continued in an effort to prevent more serious adverse sequelae.

The statement of the Committee on Youth of the American Academy of Pediatrics in 1979 underscores the need of the teenage unwed mothers for continuing support and guidance, including contraceptive advice and other rehabilitative measures. Teenagers tend to deny the need for contraceptive measures even following an abortion. Postabortion group therapy, with small groups of teenagers and some older women led by a psychiatrist-gynecologist team, has helped patients cope with guilt feelings and to clear up any misconception they had about sexual functioning and contraception.

In my opinion, psychotherapy is necessary for many teenage mothers—and fathers—before an abortion is done and often after it is done.

Juvenile Delinquency. The term delinquency is a legal one not a medical one. Juvenile delinquency may be defined as repeated acts that violate the community's written code and for which the young person has been adjudicated a delinquent by a court. Delinquent acts include some acts that would constitute a crime if they were done by an adult. Other acts include those which are violations of laws only when they are done by juveniles, such as running away from home, truancy, and out-of-wedlock pregnancies.* Unfortunately, the

---

*Children who commit such acts are often called Children in Need of Supervision. In some states, these children are handled not in the juvenile court system but in social services and mental health systems, as they should be.

determination of what acts are delinquent is affected by the neighborhood in which they are committed and the social class of the people involved. Many acts that are regarded by the authorities as delinquent in lower socioeconomic and disadvantaged neighborhoods, particularly ghettos or barrios, are "swept under the rug" or regarded simply as disturbed behavior in suburbs populated by the well-to-do and influential. Such factors help determine whether the adolescent winds up in the juvenile court or in other systems.[261]

However it is defined, delinquency has increased in recent years.[86] In general, the delinquent acts of boys are more aggressive and destructive, while delinquent girls are more commonly apprehended for stealing and sexual acting out. Boys 15 years old commit the greatest number of delinquent acts. No more than 2% of teenagers are involved in serious crime, and less than 10% of arrests for violent crimes involve adolescents. Studies indicate that both lower- and middle-class delinquents develop self-critical guilt reactions later than do nondelinquents.

A number of causative factors are involved in juvenile delinquency.[325] Some children resort to delinquent acting-out behavior to compensate for chronic handicaps, that make them feel inadequate. Children who have definitive brain damage may have trouble developing impulse controls, and children who have developmental lags in perceptual-motor functioning and learning problems may act out their frustrations in antisocial ways. Mentally retarded children may become delinquent, and psychotic children may be involved in bizarre delinquent acts.[233,264] Children who have reactive disorders may commit certain kinds of crimes (e.g., stealing), and certain neurotic children may steal or tell lies (which are really self-compensatory or at times self-punitive fantasies). Even healthy teenagers may get into trouble with the law for speeding or for experimenting with drugs. (Runaway children and ado-

lescents, children who are involved in various kinds of sexual acts, children and adolescents who commit homicide, and children who set fires are discussed elsewhere in the book.)

In a larger group of young persons who repeatedly commit delinquent acts, family psychopathology seems to be principally involved. The childrearing patterns of the families of such *individual* delinquents are viewed somewhat differently by various investigators. Their parents, especially their mothers, seem to be less warm, more inconsistent in their discipline, and more neglectful than the parents of nondelinquents.[24,37] The fathers also tend to use more physical punishment and to use it erratically. Delinquent boys tend to have overtly hostile relationships with their fathers, a phenomenon that cuts across all social classes although it occurs predominantly in the middle class.[103] The parent-child relationship tends to be a reflection of a larger pattern of moral deviance in the family[353] (occasionally criminality[262]), of subtler defects in moral judgment and attitudes the parents "project" onto their children, or, often, of family disorganization.[223] The incidence of the loss of a parent through death, divorce, or desertion, is higher in these children than in the general population, and some of these children have suffered emotional deprivation because they have been in a great number of foster homes or because they have had unfortunate experiences in other institutional settings.

Such family environments seem to militate against healthy personality development and moral learning.[354,429] The children of these families are permitted or unconsciously encouraged[222] to experience a "developmental arrest" at a premoral stage. They often view their parents' frustrations with them as arising out of the parents' selfish impulses or motives. They exhibit little conscience development, and they either become amoral or express the idea that their delinquent acts are retaliations against their parents and the world, which they perceive as a cold, hostile place. As adolescents, they have serious difficulty in achieving a positive identity, which includes their playing a constructive role in the world as they perceive it. Diagnostically, the majority of these young people would be classified as having personality disorders of the impulse-ridden type. Those who have progressed to the point where they feel some guilt about their behavior may exhibit neurotic personality disorders, with an unconscious need to be caught and controlled. As indicated earlier, there is some overlapping of these two categories. Some of these young people remain in conflict with society and the law for many years although the majority "burn out" by age 25 and acquire at least partial control of their impulses, which permits them to stay out of trouble with the law.[24]

Often these children begin to show antisocial behavior in the late preschool-age stage. That fact and the fact that a number have problems in school performance, as well as apparent abnormalities in their EEG tracings, have led some to feel that "minimal brain damage" or some other biologic factor, such as hyperactivity,[79] may be involved. The limitations in the concept of minimal brain damage have already been discussed, as has the looseness of the terms hyperactivity and EEG abnormality. A recent study shows that there is little evidence to correlate true EEG abnormalities and continued delinquent behavior. Most of the school problems in this group seem to be related to problems in motivation, concentration, and self-discipline although some of the school problems may involve developmental lags in perceptual-motor functioning without brain damage. One study suggests that these and certain other children may be biologically and temperamentally predisposed to deal with tensions through motor discharge rather than through fantasy or other ways and that family psychopathology determines which children develop a pattern of acting out

conflicts. Hormonal studies have not provided the answer.[129,309]

Other factors (e.g., poverty, unemployment, inadequate housing, frequent absence of the father, broken homes, gross disorganization in the family, lack of recreational facilities, community instability or disorganization, a tendency to turn to the use of drugs out of hopelessness, and a feeling of alienation from society) underlie the higher incidence of *gang delinquency* among young people in lower socioeconomic groups in disadvantaged neighborhoods. Such forces affect especially young people from minority backgrounds, who also encounter racial and ethnic discrimination and segregation. Under such circumstances, some acts that would be defined as delinquent in suburban areas are coping behaviors in disadvantaged neighborhoods.

The gang subculture in deprived areas is complex. "Conflict" gangs are the most common type; their purpose seems to be to give the individual status distinct from the status of individuals in other gangs. "Fighting" gangs compete with each other for such things as territory, reputation, and goods that are scarce. "Retreatist" gangs also exist, however; they often use drugs in group situations. "Criminal cliques" have also been described; they commit specialized acts among and within gangs.[95,97,388] Not all gang members are delinquent, however, even when the gang's specialization tends toward delinquency, and most gang members are not delinquent when by themselves.[307] Gangs were largely male until recently; female gangs have begun to appear in larger numbers.

Blocked from taking legitimate avenues to social and material success, gang members generally are deficient in social skills and tend to do poorly in school. Gangs offer their members protection, status, and a sharing of exploits. They tend to harden new members against feelings of sympathy, fear, disapproval, or guilt, and they are not conducive to the development of warmth, true loyalty, or trustworthiness. Gang members tend to be more conflicted and anxious about being dependent on others than are nongang youths. For the boy, there is also the danger of being killed, and for the girl the danger of becoming pregnant.

Neither ethnic background nor race can be assumed to be in itself a cause of high delinquency or gang behavior. Culture conflict may be involved in gang behavior, as may the process of social disorganization. Black and Puerto Rican groups have been more seriously kept from achieving social assimilation than have the various waves of immigrants in the past.

The absence of legitimate opportunities for advancement often leads boys to develop a disciplined criminal subculture that is based on the example of their elders and that seeks legitimation in the eyes of powerful adults. Those who fail to achieve even in the criminal subculture may use drugs and other "kicks" more heavily as escapist reactions and they show severe personality disorders more often than do those outside the criminal subculture. Some people remain locked in the criminal subculture as adults; some are able to break out.

Gang behavior began to decline in the late 1950s. In the last 15 years, however, it has shown a steady rise, and gang violence has increased.[462] The increase seems to be related to a growing rage among young people (especially those in minority groups) about their poor living conditions in a culture which emphasizes material comfort and to their despair about ever achieving success or even having a voice in their future.

Individuals or gang members who become delinquent as a result of sociocultural forces are responding to a combination of the forces mentioned earlier, as the study carried out by the Gluecks[179] indicates. There is also some overlapping of those forces with family psychopathology. The Gluecks studied 500 delinquent boys and 500 boys in a matched control group. The delinquent boys came from less stable, less organized, more crowded, and poorer homes. More of them came from broken homes, and their parents suffered more often from alcoholism, physical disorders, and mental disorders. Their parents and siblings showed them less affection, and their families were less cohesive. The delinquents showed less coping capacity, poorer school performances, less sense of values, more defiance, and more unrealistic thinking. Delinquents from the socioeconomic background just described tend to be placed in training schools, public shelters, or other correctional facilities, in contrast to middle-class delinquents, whose parents can pay for treatment in clinics or residential treatment facilities. Even when they manage to break out of the juvenile justice system, such deprived delinquent children have a high risk as parents of having children like themselves and thus perpetuating the problem.

A number of attempts have been made to make possible the early identification of delinquents. The best known attempt is that of the Gluecks[180] who assigned a score of probable delinquency based on the following 5 factors: (1) the father's discipline of the child, (2) the mother's supervision of the child, (3) the father's affection for the child, (4) the mother's affection for the child, and (5) the cohesiveness of the child's family. Kvaraceus[251] has also devised a "delinquency-proneness" scale. It is made up of multiple-choice items based on home and family backgrounds, differences in personal make-up, and the school experience of delinquents and nondelinquents. Other indices have also been devised. Long-term testing of the Gluecks' Predictive Index has demonstrated that later delinquency can be successfully predicted in individual children in their early school years. Controlled attempts to prevent such an outcome have not been successful. It should be mentioned, however, that the danger of "labeling" a child as a future delinquent is real.

A number of approaches are used to deal with delinquency. The traditional approach, which is used for the largest group of delinquents, is essentially a punitive one; the delinquents are put in reformatories, correctional institutions (such as training schools), and even adult jails or prisons. Often little attempt is made to rehabilitate the delinquents. Thousands of children and adolescents languish for many months in detention centers or public shelters. The conditions in many such institutions are abominable. The food is poor, and physical abuse is common. The incidence of homosexuality in sex-segregated institutions for adolescents has been estimated to be as high as 60% to 70% (many delinquents probably do not continue homosexual behavior after they have been discharged). No follow-up information is available about adolescents who were subjected to homosexual assault in adult prisons. The incidence of recidivism in delinquents placed in reform schools has been as high as 60% to 80%.

The juvenile court movement, which began in the early 1900s, has curbed some of these abuses, with intake studies, the judicious use of probation, and recommendations for treatment in appropriate situations. Although the results of Robins'[363] long-term follow-up study of relatively untreated delinquents were not cause for optimism, various modifications of traditional psychotherapy for delinquents have been relatively successful in the hands of Aichhorn,[3] Redl,[352] Slavson,[144] and others[276,311] on an inpatient basis. Eissler,[138] Kaufman[233] Rexford,[354] Schmideberg,[380] and others have treated delinquents individually on an outpatient basis, working also with parents. Group therapy has been used by Peck[333] and Kinsey,[247] while Cutter and Hallowitz[109] and others have used modifications of family therapy. Behavior modification therapy[67] has been helpful in residential settings. Mandated therapy on an individual family or group basis for families who do not voluntarily follow recommendations for ther-

apy has been carried out in clinics in the juvenile court setting. Such therapy has been given for more than 20 years in the pioneering court clinic operated by Russell[371] out of the Judge Baker Guidance Center in Boston.

In the legal profession, Bazelton has been a leader in calling for treatment rather than punishment for delinquents. At present, many juvenile court judges still have little special training in understanding the needs of children and adolescents, and many communites have inadequate or no facilities either for placing delinquents in other than institutional settings or for treating delinquents.[191] The American Academy of Pediatrics has recently worked out health standards for residential facilities for juvenile delinquents. The standards were endorsed by the National Council of Juvenile Court Judges, but many such facilities still have few or no health personnel or programs.

Other creative and innovative steps have been taken more recently within the juvenile justice system. Mental health personnel have been added to the staffs of some correctional institutions in order to develop more treatment-oriented programs.[263] Work camps designed to provide a rehabilitative climate and individual and group counseling have been used successfully in many states. Peer-confrontation groups that emphasize responsibility and use rewards have been of value in detention centers. Work-release programs and halfway houses have helped delinquents who have been discharged from institutions. Recently group homes and psychotherapy for the child and his parents and other alternatives to institutional placement have become more popular.

Mental health consultation has been offered to juvenile probation departments by a number of workers. The staffs of the departments are helped to deal with their own frustrations[246,342] as well as their caseloads. A comprehensive, community-based, vocationally oriented psychotherapeutic program was developed by Shore and Massimo. It emphasizes job placement, remedial education, and psychotherapy, and it has resulted in a significantly better overall adjustment for a group of adolescent delinquent boys than for a group of untreated controls. The results of the program have held up after 15 years.[387]

In some settings, special training in the handling of juveniles, particularly those from minority groups, has been offered to police officers. Also, there has been a gradual increase in the number of police from minority groups. "Detached" ("street") workers are trained to mediate and manipulate gang actions away from conflict and toward constructive behavior. When correctional services are offered in conjunction with family casework services ("reaching out" services), juvenile court consultation, and other community services, such as the development of recreational programs, the total costs of the correctional services are startlingly lower than the costs for handling delinquents in "unserviced" groups—and lower than the costs of handling unserviced younger brothers of "full-serviced" boys. (It costs over $300,000 to handle the case of a delinquent placed in the traditional institutional system.) The effects of large-scale experimental government programs must still be evaluated. Some of these programs aim at the rehabilitation of delinquents and the prevention of delinquency, and some are concerned with the more fundamental processes of socialization, motivation, stimulation, education, vocational training, and community organization. Some encouraging results can be cited, but there must be more emphasis on coordination among the workers in such programs and with comprehensive health and mental health programs.

Since the early 1960s there has been more emphasis on the need for services of all types to be based in the community and to reflect the community's needs and expectations. A companion need is the need for a spectrum of services to children, adolescents, and their families. Ideally and ultimately, children's services would include prenatal and well-child care, enrichment programs, day care, community schools, mental health programs, and work-release programs. In regard to youth services, comprehensive services would include reception and evaluation facilities in collaboration with community mental health centers and youth service bureaus, shelter facilities for runaways and "cast outs," group and foster placement services, volunteer probation and Big Brother and Big Sister type services, better probation staffs, alternative detention arrangements, and sophisticated detention and treatment facilities, including closed psychiatric centers for recidivists, runaways, and chronic offenders. In addition, more residential treatment facilities are needed for those youths who do not fit the delinquent pattern.

The pediatrician can help in the management of delinquency in various ways. As Deisher[118] has pointed out, if a child or adolescent who has a physical defect or chronic handicap is engaging in delinquent acts to compensate for a feeling of inadequacy or for a poor self-image, the physician can try to correct the disability. If he cannot correct it, he can help the young person (and his parents) adjust to his disability. The pediatrician may help treat the drug problems, sex problems, brain damage, mental retardation, or other difficulties of delinquent adolescents. Richmond[357] has indicated that the pediatrician can also identify predelinquent behavior in early school-age children (e.g., repeated minor thefts, truancy, or aggressive behavior), as well as problems in parental supervision and parent-child relationships, and he can offer pediatric counseling to the child and his parents. If the family is unable to use the pediatrician's help effectively, he may obtain psychiatric consultation for them, or he may refer the family to a mental health facility or family agency. Older children who have established personality disorders of impulse-ridden or other types will require referral for intensive long-term psychotherapeutic efforts and sometimes residential treatment. Through his approach to a child who has a learning problem, the pediatrician may be able to help prevent delinquency; such a child may be vulnerable and at high risk, especially if he drops out of school. Through anticipatory guidance and counseling in health supervision, the pediatrician may help the parents deal with problems in discipline or handle aggressive behavior in preschool-age children that might predispose those children to delinquent behavior later.

In the context of his relationship with an adolescent, the pediatrician may learn of delinquent acts which have been committed or are being planned. If these acts are of major significance, it is the pediatrician's responsibility to encourage the adolescent to tell his parents about them. If that is not possible, the pediatrician must inform the parents, ideally with the adolescent's consent but without it if necessary. If the latter course has to be taken, the pediatrician should tell the adolescent exactly what he is going to tell the parents. It sometimes happens that an adolescent who is afraid to tell his parents of his behavior confides in the pediatrician, half hoping that the pediatrician will tell his parents or will help him tell his parents. If, as occasionally happens, the parents take no action in regard to a serious offense, it is the responsibility of the pediatrician to call the problem to the attention of the Child Protection Division of the Welfare Department or of a private agency or to get assistance from the juvenile court.

The pediatrician should be familiar with the programs in his community that aim to prevent delinquency or rehabilitate delinquents—programs in neighborhood youth centers, school work-study programs, and vocational and day treatment programs. He should be prepared to make use of those programs by referring patients to them and by working with their staffs. He can also offer his services as a health consultant to agencies engaged in the treatment of delinquents (e.g., child psychiatry clinics, family services agencies, and correctional facilities), as well as to preventive programs. Finally, as an informed citizen and as a knowledgeable professional concerned with children's needs, the pediatrician should participate in the community's efforts to set up programs and coordinate existing ones and to maintain standards in their medical components.

Running Away. Running away from home in the school-age period is uncommon although school-age children often threaten to do so. Parents may take a child's threats to run away too seriously. Adolescents or even postadolescents may run away to seek excitement, to see the world, to respond to a sudden loss of self-esteem, to express rebellion, to deal with depressed feelings, to find themselves, or to help earn money for the family. It is much harder for the adolescent to survive on his own today than when he could run away to sea, and a number of parents are subsidizing their wandering youngsters. Many runaways are simply having a *Wanderjahr*, but others (particularly girls) may get into serious difficulty because they are not ready for such freedom.[443] Most middle-class adolescents who run away wish to be found; they are testing their parents' interest in them or they are expressing anger or rebellion.[442] Most of them return home fairly promptly, or they at least leave clues for their parents to follow.

Some adolescent girls run away to avoid the unconscious threat of an incestuous or overly seductive relationship with their fathers, other relatives, or their mothers' lovers. Underprivileged adolescents who receive inadequate warmth and supervision at home may simply drift away into a gang, and the likelihood that later they will have trouble with the law is great. Repeated running away often begins in early childhood as a response to conflicts in the parent-child relationship or as a sign of difficulty. Follow-up care usually shows continued difficulty in adjustment, problems with impulse control, and a high incidence of deep personality disorders of the tension-discharge type.[364] Psychiatric consultation is often called for. Some adolescents require intensive psychotherapy with their parents. Adolescents who run away repeatedly often need residential treatment, sometimes in a closed setting.

Fire Setting. Many early school-age children play with matches. Their fascination with fire leads a number of normal early school-age children to set small fires, usually only one if the parents have set firm limits. Some school-age children set fires repeatedly; they often have problems with impulse control associated with other signs of developmental lags in maturational patterns.[464] Resentment toward adults, sexual symbolism, and struggles to control enuretic tendencies are frequently present. These children may gain control of their impulses as they develop, but most children who set fires repeatedly require intensive psychotherapy, and some require residential treatment.[430]

If fire setting continues beyond the prepubescent period, a more serious personality disturbance is invariably involved. Fires are usually set on a conscious, planned basis; they do not represent a temporary yielding to impulse. Boys, who make up the majority of fire setters, may turn in the fire alarm themselves. They often linger or return to see the consequences, and they sometimes attempt to put out the fire. Fire setters may operate in pairs, with an aggressive member and a passive member. Although some adolescent fire setters are mentally retarded, the majority are disturbed to near psychotic or psychotic proportions, exhibiting revengeful fantasies of destroying the world or attempts to master their impulses by putting out a fire they have started.[234] Gang fire setting usually involves group contagion or excitement. Adolescent fire setters usually require long-term psychiatric treatment in closed residential settings.

Homicide and Other Crimes of Violence. Children and adolescents rarely commit homicide. Homicide is committed predominantly by adolescent males and more frequently under conditions of poverty and social oppression. Gang violence can escalate into murder. Bender[33] first described children and adolescents who kill; most often they do so in situations involving intense family rivalry and in families with highly aggressive or violent behavior patterns. Bender and Kaufman and his colleagues[233] later came to feel that there was a relationship between crimes of violence, so-called childhood schizophrenia, and fire setting that centered around both uncontrolled rage and a striking out against feared annihilation.

More recently, cases of murder in the family have been described[339] in which an adolescent's abrupt loss of control has been associated with a change in his relationship with the victim, together with a sequence of events that became progressively more unbearable to him and less controllable by him. In most cases, an act of homicide is a culmination of events that developed in the previous few days and alternatives are not available or have been tried and failed. The risk of homicide seems to be greater if the adolescent believes a homicidal act would benefit others as well as himself, as in an attempt to protect one parent from an assault by another. Some adolescents show episodic violent behavior related to unconscious transmission from the parents of unhealthy attitudes about aggression,[201] and accidental homicide may occur in similar families.[160]

Violence seems to breed violence, and adolescents who kill have often met extreme violence or brutality at the hands of their parents. Often the adolescent has run away or contacted the police in an attempt to get help for himself or his parents. Suicide thoughts or suicide attempts may precede the act. Several studies[374] have described the unconscious and intense fostering of murderous aggression in the adolescent by the parents of an adolescent who killed.

No common pattern of personality disturbance has been identified in adolescent homicide. Most of these adolescents are not psychotic; some have been described as having personality disorders which would appear to be of the impulse-ridden, neurotic, isolated, or mixed types. I have seen in consultation two boys in early adolescence, one of whom had killed his sister and one of whom had killed his father. Both showed little gross psychopathology, and both had adjusted well superficially. They were cold and aloof, however, and had no close friends. Previously they had shown some sadistic tendencies in their treatment of animals, and they showed little guilt or remorse over their acts. Their clinical pictures could be said to resemble most closely moderate-to-severe isolated personality disorders. The parents of both boys had also showed little warmth. They had beaten the boys and had encouraged violence within the family. Neurologic problems, such as psychomotor seizures, were not involved, as some have alleged.[337] Treatment was recommended by a physician, but not required by the court, nor was it wished by the boys' families. After brief periods in correctional institutions, both boys were released to their parents. Both families left the state; follow-up by correspondence over several years indicated that the parents felt their adolescents were adjusting adequately. Most adolescents who kill do not kill again, but I remain concerned about violence in the adult lives of these two adolescents.

A detailed case report has been offered recently by Scherl and Mack[379]. It dealt with a 14$^{1}/_{2}$-year-old boy who killed his mother. The mother had established a pattern of relentless mutual provocation in the boy's early childhood that gave him no chance to form meaningful human relationships or to discharge tension outside his family. The boy ran away repeatedly. The local community failed to help him, however, and several agencies did not comprehend his efforts to obtain help. The matricide occurred after a build-up of events that involved especially sadistic behavior by the boy's mother and father. At the time of the matricide, the boy felt that killing his mother was the only way he could relieve the unbearable tensions which the sexualized relationship with his mother had aroused in him. To give himself the necessary inner permission for the matricide, the boy had to totally devalue his mother, and thus "justify" the murder.

In a correctional setting, the boy later developed dizziness and conversion pains as well as brief paralyses of his limbs. These phenomena were followed by a transient hallucination (of his mother's return as a witch), together with assaultive behavior and a brief breakdown in reality testing. Initially he showed amnesia for the matricide, and he showed no guilt about the act. No physical or neurologic abnormalities were found during a brief hospitalization, and a diagnosis of personality disorder of mixed type, with conversion and dissociative features, was made. The boy showed continuing assaultive behavior, and he was transferred to a closed correctional setting. After nearly two years in the institution, treatment was undertaken by a psychiatrist. At first, the boy could not talk easily or trust his therapist. In a year and a half of treatment, he became more trustful, began to fear loss of control of his anger, and began to express rage at the mother and then guilt about the matricide. At the time of his parole at 18 years of age, he continued his therapy but he remained a rather isolated person who had superficial relationships with members of both sexes. His prognosis remains guarded. Prugh and others believe, however, that such people may be treated in a closed psychiatric setting over a number of years.

Monahan[315] has summarized the research that has been done on the prediction of violent behavior. He concludes that such factors as homicidal threats, history of loss of control over aggressive impulses, situational factors (e.g., provocation by an intended victim and the availability of weapons) are not as accurate predictors of violent behavior as some have believed them to be and that reliance on them may have led to overprediction. If a person is diagnosed as being mentally ill and potentially dangerous, the presence of such factors as those just listed may, with psychiatric consultation, justify a brief, involuntary hospitalization. Even in the case of a violent crime, it is difficult to predict whether the person will commit a violent crime again. How to protect both society and the individual is a problem.

The pediatrician can help identify patterns of violent behavior in individual children and adolescents, and he can offer pediatric counseling, psychiatric consultation, or referral to a mental health facility. Through anticipatory guidance and pediatric counseling, he can help parents help their children control their aggression. Violence in our society, as reflected on television, is a problem with which pediatricians (e.g., Brazelton and Rothenberg) have struggled for years. A little progress has been made.

Bibliography

1. Adams, M.S., and Neel, J.V.: Children of incest. Pediatrics, *40*:55, 1967.
2. Addis, R.S.: A statistical study of nocturnal enuresis. Arch. Dis. Child., *10*:169, 1935.
3. Aichhorn, A.: *Wayward Youth*. New York, Viking, 1935.
4. Aleksandrowicz, M.A., and Mares, A.J.: Trichotillomania and trichobezoar in an infant. J. Am. Acad. Child Psychiatry, *17*:533, 1978.
5. Alpert, A.: Reversibility of pathological fixations associated with maternal deprivation in infancy. Psychoanal. Study Child., *14*:169, 1959.
6. Altman, M.: Admitting babies with mothers to psychiatric hospitals. J. Hosp. Comm. Psychiatry, *19*:356, 1968.
7. Altman, M., Garrity, C., and Hamlett, G.: The mental health curriculum: A technique of classroom consultation. Unpublished material.
8. American Academy of Pediatrics, Committee on Adolescence: Statement on teenage pregnancy. Pediatrics, *63*:795, 1979.
9. American Academy of Pediatrics, Committee on Adoption and Dependent Care: Statement on Rights of Putative Fathers. Evanston, Ill., American Academy of Pediatrics, 1973.
10. American Academy of Pediatrics, Committee on Adoption and Dependent Care: The role of the pediatrician in adoption with reference to the "right to know." Pediatrics, *60*:378, 1977.
11. American Academy of Pediatrics, Committee on Environmental Hazards: Effects of cigarette-smoking on the fetus and child. Pediatrics, *57*:411, 1976.
12. Amsterdam, B.: Chronic Encopresis: A system based psychodynamic approach. Child Psychiatry Hum. Dev., *9*:137, 1979.
13. Anastiow, N.J., et al.: Improving teenage attitudes toward children, child handicaps, and hospital settings: A child development curriculum for potential parents. Am. J. Orthopsychiatry, *48*:663, 1978.
14. Anthony, E.J.: The influence of maternal psychosis on children: Folie à Deux. In: *Parenthood: Its Psychology and Psychopathology* (E.J. Anthony and T. Benedek, Eds.). New York, Little, 1970.
15. Anthony, E.J.: An experimental approach to the psychopathology of childhood: encopresis. Br. J. Med. Psychol., *30*:146, 1957.
16. Anthony, E.J.: Clinical evaluation of children with psychotic parents. Am. J. Psychiatry, *126*:177, 1969.
17. Anthony, E.J.: Naturalistic studies of disturbed families. In: *Explorations in Child Psychiatry* (E.J. Anthony, Ed.). New York, Plenum, 1975.
18. Arnold, L.E., Ed.: *Helping Parents Help Their Children*. New York, Brunner/Mazel, 1978.
19. Arthur, G.: *Tutoring As Therapy*. New York, Commonwealth Fund, 1946.
20. Bajda, L.A.: A survey of smoking habits of students at Newton high school—A cooperative project. Am. J. Public Health, *54*:441, 1964.
21. Bakwin, H.: Enuresis in children. J. Pediatr., *58*:806, 1961.
22. Bakwin, H.: Suicide in children and adults. J. Am. Med. Women Assoc., *19*:489, 1964.
23. Bakwin, H., and Bakwin, R.M.: *Clinical Management of Behavior Disorders in Children*. 3rd Ed., Philadelphia, Saunders, 1967.
24. Bandura, A., and Walters, R.H.: *Adolescent Aggression: A Study of the Influences of Child-Training Practices and Family Interrelationship*. New York, Ronald, 1959.
25. Barbour, R.F.: Enuresis as a disorder of development. Br. Med. J., *2*:787, 1963.
26. Barnett, C.R., et al.: Neonatal separation: The maternal side of interactional deprivation. Pediatrics, *45*:197, 1978.
27. Barter, J.T., Swaback, P.O., and Todd, D.: Adolescent suicide attempts. Arch. Gen. Psychiatry, *19*:523, 1968.
28. Battaglia, F.C., et al.: Obstetric and pediatric complications of juvenile pregnancy. Pediatrics, *32*:902, 1963.

29. Becker, D., and Margolin, F.: How surviving parents handled their young children's adaptation to the crisis of loss. Am. J. Orthopsychiatry, *37*:753, 1967.

30. Bellman, M.: Studies on encopresis. Acta Paediatrica Scand., (Suppl.) *170*:17, 1966.

31. Bemporad, J.R., et al.: Characteristics of encopretic patients and their families. J. Am. Acad. Child Psychiatry, *10*:272, 1971.

32. Bender, L.: Children's reaction to death in the family. In: *Dynamic Psychopathology of Childhood* (L. Jessner and E. Pavenstedt, Eds.). Springfield, Ill., Thomas, 1944.

33. Bender, L.: Children and adolescents who have killed. Am. J. Psychiatry, *116*:510, 1959.

34. Benedek, T.: Parenthood as a developmental phase. J. Am. Psychoanal. Assoc., *7*:389, 1959.

35. Benedek, R.S., and Benedek, E.: Postdivorce visitation: A child's right. J. Am. Acad. Child Psychiatry, *15*:256, 1976.

36. Benjamin, J.D.: Developmental biology and psychoanalysis. In: *Psychoanalysis and Current Biological Thought* (N. Greenfield and W. Lewis, Eds.). Madison, University of Wisconsin Press, 1965.

37. Bennett, I.: *Delinquent and Neurotic Children: A Comparative Study*. London, Tavistock, 1960.

38. Bennett, V.C., and Bardon, J.J.: The effects of a school program on teenage mothers and their children. Am. J. Orthopsychiatry, *47*:671, 1977.

39. Bentzen, F.: Sex ratios in learning and behavior disorders. Am. J. Orthopsychiatry, *33*:92, 1963.

40. Berg, B.R.: Separating siblings in placement. Child Welfare, *36*:7, 1957.

41. Berk, R.L., and Feldman, A.S.: Functional hearing loss in children. N. Engl. J. Med., *259*:214, 1958.

42. Berlin, J.I.: Preventive aspects of mental health consultation to schools. Mental Hygiene, *51*:34, 1967.

43. Bernard, V.W.: Some principles of dynamic psychiatry related to poverty. Am. J. Psychiatry, *122*:254, 1965.

44. Bernstein, N., and Robey, J.S.: Detection and management of pediatric difficulties created by divorce. Pediatrics, *30*:950, 1962.

45. Beverly, B.I.: Incontinence in children. J. Pediatr., *2*:718, 1933.

46. Bibliography: *The Psychological Approach to the Cause of Stuttering*. Baltimore, Johns Hopkins University, Information Center for Hearing, Speech, and Disorders of Human Communication, 1969.

47. Bibring, G., et al.: A study of the psychological processes in pregnancy and the earliest mother-child relationship. Psychoanal. Study Child, *16*:9, 1961.

48. Birch, H.G., and Gussow, J.D.: *Disadvantaged Children: Health, Nutrition, and School Failure*. New York, Grune & Stratton, 1970.

49. Bissell, J.S.: *Implementation of Planned Variation in Head Start. I. Review and Summary of Stanford Research Institute Interim Report: Final Year of Evaluation*. Department of Health, Education, and Welfare, Washington, Government Printing Office, 1971.

50. Blaker, E., Demone, H.W., Jr., and Freeman, H.E.: Drinking behavior of delinquent boys. Q. J. Stud. Alcohol, *26*:223, 1965.

51. Bland, M., et al.: Effect of children's and parents' smoking on respiratory symptoms. Arch. Dis. Child., *53*:112, 1978.

52. Blane, H.T., and Hewitt, L.E.: *Alcohol and Youth: An Analysis of the Literature 1960–1975, Final Report*. WIAA Contract ADM-281-75-0026, Pittsburgh, University of Pittsburgh, 1977.

53. Blau, A.: *The Master Hand*. Research monograph of Society for Research in Child Development. American Orthopsychiatric Association, New York, 1946.

54. Blau, A., et al.: The psychogenic etiology of premature births: A preliminary report. Psychosom. Med., *25*:201, 1963.

55. Bloomquist, E.R.: *Marijuana*. Beverly Hills, Calif., Glencoe Press, 1969.

56. Bostwick, J., and Shackleton, M.G.: Enuresis and toilet training. Aust. Med. J., *2*:110, 1951.

57. Bower, E.M.: *Early Identification of Emotionally Disturbed Children in School*. Springfield, Ill., Thomas, 1960.

58. Bowlby, J.: *Maternal Care and Mental Health*. Geneva, World Health Organization, 1951.

59. Bowlby, J.: Grief and mourning in infancy and early childhood. Psychoanal. Study Child, *15*:9, 1960.

60. Bowlby, J.: Childhood mourning and its implications for psychiatry. In: *Childhood Psychopathology: An Anthology of Basic Readings*. New York, International Universities Press, 1972.

61. Boyd, M.M.: The depth of sleep in enuretic school children and in nonenuretic controls. J. Psychosom. Res., *4*:274, 1960.

62. Bradley, J.E., and Bessman, S.P.: Poverty, pica, and poisoning. Pat. Health Rep., *73*:467, 1958.

63. Brazelton, T.B.: A child-oriented approach to toilet training. Pediatrics, *29*:121, 1962.

64. Brazelton, T.B.: Crying in infancy. Pediatrics, *29*:579, 1962.

65. Brazelton, T.B.: Effect of drugs on the behavior of the neonate. Am. J. Psychiatry, *126*:1, 1970.

66. Breger, E.: Etiologic factors in enuresis: A psychobiologic approach. J. Am. Acad. Child Psychiatry, *4*:667, 1963.

67. Burchard, J., and Tyler, V., Jr.: The modification of delinquent behavior through operant conditioning. Behav. Res. Ther., *2*:245, 1965.

68. Burton, L.: *Vulnerable Children: Three Studies of Children in Conflict: Accident Involved Children, Sexually Assaulted Children, and Children with Asthma*. London, Routledge and Kegan Paul, 1968.

69. Buxbaum, E.: Hair pulling and fetishism. Psychoanal. Study Child, *15*:243, 1960.

70. Cain, A.C.: Children's disturbed reactions to their mother's miscarriage. Psychosom. Med., *26*:58, 1964.

71. Cain, A.C.: *Survivors of Suicide*. Springfield, Ill., Thomas, 1972.

72. Cain, A.C., and Fast, J.: Children's disturbed

reactions to parent's suicide. Am. J. Orthopsychiatry, 36:873, 1966.

73. Cain, A.C., Fast, J., and Erickson, M.E.: Children's disturbed reactions to the death of a sibling. Am. J. Orthopsychiatry, 34:741, 1964.

74. Caldwell, B.M.: The effects of psychosocial deprivation on human development in infancy. Merrill Palmer Q., 16:260, 1970.

75. Caldwell, B.B., and Richmond, J.B.: The children's center in Syracuse, New York. In: *Early Child Care: The New Perspective* (L.L. Dittman, Ed.). New York, Atherton, 1968.

76. Caldwell, B.C., et al.: Infant day care and attachment. Am. J. Orthopsychiatry, 40:397, 1970.

77. Call, J.D., et al.: Psychogenic megacolon in three preschool boys. Am. J. Orthopsychiatry, 33:923, 1963.

78. Cantwell, D.P., Ed.: *The Hyperactive Child.* New York, Spectrum, 1975.

79. Cantwell, D.P.: Hyperactivity and antisocial behavior. J. Am. Acad., Child Psychiatry, 17:252, 1978.

80. Caplan, G.: Mental health consultant in schools. In: *The Elements of a Community Health Program.* New York, Milbank Memorial Fund, 1956.

81. Caplan, G.: Patterns of parental response to the crisis of premature births. Psychiatry, 23:365, 1960.

82. Caplan, H., Bibace, R., and Rabinovitch, M.S.: Paranatal stress, cognitive organization and ego function: A controlled follow-up study of children born prematurely. J. Am. Acad. Child Psychiatry, 2:434, 1963.

83. Cardinal, M.H.: Anxiety among displaced children. Bull. World Fed. Ment. Health, 2:27, 1950.

84. Carey, W.: Measurement of infant temperament in pediatric practice. In: *Individual Colic Differences in Children.* (J.C. Westman, Ed.). New York, Wiley, 1973.

85. Chafetz, M.E., and Blaine, T.: High school drinking practices and problems. Psychiatr. Opinion, 17: March, 1979.

86. The Challenge of Crime in a Free Society: A Report by the President's Commission on Law Enforcement and Administration of Justice. Washington, Government Printing Office, 1967.

87. Chambers, C.D., and Brill, A.A.: *Drug Abuse, Methadone: Experiences and Issues.* New York, Behavioral Publications, 1972.

88. Chess, S.: Developmental language disability as factor in personality distortion. Am. J. Orthopsychiatry, 49:483, 1944.

89. Child Welfare League of America: *Adoption of Oriental Children by American White Families.* New York, Child Welfare League of America, 1959.

90. Child Welfare League of America: *New Approaches to Homemaker Service.* New York, Child Welfare League of America, 1968.

91. Child Welfare League of America: *Standards for Adoption Service.* New York, Child Welfare League of America, 1973.

92. Child Welfare League of America: *Black Children–White Parents: A Study of Transracial Adoption.* New York, Child Welfare League of America, 1974.

93. Christie, R., and Jahoda, M. Eds.: *Studies in the Scope and Method of "The Authoritarian Personality."* Glencoe, Ill., Free Press, 1954.

94. Clausen, J.: Family structure, socialization, and personality. In: *Review of Child Development Research* (L.W. Hoffman and M.L. Hoffman, Eds.). New York, Russell Sage Foundation, 1966.

95. Cloward, R.A., and Ohlin, L.E.: *Delinquency and Opportunity: A Theory of Delinquent Gangs.* New York, Free Press, 1960.

96. Cobrink, R.W., Hood, R.T., and Chusid, E.: The effect of maternal narcotic addiction on the newborn infant: Review of literature and report of 22 cases. Pediatrics, 24:288, 1959.

97. Cohen, A.K.: *Delinquent Boys: The Culture of the Gang.* New York, Free Press, 1955.

98. Cohen, D.J., and Zigler, E.: Federal day care standards: Rationale and recommendations. Am. J. Orthopsychiatry, 47:456, 1977.

99. Cole, S.O.: Hyperkinetic children: The use of stimulant drugs evaluated. Am. J. Orthopsychiatry, 45:28, 1975.

100. Coles, R.: Privileged American Children. Pediatrics, 60:381, 1977.

101. Comer, J., and Poussaint, A.: *Black Child Care.* New York, Simon & Schuster, 1975.

102. Comly, H.H., and Hadjisky, M.: One clinic's response to Head Start: A program of mental health appraisals. J. Am. Acad. Child Psychiatry, 6:398, 1967.

103. Conger, J.J.: *Personality, Social Class and Delinquency.* New York, Wiley, 1966.

104. Coolidge, J.C., et al.: School phobia in adolescence: A manifestation of severe character disorder. Am. J. Orthopsychiatry, 30:599, 1960.

105. Cooper, H.A.: Hallucinogenic drugs. Lancet, 268:1078, 1955.

106. Cooper, M.M.: *Pica.* Springfield, Ill., Thomas, 1957.

107. Coppolillo, H.P.: A conceptual model for study of some abusing parents. In: *The Child in His Family: Vulnerable Children.* (E.J. Anthony, C. Koupernik, and C. Chiland, Eds.). New York, Wiley, 1978.

108. Critchley, M.: *Developmental Dyslexia.* London, Heinemann, 1964.

109. Cutter, A.V., and Hallowitz, D.: Diagnosis and treatment of the family unit with respect to the character-disordered youngster. J. Am. Acad. Child Psychiatry, 1:605, 1962.

110. Dann, M., Levine, S.Z., and New, E.V.: A long-term follow-up of small premature infants. Pediatrics, 33:945, 1964.

111. Davidson, M.: Constipation and fecal incontinence. Pediatr. Clin. North Am., 5:749, 1958.

112. Davidson, M., Kugler, M.M., and Bauer, C.H.: Diagnosis and management in children with severe and protracted constipation and obstipation. J. Pediatr., 62:261, 1963.

113. DeBakey, M., and Ochsner, A.: Bezoars and concretions. Surgery, 4:934, 1938.

114. DeFries, J., Jenkins, S., and Williams, E.C.: Treatment of disturbed children in foster care. Am. J. Orthopsychiatry, 34:615, 1964.

115. DeHaan, R.F., and Havighurst, R.J.: Educating

Gifted Children. Chicago, University of Chicago Press, 1957.

116. DeHirsch, K., Jansky, J., and Langford, W.: Comparisons between prematurely and maturely born children at three age levels. Am. J. Orthopsychiatry, *36*:616, 1966.

117. DeHirsch, K., Jansky, J.J., and Langford, W.S.: *Predicting Reading Failure.* New York, Harper & Row, 1967.

118. Deisher, R.W., and O'Leary, J.F.: Early medical care of delinquent children. Pediatrics, *25*:329, 1950.

119. Deisher, R.W., et al.: Drug abuse in adolescence: The use of harmful drugs—A pediatric concern. Pediatrics, *44*:131, 1969.

120. Derdeyn, A.P.: Children in divorce: Intervention in the phase of separation. Pediatrics, *60*:20, 1977.

121. Dinello, F.A., and Champelli, J.: The use of imipramine in the treatment of enuresis: A review of the literature. Can. Psychiatr. Assoc. J., *13*:237, 1968.

122. Dixon, K.N., Arnold, L.E., and Calestro, K.: Father-son incest: Underreported psychiatric problem? Am. J. Psychiatry, *135*:835, 1978.

123. Dizmang, L.H., et al.: Adolescent suicide at an Indian reservation. Am. J. Orthopsychiatry, *44*:43, 1974.

124. Dodds, J., and Santostefano, S.: A comparison of the cognitive functioning of gluesniffers and nonsniffers. J. Pediatr., *64*:565, 1964.

125. Drew, A.L.: A neurological appraisal of familial congenital word blindness. Brain, *79*:440, 1956.

126. Drillien, C.: *The Growth and Development of the Prematurely Born Infant.* Baltimore, Williams & Wilkins, 1964.

127. Dwyer, J.F.: Teenage pregnancy. Am. J. Obstet. Gynecol., *118*:373, 1974.

128. Edlund, C.V.: A reinforcement approach to the elimination of a child's school phobia. Ment. Hygiene, *55*:433, 1971.

129. Ehrenbranz, J., Bliss, E., and Sheard, M.H.: Plasma testosterone: Correlation with aggressive behavior and social dominance in man. Psychosom. Med., *36*:469, 1974.

130. Eideson, B.T., and Lifermore, J.B.: Complications in therapy with adopted children. Am. J. Orthopsychiatry, *23*:795, 1953.

131. Eisenberg, L.: School phobia: A study in the communication of anxiety. Am. J. Psychiatry, *114*:712, 1958.

132. Eisenberg, L.: The pediatric management of school phobia. J. Pediatr., *35*: 758, 1959.

133. Eisenberg, L.: The sins of the fathers: Urban decay and social pathology. Am. J. Orthopsychiatry, *32*:5, 1962.

134. Eisenberg, L.: Deprivation and foster care. J. Am. Acad. Child Psychiatry, *4*:243, 1965.

135. Eisenberg, L.: Reading retardation. I. Psychiatric and sociological aspects. Pediatrics, *37*:352, 1966.

136. Eisenberg, L.: Hyperkinesis revisited. Pediatrics, *61*:319, 1978.

137. Eisenberg, L., Marlowe, B., and Hastings, M.: Diagnostic services for maladjusted foster children: An orientation toward an acute need. Am. J. Orthopsychiatry, *28*:750, 1958.

138. Eissler, K.R.: Ego-psychological implications of the psychoanalytic treatment of delinquents. Psychoanal. Study Child, *4*:97, 1950.

139. Ekdahl, M.C., Rice, E.P., and Schmidt, W.M.: Children of parents hospitalized for mental illness. Am. J. Public Health, *52*:15, 1962.

140. Elmer, E., and Gregg, G.: Developmental characteristics of abused children. Pediatrics, *40*:596, 1967.

141. Elmer, E.: Failure to thrive: Role of the mother. Pediatrics, *25*:725, 1960.

142. Emde, R.N., Gainsbauer, T.J., and Harmon, R.J.: *Emotional Expression in Infancy: A Biobehavioral Study.* Psychol. Iss., *10*:Mon. No. 37, 1976.

143. Engel, M.: Public education and the "emotionally disturbed" child. J. Am. Acad. Child Psychiatry, *3*:617, 1964.

144. Epstein, N., and Slavson, S.R.: Further observations on group psychotherapy with adolescent delinquent boys in residential treatment. I. "Breakthrough" in delinquent adolescent boys. Int. J. Psychother., *12*:199, 1962.

145. Erikson, E.: *Childhood and Society.* Rev. Ed., New York, Norton, 1963.

146. Evans, N.S.: Mourning as a family secret. J. Am. Acad. Child Psychiatry, *15*:502, 1976.

147. Ewing, J.A., and Rouse, B.A.: Therapeutic abortion and a prior psychiatric history. Am. J. Psychiatry, *130*:37, 1973.

148. Falek, A.: Handedness: A family study. Am. J. Hum. Genet., *11*:52, 1959.

149. Fanaroff, A.A., Kennell, J.H., and Klaus, M.H.: Follow-up of low birth weight infants—the predictive value of maternal visiting patterns. Pediatrics, *49*:287, 1972.

150. Fanshiel, D.: The pediatrician and children in foster care. Pediatrics, *60*:255, 1977.

151. Farnsworth, D.L.: *Psychiatry, Education and the Adult.* Springfield, Ill., Thomas, 1966.

152. Farraghu, M.E.: Therapeutic tutoring as an approach to psychogenic learning disturbances. J. Spec. Ed., *2*:117, 1968.

153. Finch, S.M.: Sexual activity of children with other children and adults. Clin. Pediatr., *6*:1, 1967.

154. Fineman, J.B., Kuniholm, P., and Sheridan, S.: Spasmus nutans: A syndrome of auto-arousal. J. Am. Acad. Child Psychiatry, *10*:136, 1971.

155. Fink, M., et al.: Prolonged adverse reactions to LSD in psychotic subjects. Arch. Gen. Psychiatry, *15*:450, 1966.

156. Fischoff, J., Whitten, C.F., and Petit, M.G.: A psychiatric study of mothers and infants with growth failure secondary to maternal deprivation. J. Pediatr., *79*:209, 1971.

157. Fleisher, D.R.: Diagnosis and treatment of disorders of defecation in children. Pediatr. Ann., *5*:70, 1976.

158. Folland, D.S., et al.: Gonorrhea in preadolescent children: An inquiry into source of infection and mode of transmission. Pediatrics, *60*:153, 1977.

159. Fontana, V.J., and Schneider, C.: Help for abusing parents. In: *Helping Parents Help Their Children* (L.E. Arnold, Ed.). New York, Brunner/Mazel, 1978.

160. Fordman, A., and Estrada, C.: Adolescents who

commit accidental homicide: The emotional consequences to the individual, family and community. J. Am. Acad. Psychiatry, *16*:314, 1970.

161. Frankl, L.: Self-preservation and the development of accident-proneness in children and adolescents. Psychoanal. Study Child, *18*:464, 1963.

162. Freedman, A., and Wilson, E.: Childhood and adolescent addictive disorders. I. Pediatrics, *34*:254, 1964.

162a. Freedman, A., and Wilson, E.: Childhood and adolescent addictive disorders. II. Pediatrics, *34*:283, 1964.

163. Friedman, S.B.: Management of death of a parent or sibling. In: *Ambulatory Pediatrics* (M. Green and R.J. Haggerty, Eds.). Philadelphia, Saunders, 1968.

164. Furman, E.: *A Child's Parent Dies: Studies in Childhood Bereavement.* New Haven, Yale University Press, 1974.

165. Furstenberg, F.F.: *Unplanned Parenthood: The Social Consequences of Teenage Childbearing.* New York, Free Press, 1976.

166. Gaddini, R.D., and Gaddini, E.: Rumination in infancy. In: *Dynamic Psychopathology in Childhood* (L. Jessner, and E. Pavenstedt, Eds.). New York, Grune & Stratton, 1959.

167. Gardner, R.A.: *Psychotherapy with Children of Divorce.* New York, Jason Aronson, 1976.

168. Garrard, S.D., and Richmond, J.B.: Psychogenic megacolon manifested by fecal soiling. Pediatrics, *10*:474, 1952.

169. Gebber, H., and Meyer, V.: Behavior therapy and encopresis: The complexities involved in treatment. Behav. Res. Ther., *2*:227, 1965.

170. Gebhard, P.H., et al.: *Sex Offenders.* New York, Harper & Row, 1965.

171. Geist, R.A.: Some observations on adolescent drug use: Therapeutic implications. J. Am. Acad. Child Psychiatry, *13*:54, 1974.

172. Geleerd, E.R.: Observations on temper tantrums in children. Am. J. Orthopsychiatry, *15*:238, 1945.

173. Gerard, M.: Enuresis: A study in etiology. Am. J. Orthopsychiatry, *9*:48, 1939.

174. Gerard, M.W., and Dukette, R.: Techniques for preventing separation trauma in child placement. Am. J. Orthopsychiatry, *20*:293, 1950.

175. Glaser, K.: Attempted suicide in children and adolescents. Am. J. Psychotherapy, *19*:220, 1965.

176. Glaser, K.: Masked depression in children and adolescents. Am. J. Psychotherapy, *21*:565, 1967.

177. Glicklich, L.B.: An historical account of enuresis. Pediatrics, *8*:859, 1951.

178. Glidewell, J., and Swallow, C.: *The Prevalence of Maladjustment in Elementary Schools.* Report prepared for the Joint Commission on Mental Health of Children, Chicago, University of Chicago Press, July 26, 1968.

179. Glueck, S., and Glueck, E.T.: *Unraveling Juvenile Delinquency.* Cambridge, Mass., Harvard University Press, 1950.

180. Glueck, S., and Glueck, E.T.: *Predicting Delinquency and Crime.* Cambridge, Mass., Harvard University Press, 1959.

181. Goldfarb, W.: Effects of psychological depriva-tion in infancy and subsequent stimulation. Am. J. Psychiatry, *102*:18, 1945.

182. Goldstein, J., Freud, A., and Solnit, A.J.: *Beyond the Best Interests of the Child.* New York, Free Press, 1973.

183. Graffagnino, P.N.: A Head Start school in a child psychiatric clinic: Cornerstone of a collaborative program. J. Am. Acad. Child Psychiatry, *6*:415, 1967.

184. Gray, J.D., et al.: Prediction and prevention of child abuse and neglect. Child Abuse Neglect, *1*:45, 1977.

185. Green, A.H.: Psychiatric treatment of abused children. J. Am. Acad. Child Psychiatry, *17*:356, 1978.

186. Green, A.H.: Psychopathology of abused children. J. Am. Acad. Child Psychiatry, *17*:92, 1978.

187. Greenberg, M., et al.: A study of pica in relation to lead poisoning. Pediatrics, *22*:756, 1958.

188. Greenberg, N.H.: Origins of head-rolling (spasmus nutans) during early infancy: Clinical observations and theoretical implications. Psychosom. Med., *26*:162, 1964.

189. Greenberg, N.H., Loesch, J.G., and Lakin, M.: Life situation associated with the onset of pregnancy. I. The role of separation in a group of unmarried pregnant women. Psychosom. Med., *21*:296, 1959.

190. Grunebaum, M.G., et al.: Fathers of sons with primary neurotic learning inhibitions. Am. J. Orthopsychiatry, *32*:462, 1962.

191. Guides for Juvenile Court Judges. National Council on Crime and Delinquency, New York, 1963.

192. Guttmacher, A.F.: Unwanted pregnancy: A challenge to mental health. Ment. Hygiene, *51*:512, 1967.

193. Haggard, E.: Socialization, personality, and academic achievement in gifted children. School Rev., *14*:388, 1957.

194. Haggerty, R.J.: Home accidents in childhood. N. Engl. J. Med., *13*:22, 1959.

195. Hallgren, B.: Enuresis. I. A study with reference to the morbidity risks and symptomatology. Acta Psychiatr. Neurol. Scand., *31*:379, 1956.

196. Hallgren, B.: Enuresis. II. A study with reference to certain physical, mental, and social factors possibly associated with enuresis. Acta Psychiatr. Neurol., *31*:405, 1956.

197. Hallgren, B.: Enuresis: A clinical and genetic study. Acta Psychiatr. Neurol. Scand., *32*:1, 1957.

198. Hallinan, Helen W.: Adoption for older children. Soc. Casework, *33*:277, 1952.

199. Hamilton, J.A.: *Post-partum Psychiatric Problems.* St. Louis, Mosby, 1962.

200. Hanson, F.N., and Rock, J.: The effect of adoption on fertility and other reproductive functions. Am. J. Obstet. Gynecol., *59*:311, 1950.

201. Harbin, H.T.: Episodic dyscontrol and family dynamics. Am. J. Psychiatry, *134*:1113, 1977.

202. Harper, P.A., et al.: Neurological and intellectual status of prematures at three to five years of age. J. Pediatr., *55*:679, 1959.

203. Hatherington, E.M.: Girls without fathers. Psychol. Today, *6*:47, 1973.

204. Havighurst, R.J., and Davis, A.A.: A comparison of the Chicago and Harvard studies of social class differences in child rearing. Am. Sociol. Rev., *20*:438, 1955.

205. Heckel, R.V.: The effects of fatherlessness on the preadolescent female. Ment. Hygiene, *47*:69, 1962.

206. Heinecke, C.M., et al.: The organization of day care: Considerations relating to the mental health of the child and family. Am. J. Orthopsychiatry, *43*:8, 1973.

207. Helfer, R.E., and Kempe, C.H.: *The Battered Child.* 2nd Ed., Chicago, University of Chicago Press, 1974.

208. Helfer, R.E., and Schmitt, B.D.: The community-based child abuse and neglect program. In R.E. Helfer and C.H. Kempe, Eds.: *Child Abuse and Neglect. The Family and the Community.* Cambridge, Mass., Ballinger, 1976.

209. Heller, J.R., and Derdeyn, A.P.: Child custody evaluation in abuse and neglect: A practical guide. Child Psychiatry Hum. Dev., *9*:171, 1979.

210. Hellman, I.: Some observations on mothers of children with intellectual inhibitions. Psychoanal. Study Child., *9*:259, 1954.

211. Herzog, E., and Sudia, C.E.: Children in fatherless families. In: *Review of Child Development Research.* Chicago, University of Chicago Press, 1973, Vol. 3.

212. Hilgard, J.R.: Strength of adult ego following childhood bereavement. Am. J. Orthopsychiatry, *30*:788, 1960.

213. Hitschman, M.: Unpublished material.

214. Hodge, K.S., and Hutchings, H.M.: Enuresis: A brief review, a tentative theory, and a suggested treatment. Arch. Dis. Child., *27*:498, 1952.

215. Holinger, P.C.: Adolescent suicide. An epidemiological study of recent trends. Am. J. Psychiatry, *135*:754, 1978.

216. Holter, J.C., and Friedman, S.B.: Child abuse: Early case finding in the emergency department. Pediatrics, *42*:128, 1968.

217. Hunter, R.S., et al.: Antecedents of child abuse and neglect in premature infants: A prospective study in a newborn intensive care unit. Pediatrics, *61*:629, 1978.

218. Husband, P., and Hinton, P.E.: Physical, psychiatric illness found in families of accident prone children. Arch. Dis. Child., *47*:396, 1972.

219. Huschka, M.: The child's response to coercive bowel training. Psychosom. Med., *4*:301, 1942.

220. Illingworth, R.S.: Three months colic. Arch. Dis. Child., *29*:165, 1954.

221. Jacobs, J., and Teicher, J.: Broken homes and social isolation in attempted suicides of adolescents. Int. J. Psychiatry, *13*:139, 1967.

222. Johnson, A.M.: Sanctions for superego lacunae of adolescents. In: *Searchlights on Delinquency* (K.R. Eisler, Ed.). New York, International Universities Press, 1949.

223. Johnson, A.M., and Szurek, S.: The genesis of antisocial acting out in children and adults. Psychoanal. Q., *21*:323, 1952.

224. Johnson, W.: *Stuttering in Children and Adults.* Minneapolis, University of Minnesota Press, 1958.

225. Jones, H.G.: The behavioral treatment of enuresis nocturne. In: *Behavior Therapy and the Neuroses* (H.J. Eysenck, Ed.). New York, Pergamon, 1960.

226. Jones, K.L., and Smith, D.: Recognition of the fetal alcohol syndrome in early infancy. Lancet, *2*:999, 1973.

227. Kanner, L.: *Child Psychiatry.* Springfield, Ill., Thomas, 1957.

228. Kaplan, D., and Mason, E.: Maternal reactions to premature birth viewed as an acute emotional disorder. Am. J. Orthopsychiatry, *30*:539, 1960.

229. Kaplan, L.K., and Turtz, L.: Treatment of severely emotionally traumatized young children in foster home setting. Am. J. Orthopsychiatry, *27*:271, 1957.

230. Kaplan, M.: The suicide prevention center. Soc. Work Papers, *10*:32, 1963.

231. Karlin, I.W.: Incidence of spina bifida occulta in children with and without enuresis. Am. J. Dis. Child., *49*:19, 1935.

232. Katan, A.: Experience with enuretics. Psychoanal. Study Child., *2*:241, 1946.

233. Kaufman, I.: Crimes of violence and delinquency in schizophrenic children. J. Child Psychiatry, *1*:269, 1962.

234. Kaufman, I., Heims, L.W., and Reiser, D.E.: A re-evaluation of the psychodynamics of firesetting. Am. J. Orthopsychiatry, *31*:123, 1961.

235. Kaufman, I., Tagiuri, C., and Peck, A.: The family constellation and overt incestuous relations between father and daughter. Am. J. Orthopsychiatry, *24*:266, 1954.

236. Kaufman, P.N., and Deutsch, A.L.: Group therapy for pregnant unwed adolescents in the prenatal clinic of a general hospital. Int. J. Group Psychother., *17*:309, 1967.

237. Kellam, S.G., et al.: Psychiatric aspects of child day care programs. In: *Comprehensive Textbook of Psychiatry.* 2nd Ed. (A. Freedman, H. Kaplan, and B. Sadock, Eds.). Baltimore, Williams & Wilkins, 1975, Vol. 2.

238. Kellerman, J.: *Childhood Encopresis: A Multimodal Therapeutic Approach.* Bull. Child. Hosp., Los Angeles, May–June, 1977.

239. Kelly, J.B., and Wallerstein, J.S.: The effects of parental divorce: Experiences of the child in early latency. Am. J. Orthopsychiatry, *46*:20, 1976.

240. Kempe, C.H.: Sexual abuse, another hidden pediatric problem. The 1977 C. Anderson Aldrich Lecture. Pediatrics. *62*:382, 1978.

241. Kempe, C.H., et al.: The Battered Child Syndrome. JAMA, *181*:17, 1962.

242. Kennell, J.H., Slyter, H., and Klaus, M.H.: The mourning response of parents to the death of a newborn infant. N. Engl. J. Med., *283*:344, 1970.

243. Kenny, T.J., and Clemmens, R.L.: Medical and psychological correlates in children with learning disabilities. Pediatrics, *78*:273, 1971.

244. Kephart, V.C.: *The Slow Learner in the Classroom.* Springfield, Ohio, Merrill, 1960.

245. Kerr, M.A.D., Bogries, J.L., and Kerr, D.S.: Psy-

chosocial functioning of mothers of malnourished children. Pediatrics, *62*:778, 1978.

246. King, C.H.: Counter-transference and counterexperience in the treatment of violence-prone youth. Am. J. Orthopsychiatry, *46*:43, 1976.

247. Kinsey, L.R.: Outpatient group therapy with juvenile delinquents. Dis. Nerv. System, *30*:472, 1969.

248. Klaus, M.H., et al.: Maternal attachment: Importance of the first postpartum days. N. Engl. J. Med., *286*:460, 1972.

249. Koel, B.S.: Failure to thrive and fatal injury as a continuum. Am. J. Dis. Child., *118*:565, 1969.

250. Kravitz, H., et al.: A study of head-banging in infants and children. Dis. Nerv. Syst., *21*:203, 1960.

251. Kvaraceus, W.C.: *Delinquent Behavior: Culture and the Individual*. Washington, D.C., National Education Association, 1959.

252. Langford, W.S.: Disturbances in mother-infant relationship leading to apathy, extra-nutritive sucking and hairball. In: *Emotional Problems of Early Childhood*. G. Caplan, Ed. New York, Basic Books, 1955.

253. Laufer, M., and Denhoff, E.: Hyperkinetic behavior syndrome in children. J. Pediatrics, *50*:463, 1957.

254. Lehman, E.: Psychogenic incontinence of feces (encopresis) in children: Report of recovery of four patients following psychotherapy. Am. J. Dis. Child., *68*:190, 1944.

254a. Leifer, A.W., Leiderman, P.H., et al.: Effects of mother-infant separation on maternal attachment behavior. Child Dev., *43*:1203, 1972.

255. Leonard, M.: Failure to thrive in infants. Am. J. Dis. Child., *3*:608, 1966.

256. Leonard, M.F.: The significance of pica in children. Community Med., *35*:479, 1971.

257. Lesser, L.: Hyperkinesis in children. Clin. Pediatr., *9*:548, 1970.

258. Levenson, E.A., Stockhamer, N., and Feiner, A.H.: Family transactions in the etiology of dropping out of college. Contemp. Psychoanal., *3*:134, 1967.

259. Levine, M.D., and Bakow, H.: Children with encopresis: A study of treatment outcome. Pediatrics, *58*:845, 1976.

260. Levine, M.D., and Bell, A.J.: The treatment of "colic" in infancy by the use of the pacifier. J. Pediatr., *37*:750, 1950.

261. Lewis, D.O., and Balla, D.: *Delinquency and Psychopathology*. New York, Grune & Stratton, 1976.

262. Lewis, D.O., et al.: Delinquency, parental psychopathology, and parental criminality: Clinical and epidemiological findings. J. Am. Acad. Child. Psychiatry, *15*:665, 1976.

263. Lewis, D.O., et al.: Introducing a child psychiatric service to a juvenile justice setting. J. Child Psychiatr. Hum. Dev., *42*:98, 1973.

264. Lewis, D.O., and Shanok, S.S.: Delinquency and the schizophrenic spectrum of disorders. J. Am. Acad. Child Psychiatry, *17*:263, 1978.

265. Lewis, M., and Solnit, A.: The adolescent in a suicidal crisis: Collaborative care on a pediatric ward. In: *Modern Perspectives in Child Development*

(A. Solnit and S. Provence, Eds.). New York, International Universities Press, 1963.

266. Lewis, M., et al.: An exploratory study of accidental ingestion of poison in young children. J. Am. Acad. Child. Psychiatry, *5*:235, 1966.

267. Lewis, M., and Sorrel, P.M.: The management of sexual assault upon children. In: *Ambulatory Pediatrics* (M. Green and R.J. Haggerty, Eds.). Philadelphia, Saunders, 1968.

268. Lewis, C.: *Children of the Cumberland*. New York, Columbia University Press, 1946.

269. Lindemann, E., and Ross, A.: A follow-up study of a predictive test of social adaptation in preschool children. In: *Emotional Problems of Early Childhood* (G. Caplan, Ed.). New York, Basic Books, 1955.

270. Lindemann, E., Vaughn, W.T., Jr., and McGinnis, M.: Preventive intervention in a four-year-old child whose father committed suicide. In: *Emotional Problems of Early Childhood* (G. Caplan, Ed.). New York, Basic Books, 1955.

271. Litt, I.F., Edberg, S., and Finberg, L.: Gonorrhea in children and adolescents: A current review. J. Pediatr., *85*:595, 1974.

272. Littner, N.: The child's need to repeat his past: Some implications for placement. In: *Changing Needs and Practices in Child Welfare*. New York, Child Welfare League of America, 1960.

273. Loesch, J.G., and Greenberg, N.H.: Some specific areas of conflicts observed during pregnancy: A comparative study of married and unmarried mothers. Am. J. Orthopsychiatry, *32*:624, 1962.

274. Lombroso, C.T., and Lerman, P.: Breathholding spells (cyanotic and pallid infantile syncope). Pediatrics, *39*:563, 1967.

275. Loof, D.H.: *Appalachia's Children*. Lexington, Kentucky, University of Kentucky Press, 1971.

276. Loughmiller, C.: *Wilderness Road*. Austin, Texas, The Hogg Foundation, University of Texas, 1965.

277. Lourie, R.: Personal communication.

278. Lourie, R.: The role of rhythmic patterns in childhood. Am. J. Psychiatry, *106*:653, 1949.

279. Low, M.B.: The Education for All Handicapped Children Act of 1975: A pediatrician's viewpoint. Pediatrics, *62*:271, 1978.

280. Lubchenko, L., et al.: Sequelae of premature birth. Am. J. Dis. Child., *106*:101, 1963.

281. Luepker, E.T.: Joint admission and evaluation of postpartum psychiatric patients and their infants. Hosp. Community Psychiatry, *23*:284, 1972.

282. Machotka, P., Pittman, F.S., and Flomenhaft, K.: Incest as a family affair. Fam. Process, *6*:98, 1967.

283. Main, T.F.: Mothers with children in a psychiatric hospital. Lancet, *2*:845, 1958.

284. Malmquist, C.P.: School phobia: A problem in family neurosis. J. Am. Acad. Child Psychiatry, *4*:293, 1965.

285. Malmquist, C.P.: The role of parental mental illness in custody proceedings. Fam. Law Q., *21*:360, 1968.

286. Malmquist, C.P.: Depressions in childhood and adolescence. N. Engl. J. Med., *284*:887, 1971.

287. Mann, E.C.: The role of emotional determinants in habitual abortion. Surg. Clin. North Am., *37*:447, 1957.

288. Mann, E.C., et al.: Habitual abortion: A report in two parts on 160 patients. Am. J. Obstet. Gynecol., *77*:706, 1959.

289. Mannino, F.V., and Delgado, R.A.: Trichotillomania in children. Am. J. Psychiatry, *126*:505, 1969.

290. Martin, H.L.: Antecedents of burns and scalds in children. Br. J. Med. Psychol., *43*:39, 1970.

291. Martin, H.P.: Development of the battered child. In: *Helping the Battered Child and his Family*. Philadelphia, Lippincott, 1972.

292. Martin, H.P.: A child-oriented approach to prevention of abuse. In: *Child Abuse: Prediction, Prevention, and Follow-up*. New York, Churchill Livingstone, 1977.

293. Massengale, O.N., et al.: Physical and psychological factors in glue sniffing. N. Engl. J. Med., *269*:121, 1963.

294. Mason, E.A.: A method of predicting crisis outcome for mothers of premature babies. Public Health Rep., *78*:1031, 1963.

295. Mass, H.S., and Engler, R.E.: *Children in Need of Parents*. New York, Columbia University Press, 1959.

296. Mattsson, A., Seese, L.R., and Hawkins, J.W.: Suicidal behavior as a child psychiatric emergency. Arch. Gen. Psychiatry, *20*:100, 1969.

297. McAlister, A.L., Perry, C., and Maccoby, N.: Adolescent smoking: Onset and prevention. Pediatrics, *63*:650, 1979.

298. McAnarney, E.R., et al.: Obstetric, neonatal, and psychosocial outcome of pregnant adolescents. Pediatrics, *61*:199, 1978.

299. McCord, W., et al.: Early familial experiences and bigotry. Am. Soc. Review, *25*:717, 1960.

300. McDermott, J.F., Jr.: Divorce and its psychiatric sequelae in children. Arch. Gen. Psychiatry, *23*:421, 1970.

301. McDonald, J.M.: *Rape: Offenders and their Victims*. Springfield, Ill., Thomas, 1977.

302. McDonald, R.L.: The role of emotional factors in obstetric complications: A review. Psychosom. Med., *30*:222, 1968.

303. McDonald, R.L., and Parham, K.J.: Relation of emotional changes during pregnancy to obstetrical complications in unmarried primigravidas. Am. J. Obstet. Gynecol., *90*:195, 1964.

304. McFadden, M., and Wechsler, H.: Minimum drinking age laws and teenage drinking. Psychiatr. Opinion, *16*:22, 1979.

305. McWhinnie, A.M.: The adopted child in adolescence. In: *Adolescence: Psychosocial Perspectives*. New York, Basic Books, 1969.

306. Mednick, S.A., and Schulsinger, F.: Some premorbid characteristics related to breakdown in children with schizophrenic mothers. In: *The Transmission of Schizophrenia* (D. Rosenthal and S. Vetz, Eds.). London, Pergamon, 1965.

307. Meeks, J.E.: Group delinquent reaction. In: *Comprehensive Textbook of Psychiatry* (A. Freedman, H. Kaplan, and B. Saddock, Eds.). Baltimore, Williams & Wilkins, 1975, Vol. 2.

308. Meyer, R.J., et al.: Accidental injury to the preschool child. J. Pediatr., *63*:95, 1963.

309. Meyer-Bahlburg, H.F.L., et al.: Aggressiveness and testosterone measures in man. Psychosom. Med., *36*:269, 1974.

310. Michaels, J.J.: Parallels between persistent enuresis and delinquency in the psychopathic personality. Am. J. Orthopsychiatry, *11*:260, 1941.

311. Miller, D.: *Growth to Freedom: The Psychosocial Treatment of Delinquent Youth*. London, Travistock, 1964.

312. Millikan, F.K., et al.: Emotional factors in the etiology and treatment of lead poisoning. Am. J. Dis. Child., *91*:144, 1966.

313. Milowe, I.D., and Lourie, R.S.: The child's role in the battered child syndrome. J. Pediatr., *65*:1079, 1964.

314. Minuchin, S., et al.: *Families of the Slums*. New York, Basic Books, 1967.

315. Monahan, J.: Prediction research and the emergency commitment of dangerously mentally ill persons: A reconsideration. Am. J. Psychiatry, *135*:198, 1978.

316. Morrison, G.C., and Collier, J.C.: Family treatment approaches to suicidal children and adolescents. J. Am. Acad. Child Psychiatry, *8*:140, 1969.

317. Mudd, E.H., et al.: Adolescent health services and contraceptive use. Am. J. Orthopsychiatry, *48*:495, 1978.

318. Muellner, S.R.: Development of urinary control in children: Some of the causes and treatment of primary enuresis. JAMA, *172*:1256, 1960.

319. Murphy, S., Nickols, J., and Hammer, S.: Neurological evaluation of adolescent enuretics. Pediatrics, *45*:269, 1970.

320. Nadelson, C.C., and Notman, M.T.: Psychological responses to rape. Psychiatr. Opinion, *14*:13, 1977.

321. Nakashima, I.J., and Zakus, G.E.: Incest: Review and clinical experience. Pediatrics, *60*:696, 1977.

322. Nakashima, I.: Teenage pregnancy—Its causes, costs, and consequences. Nurse Practitioner, *2*:10, 1977.

323. Neubauer, P.B.: The one-parent child and his Oedipal development. Psychoanal. Study Child, *15*:286, 1960.

324. Newman, M.B., and San Martino, M.R.: The child and the seriously disturbed parent: Patterns of adaptation to parental psychosis. J. Am. Acad. Child Psychiatry, *10*:358, 1971.

325. Noshpitz, J.D., and Spielman, P.: Diagnosis: Study of the differential characteristics of hyperaggressive children. Am. J. Orthopsychiatry, *31*:111, 1961.

326. Oppel, W.C., Harper, P.A., and Rider, R.V.: The age of attaining bladder control. Pediatrics, *42*:614, 1968.

327. Orton, S.T.: *Reading, Writing, and Speech Problems in Children*. New York, Norton, 1937.

328. Osofsky, J.D., and Osofsky, H.J.: The psychological reactions of patients to legalized abortion. Am. J. Orthopsychiatry, *42*:48, 1972.

329. Paradise, J.L.: Maternal and other factors in the etiology of infantile colic. JAMA, *197*:191, 1966.

330. Parcel, G.S., Nader, P.R., and Meyer, M.P.: Adolescent health concerns, problems, and patterns of utilization in a triethnic urban population. Pediatrics, *60*:157, 1977.

331. Pavenstedt, E.: A comparison of the child-rearing environment of upper-lower and very low-lower class families. Am. J. Orthopsychiatry, *35*:89, 1965.

332. Pavenstedt, E.: *The Drifters: Children of Disorganized Lower-Class Families.* Boston, Little, Brown, 1972.

333. Peck, H.B.: *Treatment of the Delinquent Adolescent; Group and Individual Therapy with Parent and Child.* New York, Family Service Association of America, 1954.

334. Pediatrician's Role in Day Care of Children. Report of Committee on Community Health Services, American Academy of Pediatrics. Pediatrics, *52*:746, 1973.

335. Pierce, C.: Effects of Racism on Kids. In I.N. Berlin, Ed.: *Advocacy for Child Mental Health.* New York, Brunner-Mazel, 1975.

336. Pierce, C.M., et al.: Enuresis and dreaming. Arch. Gen. Psychiatry, *4*:166, 1961.

337. Pincus, J.H., and Tucker, G.J.: Violence in children and adults: A neurological view. J. Am. Acad. Child Psychiatry, *17*:277, 1978.

338. Pinkerton, P.: Psychogenic megacolon in children: The implications of bowel negativism. Arch. Dis. Child., *33*:371, 1958.

339. Podolsky, E.: Children who kill. G.P., *31*:98, 1965.

340. Poznanski, E.O., Korahenbuhl, V., and Zrull, J.P.: Childhood depression—A longitudinal perspective. J. Am. Acad. Child Psychiatry, *15*:491, 1976.

341. Poznanski, E., Maxey, A., and Marsden, G.: Clinical implications of maternal employment: A review of research. J. Am. Acad. Child Psychiatry, *9*:741, 1970.

342. Proctor, J.T.: Countertransference phenomena in the treatment of severe character disorders in children and adolescents. In: *Dynamic Psychopathology in Childhood* (Jessner, L., and Pavenstedt, E., Eds.). New York, Grune & Stratton, 1959.

342a. Proskauer, S., and Rolland, R.S.: Youth who use drugs. J. Am. Acad. Child Psychiatry, *12*:32, 1973.

343. Provence, S.: *Guide for the Care of Infants in Groups,* New York, Child Welfare League of America, 1967.

344. Provence, S., and Coleman, R.: Environmental retardation (Hospitalism) in infants living in families. Pediatrics, *19*:285, 1957.

345. Provence, S., and Lipton, R.: *Infants in Institutions.* New York, International Universities Press, 1962.

346. Prugh, D.G.: Childhood experience and colonic disorder. Ann. N.Y. Acad. Sci., *58*:355, 1954.

347. Prugh, D.G., and Eckhardt, L.O.: Guidance by physicians and nurses: A developmental approach. In: *Helping Parents Help Their Children* (L.E. Arnold, Ed.). New York, Brunner/Mazel, 1978.

348. Prugh, D.G., and Harlow, R.G.: "Masked deprivation" in infants and young children. In: *Deprivation of Maternal Care. A Reassessment of its Effects.* Public Health Papers No. 14. Geneva, World Health Organization, 1962.

349. Prugh, D.G., Wermer, H., and Lord, J.: The significance of the anal phase for pediatrics and child psychiatry. In: *Case Studies in Childhood Emotional Disabilities* American Orthopsychiatric Association, 1956, Vol. 2.

350. Rapaport, J.: The psychopathology of learning difficulties. N. Y. State J. Med., *57*:382, 1951.

351. Rechtschaffen, A., Goodenough, D.R., and Shapiro, A.: Patterns of sleep talking. Arch. Gen. Psychiatry, *7*:418, 1962.

352. Redl, F., and Wineman, D.: *Controls from Within: Techniques for the Treatment of the Aggressive Child.* Glencoe, Ill., Free Press, 1952.

353. Reiner, B.S., and Kaufman, I.: *Character Disorders in Parents of Delinquents.* New York, Family Service Association of America, 1959.

354. Rexford, E.N.: *A Developmental Approach to Problems of Acting Out: A Symposium.* New York, International Universities Press, 1966.

355. Rice, E.P., Eckdahl, M.C., and Mitler, L.: *Children of Mentally Ill Parents.* New York, Behavioral Publications, 1971.

356. Richmond, J.B.: Some psychologic considerations in adoption practice. Pediatrics, *20*:377, 1957.

357. Richmond, J.B.: The pediatrician and the individual delinquent. Pediatrics, *26*:126, 1960.

358. Richmond, J.B., Eddy, E.J., and Garrard, S.D.: The syndrome of fecal soiling and megacolon. Am. J. Orthopsychiatry, *24*:391, 1954.

359. Richmond, J.B., Eddy, E., and Green, M.: Rumination: A psychosomatic syndrome of infancy. Pediatrics, *22*:49, 1958.

360. Ringrose, C.A.D.: Further observations on the psychosomatic character of toxemia of pregnancy. Can. Med. Assoc. J., *84*:1064, 1961.

361. Roberts, K.E., and Schoelkopf, J.A.: Eating, sleeping, and elimination practices of a group of two and one-half year old children. I. Introduction. Am. J. Dis. Child., *82*:121, 1951.

362. Robey, J.S.: Divorce. In: *Ambulatory Pediatrics* (M. Green and R.J. Haggerty, Eds.). Philadelphia, Saunders, 1968.

363. Robins, L.: *Deviant Children Grown Up.* Baltimore, Williams & Wilkins, 1966.

364. Robins, L.N., and O'Neal, P.: The adult prognosis for runaway children. Am. J. Orthopsychiatry, *29*:752, 1959.

365. Rosenblum, G.: A community mental health center's interaction with the project head program. J. Am. Acad. Child Psychiatry, *6*:410, 1967.

366. Rosenfeld, A.A., et al.: Incest and sexual abuse of children. J. Am. Acad. Child. Psychiatry, *16*:327, 1977.

367. Rosenwald, G.C., and Stonehill, M.W.: Early and late postpartum illnesses. Psychosom. Med., *34*:129, 1972.

368. Ross, A.O.: *Psychological Aspects of Learning Dis-*

abilities and Reading Disorders. New York, McGraw-Hill, 1974.

369. Rowe, D.S., et al.: A hospital program for the detection and registration of abused and neglected children. N. Engl. J. Med., *282*:950, 1970.

370. Rowntree, G.: Accidents among children under two years of age in Great Britain. J. Hyg., *48*:323, 1950.

371. Russell, D.: Personal communication.

372. Rutter, M.: Parent-child separation: Psychological effects on the child. J. Child Psychol. Psychiatry, *12*:233, 1971.

373. Sander, L., et al.: Effects of alcohol intake during pregnancy on newborn state regulation: A progress report, alcoholism. Clin. Exp. Res., *1*:233, 1977.

374. Sargent, D.: Children Who Kill— A family conspiracy. In: *Theory and Practice of Family Psychiatry* (J.G. Howells, Ed.). New York, Brunner-Mazel, 1971.

375. Sarles, R.M.: Incest: Symposium on behavioral pediatrics. Pediatr. Clin. North Am., *22*:633, 1975.

376. Scham, M.: Poverty, illness, and the Negro child. Pediatrics, *46*:305, 1970.

377. Schecter, M.: Observations on adopted children. Arch. Gen. Psychiatry, *3*:21, 1960.

378. Scheifele, M.: *The Gifted Child in the Regular Classroom*. New York, Teachers College, Columbia University, 1953.

379. Scherl, D.J., and Mack, J.E.: A study of adolescent matricide. J. Child Psychiatry, *5*:569, 1966.

380. Schmideberg, M.: Making the patient aware. Crime Delinq., *6*:255, 1960.

381. Schmitt, B.D.: *The Child Protection Team Handbook: A Multidisciplinary Approach to Managing Child Abuse and Neglect*. New York, Garland, 1978.

382. Schmitt, B.D.: School phobia—The great imitator: A pediatrician's viewpoint. Pediatrics, *48*:433, 1971.

383. Schmitt, B.D., et al.: The hyperactive child. Clin. Pediatr., *12*:154, 1973.

384. Shaw, R., and Eagle, C.: A clinic as catalyst in a Head Start program. J. Am. Acad. Child Psychiatry, *6*:388, 1967.

385. Shechter, M.: About adoptive parents. In: *Parenthood: Its Psychology and Psychopathology* (E.J. Anthony and T. Benedek, Eds.). Boston, Little, Brown, 1970.

386. Shoor, M., Speed, M.H., and Bartelt, C.: Syndrome of the adolescent child molester. Am. J. Psychiatry, *122*:783, 1966.

387. Shore, M.F., and Massimo, J.L.: Fifteen years after treatment: A follow-up study of comprehensive vocationally oriented psychiatry. Am. J. Orthopsychiatry, *49*:240, 1979.

388. Short, J.F.: Juvenile delinquency: The sociocultural context. In: Review of Child Development Research (L. Hoffman and M. Hoffman, Eds.). New York, Russell Sage Foundation, 1966, Vol. 2.

389. Silver, A.A., and Hagin, R.A.: Specific reading disability. Compr. Psychiatry, *1*:126, 1960.

390. Snyder, R.D.: Personal communication.

391. Snyder, R.D.: The right not to read. Pediatrics, *63*:71, 1979.

392. Sobel, R.: Psychiatric implications of accidental poisoning in childhood. Pediatr. Clin. North Am., *17*:653, 1971.

393. Sobel, R., and Margolis, J.A.: Repetitive poisoning in children: A Psychosocial Study. Pediatrics, *35*:141, 1965.

394. Solnit, A.J., and Stark, M.H.: Pediatric management of school learning problems of underachievement. N. Engl. J. Med., *261*:988, 1959.

395. Sours, J.A., et al.: Somnambulism. Arch. Gen. Psychiatry, *112*:400, 1963.

396. Spaulding, J.G., and Cavenar, J.O.: Psychosis following therapeutic abortion. Am. J. Psychiatry, *135*:364, 1978.

397. Sperling, M.: Dynamic considerations and treatment of enuresis. J. Am. Acad. Child Psychiatry, *4*:19, 1955.

398. Sperling, M.: Pavor nocturnus. J. Am. Acad. Child Psychiatry, *6*:79, 1958.

399. Sperry, B., et al.: Renunciation and denial in learning difficulties. Am. J. Orthopsychiatry, *28*:98, 1958.

400. Spitz, R.A.: The role of ecological factors in emotional development in children. Child Dev., *20*:145, 1949.

401. Spitz, R.: Psychiatric therapy in infancy. Am. J. Orthopsychiatry, *21*:623, 1950.

402. Spock, B., and Bergen, M.: Parents' fear of conflict in toilet training. Pediatrics, *34*:112, 1964.

403. Spurlock, J.: Problems of identification in young black children. J. Natl. Med. Assoc., *61*:504, 1969.

404. Stanley, E.J., and Barter, J.T.: Adolescent suicidal behavior. Am. J. Orthopsychiatry, *40*:87, 1970.

405. Statement on Parent and Newborn Interaction, Committee on Maternal and Child Care: Chicago, American Medical Association, House of Delegates, December, 1977.

406. Steele, B.F., and Pollock, C.B.: A psychiatric study of parents who abuse infants and small children. In: *The Battered Child*. 2nd Ed. (R.E. Helfer and C.H. Kempe, Eds.). Chicago, University of Chicago Press, 1974.

407. Stein, M.L., Rausen, A.R., and Blau, A.: Psychotherapy of an infant with rumination. JAMA, *171*:2309, 1959.

408. Stein, Z.A., and Susser, M.W.: Socio-medical study of enuresis among delinquent boys. Br. J. Prev. Soc. Med., *19*:174, 1965.

409. Stein, Z.A., Susser, M.W., and Wilson, A.E.: Families of enuretic children. I. Family type and age. II. Family culture, structure and organization. Dev. Med. Child. Neurol., *7*:658, 1968.

409a. Sterritt, G.: Personal communication.

410. Stewart, A.H., et al.: Excessive infant crying (colic) in relation to parent behavior. Am. J. Psychiatry, *110*:687, 1954.

411. Stierlin, H.: A family perspective on adolescent runaways. Arch. Gen. Psychiatry, *29*:56, 1973.

412. Stockwell, L., and Smith, C.K.: Enuresis: A study of causes, types, and therapeutic results. Am. J. Dis. Child., *59*:1013, 1940.

413. Stringer, L., and Glidewell, J.: *Final Report for*

Early Detection of Emotional Illness in School Children. Report to National Institute of Mental Health. St. Louis, County Health Dept., 1967.

414. Swift, J.: Effects of early group experience: The nursery school and day nursery. In: *Review of Child Development Research* (M. Hoffman, and L.W. Hoffman, Eds.). New York, Russell Sage Foundation, 1964.

415. Switzer, J.: A genetic approach to the understanding of learning problems. J. Am. Acad. Child Psychiatry, 2:653, 1963.

416. Talbott, J.A., and Teague, J.W.: Marihuana Psychosis. JAMA, 210:299, 1968.

417. Teicher, J., and Jacobs, J.: Adolescents who attempt suicide: Preliminary findings. Am. J. Psychiatry, 122:1748, 1966.

418. Tennes, K., et al.: The stimulus barrier in early infancy: An exploration of some formulations of John Benjamin. Psychoanal. Contemp. Sci., 1:206, 1972.

419. Tennes, K.H., and Lampl, E.E.: Stranger and separation anxiety in infancy. J. Nerv. Ment. Dis., 139:247, 1964.

420. Tennes, K.H., and Lampl, E.E.: Some aspects of mother-child relationship pertaining to infantile separation anxiety. J. Nerv. Ment. Dis., 143:426, 1966.

421. Teplitz, Z.: The ego and motility in sleepwalking. J. Am. Psychoanal. Assoc., 6:95, 1958.

422. Timmons, F.R.: Freshman withdrawal from college: A positive step toward identity formation? A follow-up study. J. Youth Adolesc., 8:2, 1978.

423. Toolan, J.M.: Suicide and suicidal attempts in children and in adolescents. Am. J. Psychiatry, 118:719, 1962.

424. Tooley, K.: Antisocial behavior and social alienation post divorce: The "man of the house" and his mother. Am. J. Orthopsychiatry, 46:33, 1976.

425. Towne, R.D., and Afterman, J.: Psychosis in males related to parenthood. Bull. Menninger Clin., 19:19, 1955.

426. Turitz, Z.R.: Foster care. In: *Ambulatory Pediatrics* (M. Green and R.J. Haggerty, Eds.). Philadelphia, Saunders, 1968.

427. Turner, R.M., and Clanian, L.: Teaching strategies in a public school class for emotionally disturbed children. J. Am. Acad. Child Psychiatry, 6:86, 1967.

428. Ullman, D.G., Barkley, R.A., and Brown, H.W.: The behavioral symptoms of hyperkinetic children who successfully responded to stimulant drug treatment. Am. J. Orthopsychiatry, 48:425, 1978.

429. van Amerongen, S.T., and Schleifer, M.J.: Families of antisocial young children. Ment. Hygiene, 40:196, 1956.

430. Vandersall, T.A., and Wiener, J.M.: Children who set fires. Arch. Gen. Psychiatry, 22:63, 1970.

431. Vincent, C.E.: *Unmarried Mothers.* New York, Free Press, 1964.

432. Wahl, C.W.: The psychodynamics of consummated maternal incest. Arch. Gen. Psychiatry, 3:188, 1960.

433. Waldfogel, S., Coolidge, J.C., and Hahn, P.B.: The development, meaning, and management of school phobia. Am. J. Orthopsychiatry, 27:754, 1957.

434. Waldfogel, S., Tessman, E., and Hahn, P.B.: A program for early intervention in school phobia. Am. J. Orthopsychiatry, 29:324, 1959.

435. Wallerstein, J.S., and Kelly, J.B.: The effects of parental divorce: The adolescent experience. In: *The Child in His Family: Children at Psychiatric Risk* (E.J. Anthony and C. Koupernik, Eds.). New York, Wiley, 1974.

436. Wallerstein, J.S., and Kelly, J.B.: The effects of parental divorce: Experiences of the preschool child. J. Am. Acad. Child Psychology, 14:600, 1975.

437. Wallerstein, J.S., and Kelly, J.B.: The effects of parental divorce: Experiences of the child in later latency. Am. J. Orthopsychiatry, 46:20, 1976.

438. Wallerstein, J.S., and Kelly, J.B.: Divorce counselling: A community service for families in the middle of divorce. Am. J. Orthopsychiatry, 47:23, 1977.

439. Walker, C.H.M., and Langeth, P.R.: Developmental speech abnormalities in apparently normal children. Br. Med. J., 2/2:1455, 1956.

440. Webb, G., et al.: A comprehensive adolescent maternity program in a community hospital. Am. J. Obstet. Gynecol., 113:511, 1972.

441. Weinberg, S.: Suicidal attempt in adolescence: A hypothesis about the role of physical illness. J. Pediatr., 77:579, 1970.

442. Weinreb, J.: The treatment of a runaway adolescent girl through treatment of the mother. Am. J. Orthopsychiatry, 28:188, 1958.

443. Weinreb, J., and Counts, R.M.: Impulsivity in adolescents and its therapeutic management. Arch. Gen. Psychiatry, 2:548, 1960.

444. Weinstein, E.A.: *The Self-Image of the Foster Child.* New York, Russell Sage Foundation, 1960.

445. Weiss, J.L., Grunebaum, H.U., and Schell, R.: Psychotic mothers and their children. Arch. Gen. Psychiatry, 11:90, 1964.

446. Werkman, S.L.: Adolescent drug addiction. In: *Behavioral Disorders of Adolescence* (S. Copel, Ed.). New York, Basic Books, 1977.

447. Werman, D.S., and Raft, D.: Some psychiatric problems related to therapeutic abortion. N. C. Med. J., 34:274, 1973.

448. Werry, J.S., and Cohrssen, J.: Enuresis: An etiologic and therapeutic study. J. Pediatr., 67:423, 1965.

449. Wessel, M.: Death of an adult—And its impact upon the child. Clin. Pediatr., 12:28, 1973.

450. Wessel, M.A., et al.: Paroxysmal fussing in infancy, sometimes called colic. Pediatrics, 14:421, 1954.

451. Wessel, M.A.: The pediatrician and adoption. N. Engl. J. Med., 262:446, 1960.

452. Weston, D., and Irwin, J.: Preschool child's response to death of infant sibling. Am. J. Dis. Child., 106:564, 1963.

453. Wiener, G.R., et al.: Correlates of low birth weight: Psychological status at six to seven years of age. Pediatrics, 35:434, 1965.

454. Wikler, A.: Present status of the concept of drug dependence. Psychol. Med., 1:377, 1971.

455. Wildy, L.: The professional foster home. In: *Foster Care for Emotionally Disturbed Children*. New York, Child Welfare League of America, 1962.
456. Williams, C.P.S., and Oliver, T.K., Jr.: Nursery routines and Staphylococcal colonization of the newborn. Pediatrics, *44*:640, 1969.
457. Williams, H.R., and Prugh, D.G.: School phobia. In: *Ambulatory Pediatrics* (M. Green and R.J. Haggerty, Eds.). Philadelphia, Saunders, 1968.
458. Wilson, G.S., et al.: The development of preschool children of heroin-addicted mothers. Pediatrics, *63*:135, 1979.
459. Woodmansey, A.C.: Emotion and the motions: An inquiry into the causes and prevention of functional disorders of defecation. Br. J. Med. Psychol., *40*:207, 1967.
460. Wyatt, G.L.: *Language Learning and Communication Disorders in Children*. New York, Free Press, 1969.
461. Wyatt, G., and Herzan, H.: Therapy with stuttering children and their mothers. Am. J. Orthopsychiatry, *32*:645, 1962.
462. Yablonsky, L.: *The Violent Gang*. New York, Macmillan, 1962.
463. Yalom, J.D., et al.: Postpartum blues syndrome. Arch. Gen. Psychiatry, *18*:16, 1968.
464. Yarnell, H.: Firesetting in children. Am. J. Orthopsychiatry, *10*:262, 1970.
465. Yarrow, L.J.: Separation from parents during early childhood. In: *Review of Child Development Research* (M.L. Hoffman and L.W. Hoffman, Eds.). New York, Russell Sage Foundation, 1964, Vol. 1.
466. Youngs, D.D., and Niebyl, J.R.: Teenage pregnancy. J. Maine Med. Assoc., *67*:296, 1976.
467. Zackler, J., and Brandstedt, W., Eds.: *The Teenage Pregnant Girl*. Springfield, Ill., Thomas, 1975.
468. Zax, M., et al.: Identifying emotional disturbance in the school setting. Am. J. Orthopsychiatry, *24*:447, 1964.
469. Zelson, C., Rubio, E., and Wasserman, E.: Neonatal narcotic addiction: 10 year observation. Pediatrics, *48*:178, 1971.
470. Zimmering, P., et al.: Heroin addiction in adolescent boys. J. Nerv. Ment. Dis., *114*:19, 1957.

General References

Anthony, E.J.: Children at risk from divorce: A review. In: *The Child in His Family: Children at Psychiatric Risk* (E.J. Anthony and C. Koupernik, Eds.). New York, Wiley, 1974.
Anthony, E.J., Koupernik, C., and Chiland, C., Eds.: *The Child in His Family: Vulnerable Children*. New York, Wiley, 1978.
Auerbach, A.B.: *Parents Learn Through Discussion: Principles and Practices of Group Education*. New York, Wiley, 1968.
Barbara, D.A.: *Psychological and Psychiatric Aspects of Speech and Hearing*. Springfield, Ill., Thomas, 1960.
Barnes, H.V.: The teenager with pubertal delay. Primary Care, *3*:215, 1967.

Bender, L.: *Aggression, Hostility and Anxiety in Children*. Springfield, Ill., Thomas, 1953.
Berlin, I.N.: Psychiatry and the school. In: *Comprehensive Textbook of Psychiatry* 2nd Ed. (A. Freedman, H. Kaplan, and B. Saddock, Eds.). Baltimore, Williams & Wilkins, 1975, Vol. 2.
Berlin, I.N., et al.: *Learning and Its Disorders*. Palo Alto, Calif., Science and Behavior Books, 1965.
Bibliography: *The Relationship Between Emotion and Speech*. Baltimore: Johns Hopkins University. Information Center for Hearing, Speech, and Disorders of Human Communication, 1969.
Bleiberg, N., and Forrest, S.: Group discussions with mothers in the child health conference. Pediatrics, *24*:117, 1959.
Blos, P.: *The Adolescent Personality: A Study of Individual Behavior*. New York, Appleton-Century-Crofts, 1941.
Blos, P.: *On Adolescence: A Psychoanalytic Interpretation*. New York, Free Press, 1962.
Blos, P.: The initial stage of male adolescence. Psychoanal. Study Child., *20*:145, 1965.
Bowlby, J.: Childhood mourning and its implications for psychiatry. Am. J. Psychiatry, *118*:481, 1965.
Bowlby, J.: *Maternal Care and Mental Health*. World Health Organization Monograph Series. No. 2. Geneva, 1952.
Brazelton, T.B.: *Infants and Mothers*. New York, Dell, 1969.
Brazelton, T.B.: The post-partum period: The pediatrician's role. In: *Ambulatory Pediatrics* (M. Green and R. Haggerty, Eds.). Philadelphia, Saunders, 1968.
Brazelton, T.B.: *Toddlers and Parents*. New York, Dell, 1974.
Brim, O.J., Jr.: *Education for Child Rearing*. New York, Russell Sage Foundation, 1959.
Brody, S.: *Patterns of Mothering: Maternal Influences During Pregnancy*. New York, International Universities Press, 1954.
Burgess, L.C.: *The Art of Adoption*. Washington, D.C., Acropolis Books, 1977.
Caplan, G., Ed.: *Prevention of Mental Disorders in Children*. New York, Basic Books, 1971.
Caplan, G., Mason, E., and Kaplan, D.: Four studies of crisis in parents of prematures. Community Ment. Health J., *1*:149, 1965.
Chess, S.: Individuality in children: Its importance to the pediatrician. J. Pediatr., *69*:676, 1966.
Children and the Threat of Nuclear War. New York, Child Study Association of America, 1964.
Cohen, A.K.: The study of social disorganization and deviant behavior. In: R. Merton, L. Broom, and L. Cottrell, Eds.: *Sociology Today*. New York, Basic Books, 1959.
Cohen, D.J., and Caparulo, B.K., Eds.: Symposium: Language development and its disorders. J. Am. Acad. Child Psychiatr., *16*:5615, 1977.
Coles, R.: *Children of Crisis: A Study of Courage and Fear*. Boston, Little, Brown, 1967.
Comer, J.: The black American child in school. In: *The Child in His Family: Children at Psychiatric Risk* (E.J. Anthony and C. Koupernik, Eds.). New York, Wiley, 1974.

Comer, J., and Poussaint, A.: *Black Child Care.* New York, Simon & Schuster, 1975.

Conger, J.J.: *Adolescence and Youth: Psychological Development in a Changing World.* 2nd Ed. New York, Harper & Row, 1977.

Cooper, M.M.: Evaluation of the mother's advisory service. Monogr. Soc. Res. Child Dev. No. 12, 1947.

Cruickshank, W.M.: Learning disabilities in school, home, and community. Englewood Cliffs, Prentice-Hall, 1971.

Davis, A.: *Social-Class Influences upon Learning.* The Inglis Lecture, 1948. Cambridge, Harvard University Press, 1952.

Derdey, A.P., and Waddington, W.J., III: Adoption: The rights of parents versus the best interests of their children. J. Am. Acad. Child Psychiatry, 15:238, 1976.

Despert, J.L.: *Children of Divorce.* Garden City, N.J., Doubleday, 1962.

Eisenberg, L.: If not now, when? Am. J. Orthopsychiatry, 32:781, 1962.

Eissler, K.R., Ed.: *Searchlights on Delinquency.* New York, International Universities Press, 1949.

Ekstein, R., and Motto, R.L.: *From Learning for Love to Love of Learning: Essays on Psychoanalysis and Education.* New York, Brunner/Mazel, 1969.

Emde, R.N., Gainsbauer, T.J., and Harmon, R.J.: *Emotional Expression in Infancy: A Bio-behavioral Study.* Psycholog. Iss., 10:Mon. N. 37, 1976.

Erickson, E.H.: The Problem of Ego Identity. J. Am. Psychoanal. Assoc., 4:56, 1956.

Feinstein, S.C., and Giovacchini, P., Eds.: *Adolescent Psychiatry.* Chicago, Basic Books, 1973, Vols. 1–5.

Finch, S.M., and Poznanski, E.O.: *Adolescent Suicide.* Springfield, Ill., Thomas, 1971.

Fine, L.L.: *After All We've Done for Them: Understanding Adolescent Behavior.* Englewood, Cliffs. N.J., Prentice-Hall, 1977.

Fraiberg, S., Adelson, E., and Shapiro, V.: Ghosts in the nursery: A psychoanalytic approach to the problem of impaired infant-mother-relationships. J. Am. Acad. Child Psychiatry, 14:387, 1975.

Freud, A.: *The Ego and the Mechanisms of Defense.* New York, International Universities Press, 1946.

Friedlander, K.: *The Psychoanalytic Approach to Juvenile Delinquency.* New York, International Universities Press, 1947.

Gallagher, J.R., and Harris, H.I.: *Emotional Problems of Adolescence.* 3rd Ed. New York, Oxford University Press, 1976.

Gardner, R.: *The Boys' and Girls' Book About Divorce.* New York, Science House, 1970.

Glasscote, R., and Fishman, H., Eds.: *Mental Health Programs for Preschool Children: A Field Study.* Washington, D.C., American Psychiatric Association, 1974.

Group for the Advancement of Psychiatry: *Promotion of Mental Health in the Primary and Secondary Schools.* New York, Group for the Advancement of Psychiatry, 1951, Report No. 18.

Group for the Advancement of Psychiatry: *Sex and the College Students.* New York, Group for the Advancement of Psychiatry, 1965, Report No. 60.

Hader, M.: The importance of grandparents in family life. Fam. Process, 4:2, 1965.

Harlow, H.F.: The nature of love. Am. Psychol., 13:673, 1958.

Havighurst, R.J., and Neugarten, B.L.: *American Indian and White Children. A Sociopsychological Investigation.* Chicago, University of Chicago Press, 1969.

Herzog, E., and Lewis, H.: Children in poor families: Myths and realities. Am. J. Orthopsychiatry, 40:375, 1970.

Holmes, D.: *The Adolescent in Psychotherapy.* Boston, Little, Brown, 1969.

Jackson, E.B., and Trainham, G., Eds.: Family centered maternity and infant care. In: *Problems of Infancy and Early Childhood* (M.J.E. Senn, Ed.). New York, Macy Foundation, 1948.

Jenkins, S., and Morrison, B.: *Ethnicity and Child Welfare: An Annotated Bibliography.* New York, Columbia University School of Social Work, 1974.

Joint Commission on Mental Health of Children: Report of the Committee on Children in Minority Groups. In: *Social Change and the Mental Health of Children.* New York, Harper & Row, 1971.

Jones, H.W., and Heller, R.H.: *Pediatric and Adolescent Gynecology.* Baltimore, Williams & Wilkins, 1966.

Josselyn, I.M.: The psychoanalytic psychology of the adolescent. In: *Readings in Psychoanalytic Psychology.* (M. Levitt, Ed.). New York, Appleton-Century-Crofts, 1959.

Keith, P.R.: Night terrors: A Review of the psychology, neurophysiology, and therapy. J. Am. Acad. Child Psychiatry, 14:477, 1975.

Kempe, C.H., and Helfer, R.E.: *Helping the Battered Child and his Family.* Philadelphia, Lippincott, 1972.

Kennell, J.H., and Rolnick, A.R.: Discussing problems in newborn babies with their parents. Pediatrics, 26:832, 1960.

Kirchner, A.: Parents' classes in a maternity program. Am. J. Public Health, 43:896, 1953.

Klaus, M.H., and Kennell, J.H.: *Maternal-Infant Bonding.* St. Louis, Mosby, 1976.

Konopka, G.: *The Adolescent Girl in Conflict.* Englewood Cliffs, N.J., Prentice-Hall, 1966.

Levin, T.M., and Zegans, L.S.: Adolescent identity crisis and religious conversion: Implications for psychotherapy. Br. J. Med. Psychol., 47:73, 1974.

Lewis, H.: The psychiatric aspects of adoption. In: *Modern Perspectives in Child Psychiatry.* London, Oliver & Boyd, 1965.

Loof, D.: Psychiatric perspectives on poverty. In: *Poverty: New Interdisciplinary Perspectives* (T. Weaver and A. Magid, Eds.). San Francisco, Chandler, 1969.

Lorand, S., and Schneer, H.T.: *Adolescents.* New York, Hoeber, 1961.

Lourie, R.S., and Millikan, F.K.: Pica. In: *Modern Perspectives in International Child Psychiatry* (J.G. Howells, Ed.). Edinburgh, Oliver and Boyd, 1969.

Ludwig, E., and Santibanez, J.: *The Chicanos.* Baltimore, Penguin, 1971.

Masterson, J.F.: *The Psychiatric Dilemma of Adolescence.* Boston, Little, Brown, 1967.

Mattick, J.: Adaptation of nursery techniques to deprived children. J. Am. Acad. Child. Psychiatry, 4:670, 1965.

McCarthy, D.: Language disorders and parent-child relationships. J. Speech Hear. Dis., 19:514, 1954.

McDermott, J.F., et al.: Child custody decision making: The search for improvement. J. Am. Acad. Child Psychiatry, 17:104, 1978.

Mead, M.: Adolescence in primitive and modern society. In: *Readings in Social Psychology*. New York, Holt, 1947.

Mechanic, D.: The influence of mothers on their children's health attitudes and behavior. Pediatrics, 33:444, 1964.

Miller, D.: *Adolescence: Psychology, Psychopathology and Psychotherapy*. New York, Aronson, 1974.

Montiel, M.: The chicano family: A review of research. Social Work, 18:22, 1973.

Murphy, L., and Moriarty, A.: *Vulnerability, Coping, and Growth*. New Haven, Yale University Press, 1976.

Oakland, T., and Beeman, P., Eds.: *Assessing Minority Group Children*. New York, Behavioral Publications, 1974.

Offer, D., and Offer, J.B.: *From Teenage to Young Manhood*. New York, Basic Books, 1975.

Oster, J., and Nielsen, A.: Growing Pains. Acta. Paediatr. Scand., 61:329, 1972.

Palmer, J.: Treating prolonged mourning in Spanish-speaking patients. Hosp. Community Psychiatry, 24:337, 1973.

Parmalee, A.H., and Schulte, F.J.: Developmental testing of pre-term and small-for-dates infants. Pediatrics, 45:21, 1970.

Pratt, K.C.: The Neonate. In: *Manual of Child Psychology*. (L. Carmichael, Ed.). New York, Wiley, 1954.

Provence, S.: Psychoanalysis and the treatment of psychological disorders of infancy. In: *Handbook of Child Psychoanalysis* (B.B. Wolman, Ed.). New York, Van Nostrand Reinhold, 1972.

Prugh, D.: Emotional problems of the premature infant's parents. Nurs. Outlook, 1:461, 1953.

Prugh, D.G.: Children at school. Tipta Yenlikler (Turkey), 7:68, 1962.

Redl, F.: *The Aggressive Child*. Glencoe, Ill., Free Press, 1957.

Reiter, E.O., and Root, A.W.: Hormonal changes of adolescence. Med. Clin. North Am., 59:1289, 1975.

Rexford, E.N., Sander, L.W., and Shapiro, T.: *Infant Psychiatry: A New Synthesis*. New Haven, Yale University Press, 1976.

Robson, K.S., and Moss, H.A.: Patterns and determinants of maternal attachment. J. Pediatr., 77:976, 1970.

Rowe, D.S., et al.: A hospital program for the detection and registration of abused and neglected children. N. Engl. J. Med., 282:950, 1970.

Rutter, M., Tizard, J., and Whitemore, K.: *Education, Health and Behavior*. London, Longmans, 1970.

Schmitt, B.D.: The pediatrician's role in child abuse. Curr. Probl. Pediatr., 5:3, 1975.

Schmitt, B.D., Jordan, K., and Hamburg, F.L.: The role of the pediatrician in helping children develop a sense of responsibility: Suggestions on prevention of irresponsibility. Clin. Pediatr., 11:509, 1972.

Schmitt, B.D., and Kempe, C.H.: The pediatrician's role in child abuse and neglect. In: *Current Problems in Pediatrics*. (J. Gluck, Ed.). Chicago, Year Book, 1975.

Schwartz, J.L., and Schwartz, L.H.: *Vulnerable Infants: A Psychosocial Dilemma*. New York, McGraw-Hill, 1977.

A Selective Bibliography of Writings on Poverty in the United States. Printed with the permission of the Washington Center for Metropolitan Studies by Department of Health, Education, and Welfare, Washington, Government Printing Office, 1964.

Sperling, O.E.: A psychoanalytic study of hypnagogic hallucinations. J. Am. Psychoanal. Assoc., 5:115, 1957.

Spiegel, L.A.: Comments on the psychoanalytic psychology of adolescence. Psychoanal. Study Child, 13:296, 1958.

Spitz, R.: Psychiatric therapy in infancy. Am. J. Orthopsychiatry, 20:623, 1950.

Spock, B.: The middle-aged child. Penn. Med. J., 50:1045, 1947.

Spurlock, J.: Should the poor get none? J. Am. Acad. Child Psychiatry, 8:16, 1969.

Stuart, H., and Prugh, D.G., Eds.: *The Healthy Child: His Physical, Psychological, and Social Development*. Cambridge, Harvard University Press, 1960.

Stubblefield, R.L.: Antisocial personality in children and adolescents. In: *Comprehensive Textbook of Psychiatry*. (A. Freedman, H. Kaplan, and B. Saddock, Eds.). Baltimore, Williams and Wilkins, 1975, Vol. 2.

Swigar, M.E., Bowers, M.D., and Fleck, S.: Grieving and unplanned pregnancy. Psychiatry, 39:72, 1976.

Trouern-Trend, J., and Leonard, M.F.: Prevention of child abuse: Current progress in Connecticut. I. The problem. Conn. Med., 36:135, 1972.

Watson, A.S.: The children of Armageddon: Problems of custody following divorce. Syracuse Law Rev., 21:55, 1972.

Werkman, S.L.: The child or adolescent in court. Clin. Proc. Child. Hosp. D.C., 19:82, 1963.

Werkman, S.L.: Sex education in adolescence. In: *Adolescent Gynecology* (F. Heald, Ed.). Baltimore, Williams & Wilkins, 1966.

Werkman, S.L.: Psychiatric disorders of adolescence. In: *American Handbook of Psychiatry* (G. Caplan, Ed.). New York, Basic Books, 1974.

Werner, E.E.: *The Kauai Study: Follow-up at Adolescence*. Davis, Calif., University of California Press, 1974.

Werner, E., Bierman, J., and French, F.: *The Children of Kauai*. Honolulu, University of Hawaii Press, 1971.

Wessel, M.A., and La Camera, R.G.: The pediatrician and the adolescent: An extraordinary opportunity to be helpful. Clin. Pediatr., 6:227, 1967.

Westman, J.C.: The psychiatrist and child custody contests. Am. J. Psychiatry, 127:123, 1971.

Westman, J.C.: *Individual Differences in Children*. New York, Wiley, 1976.

Westman, J.D., et al.: The role of child psychiatry in divorce. Arch. Gen. Psychiatry, 23:416, 1970.

Whittington, H.G.: *Psychiatry on the College Campus.* New York, International Universities Press, 1964.

Wiener, G.: Psychological correlates of premature birth: A review. J. Nerv. Ment. Dis., *134*:129, 1962.

Wilson, R.S., et al.: Emergence and persistence of behavioral differences in twins. Child Dev., *42*:1381, 1971.

Wishik, S.M.: Parents' group discussions in a child health conference. Am. J. Public Health, *43*:888, 1953.

Wolff, H.G., Wolf, S.G., and Hare, C.C., Eds.: *Life Stress and Bodily Disease.* Baltimore, Williams & Wilkins, 1950.

Work, H.H.: Parent-child centers: A working reappraisal. Am. J. Orthopsychiatry, *42*:582, 1972.

Wortis, H., et al.: Children who eat noxious substances. J. Am. Acad. Child Psychiatry, *1*:536, 1962.

IV
Considerations for Planning

The [U.S. National] Commission [for the International Year of the Child] will reaffirm our obligation to help each child gain:
- affection, love and understanding;
- adequate nutrition and medical care;
- free education;
- opportunity for play and recreation;
- a name and citizenship;
- special care, if handicapped;
- a chance to become a useful member of society and
- to develop individual abilities;
- peace and universal brotherhood;
- enjoyment of these rights, regardless of race, color, sex, religion, national or social origin. (From the Preliminary Report of the U.S. National Commission on the International Year of the Child, 1979)

Medicine has imperceptibly led us into a position to deal with the great social problems of our time. Doctors are the natural advocates of the poor, and social problems are very largely within their jurisdiction.
Rudolf Virchow

29

Trends of the Future

*If we paid no more attention to plants than we
do to our children, we would be living in a
jungle of weeds.*
(Luther Burbank)

In 1970, in *Lengthening Shadows: A Report
on the Delivery of Health Care to Children,*[3] the
Council on Pediatric Practice of the American Academy of Pediatrics addressed itself
to the problems of the health care system
in the United States. The report indicated
that large numbers of children, particularly
those who live in urban ghettos or in remote rural areas, do not receive the continuous, comprehensive care that middle-
class children receive. At best, those children receive only episodic health care—for
acute and serious illnesses—and that only
with difficulty. The report listed the social
and economic factors involved in the lack
of health care:

1. Poverty—and its associated problems
(among them malnutrition and inadequate
housing)

2. The child's race or place of origin

3. The child's place of residence such as
a ghetto or a rural area, a foster home, or
an institution for the delinquent, mentally
ill, or mentally retarded

4. The child's lack of legal residence (as
with a child of migrant workers)

5. A chronic illness or handicap

6. The dearth and maldistribution of
physicians, allied health personnel, and
medical facilities and

7. The reluctance of the taxpayer to support the necessary programs, often because of lack of knowledge or awareness
of their importance.

It has been estimated that 20 to 30 million
children and adolescents suffer from acute
and chronic illness or handicaps, including
mental and emotional problems and mental retardation (see Chap. 25). The majority
of these children are from poor families who
live in ghettos, barrios, and rural areas.
High incidences of infant mortality, death
by accident, drug problems, child abuse
and neglect, pregnancy among unmarried
girls, and suicide are other factors which
increasingly affect the young in highly mobile families in urban areas.

The Relationship of the Pediatrician to the Community

In 1972 the report of the Committee on Standards of Child Health Care of the Academy of Pediatrics[5] discussed the community responsibilities of the pediatrician, particularly in his role as a consultant to the newly developing maternal and infant care projects, neighborhood health centers, Head Start programs, parent-child centers, day care centers, child adoption agencies, public schools, and other state and local health and welfare agencies. The report stressed that the pediatrician needed to work closely with new kinds of health personnel (e.g., pediatric nurse associates, health associates, office assistants) and other allied health personnel, and it called on the pediatrician to continue his education to keep up with new developments.

The report also discussed several trends in facilities and in the delivery of health services. It stated that the family, not just one individual, is the basic unit to receive consideration. It supported the maintenance of life-long health as well as the keeping of a complete and life-long health record for each patient. Yet the report has reservations about the future of family practice, and the American Academy of Pediatrics has shown opposition to the trend toward family practice residencies.

The report is in favor of locating all medical care in one setting and developing facilities and methods to make continuous comprehensive care possible. The report encourages group practices, both multidisciplinary and single-specialty practices, the clustering of private offices around hospitals, the development of neighborhood health centers, the incorporation of other health workers into the framework of the health facility, and the avoidance of fragmenting services by incorporating separate facilities into more inclusive ones. Yet the report questioned the value of coordination or the "team approach" in other than chronic illnesses, saying that, if the team

approach is overused, it "consumes much time of scarce professional people, is extremely expensive, and may yield personality clashes."

The obvious inconsistencies in the statements just quoted are not confined to the American Academy of Pediatrics. Ambivalence toward other disciplines is characteristic of virtually every professional association that represents a single discipline. The failure of community mental health centers (a failure that is sanctioned by the American Psychiatric Association) to include pediatricians on their staffs is another case in point. Planning is going on, but the planning groups rarely talk to each other, and they fail to plan in a coordinated fashion.

These problems and inconsistencies have begun to be recognized by the American Academy of Pediatrics. In April, 1972, a conference was held to discuss the special problems of child health care in the ghetto. It was co-sponsored by the American Academy of Pediatrics, the Section on Pediatrics of the National Medical Association, and the department of pediatrics at Howard University. Dr. Jay Arena, the president of the American Academy of Pediatrics in 1972, said, "We must produce more pediatricians interested in the primary and general care of children, and provide a more equitable distribution of these physicians to areas of need." The American Academy of Pediatrics has appointed a committee on community health services and created a department of community services. It called for a new action program for children who did not receive adequate health care. The program aims to produce comprehensive, personalized health care, including preventive services. Yet adult programs in ambulatory medicine have developed even more slowly than those in pediatrics—and both have received little real support from the American Medical Association.

The American Psychiatric Association has for some time supported the development of community mental health centers. But only 1 in 8 of these centers had adequate specialized services for children, a fact that was pointed out by the Joint Commission on Mental Health of Children in 1970.[34] The National Institute of Mental Health has attempted to remedy the situation, with the recent support of the American Academy of Child Psychiatry and other professional associations from other fields. Although a survey in Massachusetts indicated that pediatricians are interested in being involved in local community planning for mental health and mental retardation, very little coordinated planning involving physicians has taken place.[19] The American Academy of Pediatrics has supported the concept of family planning and has endorsed the statement of the American College of Obstetrics and Gynecology regarding contraception for sexually active teenagers.

Despite the development of such services and concepts as child advocacy, family planning, consumerism, community health and mental health services, day care, child care, self-evaluation, Head Start and "health start," public education, accountability, built-in evaluation, and quality assurance, child health and welfare has still not been established as a national priority, and there is no national policy for children. The health system is still a nonsystem, and, because of the lack of coordinated planning, many children and young people, especially those from poor and minority groups, are allowed to go "down the drain."

Developmental Child Care

Despite the relative lack of professional involvement and coordination at the national level, important developments have taken place on the local level in regard to programs that have received federal support and, to some extent, state support. Many of these programs are threatened by recent budget cuts. The Office of Economic Opportunity led with the Head Start program, which was helped by the American Academy of Pediatrics. In some Head Start programs, health and mental health screening has been available, and parents from poverty and ghetto areas have been successfully involved. Communication between Head Start programs and kindergarten or first-grade programs has failed to take place (except in those cases in which a public health nurse has offered to give screening information to the elementary school teacher), and enrichment has only recently been continued into the early grades.

The recent development of well-staffed and well-run community day care centers for infants and children of working mothers (as opposed to the custodial programs of the past) is encouraging. However, the day care programs have not been coordinated with the Head Start programs or the programs in the Parent-Child centers. (The programs in the Parent-Child centers include home-based enrichment programs for infants and very young children.)

Neighborhood health centers, which often have satellite health stations, have generally succeeded in "taking the clinic into the community," as have Children's Bureau programs for mothers, infants, children, and youths, health clinics for migrant workers, centers for children who have developmental disabilities and congenital anomalies, home care programs for chronically ill children, and other special clinics provided for by the Comprehensive Health Planning Act. But coordination of the services offered has been a problem in these programs, as well as in clinics sponsored by community groups, medical societies, medical students, industries, and insurance companies. More flexible schedules are needed to accommodate poor families and fathers and mothers who cannot take time off from the job and who therefore must come at night. The relationship of these clinics to "back-up" public and private hospitals has not always been clearly defined, and clinic physicians may not have full staff privileges, as Haggerty and his associates[19] have pointed out. Continuity of care is difficult under these circumstances, and the relationship of clinic services to other neighborhood based services is unclear. (The services include legal services, job counseling and employment services, youth services, delinquency prevention programs, alcoholism programs, and action council programs. A number of these programs are also threatened by recent budget cuts.) Consumer participation in the programs has been uneven, and at times the "establishment" has totally ignored the residents' perceptions of their needs or their children's needs, and bitter and destructive fights have resulted. The "target population" has not always been clearly defined; often it has been different for different services. The health, mental health, mental retardation, welfare, educational, and delinquency prevention "maps" of the community have often been different, and little communication has taken place among the groups involved. "We hear but we do not listen; we talk but we do not communicate," Doris Howell, chairperson of pediatrics at the Medical College of Pennsylvania, was quoted as saying.

In Rochester, New York, the number of emergency visits made by children to hospitals dropped significantly when a neighborhood health center was established. The center emphasizes comprehensive medical care.[22] Where such a center is operating successfully, infant mortality has decreased, hospital admissions have dropped, and patient acceptance of the center has generally been good. In some areas (e.g., Denver) inadequate transportation has been overcome by the use of small buses to transport patients from satellite health stations to the health center and to the back-up hospital. Mobile health vans have been used effectively in neighborhood outreach projects (e.g., in Chicago); they offer immunization programs, sickle cell anemia detection programs, lead poisoning prevention programs, and other services. Advertising those programs and training college students and others for volunteer work, often those from ghettos, has been helpful.

In rural areas (e.g., in Colorado and Vermont) family counseling programs as well as child development programs are being developed. "Reaching out" to often mistrusting Spanish-surnamed families through home-based programs offered by Spanish-speaking staff or to isolated, poor but independent farming families through the development of "skill and repair centers" is needed first to involve parents and family members before family counseling about child care and other available services can be considered. Group rural-neighborhood Health Maintenance Organization programs and the National Health Corps programs show promise although there are serious problems in recruiting workers. The need to recognize particular sociocultural attitudes toward Anglo medical and nursing staffs has been too little emphasized, as has the need for cooperative work with *curanderos* in rural Spanish-surnamed areas and with medicine men on Indian reservations.

As Freedman[12] has stressed, the cost of not providing good developmental child care is prohibitive, leading as it does to the huge costs of dealing with the problems caused by poor physical and mental health, drug problems, and crime, which might otherwise be prevented—not to mention the more fundamental problems of human suffering.

Although pending a final evaluation such community health programs can be said to have had good results (despite the coordination difficulties mentioned), the underlying problems of a separate health system for the poor have not been faced squarely. Ghettos, barrios, and rural areas of poverty exist, and the people living in those areas need good health care now. But will delivery of that health care perpetuate the separate housing, social, economic, and employment patterns? Or can the demeaning segregation of minority groups and poor people be broken up (by breaking down prejudice, desegregating schools, developing low-cost housing in the suburbs, and taking other steps) so that there is one health care delivery system for all? Some, including myself, believe that a unified system can be achieved, but others think it cannot. In December, 1974, Congress passed a law dealing with health planning and resource development that would require state regional planning for rural as well as urban areas. That law is a step in the right direction although the planning has been generally slow and uneven.

The New Nontraditional Professionals

Mention was made elsewhere of the people who have made new and significant contributions to physical and mental health, welfare, and educational programs for children. Although these workers are sometimes referred to as para-professionals and nonprofessionals, many of them have a professional attitude toward their jobs and the people they serve. These workers include foster-grandmothers, indigenous neighborhood or family health workers, child development specialists, community mental health workers or health aides, teachers' aides, street workers, advocates, and "partners" in delinquency programs, judicial aides in juvenile courts, infant care workers and child care workers in day care programs, social work case aides, sociotherapists in residential or inpatient treatment programs, homemakers, office assistants or health aides, dental hygienists, health visitors, and many other allied health workers (who number 12 to 14 per physician). Some nontraditional paraprofessional groups have an educational curriculum, a career ladder, and different types of certification. Licensed practical nurses, psychiatric technicians, nurse practitioners, child health associates, and

certain community workers are among those groups, and other groups are moving in the same direction. Community colleges have often collaborated with medical centers in developing training programs. Besides the various allied health workers, dedicated volunteers have made a number of contributions that extend beyond their traditional hospital duties. Besides VISTA volunteers, trained volunteers have helped in day care programs, and high-school students have been trained as tutors for ghetto children—to mention a few contributions.

In regard to the pediatrician, the most significant developments have been those involving pediatric office assistants and the wider and more intensive training of certain established professionals, such as the nurse practitioner and the school nurse practitioner, as well as the emergence of a truly new type of worker, the child health associate. Under medical supervision, all these people can perform some of the functions involved in screening, prevention, diagnosis, treatment, and referral.

The pediatrician must also collaborate in community programs with dentists, psychiatrists, psychologists, social workers, speech therapists, audiologists, and members of other disciplines.

The Changing Role of the Pediatrician

As the disciplines just described have evolved, the pediatrician has found himself less often cast in the role of a practitioner. He still may be on the front lines, functioning as one of the members of the first echelon of comprehensive primary care and acting as a casefinder or referral source for psychiatric and other facilities. More and more often he is asked to act as a supervisor of nurse practitioners who run satellite health stations and nurse practitioners in schools, and to act as a consultant to other individuals and community agencies, including developmental child care agencies, community mental health facilities, and adoption agencies.

The pediatrician may be asked to be the director or coordinator of a health team which offers comprehensive health services and which is composed of a number of people from traditional and nontraditional backgrounds. That role may be difficult for some pediatricians because many pediatricians have had little training in collaboration and coordination. Also, the pediatrician cannot always be the captain of the team in the community, as he would ordinarily be in a pediatric hospital or a traditional clinic program. He may find that someone from another discipline (e.g., a child psychiatrist, a psychologist, a social worker, or an administrator) is in charge of the program and that his role is that of a collaborator. For example, he might be a part-time or full-time staff member of a community mental health program that involves children or of an inpatient unit for disturbed children and adolescents. Unfortunately, many such programs have only minimal pediatric consultation. *Standards for Psychiatric Facilities Serving Children and Adolescents,* published in 1972 by the American Psychiatric Association, calls for a pediatrician to be a full-time or part-time member of such facilities. Only in this way can the pediatrician learn firsthand the problems workers in these facilities face and come to offer his pediatric knowledge in a meaningful way.

Finally, the pediatrician can contribute importantly to the community in his role as an informed person, a professional who knows children and knows how environment and experience affect their development. As such the pediatrician can and should take his place on the boards of community agencies that deal with poverty, delinquency, and other matters of social concern that go far beyond his usual professional concerns. As an influential person in the community, he can and should work with child psychiatrists and other physical and mental health, educa-

tion, and welfare professionals to formulate policy at neighborhood, urban, state and national levels (as the American Academy of Pediatrics has recommended). Sophisticated pediatricians (e.g., Senn and Richmond) have been leaders in the Head Start program, in the Joint Commission on Mental Health of Children, and in many other important movements in recent years.

The Relationship of Pediatric Services to Community Mental Health Programs

There are other things to consider besides the provision of pediatric consultant and staff services to the programs of psychiatric facilities for children and adolescents. Bullard[8] has discussed the relationship of the urban pediatric hospital to community mental health programs. He has pointed out that the hospital's expanded role in the delivery of comprehensive medical care has been accompanied by increasing numbers of referrals of patients who have social and emotional problems. In Bullard's study, most referrals by pediatricians to the general medical clinic at the Children's Hospital Medical Center in Boston came from suburban areas or other areas outside the metropolitan area. Of these, 25% of the patients referred had chief complaints of emotional or behavior problems. The initial pediatric evaluations indicated that (1) 20% of the children's problems were considered to be emotional or behavior disorders, (2) 11% were psychophysiologic disorders, and (3) 10% (or a total of 41% of the group referred) had a primary diagnosis which ordinarily implied that their problems had psychosocial components.

As Bullard indicated, these emotional disorders were not unusual or obscure but rather were problems commonly dealt with in pediatric and child psychiatric practice. After the initial pediatric evaluation, about 25% of these patients were seen in psychiatric consultation, and 50% of this group were referred to mental health clinics, family service organizations, or to the pediatrician in their local community for follow-up. The other 50% of the group seen in consultation underwent a full psychiatric diagnostic evaluation, and 30% of those who had a full evaluation were referred to local facilities for treatment. Thus a "circular" route was followed by patients—from a practicing pediatrician to a hospital pediatrician, to a psychiatric consultant, with some receiving a full psychiatric diagnostic evaluation, to a mental health clinic. Bullard points out that schools, like pediatricians, often took the circular route, either because they did not know about local mental health facilities or because they felt that there were not enough facilities to meet the demand.

Bullard's experience is similar to mine and that of others. Pediatricians use the modern urban pediatric hospital for help with emotional and behavioral problems, and many families living near these hospitals use them as the "family doctor," often making sporadic visits for acute illness or crisis needs. There is often little continuity of contact with physicians or other staff members. The problem is one of clear assignment of responsibility. As Bullard indicated, chronic physical illness or disability and psychophysiologic disorders in children require the close coordination of medical and psychiatric treatment in the hospital setting. Such disorders as psychoneurotic disorders, problems in learning, tension-discharge disorders, and those associated with multiproblem families are better handled by the staff of a local mental health facility working closely with either individuals or the staffs of other facilities in the area.

The urban pediatric hospital can thus give up its "Mecca" policy without abandoning its open door policy. It can screen referred patients, using curbstone psychiatric consultations or social service intake procedures, thus educating the pediatric staff while directing the patients to the appropriate resource. Ideally, "catchment areas" for medical and psychiatric care should correspond, but that is often not the case, and there is a lack of coordination among the various programs. If the facilities for handling school problems, psychoneurotic disorders, and the like are not adequate at the local level, that defect should be corrected with a community coordinational plan that avoids duplication and overlapping of services, fragmentation of families, and "cracks" between which certain patients fall. As Bullard emphasized, referrals from an urban pediatric hospital to a local mental health facility should be "open"; that is, the particular type of treatment should be decided on by the local facility, thus avoiding uncertainty and confusion for the family and the staff. In children's hospitals that are associated with university programs, the department of child psychiatry can offer direct treatment for a spectrum of psychosocial disorders. Some pediatricians of course refer children and families directly to child psychiatric or other child mental health facilities in the community.[41]

Other problems in community coordination can be identified easily. Although planning for community mental health services proceeded earlier, it often failed to include pediatricians and specialized child psychiatric services; and planning for comprehensive health centers generally failed to include mental health services for children or adults. That was especially true in the "poverty program" neighborhood health centers in rural areas. The people served by the health centers made up only a part of the people under county jurisdiction. It offered comprehensive medical and social services, together with organized field projects yielding demographic information about families, including nutritional and obstetrical histories. Its educational approach led to the organization of small local community meetings, which ultimately produced several small health councils. Despite the positive effects of the approach, which was supported by university medical centers, no attempt was made to take a coordinated approach to planning for dealing with mental health, educational, or welfare problems.

The community mental health movement in the United States began in the early 1960s after the publication of the report of the Joint Commission on Mental Health and Illness. The movement was based on the concept of comprehensive care for a geographically defined population. Outpatient and inpatient services, partial hospitalization or day (or night) treatment programs, and consultation and community education offered by a multidisciplinary staff were the services through which care was to be delivered. Reaching out to people in minority and poverty neighborhoods with the help of specially trained community mental health workers was emphasized, and early intervention, crisis intervention, family therapy, and group therapy were used heavily. A move away from large state hospital inpatient programs coincided with the community mental health movement, partly because of developments in England and other countries and partly because of the development of tranquilizers; and important attempts were made to shorten the hospitalization time and keep patients in the community.

About 400 of a projected network of 2000 community health centers have been funded since the passage of the Mental Health Act of 1966. Although major benefits have been realized, major problems must be solved. The community mental health center is now considered a program[31]—not a building—and the goals of such a program demonstrated large gaps in technology, manpower, and organization.[32] As adult patients were discharged in large numbers from state mental hospitals, budgets were often cut despite the lack of immediately available follow-up programs in the community.

Even the problem of defining mental ill-ness became more complex, as different professional groups took different and sometimes competing professional and philosophical stances. The question of whether emotional and behavioral problems are illnesses or are psychosocial disorders or deviations has been hotly debated. The answer, of course, affects what professional disciplines should offer treatment, what programs should be funded, and for what disorders and to whom third-party insurance payments should be made. As mentioned earlier, I drew up for the Joint Commission on Mental Health of Children a classification[29] based on the child's levels of psychosocial functioning. The classification is a step toward solving some of the problems; it includes a survey of all the services required for the child at different levels of his development and functioning. This approach has been elaborated by the Group for the Advancement of Psychiatry.[15] The GAP Ad Hoc Committee expressed my concept in the form of a "mental health grid," which has been congently expanded and developed by Noshpitz.[27a]

Although outreach services, early intervention, and group methods of treatment are important developments, some community programs have so heavily deemphasized long-term intensive psychotherapy and one-to-one relationships that they fail to offer adequate services for patients who require more intensive care, as well as adequate specialized services for children.[32] As a result the person or the family has often been forced to fit the available therapeutic mold rather than the mold made to fit the person or the family.

I think that mental health professionals who work with children (psychiatrists, psychologists, social workers, nurses, and others) can play constructive roles in community health and mental health programs only if they collaborate with pediatric, nursing, educational, and other personnel. Child mental health cannot be separated from the health, education, and cultural forces that affect child development. Thus I support a community center (rather than a health or mental health center), where all services can be coordinated.[35] Whether in large communities all such services could be housed in a school setting[21] as an educational, service and social center remains to be seen. Certainly, that goal could be achieved in smaller communities, with the face-to-face smaller group contact which is so important—and so difficult to achieve—in large, impersonal urban settings.

Patterns of Pediatric Practice

Until recently, in many teaching hospitals the outpatient or ambulatory care division has been a stepchild. As a result, the physician often has had little interest in and has had little training in office management. As Yankauer and his associates have pointed out, the kinds of settings in which pediatricians work—private offices, clinics, and health centers—tend to be run inefficiently. Physicians and nurses spend much of their time performing managerial, technical, and clerical duties. Financial barriers to care still exist, and home visits are rare. Yankauer and Connolly estimate that pediatricians could serve twice as many children if a large number of nurse practitioners or health associates were trained and used, if medical groups replaced solo practices, and if automation concepts were used to improve efficiency.[43] Ambulatory clinics are beginning to grow stronger, with better balance in their relationships to emergency clinics.[7]

Changes are going on, of course; the development of allied health workers and the movement toward reaching out into the community have been mentioned. Small groups of pediatricians who provide 24-hour coverage and mixed-specialty groups, in which the pediatrician is one of a number of physicians, are becoming more popular and solo pediatric practice is declining.[28] Some pediatric groups include a part-time or even a full-time social worker[42] or a part-time psychologist, who enhances their effectiveness in dealing with psychosocial problems, and some pediatric groups have consultant arrangements with child psychiatrists. Many pediatric practitioners and medical centers are beginning to use Weed's problem-oriented system of recordkeeping, which can help establish a better patient profile, help analyze the patient's problems, and permit better follow-up care. Prepaid health programs that include mental health services[14] are becoming more acceptable to physicians and families. Some pediatric centers offer television consultations to physicians in isolated rural areas.

Many hospitals and medical schools, however, have still not addressed themselves to the problems of the city and the community. The concept of "echelons of service" is being accepted in community mental health centers and neighborhood health centers, which have satellite health stations and back-up hospitals. But the concept is not widely discussed, in many pediatric teaching centers and in some departments of psychiatry. Even the allied health workers are not yet fully accepted by some pediatricians—and some psychiatrists.

Although in England, New Zealand, and many other countries, the pediatrician does not offer primary child care but acts as a consultant to general practitioners, in the United States pediatricians, despite their limited numbers, tend to act as general practitioners for children. That may change as more physicians establish family practices. Today only 6% of nonacademic pediatricians list themselves as subspecialists, and only 10% of all pediatricians are certified by a subspecialty board.[4] Most pediatricians devote most of their time to "general pediatrics," but many of them have special interests. As Kempe[23] pointed out, pediatricians are increasingly interested in the biosocial, developmental, school health, and community health aspects of pediatrics, as well as in adolescent problems.

Pediatric Education: Implications of Change

The recent changes in pediatric practice are beginning to affect educational programs. The growing interest in ambulatory pediatrics is highlighted by a number of developments. Child development is becoming important as a basic science for pediatrics.[36] The earlier approach of Senn and Solnit[40] and others to the teaching of comprehensive pediatrics in an outpatient setting is bearing a variety of fruits. Prugh[30] has summarized the history of these and other teaching approaches in pediatric residency training, in the context of the evolving relationship between child psychiatry and pediatrics. Recently, the Robert Wood Johnson Foundation has offered program grants to departments of pediatrics to improve the teaching of ambulatory pediatrics. The few university-based scholarships in the psychosocial aspects of pediatrics offered for years by Senn, Lourie, Richmond, Prugh, and others are now increasing in number, as are those in maternal and child health, and are being rounded out by newer fellowships in developmental pediatrics and adolescent medicine, as funds become available from private sources. (Recent cutbacks in federal funding may change these patterns.)

With the increasing awareness of the health problems of children from low-income families and of children of migrant workers, university training programs include fellowships in community pediatrics (under the leadership of Haggerty[19] and others). As acute disability becomes less frequent and chronic illness becomes more visible, more fellowships are being offered in pediatric rehabilitation and mental retardation.

Along with those areas of special interest, the organized teaching of individual[11] and family[38] interviewing techniques and the psychosocial aspects of child health supervision[25] to pediatric residents is becoming more common, and controlled studies show evidence of the effectiveness of such teaching.[16] Other teaching approaches are being experimented with (e.g., a required period of supervised work with patients who have psychosocial problems). Somewhat similar approaches are being taken more often with medical students[18] and postgraduate fellows,[33] some in family medicine. And a new journal, *Advances in Behavioral Pediatrics*, has recently begun publication.

In 1978, the Task Force on Pediatric Education[2] of the American Academy of Pediatrics identified the changing health needs of infants, children, and adolescents, including those associated with poverty, changing family structures, and other social and psychologic factors. Underemphasis in pediatric education was found to exist in the teaching of the biosocial and developmental aspects, adolescent medicine, pharmacology and toxicology, community pediatrics, handicaps, health maintenance, and medical ethics. The reforms recommended included the drawing up of a national policy for the periodic assessment of the health status of children and adolescents, flexible residencies of suitable length, preparation for group practice, and commitment by pediatricians to their own continuing education. Prominent among the reforms suggested was the provision of better education in areas of biosocial concern. Collaboration with family physicians and other health care professionals, including mental health professionals, was also recommended. A recent survey by Anders[6] indicates that although child psychiatry has much to contribute to the pediatric reforms, the relationship between child psychiatry and pediatrics is still in an evolutionary stage.

Evidence of change is accumulating.[13] A new subspecialty is emerging, that of behavioral pediatrics, which draws on new knowledge in the psychosocial and child development areas. Senn, Spock, Bakwin, and Richmond were among the early leaders in this direction, and Korsch, Provence, Green, Freedman, Friedman, and others have joined them more recently, as have the graduates of the training programs in the psychosocial aspects of pediatrics mentioned earlier. The increase in the number of training programs in behavioral pediatrics (some have recently been supported by the Grant Foundation), the recent emphasis on psychiatric liaison programs at the National Institute of Mental Health (an emphasis that remains, despite decreasing federal support), and the recognition by the President's Task Force on Mental Health of the needs of children and the need to train more child psychiatrists are other timely developments. Child psychiatrists must participate in such programs for pediatricians; they should recognize that pediatricians can help many children who have milder emotional and developmental problems.

Finally, affirmative action programs in medical schools have resulted in more women students and more students from ethnic minority groups. More physicians from minority groups will serve on university faculties and will be role models for minority students. And those students will someday deliver the medical services more effectively to children and families in ghettos and barrios.

Developments in Research

Certain developments in the psychosocial and psychophysiologic aspects of research deserve comment. Earlier in the book, it was pointed out that interdisciplinary psychophysiologic research had become a respected part of adult medicine, but not yet of pediatric medicine, despite the opportunities in a number of centers for the collaboration of pediatricians, child psychiatrists, and mental health workers.

Many child psychiatrists and pediatricians need training in investigative techniques.[9]

Clinical investigation in general should be given more emphasis in medical centers. It should be stressed that the distinction between basic and applied research does not necessarily apply to laboratory research as opposed to clinical research. Clinical research can be basic, and laboratory research can be applied. Many of the hypotheses tested in the laboratory came from the "hunches" of clinical investigators. Clinical investigation can generate as well as confirm hypotheses, in behavioral, psychophysiologic, and other areas. Many of Freud's ideas were not couched in formal hypotheses, but many clinical investigators have set up systematic studies that have confirmed some—and failed to confirm some—of Freud's ideas. Clinical research, like laboratory research, can be systematic and rigorous. Clinical research is more difficult than animal laboratory research, because for ethical reasons, the same kinds of experiments cannot be set up. Animal research supports but does not absolutely confirm clinical research since it is impossible to transfer conclusions directly from one species to another. Much clinical research is needed in the behavioral and developmental areas especially. Collaborative research can be carried out in private practice, as Haggerty[17] has indicated.

There is a need for anterospective research, because of the limitations of retrospective research, especially in regard to child-rearing data. What is needed is not the shotgun approach of some past-longitudinal studies but hypothesis-testing research based on biologic "tags" which permit the identification of populations who may develop a particular psychophysiologic disorder. Some biologic tags (e.g., increased or decreased serum pepsinogen levels), are known. The discovery of others will take time as (for example) new biochemical methods are used to identify minute amounts of hormones which may be effective in producing physiologic changes.

Of course, there is a need for "short" longitudinal studies in many areas.

Although some research in the area of primary prevention has been done (e.g., on reactions to hospitalization and illness), much more is needed in order to permit interventions with children at risk for the development of emotional and behavioral problems.[10]

Evaluation research in community programs has recently received a "must" priority from the Department of Health and Human Services. "High-falutin" evaluative research is not easy, however, as Herzog[20] has commented. "Low-falutin" research (e.g., simple counting methods) based on systems analysis have been too much neglected. Health services research in general received little emphasis until recently, when research in the approach to ambulatory care[1] and other areas have been explored.[39] The field deserves much more interest and support, as does measuring the effectiveness of teaching methods. Some teachers have used videotapes and standardized measures to evaluate any changes over a period of time in the attitudes of medical students toward mental illness and thus to evaluate the effects of the teaching programs.

Changes in research support from the National Institutes of Health are pertinent. Recently, the trend has been toward cutting support. Private foundations also have been affected by inflation. In addition, pressures have arisen to decrease basic research and to put more emphasis on practical results or applications. But many outstanding scientists have warned that applied research should not be emphasized at the expense of the research of individual scientists, whose work may seem not directly related to the desired ends. The results of concentrated research resources runs headlong against a "history of evidence" that major breakthroughs come from the work of individuals and small groups that arises out of their own experience and reflects their personal creativities.

The problem of social research is real. Social research is important, and it needs major financial support from the government. But care must be taken that the government does not use the results of such research to manipulate behavior through propaganda, psychologic warfare, or in other ways. In addition, major ethical issues confront scientists in the behavioral and other areas.

Finally, the computer is a promise and a problem. The difficulties in programming computers for handling medical record data are great. The research team often finds it hard to agree on what data are to be fed into the computer. The adage, Garbage in, garbage out, is still pertinent, despite the help a properly programmed computer can give in the statistical analysis of data and in the handling of demographic and other types of material. Computers have been used to conduct interviews in the absence of the physician—in my opinion an inhuman, unemotional, and invalid approach. As mentioned earlier, computer diagnosis can be of little help in handling psychosocial disorders. Collecting and storing data about patients in state and community mental health programs is helpful statistically, but it runs the risk of invading privacy if measures are not taken to avoid identifying patients and transmitting the data collected to data banks kept by the military, the police, credit agencies, and others.

Comprehensive Planning for Children

Almost all planning groups agree that the United States has a health care crisis, one marked by inadequate, fragmented, overlapping, poorly distributed, and uncoordinated services. Those groups agree that the present health care delivery system (nonsystem?) is too costly for the patient. They think that most Americans, particularly the poor, who have the most illnesses, do not have access to the health services they need. They believe that federal, state, and local services must be coordinated to guarantee adequate health care for all people, as is the case in many other countries. Most people agree that a health care delivery system must be available, accessible, and responsive.

Today politicians and the general public support the concept of national health insurance, a concept long ago implemented in many countries (e.g., New Zealand, Britain, and the Scandinavian countries) but until recently considered somewhat subversive in the United States. (Recently, concern about funding unfortunately has diminished this support.) The present controversy centers on costs and methods of support, whether through payroll and federal taxes, a combination of private and public insurance, or some other method. The need to protect human values in such a plan has been expressed by the American Public Health Association; and other organizations have been concerned about quality control.

An attempt to coordinate delivery of health care services was made by the federal Comprehensive Health Planning Program over a number of years. Secretary Richardson of the Department of Health, Education, and Welfare admitted that the attempt had been unsuccessful because of the welter of federal authorities and agencies, which inhibited rather than enhanced planning. Richardson felt that state and local planning bodies must have greater authority and freedom in using federal money. (A recent survey indicated that within the Department of Health, Education, and Welfare there are more than 200 programs which deal with the problems of children and adolescents. Lourie[26] has remarked that except for the Bureau of Mines every department of government, from the Department of Commerce to the Department of Labor, has programs that deal with

the problems of children and youth.) The Health Resources Planning and Delivery Act of 1974 requires that the state plan around regional health services. That approach (if fully implemented) should help in the planning and development of services needed for a national health insurance system.

A number of groups have evaluated the problems of children and youth in the United States and have made suggestions for a national policy for children in the context of the family. Two of the most important evaluations have come from the National Academy of Sciences[27] and the Carnegie Council on Children.[24] Although many creative recommendations have been made, no recommendations have been made for a coordinated system to solve the problems faced by children and adolescents, who cannot vote. Voluntary groups have been formed at the state level, such as ACY (Advocacy for Children and Youth–Colorado Coalition), which involved professionals, laypersons, and youth and which established regional and local councils with the help of funds for child advocacy from the National Institute of Mental Health. Although valuable coordinating efforts were made, the lack of a quasi-official status meant that most of its activities stopped when funds ran out.

The Joint Commission on Mental Health of Children tried to solve the problem of coordinating the existing and the new programs. The Commission's report, Crisis in Child Mental Health: A Challenge for the 70's,[34] stressed the importance of having a system of child advocacy as well as of developing more numerous and more innovative services concentrating on preventing mental illness and other problems in infancy and the preschool-age period. Citizen advocacy has existed in Denmark for 70 years; the ombudsman system in Sweden is familiar, as are advocate programs in France and physical and mental health advocacy programs in Holland.

The Joint Commission on Mental Health

of Children, which had been set up in 1965 by Senator Ribicoff, recommended in 1970 that a system of child (and youth) advocacy be established with, at the top, a presidential commission on child and youth advocacy. It also recommended that there be an assistant secretary for child and youth advocacy in the Department of Health, Education, and Welfare and a system of coordinating councils on child and youth advocacy at state levels, as well as regional, urban, and neighborhood councils. The Joint Commission saw these councils as made up of not only representatives of health, mental health, mental retardation, welfare, education, day care, and other programs but also of the people to be served. The Joint Commission saw these councils as planning bodies which would survey needs at different levels, would identify problems, would recommend new or intensified services, would follow up and evaluate programs, and generally would provide a coordinating function not now available. In this way, individuals and agencies could cooperate, rather than compete for existing funds, as now happens. The Joint Commission also recommended that since children and youth comprise almost 50% of the population, programs for their needs receive proportional funding, along with the elderly, rather than the 10% on a national basis they now receive (the percentages in some states for mental health programs in particular are much lower).

Partly as a result of the report of the Joint Commission, the Office of Child Development was set up in the Department of Health, Education, and Welfare, as was a suboffice of Child Advocacy. These offices were to coordinate programs within the department and with other departments. A presidential commission has not been established and Senator Ribicoff's bill to establish a national system of child advocacy was somehow transmuted into a bill for day care, which was vetoed. Demonstration projects in child advocacy have been set up by the National Institute of Mental Health and the Office of Child Development in urban and rural settings and in settings involving different ethnic groups. One of the most innovative of these demonstration projects has been undertaken by COPAS, in Sante Fe. COPAS works in the barrio, using indigenous child advocates who work with youths and parents, educating the barrio people about their needs and about ways of meeting them. COPAS has an advisory board made up of professionals and an elected "ethnic" board, which sets policy.

The mental health of children, particularly children from minority backgrounds, was designated as having top priority by Bert Brown, then director of the National Institute of Mental Health.

Recently a number of states have been working on legislation to set up systems of child advocacy that would embrace all the needs of young people. Massachusetts and Connecticut, for example, have set up departments for children at the state government level, where funds spent for children are concentrated, and they have established regional and local councils, with citizen involvement, which have a quasilegal role in the review of fiscal planning for all services for children. Other states have moved in similar directions in varying degrees. It is too early to see how such state planning will go and whether it can be tied in with federal planning. Among others, Julius Richmond, until recently Assistant Secretary for Health of the Department of Health and Human Resources and Surgeon General, has said[37] that the time has come when the government and the private sector can collaborate effectively in addressing themselves to the health problems of children and others. I think so too. (Recent changes in political attitudes and funding patterns raise questions about the immediate future in this area.)

The United States must not forget children in underdeveloped countries, who face nutritional, infectious, and other medical problems, as well as mental illness and mental retardation. The national preoccupation with war and defense must be controlled, so that the nation can address itself to the problems of children and youth—who comprise half of our population and all of our future.

Bibliography

1. Alpert, J.J.: Research in ambulatory care. In: *Ambulatory Pediatrics* (R.J. Haggerty and M. Green, Eds.). Philadelphia, Saunders, 1968.
2. American Academy of Pediatrics: *The Future of Pediatric Education: A Report by the Task Force on Pediatric Education.* Evanston, Ill., American Academy of Pediatrics, 1978.
3. American Academy of Pediatrics: *Lengthening Shadows: A Report on the Delivery of Health Care to Children.* Prepared by the Council on Pediatric Practice. Evanston, Ill., American Academy of Pediatrics, 1970.
4. American Academy of Pediatrics: Projecting pediatric practice patterns: report of survey by pediatric manpower committee. Pediatrics, (Suppl.), 62:625, 1978.
5. American Academy of Pediatrics, Committee on Standards of Health Care: *Standards of Child Health Care.* 2nd Ed. Evanston, Ill., American Academy of Pediatrics, 1972.
6. Anders, T.F.: Child psychiatry and pediatrics: The state of the relationship. Pediatrics (Suppl.), 60:616, 1977.
7. Bergman, A., and Haggerty, R.J.: The emergency clinic: A study of its role in a teaching hospital. Am. J. Dis. Child., 104:36, 1962.
8. Bullard, D.M.: Some aspects of the relationship of the urban pediatric hospital to community mental health programs. Am. J. Psychiatry, 124:944, 1968.
9. Call, J.D.: Some problems and challenges in the geography of scholarship for child psychiatry. J. Am. Acad. Child Psychiatry, 15:139, 1976.
10. Escalona, S.K.: Intervention programs for children at psychiatric risk: The contribution of child psychiatry and development theory. In: *The Child in His Family: Children at Psychiatric Risk.* (E.J. Antony and C. Coupernik, Eds.). New York, Wiley, 1974.
11. Farsad, P., et al.: Teaching interviewing skills to pediatric house officers. Pediatrics, 61:384, 1978.
12. Freedman, D.B.: Personal communication.
13. Friedman, S.B., Ed.: Symposium on behavioral pediatrics. Pediatr. Clin. North Am., 22:517, 1975.
14. Goldensohn, S.S., Fink, R., and Shapiro, S.: The delivery of mental health services to children in a prepaid medical care program. Am. J. Psychiatry, 127:1357, 1971.
15. Group for the Advancement of Psychiatry: *Crisis in Child Mental Health: A Critical Assessment.* Formulated by the Ad Hoc Committee. New York,

Group for the Advancement of Psychiatry, 1972, Report No. 82.
16. Gutelins, M.F., et al.: Controlled study of child health supervision: Behavioral results. Pediatrics, 60:294, 1977.
17. Haggerty, R.J.: Collaborative research in pediatric practice. Pediatrics, 40:1957, 1967.
18. Haggerty, R.J.: Patient care and student learning in a pediatric clinic. Pediatrics, 50:847, 1972.
19. Haggerty, R.J., Roghmann, K.J., and Pless, I.B.: *Child Health and the Community.* New York, Wiley, 1975.
20. Herzog, E.: *Some Guidelines for Evaluative Research.* Department of Health, Education, and Welfare. Washington, Government Printing Office, 1959.
21. Hobbs, N., Ed.: *The Futures of Children: Recommendations of the Project on Classification of Exceptional Children.* San Francisco, Jossey-Bass, 1975.
22. Hochheiser, L.J., Woodward, K., and Charney, E.: Effect of the neighborhood health center on the use of pediatric emergency departments in Rochester, New York. N. Engl. J. Med., 285:148, 1971.
23. Kempe, C.H.: The 1978 presidential address of the American Pediatric Society. Pediatr. Res., 12:1149, 1978.
24. Keniston, K., for the Carnegie Council on Children: *All Our Children: The American Family Under Pressure.* New York, Harcourt Brace Jovanovich, 1977.
25. Liptak, G.S., Hulka, B.S., and Cassel, J.C.: Effectiveness of physician-mother interactions during infancy. Pediatrics, 60:186–192, 1977.
26. Lourie, R.: Personal Communication.
27. National Academy of Sciences: *Toward a National Policy for Children and Families.* Advisory Committee on Child Development, Assembly of Behavioral and Social Sciences. National Research Council. Washington, D.C., National Academy of Sciences, 1976.
27a. Noshpitz, J.D.: The Child Mental Health Grid. In *Basic Handbook of Child Psychiatry.* J.D. Noshpitz, Editor-in-Chief. Volume IV. (I.Z. Berlin and L.A. Stone, Eds.) New York, Basic Books, 1979.
28. Olmsted, R.W.: A perspective: pediatrics today and tomorrow. Am. J. Dis. Child., 132:962, 1978.
29. Prugh, D.G.: Psychosocial disorders in childhood and adolescence: Theoretical considerations and an attempt at classification. (Reports of Task Forces IV and V and Report of the Committee on Clinical Issues by the Joint Commission on Mental Health of Children.) In: *The Mental Health of Children: Services, Research, and Manpower.* New York, Harper & Row, 1973.
30. Prugh, D.G., and Eckhardt, L.O.: Child psychiatry and pediatrics. In: *Basic Handbook of Child Psychiatry.* (J. Noshpitz, et al. Eds.). New York, Basic Books, 1979.
31. Prugh, D.G., and Leon, R., Eds.: *Planning Children's Psychiatric Services in the Community Mental Health Program.* Washington, D.C., American Psychiatric Association, 1964.
32. Rafferty, F.T.: Community mental health centers and the criteria of quantity and universality of

services for children. J. Am. Acad. Child. Psychiatry, *14*:5, 1975.

33. Reichsman, F.: Teaching psychosomatic medicine to medical students, residents, and postgraduate fellows. Int. J. Psychiatry Med., *6*:307, 1975.

34. Report of the Joint Commission on Mental Health of Children: *Crisis in Child Mental Health—A Challenge for the 1970's.* New York, Harper & Row, 1970.

35. Richmond, J.B.: Some observations on the sociology of pediatric education and practice. Pediatrics, *23*:1175, 1959.

36. Richmond, J.B.: Child development: A basic science for pediatrics. Pediatrics, *39*:649, 1967.

37. Richmond, J.B.: *Government and the Pediatrician: The Challenge of Partnership.* Keynote address delivered at the annual meeting of the American Academy of Pediatrics, New York, 1978.

38. Russak, S., and Friedman, D.B.: Family interviewing and pediatric training. Clin. Pediatr., *9*:594, 1970.

39. Schulberg, H.C., Sheldon, A., and Baker, F.: *Program Evaluation in the Health Fields.* New York, Behavioral Publications, 1970.

40. Solnit, A.J., and Senn, M.J.E.: Teaching comprehensive pediatrics in an outpatient clinic. Pediatrics, *12*:547, 1954.

41. Thorpe, H.S., and Halpern, W.J.: Pediatricians and a community child guidance clinic. Pediatrics, *36*:773, 1965.

42. Townsend, E. Jr.: The social worker in pediatric practice: An experiment. Am. J. Dis. Child., *107*:77, 1963.

43. Yankauer, A., Connelly, J.P., and Feldman, J.J.: Pediatric practice in the United States: With special attention to utilization of allied health worker services. Pediatrics (Suppl.), *45*:521, 1970.

General References

American Academy of Pediatrics: *Child Health and Community Health Centers in the Americas.* Evanston, Ill., American Academy of Pediatrics, 1969.

Bergstrom, W.H., and Devlin, L.B.: Pediatric care for migrant workers: An opportunity for teaching and investigation. Pediatrics, *30*:284, 1962.

Berlin, I.N., Ed.: *Advocacy for Mental Health of Children.* New York, Brunner/Mazel, 1974.

Breslow, L.: Some essentials in a national program for child health. Pediatrics, *44*:327, 1969.

Caplan, G., Ed.: *Prevention of Mental Disorders in Children.* New York, Basic Books, 1961.

Caplan, G.: *Principles of Preventive Psychiatry.* New York, Basic Books, 1964.

Caplan, G.: The role of pediatricians in community mental health. In: *Handbook of Community Psychiatry and Community Mental Health* (L. Bellak, Ed.). New York, Grune & Stratton, 1964.

Charney, E.: Primary care pediatrics. Pediatr. Clin. North Am., *21*:3, 1974.

David, H.P.: Mental health and social action problems for children in international perspective. Ment. Hygiene, *54*:503, 1978.

Dimond, E.G.: The physician and the quality of life. JAMA, *228*:1117, 1974.

Eisenberg, L.: Possibilities for a preventive psychiatry. Pediatrics, *30*:815, 1962.

Eisenberg, L., and Gruenberg, E.M.: The current status of secondary prevention in child psychiatry. Am. J. Orthopsychiatry, *31*:355, 1961.

Fost, N.C.: Ethical problems in pediatrics. Current Problems in Pediatrics, *6*:97, 1976.

Fraad, L.M.: Doctor, patient, and family in comprehensive pediatric care. Pediatrics, *43*:2, 1969.

Franklin, A.W.: *Widening Horizons in Child Health.* Flemington, N.J., Medical Media Corporation, 1977.

Garland, J.E.: Social leadership—The fourth function of the teaching hospital. N. Engl. J. Med., *266*:762, 1962.

Gliedman, J., and Roth, W., for the Carnegie Council for Children: The Unexpected Minority: Handicapped Children in America. New York, Harcourt Brace Jovanovich, 1980.

Haggerty, R.J., Roghmann, K.J., and Pless, I.B.: *Child Health and the Community.* New York, Wiley, 1975.

Hammond, K.R., et al.: *Teaching Comprehensive Medical Care: A Psychological Study of a Change in Medical Education.* Commonwealth Fund, Cambridge, Mass., Harvard University Press, 1959.

Hetznecker, W., and Forman, M.A.: *On Behalf of Children.* New York, Grune & Stratton, 1974.

Hoekelman, R.A.: What constitutes adequate well-baby care? Pediatrics, *55*:313, 1975.

Kempe, C.H.: Family intervention: The right of all children. Pediatrics, *56*:693, 1975.

Kenny, T.J., and Clemmens, R.L.: *Behavioral Pediatrics and Child Development.* Baltimore, Williams & Wilkins, 1975.

Kretchmer, N.: Child health in the developing world. Pediatrics, *43*:4, 1969.

Marshall, C.L., et al.: Attitudes toward health care among children of different races and socioeconomic status. Pediatrics, *46*:422, 1970.

Moore, T.D., Ed.: *A Search for a Better Way: The Future of Child Health Services.* Report of the Sixty-Third Ross Conference on Pediatric Research, Columbus, Ohio, Ross Laboratories, 1972.

Naylor, K.A., and Mattsson, A.: For the sake of the children. Psychiatr. Med., *4*:389, 1973.

Newberger, E., Newberger, C., and Richmond, J.: Child health in America: Toward a rational public policy. Milbank Mem. Fund Q. Health Society, *54*:249, 1976.

Primary Care: Special issue. Pediatrics, *60*:259, 1977.

Reader, G.G., and Goss, M.E.W.: *Comprehensive Care and Teaching.* Ithaca, New York, Cornell University Press, 1967.

Richmond, J.B., and Eisenberg, L.: The needs of children. In: *Doing Better and Feeling Worse* (J. Knowles, Ed.). New York, Norton, 1977.

Senn, M.J.E.: *Speaking Out for America's Children.* New Haven, Yale University Press, 1977.

Silver, H.K., and McAtee, P.R.: The essentials of primary health care. J. Fam. Pract., *4*:151, 1977.

Sonis, M., and Sonis, A.C.: Children, youth, and their gatekeepers. J. Am. Acad. Child Psychiatry, *14*:95, 1975.

Ullman, R., Kotak, F., and Tobin, J.R.: Hospital-based group practice and comprehensive care for children of indigent families. Pediatrics, *60*:873, 1977.

Veatch, R.M., and Branson, R., Eds.: *Ethics and Health Policy.* Cambridge, Mass., Ballinger, 1976.

Appendix A: Form for History and Physical Examination*

Identification of Informant(s)

Initial description of parent or informant (if not parent, state relationship to patient), manner of giving data, and apparent accuracy. Evaluation of emotional state or other factors which might bear on accuracy of data.

Chief Complaint or Presenting Problem

In terms of parent or child

Present Illness or Disorder

Date of onset and initial symptoms. Careful description of kind, duration, and degree of symptoms. Chronologic progress or change in symptoms, including details of any therapy. Correlation with significant life events. Health prior to onset. Pertinent epidemiologic information (exposure to illness, potential carriers, animal or insect vectors). Effect of illness on behavior or adjustment of patient and family. Pertinent negative data.

Past History

1. Developmental Survey
   a. **Prenatal.** Health, medical supervision, nutrition, attitudes and emotional state of mother during pregnancy. Illnesses during pregnancy, toxemia, diabetes, cardiac disease, depression. Health and attitudes of father during pregnancy. Living circumstances of family during pregnancy. Fetal activity, including response of parents to fetal activity.
   b. **Birth.** Date, weight, premature (cause if known) or term, birth order. Nature of birth, presentation, use of forceps, cesarean section, length of labor and delivery, degree of difficulty.
   c. **Neonatal Condition.** Spontaneous or delayed respiration, difficulty in resuscitation, respiratory distress, degree of activity, jaundice, cyanosis, convulsions, paralysis, hemorrhage, stupor, difficulty in sucking, rashes, sniffles, congenital anomalies, intractable crying. Mother's condition. Mother's reaction to baby. Blood group incompatibility.
   d. **Feeding**
      (1) *Infancy.* Breast fed or bottle fed. If bottle fed, when started, type, frequency, amount taken, appetite, changes in formula and reasons for changes, relationship of feeding to stools, infant's response to feeding, paroxysmal

*The organization and content of this history form are based in part on D. Prugh: Clinical appraisal of infants and children. In: *Textbook of Pediatrics*, 9th Edition (W.E. Nelson, V.C. Vaughn, and R.J. McKay, Eds.). Philadelphia, Saunders, 1969.

fussing (colic), sleep, vomiting, regurgitation, mother's feelings about feeding of infant, father's attitudes and degree of participation. Amount of medical supervision.

(2) *Supplementary Vitamins.* Age when begun, type, regularity of administration, amount taken, length of time taken.

(3) *Solid Foods.* Time various items started, infant's response, rashes, feeding difficulties (nature, time of onset).

(4) *Weaning.* Breast to bottle, breast to cup, or bottle to cup, reason weaned, time started, length of time required, infant's response, negative reactions, mother's attitudes.

(5) *Childhood.* Appetite, food likes or dislikes, feeding difficulties, struggles over feeding, parents' attitudes toward food and feeding.

e. **Growth and Development**
(1) *Psychomotor.* Age of control of head, hand-to-mouth coordination, social response, sitting (with support and alone), creeping, differentiation between parents and strangers (stranger and separation anxiety), standing, walking (with support and alone), speech, babbling, first words, brief sentences, complicated expressions, disturbances in growth patterns, delay, regression, difficulties in coordination, speech disturbances, hesitation, stammering, infantile speech, aphasia.

(2) *Growth Patterns:* (if known). Approximate weights at birth, at 1 year, 2 years, 5 years, 10 years, steadiness of gain, growth spurts, growth disturbances, obesity, weight loss, growth lags, child's and parents' attitudes toward growth lags. Age at eruption of first tooth, abnormal dentition.

(3) *Sleeping Patterns.* Amount of sleep at various ages, nightmares, night terrors, disturbances in sleep rhythm, child's and parents' attitudes toward sleep and sleep disturbances.

(4) *Bowel and Bladder Training.* Time begun, methods used, age control achieved, difficulties, relapses in control, enuresis, encopresis, parents' attitudes toward toilet training and disturbances in control.

(5) *Sexual Development.* Questions about conception, pregnancy, differences between boys and girls, information given, exploratory activities (e.g., playing doctor), preparation for menarche, age at menarche, secondary sex characteristics, girl's reaction to menarche, preparation of boy for puberty, age at onset, secondary sex characteristics, boy's reaction to puberty, parents' attitudes and feelings, relationship with opposite sex, acceptance of male or female role, masturbation, difficulties in sexual adjustment, child's and parents' attitudes toward dating.

f. **Discipline.** Methods (rules, chores, dos and don'ts, limits, deprivation, punishment), use of praise, child's acceptance, negativism, tantrums, rebelliousness, aggressive or destructive behavior, withdrawal, running away, comparison of approach with child and siblings.

g. **Habit Disturbances.** Age of occurrence, degree, duration of nail biting, thumb sucking, rocking, head banging, rumination, pica, rituals, other habits.

h. **School Adjustment.** Preschool experience, age at entrance into school, adjustment, child's and parents' attitudes and reactions toward separation, child's adjustment (school phobia, withdrawal, disciplinary problems, aggressive behavior, daydreaming), child's and parents' attitudes toward school programs, achievement test or I.Q. test scores, child's progress, general academic performance, easiest and hardest subjects, study habits, attendance record, participation in class and on playground, relationship with teachers.

i. **Social Adjustment.** Early response to separation from mother, child's relationship to peers in neighborhood and at school, relationship to adults, degree of independence, adjustment in group situations (leader, follower, or loner), degree and nature of participation in scouting and other group activities, hobbies, sports, special interests and skills, difficulties in adjustment (aggressive, withdrawn, oversubmissive), attitudes of child and parents toward other people and groups, changes in attitudes during adolescence (including adjustment to peer group and parental authority), plans for college or work.

2. Medical Survey
   a. **Prophylaxis.** Immunizations against smallpox, pertussis, diphtheria, tetanus, poliomyelitis, measles, (typhoid fever, Rocky Mountain spotted fever, yellow fever, if done). Age at immunizations, number of injections, booster shots. Untoward reactions, evidence of artificially induced immunity, scar of smallpox vaccination, Dick and Schick reactions (if done), tuberculin tests, chest x-rays.
   b. **Specific Illnesses**
      (1) *Contagious Diseases.* Measles, rubella, exanthem subitum, pertussis, chickenpox, smallpox, scarlet fever, diphtheria, mumps, poliomyelitis, others. Age at illness,

degree of severity, behavioral reaction, complications.
      (2) *Other Illnesses.* Listed according to system involved or in regard to disturbance in behavior. Age, severity, treatment, sequelae, reactions of child and parents to treatment, hospitalization, or any continuing disability or treatment. Reactions to administration of serum, blood, blood derivatives, chemotherapeutic agents, antibiotic agents.
      (3) *Allergic Reactions.* Eczema, asthma, hay fever, urticaria, hypersensitivity reactions to inhalants, food, drugs, contact with cloth, soaps, age at onset, treatment, complications.
      (4) *Operations.* Dates, nature, results, complications or sequelae, child's and parents' reaction. Preoperative preparation.
      (5) *Injuries.* Dates, nature and circumstances of significant accidents, frequency, sequelae, evaluations and treatments. Child's and parents' reactions.
      (6) *Review of Body Parts and Systems*
         a. *Head.* Headache, trauma.
         b. *Eyes.* Vision, glasses, strabismus, pain, inflammation, diplopia, other disturbances.
         c. *Ears.* Hearing, pain, discharge, tinnitus.
         d. *Nose.* Discharge, epistaxis, obstruction, disturbances in olfactory sense.
         e. *Teeth.* Extractions, disorders in dentition, abscesses, general condition, child's reaction.
         f. *Mouth.* Mouth-breathing, sore mouth, sore tongue, caries, bleeding gums, taste disturbances.
         g. *Throat.* Pain, infections, tonsillitis, difficulty in swallowing, hoarseness.

h. *Neck.* Masses, pain, stiffness, cervical adenitis, thyroid enlargement.

i. *Respiratory.* Frequency and nature of colds, cough, sputum, hemoptysis, stridor, foreign bodies, croup, bronchitis, asthma.

j. *Gastrointestinal.* Appetite, food idiosyncrasies, vomiting, abdominal discomfort or pain, constipation, diarrhea, encopresis, character of stools, jaundice.

k. *Cardiovascular.* Dyspnea, cyanosis, edema, precordial pain, palpitation, syncope.

l. *Genitourinary.* Enuresis (diurnal or nocturnal), frequency, urgency, dysuria, circumcision, vaginal discharge, menstrual disturbances.

m. *Musculoskeletal.* Weakness, joint or muscular pain or swelling, posture, muscular coordination, deformities, fractures.

n. *Nervous.* Sleep disturbances, tics, tremors, vertigo, twitchings, convulsions, ataxia, paralysis, projectile vomiting, shortened attention span, distractibility. (The approach to the mental status examination is discussed in Chapter 7.)

o. *Skin.* Eruptions, congenital anomalies, itching, pigmentation, erythema, blushing, bruising, petechiae.

3. Family Survey

a. *Parents.* Age, occupation, state of physical and emotional health of each parent or parent substitute, currently and at important points in patient's illness. (If parents not living, age at death, cause of death if known, nature of symptoms, age of patient at time of parents' death.) Marital relationship. Attitudes of each parent toward patient and toward child-rearing practices. Previous pregnancies of mother (outcome, abnormality). Brief summary of family's circumstances. Sociocultural and ethnic backgrounds of each parent. Current health of grandparents. (If grandparents not living, age at death, cause of death if known, nature of symptoms, age of patient at time of grandparents' death.) Cohesiveness of family. External integration of family into community. Patterns of communication, leadership. Sharing of pleasurable activities.

b. *Siblings.* Age, place of residence, health. (If not living, age at death, cause of death if known, nature of symptoms, age of patient at time of siblings' death.) School and social performance. Relationship to patient. Attitudes of parents toward patient compared with attitudes toward siblings.

c. *Living Circumstances.* Place and type of residence. Sleeping arrangements. Number of persons living in home in addition to parents and children. Relationships of these persons to family members. Members of family who work, working hours (if unusual), general level of economic independence, financial support from community agencies. Type of neighborhood. Recreational resources.

d. *Familial Illnesses or Anomalies if known.* Tuberculosis, syphilis, diabetes, cancer, epilepsy, rheumatic fever, allergy, hereditary blood dyscrasias, Rh status, mental illness, mental retardation, dystrophies, congenital anomalies, heredodegenerative diseases.

Summary

A brief recapitulation of the essential features of the present illness or the current state of health if the child is being seen for a health examination. Significant correlations between features of past development or illness and significant life events or family circumstances. Essentially an organization and synthesis of the historical data into meaningful trends so far as they can be seen up to this point. The problem-oriented record can be most helpful. (See Chapter 7 for a discussion of the use of this form.)

Appendix B: Identifying High-Risk Parent-Infant Relationships: The "Five Questions" Approach

The Five Questions approach is designed to elicit information from a woman who has just delivered a baby that aids in the identification of high-risk parent-infant relationships in about 20 minutes. The questions used in this approach have not been standardized or validated as yet. Harmon (personal communication), however, has recently demonstrated their reliability. They are offered simply as a clinical instrument for use in screening and in planning management. Social work, psychiatric, or other types of consultations may be used as indicated.

I have demonstrated the use of the Five Questions approach to groups of pediatric house staff members, nurses, medical students, nurse practitioners, child health associates, and other professionals.

Before the interview, the mother is asked whether she wishes to be interviewed, and she is prepared for the interview. She is told that information about parents' experiences will help the hospital staff in their work and that a child psychiatrist will interview her in front of a group. To my knowledge, very few mothers have refused to be interviewed and no mothers have been upset by the interview. Some mothers have brought out feelings or facts during the interview that they had not previously mentioned, and they felt that they were helped by having done so. The mother is encouraged to hold and to feed her baby during the interview, a practice that enables the observers to get valuable information about how the mother and infant interact. Observing marital and other family interactions can also be revealing, as with the husband or the grandmother who takes over the care or feeding of the baby. (Fathers and grandparents are encouraged to participate, if available.)

The Five Questions are really five clusters of short questions the mother is to be asked on the interviewer's first contact with her after the birth of her child. The questions can be used in any order (although the order in which they are presented has a certain inherent logic), and they can be modified to fit the mother's response. Other questions may also be asked at the interviewer's discretion. Such questions may lead to other interviews.

Question No. 1: "How are you feeling?"

Question No. 1 focuses attention on the mother at the outset of the interview and sets the stage for a relaxed, informal interview. It indicates concern for the mother's condition as well as the baby's (usually the first question put to a women who has just had a baby is, "How is the baby?"). Most mothers get relief or even pleasure in talking about their own condition, and they often spontaneously talk about the delivery and their feelings of elation, depression, or apprehension. The mother who says, "I feel terrible, and my husband doesn't believe it" is giving a significant glimpse into her marriage. She can be asked further questions to draw her out in that direction.

If the mother responds in a conventional way to Question No. 1 (e.g., "Fine"), the interviewer can ask, "How is the baby's father taking it?" This question often produces further significant information (e.g., "He hasn't even been in to see me yet," a statement that can also be followed up with revealing results). "How about your families?" may open up other aspects of the parent-infant relationship, including the mother's model for mothering, unwed motherhood, and the loss of a parent.

The mother's answer to Question No. 1 may also reveal how she responds to stressful situations and how she handles her need to be helped. For example, the mother might describe the labor and delivery as a difficult but manageable experience during which she got the help she needed. Or she might describe the labor and delivery as a horrendous experience during which she got no help. If the father or a grandparent is present, they might be drawn into the discussion. Sometimes the results are startling (as with the father who says in front of his wife, "My wife is always complaining. I won't be able to shut her up when the baby comes home"). Such a response signals that troubles are ahead. Other kinds of responses may quickly tell the observer that the marital and other family relationships are sympathetic and supportive ones.

Question No. 2

Question No. 2 has to do with the "maternal time lag" (a phenomenon described by Benedek and Caplan), and it requires that the interviewer start with a generalization. If the interviewer asks directly, "Does it seem as if the baby is real?" or "Do you feel like a mother yet?" a primiparous woman is socially bound to say, "Of course." But if the interviewer says first, "You know, most mothers who have a baby for the first time have thought that they will right away feel, 'This is my baby.' But then they find that for the first little while it's hard to believe that it's all real," the mother usually gives an eager and open reply. The reply may range from, "That's not how I feel. I know he's mine" to "Nothing seems real. It's like a dream. I can't believe I'm a mother already and that that's my baby." (The interviewer may ask women who have given birth before about their first pregnancy. Some mothers experience the maternal time lag with decreasing intensity over several pregnancies.)

Replies such as these usually give relief from feelings of guilt or worry, especially when the interviewer reinforces the idea that such reactions are normal and that after a "little while" or in "several days" the baby's birth will be easy to believe. Occasionally a mother will respond to Question No. 1 ("How are you feeling?") by bursting out with "I'm feeling OK, but I just can't believe all that has happened and that I really have a baby." Her response may change the order of the questions since it indicates that she needs extra and immediate reassurance.

The maternal time lag normally lasts from a few hours to several days. It seems to be shorter when rooming-in and related approaches are taken, and it may not occur in women from certain subcultures. If such adverse factors as conflicts about pregnancy, physical defects, and prematurity are present, the maternal time lag may last for weeks, and it may interfere with the mother's attachment or bonding.

Question No. 3: "How is the baby?" Later, "What is the baby's name?"

In response to question No. 3, the mother may bring up any concerns she has about her baby (e.g., about blemishes, birthmarks, or forceps marks). If she does not, the interviewer may ask her whether she has any concerns about the baby. He can ask her also how the baby seemed to her at birth, indicating that every mother counts her newborn's fingers and toes. That assurance may elicit some fears the mother had during pregnancy about possible defects in her baby, or it may elicit some current concerns that she had not mentioned before.

If in answer to the question about the baby's name, the mother says that a name has not yet been chosen, the interviewer can infer that problems are ahead (except in the case of Native American families, who may wait for some time after the baby's birth to choose a name). The interviewer may be able to discover the reason for the delay; it may be that the parents simply could not agree on a name. Such a reason gives a glimpse of the family's decision-making ability (or lack of it), and it may quickly lead to the revelation that a serious marital problem exists. The mother's answer to the question about the name may also point to serious problems during the pregnancy (as with a teenage or an unwed mother). If the mother tells the interviewer the baby's name, the interviewer can ask at what point in the pregnancy the name was chosen. If the mother says that it was chosen very late in the pregnancy, perhaps even the day before the birth, that information can lead to the revelation of a marital problem or other conflict, and it may be predictive of problems later in regard to the parents' child-rearing practices.

The interviewer can also ask the parents whether they had chosen a name for a baby of the opposite sex. Even if the name was chosen early in the pregnancy, this can open up a picture of which sex the parents hoped their baby would be, a fact that might not emerge if the interviewer questioned the parents more directly. If the mother says, "My husband had his heart so set on a boy that he wouldn't even talk about a girl, and I went along with him," the interviewer can not only see who may be the dominant parent in regard to child-rearing but he may also get a hint that the wife will not always give in to her husband. Most women feel more comfortable about the idea of rearing a girl as the first baby. If a mother says, "I wanted a boy because he's going to have to be strong to face life in this world," the interviewer gets a good idea of how the mother sees life and possibly that she envies men.

Question No. 4: "Do you remember, during your pregnancy, how you felt when the baby began to move?" Later, "Could you picture him or her in your mind?"

Question No. 4 tries to establish the nature of the mother's relationship with her unborn fetus, described by Benedek and Caplan. They believe that the acceptance of motherhood begins during pregnancy, and I believe that maternal attachment begins then, or even earlier in a psychologic sense.) If the parents' marriage was sound and if other psychosocial aspects of the pregnancy were healthy, the interviewer would generally expect to get positive answers about the pregnant woman's response (and her husband's response) to quickening (e.g., "We both loved to feel the baby moving; it made the baby seem real"). But if the mother says, "It was terrible. The baby kept kicking me all the time so that I couldn't sleep at all," the interviewer can infer that she was not comfortable at that point with her coming motherhood. If the mother says, "It wasn't bad, but my husband didn't like it," that response may fit with other responses that indicate that the marriage is shaky. Some of these questions can be asked during pregnancy, and any necessary supportive action taken then.

The interviewer can ask the parents whether they had a pet name for their unborn child. A healthy mother might make such a remark as, "We called him Junior" or "We called the baby Sally, after my little sister, who is so active." If a mother makes such a response as, "we just called it 'it' " or "It didn't like me, it kept banging me all the time," problems were involved.

The interviewer might ask the mother about any dreams she had about the baby. If the mother had no good dreams, or dreams that the baby had no face (for example), or recurrent frightening dreams, that fact may be significant.

A corollary question is involved with No. 4 if the mother has not already given a spontaneous response, such as "I used to love to imagine what the baby would look like." The interviewer can ask: "When the baby began to move, were you able to form a picture in your mind of what the baby would look like?" A healthy response would be an affirmative answer (e.g., "Yes, I could even see the color of his eyes and hair although he looks different now that he's here"). The mother might add, "I could see myself feeding him." A negative answer (e.g., "I couldn't see the baby in my mind. I didn't even want to think about it") may point to marital problems or conflicts about the pregnancy or about motherhood that further questioning will uncover. The mother who says, "I didn't dare think about the baby. I was too worried. I lost my first baby, you know," may be referring for the first time to a miscarriage or a longstanding fertility problem, and, perhaps, associated marital problems.

Such a question may also elicit other kinds of previously unmentioned psychosocial information, as with the mother who says, "I couldn't think about anything during the pregnancy. I was depressed the whole time because my mother was sick. She died just last week. I'll miss her so, because she helped me with everything."

Problems are ahead for such a dependent woman, who has become a mother just after losing her own mother.

Question No. 5: "What kind of plans have you made for someone to help you after you get home from the hospital?" Later, "How do you see your baby's future?" (If appropriate, "How will your other children react to the arrival of this child?")

Question No. 5 is designed to elicit information about the nature of the marital relationship, about how much help the mother has received or anticipates receiving from relatives and friends, and about her attitudes about accepting help. If the mother answers happily, "My husband is going to take his vacation to help me with things around the house," obviously the parents have made some plans and have a supportive relationship with each other. The mother who answers, "My girlfriend will help. My husband wouldn't think of it. He's too busy drinking beer" is obviously painting a picture of a different kind of marital relationship. If a mother says that her mother is coming to help her, the interviewer might ask, "How's her advice?" The mother's answers may range from, "She lets me make my own decisions" to "She's always bossed me around; I don't know how long I can stand having her with me."

If the mother does not mention her mother spontaneously, the interviewer might bring up the subject. The question, "Would you like your mother to help?" often elicits important information about the mother's experience with being mothered and with parenting in general.

The mother may show attitudes toward being helped that indicate that she will have difficulties later. The mother who says grimly, "I've never asked anyone for help, and no one ever offered it" is telling a good deal about her earlier life. She will probably not ask the physician or nurse for help, even when she needs it. Such a mother may need someone to reach out gently to her during brief visits later to her home.

In talking about her child's future, a healthy mother might say, "I just want my child to grow up to be a happy person." Problems loom for the mother who says, "She will have to be independent" or "He'll have to toe the line."

How the mother thinks her other children will react (or are reacting) to the birth often gives a glimpse into the mother's ability to perceive her children's needs, to anticipate problems, to tolerate any regression in them, and related matters.

The Five Questions approach often elicits a pattern of response. The mother who says that she feels "lousy," who can't believe she is really a mother, who chose the baby's name very late, who did not enjoy the movements of her unborn baby, who could not imagine what her unborn baby would look like, and who has made no plans for help when she takes her baby home will have problems later even if she gives no further information about her marriage or other pertinent psychosocial factors. But the interviewer should remember that a healthy pattern is not always completely consistent; a young mother who enjoyed sharing the movements of her unborn baby with her husband may not have been able to imagine what the baby would look like. Nevertheless, the pattern seems to be fairly predictive, especially when considered along with the clinical information and with the observations of family interactions that were made during the interview or entered into the nurse's report.

On the basis of the picture obtained from this brief screening interview, the interviewer can determine what families have high-risk situations and can decide how to help them. For example, if an anxious, dependent mother and an immature husband have made no plans for help following the mother's discharge from the hospital, it can be arranged that she will stay in the hospital for a day or two longer while some help in planning is offered. Or it can be arranged that a child health associate or nurse practitioner will make a home visit during the first week to make sure that the parents get to a well-child clinic for pediatric counseling or to offer additional counseling and support. Supportive psychotherapy by a mental health professional can be undertaken immediately in the hospital setting, or a referral to a mental health facility or some other agency (e.g., one that provides public health nursing services or homemaker services) can be arranged.

The Five Questions approach does not of itself predict child battering. (Dr. C. Henry Kempe and the child protection team at the University of Colorado Medical Center are attempting to do so, using a much longer and more detailed questionnaire and other methods. Their technique covers some of the items covered in the Five Questions approach, but it also includes questions about attitudes toward discipline and other matters.) With the Five Questions approach, however, the interviewer can often find out whether the parents had themselves been battered as children. That information, together with a current situation involving impending mother-infant separation (because of prematurity or illness) represent the most helpful partially predictive items so far available. The parents' attitudes toward discipline also often emerge in the Five Questions approach, particularly when the interviewer asked the parents how the siblings are responding to the new baby's birth. The parents may answer in a way that indicates that they have a rigid, punitive attitude toward jealous siblings. Also, the interviewer can obtain a glimpse of severe psychopathology in a parent or a picture of a helpless, dependent parent, who needs special support whether or not she or he is likely to strike out at the infant when frustrated.

Index